CLINICAL HANDBOOK OF COUPLE THERAPY

Clinical Handbook of Couple Therapy

FOURTH EDITION

EDITED BY

ALAN S. GURMAN

THE GUILFORD PRESS
New York   London

©2008 The Guilford Press
A Division of Guilford Publications, Inc.
72 Spring Street, New York, NY 10012
www.guilford.com

Printed in the United States of America

This book is printed on acid-free paper.

Last digit is print number: 9 8 7 6 5 4 3

The authors have checked with sources believed to be reliable in their efforts to provide information that is
complete and generally in accord with the standards of practice that are accepted at the time of publication.
However, in view of the possibility of human error or changes in medical sciences, neither the authors, nor
the editor and publisher, nor any other party who has been involved in the preparation or publication of this
work warrants that the information contained herein is in every respect accurate or complete, and they are
not responsible for any errors or omissions or the results obtained from the use of such information. Readers
are encouraged to confirm the information contained in this book with other sources.

Library of Congress Cataloging-in-Publication Data

Clinical handbook of couple therapy / edited by Alan S. Gurman.—4th ed.
   p. ; cm.
   Includes bibliographical references and index.
   ISBN 978-1-59385-821-6 (hardcover : alk. paper)
   1. Marital psychotherapy—Handbooks, manuals, etc. I. Gurman, Alan S.
   [DNLM: 1. Marital Therapy—methods. 2. Couples Therapy—methods. WM 430.5.M3 C641 2008]
   RC488.5.C584 2008
   616.89′1562—dc22

                                                          2008010079

To Jim Framo, Cliff Sager, and Robin Skynner—
who understood a thing or two about couples,

and, of course, to Neil Jacobson—
who is still a part of this

About the Editor

Alan S. Gurman, PhD, is Emeritus Professor of Psychiatry and Director of Family Therapy Training at the University of Wisconsin School of Medicine and Public Health. He has edited and written many influential books, including *Theory and Practice of Brief Therapy* (with Simon H. Budman), the *Handbook of Family Therapy* (with David P. Kniskern), and *Essential Psychotherapies* (with Stanley B. Messer). A past two-term Editor of the *Journal of Marital and Family Therapy* and former President of the Society for Psychotherapy Research, Dr. Gurman has received numerous awards for his contributions to marital and family therapy, including awards for "Distinguished Contribution to Research in Family Therapy" from the American Association for Marriage and Family Therapy, for "Distinguished Achievement in Family Therapy Research" from the American Family Therapy Academy, and for "Distinguished Contributions to Family Psychology" from the American Psychological Association. More recently, he received a national teaching award from the Association of Psychology Postdoctoral and Internship Centers for "Excellence in Internship Training/Distinguished Achievement in Teaching and Training." A pioneer in the development of integrative approaches to couple therapy, Dr. Gurman maintains an active clinical practice in Madison, Wisconsin.

Contributors

Donald H. Baucom, PhD, Professor, Psychology Department, University of North Carolina–Chapel Hill, Chapel Hill, North Carolina

Steven R. H. Beach, PhD, Professor, Department of Psychology, and Director, Institute of Behavioral Research, University of Georgia, Athens, Georgia

Gary R. Birchler, PhD, Retired, formerly Clinical Professor of Psychiatry, University of California–San Diego, San Diego, California

Nancy Boyd-Franklin, PhD, Professor, Graduate School of Applied and Professional Psychology, Rutgers, The State University of New Jersey, New Brunswick, New Jersey

James H. Bray, PhD, Associate Professor, Departments of Family and Community Medicine and Psychiatry, Baylor College of Medicine, Houston, Texas

Andrew Christensen, PhD, Professor, Department of Psychology, University of California–Los Angeles, Los Angeles, California

Audrey A. Cleary, MS, PhD candidate, Department of Psychology, University of Arizona, Tucson, Arizona

Gene Combs, MD, Director of Behavioral Science Education, Loyola/Cook County/Provident Hospital Combined Residency in Family Medicine, Chicago, Illinois

Sona Dimidjian, PhD, Assistant Professor, Department of Psychology, University of Colorado–Boulder, Boulder, Colorado

Lee J. Dixon, MA, PhD candidate, Department of Psychology, University of Tennessee–Knoxville, Knoxville, Tennessee

Jessica A. Dreifuss, BS, PhD candidate, Department of Psychology, University of Georgia, Athens, Georgia

Jennifer Durham, PhD, President, Omolayo Institute, Plainfield, New Jersey

Norman B. Epstein, PhD, Professor, Department of Family Science, and Director, Marriage and Family Therapy Program, University of Maryland–College Park, College Park, Maryland

William Fals-Stewart, PhD, Director, Addiction and Family Research Group, and Professor, School of Nursing, University of Rochester, Rochester, New York

Barrett Fantozzi, BS, PhD candidate, and Research Coordinator, DBT Couples and Family Therapy Program, Department of Psychology, University of Nevada–Reno, Reno, Nevada

Kameron J. Franklin, BA, PhD candidate, Department of Psychology, University of Georgia, Athens, Georgia

Jill Freedman, MSW, Director, Evanston Family Therapy Center, Evanston, Illinois

Alan E. Fruzzetti, PhD, Associate Professor and Director, Dialectical Behavior Therapy and Research Program, Department of Psychology, University of Nevada–Reno, Reno, Nevada

Barbara Gabriel, PhD, Research Scholar, Graduate Study Research Center, University of Georgia, Athens, Georgia

Kristina Coop Gordon, PhD, Associate Professor, Department of Psychology, University of Tennessee–Knoxville, Knoxville, Tennessee

Michael C. Gottlieb, PhD, FAFP, Clinical Professor, Department of Psychiatry, University of Texas Health Science Center, Dallas, Texas

John Mordechai Gottman, PhD, Emeritus Professor, Department of Psychology, University of Washington, and Director, Relationship Research Institute, Seattle, Washington

Julie Schwartz Gottman, PhD, Cofounder and Clinical Director, The Gottman Institute, and Cofounder and Clinical Director, Loving Couples/Loving Children, Inc., Seattle, Washington

Robert-Jay Green, PhD, Executive Director, Rockway Institute for LGBT Research and Public Policy, and Distinguished Professor, California School of Professional Psychology, Alliant International University–San Francisco, San Francisco, California

Alan S. Gurman, PhD, Emeritus Professor and Director of Family Therapy Training, Department of Psychiatry, University of Wisconsin School of Medicine and Public Health, Madison, Wisconsin

Michael F. Hoyt, PhD, Staff Psychologist, Kaiser Permanente Medical Center, Department of Psychiatry, San Rafael, California

Susan M. Johnson, EdD, Professor, Department of Psychology, University of Ottawa, Ottawa, Ontario, Canada, and Research Professor, Alliant University–San Diego, San Diego, California

Charles Kamen, MS, PhD candidate, Department of Psychology, University of Georgia, Athens, Georgia

Shalonda Kelly, PhD, Associate Professor, Graduate School of Applied and Professional Psychology, Rutgers, The State University of New Jersey, New Brunswick, New Jersey

Jennifer S. Kirby, PhD, Research Assistant Professor, Psychology Department, University of North Carolina–Chapel Hill, North Carolina

Carmen Knudson-Martin, PhD, Professor and Director, PhD Program in Marital and Family Therapy, Department of Counseling and Family Sciences, Loma Linda University, Loma Linda, California

Jon Lasser, PhD, Assistant Professor, Department of Educational Administration and Psychological Services, Texas State University–San Marcos, San Marcos, Texas

Jaslean J. LaTaillade, PhD, Assistant Professor, Department of Family Science, University of Maryland–College Park, College Park, Maryland

Jay Lebow, PhD, Clinical Professor of Psychology, The Family Institute at Northwestern and Northwestern University, Evanston, Illinois

Christopher R. Martell, PhD, ABPP, Independent Practice and Clinical Associate Professor,

Department of Psychiatry and Behavioral Sciences and Department of Psychology, University of Washington, Seattle, Washington

Barry W. McCarthy, PhD, Professor, Department of Psychology, American University, and Partner, Washington Psychological Center, Washington, DC

Susan H. McDaniel, PhD, Professor, Departments of Psychiatry and Family Medicine, and Director, Wynne Center for Family Research, University of Rochester School of Medicine and Dentistry, Rochester, New York

Alexandra E. Mitchell, PhD, Professor, Department of Psychology, Texas A&M University, College Station, Texas

Valory Mitchell, PhD, Professor, Clinical Psychology PsyD Program, Fellow at the Rockway Institute for LGBT Research and Public Policy, and California School of Professional Psychology, Alliant International University–San Francisco, San Francisco, California

Timothy J. O'Farrell, PhD, Professor, Department of Psychology, and Chief, Families and Addiction Program, Department of Psychiatry, Harvard Medical School, VA Boston Healthcare System, Boston, Massachusetts

K. Daniel O'Leary, PhD, Distinguished Professor and Director of Clinical Training, Department of Psychology, State University of New York–Stony Brook, Stony Brook, New York

Laura Roberto-Forman, PsyD, Professor, Department of Psychiatry and Behavioral Sciences, Eastern Virginia Medical School, Norfolk, Virginia

Michael J. Rohrbaugh, PhD, Professor, Departments of Psychology and Family Studies, University of Arizona, Tucson, Arizona

Nancy Breen Ruddy, PhD, Behavioral Science Faculty, Hunterdon Family Practice Residency Program, Hunterdon Medical Center, Flemington, New Jersey

David E. Scharff, MD, Codirector, International Psychotherapy Institute, and Clinical Professor, Department of Psychiatry, Georgetown University, Washington, DC, and the Uniformed Services University of the Health Sciences, Bethesda, Maryland

Jill Savege Scharff, MD, Codirector, International Psychotherapy Institute and Clinical Professor, Department of Psychiatry, Georgetown University, Washington, DC

Varda Shoham, PhD, Professor and Director of Clinical Training, Department of Psychology, University of Arizona, Tucson, Arizona

George M. Simon, MS, Faculty, The Minuchin Center for the Family, New York, New York

Georganna L. Simpson, JD, Attorney at Law, Owner, Law Offices of Georganna L. Simpson, Dallas, Texas

Douglas K. Snyder, PhD, Professor and Director of Clinical Psychology Training, Department of Psychology, Texas A&M University, College Station, Texas

Maria Thestrup, MA, PhD candidate, Department of Psychology, American University, Washington, DC

Contents

Social Constructionist Approaches

Systemic Approaches

Integrative Approaches

PART II. APPLICATIONS OF COUPLE THERAPY:
SPECIAL POPULATIONS, PROBLEMS, AND ISSUES

Rupture and Repair of Relational Bonds: Affairs, Divorce, Violence, and Remarriage

Couple Therapy and the Treatment of Psychiatric and Medical Disorders

CHAPTER 1

A Framework for the Comparative Study of Couple Therapy

History, Models, and Applications

ALAN S. GURMAN

This volume presents the core theoretical and applied aspects of couple therapy in modern clinical practice. These core couple therapies are those that form the conceptual and clinical bedrock of therapeutic training, practice, and research. There are two quite distinct categories of such couple therapies (Gurman & Fraenkel, 2002). First, there are those whose origins are to be found in the earliest phases of the history of the broad field of family and couple therapy. Although central attributes of these methods have largely endured across several generations of systems-oriented therapists, they have been revised and refined considerably over time. Examples of such time-honored approaches are structural and brief strategic approaches, and object relations and transgenerational (e.g., Bowenian, Contextual, and Symbolic–Experiential) approaches. Second, core couple therapies include several visible and increasingly influential approaches that have been developed relatively recently; have had undeniably strong effects on practice, training and research; and are likely to endure long into the future. Examples in this category are cognitive and behavioral, narrative and emotion-focused, and integrative approaches.

As intended in its first edition in 1985, this *Handbook* has become a primary reference source for comprehensive presentations of the most prominent contemporary influences in the field of couple therapy. Although one could identify large numbers of differently labeled couple therapies, there appear to be only about a dozen genuinely distinguishable types. Some among these are obviously closely related in their conceptual and historical bloodlines, though having enough significant differences to warrant separate coverage here.

In all these cases, whether involving earlier or later generation approaches, the authors contributing to this fourth edition have brought us what is not only basic and core to their ways of thinking about and working with couples but also new and forward-looking. These contributors, all eminent clinical scholars (all practicing clinicians, as well) have helped to forge a volume that is well suited to exposing advanced undergraduates, graduate students at all levels, and trainees in all the mental health professions to the major schools and methods of couple therapy. Because all the chapters were written by cutting-edge representatives of their approaches, there is something genuinely new to these presentations that will be of value to more experienced therapists as well.

Offering these observations here is not motivated by self-congratulatory puffery. Rather, it is a way of acknowledging to the reader that there is a

1

lot in these pages, a lot to be considered and absorbed, whether by novices or seasoned veterans. And that is perhaps the main reason for this introductory chapter, which is to provide a comprehensive framework for the study of any given "school" of couple therapy, and for the comparative study of different couple therapies.

As in earlier editions of the *Handbook*, each of the chapters in Part I ("Models of Couple Therapy") offers a clear sense of the history, current status, assessment approach, and methods of therapy being discussed, along with its foundational ideas about relational health and dysfunction. The old adage that "there is nothing so practical as a good theory" is still valid, and so each chapter balances the discussion of theory and practice, and emphasizes their interplay. And since this is the 21st century, in which testimonials no longer are acceptable as adequate evidence of the efficacy or effectiveness of psychotherapeutic methods, each chapter addresses the evidence base, whatever its depth or nature, of its approach.

Part II of the *Handbook* ("Applications of Couple Therapy: Special Populations, Problems, and Issues") includes nine chapters that focus on very specific, clinically meaningful problems that on the one hand are either inherently and self-evidently relational (affairs, separation and divorce, intimate partner violence, and remarriage) or, on the other, are still often viewed (even in the year 2008) as the problems of individuals (alcoholism and drug abuse, depression, personality disorders, sexual dysfunction, and illness).

To facilitate the study of both the major models of couple therapy and the application of these approaches to significant and common clinical problems, this edition of the *Handbook*, like its predecessors, was organized around a set of expository guidelines for contributing authors. These guidelines represent a revised version of similar guidelines originally set forth in the Gurman and Kniskern's (1991) *Handbook of Family Therapy*. Teachers and students have found these guidelines to be a valuable adjunctive learning tool. They are presented here along with contextualizing discussion of the rationale for inclusion of the content addressed within each broad section of these chapters.

The various models of couple therapy appearing here have grown out of different views of human nature and intimate adult relationships, about which there is nothing approaching universal agreement. These therapy approaches call for many fundamentally different ways of getting to know clients, and encompass rather distinctly dif-

ferent visions of both relational "reality" and therapeutic coherence. They also differ in the degree to which they assume that fundamental change is possible, and even what should constitute clinically relevant change with couples.

Given this diversity and variety of views on such cornerstone issues, it is important for the field to continue to respect the different perspectives each model of couple therapy exemplifies, even while there appears to be more and more interest in the identification, elucidation, and application of common principles in theory and practice.

In this ecumenical spirit, a brief note on the organization of the chapters in Part I of the *Handbook* ("Models of Couple Therapy") is in order. The sequence of these chapters was not determined according to some complex and very arbitrary dimensional or categorical scheme, or according to some midlevel distinguishing characteristics of the models (e.g., "Traditional," "Integrative," "Postmodern," as appeared in the third edition of the *Handbook*). Instead, they are sequenced by the most unbiased method available: alphabetical order (granted, random sequencing by drawing names out of a hat could be argued to have been inherently less biased, but no matter the results of such a series of "draws," inevitably some readers would have inferred from the outcome some telling significance). Although it is true that the very naming of these six "types" of couple therapy (Behavioral, Humanistic–Existential, Psychodynamic–Transgenerational, Social Constructionist, Systemic, and Integrative) itself may reveal the unconscious biases, predilections, and favoritisms of the editor (not to mention his ignorance and/or linguistic deficits), this appeared to be the most "level playing field" at hand.

THREE FOUNDATIONAL POINTS

Why Couple Therapy Is Important

Significant cultural changes in the last half-century have had an enormous impact on marriage, and the expectations and experiences of those who marry or enter other long-term committed relationships. Reforms in divorce law (e.g., no-fault divorces), more liberal attitudes about sexual expression, the increased availability of contraception, and the growth of the economic and political power of women have all increased the expectations and requirements of marriage to go well beyond maintaining economic viability and ensuring procreation. For most couples nowadays, marriage is also expected to be the primary source of adult intimacy, support, and companionship. and a facilitative context for personal growth. At the same time, the "limits of human pair-bonding" (Pinsof, 2002, p. 135) are increasingly clear, and the transformations of marital expectations have led the "shift from death to divorce" as the primary terminator of marriage (p. 139). With changing expectations of not only marriage itself but also of the permanence of marriage, the public health importance of the "health" of marriage has understandably increased. Whether through actual divorce or chronic conflict and distress, the breakdown of marital relationships exacts enormous costs.

Recurrent marital conflict and divorce are associated with a wide variety of problems in both adults and children. Divorce and marital problems are among the most stressful conditions people face. Partners in troubled relationships are more likely to suffer from anxiety, depression and suicidality, and substance abuse; from both acute and chronic medical problems and disabilities, such as impaired immunological functioning and high blood pressure; and from health risk behaviors, such as susceptibility to sexually transmitted diseases and accident-proneness. Moreover, the children of distressed marriages are more likely to suffer from anxiety, depression, conduct problems, and impaired physical health.

Why Couples Seek Therapy

Although physical and psychological health are affected by marital satisfaction and health, there are more common reasons why couples seek, or are referred for, conjoint therapy. These concerns usually involve relational matters, such as emotional disengagement and waning commitment, power struggles, problem-solving and communication difficulties, jealousy and extramarital involvements, value and role conflicts, sexual dissatisfaction, and abuse and violence (Geiss & O'Leary, 1981; Whisman, Dixon, & Johnson, 1997). Generally, couples seek therapy because of threats to the security and stability of their relationships with the most significant attachment figures of adult life (Johnson & Denton, 2002).

Common Characteristics of Couple Therapy

Modern approaches to couple therapy include important concepts from general systems theory (the study of the relationship between and among interacting components of a system that exists over time), cybernetics (the study of the regulatory mechanisms that operate in systems via feedback loops), and family development theory (the study of how families, couples, and their individual members adapt to change while maintaining their systemic integrity over time). In addition, extant models of couple therapy have been significantly influenced, to varying degrees, by psychodynamic (especially object relations) theory, humanistic theory, and cognitive and social learning theory (see Gurman [1978] for an extensive comparative analysis of the psychoanalytic, behavioral, and systems theory perspectives), as well as more recent perspectives provided by feminism, multiculturalism, and postmodernism (Gurman & Fraenkel, 2002).

Despite this wide array of significant influences on the theory and practice of couple therapy, a number of central characteristics are held in common by almost all currently influential approaches to conjoint treatment. Gurman (2001) has identified the dominant attitudes and value systems of couple (and family) therapists that differentiate them from traditional individual psychotherapists, as well as four central technical factors common to most models of couple therapy. Most couple therapists value (1) clinical parsimony and efficiency; (2) the adoption of a developmental perspective on clinical problems, along with attention to current problems; (3) a balanced awareness of patients' strengths and weaknesses; and (4) a deemphasis on the centrality of treatment (and the therapist) in patients' lives. These common attitudes significantly overlap the core treatment attitudes of brief individual therapists (cf. Budman & Gurman, 1988) and help most couple therapy to be quite brief.

Gurman also identified four central sets of technical factors that regularly characterize couple (and brief) therapy. First, the meaning of time is manifest in three particular ways. Although couple therapists generally adopt a developmental perspective on clinical problems, they see an understanding of the *timing of problems* (i.e., "Why now?") as essential to good clinical practice, but with little attention paid to traditional history taking. As Aponte (1992) stated, "A therapist targets the residuals of the past in a (couple's) experience of the present" (p. 326). In addition, most marital therapists do not expend a great deal of effort in formal assessment; thus, the *timing of intervention* usually seems quite early by traditional individual psychotherapy standards, with active, change-oriented interventions often occurring in the first session or two. Moreover, the *timing of termination* in most couple therapy is typically handled rather differently than the ending of traditional individual psychotherapy, in that it is uncommon for couple therapists to devote much time to a "working through" phase of treatment. Couples in therapy rarely find termination to be as jarring an event as do patients in individual therapy, in part because the intensity of the patient–therapist relationship in couple therapy is usually less than that in individual therapy.

Second, the clear establishment of treatment focus is essential to most couple therapists (Donovan, 1999). Many couple therapists emphasize the couple's presenting problems, with some even limiting their work to these problems, and all couple therapists respect them. Couple therapists typically show minimal interest in a couple's general patterns of interaction and tend to emphasize the patterns that revolve around presenting problems, that is, the system's "problem-maintenance structures" (Pinsof, 1995).

Third, couple therapists tend to be eclectic, if not truly integrative, in their use of techniques; to be ecumenical in the use of techniques that address cognitive, behavioral, and affective domains of patients' experience; and increasingly, to address both the "inner" and "outer" person. Moreover, couple therapists of varying therapeutic persuasions regularly use out-of-session "homework" tasks in an effort to provoke change that is supported in the natural environment.

Fourth, the therapist–patient relationship in most couple therapy is seen as far less pivotal to the outcome of treatment than in most individual therapy because the central healing relationship is the relationship between the couple partners. Moreover, the usual brevity of couple therapy tends to mitigate the development of intense transferences to the therapist. In contrast to much traditional individual psychotherapy, the classical "corrective emotional experience" is to be found within the couple-as-the-patient.

A FRAMEWORK FOR COMPARING COUPLE THERAPIES

Our theories are our inventions; but they may be merely ill-reasoned guesses, bold conjectures, hypotheses. Out of these we create a world, not the real world, built our own notes on which we try to catch the real world.
                                    —Karl Popper

The guidelines that follow include the basic and requisite elements of an adequate description of any approach to couple therapy or discussion of its application to particular populations. In presenting these guidelines, the intent was to steer a middle course between constraining the authors' expository creativity, and providing the reader with sufficient anchor points for comparative study. Contributors to the *Handbook* succeeded in following these guidelines, while describing their respective approaches in an engaging way. Although authors were encouraged to sequence their material within chapter sections according to the guidelines provided, some flexibility was allowed. Authors were not required to limit their presentations to the matters raised in the guidelines, and certainly did not need to address every point identified in the guidelines, but they were urged to address these matters if they were relevant to the treatment approach being described. Authors were also allowed to merge sections of the guidelines, if doing so helped them communicate their perspectives more meaningfully.

BACKGROUND OF THE APPROACH

History is the version of past events that people have decided to agree on.
                                    —Napoleon Bonaparte

Purpose

To place the approach in historical perspective both within the field of psychotherapy in general and within the domain of couple–family therapy in particular.

Points to Consider

1. The major influences contributing to the development of the approach—for example, people, books, research, theories, conferences.
2. The therapeutic forms, if any, that were forerunners of the approach. Did this approach evolve from a method of individual therapy? Family therapy?
3. Brief description of early theoretical principles and/or therapy techniques.
4. Sources of more recent changes in evolution of the model (e.g., research findings from neuroscience).

People's experience and behavior can be changed for the better in an inestimable variety of ways that have a major, and even enduring, impact on both their individual and relational lives. And although many naturally occurring experiences can be life-altering and even healing, none of these qualify as "psychotherapeutic." "Psychotherapy" is not defined as any experience that leads to valued psychological outcomes. Rather, it refers to a particular type of socially constructed process. Though written almost four decades ago in the context of individual psychotherapy, Meltzoff and Kornreich's (1970) definition of psychotherapy probably has not yet been improved upon:

> Psychotherapy is … the informed and planful application of techniques derived from established psychological principles, by persons qualified through training and experience to understand these principles and to apply these techniques with the intention of assisting individuals to modify such personal characteristics as feelings, values, attitudes and behaviors which are judged by the therapist to be maladaptive or maladjustive. (p. 4)

Given such a definition of (any) psychotherapy, it follows that developing an understanding and appreciation of the professional roots and historical context of psychotherapeutic models is an essential aspect of one's education as a therapist. Lacking such awareness, the student of couple therapy is likely to find such theories to be rather disembodied abstractions that seem to have evolved from nowhere, and for no known reason. Each therapist's choice of a theoretical orientation (including any variation of an eclectic or integrative mixture) ultimately reflects a personal process (Gurman, 1990). In addition, an important aspect of a therapist's ability to help people change lies not only in his or her belief in the more technical aspects of the chosen orientation but also the worldview implicit in it (Frank & Frank, 1991; Messer & Winokur, 1984; Simon, 2006). Having some exposure to the historical origins of a therapeutic approach helps clinicians comprehend such an often only-implicit worldview. Moreover, having some exposure to the historical origins and evolving conceptualizations of couple therapy more broadly is an important component of a student's introduction to the field.

In addition to appreciating the professional roots of therapeutic methods, it is enlightening to understand why particular methods, or sometimes clusters of related methods, appear on the scene in particular historical periods. The intellectual, economic, and political contexts in which therapeutic approaches arise often provide meaningful clues

about the emerging social, scientific, and philosophical values that frame clinical encounters. Such values may have subtle but salient impact on whether newer treatment approaches endure. Thus, for example, postmodernism, a modern, multinational intellectual movement that extends well beyond the realm of couple therapy into the worlds of art, drama, literature, political science, and so forth, questions the time-honored notion of a fully knowable and objective external reality, arguing that all "knowledge" is local, relative, and socially constructed. Likewise, integrative approaches have recently occupied a much more prominent place in the evolving landscape of couple therapy, partly in response to greater societal expectations that psychotherapy demonstrate its efficacy and effectiveness, and partly as a natural outgrowth of the practice of couple and family therapy having become commonplace in the provision of "mainstream" mental health services to a degree that even a couple of decades ago could only have been imagined.

A brief historical review of the evolution of the history of couple therapy may help to put a great deal of the rest of this volume in context. Readers interested in a more detailed and nuanced discussion of the history of the field are referred to Gurman and Fraenkel's (2002) "The History of Couple Therapy: A Millennial Review," which describes the major conceptual and clinical influences and trends in the history of couple therapy, and chronicles the history of research on couple therapy as well. But, as urged by Alice when she was adventuring in Wonderland, we "start at the beginning" before proceeding to the middle (or end).

Every chronicler of the history of couple therapy (present company included, e.g., Gurman & Fraenkel, 2002) notes that as recently as 1966, couple therapy (then usually referred to as "marriage counseling") was considered "a technique in search of a theory" (Manus, 1966), a "hodgepodge of unsystematically employed techniques grounded tenuously, if at all, in partial theories at best" (Gurman & Jacobson, 1985, p. 1). By 1995, the field had evolved and matured to such a degree that Gurman and Jacobson saw adequate evidence to warrant asserting that couple therapy had "come of age" (p. 6). Although this assessment was thought by some (Johnson & Lebow, 2000) to be "premature," certainly the last decade of both conceptual and scientific advances in the understanding and treatment of couple and marital problems has included some of the most significant, coherent, and empirically grounded developments of the last 20 years in any branch of the broad world of psychotherapy (Gurman & Fraenkel, 2002), as a reading of this volume demonstrates.

A Four-Phase History of Couple Therapy

Couple therapy has evolved through four quite discernibly different phases. The first phase, from about 1930 to 1963, was the "Atheoretical Marriage Counseling Formation" phase. "Marriage counseling," practiced by many service-oriented professionals who would not be considered today to be "mental health experts" (e.g., obstetricians, gynecologists, family life educators, clergymen), was regularly provided to consumers who were neither severely maladjusted nor struggling with diagnosable psychiatric/psychological disorders, often with a rather strong value-laden core of advice giving and "guidance" about proper and adaptive family and marital roles and life values. Such counseling was typically very brief and quite didactic, present-focused, and limited to conscious experience.

Of tremendous significance, conjoint therapy, the almost universally dominant format in which couple therapy is practiced nowadays, did not actually begin to be regularly practiced until the middle to late 1960s, during the second phase (c. 1931–1966) of couple therapy, which Gurman and Fraenkel (2002) call "Psychoanalytic Experimentation." "Marriage counseling," having no theory or technique of its own to speak of, grafted onto itself a sort of loosely held together array of ideas and interventions from what was then the only influential general approach to psychotherapeutic intervention, that is, psychoanalysis, in its many shapes and varieties, including less formal psychodynamic methods. Novices to the current world of couple therapy may find it more than difficult to imagine a world of practice and training in which there were no cognitive-behavioral, narrative, structural, strategic, solution-focused, or humanistic–experiential, let alone "integrative" or "eclectic" approaches from which to draw.

A few daring psychoanalysts, recognizing what now seem like such self-evident, inherent limitations of trying to help dysfunctional couples by working with individuals, had begun in this phase to risk (and often suffered the consequence of) professional excommunication from psychoanalytic societies by meeting jointly with members of the same family, a forbidden practice, of course. In a phrase, the focus of their efforts was on the "interlocking neuroses" of married partners. And now, marriage counselors, completely marginalized by the world of psychoanalysis, and even by the field of clinical psychology that emerged post–World War II, was understandably attempting to attach itself to the most prestigious "peer" group it could. Unfortunately for them, marriage counseling had "hitched its wagon not to a rising star, but to the falling star of psychoanalytic marriage therapy" (Gurman & Fraenkel, 2002, p. 207) that was largely about to burn out and evaporate in the blazing atmosphere that would begin with the rapid emergence of the revolutionary psychotherapeutic movement known as "family therapy."

The third phase of couple therapy's history, "Family Therapy Incorporation" (c. 1963–1985) was deadly for the stagnating field of marriage counseling. The great majority of the early pioneers and founders of family therapy (e.g., Boszormenyi-Nagy, Bowen, Jackson, Minuchin, Whitaker, Wynne) were psychiatrists (many, not surprisingly, with formal psychoanalytic training) who had become disaffected with the medical/psychiatric establishment because of its inherent conservatism, in terms of its unwillingness to explore new models of understanding psychological disturbance and new methods to help people with such difficulties. These leaders railed against the prevailing, individually oriented zeitgeist of almost all psychoanalytic thought and what they viewed philosophically as unwarranted pathologizing of individuals in relational contexts. And so, in distancing themselves from the psychoanalytic circle, they inevitably left the marriage counselors behind. Haley (1984) has caustically argued, moreover, that there was not "a single school of family therapy which had its origin in a marriage counseling group, nor is there one now" (p. 6). Going still further, and capturing the implicit views of other leaders within family therapy, Haley noted tersely that "marriage counseling did not seem relevant to the developing family therapy field" (pp. 5–6). As family therapy ascended through its "golden age" (Nichols & Schwartz, 1998, p. 8) from about 1975 to 1985, marriage counseling and marriage therapy (e.g., Sager, 1966, 1976), while certainly still practiced, receded to the end of the line.

Four Strong Voices

Four especially influential voices arose in family therapy in terms of influence, both short and long-term, on clinical work with couples. Don Jackson (1965a, 1965b), a psychiatrist trained in Sullivanian psychoanalysis, and a founder of the famous Mental Research Institute in Palo Alto, California, made household names of such influential concepts as the "report" and "command" attributes of communication, the "double bend," "family homeostasis," and "family rules." And the "marital quid pro quo" became a cornerstone concept in all of couple therapy. This notion, linking interactional/systemic dimensions of couple life with implicit aspects of individual self-definition and self-concept, was a very powerful one. Its power on the field at large, unfortunately, was limited to a major degree because of the untimely death of its brilliant creator in 1969, at the age of 48. Had Jackson lived much longer, he no doubt would have been the first significant "integrative" couple therapist. In this sense, his premature death certainly delayed the advent of such integrative ideas for at least a decade (cf. Gurman, 1981).

Another seminal clinical thinker in the third phase of the history of couple therapy, whose work was decidedly eclectic and collaborative with new ideas, was Virginia Satir (1964). Her work, like many current approaches to couple therapy, emphasized both skills and connection, always aware of what Nichols (1987) would many years later, in a different context, refer to as "the self in the system." She was both a connected humanistic healer and a wise practical teacher with couples, urging self-expression, self-actualization, and relational authenticity. Sadly for the field of couple (and family) therapy, Satir, the only highly visible woman pioneer, was soon marginalized by decidedly more "male" therapeutic values such as rationality and attention to the power dimension of intimate relating. Indeed, Satir was even referred to by a senior colleague in family therapy as a "naive and fuzzy thinker" (Nichols & Schwartz, 1998, p. 122). Not for about 20 years, following a 1994 debate with one of the world's most influential family therapists, who criticized Satir for her humanitarian zeal, would there emerge new approaches to couple therapy that valued, indeed privileged, affect, attachment, and connection (Schwartz & Johnson, 2000).

Murray Bowen was the first family therapy clinical theorist to address multigenerational and transgenerational matters systematically with couples. Although his early forays into the field of family disturbance emphasized trying to unlock the relational dimensions of schizophrenia, in fact, his most enduring contributions probably center on the marital dyad, certainly his central treatment unit. His emphasis on blocking pathological multigenerational transmission processes via enhancing partners' self-differentiation was not entirely individually focused, and, indeed, placed a good deal of clinical attention on the subtle ways in which distressed couples almost inevitably seemed to be able intuitively to recruit in ("triangulate") a third force (whether an affair partner, family member, or even abstract values and standards) to stabilize a dyad in danger of spinning out of control. Unlike Satir, Bowen (1978) operated from a therapeutic stance of a dispassionate, objective "coach," believing that "conflict between two people will resolve automatically if both remain in emotional contact with a third person who can relate actively to both without taking sides with either" (p. 177). Bowen died in 1990, leaving behind a rich conceptual legacy, but a relatively small number of followers and adherents to his theories.

Without doubt, the "golden age" family therapist whose work most powerfully impacted the practice of couple therapy was Jay Haley. His 1963 article, efficiently entitled "Marriage Therapy," undoubtedly marked *the* defining moment at which family therapy incorporated and usurped what little was left in the stalled-out marriage counseling and psychodynamic marriage therapy domains. Haley's ideas are considered here in some detail because they were, and continue to be, the most pervasively influential and broad-scope clinical perspective on couple functioning and couple therapy to have emerged from the family therapy movement.

Beyond its very substantial content, Haley's (1963) article (and many subsequent publications) challenged virtually every aspect of extant psychodynamic and humanistic therapy principles. It disavowed widespread beliefs about the nature of marital functioning and conflict, about what constituted the appropriate focus of therapy and the role of the therapist, and what constituted appropriate therapeutic techniques.

For Haley, the central relational dynamic of marriage involved power and control. As he put the matter, "The major conflicts in marriage center in the problem of who is to tell whom what to do under what circumstances" (Haley, 1963, p. 227). Problems arose in marriage when the hierarchical structure was unclear, when there was a lack of flexibility, or when the relationship was marked by rigid symmetry or complementarity. When presenting complaints centered explicitly on the marital relationship, control was seen by Haley as the focal clinical theme. More subtly, though, Haley also believed that even when the presenting problem was the symptom of one person, power was at issue: The hierarchical incongruity of the symptomatic partner's position was central, in that the symptom bearer was assumed to have gained and maintained an equalization of marital power through his or her difficulties. Symptoms of individuals, then, became ways to define relationships, and they were seen as both metaphors for and diversions from other problems that were too painful for the couple to address explicitly.

In this way, symptoms of individuals in a marriage, as well as straightforwardly relational complaints, were mutually protective (Madanes, 1980), and were significantly seen as serving functions for the partners as a dyad. Because symptoms and other problems were seen as functional for the marital unit, resistance to change was seen as almost inevitable, leading Haley (1963) to formulate his "first law of human relations"; that is, "when one individual indicates a change in relation to another, the other will respond in such a way as to diminish that change" (p. 234, original emphasis omitted).

Such a view of the almost inherent property of marital (and family) systems to resist change was not limited to the husband–wife interaction. This view necessarily led to the position that the therapist, in his or her attempts to induce change, must often go about this task indirectly. Thus, for Haley (1963), the therapist "may never discuss this conflict (who is to tell whom what to do under what circumstances) explicitly with the couple" (p. 227). Haley (1976) believed that "the therapist should not share his observations ... that action could arouse defensiveness" (p. 18). Achieving insight, although not entirely dismissed, was enormously downplayed in importance, in marked contrast to psychodynamic models.

Also viewed negatively by Haley (1976) were such commonplace and previously unchallenged clinical beliefs as the possible importance of discussing the past ("It is a good idea to avoid the past ... because marital partners are experts at debating past issues. ... No matter how interested a therapist is in how people got to the point where they are, he should restrain himself from such explorations" [p. 164]); the importance of making direct requests ("The therapist should avoid forcing a couple to ask explicitly for what they want from each other. ... This approach is an abnormal way of communicating" [p. 166, original emphasis omitted]); and the possible usefulness of interpretation ("The therapist should not make any interpretation or

comment to help the person see the problem differently" [p. 28]). Nor was the expression of feelings, common to other couple treatment methods, valued by Haley:

> When a person expresses his emotion in a different way, it means that he is communicating in a different way. In doing so, he forces a different kind of communication from the person responding to him, and this change in turn requires a different way of responding back. When this shift occurs, a system changes because of the change in the communication sequence, but this fact has nothing to do with expressing or releasing emotions [in the sense of catharsis]. (p. 118)

Nor did Haley value expression of feelings for the enhancement of attachment or to foster a sense of security through self-disclosure. Indeed, feeling expression in general was of no priority to Haley ("He should not ask how someone feels about something, but should only gather facts and opinions" [p. 28]).

In contrast, Haley's preferred therapeutic interventions emphasized planned, pragmatic, parsimonious, present-focused efforts to disrupt patterns of behavior that appeared to maintain the major problem of the couple. The strategic therapist was very active and saw his or her central role as finding creative ways to modify problem-maintaining patterns, so that symptoms, or other presenting problems, no longer served their earlier maladaptive purposes. Directives were the therapist's most important change-inducing tools. Some directives were straightforward, but Haley also helped to create a rich fund of indirect, and sometimes resistance-oriented, paradoxical directives (e.g., reframing, prescribing the symptom, restraining change, and relabeling: "Whenever it can be done, the therapist defines the couple as attempting to bring about an amiable closeness, but going about it wrongly, being misunderstood, or being driven by forces beyond their control" [Haley, 1963, p. 226]).

Haley's theoretical and technical contributions were enormously influential in the broad field of family and couple therapy. More than any other individual, Haley influenced sizable portions of at least an entire generation of marital (and family) therapists to see family and couple dynamics "as products of a 'system,' rather than features of persons who share certain qualities because they live together. Thus was born a new creature, 'the family system'" (Nichols & Schwartz, 1998, pp. 60–61). The notion of symptoms serving functions "for the system" was a hallmark of the strategic approach that pervaded clinical discussions, presentations, and practices in the late 1960s through the 1970s and beyond. The anthropomorphizing of the family or couple "system" seemed to "point to an inward, systemic unity of purpose that rendered 'the whole' not only more than the sum of its parts ... [but] somehow *more important than its parts*" (Bogdan, 1984, pp. 19–20).

In summary, Haley urged clinicians to avoid discussing the past, to resist temptations to instill insight, and to downplay couples' direct expression of wishes and feelings. As Framo (1996) would venture three decades after Haley's (1963) concept-shifting marriage therapy article, "I got the impression that Haley wanted to make sure that psychoanalytic thinking be prevented from ruining the newly emerging field of family therapy" (p. 295).

Treading Water

Family therapy had now not merely incorporated, merged with, or absorbed marriage counseling and psychoanalytic couple therapy; it had engulfed, consumed, and devoured them both. Although none of these four family therapy perspectives ever resulted in a separate, discernible "school" of couple therapy, the central concepts in each have trickled down to and permeated the thinking and practices of most psychotherapists who work with couples.

The conceptual development of couple therapy, it must be said, remained quite stagnant during family therapy's "golden age." The most influential clinical thinkers during that period were Clifford Sager (1966, 1976) and James Framo (1981, 1996), whose contributions were in the psychodynamic realm. Although neither Sager, a psychiatrist, nor Framo, a clinical psychologist, were in marginalized professions, their work, though highly respected in some circles, never had the impact it deserved in the overwhelmingly "systems–purist" (Beels & Ferber, 1969) *zeitgeist* of family therapy. And, as noted, Satir's humanistic–experiential emphasis struggled to maintain its currency. The antagonistic attitude of many pioneering family therapists toward couple therapy was all the more bizarre when considered in the context of the unabashed assertion by Nathan Ackerman (1970), the unofficial founder of family therapy, that "the therapy of marital disorders (is) the core approach to family change" (p. 124).

Renewal

By the mid-1980s, couple therapy began to re-emerge with an identity rather different from that of family therapy. This beginning period of sustained theory and practice development and advances in clinical research on couples' relationships and couple therapy signaled the onset of the fourth phase in the history of couple therapy, "Refinement, Extension, Diversification, and Integration" (c. 1986–present).

The attribute of "refinement" in couple therapy of the last two decades has been highlighted primarily by the growth of three treatment traditions in particular: behavioral/cognitive-behavioral couple therapy, attachment-oriented emotionally focused couple therapy, and psychodynamic couple therapy. Details of these clinical methods aside, their most noteworthy commonality is that they all fundamentally derive from longstanding psychological traditions (i.e., social learning theory, humanism–existentialism, and psychodynamicism) that were never core components of the earlier family therapy movement.

Behavioral couple therapy (BCT), launched by the work of Stuart (1969, 1980) and Jacobson (Jacobson & Margolin, 1979; Jacobson & Martin, 1976), has itself passed through quite distinct periods. The "Old BCT" phase emphasized skills training (e.g., communication and problem solving) and change in overt behavior (e.g., behavioral exchanges), and the therapist's role was highly psychoeducational and directive. The second or "New BCT" phase, marked by the development of "Integrative Behavioral Couple Therapy" (Christensen, Jacobson, & Babcock, 1995) shifted a former emphasis on changing the other to a more balanced position of changing self as well, marked by new interventions to facilitate the development of greater mutual acceptance, especially around repetitive patterns of interaction and persistent partner characteristics (e.g., broad personality style variables), or what Gottman (1999) called "perpetual issues." The third BCT evolutionary phase, the "Self-Regulation Phase," focused on the very salient impact of partners' affective self-regulation capacity, as sometimes highlighted in clinical work with volatile, "difficult" couples, in which, for example, one of the partners has with a demonstrably significant personality disorder, often, but not always, borderline personality disorder. Indeed, this self-regulation phase overlaps with the very current phase of BCT's evolution, which has made significant contributions to the treatment of a wide variety of psychological/psychiatric disorders in their intimate relational context (e.g., alcoholism and drug abuse, sexual dysfunction, depression, and bipolar disorder).

The reascendance of the humanistic tradition in psychology and psychotherapy has been heralded by the development and dissemination of the attachment theory–oriented approach known as emotionally focused couple therapy (Johnson & Denton, 2002), and it has not been without the influence of Satir's clinical epistemology and methodology. This approach, which includes a mixture of client-centered, Gestalt, and systemic interventions, fosters affective expression and immediacy, and relational availability and responsiveness. Beyond its initial use with generic couple conflicts, this approach, like some BCT approaches, has been applied recently to the treatment of "individual" problems and disorders, especially those thought to be likely to be influenced positively by an emphasis on secure interpersonal attachment, such as posttraumatic stress disorder. At a more "macro" level, this approach has led the way in the field's "shaking off its no-emotion legacy" (Schwartz & Johnson, 2000, p. 32), and is reminiscent of Duhl and Duhl's (1981) telling comment, "It is hard to kiss a system" (p. 488).

Psychodynamically oriented approaches have reascended in recent years via two very separate pathways. First, object relations theory (e.g., Dicks, 1967; Scharff & Bagnini, 2002) has been undergoing slow but consistent development both in the United States and abroad, and has reestablished a connection with a conceptual thrust in couple and family therapy (e.g., Framo, 1965; Skynner, 1976, 1980, 1981) that had, as noted earlier, largely died out, or at least had gone well underground, in earlier times. Second, psychodynamic concepts have reemerged in couple therapy through their incorporation into more recently developing integrative (e.g., Gurman, 1981, 1992, 2002) and pluralistic (e.g., Snyder, 1999; Snyder & Schneider, 2002) models of treatment, paralleling the very strong movement in the broader world of psychotherapy fostering the process of bringing together both conceptual and technical elements from seemingly incompatible, or at least historically different, traditions to enhance the salience of common mechanisms of therapeutic change and to improve clinical effectiveness.

The "Extension" phase of couple therapy in recent years refers to efforts to broaden its purview beyond helping couples with obvious relationship conflict to the treatment of individual psychiatric disorders, some of which were mentioned earlier. Although family therapy was initially developed, to an important degree, in an effort to understand major mental illness (Wynne, 1983), the political fervor that characterized much of family therapy's "golden age" seriously curtailed attention to the study and treatment of individual psychiatric problems, even (ironically, to be sure) in familial–relational contexts. A great deal of study in recent years has focused on the role of couple/marital factors in the etiology and maintenance of such problems on the one hand, and the use of couple therapy intervention in the management and reduction of the severity of such difficulties on the other.

"Diversification" in couple therapy has been reflected by the broadening perspectives brought to bear by feminism, multiculturalism, and postmodernism. The feminist perspective has cogently drawn attention to the many subtle and implicit ways the process of couple therapy is influenced by gender stereotypes of both therapists and patients/clients (e.g., the paternalistic aspects of a hierarchical, therapist-as-expert, therapy relationship; differing partner experiences of their relationship based on differential access to power, and different expectations regarding intimacy and autonomy).

Multiculturalism has provided the base for couple therapists' broader understanding of the diversity of couples' experience as a function of differences in race, ethnicity, religion, social class, sexual orientation, age, and geographic locale. A modern multicultural perspective has also emphasized that the norms relative to intimacy, the distribution and use of power, and the role of various others in the couple's shared life vary tremendously across couples depending on many of the sociocultural variables noted earlier. The influence of both feminist and multicultural perspectives has no doubt made couple therapy a more collaborative experience than was likely in earlier times.

Finally, the postmodern perspective has introduced profoundly interesting and important practical critiques of how people come to know their reality, with a strong emphasis on the historical and social construction of meaning embodied in many important aspects of being a couple in a long-term relationship. Like feminism and multiculturalism, postmodernism has pushed therapists to recognize the multiplicity of ways in which it is possible to be "a couple."

"Integration" is the final component of this fourth phase in the development of couple therapy. Significant in its emphasis on bringing to bear on clinical practice the best the field has to offer in terms of using validated clinical theories and treatment methodologies and interventions, this dimension of couple therapy has been aptly described (Lebow, 1997) as a "quiet revolution" (p. 1). The integrative movement began in response to the recognition of the existence of common factors that affect treatment outcomes (Sprenkle & Blow, 2004) and the limited evidence of differential effectiveness and efficacy of various couple therapies (Lebow & Gurman, 1995). Proponents of integrative positions (e.g., Gurman, 1981, 2002; Lebow, 1997) assert that a broad base for understanding and changing human behavior is necessary, and that evolving integrative approaches allow for greater treatment flexibility and thereby improve the odds of positive therapeutic outcomes.

The Three-Phase History of Research in Couple Therapy

Statistics are like bikinis ... what they reveal is interesting, what they conceal, vital.

—PAUL WATZLAWICK

Despite the increasing recent importance of the scientific study of therapeutic processes and outcomes in working with couples, research on couples' clinically relevant interaction patterns and on clinical intervention itself has not always been a hallmark of this domain within psychotherapy. Just as Manus (1966) called marriage counseling a "technique in search of a theory," Gurman and Fraenkel (2002) described the period from about 1930 to 1974 as "a technique in search of some data" (p. 240). In a 1957 article, Emily Mudd, a marriage counseling pioneer, discussed the "knowns and unknowns" in the field and, in a word, concluded that there were none of the former and a plethora of the latter. By 1970, Olson reported that the majority of marriage counseling research publications were "mostly descriptive" (p. 524), and what little had appeared on treatment outcomes largely comprised single author–clinicians reporting on their own (uncontrolled) clinical experiences with couples.

In its second phase (c. 1975–1992), beginning in the mid- to late 1970s, there was a decidedly upbeat tone (which Gurman and Fraenkel [2002] called the period of "Irrational Exuberance"), in the field, justified, if not overly justified, by the appearance of the earliest comprehensive reviews of (actual) empirical research on the outcomes of couple therapy (Gurman, 1971, 1973; Gurman

& Kniskern, 1978a, 1978b; Gurman, Kniskern, & Pinsof, 1986). Couple therapy had now established a reasonable empirical base to warrant assertions of its efficacy.

The third phase of the research realm (c. 1993–present), also known as the period of "Caution and Extension," has evidenced attention to a wide variety of much more sophisticated and clinically relevant questions about couple therapy than older "Does it work?" inquiries. Such matters investigated in the last 15 years address questions such as

1. How powerful is couple therapy? (i.e., how "large" are its positive effects in terms of its impact on couples and the percentages of couples whose relationships improve from treatment?)
2. How durable are the effects of change from couple therapy?
3. Does couple therapy ever bring about "negative effects," also known as "deterioration"?
4. What is the relative efficacy and effectiveness of different methods of couple therapy?
5. What therapist factors and what couple factors predict responsiveness to treatment (or, to which treatments)?
6. Is couple therapy helpful in the treatment of "individual" problems and disorders?
7. By what mechanisms do couples' relationships improve in therapy, when they do improve?
8. What are the most essential, core therapeutic change processes that, in general, should be fostered in therapy with couples?

Many of these theoretically and practically important questions had not even been formulated within the field of couple therapy early in the previous decade.

Four Profound Shifts

None of us understand psychotherapy well enough to stop learning from all of us.

—FRANK PITTMAN

Four major shifts in couple therapy that have occurred over time constitute not simply "trends" in the field, but an altered shape of the field that is profound. First, there has been a reinclusion of the individual, a renewed interest in the psychology of the individual that complements the rather unilateral emphasis on relational systems that marked the field for many years. In this sense, couple therapy has become more genuinely "systemic." Second, there has been greater acknowledgment of the reality of psychiatric/psychological disorders, and of the reality that such problems, although both influenced enormously by and influencing core patterns of intimate relaxing, are not reducible to problems at systemic levels of analysis. Third, the major energies that have fueled the growth of couple therapy in the last two decades in terms of both clinical practice and research have come not from the broader field of family therapy, but from the more "traditional" domains of psychological inquiry of social learning theory, psychodynamic theory, and humanistic–experiential theory. This third shift, at once lamentable and renewing, carries profound implications for the field of couple therapy, and nowhere more notably than in the domain of clinical teaching and training.

The final, and ironic, shift identified by Gurman and Fraenkel (2002) in their millennial review of the history of couple therapy, was described as follows:

> No other collective methods of psychosocial intervention have demonstrated a superior capacity to effect clinically meaningful change in as many spheres of human experience as the couple therapies, and many have not yet even shown a comparable capacity. Ironically, *despite its long history of struggles against marginalization and professional disempowerment, couple therapy has emerged as one of the most vibrant forces in the entire domain of family therapy and of psychotherapy-in-general.* (p. 248, emphasis in original)

It is this vibrancy that this *Handbook* is intended to convey.

THE HEALTHY/WELL-FUNCTIONING VERSUS PATHOLOGICAL/DYSFUNCTIONAL COUPLE/MARRIAGE

A successful marriage requires falling in love many times, always with the same person.
                                    —MIGNON MCLAUGHLIN

A healthy marriage is one in which only one person is crazy at a time.
                                    —HEINZ KOHUT

Do married people really live longer, or does it just seem that way?
                                    —STEVEN WRIGHT

Purpose

To describe typical relationship patterns and others factors that differentiate healthy/well-functioning and pathological/dysfunctional couples/marriages.

Points to Consider

1. Does your approach have an explicit point of view on the nature of romantic love?
2. What interaction patterns, or other characteristics, differentiate healthy/satisfied from unhealthy/dissatisfied couples? (Consider relationship areas such as problem solving, communication, expression of affect, sexuality, the balance of individual and couple needs, and the role of individual psychological health.)
3. How do problematic relationship patterns develop? How are they maintained? Are there reliable risk factors for couple functioning and/or couple longevity?
4. Do sociocultural factors, such as ethnicity, class, and race, figure significantly in your model's understanding of couple satisfaction and functioning? Gender factors?
5. How do healthy versus dysfunctional couples handle life-cycle transitions, crises, and so forth? How do they adapt to the inevitable changes of both individuals and relationships?

"Couples" and "Marriages"

The term "couple therapy" has recently come to replace the historically more familiar term "marital therapy" because of its emphasis on the bond between two people, without the associated judgmental tone of social value implied by the traditional term. In the therapy world, the terms are usually used interchangeably. Whether therapeutic methods operate similarly with "marriages" and with "couple" relationships in which there is commitment but no legal bond is unknown but is assumed here. Although there are philosophical advantages to the term "couple therapy," the more familiar term "marital therapy" is still commonly used, and both terms are intended to refer to couples in long-term, committed relationships.

Clarifying the sociopolitical meaning of "couple" versus "marriage" points to a much larger issue; that is, psychotherapy is not only a scientific and value-laden enterprise but is also part and parcel of its surrounding culture. It is a significant source of our current customs and worldviews, thus possessing significance well beyond the interactions between clients and therapists.

At the same time, psychotherapy is a sensitive barometer of those customers and outlooks that the different modes of practice respond to and incorporate within their purview. The relationship between culture and psychotherapy, including couple therapy, to be sure, then, is one of reciprocal influence. For example, a currently important cultural phenomenon affecting the practice of all psychotherapy, couple therapy not excepted, is the medicalization of the treatment of psychological distress and disorder. Thus, the language of medicine has long been prominent in the field of psychotherapy. We talk of "symptoms," "diseases," "disorders," "psychopathology" and "treatment." As Messer and Wachtel (1997) remarked, "It is a kind of new narrative that reframes people's conflicts over value and moral questions as sequelae of 'disease' or 'disorder,' thereby bringing into play the prestige (and hence curative potential) accruing to medicine and technology in our society" (p. 3). Thus, the spread of the biological way of understanding psychopathology, personality traits, and emotional suffering in general, as well as the biological mode of treating emotional disorders, have had their effects on the practice of psychotherapy. Couple therapy is not immune to such cultural phenomena. Clients and therapists are more likely to consider having medication prescribed. Psychologists and other nonmedical therapists, including couple therapists, are collaborating more frequently with physicians in treating their patients. Courses in psychopharmacology that are now routinely offered or even required in clinical and counseling psychology and psychiatric social work training programs are at times also available in programs dedicated to the training of couple and family therapists. Most of the work of couple therapy, of course, is not readily reducible to psychopharmacological therapeusis.

Moreover, any method of couple therapy probably implicitly reveals its aesthetic and moral values by how it conceptualizes mental health and psychological well-being, including relational well-being. As Gurman and Messer (2003, p. 7) have put it,

> The terms of personality theory, psychopathology and the goals of psychotherapy are not neutral. ... They are embedded in a value structure that determines what is most important to know about and change in an individual, couple, family or group. Even schools of psychotherapy that attempt to be neutral with regard to what constitutes healthy (and, therefore, desirable) behavior, and unhealthy (and, therefore, undesirable) behavior inevitably, if unwittingly, reinforce the acceptability of some kinds of client strivings more so that others.

Interestingly, while all approaches to couple therapy are attempts to change or improve some aspect of personality or problematic behavior, the majority of these theories of therapy neither include a concept of personality nor are they closely linked, or at times even linked at all, to a specific theory of personality. In the world of couple therapy, the de facto substitute for personality theory is usually a theory that defines the "interactive personality" of the couple dyad (and its contextual qualifiers). The old family therapy saw that captures this position is the notion that "a system is its own best explanation."

Given the variety of theoretical approaches to couple therapy discussed in this volume, it is hardly surprising that therapists of different theoretical orientations define the core problems of the couples they treat quite differently. These range from whatever the couple presents as its problem to relationship skills deficits, to maladaptive ways of thinking and restrictive narratives about relationships, to problems of self-esteem, to unsuccessful handling of normal life cycle transitions, to unconscious displacement onto the partner of conflicts with one's family of origin, to the inhibited expression of normal adult needs, to the fear of abandonment and isolation.

Despite these varied views of what constitutes the core of marital difficulties, marital therapists of different orientations in recent years have sought a clinically meaningful description and understanding of functional versus dysfunctional intimate relationships that rests on a solid research base. Quite remarkably, and perhaps uniquely in the world of psychotherapy, there has accumulated a very substantial body of research (on couple interaction processes) that has been uniformly praised by and incorporated into the treatment models of a wide range of couple therapies. These findings, on aggregate (Cassidy & Shaver, 1999; Gottman, 1994a, 1994b, 1998, 1999; Johnson & Whiffen, 2003), provide a theoretically and clinically rich and credible description of the typical form and shape of "healthy" and "unhealthy" couple–marital interactions. They are cited as having influenced several of the models of therapy presented in this *Handbook*.

THE PRACTICE OF COUPLE THERAPY

All knowledge is sterile which does not lead to action and end in charity.

—Cardinal Mercier

The Structure of the Therapy Process

Who forces time is pushed back by time; who yields to time finds time on his side.

                 —THE TALMUD

Purpose

To describe the treatment setting, frequency, and duration of treatment characteristic of your approach.

Points to Consider

1. How are decisions made about whom to include in therapy? For example, besides the couple, are children or extended family members ever included?
2. Are psychotropic medications ever used within your method of couple therapy? What are the indications–contraindications for such use? Within your approach are there any particular concerns about a couple therapist referring a patient to a medical colleague for medication evaluation?
3. Are individual sessions with the partners ever held? If "yes," under what conditions? If "no," why not?
4. How many therapists are usually involved? From your perspective, what are the advantages (or disadvantages) of *using* cotherapists?
5. Is therapy typically time-limited or unlimited? Why? Ideal models aside, how long does therapy typically last? How often are sessions typically held?
6. If either partner is in concurrent individual therapy (with another therapist), does the couple therapist regularly communicate with that person about the couple?
7. How are out-of-session contacts (e.g., phone calls) handled? Are there any especially important "ground rules" for proceeding with therapy?

    The two central matters involved in the structure of couple therapy are (1) who participates and (2) for how long (and how often?). As noted earlier, "couple therapy" is nowadays considered to be redundant with the term "conjoint," that is, therapy with an individual that focuses on that person's marital issues is individual therapy focused on marital issues. It is not couple therapy, though it certainly may be conducted in such a way as to reasonably be considered "systematically aware" or "contextually sensitive." Still, it is not

couple therapy. Therapy *about* the couple is not synonymous with therapy *of* the couple.

    And although nonpartners (e.g., parents, children) are not commonly included (cf. Framo, 1981) in therapy sessions during couple therapy, configurations other than the obvious two partners plus one therapist (or two therapists, if there is a cotherapist) are hardly rare. Specifically, many approaches to couple therapy, with a very cogent rationale, and as a matter of standard protocol, arrange for individual meetings with each partner during the early (assessment) phase of the work. Other approaches are very open to intermittent individual meetings for very focused and clear reasons, albeit usually only quite briefly, for very specific strategic purposes (e.g., to help calm down each partner in a highly dysregulated, volatile marriage when little is being accomplished in three-way meetings). At the other end of the continuum are couple therapy models that, for equally compelling reasons, never, or almost never, allow the therapist to meet with individual partners.

    This specific aspect of the structure of couple therapy regarding whether, and under what conditions, individual sessions may occur is one of the most important practical decisions to be made by couple therapists, regardless of their preferred theoretical orientations. Although a seemingly simple matter on the surface, therapist policies and procedures about how the decision is addressed and implemented can carry truly profound implications for the establishment and maintenance of working therapeutic alliances, therapeutic neutrality–multilaterality, and even basic positions on what (or who) is (or has) "the problem." It is a recurrent clinical situation that each therapist working with couples must think through carefully and about which it is important to maintain consistency.

    As to the matter of the length of couple therapy, it is clear, as discussed earlier, that couple therapy is overwhelmingly brief by any temporal standards in the world of psychotherapy. Three decades ago, Gurman and Kniskern (1978b, 1981) found that well over two-thirds of the courses of couple therapy were less than 20 sessions, and almost 20 years later, Simmons and Doherty (1995; Doherty & Simmons, 1996) found reliable evidence that the mean length of couple therapy is about 17–18 sessions. In contrast to the history of individual psychotherapy, the dominant pattern in couple (and family) therapy has been that "brief" treatment by traditional standards is "expected, commonplace, and the norm" (Gurman, 2001).

Couple (and family) therapies were brief long before managed care administratively truncated therapy experiences, as Gurman has demonstrated.

It is important and interesting to note, moreover, that most of this naturally (vs. administratively) occurring brevity of couple therapy has not included planned, time-limited practice. In no small measure this has occurred not because of arbitrarily imposed treatment authorization limits, but because of the dominant treatment values of most couple (and family) therapists (e.g., valuing change in presenting problems, emphasizing couples' resourcefulness and resilience; focusing on the "Why now?" developmental context in which couple problems often arise; viewing symptoms as relationally embedded; and emphasizing change in the natural environment).

The Role of the Therapist

Some people see things as they are and ask, "Why?"; others see things as they could be and ask, "Why not?"
—GEORGE BERNARD SHAW

We need different thinks for different shrinks.
—A. C. R. SKYNNER

Purpose

To describe the stance the therapist takes with the couple.

Points to Consider

1. What is the therapist's essential role? Consultant? Teacher? Healer?
2. What is the role of the therapist–couple alliance? How is a working alliance fostered? In your approach, what are the most common and important errors the therapist can make in building early working alliances?
3. To what degree does the therapist overtly control sessions? How active/directive is the therapist? How should the therapist deal with moments of volatile emotional escalation or affective dysregulation in sessions?
4. Do patients talk predominantly to the therapist or to each other?
5. Does the therapist use self-disclosure? What limits are imposed on therapist self-disclosure?
6. Does the therapist's role change as therapy progresses? As termination approaches?
7. What clinical skills or other therapist attributes are most essential to successful therapy in your approach?

In the last couple of decades, a great deal of effort has been put into identifying empirically supported treatments (ESTs) among the many existing forms of psychotherapy, including couple therapy. Although such efforts are helpful for public policy-making, they tend to focus heavily on one particular domain of the therapy experience, the role and power of therapeutic techniques. Increasingly, but only quite recently, EST-oriented efforts have been counterbalanced by attempts to investigate and understand the essential characteristics of ESRs (i.e., empirically supported therapeutic relationships; Norcross, 2002). Indeed, such efforts now rest on a solid empirical base for arguing that the therapist as a person exerts large effects on the outcome of psychotherapy, and that these effects often outweigh the effects attributable to treatment techniques per se; in addition, the relationship established between therapist and patient may be more powerful than particular interventions (Wampold, 2001). Even very symptom-focused and behavior-focused therapy encounters, which emphasize the use of clearly defined change-inducing techniques, occur in the context of human relationships characterized by support and reassurance, persuasion, and the modeling of active coping.

The kind of therapeutic relationship required by each approach to couple therapy includes the overall "stance" the therapist takes toward the experience (how working alliances are fostered and how active, how self-disclosing, how directive, and how reflective, etc., the therapist is). Different models of couple therapy may call forth and call for rather different therapist attributes and interpersonal inclinations. Thus, therapists with a more or less "take charge" personal style may be better suited to therapy approaches that require a good deal of therapist activity and structuring than to those requiring a more reflective style.

Given the presumed effectiveness equivalence of the major methods of psychotherapy and the absence within couple therapy of any evidence (Lebow & Gurman, 1995) deviating from this recurrent pattern of research findings, it is not surprising that idiosyncratic personal factors influence therapists' preferred ways of practicing. Thus, Norcross and Prochaska (1983) found that therapists generally do not advocate different approaches on the basis of their relative scientific status, but are more influenced by their own direct clinical experience, personal values and philosophy, and life experiences.

The therapist's role in couple therapy varies along several dimensions, most noticeably in terms of emotional closeness–distance relative to the couple. Three gross categories of the therapist's emotional proximity can be discerned: the educator/coach, the perturbator, and the healer. These relational stances vary as a function of the degree to which the therapist intentionally and systematically uses his or her "self" (e.g., by self-disclosure of fantasy material, personal or countertransferential reactions, or factual information) or explicitly addresses the nature and meaning of the therapist–partner relationship. The therapist as educator/coach sees him- or herself as possessing expert, professional knowledge about human relationships and change processes, and attempts to impart such knowledge to couples as a basis for inducing change. The couple therapist as perturbator possesses expert understanding of problematic family processes, but tends to use this awareness more from an outside stance to induce change in the couple system, without giving partners information, concepts, or methods they can take away from therapy for future use. The couple therapist as healer places special value on the transformative power of the personal relationships in treatment.

Assessment and Treatment Planning

If you are sure you understand everything that is going on, you are hopelessly confused.

—WALTER MONDALE

Purpose

To describe the methods used to understand a couple's clinically relevant patterns of interaction, symptomatology and adaptive resources.

Points to Consider

1. Briefly describe any formal or informal system (including tests, questionnaires) for assessing couples, in addition to the clinical interview.
2. In addition to understanding the couple's presenting problem(s), are there areas/issues that you routinely assess (e.g., violence, substance abuse, extramarital affairs, sexual behavior, relationships with extended family, parenting, etc.)?
3. At what unit levels (e.g., intrapsychic, behavioral) and psychological levels (e.g., intrapsychic, behavioral) is assessment done?
4. What is the temporal focus of assessment (i.e., present vs. past); for example, is the history

of partner/mate selection useful in treatment planning?
5. To what extent are issues involving gender, ethnicity, and other sociocultural factors included in your assessment? Developmental/life cycle changes?
6. Are couple strengths/resources a focus of your assessment?
7. Is the assessment process or focus different when a couple presents with problems about both relational and "individual" matters (e.g., depression, anxiety)?
8. Likewise, is the assessment process or focus different when the therapist perceives the presence of individual psychopathology in either–both partners, even though such difficulties are not identified by the couple as central concerns?

The practicality of a coherent theory of couple therapy, including ideas about relationship development and dysfunction, becomes clear as the therapist sets out to make sense of both problem stability (how problems persist) and problem change (how problems can be modified). As indicated earlier in Meltzoff and Kornreich's (1970) definition of psychotherapy, couple therapists are obligated to take some purposeful action in regard to their understanding of the nature and parameters of whatever problems, symptoms, complaints or dilemmas are presented. They typically are interested in understanding what previous steps patients have taken to resolve or improve their difficulties, and what adaptive resources the couple, and perhaps other people in the couple's world, has for doing so. They also pay attention to the cultural (ethnic, racial, religious, social class, gender) context in which clinically relevant concerns arise. Such contextualizing factors can play an important role in how therapists collaboratively both define the problem at hand and select a general strategy for addressing the problem therapeutically. As Hayes and Toarmino (1995) have emphasized, understanding the cultural context in which problems are embedded can serve as an important source of hypotheses about what maintains problems, and what types of interventions may be helpful.

How couple therapists actually engage in clinical assessment and treatment planning vary from approach to approach, but all include face-to-face clinical interviews. The majority of couple therapists emphasize the therapist–patient conversation as the source of such understanding. Couple therapists also inherently complement such conversations with direct observations of the problem as it occurs between the couple partners in the clinical interview itself. Multigenerationally oriented therapists may also use genograms to help discern important transgenerational legacies. In addition, some therapists regularly include in the assessment process a variety of patient self-report questionnaires or inventories, and a smaller number may also use very structured interview guides, which are usually research-based instruments. Generally, therapists who use such devices have very specialized clinical practices (e.g., focusing on a very particular set of clinical disorders, in their relational context) for which such measures have been specifically designed (e.g., alcoholism and drug abuse, sexual dysfunction).

The place of standard psychiatric diagnosis in the clinical assessment phase of psychotherapy varies widely. The majority of couple therapists of different theoretical orientations routinely consider the traditional diagnostic psychiatric status of patients according to the criteria of the *Diagnostic and Statistical Manual of Mental Disorders* (DSM-IV; American Psychiatric Association, 1994), at least to meet requirements for financial reimbursement, maintenance of legally required treatment records, and other such institutional contingencies. Although considering such diagnostic dimensions may provide a useful general orientation to concerns of a subset of couples seen in therapy, proponents of every method of couple therapy develop their own idiosyncratic ways of understanding each couple's problem. Moreover, proponents of some newer approaches to couple therapy argue that "diagnoses" do not exist "out there" in nature, but merely represent the consensual labels attached to certain patterns of behavior in particular cultural and historical contexts. Such therapists consider the use of diagnostic labeling as an unfortunate and unwarranted assumption of the role of "expert" by therapists, which may inhibit genuine collaborative exploration between therapists and "patients" (or "clients"). For such therapists, what matters more are the more fluid issues with which people struggle, not the diagnoses they are given.

The major differences among couple therapists are more likely to appear in their conceptualizations of what they experience and observe. Therapists of different theoretical orientations can be rather reliably differentiated in terms of the levels of assessment on which they focus. Two dimensions of these levels may be identified—the unit level and the experiential level. The "unit level" refers to the composition of the psychosocial unit(s) on which the assessment focuses. The individual, the couple, the parental subsystem, the whole family, and the family plus nonnuclear family social entities (grandparental subsystem, school system, etc.) may all be given attention. Psychodynamic, experiential–humanistic, and intergenerational therapists tend to be interested in assessing the potential treatment-planning role (even if only by reference, rather than face-to-face) of a larger number of units, whereas proponents of orientations that focus more on resolving presenting problems (e.g., cognitive-behavioral, narrative, structural, and strategic approaches) tend to assess a less complex array of these units. The "experiential level" refers to the level of organization at which assessment occurs (e.g., molecular/biological, unconscious, conscious, interpersonal, and transpersonal), and couple therapists also differ quite significantly on the related dimension of past- versus present-centeredness. The more pragmatic (Keeney & Sprenkle, 1982) therapists, who focus more on presenting problems (e.g., cognitive-behavioral, strategic, and structural approaches), tend to show little to no significant interest in either unconscious psychological processes, or the couple's or its individual members' past. By contrast, more aesthetically oriented (Keeney & Sprenkle, 1982) therapists (e.g., psychodynamic–object relations, humanistic, and symbolic–experiential therapists), who tend to espouse a more relationship-based style of intervention in which the "real" problem is believed initially to be hidden, are more attuned to psychological events that are not so immediate. Such therapists' assessments tend to emphasize inference, whereas the more pragmatic therapists' assessments tend to emphasize observation.

Of course, it is essential for couple therapists to cast a fairly wide net in the opening assessment–treatment planning phase of the work, routinely raising questions about the possible presence in the couple's relationship of patterns and problems that in fact often go unstated by couples, even though they might become essential treatment foci (e.g., substance abuse), or that might even preclude couple therapy (e.g., severe physical or verbal aggression).

Goal Setting

Every calling is great when greatly pursued.
—OLIVER WENDELL HOLMES

Purpose

To describe the nature of therapeutic goals and the process by which they are established.

Points to Consider

1. Are there treatment goals that apply to all or most cases for which your approach is appropriate regardless of between-couple differences or presenting problem? Relatedly, does a couple's marital status influence your goal setting?
2. How are the central goals determined for/with a given couple? How are they prioritized?
3. Who determines the goals of treatment? Therapist, couple, other? How are differences in goals resolved? To what extend and in what ways are therapist values involved in goal setting?
4. Are treatment goals discussed with the couple explicitly? If "yes," why? If "no," why not?
5. How are the goals (initial and longer-term) of therapy affected when the couple's presenting problems focus on matters of violence, infidelity, or possible separation/divorce?

Different theoretical orientations to couple therapy emphasize different types of typical goals, but a number of goals are also shared across couple therapy approaches. Most couple therapists would endorse most of the following ultimate goals (desired end states), regardless of the nature of the presenting problem: (1) reduction of psychiatric symptoms, or, when such symptoms are not a major focus of treatment, reduction of other presenting problem behavior or experience, especially in relation to interactional patterns that maintain the problem(s); (2) increased couple resourcefulness (e.g., improved communication, problem-solving, and conflict resolution skills, and enhanced coping skills and adaptability); (3) improvement in the fulfillment of individual psychological needs for attachment, cohesion, and intimacy; increased trust and equitability; and enhanced capacity to foster the development of individual couple members; (4) increased ability to interact effectively with important, larger social systems; and (5) increased awareness and understanding of how couples' patterns of interaction influence their everyday effectiveness in living, as well as how such patterns affect, and are affected by, the psychological health and satisfaction of individuals.

Within some approaches to couple therapy, certain specific *ultimate goals* are considered impor-tant in all cases, regardless of differences among couples. For example, in Bowen family systems therapy, a universal goal is the differentiation of the self from the system. Other approaches (e.g., brief strategic and solution-focused approaches) aim almost exclusively at solving the presenting problem.

In addition to ultimate goals, a variety of *mediating goals* are emphasized in the various couple therapy approaches. Mediating goals are shorter-term and include changes in psychological processes through which it is presumed an individual or couple go to reach treatment objectives. They are sometimes referred to as "process goals." Common forms of mediating or process goals are the achievement of insight; the teaching of various interpersonal skills, such as communication and problem solving; and the description of interlocking pathologies or blocking of rigid symptom and problem-maintaining patterns of behavior to allow opportunities to experiment with more adaptive responses. Mediating goals may also be more abstract and, in any case, are not necessarily made explicit by the therapist. Mediating goals are particularly unlikely to be discussed between the couple and therapist in a wide variety of approaches, and even the extent of the discussion of ultimate goals of treatment varies enormously across the many influential methods of couple therapy.

Process and Technical Aspects of Couple Therapy

It is only an auctioneer who can equally and impartially admire all schools of art.

—OSCAR WILDE

Purpose

To describe techniques and strategies always or frequently used in your approach to couple therapy, and their tactical purposes.

Points to Consider

1. How structured are therapy sessions? Is there an ideal (or typical) pacing or rhythm to sessions?
2. What techniques or strategies are used to join the couple or to create a treatment alliance? How are "transference"–"countertransference" reactions dealt with?
3. What techniques or strategies lead to changes in structure or transactional patterns? Iden-

tify, describe, and illustrate major commonly used techniques.

4. How is the decision made to use a particular technique or strategy at a particular time? Are some techniques more or less likely to be used at different stages of therapy?
5. Are different techniques used with different types of couples? For example, different or additional techniques called upon when the therapy in addressing problems involving individual psychopathology, difficulties, or disabilities, and so forth, in addition to interactional/relational problems, or, alternatively, with more dysfunctional, distressed, or committed couples?
6. Are "homework" assignments or other out-of-session tasks used?
7. Are there techniques used in other approaches to couple therapy that you would probably never use?
8. What are the most commonly encountered forms of resistance to change? How are these dealt with?
9. If revealed to the therapist outside conjoint sessions, how are "secrets" (e.g., extramarital affairs) handled?
10. What are both the most common and the most serious technical or strategic errors a therapist can make operating within your therapeutic approach?
11. On what basis is termination decided, and how is termination effected? What characterizes "good" versus "bad" termination?

To a newcomer to the world of couple therapy, the variety and sheer number of available therapeutic techniques no doubt seem daunting and dizzying to apprehend: acceptance training, affective downregulation, affective reconstruction, behavioral exchange, boundary marking, communication training, circular questioning, dream analysis, enactment, empathic joining, exceptions questioning, exposure, externalizing conversations, family-of-origin consultation, genogram construction, interpretation of defenses, jamming, joining, meta-emotion training, ordeal prescription, paradoxical injunction, positive connotation, problem-solving training, reattribution, reframing, scaling, sculpting, Socratic questioning, softening, unbalancing, unified detachment training, unique outcomes questioning, witnessing (all used, of course, with *zeal*).

Yet, appearances to the contrary notwithstanding, there is actually less technique chaos than might be obvious at first to a newly arrived

Martian. Overall, behavior change is probably the dominant mode of change induction in couple therapy, in contrast to insight–reflection. "Behavior change techniques" refer to any therapeutic techniques used to modify observable behavior, whether at the level of the individual or the dyad (or larger family), whereas "insight-oriented techniques" refer to those techniques that lead to change in awareness or perhaps affective experience, without any automatic change in overt behavior. In contrast to much traditional individual psychotherapy, in which insight is generally assumed to precede therapeutic change, the opposite sequence is often preferred in most couple therapy. In addition, couple therapists are usually more bidirectional in their thinking; that is, they believe that change can be initiated in any domain of psychosocial organization. For pragmatic reasons, though, initial change is more often sought at the interactional, public level of experience.

We can furthermore distinguish between couple therapy techniques that focus on in-session versus out-of-session experience. The wide use of techniques that emphasize patients' experiences away from the consultation room reflects couple therapists' respect for the healing power of intimate relationships and their belief that change that endures and generalizes to everyday life is not achieved primarily in the substitutive relationship between therapists and their patients but, rather, between relationship partners in their natural environment. What is especially striking about the centrality of out-of-session techniques in couple therapy is that it also reflects the modal couple therapist's view that the dominant site of action in therapy change is within the couple relationship.

Therapeutic techniques in couple therapy are heavily influenced by techniques focused on cognitive dimensions of experience, such as meaning and attribution, and those focused on action. The former may emphasize a therapist's attempts to *change meaning*, to *discover meaning*, or to *co-create meaning*. Such efforts can range, for example, from one therapist's attempts to influence a partner to see that his or her partner's general inexpressiveness reflects not that person's lack of loving feeling but internal discomfort regarding intimate conversation, to another therapist's "positive reframing" of such inexpressiveness as an understandable attempt to maintain a tolerable level of affective arousal in a marriage to a highly expressive mate, even with the unfortunate self-sacrifice that it requires. Some meaning-oriented interventions in couple therapy assume that the therapist's meaning is correct and reflects a "knowable reality" and psychological truth. Others are 180 degrees from this position, and believe that because there is no knowable external reality, all of therapy involves the making of meanings ("co-construction of reality") rather than their discovery. For these latter approaches, "truth" is pragmatic—in other words, it is a meaning or explanatory framework that leads to clinically relevant change.

Action-oriented techniques can be further meaningfully divided into techniques that assume couple partners already have the requisite behaviors in their repertoire and those that assume that they presently lack such skills or knowledge. Action-oriented techniques involve either therapeutic directives or skills training. Directives can involve either in-session or out-of-session (often referred to as "homework tasks") actions.

Since the 1990s, there has been a strong movement within couple therapy toward combining elements of different methods, leading to the increased borrowing of techniques across scholastic lines. Some of this borrowing has been in the form of technical eclecticism—that is, using techniques presumed to be relevant and effective, without regard to the originating theories' basic assumptions or the contradictions therein contained. Other borrowing has grown out of the search for the so-called "common ingredients" of effective therapy, as discussed earlier, and has paid considerable attention to matters of conceptual clarity and coherence. In addition, the general practice of couple therapy has become increasingly more comprehensive and increasingly less doctrinaire (in the use of individual therapy plus couple therapy, couple therapy plus [child-focused] family therapy, etc.). Moreover, the field's early history of disdain for psychiatric and psychodiagnostic perspectives and practices has perceptibly changed as clinicians increasingly coordinate the use of psychopharmacological agents with flexible psychosocial treatment plans. As couple therapy has generally become more accepted in mainstream health and mental health care treatment systems, its varied methods have been increasingly combined with both other psychosocial interventions (e.g., individual psychotherapy) and other sorts (e.g., psychopharmacological) of intervention.

Curative Factors/Mechanisms of Change

You can do very little with faith, but you can do nothing without it.
                                              —SAMUEL BUTLER

Purpose

To describe the factors, that is, mechanisms of change, that lead to change in couples and to assess their relative importance.

Points to Consider

1. Do patients need insight or understanding to be able to change? (Differentiate between historical-genetic insight and interactional insight.)
2. Is interpretation of any sort important and, if so, does it take history into account? If interpretation is used, is it seen as reflecting a psychological "reality" or is it viewed rather as a pragmatic tool for effecting change, shifting perceptions or attributions, and so forth?
3. Is the learning of new interpersonal skills seen as important? If so, are these skills taught in didactic fashion, or are they shaped as approximations occur naturalistically in treatment?
4. Does the therapist's personality or psychological health play an important part in the process and outcome of therapeutic approach?
5. What other therapist factors are likely to influence the course and outcome of your approach? Are certain kinds of therapists ideally suited to work according to this approach? Are there others for whom the approach is probably a poor "fit"?
6. What other factors influence the likelihood of successful treatment in your approach?
7. How important are techniques compared to the patient–therapist relationship?
8. Must each member of the couple change? Is change in an "identified patient" (where relevant) possible without interactional or systemic change? Does systemic change necessarily lead to change in symptoms and vice versa?

A major controversy in individual psychotherapy and, more recently, in couple therapy (Simon, 2006; Sprenkle & Blow, 2004) is whether change is brought about more by specific ingredients of therapy or factors common to all therapies. "Specific ingredients" usually refer to specific technical interventions, such as communication training, paradoxical injunctions, cognitive reframing, interpretations, or empathic responding, which are said to be the ingredient(s) responsible for clinical change. At times, these techniques are detailed in manuals to which the clinician is expected to adhere to achieve the desired result. The specific ingredient approach is in keeping with a more "medical" model of therapy, insofar as one treats a particular disorder, or particular interaction pattern, with a psychological technique (akin to administering a pill), producing the psychological rough equivalent of a biological effect. Followers of the EST movement are typically adherents of this approach, advocating specific modes of intervention for different forms of psychopathology.

"Common factors" refers to features of couple therapy that are not specific to any one approach. Because outcome studies comparing different therapies have found few differences among the common different extant therapies, it has been inferred that this finding is due to the importance of therapeutic factors common to the various therapies. Thus, instead of running "horse race" research to discern differences among the therapies, proponents argue that effort should be redirected to their commonalities. These include client factors, such as positive motivation and expectation for change; therapist qualities, such as warmth, ability to form good alliances, and empathic attunement; and structural features of the treatment, such as the provision of a rationale for a person's suffering and having a coherent theoretical framework for interventions.

Moreover, as Sexton et al. (2008) have recently emphasized, there is a very great need within both the research and conceptual realms of couple therapy to further our understanding of core intervention principles that "transcend the treatment methods that are available today for classification" as has been attempted within individual psychotherapy (Beutler, 2003). These core principles "facilitate meaningful change across therapeutic methods" (Sexton et al., 2008). For example, a core change mechanism in couple therapy may involve a changed experience of one's partner that leads to an increased sense of emotional safety and collaboration. Such a change might be activated by the use of techniques from such varied therapy models as cognitive-behavioral (e.g., reattribution methods), object relations (e.g., interpretations used to disrupt projective processes), and emotionally focused therapy (e.g., restructuring interactions by accessing unacknowledged emotions in problematic partner cycles).

Treatment Applicability and Empirical Support

If all the evidence as you receive it leads to but one conclusion, don't believe it.
                                    —MOLIÈRE

All who drink this remedy recover in a short time, except those whom it does not help, who all die and have no relief from any other medicine. Therefore, it is obvious that it fails only in incurable cases.
                                    —GALEN

Purpose

To describe those couples for whom your approach is particularly relevant and to summarize existing research on the efficacy and/or effectiveness of your approach.

Points to Consider

1. For what couples is this approach particularly relevant? For example, is it relevant for couples in which one partner has a medical or psychiatric disorder as well as for couples with primarily "relational" concerns?
2. For what couples is this approach either not appropriate or of uncertain relevance (e.g., is it less relevant for severely disturbed couples or couples with a seriously disturbed member, for couples with nontraditional relationship structures, etc.)? Why?
3. When, if ever, would a referral be made for either another (i.e., different) type of couple therapy, or for an entirely different treatment (e.g., individual therapy, drug therapy)?
4. Are there aspects of this approach that raise particular ethical and/or legal issues that are different from those raised by psychotherapy in general?
5. How is the outcome of therapy in this model usually evaluated in clinical practice? Is there any empirical evidence of the efficacy or effectiveness of your approach?

In the end, questions about the applicability, relevance, and helpfulness of particular couple therapy approaches to particular kinds of problems, issues, and symptoms are best answered through painstaking research on treatment efficacy (as determined through randomly controlled trials) and treatment effectiveness (field studies). Testimonials, appeals to established authority and tradition, and similar unsystematic methods, are insufficient to the task. Couple therapy is too complex to track the interaction among, and impact of, the most relevant factors in therapeutic outcomes via individuals' participation in the process alone. Moreover, the contributions to therapeutic outcomes of therapist, patient, and technique factors probably vary from one approach to another.

If Galen's observations about presumptively curative medicines are applied to couple therapy nowadays, they are likely to be met with a knowing chuckle and implicit recognition of the inherent limits of all of our treatment approaches. Still, new therapy approaches rarely, if ever, make only modest and restrained claims of effectiveness, issue "warning labels" to "customers" for whom their ways of working are either not likely to be helpful or may possibly be harmful, or suggest that alternative approaches may be more appropriate under certain conditions.

If couple therapy methods continue to grow in number, the ethical complexities of the field may also grow. There are generic kinds of ethical matters that couple therapists of all persuasions must deal with (confidentiality, adequacy of record keeping, duty to warn, respecting personal boundaries regarding dual relationships, etc.). Multiperson therapies, such as couple therapy, raise practical ethical matters that do not emerge in more traditional modes of practice, for example, balancing the interests and needs of more than one person against the interests and needs of another person, all the while also trying to help maintain the very viability of the patient system (e.g., marriage) itself.

Such potential influences of new perspectives on ethical concerns in psychotherapy are perhaps nowhere more readily and saliently seen than when matters involving cultural diversity are considered. Certainly, all couple therapists must be sensitive in their work to matters of race, ethnicity, social class, gender, sexual orientation, and religion, adapting and modifying both their assessment and treatment-planning activities, and perspectives and intervention styles as deemed functionally appropriate to the situation at hand (Hayes & Toarmino, 1995). To do otherwise would risk the imposition, wittingly or unwittingly, of the therapist's own values onto the patient (e.g., in terms of the important area of setting goals for their work together).

A culture-sensitive/multicultural theoretical orientation has been predicted by experts in the field of psychotherapy (Norcross, Hedges, & Prochaska, 2002) to become one of the most widely employed points of view in the next decade. And feminism, which, as noted earlier, shares many philosophical assumptions with multiculturalism, is also predicted to show an increasing impact on psychotherapy (Norcross et al., 2002). Together,

these modern perspectives have usefully challenged many normative assumptions and practices in the general field of psychotherapy, forcing the field to recognize the diversity of social and psychological experience and the impact of relevant broader social beliefs that often confuse clinical description with social prescription. Critiques of various psychotherapies from these contemporary perspectives have sensitized the therapist to the potential constraining and even damaging effects of a failure to recognize the reality of one's own necessarily limited perspective. Certainly, couple therapists have also become deeply involved in such social and therapeutic analyses and critiques, as discussed in the earlier historical overview of the field.

It must be recognized, nonetheless, that such critiques of established therapeutic, including couple therapeutic, worldviews do not necessarily provide clear guidelines about the ways in which culture-sensitive and gender-sensitive therapists should actually practice couple therapy. As Hardy and Laszloffy (2002) noted, a multicultural perspective "is not a set of codified techniques or strategies ... but rather a philosophical stance that significantly informs how one sees the world in and outside of therapy" (p. 569). Relatedly, Rampage (2002) has stated that "how to *do* feminist therapy is much less well understood than is the critique of traditional ... therapy" (p. 535).

Like other attitudes, perspectives and worldviews, multiculturalism and feminism, then, are not clinical couple methodologies to be taught and refined. As couple therapists of all theoretical orientations strive to enhance their awareness of and sensitivity to the kinds of societal concerns brought to their attention by such modern perspectives, it is ethically incumbent on them to focus on the larger lesson of these perspectives. This larger lesson is that their responsibility and primary loyalty are to their clients, not their theories, strategies, or techniques.

COUPLE THERAPY AND THE PROBLEMS OF INDIVIDUALS

This last point about the primary clinical responsibility of couple therapists leads to a brief consideration of another extremely important issue.

Given that couple therapists generally have had little to say about the treatment of many common, diagnosable adult psychiatric/psychological disorders, it is ironic that these disorders have recently come to comprise one of the most scientifically based areas of clinical practice in the entire couple–family therapy field. Recognizing the existence of real psychiatric disorders has not, as some in the couple–family therapy field feared, led to a negation of the relevance of couple therapy. Rather, as discussed in the earlier historical overview, by drawing upon the canons of traditional scientific methodology, clinical researchers have actually enhanced the credibility of couple therapy interventions for these problems.

Research on the couple treatment of such disorders in the last decade has shown strikingly that individual problems and relational problems influence each other reciprocally. These data have important implications for what is still perhaps the most controversial issue in the realm of systems-oriented treatment of psychiatric disorders, that is, whether individual problems are functional for relationships. Neil Jacobson and I suggested in the first edition of this *Handbook* that the more appropriate form of the question might be "*When* do symptoms serve such functions?" A thoughtful reading of several of the chapters in this volume seems to confirm, as suggested earlier, that some individual symptoms (1) seem often to serve interpersonal functions; (2) seem rarely to serve interpersonal functions; and (3) are quite variably interpersonally functional. Recent research has confirmed what some of us in the field (e.g., Gurman et al., 1986) have long asserted, against prevailing clinical wisdom, that functions are dangerously confused with consequences.

The Science and Practice of Couple Therapy

The process of being scientific does not consist of finding objective truths. It consists of negotiating a shared perception of truths in respectful dialogue.
—Robert Beavers

As in the broader world of psychotherapy, there is a long history of disconnection between couple therapy practitioners and couple therapy researchers. Researchers typically criticize clinicians for engaging in practices that lack empirical justification, and clinicians typically criticize researchers as being out of touch with the complex realities of working with couples. Though reflecting caricatured positions, such characterizations on both sides are unfortunately not entirely unwarranted.

The broader world of psychotherapy has seen an increased pressure placed on the advocates of particular therapeutic methods to document both the efficacy of their approaches through carefully controlled clinical research trials and the effectiveness of these methods via patient evaluations in uncontrolled, naturalistic clinical practice contexts. This movement to favor ESTs has even more recently been challenged by a complementary movement of psychotherapy researchers who assert the often overlooked importance of ESRs (Norcross, 2002).

At the risk of oversimplification, ESTers tend to be associated with certain theoretical orientations (e.g., behavioral, cognitive, cognitive-behavioral) and styles of practice (brief), whereas ESRers tend to be associated with other theoretical orientations (e.g., object relations, person-centered, experiential, existential–humanistic), with still other influential approaches (e.g., integrative, pluralistic) standing somewhere in the middle.

The questions raised by such unfortunately competing points of view are not at all insignificant:

1. Will ESTs, which tend to emphasize technical refinement, symptomatic change, and changes in presenting problems, not only survive, but thrive?
2. Will ESR-oriented approaches, which tend to emphasize enhancing client resources and resilience, and self-exploration and personal discovery, fade from view?
3. Will the influence of brief approaches continue to expand, while the influence of long-term approaches continues to contract?
4. Can research better inform us how not only to disseminate effective couple therapy methods, but also to better identify effective couple therapists?
5. Can both qualitative and quantitative research methods be brought to bear on theoretically and clinically important questions, or will they, like researchers and clinicians, tend to operate quite independently?

In the end, the field of couple therapy will benefit by fostering more evidence-based practice, without prematurely limiting the kinds of evidence that may help to inform responsible practice.

CONCLUSION

Start at the beginning, proceed through the middle, and stop when you get to the end.
—Lewis Carroll, *Alice in Wonderland*

REFERENCES

Ackerman, N. W. (1970). Family psychotherapy today. *Family Process, 9,* 123–126.

American Psychiatric Association. (1994). *Diagnostic and statistical manual of mental disorders* (4th ed.). Washington, DC: Author.

Aponte, H. (1992). The black sheep of the family: A structural approach to brief therapy. In S. H. Budman, M. Hoyt, & S. Friedman (Eds.), The first session in brief therapy (pp. 324–341). New York: Guilford Press.

Beels, C. C., & Ferber, A. (1969). Family therapy: A view. *Family Process, 8,* 280–318.

Beutler, L. E. (2003). David and Goliath: When empirical and clinical standards of practice meet. *American Psychologist, 55,* 997–1007.

Bogdan, J. (1984). Doctor Pangloss as family therapist. *Family Therapy Networker, 8*(2), 19–20.

Bowen, M. (1978). *Family therapy in clinical practice.* New York: Aronson.

Budman, S. H., & Gurman, A. S. (1988). *The theory and practice of brief therapy.* New York: Guilford Press.

Cassidy, J., & Shaver, P. (Eds.). (1999). *Handbook of attachment: Theory, research, and clinical applications.* New York: Guilford Press.

Christensen, A., Jacobson, N. S., & Babcock, J. (1995). Integrative behavioral couple therapy. In N. S. Jacobson & A. S. Gurman (Eds.), *Clinical handbook of couple therapy* (2nd ed., pp. 31–64). New York: Guilford Press.

Dicks, H. V. (1967). *Marital tensions.* New York: Basic Books.

Doherty, W. J., & Simmons, D. S. (1996). Clinical practice patterns of marriage and family therapists: A national survey of therapists and their clients. *Journal of Marital and Family Therapy, 22,* 9–25.

Donovan, J. (Ed.). (1999). *Short-term couple therapy.* New York: Guilford Press.

Duhl, B. S., & Duhl, F. D. (1981). Integrative family therapy. In A. S. Gurman & D. P. Kniskern (Eds.), *Handbook of family therapy* (pp. 483–513). New York: Brunner/Mazel.

Framo, J. L. (1965). Rationale and techniques of intensive family therapy. In I. Boszormenyi-Nagy & J. L. Framo (Eds.), *Intensive family therapy* (pp. 143–212). New York: Harper & Row.

Framo, J. L. (1981). The integration of marital therapy with sessions with family of origin. In A. S. Gurman & D. P. Kniskern (Eds.), *Handbook of family therapy* (pp. 133–158). New York: Brunner/Mazel.

Framo, J. L. (1996). A personal retrospective of the family therapy field: Then and now. *Journal of Marital and Family Therapy, 22,* 289–316.

Frank, J. D., & Frank, J. B. (1991). *Persuasion and healing.* Baltimore: Johns Hopkins University Press.

Geiss, S. K., & O'Leary, K. D. (1981). Therapist ratings of frequency and severity of marital problems: Implications for research. *Journal of Marital and Family Therapy, 9,* 515–520.

Gottman, J. M. (1994a). *What predicts divorce?* Hillsdale, NJ: Erlbaum.

Gottman, J. M. (1994b). *Why marriages succeed or fail.* New York: Simon & Schuster.

Gottman, J. M. (1998). Psychology and the study of marital processes. *Annual Review of Psychology, 49,* 169–197.

Gottman, J. M. (1999). *The marriage clinic: A scientifically based marital therapy.* New York: Norton.

Gurman, A. S. (1971). Group marital therapy: Clinical and empirical implications for outcome research. *International Journal of Group Psychotherapy, 21,* 174–189.

Gurman, A. S. (1973). The effects and effectiveness of marital therapy: A review of outcome research. *Family Process, 12,* 145–170.

Gurman, A. S. (1978). Contemporary marital therapies: A critique and comparative analysis of psychoanalytic, behavioral and systems theory approaches. In T. Paolino & B. McCrady (Eds.), *Marriage and marital therapy* (pp. 445–566). New York: Brunner/Mazel.

Gurman, A. S. (1981). Integrative marital therapy: Toward the development of an interpersonal approach. In S. H. Budman (Ed.), *Forms of brief therapy* (pp. 415–462). New York: Guilford Press.

Gurman, A. S. (1990). Integrating the life of an integrative family psychologist. In F. Kaslow (Ed.), *Voices in family psychology* (Vol. 2, pp. 250–266). Newbury Park, CA: Sage.

Gurman, A. S. (1992). Integrative martial therapy: A time-sensitive model for working with couples. In S. Budman, M. Hoyt, & S. Friedman (Eds.), *The first session is brief therapy* (pp.186–203). New York: Guilford Press.

Gurman, A. S. (2001). Brief therapy and family/couple therapy: An essential redundancy. *Clinical Psychology: Science and Practice, 8,* 51–65.

Gurman, A. S. (2002). Brief integrative marital therapy: A depth-behavioral approach. In A. S. Gurman & N. S. Jacobson (Eds.), *Clinical handbook of couple therapy* (pp. 180–220). New York: Guilford Press.

Gurman, A. S., & Fraenkel, P. (2002). The history of couple therapy: A millennial review. *Family Process, 41,* 199–260.

Gurman, A. S., & Jacobson, N. S. (1985). Marital therapy: From technique to theory, back again, and beyond. In N. S. Jacobson & A. S. Gurman (Eds.), *Clinical handbook of marital therapy* (pp. 1–9). New York: Guilford Press.

Gurman, A. S., & Jacobson, N. S. (1995). Therapy with couples: A coming of age. In N. S. Jacobson & A. S. Gurman (Eds.), *Clinical handbook of couple therapy* (2nd ed., pp. 1–6). New York: Guilford Press.

Gurman, A. S., & Kniskern, D. P. (1978a). Deterioration in marital and family therapy: Empirical, clinical and conceptual issues. *Family Process, 17,* 3–20.

Gurman, A. S., & Kniskern, D. P. (1978b). Research on marital and family therapy: Progress, perspective and prospect. In S. L. Garfield & A. E. Bergin (Eds.),

Handbook of psychotherapy and behavior change (2nd ed., pp. 817–901). New York: Wiley.

Gurman, A. S., & Kniskern, D. P. (1981). Family therapy outcome research: Knowns and unknowns. In A. S. Gurman & D. P. Kniskern (Eds.), *Handbook of family therapy* (pp. 742–773). New York: Brunner/Mazel.

Gurman, A. S., & Kniskern, D. P. (Eds.). (1991). *Handbook of family therapy*. New York: Brunner/Mazel.

Gurman, A. S., Kniskern, D. P., & Pinsof, W. (1986). Process and outcome research in family and marital therapy. In A. E. Bergen & S. L. Garfield (Eds.), *Handbook of psychotherapy and behavior change* (3rd ed., pp. 565–624). New York: Wiley.

Gurman, A. S., & Messer, S. B. (2003). Contemporary issues in the theory and practice of psychotherapy. In A. S. Gurman & S. B. Messer (Eds.), *Essential psychotherapies* (2nd ed., pp. 1–23). New York: Guilford Press.

Haley, J. (1963). Marriage therapy. *Archives of General Psychiatry, 8*, 213–234.

Haley, J. (1976). *Problem-solving therapy*. San Francisco: Jossey-Bass.

Haley, J. (1984). Marriage or family therapy. *American Journal of Family Therapy, 12*, 3–14.

Hardy, R. V., & Laszloffy, T. A. (2002). Couple therapy using a multicultural perspective. In A. S. Gurman & N. S. Jacobson (Eds.), *Clinical handbook of couple therapy* (3rd ed., pp. 569–593). New York: Guilford Press.

Hayes, S. C., & Toarmino, D. (1995, February). If behavioral principles are generally applicable, why is it necessary to understand cultural diversity? *Behavior Therapist*, pp. 21–23.

Jacobson, N. S., & Margolin, G. (1979). *Marital therapy: Strategies based on social learning and behavior exchange principles*. New York: Brunner/Mazel.

Jacobson, N. S., & Martin, B. (1976). Behavioral marriage therapy: Current status. *Psychological Bulletin, 83*, 540–566.

Jackson, D. D. (1965a). Family rules: The marital quid pro quo. *Archives of General Psychiatry, 4*, 589–594.

Jackson, D. D. (1965b). The study of the family. *Family Process, 4*, 1–20.

Johnson, S. M., & Denton, W. (2002). Emotionally focused couple therapy: Creating secure connections. In A. S. Gurman & N. S. Jacobson (Eds.), *Clinical handbook of couple therapy* (3rd ed., pp. 221–250). New York: Guilford Press.

Johnson, S. M., & Lebow, J. (2000). The "coming of age" of couple therapy: A decade review. *Journal of Marital and Family Therapy, 26*, 23–28.

Johnson, S. M., & Whiffen, V. (Eds.). (2003). *Attachment processes in couple and families*. New York: Guilford Press.

Keeney, B. P., & Sprenkle, D. H. (1982). Eco-systemic epistemology: Critical implications for aesthetics and pragmatics of family therapy. *Family Process, 21*, 1–19.

Lebow, J. (1997). The integrative revolution in couple and family therapy. *Family Process, 36*, 1–17.

Lebow, J. L., & Gurman, A. S. (1995). Research assessing couple and family therapy. *Annual Review of Psychology, 46*, 27–57.

Madanes, C. (1980). Marital therapy when a symptom is presented by a spouse. *International Journal of Family Therapy, 2*, 120–136.

Manus, G. (1966). Marriage counseling: A technique in search of a theory. *Journal of Marriage and the Family, 28*, 449–453.

Meltzoff, J., & Kornreich, M. (1970). *Research in psychotherapy*. New York: Atherton.

Messer, S. B., & Wachtel, P. L. (1997). The contemporary psychotherapeutic landscape: Issues and prospects. In P. C. Wachtel & S. B. Messer (Eds.), *Theories of psychotherapy: Origins and evolution* (pp. 1–38). Washington, DC: American Psychological Association.

Messer, S. B., & Winokur, M. (1984). Ways of knowing and visions of reality in psychoanalytic therapy and behavior therapy. In H. Arkowitz & S. B. Messer (Eds.), *Psychoanalytic therapy and behavior therapy: Is integration possible?* (pp. 53–100). New York: Plenum.

Mudd, E. H. (1957). Knowns and unknowns in marriage counseling research. *Marriage and Family Living, 19*, 75–81.

Nichols, M. P. (1987). *The self in the system*. New York: Brunner/Mazel.

Nichols, M. P., & Schwartz, R. C. (1998). *Family therapy: Concepts and methods*. Boston: Allyn & Bacon.

Norcross, J. C. (Ed.). (2002). *Psychotherapy relationships that work*. New York: Oxford University Press.

Norcross, J. C., Hedges, M., & Prochaska, J. (2002). The face of 2010: A Delphi poll on the future of psychotherapy. *Professional Psychology, 33*, 316–322.

Norcross, J. C., & Prochaska, J. (1983). A study of eclectic (and integrative) views revisited. *Professional Psychology, 19*, 170–174.

Olson, D. H. (1970). Marital and family therapy: Integrative review and critique. *Journal of Marriage and the Family, 32*, 501–538.

Pinsof, W. M. (1995). *Integrative problem-centered therapy*. New York: Basic Books.

Pinsof, W. M. (2002). The death of til death do us part: The twentieth century's revelation of the limits of human pair-bonding. *Family Process, 41*, 133–157.

Rampage, C. (2002). Working with gender in couple therapy. In A. S. Gurman & N. S. Jacobson (Eds.), *Clinical handbook of couple therapy* (3rd ed., pp. 533–545). New York: Guilford Press.

Sager, C. J. (1966). The development of marriage therapy: An historical overview. *American Journal of Orthopsychiatry, 36*, 458–467.

Sager, C. J. (1976). *Marriage contracts and couple therapy*. New York: Brunner/Mazel.

Satir, V. (1964). *Conjoint family therapy*. Palo Alto, CA: Science and Behavior Books.

Scharff, J. S., & Bagnini, C. (2003). Object relations couple therapy. In A. S. Gurman & N. S. Jacobson (Eds.), *Clinical handbook of couple therapy* (3rd ed., pp. 59–85). New York: Guilford Press.

Schwartz, R., & Johnson, S. M. (2000). Commentary: Does couple and family therapy have emotional intelligence? *Family Process, 39*, 29–33.

Sexton, T. L., Gordon, K. C., Gurman, A. S., Lebow, J. C., Holtzworth-Munroe, A., & Johnson, S. M. (2008). *Guidelines for evidence-based treatments in family psychology.*

Simmons, D. S., & Doherty, W. J. (1995). Defining who we are and what we do: Clinical practice patterns of marriage and family therapists in Minnesota. *Journal of Marital and Family Therapy, 21*, 3–16.

Simon, G. M. (2006). The heart of the matter: A proposal for placing the self of the therapist at the center of family therapy research and training. *Family Process, 45*, 331–344.

Skynner, A. C. R. (1976). *Systems of family and marital psychotherapy.* New York: Brunner/Mazel.

Skynner, A. C. R. (1980). Recent developments in marital therapy. *Journal of Family Therapy, 2*, 271–296.

Skynner, A. C. R. (1981). An open-systems, group analytic approach to family therapy. In A. S. Gurman & D. P. Kniskern (Eds.), *Handbook of family therapy* (pp. 39–84). New York: Brunner/Mazel.

Snyder, D. K. (1999). Affective reconstruction in the context of a pluralistic approach to couple therapy. *Clinical Psychology: Science and Practice, 6*, 348–365.

Snyder, D. K., & Schneider, W. J. (2002). Affective reconstruction: A pluralistic, developmental approach. In A. S. Gurman & N. S. Jacobson (Eds.), *Clinical handbook of couple therapy* (3rd ed., pp. 151–179). New York: Guilford Press.

Sprenkle, D. H., & Blow, A. J. (2004). Common factors and our sacred models. *Journal of Marital and Family Therapy, 30*, 113–129.

Stuart, R. B. (1969). Operant–interpersonal treatment of marital discord. *Journal of Consulting and Clinical Psychology, 33*, 675–682.

Stuart, R. B. (1980). *Helping couples change: A social learning approach to marital therapy.* New York: Guilford Press.

Wampold, B. E. (2001). *The great psychotherapy debate: Models, methods and findings.* Mahwah, NJ: Erlbaum.

Whisman, M. A., Dixon, A. E., & Johnson, B. (1997). Therapists' perspectives of couple problems and treatment issues in couple therapy. *Journal of Family Psychology, 11*, 361–366.

Wynne, L. C. (1983). Family research and family therapy: A reunion? *Journal of Marital and Family Therapy, 9*, 113–117.

PART I

MODELS OF COUPLE THERAPY

Behavioral Approaches

CHAPTER 2

Cognitive-Behavioral Couple Therapy

Donald H. Baucom
Norman B. Epstein
Jaslean J. LaTaillade
Jennifer S. Kirby

BACKGROUND OF COGNITIVE-BEHAVIORAL COUPLE THERAPY

Cognitive-behavioral couple therapy (CBCT) has developed from the confluence of three major influences: (1) behavioral couple therapy (BCT), (2) cognitive therapy (CT), and (3) basic research on information processing in the field of cognitive psychology. CBCT is a relatively new development in couple therapy, emerging in the early 1980s, although its precursors all have longer histories, and CBCT clinical assessment and intervention strategies have adopted major components of both BCT and CT.

Roots of CBCT
in Behavioral Couple Therapy

BCT emerged in the late 1960s as a branch of behavior therapies that were based on applications of basic learning principles (in particular, reinforcement principles of operant conditioning) to clinical problems. Stuart (1969) presented the first published application of behavioral principles to couple problems. Based on social exchange theory (Thibaut & Kelley, 1959), Stuart hypothesized that successful marriages could be distinguished

from unsuccessful ones by the frequency and range of positive acts exchanged reciprocally by the partners. As such, distressed relationships were characterized by a scarcity of positive outcomes available for each member, particularly in relation to the frequency of negative outcomes. Social exchange theory predicted that individuals' satisfaction with their relationships would be based on the ratio of benefits to costs received in the form of positive and negative behaviors from their partners. In addition, operant conditioning principles suggested that partners would be more likely to behave in positive ways toward each other if they received positive consequences from each other for those actions. Stuart's (1969) treatment consisted of obtaining a list of positive behaviors that each person desired from the partner and instituting an agreement for the two individuals to exchange tokens as rewards for enacting the desired behaviors. Although his "token economy" has since been replaced in BCT with written contracts, as well as communication and problem-solving skills training, his use of an operant conditioning paradigm was a milestone in the development of BCT and family therapies (Falloon, 1991).

Liberman (1970) also utilized behavioral principles in his work with couples and families, applying a social learning framework (Bandura, 1977; Bandura & Walters, 1963). Liberman added the strategies of role rehearsal and modeling of alternative interpersonal communication patterns to his treatment of dysfunctional family relationships (Falloon, 1991). His approach involved an extensive behavioral analysis of the presenting problems and family interaction patterns; for example, identifying instances in which responses by other family members actually reinforced an individual's undesirable behavior. Liberman advocated the use of behavioral analysis throughout the course of therapy, allowing the treatment to be modified as needed.

The use of operant conditioning in the modification of children's behavior also had a strong influence on the development of BCT. Patterson and his colleagues (Patterson, 1974; Patterson & Hops, 1972) described "coercive family systems" in which the parents and children mutually used aversive behavior to try to influence each other's actions. Therapists emphasized operant principles in which parents were trained to use reinforcers and punishers selectively to increase a child's desired behaviors and decrease negative behavior. Weiss, Hops, and Patterson (1973) extended the use of operant principles from parent–child relationships to the treatment of couple relationship discord. In addition to developing systematic, learning-based interventions for distressed couples, Weiss et al. made a major contribution to establishing a tradition of empiricism in BCT, in which therapists and clinical researchers collect data to identify couples' behavioral strengths and problems, and also assess the degree to which specific behaviors change as a function of treatment.

The early writings on BCT principles and methods were not comprehensive and specific in terms of clinical techniques. The integration of social exchange and learning principles, and the elaboration of clinical intervention procedures did not occur until the late 1970s and early 1980s, when the first detailed treatment manuals were published (Jacobson & Margolin, 1979; Stuart, 1980). These texts provided both a clear presentation of behavioral principles as they apply to the processes occurring in intimate relationships and a guide for using specific techniques to treat couple distress.

Several principles characterize the theory and treatment strategies used in BCT. A traditional behavioral model posits that the behaviors of both members of a couple are shaped, strengthened, weakened, and can be modified in therapy by consequences provided by environmental events, particularly those involving the other partner. Based on social exchange principles (Thibaut & Kelley, 1959), BCT also proposes that partners' subjective satisfaction with their relationship is a function of the ratio of rewards derived to costs incurred from being in the relationship. However, satisfaction also is influenced by events outside the relationship (e.g., a relationship with an outside individual who provides a member of the couple more positive reinforcement than does the person's partner; Jacobson & Margolin, 1979). The BCT model also proposes that couples are distressed in part because they have not developed or maintained the skills necessary to produce interactions that result in feelings of closeness in their relationship. These include skills for conflict resolution, behavior change, constructive communication, intimacy, and mutual social support. Difficulties with such skills are presumed to result either from a skills deficit (i.e., the partners have not learned particular skills) or partners' failure to perform skills they know, due to a variety of factors, such as anger or fear. The early BCT manuals placed heavy emphasis on teaching couples effective relationship skills.

The traditional BCT model also posits that a couple's relationship consists of reciprocal and circular sequences in which each partner's behavior simultaneously affects and influences that of the other. This dependence of each partner on the reinforcing and punishing behaviors of the other dictates the terms of a functional analysis of the couple's behavior patterns, in which events occurring within the couple's interactions and in their broader environment (eliciting stimuli and consequences) control the frequencies of positive and negative actions by each partner. Although social learning theory (Bandura, 1977) suggests that partners' behaviors toward each other may be influenced by each individual's prior learning experiences (e.g., in family of origin relationships), the emphasis in BCT tends to be on a functional analysis of the specific patterns that have developed and are operating currently in the couple's own relationship. An idiographic functional analysis prevents behavioral couple therapists from assuming the relevance of universal truths in explaining a particular couple's interaction patterns, and it emphasizes an empirical perspective in examining couples' presenting concerns, tailoring interventions to each couple's needs, and assessing change on specific behaviors that have been targeted for improvement (LaTaillade & Jacobson, 1995).

Across numerous investigations, BCT has consistently been found to be effective (Baucom, Shoham, Mueser, Daiuto, & Stickle, 1998; Hahlweg & Markman, 1988); even so, this approach is not without notable limitations. Results of BCT outcome studies have demonstrated that increases in partners' exchanges of positive behavior and improved communication skills in many instances have not resulted in commensurate improvement in relationship satisfaction (Halford, Sanders, & Behrens, 1993; Iverson & Baucom, 1988). In addition, comparisons of BCT with other treatment approaches that do not emphasize the modification of behavioral exchanges and skills training have found these interventions to be equally efficacious in alleviating marital distress, indicating that pure behavioral interventions may not be necessary or sufficient for positive treatment outcomes (Baucom, Epstein, & Gordon, 2000; Baucom et al., 1998). Furthermore, clinical research indicated marked discrepancies between not only spousal reports about the types of positive and negative behavior in their relationship but also between spousal and trained observers' reports of couples' behavior. Such findings emphasized the subjectivity of individuals' experiences of their own and their partners' behavior; thus, it could not be assumed that one partner's efforts to behave positively would be perceived as positive behavior by the other partner (Fincham, Bradbury, & Scott, 1990). These findings indicated that a behavioral skills deficit model was too restrictive in the treatment of couple distress, and highlighted the need to attend not only to partners' behavior but also to their *interpretations* and *evaluations* of their own and each other's behavior (Baucom & Epstein, 1990; Epstein & Baucom, 2002; Fincham et al., 1990).

Influences of Cognitive Therapies on CBCT

The second major influence on the development of CBCT was the rise of cognitive models of individual psychopathology (Beck, Rush, Shaw, & Emery, 1979; Ellis, 1962; Meichenbaum, 1977), emphasizing how an individual's emotional and behavioral responses to life events commonly are mediated by idiosyncratic interpretations that may be biased by cognitive distortions. Given that events occurring in individuals' intimate couple relationship are among the most significant of life events that they are likely to experience subjectively, cognitive therapists began to apply their conceptual model to the treatment of relationship problems, and in turn behavioral couple therapists began to integrate cognition into the BCT model. Margolin and Weiss (1978) conducted a BCT outcome study in which partners' attributions about each other's behavior were addressed, and Epstein (1982) described the application of cognitive therapy to the treatment of distressed couples.

CBCT evolved from the gradual expansion of BCT and its treatment strategies to include a major focus on cognitive factors in the onset and treatment of couple distress, while maintaining the core model and behavioral interventions of BCT. In CBCT, cognitive, behavioral, and emotional factors are all given attention (Baucom & Epstein, 1990; Epstein & Baucom, 2002; Rathus & Sanderson, 1999). A major premise of this approach is that partners' dysfunctional emotional and behavioral responses to relationship events are influenced by information-processing errors, whereby cognitive appraisals of the events are either arbitrary or distorted (e.g., "You stayed most of the day at your parents' house because they are more important to you than I am. I know that your mom has been sick and you feel responsible for helping take care of her, but you knew I was sitting here by myself, and you could have found a way to break away. I feel like you don't really love me"). Similarly, relationship events might be evaluated according to extreme or unreasonable standards of what a relationship should be (e.g., "If you really cared, you'd want to spend all your free time with me. That's what a marriage should be"). Often partners fail to evaluate the appropriateness of their cognitions, and instead trust in the validity of their own subjective, stream-of-consciousness cognitions, or automatic thoughts, in response to internal or external events in the relationship (Baucom & Epstein, 1990; Epstein & Baucom, 2002). Consequently, a major task of the CBCT therapist is to help couples become more active observers and evaluators of their own automatic thoughts, and their longstanding assumptions and standards (forms of relatively stable cognitive schemas or knowledge structures) regarding their relationship. On the one hand, cognitive-behavioral therapists assume that a major path to modifying people's negative emotions and behavior is to alter their information processing and cognitions (Epstein & Baucom, 2002). On the other hand, consistent with the traditional BCT model, CBCT therapists also assume that modifying partners' negative behavioral interactions directly can result in partners experiencing more positive cognitions and emotions about each other. Thus, CBCT has evolved a significant systemic aspect in which the mutual impacts of cognition, behavior, and emotion in couple interactions are viewed as determinants of relationship quality (Epstein & Baucom, 2002).

As noted earlier, another pathway to the development of CBCT, in contrast to expansion of BCT to include consideration of partners' cognitions, has been the application of CT procedures that initially were developed for the treatment of individual psychopathology (e.g., Beck et al., 1979). Although cognitive therapists, whose roots were primarily in individual therapy (e.g., Beck, 1988; Dattilio & Padesky, 1990; Ellis, Sichel, Yeager, DiMattia, & DiGiuseppe, 1989), incorporated some behavioral concepts and methods from BCT (in particular, communication skills training), their versions of CBCT tend to be heavily weighted toward modification of each partner's distorted and extreme cognitions, with relatively little attention to the assessment and modification of behavioral interaction patterns, and the types of inhibited and unregulated emotional responses that we focus on in our approach.

Influences of Social Cognition Research on CBCT

The third influence on the development of CBCT has been basic research by social and cognitive psychologists on information processing, particularly regarding social cognition (Baldwin, 2005; Fiske & Taylor, 1991; Fletcher & Fitness, 1996; Noller, Beach, & Osgarby, 1997). Two foci of social cognition research that have had significant impact on basic research on intimate couple relationships are *attributions* that individuals make about determinants of positive and negative events in their relationships and relatively stable *schemas* (e.g., the concept of a "caring spouse") that individuals develop on the basis of past relationship experiences and subsequently apply in understanding current relationship events. During the 1980s and 1990s, couple researchers focused on cognitive variables as a critical element in understanding the relationship between couple behavior and marital distress (Baucom, Epstein, & Rankin, 1995), and practitioners of CBCT increasingly assessed and intervened with the forms of cognition that emerged from research as important influences on couples' relationship adjustment.

Recent Enhancements of CBCT

Although CBCT has established itself as an empirically supported intervention for the treatment of distressed couples (Baucom, Sayers, & Sher, 1988), until recently it has focused on certain phenomena in intimate relationships, while deemphasizing other important aspects. First, CBCT has emphasized detailed analyses of discrete, specific "micro" relational events and behaviors, without commensurate attention to broader "macro" level patterns and core themes, such as differences between partners' desired levels of closeness and intimacy (Epstein & Baucom, 2002). A variety of different behaviors often seem to fit into a similar equivalence class. Thus, Jonathon's routine pattern of coming home and checking the mail before speaking to Catherine, engaging in little conversation at dinner, and surfing the Internet for hours each night all seemed to fit together to provide a picture of Jonathon as a quiet, contemplative person who was not comfortable with intimacy and preferred solitude. Our inclusion of broader relationship themes is consistent with a similar shift across a variety of theoretical approaches to couple therapy (e.g., emotionally focused therapy [Johnson, 2004]; integrative behavioral couple therapy [Jacobson & Christensen, 1996]; insight-oriented couple therapy [Snyder & Wills, 1989]).

Second, CBCT has tended to focus on couples' cognitive processing and behavioral interactions, while minimizing the influences of personality and other more stable individual differences between partners on couple functioning (Epstein & Baucom, 2002; Karney & Bradbury, 1995). Although attending to cognitive distortions and behavioral deficits is important in outlining the topography of relationship distress, our enhanced CBCT also addresses characteristics that each partner brings to the couple relationship, explaining *why* partners behave and interpret events in maladaptive ways. Each partner brings to the relationship a unique history, preferences, needs, and motives that shape both micro- and macro-level couple interactions. These individual contributions may be normative individual differences, whereas others may stem from individual psychological distress or psychopathology. Research demonstrates that individual differences among psychologically healthy and well-adjusted partners, as well as individual manifestations of psychopathology, often play a crucial role in relationship satisfaction and functioning (e.g., Christensen & Heavey, 1993; Karney & Bradbury, 1995), and these findings have been incorporated into current CBCT.

Third, couples are influenced by external and environmental stressors, as well as by environmental resources that are available to help them meet their personal and relationship needs (Epstein & Baucom, 2002). The demands of work and children, relationships with extended family members, physical health of both partners, and negative experiences, such as racial discrimination within the larger society, all may constitute significant relationship stressors that tax individual and relationship resources. Although cognitive-behavioral perspectives on marriage have not ignored the role of the environment in relationship functioning, it has typically been given minimal attention until relatively recently, with the influence of systems and ecological models of relationship functioning on CBCT (e.g., Bronfenbrenner, 1989).

Fourth, although CBCT has not ignored emotions in couple relationships, emotions traditionally have been given secondary status and have been viewed largely as the result of partners' relationship behaviors and cognitions, consistent with CBCT's roots in both BCT and CT (Epstein & Baucom, 2002). Attending directly to emotional components of intimate couple relationships, ranging from an individual's difficulty in experiencing and/or expressing emotions to partners who have difficulty regulating negative emotions, increases the range of available interventions that the therapist has to assist the couple. The current emphasis on emotion in CBCT is consistent with the recent trend in couple therapy to attend to emotional processes, as typified by emotionally focused couple therapy (Johnson, 2004; Johnson & Denton, 2002), as well as individual and couple therapy approaches to emotion dysregulation (e.g., Fruzzetti, 2006; Kirby & Baucom, 2007; Linehan, 1993).

Fifth, although CBCT traditionally has differentiated between positive and negative valences of specific behaviors, emotions, and cognitions, the primary focus has been on negatives and how to decrease them. However, for couples to derive optimum fulfillment from their relationships, greater emphasis must be given to the role of positive behavior, cognitions, and emotions (Epstein & Baucom, 2002). One area in which basic research on positive aspects in couple relationships has increased has been social support within marriage (e.g., Cutrona, 1996; Cutrona, Hessling, & Suhr, 1997; Pasch, Bradbury, & Davila, 1997). Our expanded cognitive-behavioral model balances the roles of positive and negative emotions, cognitions, and behaviors in interventions to improve the quality of intimate relationships.

CBCT and Integrative Behavioral Couple Therapy

While we, along with others, were expanding BCT into CBCT as described earlier, others among our behavioral colleagues shared our concerns about the shortcomings and restricted nature of the original BCT model. In the early 1990s, Jacobson and Christensen (1996) concluded that the original BCT model focused too exclusively on behavior change and, similar to the evolving CBCT model, believed that an additional focus on internal, subjective changes was critical to relationship improvement. Their broadened model emphasizes the concept of "acceptance," in which an individual shifts from distress and motivation to change particular characteristics of his or her partner to a level of comfort with the partner who continues to have those characteristics. Jacobson and Christensen have viewed this acceptance process as largely an emotional experience, including cognitive elements in their approach to both assessment and treatment. Thus, their treatment, which is called integrative behavioral couple therapy (IBCT), balances acceptance and the almost exclusive emphasis on behavior change in original BCT models with the relative attention to change versus acceptance tailored to the needs of each couple (see Dimidjian, Martell, & Christensen, Chapter 3, this volume, for a recent description of IBCT). Whereas there are notable differences between CBCT as described in this chapter and IBCT in terms of theory and specific interventions, both retain their behavioral roots and expand upon early BCT models to provide an increased emphasis on couples' internal/subjective experience of the relationship as crucial in relationship functioning.

THE HEALTHY/WELL-FUNCTIONING VERSUS DYSFUNCTIONAL COUPLE RELATIONSHIP

In describing a healthy relationship, traditional cognitive-behavioral approaches have focused on the couple as the unit of analysis, while minimizing the contributions of the couple's environment and individual partners' well-being. Our enhanced CBCT employs a broader contextual perspective in defining a healthy relationship, taking into account the individual partners, the couple, and the couple's environment (Baucom, Epstein, & LaTaillade, 2002; Epstein & Baucom, 2002). A "healthy relationship" is defined as one in that contributes to the growth and well-being of both partners, in which the partners function well together as a team and relate to their physical and social environment in an adaptive fashion (Baucom, Epstein, & Sullivan, 2004).

A healthy couple relationship is one that contributes to the growth, development, well-being, and needs fulfillment of each partner. A healthy relationship fosters partners' psychological growth and maturity, development and advancement of each other's career aspirations, and promotion of the physical health and well-being of each individual. The relationship should serve as a source of support to individual partners during difficult and stressful times (Cutrona, Suhr, & MacFarlane, 1990; Pasch, Bradbury, & Sullivan, 1997) by providing instrumental support (e.g., assisting with household tasks, getting the car serviced) or emotional support (e.g., listening empathically to the partner's concerns).

A healthy couple relationship is also one in which both partners contribute to the well-being of the relationship as a unit (Epstein & Baucom, 2002). Both partners are able to make decisions and resolve problems effectively, develop closeness and intimacy, communicate constructively, engage in mutually rewarding and pleasurable activities, reciprocate the other's positive behavior, and perceive each other in positive ways.

In addition, the healthy couple is able to adapt over time to both normative (e.g., pregnancy and childbirth, career changes) and non-normative events or stressors (e.g., unemployment, death of a family member) (Epstein & Baucom, 2002). The partners are able to collaborate in solving problems rather than operating as adversaries or in a disorganized manner.

Couples are located within a broader social and physical environment that includes, but is not limited to, their families and extended kin networks, communities, social institutions and organizations, and cultures (Baucom et al., 2004). Therefore, a healthy relationship is also one in which the partners have positive connections to their physical and social environment. For example, the couple is able to utilize environmental supports and resources, such as familial support, for the well-being of the individual partners and the couple. In addition, the couple may contribute to the community or broader society, for example,

through work in charitable organizations (Baucom et al., 2002).

As the couple's relationship progresses through dating and courtship, with development of increasing sexual and emotional intimacy toward greater engagement (which may result in marriage or a comparable form of commitment), and possibly expanding to include new family members (e.g., transitioning to parenthood), the couple encounters normative demands at each phase of the partners' life cycle (Carter & McGoldrick, 1999). Their responsiveness to these demands is influenced by individual and couple vulnerabilities, as well as individual, dyadic, and environmental resources available to them. How the couple adapts to these demands can result in enhancement, deterioration, or maintenance of the status quo for the functioning of the couple and individual partners (Epstein & Baucom, 2002). A healthy relationship is distinguished by the couple's ability to adapt to changing demands and constraints in ways that allow partners to meet important individual and relational needs.

Predictors of Relationship Distress

Traditionally, BCT approaches focused on interactive processes that distinguished between happy and unhappy couples, characterizing distressed relationships as those with a scarcity of positive outcomes available for each partner (Stuart, 1969), deficits in communication and problem-solving skills (Karney & Bradbury, 1995), and a high frequency of negative or punishing exchanges that are reciprocated by both partners (Jacobson & Margolin, 1979). Research has demonstrated that partners in distressed relationships are more likely to track negative behavior selectively in the other (Jacobson, Waldron, & Moore, 1980), to make negative attributions for such behavior (Baucom & Epstein, 1990; Fincham et al., 1990), and to reciprocate negative behavior with negative behavior (Gottman, 1979, 1994). As partners continue to engage in negative reciprocity and perceive the other in a negative way, they may develop "sentiment override," or global negative emotions, toward each other (Weiss, 1980). This sentiment override increases the likelihood of subsequent negative behavior and the development of partners' negative expectancies or predictions that the other person will engage in negative acts (Baucom & Epstein, 1990). These behavioral, cognitive, and affective patterns reflect the self-maintaining process of relationship discord that often typifies distressed couples. Once one or both partners become unhappy in the relationship, the couple becomes trapped in this self-perpetuating negative process that serves to maintain the discord.

Enhanced CBCT goes beyond performance and skills deficit models, recognizing the influences of both the couple's behavioral interaction *processes* and the major themes (*the content*) that serve as the basis for relationship discord. Such themes often stem from differences in partners' individual and relational needs that contribute to relationship distress. Epstein and Baucom (2002) outline several important needs and motives that often become problematic in couple relationships. These include communal or relationship-focused needs, such as the need to affiliate or to be part of various relationships, including a marriage; the need for intimacy with one's partner; the desire to be altruistic to one's partner; and the need to receive succor, or to be attended to by one's partner. Individually focused needs that can serve as a source of personal satisfaction but contribute to relationship distress include needs for autonomy, control, and achievement.

Differences in individual wants or needs from the relationship, even among two psychologically well-adjusted partners, can potentially lead to relationship distress. For example, partners who differ in their desire for intimacy or their personal preferences for control, organization, and planning, might respond to resulting frustrations by behaving negatively toward each other, becoming emotionally upset, and distorting interpretations of the partner's behavior as they attempt to get their needs met. The distress resulting from unmet fundamental needs is described in our enhanced CBCT model as "primary distress," or a primary basis for the partners' dissatisfaction with their relationship. In contrast, partners' use of maladaptive strategies in response to their unmet needs and desires (e.g., by withdrawing or verbally abusing each other) can create "secondary distress" (Epstein & Baucom, 2002). Often these secondary sources of distress take on a life of their own, and the couple therapist must address both primary and secondary distress in helping partners to find adaptive ways to negotiate their differences (Baucom et al., 2004; Epstein & Baucom, 2002).

In addition to normative, expected individual differences between partners, the presence of significant psychopathology or long-term, unresolved individual issues in one or both partners can create additional stressors within the relationship and potentially worsen the well-being of both partners.

For example, one partner's experience of major depression can result in an inequitable division of household responsibilities and limit opportunities for closeness.

Finally, although the couple's broader social and physical environment can provide important resources, at times environmental factors exert demands that may be beyond the couple's coping capabilities. For example, a pile-up of stressors, or the occurrence of unexpected, non-normative stressors (e.g., a natural disaster) can overwhelm a couple's coping attempts and result in severe distress and crisis in the couple relationship. In their focus on the dyad, traditional BCT therapists often overlooked or minimized the impacts of external stressors on the couple, but current CBCT approaches take them into account.

The Impact of Gender and Cultural Factors on Relationship Functioning

The influences of individual, couple, and environmental factors on relationship functioning are apt to vary based on the gender, ethnicity, and cultural backgrounds of both partners. Research has demonstrated that relationship roles, approaches to power, and ways of processing information often differ between males and females as groups, as well as within and between ethnic and cultural groups. For example, Christensen and Heavey (1990, 1993; Christensen, 1988) found that a significant number of distressed couples exhibit an interaction pattern in which one partner demands and pursues the other for interaction, while the other partner withdraws. Although the gender difference in these roles may vary depending on the importance that the female and the male attach to a topic of conflict, findings across studies indicate that females are more likely to be in the demanding role and males in the withdrawing role. These roles often reflect power and gender differences in desired styles of intimacy, because females tend to be more oriented toward achieving intimacy through mutual self-disclosure than are males (Prager & Buhrmester, 1998).

In addition to differences in demand–withdraw patterns, gender also influences how males and females organize and process information about their relationship. Females are more likely than males to engage in circular "relationship schematic processing," in which they consider both partners' contributions to couple interaction patterns, whereas males are more likely to engage in "individual schematic processing," in which they focus on linear impacts that individual partners have on the relationship (Baucom, 1999; Rankin, Baucom, Clayton, & Daiuto, 1995; Sullivan & Baucom, 2005). These differences in information processing are also associated with relationship adjustment. Male partners' increases in the quality and amount of relationship schematic processing as a result of CBCT was found to be positively associated with increases in their female partners' satisfaction with the relationship (Sullivan & Baucom, 2005); that is, females became more satisfied with the relationship as their male partners learned to process more in relationship terms.

Although CBCT approaches have made significant strides in focusing on gender issues in couple therapy, they have paid limited attention to the impact of racial, ethnic, and cultural issues, on relationship functioning and treatment. Rates of divorce vary across ethnic groups and tend to be higher among some ethnic/minority couples. Researchers have generally attributed group differences in divorce rates to several stressors that disproportionately affect ethnic/minority couples, including economic instability, joblessness, exposure to poverty and violence, and continued experiences of racism and discrimination (LaTaillade, 2006). As noted by Bradbury and Karney (2004), couples' exposure to such chronic stressors tends to be associated with concurrent relationship distress, as well as longitudinal declines in marital quality. Chronic stressors are likely to tax the couple's resources, increase vulnerability to other stressful events, increase partners' negative perceptions of each other and their relationship, decrease their expectancies that they will be able to withstand the stressors, and increase the couple's conflictual interactions (LaTaillade, 2006). For example, it is not uncommon for ethnic/minority couples, in response to racism and other social stressors, to turn their frustration against each other by engaging in mutual blaming that increases distress and perceptions of powerlessness. Furthermore, partners may internalize racist and self-blaming societal messages and stereotypes associated with individual and relationship problems (e.g., the assumption that African American males are not interested in committed relationships; Kelly, 2006).

Our enhanced CBCT uses a contextual focus that prevents adoption of a "values and culture-free" approach to assessment and treatment, recognizes the impact of social and environmental stressors on relationship functioning, fosters identification of themes that often characterize conflict in ethnically diverse couple relationships (i.e., balancing power and respect), and promotes empowerment by helping couples to build on their strengths and resources, and to generalize treatment gains (Kelly, 2006; LaTaillade, 2006). This explicit focus on fostering the couple's use of environmental supports and resources, as part of a broad approach to addressing multiple levels of the couple's environment (e.g., extended family, community, social institutions), allows treatment to elicit and employ couples' diversity-related strengths toward alleviation of distress (Kelly & Iwamasa, 2005).

THE PRACTICE OF COUPLE THERAPY

The Structure of the Therapy Process

Based partly on the basic models of BCT and CT, as well as treatment protocols used in controlled therapy outcome studies that restrict therapy to a relatively limited number of sessions with structured agendas for sessions, CBCT tends to be implemented as a brief therapy approach, ranging from several to over 20 weekly sessions. It is common for therapists to gradually phase out therapy as a couple shows evidence of substituting positive interactions for negative ones and of achieving the partners' initial goals for therapy. Given that CBCT recognizes the importance of partners' mastery of skills for managing their behavioral interactions, their cognitions, and their experience and expression of emotions, periodic "booster" sessions also may be scheduled. There are no data available on the length of CBCT in clinic and private practice settings, but the length of treatment likely varies considerably among therapists and for specific couples (depending on the severity of problems in individual and/or couple functioning). For example, if a couple has experienced trauma such as intimate partner violence or infidelity, then the length of treatment depends on the partners' abilities to manage trauma symptoms, to modify their individual and relationship characteristics that placed them at risk for the traumatic events, to deal with issues surrounding forgiveness, and to decide on the future of their relationship (Snyder, Baucom, & Gordon, 2007). Couples in which one or both members exhibit a personality disorder or severe psychopathology also may require more extended CBCT (Epstein & Baucom, 2002). Although it is not always possible to predict how long work with a couple will take, it is possible to set reasonable goals for treatment, and for the therapist and both partners to assess the amount of progress made as therapy proceeds (Epstein &

Baucom, 2002; Wood & Jacobson, 1985). Goals are set at both the "micro" level (e.g., increasing the number of meals the partners eat together) and "macro" level (e.g., increasing the couple's overall level of togetherness). If it appears that the goals of therapy might not be met in a reasonable time period, it can be useful to reassess reachable goals during the time allotted for treatment, or to negotiate for additional sessions with the couple (Wood & Jacobson, 1985).

Use of Homework Assignments in CBCT

Consistent with the traditions of both BCT and CT, CBCT therapists routinely collaborate with couples in designing homework assignments to be completed between therapy sessions. Use of homework is based on the learning principle that to replace existing (and often ingrained) dysfunctional interaction patterns with new positive ones, the couple needs to rehearse the new patterns repeatedly, particularly under "real-life" conditions that are different and often more challenging than those in the therapist's office. A common assignment is practice of expressive and listening skills at home that the couple rehearsed under the therapist's guidance during therapy sessions, to generalize their use to the home environment. It is important that the therapist explore partners' possible negative cognitions about participating in homework (e.g., "It will take up too much of my leisure time") to reduce noncompliance.

Joining with the Couple and Establishing a Treatment Alliance

There are several potential barriers to joining simultaneously with both members of a couple, and these barriers apply to orientations beyond CBCT. First, members of couples who are in conflict may desire to form an alliance with the therapist, convincing the therapist that the other partner is responsible for the relationship problems (Epstein & Baucom, 2002; 2003). It is important to respond in a manner that demonstrates to the blamed partner that the therapist is not siding with the individual attempting to form the alliance; however, the therapist simultaneously must demonstrate that he or she is taking the alliance-seeker's concerns seriously and not siding with the blamed partner (unless the blamer is behaving in an abusive manner). Use of empathic reflective listening with one partner and then the other, followed by statements summarizing the reciprocal and often

interlocking concerns of the two individuals, can help to establish the therapist as a relatively neutral party whose agenda is to help both members of the couple achieve their personal goals for their relationship. Defining relationship problems in dyadic terms, as much as possible, can facilitate this process (e.g., "The two of you have been struggling with differences in your preferences for time on your own versus time together").

A second common barrier to establishment of a therapeutic alliance is one or both partners' concerns about the safety of conjoint sessions. In such instances, we screen couples for ongoing or potential physical violence and decide whether conjoint therapy is appropriate. However, many individuals who never experience violence still want to avoid being subjected to verbal attacks from their partners during therapy sessions. Consequently, CBCT therapists establish guidelines for constructive couple interaction in sessions, formalizing them in a written agreement, if necessary, and intervene quickly to block aversive behavior whenever a member of a couple violates the guidelines (Epstein & Baucom, 2002, 2003).

A third potential barrier to formation of a treatment alliance in couple therapy is partners' concerns that changes elicited in treatment will "rock the boat," changing patterns that have been reinforcing for them. For example, an individual who receives attention from a partner in response to criticizing the partner may be concerned that agreeing to engage in the therapist's recommendations for constructive communication will reduce his or her power and receipt of solicitous behavior from the partner. Within a CBCT framework, it is important to alleviate these concerns by providing new reinforcers that replace those lost by partners when the couple interacts differently. The therapist can help individuals devise new behaviors to gain positive attention from the partner. Epstein and Baucom (2002, 2003) provide a more extensive description of potential barriers to establishment of a therapeutic alliance with both partners and strategies for joining with couples.

Inclusion of Other Individuals in Couple Sessions

Most often CBCT includes both members of a couple, although significant others who influence the functioning of the couple's relationship can be included *occasionally* (with more extensive involvement of other family members essentially shifting the modality from couple to family therapy). The rationale for including another person in a session is to give the therapist an opportunity to observe the impact that person has on the couple's interactions, as well as to allow the couple to practice interacting differently with the individual. For example, after devoting some sessions to developing the partners' abilities to collaborate in parenting behavior, the couple could bring a challenging child to a session or two to practice effective coparenting with the therapist present.

As described more in the section on intervention, CBCT considers other people in the couple's environment at several levels (children in the nuclear family, extended family, friends, neighbors, work associates, etc.), and as possible sources of demands on the couple and as possible resources for the couple in resolving problems. Whether or not other people are invited to be present physically in sessions, they are often the topics of assessment and intervention during sessions conducted with only the couple.

Medication, Individual Therapy, and CBCT

Given the common co-occurrence of individual psychopathology and relationship problems (Beach, 2001; Whisman, Uebelacker, & Weinstock, 2004), it is common for one or both members of a couple to enter CBCT on medication and/or in individual therapy. To the extent that individual psychopathology of a partner has been a stressor, placing demands on the couple's coping abilities, CBCT therapists view treatments for individual difficulties as an appropriate adjunct to couple therapy. However, it is crucial that the use of medication and/or individual therapy not result in that member of the couple being defined as the sole source of problems in the relationship, interfering with the therapist's ability to intervene in the dyadic processes that also affect the couple's adjustment and satisfaction. The therapist should make efforts to identify and intervene in the mutual, reciprocal, causal processes that commonly occur when psychopathology and relationship distress coexist (Beach, 2001; Epstein & Baucom, 2002). Furthermore, it is highly advisable for the couple therapist to obtain written consent to contact the mental health professionals who are providing medication or individual therapy for a partner, and exchange information about the partner's conditions that may be influencing the couple relationship, and vice versa.

Overall, we see minimal contraindications for the concurrent use of psychotropic medications during CBCT, as long as the types (e.g., antipsychotic medications with sedative properties) and doses do not interfere with the individual's cognitive functioning in a manner that decreases his or her ability to benefit from CBCT interventions, such as those described later for modifying negative cognitions, emotions, and behavior. Another concern regards the use of antianxiety medications for partners who experience panic attacks, in that one of the key goals of cognitive-behavioral individual and couple interventions for panic disorder is to remove "safety signals" that the anxious individual relies on to feel secure, including the presence of a significant other person and/or antianxiety medication (Baucom, Stanton, & Epstein, 2003).

Because it is important that both members of a couple view the therapist as impartial and supportive, the therapist must be mindful of any implications that one partner's use of medication or individual therapy may have for the clients' perceptions that the therapist considers that person to be "the patient." We attempt to counteract such interpretations by emphasizing to the individual (in the presence of the partner) advantages of medications and individual therapy in "helping you to be in the best condition to work on achieving your goals for your couple relationship." The therapist takes a similar stance, whether discussing other treatments that a partner was already receiving when the couple began therapy or referring a member of a couple for individual therapy or a medication evaluation.

Cotherapy

Practical considerations, particularly cost, typically result in CBCT being conducted by only one therapist, but there are rationales supported by the CBCT model for advocating cotherapy when possible. Given the centrality of learning principles in CBCT, the presence of a cotherapy dyad that can model constructive communication and other positive behavioral patterns might enhance couples' learning of such skills. In addition, as the couple rehearses new communication skills, each cotherapist can coach a member of the couple, maximizing the individual attention that each partner receives as he or she works to overcome overlearned negative responses and to produce new, constructive behavior. The same modeling and coaching processes can be used in cognitive restructuring interventions, such as those described later in this chapter. Whereas cotherapy might be helpful for particular couples, the one investigation of BCT that evaluated this issue found that a single therapist and cotherapists were equally effective in providing BCT (Mehlman, Baucom, & Anderson, 1981).

Sessions with Individual Partners

Our CBCT assessment procedures include both a joint couple interview that focuses on the history and current functioning of the relationship and an individual interview with each partner (Epstein & Baucom, 2002). During the individual interviews, the therapist collects information about the person's history in terms of experiences in family of origin and other significant relationships, educational and employment history and functioning, areas of personal strength, and past and current health and mental health status. Because clients often feel more comfortable sharing information about the past in a private interview with a clinician, we tell them that we will keep information they provide about their histories confidential even from their partners, but if we learn about a client's past experiences (e.g., having been abandoned by a former intimate partner) that might be influencing the couple's current interactions, we encourage the person to share the information in joint sessions. The same criteria regarding confidentiality apply to information about each person's current functioning, with a few notable exceptions that we describe to the couple during our initial joint interview. Specifically, if an individual reports recently being abused physically by the partner to an extent that resulted in injury and/or being afraid to live with the partner, we keep that information confidential, not sharing it with the person's allegedly abusive partner. Disclosing an individual's report of being abused to the partner identified as the perpetrator may place the abused person in danger of receiving additional abuse. Consequently, under such circumstances, we decide whether it is too risky to conduct couple therapy, and if conjoint sessions are not appropriate, we tell the partners that, based on our assessment of them through observations of their communication and their reports of how they handle conflicts, we believe that they are not ready at present for couple therapy. We suggest that at this point each partner might benefit from individual therapy sessions focusing on conflict resolution, and that a decision be made later about shifting to couple sessions. We realize the complications of handling such situations but concur with other

professionals (e.g., Holtzworth-Munroe, Meehan, Rehman, & Marshall, 2002; O'Leary, Chapter 16, this volume) that protecting the physical and psychological well-being of each individual must be given priority in the decision regarding the best modality for intervention.

In contrast our handling of a secret regarding physical abuse, we tell the couple before holding any individual interviews that we do not want to become a party to a secret about ongoing infidelity that an individual has not revealed to his or her partner, because it places us in the position of colluding with the involved partner and undermines the couple therapy goal of working to improve the relationship, if possible. We also tell the couple that if a partner chooses to reveal a secret affair during an individual session, we will strongly encourage that person to reveal the affair to the partner, so that they can consider together its implications for their relationship and decide on a course of action for therapy. If the individual reveals an ongoing affair to the therapist during an individual interview but chooses to keep it a secret from the partner, we request that he or she find a way to terminate the couple therapy, so that it does not continue under conditions in which the involved partner can seek solace with the third party when the primary relationship is stressful. It is important to note that this is our personal preference for handling secrets in couple therapy, not a principle that is specific to CBCT, and that there is no consensus among clinicians on the best approach to this issue (Glass, 2002).

Most CBCT sessions beyond the initial assessment are conducted with both partners, partly to preclude the inadvertent sharing of secrets between one member of the couple and the therapist, and partly because the CBCT model emphasizes assessing and intervening with the process of couple interactions firsthand. Planning with one member of a couple during an individual meeting how he or she might attempt to alter the couple's interaction pattern by behaving differently toward the partner during the coming week may have some success, but CBCT focuses on direct observation and modification of patterns *as they are occurring*. Nevertheless, there are circumstances in which it may be advantageous to have one or more individual sessions with a member of a couple (e.g., to coach the individual in anger management strategies when he or she has had significant difficulty regulating emotional responses in the partner's presence). The main caution is that individual sessions may unbalance the degree to which the members of the couple view the therapist as equally supportive of them both, or identify one partner as "the problem" in the relationship. Consequently, we also typically schedule an individual session with the other partner, focusing on contributions that this person can make to improve the couple's relationship.

Out-of-Session Contacts with Members of the Couple

Our guidelines for phone calls with members of a couple are based more on personal preference than on CBCT principles per se. Because rapport depends on both members of a couple perceiving the therapist as impartial and caring, we emphasize that engaging in extra interactions with the therapist by phone or e-mail should be avoided, especially if this is done without the knowledge of the partner. Occasional brief calls are acceptable, particularly if the caller needs a reminder about how to enact new behaviors that the couple had agreed on during the previous therapy session. If the caller begins to complain about the partner or raise other issues that are appropriate for treatment, the therapist suggests that these concerns be voiced early in the next conjoint session.

The Role of the Therapist

The CBCT therapist undertakes multiple roles to facilitate the structure and course of therapy. Particularly during the assessment and the early stages of therapy, the therapist assumes a didactic role, striking a balance between directiveness and collaboration with the couple in setting goals and applying cognitive-behavioral strategies toward achieving them (Epstein & Baucom, 2002). During the assessment, the therapist actively collects information to be used for case conceptualization and treatment planning. Once treatment begins, the therapist at times assumes a didactic role and provides rationales for treatment recommendations and the assignment of homework; reviews assignments and events that occurred in the relationship during the past week; models skills and coaches the partners in practicing them in and outside of sessions; and continually fosters partners' motivation. The therapist's level of directiveness varies according to the partners' presenting concerns (e.g., a high degree of directiveness is used with abusive partners); their ability to self-monitor their behaviors, emotions, and cognitions; and their preference for structure in therapy (Epstein & Baucom, 2002).

In addition to the didactic role, the CBCT therapist also sets the pace of sessions, so that the goals of treatment are addressed in a timely and reasonable fashion (Baucom et al., 2002). In collaboration with the couple, the therapist typically initiates setting the agenda for each session, contributing particular agenda items such as review of homework and practice of a particular skill, always soliciting the couple's preferences for the agenda. The therapist then monitors the use of time during the session and ensures that the agenda is followed to the degree appropriate. Because couples in distress often bring multiple concerns into sessions and are likely to get sidetracked, it is the responsibility of the therapist to stay on task and address the goals of the session, teaching the couple to self-monitor as well. From a social learning perspective, the CBCT therapist is modeling the processes of time management and systematic, collaborative problem solving for the couple.

The therapist also adopts the role of facilitator, creating a safe and supportive environment in which the couple can address difficult issues. Couples often enter therapy in a state of acute distress and have difficulty regulating their levels of emotion and displays of negative behavior both during sessions and in daily life (Epstein & Baucom, 2002). To create a safe environment for the partners to identify and resolve their concerns, the therapist must be able to maintain control of the sessions with an air of confidence and credibility. For example, in response to couples with strong and frequent emotional outbursts, the therapist actively discourages the escalation of such interactions by interrupting inappropriate and harmful behaviors, and establishes clear guidelines for constructive responses in the face of conflict. Such interventions are often a crucial step in facilitating broader positive change in the couple relationship. Although some individuals may initially be frustrated by interventions that block their usual negative ways of expressing their distress about their partner and relationship, couples more often welcome consistency on the therapist's part in maintaining the structure and ground rules of treatment.

The CBCT therapist's ability to adopt the multiple roles of director, educator, facilitator, collaborator, and advocate, as well as the ability to balance these multiple roles while providing perspective and emotional support, is critical to both the effectiveness of treatment and the maintenance of the therapeutic alliance (Baucom et al., 2002). In addition, over the course of treatment, the therapist must balance his or her alliances and interventions with the two partners, so that both feel supported and remain equally invested in improving the relationship. The therapist often must shift attention and interventions back and forth between partners, maintaining involvement with both partners. When one partner presents with significant individual psychological distress, it may be necessary for the therapist to create a temporary imbalance, focusing more on the needs of the more distressed partner. Such interventions can be beneficial as long as the intentional shifts are discussed with the couple and counterbalanced over the course of treatment (Epstein & Baucom, 2002, 2003).

Because the ultimate goal of CBCT is the couple's use of the skills learned in therapy in their natural environment as needed, it is important that the therapist's direction and imposition of structure gradually diminish over time, as the partners assume increasing responsibility for managing their concerns. This gradual decrease in the therapist's influence helps to foster the couple's confidence and competence in continuing to make positive changes in their relationship following the termination of therapy (Baucom et al., 2002). The therapist sets the stage from the beginning of therapy for the gradual shift in responsibility to the couple by emphasizing collaboration rather than simply directing the couple. The therapist encourages the partners to identify treatment goals, participate in designing their own homework assignments, and periodically assess their progress in meeting their goals.

Assessment and Treatment Planning

Within a cognitive-behavioral framework, the primary goals of a clinical assessment are (1) to identify the concerns and potential areas of enrichment/growth for which a couple has sought assistance; (2) to clarify the cognitive, behavioral, and affective factors associated with the two individuals, the couple as a dyad, and the couple's environment, that contribute to their presenting concerns; and (3) to determine the appropriateness of couple therapy in addressing these concerns. The therapist clarifies partners' goals for treatment and their respective positions and perspectives regarding the areas of concern. In addition, the therapist determines each partner's emotional investment and motivation for continuing with the relationship. Clarification of the partners' levels of commitment and goals for treatment in-

forms the therapist how to structure and guide the assessment process.

Unless couples enter therapy in a state of acute crisis, the first two or three sessions are devoted to assessment and evaluation (Epstein & Baucom, 2002; LaTaillade & Jacobson, 1995). Couples are informed that the purpose of the initial evaluation is to identify their concerns about the relationship and the factors that influence their difficulties, as well as to determine whether therapy is the best course of action for them at the present time. If the couple and therapist decide that therapy is not the optimal plan, they determine some alternative course of action (e.g., individual therapy for one or both partners to address factors that do not appear to be caused by conditions within the couple relationship).

Even though the primary focus of the assessment phase is on gathering information, this pretreatment phase often has therapeutic effects. Because the focus is on strengths, as well as problems, the questions posed by the therapist often draw partners' attention to the positive aspects of their relationship. Distressed couples entering therapy often selectively track negative behaviors and events, so refocusing on the positive can increase positive affect and offer couples a sense of hope (Epstein & Baucom, 2002; Jacobson & Holtzworth-Munroe, 1986).

Assessment of the Individual Partners, Their Relationship, and Their Environment

In conducting a thorough cognitive-behavioral assessment, the therapist attends not only to characteristics of the dyad but also to factors regarding the individual partners and their interpersonal and physical environment. Regarding individual characteristics that influence current concerns, the therapist attends to partners' respective personality styles, demonstrations of psychopathology or subclinical character traits, individually oriented needs (e.g., for autonomy) and communal needs (e.g., for intimacy), and the extent to which those are being satisfied, and ways that experiences in prior significant relationships continue to affect the individual's responses to the present relationship. Dyadic factors assessed by the therapist include macro-level patterns that are a function of the partners' individual characteristics (e.g., a partner with stronger intimacy needs commonly pursuing a partner with stronger autonomy needs), as well as patterns of couple interaction that have developed over the course of the relationship (e.g., one partner engaging in a high level of nurturance behavior when the other partner experiences periodic episodes of depression). The therapist assesses degrees of difference between partners' personalities, needs, and values, as well as ways the partners interact in response to areas of conflict. Environmental factors include demands with which the couple has had to cope over the course of the relationship (e.g., relations with nuclear and extended family members, work pressures), and broader societal factors, such as economic stresses (e.g., high inflation), racial or sexual discrimination, and threats of terrorism.

Assessment Methods

The initial assessment phase typically involves multiple strategies for information gathering, including self-report questionnaires, clinical interviews with the couple and with the individual partners, and direct observation of the couple's interaction patterns. The following common methods are used in self-report, interview, and observational approaches to assessment.

Initial joint interviews of couples typically include a developmental relationship history (e.g., how they met, what attracted them to each other, how they developed a deeper involvement and commitment, what life events had significant positive or negative influences on their relationship, and any prior experiences in couple or individual therapy) to place current concerns in some meaningful perspective (Baucom & Epstein, 1990; Epstein & Baucom, 2002). Influences of race, ethnicity, religion, and other aspects of culture on the couple's relationship are explored, for example, whether or not the couple has an interfaith or interracial relationship (Hardy & Laszloffy, 2002; LaTaillade, 2006). If the couple has immigrated from another country, the therapist explores the partners' current level of acculturation into their host culture, as well as any instances of acculturative stress. The therapist also inquires about the partners' current concerns, as well as strengths of their relationship. The therapist orients the couple to the process of therapy, describing the typical structure and course of CBCT, and the roles that the therapist and couple play. Finally, the initial interview provides the therapist's first opportunity to establish a balanced and collaborative working relationship with both partners. Given the wealth of information to be obtained, the initial joint interviews can require 2–3 hours in one extended session or a few 50- to 60-minute sessions

(Baucom & Epstein, 1990). Because couples may be *either* ambivalent about entering treatment *or* eager to begin therapeutic interventions to reduce their high level of distress, it is recommended that the evaluation be completed expediently, generally during a 1- or 2-week period. Taking a couple's history also can elicit partners' memories of earlier positive times in their relationship that may counterbalance the negativism they typically experience when they seek therapy.

In addition to focusing on historical factors, the therapist also inquires about partners' current relationship concerns, as well as individual, dyadic, and environmental factors that contribute to partners' presenting issues. Concerning current individual factors, the therapist inquires about any difficulties each partner may be experiencing associated with symptoms of psychopathology, or any vulnerability due to past traumatic experiences in prior relationships. Evidence of significant psychopathology in an individual client leads the therapist to pursue a more in-depth assessment of the individual's functioning and perhaps to make a referral for individual therapy. If the therapist identifies psychopathology in either or both partners that has not been identified as an individual problem during the assessment or initial therapy sessions, then the therapist must use tact in suggesting that the individual is experiencing symptoms that detract from his or her happiness, and recommending treatment of these symptoms, as well as the couple's presenting concerns. As we discuss later in the chapter, at times a couple-based strategy might be employed to address individual psychopathology.

With regard to dyadic factors, the therapist assesses the overall rate with which meaningful positive and negative exchanges are occurring in the relationship, and the extent to which these exchanges are organized around broader macrolevel themes, such as conflict about the balance of power in the couple's decision-making process. The therapist also ascertains the partners' perceptions of presenting problems, attributions for why the problems exist, respective standards for how the relationship should function in those areas, and behavioral and emotional responses to the problems (Baucom et al., 1995; Epstein & Baucom, 2002).

Regarding assessment of environmental factors that contribute to the couple's presenting concerns, the therapist can ask about relationships with individuals at various levels, such as friends, biological relatives and "kinship" networks, and members of larger social institutions and organizations (e.g., schools, legal, and social service agencies), and identify stressful interactions that occur at each level (Epstein & Baucom, 2002). Because the couple is also embedded within a larger societal context, broader societal influences, such as experiences of racial, ethnic, religious, and/or sexual discrimination, may influence the quality of their relationship and should be explored. In addition, the therapist inquires about physical surroundings, including the couple's immediate living conditions and surrounding neighborhood, which may place significant demands on the relationship, such as pressure on the partners to keep their children safe in a violent neighborhood (Epstein & Baucom, 2002).

The therapist imposes structure on the interview regarding the couple's current concerns, typically inquiring about each person's concerns while the partner listens (Baucom & Epstein, 1990; Epstein & Baucom, 2002). This structure decreases the likelihood of escalating conflict between partners concerning their perceptions and attributions about the source of problems. It also allows each partner an opportunity to feel both heard and respected by the therapist. Understanding that their personal feelings and viewpoints will be acknowledged contributes to partners' investment in treatment and their willingness to work collaboratively toward improving their relationship by making individual positive changes.

Because distressed couples frequently are acutely aware of the weaknesses in their relationship, the therapist seeks to balance the discussion of current problems with identification of both historical and current relationship strengths. This discussion can include positive experiences in the earlier phases of the couple's relationship, characteristics of each individual that may still be valued by the partner, available environmental resources used by the couple, and the couple's previous attempts to address relationship concerns. Prior efforts, whether successful or not, can be reframed by the therapist as evidence that the couple has some commitment and skills for working together on the relationship (Wood & Jacobson, 1985). Highlighting such strengths can foster hopefulness in the couple for positive outcomes in treatment.

COMMUNICATION SAMPLE

The therapist samples partners' communication skills by asking them to engage in a structured discussion, while he or she observes their process.

Observing partners' cognitive, emotional, and behavioral responses to each other's behaviors and/or relationship topics allows the therapist to identify broader, macro-level themes that may be central issues in the relationship and to determine what interventions may be needed. The therapist can ask the partners to engage in many kinds of tasks, including (1) discussing an area of moderate concern in their relationship, so the therapist can observe how they make decisions; (2) sharing thoughts and feelings about themselves or some aspect of the relationship, so the therapist may assess their expressive and listening skills; or (3) engaging in a task requiring partners to provide each other with instrumental or expressive support (Epstein & Baucom, 2002).

QUESTIONNAIRES

Although in clinical practice the interview provides much of the basis for assessment, self-report questionnaires can add significantly and help to guide the interviews. In general, it is recommended that the therapist selectively utilize self-report measures that assess (1) partners' satisfaction with important areas of their relationship; (2) each partner's individual and communally oriented needs, and the extent to which those needs are being satisfied; (3) the range of environmental demands experienced by the partners individually and as a couple; (4) partners' cognitions and communication patterns; (5) symptoms of psychopathology in each partner; (6) levels of physical and psychological abuse exhibited by each partner; and (7) strengths that both partners bring to the relationship (Epstein & Baucom, 2002). The following examples are reliable and valid inventories that address these areas of relationship functioning. The Dyadic Adjustment Scale (DAS; Spanier, 1976) and the Marital Satisfaction Inventory (MSI; Snyder, 1979; Snyder & Costin, 1994; Snyder, Wills, & Keiser, 1981) assess global ratings of marital satisfaction, as well as satisfaction in other areas of functioning, such as parenting, finances, sexual intimacy, leisure time, and so forth. The Areas of Change Questionnaire (ACQ; Weiss et al., 1973) asks couples to indicate the direction and degree of change that they would like to see in 34 types of partner behavior. Comparison of partners' responses to these inventories can provide the therapist with information regarding discrepancies in partner satisfaction and areas of concern.

The Need Fulfillment Inventory (Prager & Buhrmester, 1998) assesses each partner's ratings of importance and fulfillment of those needs we categorize as individually oriented (e.g., autonomy, self-actualization) or communal (e.g., nurturance, intimacy, sexual fulfillment). The Family Inventory of Life Events and Changes (FILE; McCubbin & Patterson, 1987) lists a wide range of normative and non-normative events, such as pregnancy and childbearing, changes in work status, and deaths, that may be current or prior sources of demands on the couple. The Revised Conflict Tactics Scale (CTS2; Straus, Hamby, Boney-McCoy, & Sugarman, 1996) asks each member of a couple to report the frequencies with which specific forms of physically or psychologically abusive behaviors were exhibited by the partner and by the self during the past year, whereas the Multidimensional Measure of Emotional Abuse (MMEA; Murphy & Hoover, 2001) assesses forms of psychological abuse (denigration, hostile withdrawal, domination/intimidation, and restrictive engulfment) more extensively. The Brief Symptom Inventory (BSI; Derogatis, 1993) is a 53-item scale that provides a survey of symptoms of psychopathology experienced by each partner.

Numerous measures have been developed to assess relationship cognitions, such as the Relationship Belief Inventory (Eidelson & Epstein, 1982) and the Inventory of Specific Relationship Standards (Baucom, Epstein, Daiuto, & Carels, 1996; Baucom, Epstein, Rankin, & Burnett, 1996), and communication, such as the Communication Patterns Questionnaire (CPQ; Christensen, 1987, 1988). Although these measures are often used in research, in clinical practice partners' cognitions and behaviors are assessed primarily through interviews and behavioral observation. Nevertheless, clinicians can administer these measures to help ensure a thorough assessment and/or as guidelines for clinical interviews (Epstein & Baucom, 2002). Although all of the measures we have listed tap into potential concerns and sources of conflict, they also can be used to assess areas of strength within the relationship. For example, the therapist can note areas of relationship satisfaction on which the partners agree or stressful life events that the couple handled successfully.

Often it is helpful to have couples complete the inventories individually, prior to their initial interview to afford the clinician an opportunity to review them and to generate hypotheses and questions for exploring further areas of concern in the couple and individual interviews. As such, we inform couples that, with few exceptions (e.g., individual responses to questionnaires regarding

psychological and physical abuse that may place a partner at increased risk for assault), partners' responses are not kept confidential and will be shared, as appropriate, during the couple assessment.

Although the initial pretherapy assessment is crucial in identifying targets for intervention in CBCT, assessment continues throughout the course of treatment. Continued evaluation is consistent with the empirical tradition on which CBCT is based (Baucom & Epstein, 1990). Ongoing assessment provides the therapist with opportunities not only to monitor the couple's progress in targeted treatment areas and changes in marital satisfaction, but also to test hypotheses and refine treatment conceptualizations generated as a result of the initial assessment.

Goal Setting

Based on the initial assessment, the therapist meets with the couple to provide treatment recommendations. The therapist presents to the couple his or her understanding of the relevant couple, individual, and environmental factors that significantly influence the couple's relationship (e.g., the couple's demand–withdraw pattern that impedes their ability to resolve conflicts; one partner's clinical depression; escalating job pressure). The therapist also describes behavioral, cognitive, and affective response patterns that the assessment has indicated are contributors to the couple's relationship difficulties (Epstein & Baucom, 2002). At this point the therapist asks the partners for feedback about this case conceptualization, checking to see whether it matches their views of their difficulties. The therapist then collaborates with the couple in translating descriptions of relationship problems into statements of positive goals. For example, the problem of "too little intimacy in our relationship, typified by little time spent together and little sharing of thoughts and emotions" might become a goal of "increasing intimacy in our relationship by increasing time together and communication of our thoughts and emotions." The therapist then relates these goals to specific intervention techniques designed to substitute desired patterns for the existing ones. In addition, the therapist presents the feedback in a way that models for the couple collaboration, caring, concern, openness, and honesty. The therapist also attempts to model setting realistic goals for treatment, while fostering partners' hope that treatment can be beneficial and promoting their sense of self-efficacy for improving their relationship. Again, the therapist actively seeks partners' input and perspectives on their own relationship not only during the assessment feedback session but also continually, over the course of treatment, as initial goals are addressed and additional factors influencing the couple's relationship become evident as therapy evolves.

Explicit goal setting is important for several reasons. Individual partners vary in the extent to which they have a clear understanding of the factors affecting their relationship and clear goals for treatment, and how their own contributions affect the achievement of their goals (Baucom & Epstein, 1990; Baucom et al., 2002; Epstein & Baucom, 2002). CBCT therapists underscore the importance of partners taking responsibility for their own behavior and for improving the relationship. This collaborative mind-set can be fostered if the therapist and couple have a shared conceptualization of relationship functioning, long-term goals, and strategies for achieving these goals. Helping partners understand the rationales for these tasks can increase the likelihood that they will follow through with the assignments.

In addition, because couples often present for treatment with significant distress, partners may be overwhelmed and demoralized by the current state of their relationship. By working with the couple to develop clear, explicit, and achievable goals, the therapist helps to focus the partners, decrease their anxiety, and increase their optimism regarding the outcome of treatment (Epstein & Baucom, 2002).

There may be instances in which the couple and the therapist have different goals for the relationship. For example, the partners may agree on the goal of helping the husband to feel less depressed, but they may endorse a solution that involves subjugation of the wife's needs and desires to increase the husband's self-confidence and sense of empowerment. The therapist may want to help the partners develop a more equitable and balanced relationship that allows both partners' needs to be met. In such instances, the therapist might explain to the couple why he or she believes there is a discrepancy between the goals of the couple and those of the therapist, in this case the potential negative implications that the therapist anticipates if one partner sacrifices her needs for the sake of her partner. The therapist and couple discuss these differences and attempt to develop a shared set of goals. In some circumstances a therapist may decide that he or she cannot continue

to work with a couple because the couple's goals are unattainable, or because the therapist believes that he or she would be contributing to the development of an unhealthy relationship (Baucom et al., 2002). On the other hand, the therapist can propose an empirical approach, in which the partners experiment with working toward their own goal for a trial period, and the therapist and couple agree to assess later the impacts of that strategy on their individual and joint well-being.

In addition, at times the goals of two partners may be either in conflict (e.g., differences in desires for intimacy and closeness), or mutually exclusive. In such instances, the therapist typically points out these discrepancies, with the goal of having the partners work together to resolve their differences and reach compromises, accept their differences, or decide whether to continue the relationship, if each person considers his or her goals to be of primary importance (Baucom et al., 2002).

Given that there are likely to be multiple goals in working with a couple, it is important to determine the appropriate sequence of addressing these goals in therapy. Although the particular combination of factors affecting a given couple's relationship is likely to vary, there are some general principles for addressing important issues in the relationship. First, both partners must feel that the therapist is attending to the central areas of concern that prompted them to seek treatment. If they feel that the therapist is not addressing these issues or is making insignificant progress with them, their motivation for therapy is likely to decrease.

Second, many distressed couples have a history of longstanding negative interactions that interfere with their ability to address their most central concerns at the outset of treatment. Each partner may be entrenched in the "rightness" of his or her own perspectives, and as a result be unwilling to be collaborative or share areas of vulnerability. In such instances, the therapist needs to help the partners decrease the frequency of aversive interactions and establish a safe atmosphere in which they communicate in positive, respectful, and constructive ways (Epstein & Baucom, 2002). Thus, the goal of decreasing high levels of aversive interaction is a prerequisite for working on partners' goals of addressing their central concerns about their relationship, such as conflicting beliefs regarding relationships with extended family members.

Third, some couples enter therapy rather disengaged and uninvolved, which can compromise their engagement in treatment. For such a couple, an early goal may be to help both persons become more open and emotionally expressive, and to prescribe activities that foster a sense of closeness, so that the couple can address other issues in the relationship.

Finally, some goals may be difficult or impossible to attain until other goals are addressed. This is often the case when a couple presents with a relationship trauma or an acute crisis that presents a danger to one or both partners, as well as to the couple as a unit. Addressing this event or relationship trauma takes priority over other goals of therapy. The therapist must consider whether individual therapy, couple therapy, or both are appropriate in addressing and resolving the major stressors currently affecting the couple. For example, when one or both partners reports instances of couple violence, cessation of the violence becomes the primary goal of treatment, before other goals can be addressed. Other high-risk behaviors that put an individual or couple at risk, such as substance abuse, also require immediate attention.

As treatment progresses and initial goals are addressed, the couple may still feel dissatisfied with the relationship. It is important that the therapist caution the partners that it is not unusual for additional concerns to present themselves as therapy progresses, particularly if a pressing problem has distracted them from noticing other issues. Goals for therapy often evolve over time, and the therapist helps the couple become aware of additional goals that might be pursued, while monitoring the couple's progress in addressing their original goals.

COMMONLY USED INTERVENTIONS AND THE PROCESS OF THERAPY

Cognitive-behavioral couple therapists have developed a wide variety of interventions to assist couples. In differentiating among these interventions, it is important to recognize that behavior, cognitions, and emotions are integrally related. Changes in one domain typically produce changes in the other domains. Thus, if a husband starts to think about his wife differently and understand her behavior in a more benign way, he likely will also have more positive emotional reactions to her and behave toward her in more positive ways. Furthermore, an individual's subjective experience is typically a blend of cognitions and emotions that are not clearly differentiated from each other. Therefore, as we discuss interventions focused on behavior, cognitions, and emotions, it is with

the recognition that these distinctions are made partially for heuristic purposes, and that most interventions affect all of these domains of relationship functioning. Specific interventions often are focused on one of these domains, with the explicit intent that other aspects of functioning will be altered simultaneously.

Earlier, we explained the importance of understanding the roles that individual, couple interactive process, and the environment play in a couple's relationship. Each of these domains can be addressed in terms of the behaviors, cognitions, and emotions focal to a given domain. For example, a therapist might focus upon a wife's attributions for why her husband keeps long work hours, her emotional reaction to his behaviors, and her subsequent behavior toward him. Similarly, if a couple needs assistance from the social environment outside of their relationship, then the therapist might address the partners' standards regarding the appropriateness of seeking outside support, their emotional responses to being helped by others, and specific actions they might take to receive assistance. Consequently, any of these interventions for behavioral, cognitive, or emotional factors can be focused on the individual partners, the couple as a dyad, or the couple's interaction with the environment.

Interventions for Modifying Behavior

CBCT initially focused explicitly on partners' behaviors, with little explicit attention to their cognitions and emotions. The logic behind this approach was that if partners began to behave more positively toward each other, then they would think and feel differently toward each other. Hence, there has always been a strong emphasis on helping members of couples behave in more constructive ways with each other, and this emphasis continues in our current conceptualization. The large number of specific behavioral interventions that the therapist might employ with the couple fall into two categories: guided behavior change and skills-based interventions (Epstein & Baucom, 2002).

Guided Behavior Change

"Guided behavior change" involves interventions that focus on behavior change without a skills component. At times, these interventions have been referred to as "behavior exchange interventions," but this term can be misleading. Typically these interventions do not involve an explicit exchange of behaviors in a quid pro quo fashion. In fact, it is helpful for the therapist to discuss with the couple the importance of each person committing to constructive behavior changes irrespective of the other person's behavior (Halford, Sanders, & Behrens, 1994). We might introduce interventions of this type as follows,

"I would like each of you to think about how you would behave if you were being the kind of partner you truly want to be. What does that mean you would do and not do? Behaving in this manner will likely have two very positive consequences. First, your partner is likely to be much happier. Second, you are likely to feel better about yourself. One thing that frequently happens when couples become distressed is that partners stray from the kinds of behaviors in which they themselves like to engage. So, I want you to get back to being the kind of person you enjoy being in the relationship, that brings out the best in you as an individual."

Thus, we rarely attempt to establish the rule-governed behavior exchanges that were common in the early days of BCT (Jacobson & Margolin, 1979). Instead, we work together with partners to develop a series of agreements on how they want to make changes in their relationship to meet the needs of both people, to help their relationship function effectively, and to interact positively with their environment.

These types of guided behavior changes can be implemented at two levels of specificity and for different reasons. First, a couple and therapist might decide that they need to change the overall emotional tone of the relationship. As Birchler, Weiss, and Vincent (1975) discussed, often members of couples behave more constructively when interacting with strangers than they do with their partners; this is evidenced among happy relationships, as well as distressed ones. Consequently, the therapist and couple might decide that it is important for partners to decrease the overall frequency and magnitude of negative behaviors and interactions, and to increase the frequency and magnitude of positive behaviors.

A variety of interventions have been developed to shift this overall ratio of positives to negatives. These include "love days" (Weiss et al., 1973) and "caring days" (Stuart, 1980). Although specific guidelines and recommendations vary, these interventions generally involve having each partner decide to enact a number of positive behaviors to make the other person happier. This might include small, day-to-day efforts such as bringing in the newspaper, washing dishes after dinner, making a phone call during the week to say hello, and so forth. Typically, these types of interventions are used when the therapist and couple conclude that the partners have stopped making much effort to be caring and loving toward each other, have allowed themselves to become preoccupied with other demands, and have treated their relationship as low priority. In essence, these rather broad-based interventions are intended to help couples regain a sense of relating in a respectful, caring, thoughtful manner.

Guided behavior changes also can be used in a more focal manner. As part of the initial assessment, the therapist and couple typically identify key issues and themes associated with relationship distress. For example, the couple might be struggling because the wife needs a great deal more autonomy than the relationship currently supports. She might want additional time alone to read, exercise, or take walks. However, the responsibilities of the family, along with other responsibilities, might make this difficult. In such an instance, guided behavior change might focus on her desire for increased autonomy, and her husband might seek ways during the week to provide her with these opportunities. Rather than attempting to shift the overall balance of positives to negatives, more focal guided behavior change interventions can be designed around important needs that one or both people have noted as central to their well-being.

Skills-Based Interventions

In contrast to guided behavior changes, "skills-based interventions" typically involve the therapist providing the couple instruction in the use of particular behavioral skills, through didactic discussions and/or other media (e.g., readings, videotapes). The instruction is followed by opportunities for the couple to practice behaving in the new ways. Communication training typically has involved this format. Labeling these interventions as skill-based suggests that the partners lack the knowledge or skills to communicate constructively and effectively with each other, although this often is not the case. Many partners report that their communication was open and effective earlier in their relationship, but that as frustrations mounted, they now communicate with each other in destructive ways, or they have greatly decreased the amount of communication. Regardless of whether this is a skills deficit or a performance deficit, discussing guidelines for constructive communication can be helpful to couples in providing the structure they need to interact in constructive ways. We differentiate between two major types of communication: couple discussions focused on sharing thoughts and feelings, and decision-making or problem-solving conversations (Baucom & Epstein, 1990; Epstein & Baucom, 2002).

Guidelines for these two types of communication are provided in Tables 2.1 and 2.2. These guidelines are presented as recommendations, not as rigid rules. Certain points can be emphasized, and the guidelines can be altered depending on the needs of each couple. For example, the guidelines for expressiveness emphasize sharing both thoughts and feelings. If the therapist is working with a rather intellectualized couple that avoids emotions and addresses issues on a purely cognitive level, then emphasizing the expression of emotion might become paramount. As Prager (1995) has noted, an important part of intimacy is sharing what is personal and vulnerable in an interaction within which one feels understood. If partners in this intellectualizing couple complains about a lack of closeness, then therapist emphasis on sharing their emotions is appropriate.

Similarly, during decision-making conversations, we do not routinely ask that all couples brainstorm a variety of alternative solutions before discussing each one. However, if a couple's typical pattern includes each partner presenting his or her own preferred solution, with the couple then arguing over the two proposals to the point of a stalemate, brainstorming might help the partners to avoid their restrictive approach. Likewise, in the decision-making guidelines, some attention is given to implementing the agreed-upon solution. For some couples, reaching a mutually agreed-upon solution is the difficult task. Once the partners have agreed on a solution, they effectively carry it out. Other couples reach solutions more readily but rarely implement their agreements. If the latter pattern becomes evident during the course of therapy, the therapist can pay more attention to helping the partners implement their solutions more effectively. In fact, the couple might problem-solve how to increase the likelihood that the solution will be implemented, talking at length about possible barriers to following through, and ways to remind both people about the agreement during the week.

TABLE 2.1. Guidelines for Couple Discussions

Skills for sharing thoughts and emotions

1. State your views *subjectively*, as *your own* feelings and thoughts, not as absolute truths. Also, speak for yourself, what you think and feel, not what your partner thinks and feels.
2. Express your *emotions or feelings; not just your ideas.*
3. When talking about your partner, state your feelings about your partner, not just about an event or a situation.
4. When expressing negative emotions or concerns, also include any *positive feelings* you have about the person or situation.
5. Make your statement as *specific* as possible, both in terms of specific emotions and thoughts.
6. Speak in "paragraphs"; that is, express one main idea with some elaboration, then allow your partner to respond. Speaking for a long time period without a break makes it hard for your partner to listen.
7. Express your feelings and thoughts with *tact* and *timing*, so that your partner can listen to what you are saying without becoming defensive.

Skills for listening to your partner

Ways to respond while your partner is speaking
1. Show that you *understand* your partner's statements and accept his or her right to have those thoughts and feelings. Demonstrate this *acceptance* through your tone of voice, facial expressions, and posture.
2. Try to put yourself *in your partner's place* and look at the situation from his or her perspective to determine how your partner feels and thinks about the issue.

Ways to respond after your partner finishes speaking
3. After your partner finishes speaking, *summarize* and restate his or her most important feelings, desires, conflicts, and thoughts. This is called a *reflection*.
4. While in the listener role, *do not*:
   a. ask questions, except for clarification.
   b. express your own viewpoint or opinion.
   c. interpret or change the meaning of your partner's statements.
   d. offer solutions or attempt to solve a problem, if one exists.
   e. make judgments or evaluate what your partner has said.

The guidelines for both types of conversation focus primarily on the *process* of communicating, with no particular attention to the content of conversations. However, it also is important for the therapist and couple to develop a joint conceptualization of the primary content themes in the couple's areas of concern. These major themes and issues should be taken into account while the couple engages in these conversations. For example, if a lack of intimacy is a major issue for a couple,

TABLE 2.2. Guidelines for Decision-Making Conversations

1. *Clearly and specifically state what the issue is.*
   a. Phrase the issue in terms of behaviors that are currently occurring or not occurring or in terms of what needs to be decided.
   b. Break down large, complex problems into several smaller problems, and deal with them one at a time.
   c. Make certain that both people agree on the statement of the problem and are willing to discuss it.
2. *Clarify why the issue is important and what your needs are.*
   a. Clarify why the issue is important to you and provide your understanding of the issues involved.
   b. Explain what your needs are that you would like to see taken into account in the solution; do not offer specific solutions at this time.
3. *Discuss possible solutions.*
   a. Propose concrete, specific solutions that take your own and your partner's needs and preferences into account. Do not focus on solutions that meet only your individual needs.
   b. Focus on solutions for the present and the future. Do not dwell on the past or attempt to attribute blame for past difficulties.
   c. If you tend to focus on a single or a limited number of alternatives, consider "brainstorming" (generating a variety of possible solutions in a creative way).
4. *Decide on a solution that is feasible and agreeable to both of you.*
   a. If you cannot find a solution that pleases you both, suggest a compromise solution. If a compromise is not possible, agree to follow one person's preferences.
   b. State your solution in clear, specific, behavioral terms.
   c. After agreeing on a solution, have one partner restate the solution.
   d. Do not accept a solution if you do not intend to follow through with it.
   e. Do not accept a solution that will make you angry or resentful.
5. *Decide on a trial period to implement the solution if it is a situation that will occur more than once.*
   a. Allow for several attempts of the new solution.
   b. Review the solution at the end of the trial period.
   c. Revise the solution if needed, taking into account what you have learned thus far.

the partners' conversations might emphasize taking some chances to become more intimate by discussing more personal issues with each other. Alternatively, a couple might be distressed about the distribution of power in their relationship, with one person resentful that the other typically dominates the couple's decision making by being more forceful verbally. Consequently, decision-making conversations might be central to shifting this couple dynamic. The therapist might propose that each person put forth a proposed solution when the couple discuss possible solutions, before a final decision is made. The therapist might also recommend that before the solution is accepted, each partner clarify whether it contains at least some of his or her preferences, and if not, whether that seems appropriate. Thus, the theme of power can be addressed explicitly within decision-making conversations.

In essence, during skills training, the therapist should be attentive to both the process of communication and the important themes and issues the couple addresses in the relationship. In earlier approaches to CBCT, therapists commonly restricted their role to that of a coach, focusing on the communication process and attending little to the content of what the partners were discussing. We believe that communication interventions can be more effective if the communication process and the important themes in the couple's relationship are addressed simultaneously. This perspective means that the therapist might not always be a neutral party when partners propose specific solutions to a problem. If a given solution seems contrary to the couple's overall goals, and to the thematic changes needed in the relationship, the therapist might point this out and express concern about the solution.

This approach also means that at some point during the couple's decision-making conversation, the therapist might provide educational information that helps to guide the conversation. Thus, if partners are discussing how they might support each other in addressing work stresses, the therapist might provide information about a variety of types of social support that individuals generally find helpful. The couple can then take this information into account and discuss how it applies to their relationship. Similarly, if a couple whose child has challenging behavior problems is discussing parenting issues, the therapist might present didactic information about age-appropriate behavior for children or provide reading materials about parenting strategies, which the partners can take into account in making their decisions. We believe that this important shift within cognitive-behavioral approaches provides a needed balance between addressing interactive processes and attending to the content of a couple's concerns.

Interventions That Address Cognitions

The ways people behave toward each other in committed, intimate relationships have great meaning for the participants, and a capacity to evoke strong positive and negative emotional responses in each person. For example, individuals often have strong standards for how they believe the two partners should behave toward each other in a variety of domains. If the standards are not met, the individual is likely to become displeased. Similarly, degree of satisfaction with a partner's behavior can be influenced by the attributions that the person makes about the reasons for the partner's actions. Thus, a husband might prepare a nice dinner for his wife, but whether she interprets this as a positive or negative behavior is likely to be influenced by her attribution or explanation for his behavior. If she concludes that he is attempting to be thoughtful and loving, she might experience his dinner preparation as positive. However, if she believes that he wishes to buy a new computer and is attempting to bribe her by preparing dinner, she might feel manipulated and experience the same behavior as negative. In essence, partners' behaviors in intimate relationships carry great meaning, and not considering these cognitive factors can limit the effectiveness of treatment. Elsewhere we have enumerated a variety of cognitive variables that are important in understanding couples' relationships (Baucom & Epstein, 1990; Epstein & Baucom, 2002):

- Selective attention—what each person notices about the partner and the relationship.
- Attributions—causal and responsibility inferences about marital events.
- Expectancies—predictions of what will occur in the relationship in the future.
- Assumptions—what each believes people and relationships actually are like.
- Standards—what each believes people and relationships should be like.

These types of cognitions are important, because they help to shape how each individual experiences the relationship. The therapist does not attempt to have the partners reassess their cogni-

tions simply because they are negative. Instead, the therapist is concerned if one or both partners seem to be processing information in a markedly distorted manner. Thus, an individual might selectively attend to instances when a partner is forgetful, paying little attention to other ways the partner accomplishes various tasks successfully. Similarly, this same individual might attribute the partner's failure to accomplish particular tasks to a lack of respect for his or her preferences, and a clear reflection of a lack of love. Understandably, such cognitions are likely to be related to negative emotions such as anger, and under such circumstances, the individual is likely to behave negatively toward the partner.

Therefore, at times the focus of therapy is not on changing behavior but rather emphasizes helping the partners reassess their cognitions about behaviors that occur or do not occur, and view them in a more reasonable and balanced fashion. A wide variety of cognitive intervention strategies can be used, many of which are provided in Table 2.3. Epstein and Baucom (2002) provide a detailed description of each of these intervention strategies. These interventions tend to emphasize one of two broad approaches: Socratic questioning or guided discovery.

Socratic Questioning

Cognitive therapy often has been equated with "Socratic questioning," which involves asking a series of questions to help an individual reevaluate the logic of his or her thinking, to understand the underlying issues and concerns that are not at first apparent, and so forth. In working with distressed couples, such interventions can be effective but should be used cautiously. The context

TABLE 2.3. Frequently Used Cognitive Intervention Strategies

- Evaluate experiences and logic supporting a cognition.
- Weigh advantages and disadvantages of a cognition.
- Consider worst and best possible outcomes of situations.
- Provide educational minilectures, readings, and tapes.
- Use inductive "downward arrow" method.
- Identify macro patterns from cross-situational responses.
- Identify macro-level patterns in past relationships.
- Increase relationship schematic thinking by pointing out repetitive cycles in couple interaction.

for individual therapy is quite different from that of couple therapy. In individual therapy, the individual participates alone and works with a caring, concerned therapist, with whom he or she can be open and honest in reevaluating cognitions. In couple therapy, however, the individual's partner is in the room. Often the partner has explicitly blamed the individual for their relationship problems, frequently telling the individual that his or her thinking is distorted. Consequently, if a therapist begins to question an individual's thinking in the presence of the partner, then such efforts might be unsuccessful or even counterproductive. With the partner present, an individual is more likely to be defensive and unwilling to acknowledge that his or her thinking has been selective or biased to some degree against the partner. If an individual acknowledges that he or she was thinking in an extreme or distorted way, the partner might use this against him or her in the future (e.g., "Thank goodness you finally admitted it. I've been telling you for years that your thinking is all messed up"). Therefore, asking the individual a series of questions that seem somewhat confrontational in front of a critical or hostile partner can arouse the person's defensiveness. Therefore, these interventions may be more successful with couples in which the two partners are less hostile and hurtful toward each other.

Guided Discovery

Guided discovery involves a wide variety of interventions in which the therapist creates experiences for a couple, such that one or both members begin to question their thinking and develop a different perspective on the partner or relationship. For example, whether a man notices his partner's withdrawal and interprets it as her not caring about him, the therapist can address this attribution in a variety of ways. First, the therapist could use Socratic questioning and ask the man to think of a variety of interpretations for his partner's behavior. The therapist could then ask him to look for evidence either supporting or refuting each of those possible interpretations. On the other hand, the therapist could structure an interaction in which the man obtained additional information that might alter his attributions. For example, the therapist might ask the couple to have a conversation in which the woman shares what she was thinking and feeling at the time she withdrew. During the conversation, the man might find out that his partner withdrew because she was feeling hurt and cared about him a

great deal. Her vulnerability, rather than a lack of caring, might be the basis of her withdrawal. This new understanding and experience might alter the man's perspective, without the therapist questioning his thinking directly. Similarly, a woman might develop an expectancy that her partner does not care about her perspective on a variety of issues. If, however, they agree to start having such conversations on a weekly basis, and she sees that he is attentive and interested in her perspective when she expresses her perspective, her prediction might change. Thus, the therapist, in collaboration with the couple, might devise a variety of experiences to help the partners experience their relationship differently, with or without additional behavior change.

Some cognitions involve standards for how a partner should behave in a close relationship. Standards are not addressed primarily by assessing their logic, because they are not based on logic. Instead, standards for relationships are addressed more appropriately with methods that focus on the advantages and disadvantages of living by them. Here, we provide a more detailed discussion of addressing relationship standards as one example of cognitive restructuring with couples. The standards might involve an individual's behavior (e.g., whether an individual should be allowed to curse when upset), the ways that the partners interact with each other (e.g., whether it is acceptable to express disagreement openly with each other), or how to interact with the environment (e.g., how much time one should devote to an ailing parent). In general, in addressing relationship standards, we proceed through the following steps:

- Clarify each person's existing standards.
- Discuss advantages and disadvantages of existing standards.
- If standards need alteration, help revise them to form new acceptable standards.
- Problem-solve how new standards will be taken into account behaviorally.
- If partners' standards continue to differ, discuss ability to accept differences.

In essence, we discuss how any given standard relevant to the couple usually has some positive and negative consequences. First, it is important to clarify each person's standards in a given domain of the relationship. For example, partners might differ on their standards for how to spend free time. A husband might conclude that, given the couple's lack of free time, they should spend all of it together. On the other hand, the wife might believe that partners should spend some free time together, but that it is also critical to have a significant amount of alone time away from one's partner. Once the partners are able to articulate their standards regarding time together and alone, each is asked to describe the pros and cons of conducting a relationship according to those standards. Thus, the husband would be asked to describe the good things that would result if he and his wife spent all or almost all of their time together, as well as potential negative consequences. The wife would be invited to add to his perspective. Similarly, the wife would be asked to list the pros and cons of spending some free time together and some free time apart, with the husband adding his perspective. Without intervention, couples often become polarized during this phase, with each person emphasizing the positive consequences of his or her perspective, and the other partner noting the negative consequences of that point of view. By encouraging each person to share both the positive and negative consequences of his or her standard, this polarization can be avoided or minimized.

After the partners fully discuss their different standards concerning an aspect of their relationship, they are asked to think of a moderated standard that would be responsive to both partner's perspectives and acceptable to both persons. Individuals typically cling strongly to their standards and values, so rarely is an individual likely to give up his or her standards totally. Much greater success occurs from slight alterations that make standards less extreme or more similar to the other person's standards. After the partners agree on a newly evolved standard, they are asked to reach decisions on how this new standard would be implemented in their relationship on a daily basis, in terms of concrete behaviors that each person would exhibit.

Interventions Focused on Emotions

Whereas many behavioral and cognitive interventions influence an individual's emotional responses in a relationship, at times more explicit attention needs to be paid to emotional factors in the relationship. In particular, therapists often work with couples in which one or both partners demonstrate either restricted or minimized emotions, or excessive emotional responses. Each of these broad domains includes more specific difficulties that individuals experience with emotions, with particular interventions that are appropriate.

Restricted or Minimized Emotions

Many partners in committed relationships seem to be uncomfortable with emotions in general or with specific emotions in particular. This can take a variety of forms. Some individuals have general difficulty experiencing emotions or have problems accessing specific emotions. This can typify the person's experiences in life in general, or it might be more focal to the current relationship. In some instances, these difficulties might warrant cognitive or behavioral interventions; for example, a partner who believes that it is extremely rude to express anger might suppresses expression of it and censure his or her partner for expressing anger. In other instances, a person might report experiencing minimal amounts of certain emotions. To a degree, this might reflect the individual's temperament, or it might be the result of being raised in a family or culture in which certain emotions were rarely expressed. Some individuals experience both positive and negative emotions, but their levels of emotional experience are so muted that they do not find their experiences within the relationship very gratifying. Similarly, the partner of such an individual might complain that it is unrewarding to live with someone who has such restricted emotional responses.

In addition, some individuals might have stronger emotional experiences but be somewhat limited in their ability to differentiate among different emotions. They know that they feel very good or very bad but cannot articulate the types of emotions they are experiencing. The ability to make such differentiations can be helpful both to the individual and to his or her partner. For example, if an individual can clarify that he or she is feeling sad, this can often lead both members of the couple to understand that the person is experiencing a sense of loss, which can then be addressed. More explicit differentiation and expression of emotions may help partners understand and perhaps feel closer to each other.

Likewise, some individuals experience difficulty relating emotions to their internal and external experiences. Thus, a wife might know that she is quite angry but cannot relate this to what she is thinking or to experiences that occurred in an interaction with her husband. This difficulty can make both persons feel that they have little control over the relationship and are at the mercy of the wife's emotions, which appear to occur in an unpredictable manner rather than tied to specific thoughts or behaviors.

Finally, some individuals avoid what Greenberg and Safran (1987) refer to as "primary emotions" related to important needs and motives, such as anxiety associated with concern that a partner will fail to meet one's attachment needs. Often individuals avoid the experience or expression of these emotions, because they see them as dangerous or vulnerable. As a result, Greenberg proposes that people cover these primary emotions with secondary emotions that seem safer or less vulnerable. Consequently, rather than experiencing and expressing fear and anxiety to a critical partner, an individual might experience feelings such as anger, which are less threatening and help him or her feel less vulnerable.

Table 2.4 lists a variety of strategies to help individuals access and heighten emotional experience; these interventions are drawn primarily from emotionally focused couple therapy developed by Johnson (2004; Johnson & Greenberg, 1987). These interventions are based on several broad principles. First, the therapist tries to create a safe atmosphere by normalizing the experience and expression of both positive and negative emotions. In addition, the therapist promotes this safe environment by encouraging the partner to respond to the individual in a caring and supportive manner when the person expresses various emotions. Even so, the individual might attempt to avoid an emotion or escape once the session focuses on emotions. Therefore, if the individual had shifted away from feelings, the therapist might refocus him or her on expression of an emotional experience; of course, this must be done with appropriate timing and moderation in order to avoid overwhelming the individual.

Once a safe environment is created, a variety of strategies can heighten emotional experience. These interventions might include asking an individual to recount a particular incident in detail,

in the hope of evoking the emotional aspect of this experience; encouraging the individual to use metaphors and images to express emotions, if directly labeling emotions is difficult or frightening; and using questions, reflections, and interpretations to draw out primary emotions. Although it likely involves using some trial-and-error strategies with each individual, the therapist's goal is to help the individual enrich his or her emotional experience and expression in a manner that is helpful to both the individual and couple. A decision to focus on this category of interventions should not be based on a therapist's belief that a "healthy" person should have a rich emotional life, as well as a full range of emotional expression; instead, the decision to use such interventions should be based on a careful assessment that this restriction in emotional experience or expression is interfering with this particular couple's, or the partners', well-being.

Containing the Experience/Expression of Emotions

Somewhat at the other end of the continuum, a therapist may be confronted with partners who have difficulty regulating their experience and expression of emotion. Typically this is of concern to the couple if one or both partners is experiencing and expressing high levels of negative emotion, or expressing these emotions in settings that are not appropriate. At the same time, there are couples in which one person's extreme exuberance and frequent expression of strong positive emotion can become problematic. At times, one person can feel overwhelmed being around another individual who is so excited, upbeat, and happy on an ongoing basis. Although this overall positive tone is pleasurable to most individuals, when expressed in an extreme fashion, the resulting atmosphere might not feel relaxing, and the partner might feel that it is inappropriate to express negative feelings when the other individual is so happy all the time. Even so, clinicians more typically confront couples in which one person seems to have difficulty regulating the experience and expression of negative emotions. The therapist may find such couples quite demanding, because their lives appears to revolve around a series of emotional crises, strong arguments, or extreme behaviors, including spousal abuse, which result from extreme negative emotions.

Several strategies seem to be applicable to assisting couples in such circumstances. As noted

---

**TABLE 2.4. Emotional Interventions:
Accessing and Heightening Emotional Experience**

- Normalize emotional experiences, positive and negative.
- Clarify thoughts, then relate these to emotions.
- Use questions, reflections, and interpretations to draw out primary emotions.
- Describe emotions through metaphors and images.
- Discourage attempts to distract the self from experiencing emotion.
- Encourage acceptance of the individual's experience by the partner.

earlier, often behavioral and cognitive interventions are of assistance. For example, if an individual frequently is angry because of the partner's inappropriate behavior, then the therapist likely focuses on behavioral interventions to alter the unacceptable behavior. Similarly, if an individual frequently is upset because of holding extreme standards that few partners could satisfy, then focusing on those standards is appropriate. In addition, some interventions are more focal to address extreme emotional experiences. Several of these are listed in Table 2.5.

One useful strategy is for the couple to schedule times to discuss issues that are upsetting to one or both partners. The goal of this intervention is to restrict or contain the frequency and settings in which strong emotions are expressed. If couples have not set aside times to address issues, then an individual with poor affect regulation is more likely to express strong feelings whenever they arise. Some people find that they can resist expressing strong negative feelings if they know there is a time set aside to address these concerns. This intervention can be helpful in making certain that problems and expression of strong negative affect do not intrude into all aspects of the couple's life. In particular, this can be helpful in ensuring that strong negative expression does not occur at times that are likely to lead to increasing frustration for one or both persons. For example, expressing strong anger when one person is leaving the house to go to work, or initiating a conversation with strong negative emotion once the couple has turned off the light to go to sleep, likely results in further upset for both people.

Linehan (1993) has proposed a variety of interventions to assist individuals with poor affect regulation. Although her interventions do not focus on addressing strong affect in an interpersonal context, often they are applicable. Kirby and Baucom (2007) have recently integrated principles from CBCT with such skills from dialectical behavior therapy to assist couples experiencing chronic emotion dysregulation. For example, one of these interventions involves teaching individuals to tolerate distressing emotions. Some individuals seem to assume that if they are upset, they should do something immediately to alter their emotional experience, which frequently results in strong expressions of emotion to the partner. Helping individuals become comfortable and accept being upset with their partners or their relationship, without addressing every concern or doing so immediately, can be helpful. Similarly, it can be helpful to teach the individual how to focus on the current moment. Many individuals with poor affect regulation allow upset in one domain of life to infiltrate many other aspects of their lives. We explain placing limits on this intrusion to couples as a form of "healthy compartmentalization"; that is, it is important to be upset about a given aspect of one's relationship, but to restrict that sense of upset to that one issue, and to allow oneself to enjoy other, positive and pleasurable aspects of the relationship when they occur.

Finally, it can be helpful to seek alternative ways to communicate feelings and elicit support, perhaps from individuals other than one's partner. Expressing some of one's concerns to friends, keeping a journal to express one's emotions, or other alternatives for releasing strong emotion can be productive for the individual. This approach is not intended as an alternative to addressing an individual's concerns with a partner; rather, it is a means for moderating the frequency and intensity with which the person's emotions are expressed. Attempting to teach these strategies and skills to an individual in a couple context can be difficult or at times implausible. Often, the partner serves as a strong negative stimulus to the individual who has difficulty regulating emotion. When this is the case, individual therapy for the person who has poor affect regulation might be a helpful adjunct to couple therapy.

Sources of Difficulty in Therapeutic Change

When using these interventions, the therapist may experience difficulty helping couples make progress toward a given treatment goal. This difficulty might be seen by some therapists as the couple's, or a given partner's, "resistance" to change. We avoid the term "resistance" because of the connotation that the couple is just being difficult and uncooperative, yet there are a number of reasons why a partner may be reluctant or unable to change read-

---

TABLE 2.5. Emotional Interventions: Containing Experience/Expression of Negative Emotions

- Schedule times to discuss emotions and related thoughts with your partner.
- Practice "healthy compartmentalization."
- Seek alternative means to communicate feelings and elicit support.
- Tolerate distressing feelings.

ily. First, couples learn to function as a system over time, and partners become accustomed to their roles within the relationship and broader family context. Thus, it is challenging to move away from a given role that one has had for a long time because of its familiarity and predictability, even if elements of the role are maladaptive or dissatisfying. For instance, a wife who feels overwhelmed by serving as the "family manager" may ask her husband and children to participate more in household responsibilities and to do chores without being asked. Her husband, although eager to help with these duties, may have difficulty remembering or following through on particular household tasks because he is accustomed to his wife taking care of such duties or reminding him what to do. Conversely, the wife may find it hard to "let go" of overseeing these tasks for fear that her husband will not perform them to her standards, which can undermine his sense of efficacy as he takes on these new responsibilities. The therapist must help this couple anticipate the challenges they will experience in these new roles and develop appropriate strategies to adapt to these changes (e.g., the husband updates the wife periodically on the finances; the wife, rather than double-check him, raises her concerns in a respectful manner).

Second, a partner may have a knowledge or skills deficit in a given area that blocks the individual from taking appropriate steps toward change. For example, a couple whose young child has attention and behavioral difficulties may have trouble implementing appropriate parenting interventions due to a lack of parenting knowledge or little experience in the parenting role. Teaching the couple how to respond to the child's behavioral and emotional difficulties, then coaching their use of these strategies is paramount to helping them be more effective parents with less distress within their relationship.

Third, given their high distress level, couples seeking therapy are often frustrated, angry, and at times reluctant to change given the hurt that they have experienced in the relationship. For instance, a wife who is angry and hostile toward her previously alcoholic husband may not want to be kind or to feel vulnerable toward him by sharing her thoughts and feelings in conversations. In such a case, the therapist needs to help the wife understand how she benefits from staying cold and distant, and also the cost she pays in adopting such a stance. In essence, the short-term consequences of punishing her husband are outweighing the long-term consequences of improving the relationship.

Through such an analysis, the therapist hopes, the wife will focus on the long-term consequences for her, for her husband, and for their relationship and be motivated to work toward changing how she relates to her husband.

Thus, the difficulties a therapist experiences in helping partners make needed changes in their relationship can stem from a variety of sources (habit and the comfort of predictability, skills or knowledge deficits, inappropriate focus on short-term rather than long-term consequences, etc.). The therapist must therefore conduct a thorough analysis of what is contributing to this difficulty to help the couple respond effectively and continue to progress in treatment.

Termination

Therapists and couples consider together the appropriate time and manner to terminate treatment. There are a number of indications that termination should be considered. First, as described earlier, couples often seek treatment because of the partners' different preferences, needs, and personal styles, for example, different preferences for spending versus saving money—what Epstein and Baucom (2002) call "primary distress." However, the partners responds to these differences in maladaptive ways, perhaps accusing each other, with each trying to enforce his or her own preferences, fighting, and arguing—what Epstein and Baucom label as "secondary distress," or complications caused by the ways that couples address the original concerns. CBCT may not be able to alleviate these bases of primary distress, but if couples learn to manage these differences in more respectful and adaptive ways, thus lowering secondary distress, then therapy may accomplish its major goals. By addressing the primary concerns in more caring ways, the partners may find that their individual differences are less upsetting or problematic, and in fact, that they experience less primary distress as well.

Second, termination certainly should be considered when the couple's presenting concerns have been addressed. However, this does not always signal the end of treatment, and the couple and therapist should discuss whether new or additional goals should be addressed. A typical scenario is that couples request therapy when there is a high level of negative interaction that makes them miserable or that they find intolerable. In such instances, a major focus of treatment is alleviating this high level of negative exchange. When the negative interactions have been significantly decreased, some couples elect to end treatment because they are no longer notably distressed. However, this does not necessarily mean that their relationship has reached an optimal level, and there might be ample opportunity to improve the relationship by increasing positive interactions, intimacy, and so forth. In essence, a major tenet of CBCT is that decreasing negatives is not the same as increasing positives; thus, the couple and therapist might renegotiate their therapeutic contract to focus on enhancement, even after the initial presenting complaints of distress are alleviated.

Third, termination should be considered when the couple no longer needs the therapist's assistance, even though specific areas of concern have yet to be addressed in therapy. This might be the case when the partners can now communicate effectively, make thoughtful decisions, and support one another, therefore demonstrating the ability to handle challenging areas in their relationship on their own. If they have developed an effective way of addressing issues, then doing so on their own can increase their sense of couple efficacy.

When moving toward termination, the therapist and couple might taper their treatment sessions by increasing time intervals between sessions. This strategy helps the partners to experience addressing relationship issues on their own, without the therapist's help, thus contributing to their sense of efficacy prior to termination. The therapist and partners may discuss how to replicate ways the partners worked together in therapy and successfully improved their relationship to keep them focused and on track when discussing relationship domains in their own home after termination. For some couples, therapy serves the important functions of keeping partners focused on their relationship and on what they need to do to improve it, and makes them accountable to someone for these efforts. Developing alternative ways on their own to retain focus and energy on the relationship, and maintaining accountability for doing so, is important for many couples in retaining or further enhancing their gains. Also, to facilitate the maintenance of treatment gains over time, the therapist can be available for booster sessions should the couple need additional help in the future.

Common CBCT Therapist Errors or Ways That Treatment Is Not Optimized

The most common errors of beginning couple therapists involve the use of CBCT interventions.

Beginning therapists often fail to integrate cognitive, behavioral, and emotional interventions to target a couple's treatment goals effectively, and instead overutilize a particular treatment strategy. Most frequently, CBCT therapists tend to overrely on the behavioral interventions of skills training, often believing that if the partners can share thoughts and feelings, and make decisions as a team, then their complaints as a couple will be addressed. Although we strongly believe in the value of effective communication, we consider communication training to be the vehicle by which the therapist helps the couple address more effectively the major patterns and domains within their relationship. Thus, we believe that couples need to be taught more than specific communication guidelines. In addition, couple therapists who implement behavioral interventions, skills training especially, in a rote, simplistic manner fail to individualize these interventions to a given couple's relationship dynamics and in turn underutilize these interventions.

Cognitive and emotional interventions may also prove to be challenging for beginning couple therapists, because these strategies may be difficult to implement effectively with both partners present. For example, challenging a husband's strongly believed attribution for his wife's failure to initiate physical affection may require more sensitivity and grace in a couple session than in an individual session when the wife is not present. In a similar manner, couple therapists may find it difficult to control the emotional climate of the session using emotional interventions. Therapists may struggle in establishing a safe setting for couples when emotional expression typically is not a comfortable experience for them. Also, therapists may find it difficult emotionally to support both partners in a couple (e.g., a couple in which the wife has had an affair), and may in this instance fall into a pattern of validating the husband more than the wife, and challenging/confronting the wife more than the husband. In addition, therapists who find it uncomfortable and/or challenging to manage the greater emotional intensity experienced and expressed by more distressed couples therefore run the risk of not creating a safe, controlled treatment atmosphere for these couples.

In a similar manner, less experienced therapists frequently struggle in their management of couple sessions. Given the high level of distress in couples who typically seek treatment, therapists must be comfortable and skilled in managing couples' experience and expression of intense emotions, high conflict in session, and tendency to shift focus quickly from one problem area to another. For these couples, it can be difficult, but imperative, that therapist assume the role of a "traffic cop"—stopping the partners in the middle of an argument in session to direct their focus to a particular topic area, therefore decreasing their emotional arousal. Depending on the intensity of the emotions present in session, therapists may also need to engage in strategies to help calm partners down (e.g., breathing exercises, getting a drink of water), so that they can work effectively in treatment. Taking such an active, directive stance is often challenging for beginning couple therapists, but this ability to be more structured and directive when needed is paramount to the success of therapy with distressed couples.

Beginning couple therapists also may experience difficulty in the assignment and review of homework exercises. Creating individualized homework assignments that help couples continue to move forward in treatment can be a challenge for therapists. For example, a therapist may encourage partners generally to "be supportive of one another" over the coming week rather than creating a specific, individualized, guided behavior change around emotional support within their relationship. The latter is likely to be more helpful to the couple's progress in treatment. Also, assigning these exercises in an encouraging, confident manner can be difficult for beginning therapists, who often worry that couples will not want to engage in the exercise, or will find them pointless or frustrating, and so forth. Discussing these exercises in a positive, encouraging manner is key in communicating to couples the merit of these requests, as well as the therapist's expectation that couples will complete them.

In addition to creating these exercises and asking couples to conduct them outside of session, it is important that therapists discuss the couple's experience with homework assignments in the next treatment session for a variety of reasons. First, if the therapist fails to follow up on these requests, the couple may consider these practices to be unimportant and, therefore, fail to complete future assignments. Second, homework assignments by their very nature are believed to help couples build on their work in session; thus, reviewing the partners' experiences completing the assignments may yield valuable information for the therapist and couple in addressing treatment goals, such as how partners can better generalize in the outside world how they relate to one another in session.

A frequent pattern that we observe is that experienced therapists often do not review homework exercises with couples, or they do so in a brief, superficial manner. By not reviewing homework in a detailed way, therapists fail to capitalize on the therapeutic benefits of homework exercises for couples.

Although these examples of how therapists may conduct CBCT in less than optimal ways might seem unrelated, often they stem from a common approach to treatment that is unproductive. We find that CBCT is least beneficial when it is viewed primarily as a set of skills to be taught to couples in a routine manner, without sufficient thought to the uniqueness of each couple. We believe that couples are complex systems that must be conceptualized in a rich manner, with a thoughtful treatment plan that incorporates cognitive, behavioral, and emotional factors that target individual, relationship, and environmental levels. Working effectively with a couple in a confident manner, knowing how to manage a variety of types of sessions, and generalizing these interventions to the couples' everyday world can provide them the best chance to achieve their greatest potential.

MECHANISMS OF CHANGE

Neither CBCT nor any other theoretical approach to addressing relationship distress has isolated the mediators or mechanisms of change in couple therapy. More particularly, both Iverson and Baucom (1990) and Halford et al. (1993) unexpectedly found that changes in communication skills during CBCT did not predict marital adjustment at the end of treatment. Furthermore, a review of the treatment outcome literature demonstrates that various theoretical approaches to addressing relationship distress are equally efficacious (Baucom et al., 1998). Combining these sets of findings would suggest either that (1) different specific mechanisms of change are important for different couples or (2) broader mechanisms of nonspecific change cut across different theoretical orientations. First, different couples might need different types of intervention, and mechanisms of change vary accordingly. Some partners might need to understand and experience each other in different ways. Others might need to undergo significant behavioral change in their ways of interacting with each other. Some partners might need to learn how to provide social support to a partner who experiences frequent depression. Others might need to learn how to adapt to a highly stressful external environment. Thus, a therapist likely needs to have a variety of specific interventions available to tailor to specific couples.

In addition, there may be broader mechanisms of change in couple therapy that are not specific to a given theoretical orientation. For example, Sullivan and Baucom (2005) have coined the term "relationship schematic processing" (RSP) to refer to the degree to which an individual processes information in terms of circular relationship processes. An individual with high RSP thinks about his or her own behavior and its impact on the other person and the relationship, along with anticipating the partner's needs and preferences, and balancing the partner's needs with one's own needs. Sullivan and Baucom (2002) proposed that increasing RSP might be a nonspecific mechanism of change that cuts across theoretical approaches; that is, any effective couple therapy teaches individuals to think more appropriately in relationship terms, which they then bring to bear in addressing specific relationship concerns. Consistent with this notion, they demonstrated that (1) CBCT does increase the quantity and quality of men's RSP, and (2) women's increases in marital satisfaction in response to CBCT were correlated with the degree to which their male partners increased on RSP. Stated differently, women became more satisfied with the marriage when men learned to process more effectively in relationship terms. Likewise, they demonstrated that couples receiving insight-oriented couple therapy in Snyder's outcome study (Sullivan, Baucom, & Snyder, 2002) increased in RSP as well. Whether teaching couples to think more effectively in relationship terms turns out to be a nonspecific mechanism of change that is central to all efficacious forms of couple therapy is not known at present, but it is important to continue to explore whether the specific interventions that therapists employ are the critical variables, or whether therapeutic change may be accounted for in other ways as well.

Changes that couples make in response to treatment might be related to therapist factors, in addition to the interventions that are employed. At present, little attention has been paid to isolating therapist factors that might be important in offering CBCT. Our experience in training and supervising therapists over many years suggests significant variability in how the treatment is offered by different therapists, and we can speculate on what makes an effective CBCT therapist. First, as noted earlier, therapists need to develop a rich conceptualization of a specific couple, and deliver a thoughtful treatment plan based on this conceptualization. CBCT, with its inclusion of many specific interventions, lends itself to a rote manualized approach that we believe to be ineffective. Although we have seen therapists with different styles and tempos effectively adapt CBCT to their personal styles, our experience is that therapists who are able to process information quickly and respond in the moment are most effective with this approach. When partner behaviors escalate into highly aversive, negative interaction cycles during a session, CBCT calls for the therapist to process this information quickly and intervene to stop destructive interactions. At times, this involves skills training, so therapists must be comfortable in the role of teacher, as well as coach. Thus, in a variety of ways, CBCT calls for the therapist to be active and directive, and therapists who are uncomfortable with this stance may struggle with CBCT. In addition, at times the therapist must help the couple address painful or sad experiences with an emphasis on heightening emotion, so an effective CBCT therapist must be comfortable confronting these more tender emotions, as well as strong anger. In essence, a number of both intellectual and intervention skills a therapist might have can contribute to effective delivery of CBCT.

Even if we optimize treatment by considering a variety of specific and nonspecific interventions, along with an effective therapist, we must remain realistic about what we can achieve with a given couple. Even if the partners interact with each other in the ways we described earlier, they might not wish to spend their lives with each other. As couple therapists, we do not know how to create "chemistry" between two partners. We can help partners to create healthy, adaptive ways of interacting with each other, allowing individuals and relationships to reach their potential, whatever that might be. On the one hand, this potential might lead to a rewarding, enriching relationship; on the other hand, couples might thoughtfully decide that they need to end their relationship.

TREATMENT APPLICABILITY AND EMPIRICAL SUPPORT

In current practice, cognitive interventions are rarely employed without taking behaviors into account; likewise, behavioral interventions without attention to cognitive and affective interventions are rare. Given that current evidence suggests no significant differences between strictly behavioral couple therapy and a broader CBCT (Baucom & Lester, 1986; Baucom, Sayers, & Sher, 1990; Halford et al., 1993), the empirical status of these interventions are discussed together as CBCT.

CBCT is the most widely evaluated couple treatment, having been a focus of approximately two dozen well-controlled treatment outcome studies. CBCT has been reviewed in detail in several previous publications, including findings from specific investigations (e.g., Alexander, Holtzworth-Munroe, & Jameson, 1994; Baucom & Epstein, 1990; Baucom & Hoffman, 1986; Baucom et al., 1998; Bray & Jouriles, 1995; Christensen et al., 2004; Jacobson & Addis, 1993), as well as meta-analyses (Baucom, Hahlweg, & Kuschel, 2003; Dunn & Schwebel, 1995; Hahlweg & Markman, 1988; Shadish et al., 1993). All of these reviews reached the same conclusion: CBCT is an efficacious intervention for distressed couples.

The overall findings suggest that between roughly 33 and 67% of couples are in the nondistressed range of marital satisfaction after receiving CBCT. Most couples appear to maintain these gains for short time periods (6–12 months); however, long range follow-up results are not as encouraging. In a 2-year follow-up of strictly BCT, for example, Jacobson, Schmaling, and Holtzworth-Munroe (1987) found that approximately 30% of couples who had recovered during therapy subsequently relapsed. In addition, Snyder, Wills, and Grady-Fletcher (1991) reported that 38% of couples receiving BCT had divorced during a 4-year follow-up period. Thus, brief CBCT improvements are not maintained for many couples over a number of years, although some couples maintain and even improve upon their gains.

CBCT also is applicable to a wide range of specific relationship concerns. A particular class of relationship distress involves couples who have experienced relationship trauma, such as infidelity or psychological and physical abuse (LaTaillade, Epstein, & Werlinich, 2006). Traumatic experiences within the marriage can be addressed from a CBCT perspective but require some additional consideration, as described by Gordon, Baucom, Snyder, and Dixon, Chapter 14, this volume. In addition, these same CBCT principles have been adapted to prevent distress and to enhance relationship functioning, as demonstrated in the widely used Prevention and Relationship Enhancement Program (PREP) developed by Markman, Renick, Floyd, Stanley, and Clements (1993).

Couple-based interventions employing a cognitive-behavioral approach also have been used successfully to assist couples in which one partner is experiencing individual difficulties in terms of either psychopathology or health problems. Although these two latter applications are beyond the scope of this chapter, results of investigations to date are promising, and detailed descriptions of these applications are provided elsewhere (Baucom et al., 1998; Hahlweg & Baucom, in press; Schmaling & Sher, 2000; Snyder & Whisman, 2002). Whereas CBCT has been used effectively in its current form for couples in which one partner has significant individual psychopathology, such as depression (Beach, 2001; Jacobson, Dobson, Fruzzetti, Schmaling, & Salusky, 1991), there are other ways to engage a couple to assist in addressing individual psychopathology, even in the absence of relationship distress.

Baucom et al. (1998) have differentiated among three types of couple-based interventions that can be considered in addressing psychopathology or health concerns. First is a partner-assisted intervention, in which the partner is used as a coach or surrogate therapist to help the individual experiencing some disorder make needed individual changes. In this instance, the couple's relationship is not the focus of change. Instead, one partner is mainly supporting the other person in making needed individual changes. For example, if one person has agoraphobia, the partner might encourage and reinforce that person for engaging in exposure outings that have been arranged with the therapist; the partner might also problem-solve with the individual about how to approach the exposure outing successfully. Employing the partner in this way makes no assumption about a distressed relationship or dysfunctional patterns between the partners.

Second, the therapist might employ what Baucom et al. (1998) refer to as a disorder-specific intervention. In such interventions, the couple's relationship is the focus of intervention, but only in the ways the relationship influences the individual's psychopathology or is affected by the disorder. Again, using the example of agoraphobia, the partners might alter their roles and responsibilities so that the partner of the individual with agoraphobia no longer does the grocery shopping or drives the children to music lessons or athletic practices, thus building exposure for agoraphobia into the fabric of the relationship. Similarly, as the individual with agoraphobia makes progress engaging the outside world, the couple might arrange new social engagements outside of the house and plan trips and vacations away from home, so that the individual's world remains broad and rewarding beyond the confines of home. As can be seen, the therapist in such instances helps the couple alter aspects of the relationship that are focal to the agoraphobia, making no assumption of relationship distress in employing such strategies constructively.

For all of these types of couple-based interventions, cognitive, behavioral, and emotionally focused interventions similar to those used in CBCT can be adapted as needed. Also, to the extent that the couple experiences relationship discord in addition to the individual's psychopathology, couple therapy (the third form of couple-based interventions) can be of assistance as well. In this instance, not only might CBCT be of assistance in improving the relationship, but a distressed relationship can be viewed as a chronic, diffuse stressor that can exacerbate individual psychopathology. Thus, alleviating relationship discord and enhancing the relationship can lead to less stress and a more supportive environment for the individual experiencing individual distress. Elsewhere we have used this same logic and these three types of couple-based interventions to address health concerns such as cancer (Baucom et al., 2005) osteoarthritis (Keefe et al., 1996, 1999), and heart disease (Sher & Baucom, 2001).

Thus, the principles employed in CBCT appear to have wide-ranging applicability beyond alleviating relationship distress. CBCT builds upon basic principles of healthy ways to conduct intimate relationships; therefore, it can be employed with couples confronting a variety of challenges in different phases of life if adapted sensitively to those particular contexts.

CASE ILLUSTRATION

Background

David and Catherine, a couple in their mid-30s, had been married for 9 years. Catherine called the therapist requesting couple therapy because she felt that she and David had reached an impasse. Over the past few years, she believed that they had become more distant. David had become more involved in his work, and Catherine felt overwhelmed taking care of two children below age 4. In addition to feeling distant, Catherine reported that they frequently argued, which left them frustrated and irritated with each other and their relationship. Although David believed that

he and Catherine should be able to work out their own problems, he was open to couple therapy, because he was perplexed about why Catherine was so upset, and he could no longer communicate with her.

Relationship and Individual Histories

The couple met while Catherine was in graduate school in physical therapy, and David was a medical student. After a year of dating, they moved in together, spending much of their time talking about their exciting, yet demanding, lives in the hospital. Two years later they married, with Catherine taking a full-time position in a local group practice and David beginning his residency. They described their life together as very positive during the first few years and agreed that most of their energy was focused on helping David get through an extremely demanding residency. Whatever small amount of free time they had together, they relaxed if David needed to rest, or played if he needed more fun and excitement. As a result, their relationship evolved in a manner that put a primary emphasis upon David's needs and preferences. Catherine reported that although at times this became frustrating, she did not resent it at first. Their shared goal was to help him get through his training and to begin a family.

This pattern emphasizing David's needs also was understandable as David and Catherine described themselves as individuals. David grew up as a high achiever, was popular socially, and frequently assumed leadership positions. He described himself as strong and assertive while growing up, and accustomed to being in control and "setting the agenda." As he worked his way up through the ranks in a very hierarchical medical school setting as an adult, David operated in an environment in which support staff and patients expected him to take the lead and tell them what to do. Catherine, on the other hand, described herself as a "pleaser." She also generally had performed well in school but had to try harder to be successful. Despite her success, she lacked self-confidence in general, and particularly with men, Catherine always felt that she needed to prove herself. Consequently, she typically assumed a role of focusing on what her male partner wanted in romantic relationships, routinely ignoring or not expressing her own needs and desires. She was convinced that if she put too much focus on herself or was too "demanding," her relationships would end and she would be alone. Thus, David's general tendency to be in charge and

Catherine's pattern of pleasing others united with a medical residency that placed extraordinary demands upon David, with the resulting focus upon what David needed.

Their relationship had taken a major shift 4 years earlier when their first child William was born. Both Catherine and David had always expressed that they wanted to raise their children directly. Therefore, Catherine resigned her position and became a full-time, stay-at-home mom. Two years later, their second child Melissa was born, and Catherine felt overwhelmed with child care responsibilities and isolated from adults. For the first time, she and David began to bicker over his being absent too much, and over time, their bickering escalated into loud arguments. Catherine's experience was that she and the children had formed a family, and David merely entered and exited at will. In addition to his long hours, she complained that David often brought work home with him, spending little time directly with the children or helping with chores. David's perspective was that he had little time, and they were better off hiring someone to do chores rather than his doing them himself. In addition to assistance with tasks around the house, Catherine also desperately wanted David to be a part of the family system and be involved with her and children. However, she was reluctant to become "vulnerable" by asking him to become more engaged with her. By the time they sought couple therapy, Catherine was quite angry and frustrated. She felt alone in the marriage, had withdrawn sexually due to her ongoing fatigue and resentment of David, and felt trapped, as if she had stopped growing as a person. David was somewhat perplexed by what had gone wrong. They had two lovely children; Catherine was at home with them as they both had always wanted; he was successful and respected in his profession; and though still somewhat young, they had enough money to live comfortably, whereas other couples their age were struggling. They described an increasing distance between them, punctuated by occasional blowups when they did attempt to talk about areas of concern.

Initial Conceptualization

Based upon the initial assessment, the therapist isolated several themes and domains that warranted attention. She shared these with the couple during a feedback session that resulted in a common set of goals for therapy, along with an initial treatment plan.

First, the couple had developed a style of interaction that placed a major focus on David's individual growth and well-being. Whereas this was understandable to some degree given his highly demanding training program early in their marriage, they continued to operate in this way once his residency was completed. With the birth of their children, David and Catherine reached a new developmental stage in their relationship, but they did not adjust their relationship to adapt to the new demands. Thus, a heavy emphasis on David's individual preferences became increasingly maladaptive as the children's needs became more important, and as Catherine felt increasingly stagnant in her own development. Thus, the couple needed to find a variety of strategies for providing greater balance and taking into account individual needs of all the family members, as well as the family functioning as a unit.

Second, Catherine had a longstanding belief that she was valued and desirable only if she ignored her own desires and devoted the bulk of her energy to pleasing others. Thus, she needed to question this notion and find out whether David would value her if she asserted herself with regard to her own needs. This would include Catherine expressing ways that she wanted David to be involved with her and the children, as well as ways he could contribute to and support her need for individual time and personal growth. In addition, Catherine frequently felt taken for granted, saddened that David rarely complimented her privately or bragged about her around other people. Therefore, it was important for David to develop ways to affirm that he respected and valued Catherine.

Third, David needed to understand that the leadership style he practiced at work, in a hierarchical system in which he gave directives, was not appropriate within his family. It was also important that he incorporate himself more into the family, develop relationships with each of the children, and spend time with Catherine alone and develop ways they could be together as a full family. Not only did David have a demanding profession that left him limited time with the children, but when he did interact with them, Catherine often told him what to do, criticized him in front of the children, or intruded into the interaction and put the focus on herself. Thus, it would be important for Catherine to allow David the opportunity to develop his own style of interacting with the children, recognizing that there might be some missteps as he spent more time with his young children.

The Course of Therapy

Early Sessions: Using Communication Skills and Guided Behavior Change to Create a Sense of Equity

To achieve these therapeutic goals, the therapist proposed several different treatment strategies. Like many couples, Catherine and David spent time early in treatment developing more effective communication skills, learning to share thoughts and feelings effectively and to make decisions as a couple. Whereas communication training may at times be used in a broad, general way to help couples interact more positively, typically, we employ these guidelines with more specific goals in mind. With Catherine and David, a major emphasis was to help Catherine share her own feelings, desires, and preferences during couple conversations. This was difficult for her for at least two reasons. First, given that she typically focused her energies on pleasing others, Catherine spent little time thinking about what she wanted for herself or what her own feelings were. Therefore, during sessions the therapist helped David learn to ask Catherine about her feelings and help her explore what she thought and felt—a dramatic shift from their typical interaction focusing on what David wanted. Second, Catherine was reluctant to express her thoughts and feelings, assuming that David would either not be interested or, more drastically, would disengage or leave her if he had to be responsive to what she wanted. Therefore, it was important during their conversations for David to demonstrate that he not only was not frustrated by her disclosures, but he also wanted to hear them. In these same conversations that focused on sharing thoughts and feelings, the therapist emphasized the importance of David becoming a good listener. David was facile at expressing his own wishes, desires, and preferences, but he needed to become more focused on Catherine's feelings as she spoke.

Likewise, when the couple was having decision-making or problem-solving conversations, it was important to emphasize two guidelines in particular. First, each person expressed what was important to him or herself about a given area of concern, they described which would help to ensure that Catherine expressed herself and that David heard Catherine's perspective as areas of concern. Second, the therapist encouraged them to propose possible solutions that explicitly took both people's needs into account. In the past, Catherine and David typically accepted David's preferences. This was not a pattern in which David overtly attempted to dominate the conversation. To the contrary, Catherine typically proposed solutions that she felt were what David wanted, often presenting them as her own preference. Consequently, both partners needed to take responsibility for ensuring that Catherine presented her own preferences during these conversations, rather than attempting to guess what David wanted. For this reason, the therapist typically asked Catherine to express what was important to her, before hearing David's point of view.

THERAPIST: Good, I think you have clarified that you want to develop a plan for how to accomplish weekly household chores, given that you are busy with David's demanding career and taking care of two young children. Before you start proposing specific solutions for how you might address this area, it would be very valuable for each of you to clarify what is important to you in this area and what you personally need to feel good about the way you address it as a couple. Catherine, we have talked about how easy it is for you to listen to what David wants and typically go along with it. So I think it might be important for you to take time to think about what is important to you in terms of getting the chores accomplished and share that with David. Then we will ask David to do the same thing. OK?

CATHERINE: I guess so. I'm not really sure, so maybe I'll just think aloud and then we can see if I'm thinking about it in the right way.

THERAPIST: Sure, just talking aloud about what you think and feel, and what is important to you would be great. But there's not really a right way to think about it, so we won't evaluate it. This is very subjective; we want to know what is important to *you*.

CATHERINE: Well, I'm not sure, but I think there are at least a couple of things. First, I just need some help getting things done around the house. There is just too much with the children, and I can't keep up. And I want us to do it, not hire someone. Here I am healthy and in my early 30s; if we can't take care of our own house, I will really feel like a failure. And second, I need for you to do some of it, and not just for the sake of getting it done. I feel like we're not working together as team and that the children and I have become a family, and that you come and go. I want you as a part of the team, a part of our family, and that means coming in and getting your hands dirty. But that might not be right; I might be just making that up because I'm upset and frustrated.

THERAPIST: I think you actually did a beautiful job of expressing yourself. What was it like for you saying that to David?

CATHERINE: I don't know, pretty uneasy. I'm not sure if that's what I really think, and I'm worried about how it might have come across to David. I mean, his job is so demanding, with so much pressure, and I probably don't have the right to be asking him to do more.

THERAPIST: You know, one of the things we've discussed is for you to do less mind reading and trying to anticipate how David will react and what he wants. Instead, I want you to be open and honest about your own thoughts and feelings and allow David to do the same. So, let's first make sure that David understood what you're telling him and then find out from him directly how it was to hear you express your own perspectives.

DAVID: (*First reflects reasonably well Catherine's two major emphases about the chores and continues.*) Of course, I don't exactly agree with all of your points of view, but it is so nice to know what you really think and want. Often I feel like I'm in a guessing game, asking you about your opinion and not getting it. Then, I express my own preference, and we usually accept it. Although I have to admit that it is nice to get what I want, there are times when I would really like to do what you want. Believe it or not, I'm actually a pretty decent guy who would like to make my wife happy if I knew what that was.

THERAPIST: Catherine, isn't that interesting? It sounds like David was actually pleased to hear your opinion and at times would enjoy trying to please you. What do you make of that?

By employing the communication skills in this way, the therapist also was engaging in a cognitive restructuring strategy using guided discovery. In essence, Catherine made strong predictions that David would not value what she wanted and would either disengage or perhaps even leave her if she expressed her wishes and needs. Thus, she needed to have direct interactions in which she asserted herself and experienced how David was responsive to her wishes and wanted to do what would make her happy; she needed to learn by experience that her predictions were wrong. In addi-

tion, by following the communication guidelines Catherine learned that she could identify and attend to her own preferences and needs without disregarding those of David and the children. By selecting alternative solutions to problems that emphasized the needs of everyone involved, the therapist helped to dispel the all-or-nothing thinking that Catherine typically displayed in approaching problems: "Either David gets what he wants, or I get what I want, which would be selfish."

In addition to employing communication skills to help Catherine realize that David valued her opinion, the therapist used a focused, guided behavior change exercise in which David could affirm Catherine. Each week, David was to write down and bring to the next session two or three things he had seen Catherine do during the week that he valued or appreciated. These could be small things, such as how she responded when William fell and scraped his knee, or how she skillfully initiated conversations and put other people at ease at a party. The task was not only a strategy to help Catherine see that she was valued by David, but it also helped David stay focused on Catherine as an individual and her contributions to their family. David readily acknowledged that he frequently became absorbed, thinking about his work while at home and in conversation with Catherine. Thus, this task helped David remain engaged and focus on Catherine when he was around her.

The Middle Phase of Therapy: Addressing Specific Areas of Concern That Contribute to the Couple's Overall Pattern of Interaction

Over the first 2 months of therapy, Catherine and David made considerable progress. Catherine learned to express her own preferences and wishes when talking with David, and he was receptive to listening to her points of view. With an understanding of the broad pattern of interaction that they were attempting to change, and armed with new skills, Catherine and David next approached a variety of specific concerns related to their broader themes. For example, a major goal of treatment was to engage David more in the day-to-day happenings of the family, including chores, teaching and disciplining the children, and engaging in play and recreation with Catherine and the kids. First, the couple addressed how to give David more time with the children, without Catherine being present. This would allow him to get to know the children better, one-on-one, while also giving Catherine individual time for herself.

David found that as he got to know the children and learned their idiosyncrasies, he really enjoyed them, and they seem to greatly enjoy having time with their father.

However, David and Catherine had more difficulty when they attempted to interact with the children together as a full family. Whereas Catherine very much wanted David to be involved with the children, David often felt that she criticized him for vacillating between being either too lenient or overly harsh when he became frustrated with them. David's typical response was to withdraw, become relatively silent, and let Catherine take over. Without intending to do so, Catherine was punishing the very behavior that she wanted from David. In addition, as indicated in the following discussion, changing longstanding patterns often requires more than providing skills and developing behavior change plans. As couples begin interacting in new ways, the partners may recognize that they have mixed feelings or ambivalence about the changes they have requested. When it arises, it can be helpful to label such ambivalence in a normalizing fashion, then have a problem-solving discussion about how to address the mixed feelings surrounding the new ways of interacting. At times new interaction patterns involve not only gaining much that is positive but also giving up something that one or both partners value.

THERAPIST: So it sounds like you had a difficult interaction when you took the children to the park together on Sunday afternoon. Catherine, can you clarify what you experience when you see David interacting with children in a way that you view as too lenient or permissive?

CATHERINE: It is just so difficult, and at times I can't bite my tongue. I work so hard to set limits with the children, and I think they understand them. Then David comes along and lets them get by with things that we have discussed and that are not acceptable. And consistent with what we've been talking about here in our sessions, I decide to assert myself.

DAVID: You assert yourself, all right. You tell me I'm wrong, shake your finger at me in front of the children, and totally undercut my authority and my role as a parent.

THERAPIST: It sounds like it is pretty upsetting to you. Can you be more specific with Catherine? What is it like for you when you try to be more involved with the children and feel like she is

undercutting you or putting you down in front of the children?

DAVID: It's hard, really hard. I know I'm not very good with children; I've never been around young children except for our own, but I'm doing my best. Catherine says she wants me to be more involved with the children, and most of the time I really enjoy it. But, if I do something she doesn't like, I get scolded. I suddenly feel stupid and embarrassed, and I want to just run away or clam up. And sometimes she seemed to get upset even when I'm doing well with the children. What is that about?

THERAPIST: Why don't the two of you have a conversation where you share your thoughts and feelings about these types of interactions? Let's see if we can try to understand a bit better what is going on. Catherine, David feels that you sometimes get upset even when he seems to be doing well with the children. Do know what he's talking about? Tell him what those times are like for you.

CATHERINE: I don't think I always get upset when you're doing well with the children, but I guess it does happen some of the time. That sounds weird, and I don't really understand it myself. On the one hand, I love seeing you play with and enjoy the children. And it is terrific that they're getting to know you as their father. But to be honest, at times, I think I start to feel jealous and a little resentful. I mean, the children have become the only domain where I'm in charge and where I feel special. You have your whole professional life, with people admiring you and doing exactly what you say. And then you come in and the children think you are great when you spend time with them. It starts to make me feel like they will want to be with you instead of me.

THERAPIST: David, what is Catherine telling you she experiences? Let her know.

DAVID: Well, I think you said you start to feel jealous of me with the children. I believe you if you say that is what you experience, but for me it is just so different. Here you are, this totally competent mother who is finely attuned to what is going on with both of them, responding in a way that seems so effortless. And then I enter not knowing what I'm doing, feeling like I'm banging into things and that the children are laughing because I'm so inappropriate and absurd.

THERAPIST: Sometimes it's really hard to make these changes, even when you both want them and are trying your best. David, you feel unsure around the children and worry that you don't know what you are doing. Catherine, on the one hand, you really enjoy watching David develop his relationship with the kids, but you also are worried that you might lose your special place with them as his relationship develops. Let's try to understand this a bit more, and then we can spend some time trying to help you problem-solve how to do this more successfully. It is a change that you both want, but it is raising some mixed feelings as you put it in place.

This excerpt points out a common experience in couple therapy: As one partner makes requested changes, it is not as positive or rewarding as the other partner initially anticipated. Often, this is because new, unanticipated experiences, along with the attendant thoughts and emotions are encountered as the changes occur. The couple, along with the therapist, then has the challenge of understanding these new and often unanticipated responses to promote positive, long-term change. Catherine and David were able to do just that. As David found ways to include Catherine and affirm her in front of the children, and as Catherine learned that the children's love for her did not diminish but broadened as family members enjoyed being together, her ambivalence subsided and David's confidence in interacting with the children increased. As they continued to respond positively, Catherine stopped criticizing him.

The Final Phase of Therapy: Increasing Intimacy

As therapy progressed, David and Catherine continued to improve their communication in ways that showed mutual respect for each other's wishes and desires. Likewise, David became much more invested in the family and learned to enjoy his role as a father of young children. However, when David was under a great deal of stress due to a heavy workload, or was excited and engaged by a new project, he had a tendency to become absorbed in his work and be less responsive to the family. They developed a way for Catherine to tell him this in a noncondemning fashion, and typically David responded well. Given these changes, both felt much more positively about their rela-

tionship as a couple and their role as parents. In spite of these positive changes, the heavy demands of this phase of life resulted in their still not feeling as close to each other as they would like. Consequently, the final sessions of therapy focused upon increasing intimacy for the couple.

Although not the only domain of importance to achieve this goal, the couple decided to try to improve their affectionate and sexual relationship. For most of their courtship and marriage, David had routinely initiated sex between them. However, both partners agreed that they would like for Catherine to take a more assertive and initiating role in their sex life, consistent with the overall pattern of change that they were developing in other aspects of the relationship. This was difficult for Catherine, because she primarily wanted to be responsive to David's needs, she began to initiate sexual interactions and although awkward at first for both of them, they found this rewarding over time. They also concluded that it was not realistic to expect that they would frequently have time just for themselves as a couple. But by planning ahead the could have two or three nights a month out as a couple, which they really enjoyed. Finally, for rearing the children and for their own spiritual growth, they decided to seek a church to attend as a family given that they both valued the religious upbringing in their families of origin. Although they had never done this together, both spoke about how spiritual intimacy might enhance their relationship. At the time therapy ended, they were still in the early stages of exploring how to relate to each other and build intimacy in a spiritual domain.

Concluding Comments

After 6 months of therapy, Catherine and David had made notable progress in treatment. When asked what they thought was important in helping to promote change in their relationship, both commented that having someone help them stand back and see how they had developed a pattern that focused upon David's needs was of great importance. Labeling this pattern without blaming either partner made both partners open to exploring ways to make needed changes. Catherine also reported that pushing herself to express her own desires, and finding that David was receptive to them, was fundamental to supplying a needed balance within the relationship. David commented that for his entire life, he had been reinforced for taking control and being the leader, along with being successful in his academics and his professional life. Therefore, it was easy for him to get lost in his work and disregard the rest of the world around him, even though he greatly valued and loved his family. Therefore, helping him recognize these tendencies, along with specific strategies to help him become more involved with the children and Catherine, and still be a successful professional, was central in his progress.

In working with this couple, the therapist attended to the needs of Catherine and David as individuals, how they had developed maladaptive interaction patterns as a couple, and how they engaged in their surrounding environment. All three of these domains were approached while attending to important behaviors, cognitions, and emotional responses that could help the couple approach their lives in a constructive manner, taking into account the developmental stage of their family life.

SUGGESTIONS FOR FURTHER READING

Baucom, D. H., & Epstein, N. (1990). *Cognitive-behavioral marital therapy*. New York: Brunner/Mazel.

Epstein, N., & Baucom, D. H. (2002). *Enhanced cognitive-behavioral therapy for couples: A contextual approach*. Washington, DC: American Psychological Association.

Fruzzetti, A. E. (2006). *The high conflict couple: A dialectical behavior therapy guide to finding peace, intimacy and validation*. Oakland, CA: New Harbinger.

REFERENCES

Alexander, J. F., Holtzworth-Munroe, A., & Jameson, P. B. (1994). The process and outcome of marital and family therapy: Research review and evaluation. In A. E. Bergin & S. L. Garfield (Eds.), *Handbook of psychotherapy and behavior change* (4th ed., pp. 595–630). New York: Wiley.

Baldwin, M. W. (2005). *Interpersonal cognition*. New York: Guilford Press.

Bandura, A. (1977). *Social learning theory*. Englewood Cliffs, NJ: Prentice-Hall.

Bandura, A., & Walters, P. (1963). *Social learning and personality development*. New York: Holt, Rinehart & Winston.

Baucom, D. H. (1999, November). *Therapeutic implications of gender differences in cognitive processing in marital relationships*. Paper presented at the 33rd annual meeting of the Association for the Advancement of Behavior Therapy, Toronto, Canada.

Baucom, D. H., & Epstein, N. (1990). *Cognitive-behavioral marital therapy*. New York: Brunner/Mazel.

Baucom, D. H., Epstein, N., Daiuto, A. D., & Carels, R. A. (1996). Cognitions in marriage: The relationship between standards and attributions. *Journal of Family Psychology, 10*(2), 209–222.

Baucom, D. H., Epstein, N., & Gordon, K. C. (2000). Marital therapy: Theory, practice, and empirical status. In C. R. Snyder & R. E. Ingram (Eds.), *Handbook of psychological change: Psychotherapy processes and practices for the 21st century* (pp. 280–308). New York: Wiley.

Baucom, D. H., Epstein, N., & LaTaillade, J. (2002). Cognitive-behavioral couple therapy. In A. S. Gurman & N. S. Jacobson (Eds.), *Clinical handbook of couple therapy* (3rd ed., pp. 26–58). New York: Guilford Press.

Baucom, D. H., Epstein, N., & Rankin, L. A. (1995). Cognitive aspects of cognitive-behavioral marital therapy. In N. S. Jacobson & A. S. Gurman (Eds.), *Clinical handbook of couple therapy* (pp. 65–90). New York: Guilford Press.

Baucom, D. H., Epstein, N., Rankin, L., & Burnett, C. K. (1996). Understanding and treating marital distress from a cognitive-behavioral orientation. In K. S. Dobson & K. D. Craig (Eds.), *Advances in cognitive-behavioral therapy* (pp. 210–236). Thousand Oaks, CA: Sage.

Baucom, D. H., Epstein, N., & Sullivan, L. J. (2004). Brief couple therapy. In M. Dewan, B. Steenbarger, & R. P. Greenberg (Eds.), *The art and science of brief therapies* (pp. 189–227). Washington, DC: American Psychiatric Publishing.

Baucom, D. H., Hahlweg, K., & Kuschel, A. (2003). Are waiting list control groups needed in future marital therapy outcome research? *Behavior Therapy, 34*, 179–188.

Baucom, D. H., Heinrichs, N., Scott, J. L., Gremore, T. M., Kirby, J. S., Zimmermann, T., et al. (2005, November). *Couple-based interventions for breast cancer: Findings from three continents*. Paper presented at the 39th Annual Convention of the Association for Behavioral and Cognitive Therapies, Washington, DC.

Baucom, D. H., & Hoffman, J. A. (1986). The effectiveness of marital therapy: Current status and application to the clinical setting. In N. S. Jacobson & A. S. Gurman (Eds.), *Clinical handbook of marital therapy* (pp. 597–620). New York: Guilford Press.

Baucom, D. H., & Lester, G. W. (1986). The usefulness of cognitive restructuring as an adjunct to behavioral marital therapy. *Behavior Therapy, 17*(4), 385–403.

Baucom, D. H., Sayers, S. L., & Sher, T. G. (1988, November). *Expanding behavioral marital therapy*. Paper presented at the 22nd Annual Meeting of the Association for the Advancement of Behavior Therapy, New York, New York.

Baucom, D. H., Sayers, S. L., & Sher, T. G. (1990). Supplementing behavioral marital therapy with cognitive restructuring and emotional expressiveness training: An outcome investigation. *Journal of Consulting and Clinical Psychology, 58*(5), 636–645.

Baucom, D. H., Shoham, V., Mueser, K. T., Daiuto, A.

D., & Stickle, T. R. (1998). Empirically supported couples and family therapies for adult problems. *Journal of Consulting and Clinical Psychology*, 66, 53–88.

Baucom, D. H., Stanton, S., & Epstein, N. (2003). Anxiety. In D. K. Snyder & M. Whisman (Eds.), *Treating difficult couples* (pp. 57–87). New York: Guilford Press.

Beach, S. R. H. (Ed.). (2001). *Marital and family processes in depression: A scientific foundation for clinical practice*. Washington, DC: American Psychological Association.

Beck, A. T. (1988). Cognitive approaches to panic disorder: Theory and therapy. In S. Rachman & J. D. Maser (Eds.), *Panic: Psychological perspectives* (pp. 91–109). Hillsdale, NJ: Erlbaum.

Beck, A. T., Rush, A. J., Shaw, B. F., & Emery, G. (1979). *Cognitive therapy of depression*. New York: Guilford Press.

Birchler, G. R., Weiss, R. L., & Vincent, J. P. (1975). Multimethod analysis of social reinforcement exchange between maritally distressed and nondistressed spouse and stranger dyads. *Journal of Personality and Social Psychology*, 31(2), 349–360.

Bradbury, T. N., & Karney, B. R. (2004). Understanding and altering the longitudinal course of marriage. *Journal of Marriage and the Family*, 66, 862–879.

Bray, J. H., & Jouriles, E. N. (1995). Treatment of marital conflict and prevention of divorce [Special issue]. *Journal of Marital and Family Therapy*, 21(4), 461–473.

Bronfenbrenner, U. (1989). *Ecological systems theory* (Vol. 6). Greenwich, CT: JAI.

Carter, B., & McGoldrick, M. (Eds.). (1999). *The expanded family life cycle: Individual, family, and social perspectives* (3rd ed.). Boston: Allyn & Bacon.

Christensen, A. (1987). Detection of conflict patterns in couples. In K. Hahlweg & M. J. Goldstein (Eds.), *Understanding major mental disorder: The contribution of family interaction research* (pp. 250–265). New York: Family Process.

Christensen, A. (1988). Dysfunctional interaction patterns in couples. In P. Noller & M. A. Fitzpatrick (Eds.), *Perspectives on marital interaction* (pp. 31–52). Clevedon, UK: Multilingual Matters.

Christensen, A., Atkins, D., Berns, S., Wheeler, J., Baucom, D. H., & Simpson, L. (2004). Traditional versus integrative behavioral couple therapy for significantly and stably distressed married couples. *Journal of Consulting and Clinical Psychology*, 72, 176–191.

Christensen, A., & Heavey, C. L. (1990). Gender and social structure in the demand/withdraw pattern of marital conflict. *Journal of Personality and Social Psychology*, 59(1), 73–81.

Christensen, A., & Heavey, C. L. (1993). Gender differences in marital conflict: The demand/withdraw interaction pattern. In S. Oskamp & M. Costanzo (Eds.), *Gender issues in contemporary society* (Vol. 6, pp. 113–141). Newbury Park, CA: Sage.

Cutrona, C. E. (1996). Social support in marriage: A cognitive perspective. In G. R. Pierce, B. R. Sarason,

& I. G. Sarason (Eds.), *Handbook of social support and the family* (pp. 173–194). New York: Plenum.

Cutrona, C. E., Hessling, R. M., & Suhr, J. A. (1997). The influence of husband and wife personality on marital social support interactions. *Personal Relations*, 4, 379–393.

Cutrona, C. E., Suhr, J. A., & MacFarlane, R. (1990). Interpersonal transactions and the psychological sense of support. In S. Duck & R. C. Silver (Eds.), *Personal relationships and social support* (pp. 30–45). London: Sage.

Dattilio, F. M., & Padesky, C. A. (1990). *Cognitive therapy with couples*. Sarasota, FL: Professional Resource Exchange.

Derogatis, L. R. (1993). *BSI: Brief Symptom Inventory*. Minneapolis, MN: Pearson NCS.

Dunn, R. L., & Schwebel, A. I. (1995). Meta-analytic review of marital therapy outcome research. *Journal of Family Psychology*, 9(1), 58–68.

Eidelson, R. J., & Epstein, N. (1982). Cognition and relationship maladjustment: Development of a measure of dysfunctional relationship beliefs. *Journal of Consulting and Clinical Psychology*, 50(5), 715–720.

Ellis, A. (1962). *Reason and emotion in psychotherapy*. New York: Lyle Stuart.

Ellis, A., Sichel, J. L., Yeager, R. J., DiMattia, D. J., & DiGiuseppe, R. (1989). *Rational–emotive couples therapy*. New York: Pergamon.

Epstein, N. (1982). Cognitive therapy with couples. *American Journal of Family Therapy*, 10(1), 5–16.

Epstein, N., & Baucom, D. H. (2002). *Enhanced cognitive-behavioral therapy for couples: A contextual approach*. Washington, DC: American Psychological Association.

Epstein, N., & Baucom, D. H. (2003). Overcoming roadblocks in cognitive-behavioral therapy with couples. In R. L. Leahy (Ed.), *Overcoming roadblocks in cognitive therapy* (pp. 187–205). New York: Guilford Press.

Falloon, I. R. H. (1991). *Behavioral family therapy* (Vol. 2). New York: Brunner/Mazel.

Fincham, F. D., Bradbury, T. N., & Scott, C. K. (1990). Cognition in marriage. In F. D. Fincham & T. N. Bradbury (Eds.), *The psychology of marriage: Basic issues and applications* (pp. 118–149). New York: Guilford Press.

Fiske, S. T., & Taylor, S. E. (1991). *Social cognition*. New York: McGraw-Hill.

Fletcher, G. J. O., & Fitness, J. (Eds.). (1996). *Knowledge structures in close relationships: A social psychological approach*. Mahwah, NJ: Erlbaum.

Fruzzetti, A. E. (2006). *The high conflict couple: A dialectical behavior therapy guide to finding peace, intimacy, and validation*. Oakland, CA: New Harbinger.

Glass, S. P. (2002). Couple therapy after the trauma of infidelity. In A. S. Gurman & N. S. Jacobson (Eds.), *Clinical handbook of couple therapy* (3rd ed., pp. 488–507). New York: Guilford Press.

Gottman, J. M. (1979). *Marital interaction: Experimental investigations*. New York: Academic Press.

Gottman, J. M. (1994). *What predicts divorce?* Hillsdale, NJ: Erlbaum.

Greenberg, L. S., & Safran, J. D. (1987). *Emotion in psychotherapy: Affect, cognition, and the process of change.* New York: Guilford Press.

Hahlweg, K., & Baucom, D. H. (in press). *Partnerschaft und psychische Störung* [Couples and psychopathology]. Göttingen: Hogrefe.

Hahlweg, K., & Markman, H. J. (1988). Effectiveness of behavioral marital therapy: Empirical status of behavioral techniques in preventing and alleviating marital distress. *Journal of Consulting and Clinical Psychology, 56*(3), 440–447.

Halford, W. K., Sanders, M. R., & Behrens, B. C. (1993). A comparison of the generalisation of behavioral martial therapy and enhanced behavioral martial therapy. *Journal of Consulting and Clinical Psychology, 61,* 51–60.

Halford, W. K., Sanders, M. R., & Behrens, B. C. (1994). Self-regulation in behavioral couples' therapy. *Behavior Therapy, 25*(3), 431–452.

Hardy, K. V., & Laszloffy, T. A. (2002). Couple therapy using a multicultural perspective. In A. S. Gurman & N. S. Jacobson (Eds.), *Clinical handbook of couple therapy* (3rd ed., pp. 569–593). New York: Guilford Press.

Holtzworth-Munroe, A., Meehan, J. C., Rehman, U., & Marshall, A. D. (2002). Intimate partner violence: An introduction for couple therapists. In A. S. Gurman & N. S. Jacobson (Eds.), *Clinical handbook of couple therapy* (3rd ed., pp. 441–465). New York: Guilford Press.

Iverson, A., & Baucom, D. H. (1988, November). *Behavioral marital therapy: The role of skills acquisition in marital satisfaction.* Paper presented at the 22nd annual meeting of the Association for the Advancement of Behavior Therapy, New York.

Iverson, A., & Baucom, D. H. (1990). Behavioral marital therapy outcomes: Alternative interpretations of the data. *Behavior Therapy, 21*(1), 129–138.

Jacobson, N. S., & Addis, M. E. (1993). Research on couples and couple therapy: What do we know? Where are we going? *Journal of Consulting and Clinical Psychology, 61*(1), 85–93.

Jacobson, N. S., & Christensen, A. (1996). Studying the effectiveness of psychotherapy: How well can clinical trials do the job? *American Psychologist, 51*(10), 1031–1039.

Jacobson, N. S., Dobson, K. S., Fruzzetti, A. E., Schmaling, K. B., & Salusky, S. (1991). Marital therapy as a treatment for depression. *Journal of Consulting and Clinical Psychology, 59*(4), 547–557.

Jacobson, N. S., & Holtzworth-Munroe, A. (1986). Marital therapy: A social learning/cognitive perspective. In N. S. Jacobson & A. S. Gurman (Eds.), *Clinical handbook of marital therapy* (pp. 29–70). New York: Guilford Press.

Jacobson, N. S., & Margolin, G. (1979). *Marital therapy: Strategies based on social learning and behavior exchange principles.* New York: Brunner/Mazel.

Jacobson, N. S., Schmaling, K. B., & Holtzworth-Munroe, A. (1987). Component analysis of behavioral marital therapy: 2-year follow-up and prediction of relapse. *Journal of Marital and Family Therapy, 13,* 187–195.

Jacobson, N. S., Waldron, H., & Moore, D. (1980). Toward a behavioral profile of marital distress. *Journal of Consulting and Clinical Psychology, 48*(6), 696–703.

Johnson, S. M. (2004). *The practice of emotionally focused marital therapy: Creating connection* (2nd ed.). New York: Routledge.

Johnson, S. M., & Denton, W. (2002). Emotionally focused couple therapy: Creating secure connections. In A. S. Gurman & N. S. Jacobson (Eds.), *Clinical handbook of couple therapy* (3rd ed., pp. 221–250). New York: Guilford Press.

Johnson, S. M., & Greenberg, L. S. (1987). Emotionally focused marital therapy: An overview [Special issue]. *Psychotherapy, 24*(3S), 552–560.

Karney, B. R., & Bradbury, T. N. (1995). The longitudinal course of marital quality and stability: A review of theory, methods, and research. *Psychological Bulletin, 118,* 3–34.

Keefe, F. J., Caldwell, D. S., Baucom, D. H., Salley, A., Robinson, E., Timmons, K., et al. (1996). Spouse-assisted coping skills training in the management of osteoarthritic knee pain. *Arthritis Care and Research, 9,* 279–291.

Keefe, F. J., Caldwell, D. S., Baucom, D. H., Salley, A., Robinson, E., Timmons, K., et al. (1999). Spouse-assisted coping skills training in the management of knee pain in osteoarthritis: Long-term follow-up results. *Arthritis Care and Research, 12,* 101–111.

Kelly, S. (2006). Cognitive behavioral therapy with African Americans. In P. A. Hays & G. Y. Iwamasa (Eds.), *Culturally responsive cognitive-behavioral therapy: Assessment, practice, and supervision* (pp. 97–116). Washington, DC: American Psychological Association.

Kelly, S., & Iwamasa, G. Y. (2005). Enhancing behavioral couple therapy: Addressing the therapeutic alliance, hope, and diversity. *Cognitive and Behavioral Practice, 12,* 102–112.

Kirby, J. S., & Baucom, D. H. (2007). Integrating dialectical behavior therapy and cognitive-behavioral couple therapy: A couples skills group for emotion dysregulation. *Cognitive and Behavioral Practice, 14,* 394–405.

Kirby, J. S., & Baucom, D. H. (2007). Treating emotional dysregulation in a couples context: A pilot study of a couples skills group intervention. *Journal of Marital and Family Therapy, 33,* 1–17.

LaTaillade, J. J. (2006). Considerations for treatment of African American couple relationships. *Journal of Cognitive Psychotherapy: An International Quarterly, 20,* 341–358.

LaTaillade, J. J., Epstein, N. B., & Werlinich, C. A. (2006). Conjoint treatment of intimate partner violence: A cognitive behavioral approach. *Journal of Cognitive Psychotherapy: An International Quarterly, 20,* 393–410.

LaTaillade, J. J., & Jacobson, N. S. (1995). Behavioral couple therapy. In M. Elkaim (Ed.), *Therapies familiales: Les principles approaches [Family therapies: The principal approaches]* (pp. 313–347). Paris: Editions du Seuil.

Liberman, R. P. (1970). Behavioral approaches to family and couple therapy. *American Journal of Orthopsychiatry, 40*, 106–118.

Linehan, M. M. (1993). *Cognitive-behavioral treatment of borderline personality disorder.* New York: Guilford Press.

Margolin, G., & Weiss, R. L. (1978). Comparative evaluation of therapeutic components associated with behavioral marital treatments. *Journal of Consulting and Clinical Psychology, 46*(6), 1476–1486.

Markman, H. J., Renick, M. J., Floyd, F. J., Stanley, S. M., & Clements, M. (1993). Preventing marital distress through communication and conflict management training: A 4- and 5-year follow-up. *Journal of Consulting and Clinical Psychology, 61*(1), 70–77.

McCubbin, H. I., & Patterson, J. M. (1987). FILE: Family Inventory of Life Events and Changes. In H. I. McCubbin & A. I. Thompson (Eds.), *Family assessment inventories for research and practice* (pp. 81–98). Madison: University of Wisconsin–Madison, Family Stress Coping and Health Project.

Mehlman, S. K., Baucom, D. H., & Anderson, D. (1981, November). *The relative effectiveness of cotherapists vs. single therapists and immediate treatment vs. delayed treatment in a behavioral marital therapy outcome study.* Paper presented at the 15th Annual Meeting of the Association for the Advancement of Behavior Therapy, Toronto, Canada.

Meichenbaum, D. (1977). *Cognitive-behavior modification.* New York: Plenum.

Murphy, C. M., & Hoover, S. A. (2001). Measuring emotional abuse in dating relationships as a multifactorial construct. In K. D. O'Leary & R. D. Maiuro (Eds.), *Psychological abuse in violent domestic relationships* (pp. 3–28). New York: Springer.

Noller, P., Beach, S. R. H., & Osgarby, S. (1997). Cognitive and affective processes in marriage. In W. K. Halford & H. J. Markman (Eds.), *Clinical handbook of marriage and couples interventions* (pp. 43–71). Chichester, UK: Wiley.

Pasch, L. A., Bradbury, T. N., & Davila, J. (1997). Gender, negative affectivity, and observed social support behavior in marital interaction. *Personal Relationships, 4*(4), 361–378.

Pasch, L. A., Bradbury, T. N., & Sullivan, K. T. (1997). Social support in marriage: An analysis of intraindividual and interpersonal components. In G. R. Pierce, B. Lakey, I. G. Sarason, & B. R. Sarason (Eds.), *Sourcebook of theory and research on social support and personality* (pp. 229–256). New York: Plenum.

Patterson, G. R. (1974). Interventions for boys with conduct problems: Multiple settings, treatments, and criteria. *Journal of Consulting and Clinical Psychology, 42*, 471–481.

Patterson, G. R., & Hops, H. (1972). Coercion, a game

for two: Intervention techniques for marital conflict. In R. E. Ulrich & P. Mounjoy (Eds.), *The experimental analysis of social behavior.* New York: Appleton.

Prager, K. J. (1995). *The psychology of intimacy.* New York: Guilford Press.

Prager, K. J., & Buhrmester, D. (1998). Intimacy and need fulfillment in couple relationships. *Journal of Social and Personal Relationships, 15*, 435–469.

Rankin, L. A., Baucom, D. H., Clayton, D. C., & Daiuto, A. D. (1995, November). *Gender differences in the use of relationship schemas versus individual schemas in marriage.* Paper presented at the 29th Annual Meeting of the Association for the Advancement of Behavior Therapy, Washington, DC.

Rathus, J. H., & Sanderson, W. C. (1999). *Marital distress: Cognitive behavioral interventions for couples.* Northvale, NJ: Aronson.

Schmaling, K. B., & Sher, T. G. (2000). *The psychology of couples and illness: Theory, research and practice.* Washington, DC: American Psychological Association.

Shadish, W. R., Montgomery, L. M., Wilson, P., Wilson, M. R., Bright, I., & Okwumabua, T. (1993). Effects of family and marital psychotherapies: A meta-analysis. *Journal of Consulting and Clinical Psychology, 61*(6), 992–1002.

Sher, T. G., & Baucom, D. H. (2001). Mending a broken heart: A couples approach to cardiac risk reduction. *Applied and Preventive Psychology, 10*, 125–133.

Snyder, D. K. (1979). Multidimensional assessment of marital satisfaction. *Journal of Marriage and the Family, 41*(4), 813–823.

Snyder, D. K., Baucom, D. H., & Gordon, K. C. (2007). *Getting past the affair: A program to help you cope, heal, and move on—together or apart.* New York: Guilford Press.

Snyder, D. K., & Costin, S. E. (1994). Marital Satisfaction Inventory. In M. E. Maruish (Ed.), *The use of psychological testing for treatment planning and outcome assessment* (pp. 322–351). Hillsdale, NJ: Erlbaum.

Snyder, D. K., & Whisman, M. A. (2002). Understanding psychopathology and couple dysfunction: Implications for clinical practice, training, and research. In D. K. Snyder & M. A. Whisman (Eds.), *Treating difficult couples: Helping clients with coexisting mental and relationship disorders* (pp. 1–17). New York: Guilford Press.

Snyder, D. K., & Wills, R. M. (1989). Behavioral versus insight-oriented marital therapy: Effects on individual and interspousal functioning. *Journal of Consulting and Clinical Psychology, 57*(1), 39–46.

Snyder, D. K., Wills, R. M., & Grady-Fletcher, A. (1991). Long-term effectiveness of behavioral versus insight-oriented marital therapy: A 4-year follow-up study. *Journal of Consulting and Clinical Psychology, 59*(1), 138–141.

Snyder, D. K., Wills, R. M., & Keiser, T. W. (1981). Empirical validation of the Marital Satisfaction Inventory: An actuarial approach. *Journal of Consulting and Clinical Psychology, 49*(2), 262–268.

Spanier, G. B. (1976). Measuring dyadic adjustment:

New scales for assessing the quality of marriage and similar dyads. *Journal of Marriage and the Family, 38*, 15–28.

Straus, M. A., Hamby, S. L., Boney-McCoy, S., & Sugarman, D. B. (1996). The Revised Conflict Tactics Scales (CTS2): Development and preliminary psychometric data. *Journal of Family Issues, 17*(3), 283–316.

Stuart, R. B. (1969). Operant interpersonal treatment for marital discord. *Journal of Consulting and Clinical Psychology, 33*, 675–682.

Stuart, R. B. (1980). *Helping couples change: A social learning approach to marital therapy.* New York: Guilford Press.

Sullivan, L. J., & Baucom, D. H. (2002, November). *Relationship–schematic processing and matching couples to treatment intervention.* Paper presented at the Annual Meeting of the Association for Advancement of Behavior Therapy, Reno, NV.

Sullivan, L. J., & Baucom, D. H. (2005). Observational coding of relationship–schematic processing. *Journal of Marital and Family Therapy, 31*, 31–43.

Sullivan, L. J., Baucom, D. H., & Snyder, D. K. (2002, November). *Relationship–schematic processing and rela-tionship satisfaction across two types of marital interventions.* Paper presented at the Annual Meeting of the Association for Advancement of Behavior Therapy, Reno, NV.

Thibaut, J. W., & Kelley, H. H. (1959). *The social psychology of groups.* New York: Wiley.

Weiss, R. L. (1980). Strategic behavioral martial therapy: Toward a model for assessment and intervention. In J. P. Vincent (Ed.), *Advances in family intervention, assessment and theory* (Vol. 1, pp. 229–271). Greenwich, CT: JAI.

Weiss, R. L., Hops, H., & Patterson, G. R. (1973). A framework for conceptualizing marital conflict, a technology for altering it, some data for evaluating it. In M. Hersen & A. S. Bellack (Eds.), *Behavior change: Methodology, concepts and practice* (pp. 309–342). Champaign, IL: Research Press.

Whisman, M. A., Uebelacker, U. A., & Weinstock, L. M. (2004). Psychopathology and marital satisfaction: The importance of evaluating both partners. *Journal of Abnormal Psychology, 72*, 830–838.

Wood, L. F., & Jacobson, N. S. (1985). Marital distress. In D. H. Barlow (Ed.), *Clinical handbook of psychological disorders.* New York: Guilford Press.

CHAPTER 3

Integrative Behavioral Couple Therapy

Sona Dimidjian
Christopher R. Martell
Andrew Christensen

BACKGROUND

Integrative behavioral couple therapy (IBCT), developed by Andrew Christensen and Neil S. Jacobson, has its roots in careful clinical observation and empirical research on the treatment of distressed couples. It is a contextually based behavioral treatment designed to help couples achieve improved satisfaction and adjustment. An innovative new treatment, IBCT was first presented in published form in an earlier edition of this *Handbook* (Christensen, Jacobson, & Babcock, 1995). Since then, a detailed treatment manual for therapists has been published (Jacobson & Christensen, 1998), as has a guide for use by couples (Christensen & Jacobson, 2000).

IBCT grew principally from traditional behavioral couple therapy (TBCT), a widely practiced treatment that is perhaps best summarized in the now classic text *Marital Therapy: Strategies Based on Social Learning and Behavior Exchange Principles* (Jacobson & Margolin, 1979). TBCT is a skills-based, change-oriented treatment that relies on two primary intervention components: (1) behavior exchange, and (2) communication and problem-solving training. "Behavior exchange" seeks to increase the ratio of positive to negative

couple behaviors and is intended to produce rapid decreases in couple distress; however, it is not believed to give rise to long-lasting change, because such interventions do not teach couples the necessary skills to address future problems. In contrast, the second set of interventions prescribed by TBCT, "communication and problem-solving," is designed to teach skills that couples can use long after treatment has ended. These skills are intended to help couples change fundamental relationship patterns in ways that will protect them from distress for years to come.

Since its early development (e.g., Jacobson & Margolin, 1979), TBCT has become one of the most widely investigated treatments for couple distress. Currently, its documented success is unparalleled, with over 20 studies attesting to its efficacy (Baucom, Shoham, Meuser, Daiuto, & Stickle, 1998; Christensen & Heavey, 1999; Hahlweg & Markman, 1988; Jacobson & Addis, 1993). In fact, TBCT remains the only couple therapy to date that meets the most stringent criteria for empirically supported. namely, efficacious and specific, treatments (Baucom et al., 1998).

Yet, despite such impressive acclaim, in the mid-1980s, Jacobson and colleagues grew increasingly skeptical of the success of TBCT. They were unsettled by their clinical experience with couples—and by what a careful examination of the empirical data implied. Jacobson and colleagues had begun to consider not only the statistical significance of the efficacy of TBCT, but also the clinical significance. In 1984, Jacobson et al. published what was to become a landmark paper in the field of couple therapy. A reanalysis of the outcome data on TBCT suggested that TBCT was limited in its ability to produce clinically meaningful change. Specifically, Jacobson et al. (1984) reported that, at best, only one-half of couples had improved over the course of treatment, and that only one-third of those who improved had actually moved to the nondistressed range of functioning. Moreover, among those who did improve during treatment, one-third of couples experienced a relapse of their distress during the 2-year follow-up period (Jacobson, Schmaling, & Holtzworth-Munroe, 1987). Empirical examinations of the types of couples who benefited most from TBCT were also informative. In particular, it appeared that couples were more likely to respond favorably to TBCT if they were less distressed, younger, not emotionally disengaged, not experiencing concurrent individual problems (e.g., depression), and did not have a relationship based on rigidly structured, traditional gender roles (Jacobson & Addis, 1993).

These empirical data were consistent with the clinical experiences of Jacobson and Christensen, who, in their work with couples, had noticed that TBCT did not appear to be as effective with couples who were struggling with issues of compromise, collaboration, and accommodation. Christensen and Jacobson began to wonder whether a spirit of compromise was the unifying thread among the characteristics that research had found common to couples who responded best to TBCT. They also noticed that certain types of problems did not seem to be well served by the TBCT technology. In particular, problems that represented basic and irreconcilable differences between partners appeared to be less amenable to traditional change strategies. Yet they found that many couples with such intractable problems were still committed to improving their relationships.

Thus, for some couples and some problems, it became increasingly clear that TBCT's emphasis on promoting change seemed to be a poor fit for what the couples needed. In some cases, interventions designed to promote change actually seemed to exacerbate couples' distress. Christensen and Jacobson began to hypothesize about what was missing from the available treatment technology. They suggested that that the recipe for success was not an increased emphasis on change—but an increased emphasis on acceptance. In their view, acceptance was, in effect, "the missing link" in TBCT (Jacobson & Christensen, 1998, p. 11).

What is "acceptance," and why is it so important in the resolution of couple distress? First, it is important to note what acceptance is not: Acceptance is not a grudging resignation about the state of one's relationship. It is not a woeful surrender to a miserable status quo. In contrast, acceptance provides a hopeful alternative for couples faced with problems that are not amenable to typical change strategies. Moreover, acceptance can also provide a method by which couples use problems—once experienced as divisive and damaging—as vehicles for greater intimacy and closeness.

THE HEALTHY VERSUS DISTRESSED COUPLE

IBCT is based on a fundamentally different understanding of relationship distress than that underlying TBCT and many other therapeutic models. IBCT proposes that over time, even the happiest and healthiest couples will face areas of difference and disagreement, which are assumed to be both normal and inevitable. Thus, distress is not caused by such differences, disagreements, or conflicts between partners. In contrast, distress is caused by the destructive ways that some couples respond to these inevitable incompatibilities.

In the early phases of a relationship, acceptance and tolerance of differences come easily to many couples. In fact, in many relationships, partners cite one another's differences as the source of their attraction. Lisa, for instance, recalled being enamored of Bruce's outspoken and direct nature, whereas Bruce recalled being impressed with the thoughtful way that Lisa considered issues, and her indirect and tactful way of expressing her opinions. Thus, during partners' early days together, differences are less often experienced as threatening or problematic for the relationship, and partners often find that their willingness to compromise with one another is high when such differences do create difficulty.

Differences between partners are likely to create difficulties when these differences spring from vulnerabilities within each partner rather than mere differences in preference. Consider Bruce and Lisa's differences in directness and outspokenness. Bruce had a difficult first marriage and divorce with a woman he described as passive–aggressive and likely to undermine him at every turn. When Lisa's indirectness began to resemble what Bruce had found so upsetting in his first wife, he reacted very emotionally. For her part, Lisa felt that her father often bullied others, particularly her mother. When Bruce's outspoken manner began to resemble what she found so upsetting in her father, Lisa reacted very emotionally. Thus, conflicts over their differences in expression are fueled by the vulnerabilities that Bruce and Lisa brought with them into the marriage.

Three destructive patterns frequently characterize distressed couples' conflicts over their differences: mutual coercion, vilification, and polarization. Over time, as distressed couples experience an erosion in their willingness to accept, tolerate, and compromise around one another's differences, they no longer look upon each other's styles as sources of attraction; they begin to exert efforts to change their partners. Early on these change efforts may entail direct requests and gentle persuasion. However, if these efforts fail, partners may resort to negative behaviors such as criticizing, withdrawing, yelling, inducing guilt, and so forth. According to coercion theory (Jacobson & Christensen, 1998; Patterson & Hops, 1972), these negative behaviors are often inadvertently and mutually reinforced. For example, Lisa may withdraw when Bruce's outspokenness is particularly upsetting to her; he may then respond to her withdrawal by being more solicitous with her; and Lisa may respond to his solicitous behavior by engaging with him again. Thus, her withdrawal is positively reinforced by his solicitous behavior; his solicitous behavior is in turn negatively reinforced (Lisa terminates her withdrawal). Over time, partners may shape each other into more extreme and persistent patterns of their coercive behavior. For example, Lisa does not get reinforced every time she withdraws, so she learns to persist with her efforts and to use more extreme withdrawal to get Bruce's attention. Also, both partners engage in coercion. Bruce may criticize Lisa for her indirection, and a similar pattern of mutual, intermittent reinforcement and shaping occurs. The couple creates a coercive system of interaction around their differences.

As these patterns of mutual coercion become more frequent and common, partners begin to see one another not as different but as deficient. In essence, they begin to vilify one another. Therefore, Lisa is no longer one who carefully considers things; instead, she is "controlling and withhold-ing." Bruce, on the other hand, is defined not as direct and assertive, but as "impulsive and bullying." As vilification takes hold, each partner feels increasingly justified in his or her efforts to reform the wayward other.

As the differences between partners increasingly become a source of conflict, they tend to intensify or polarize; the chasm between the two partners grows wider and wider. In the face of the troubling behavior of the other, each partner exercises more and more of the behavior at which he or she is already proficient. Bruce becomes more forceful and outspoken; Lisa more withdrawn and uncommunicative. Each becomes more extreme in his or her actions. Their conflict serves to widen rather than to bridge the differences between them. They polarize. Therefore, through these processes of mutual coercion, vilification, and polarization, distress is generated—not by the differences between partners, but by partners' attempts to eliminate such differences.

Research has provided substantial support for major components of this model of relationship distress. For example, cross-sectional research comparing distressed versus nondistressed couples (e.g., Weiss & Heyman, 1997) and longitudinal research examining the predictors of distress (e.g., Karney & Bradbury, 1995) have documented the role of reciprocal, negative, coercive interaction in relationship distress. Also, research on cognitive factors has repeatedly confirmed the role of negative views of the partner (e.g., negative attributions) in relationship distress (e.g., Noller, Beach, & Osgarby, 1997).

In contrast to distressed couples, happy couples are able to confront their differences with greater acceptance and tolerance. From a theoretical standpoint (Cordova, 2001), "acceptance" is behavior that occurs in the presence of aversive stimuli. It refers to responding to such stimuli not with behavior that functions to avoid, escape, or destroy, but with behavior that functions to maintain or to increase contact. From a couple's standpoint, acceptance means not being drawn into patterns of coercion, vilification, and polarization. Partners are able to maintain their positive connection despite and, at times, maybe even because of their differences. What promotes acceptance in happy couples? Perhaps their differences are not as great, perhaps their individual personalities are not as threatened by differences, or perhaps there is greater social support for their union. These individual and contextual factors probably interact reciprocally with greater acceptance, so that, for example, greater acceptance in the relationship leads to partners feeling less threatened by their differences, which in turn leads to greater acceptance in the relationship. Existing research says little about the processes by which couples, who, typically happy at the beginning, travel different trajectories, leading some to discord and separation, and others to stable and fulfilling unions.

THEORY OF THERAPEUTIC CHANGE

As the name indicates, IBCT is a behavioral therapy. In their writings about the approach, Christensen and Jacobson (2000; Jacobson & Christensen, 1998) acknowledge its behavioral roots. However, they also acknowledge other influences, particularly the work of Dan Wile (e.g., 1988). Some may see similarities between Wile's ideas and particular strategies in IBCT. Also, there are similarities between IBCT strategies and strategies of other approaches. For example, some of IBCT's tolerance interventions are similar to techniques in strategic therapy, and IBCT's acceptance intervention of empathic joining is similar to client-centered and emotion-focused therapy strategies. However, what marks IBCT as unique is not only that the strategies are conducted differently, and for different purposes, but also that all the strategies in IBCT come from a behavioral theoretical perspective. We call IBCT an integrative approach, because it integrates strategies for change with strategies for acceptance. However, it is also an integrative behavioral approach, because it melds a variety of interventions within a coherent behavioral approach.

Both TBCT and IBCT are distinctly behavioral theories, because each views behavior and any changes in that behavior as a function of the context in which the behavior occurs. In a romantic relationship, the primary, although by no means exclusive, context is the partner's behavior. Therefore, each partner's behavior is responsive to the context provided by the other's behavior, as well as to other significant features of the context (the larger family context that includes a critical in-law, an out of control child, etc.). The goal of TBCT is to change this context by changing the agents of behavior. If there is dissatisfaction because a husband is too negative or a wife is not affectionate enough, then the goal is to increase the husband's positivity and the wife's affection. Behavior exchange and communication and problem-solving training are the means by which TBCT achieves

those changes. Evidence has supported this theory of change (Jacobson, 1984).

In contrast to TBCT, IBCT focuses as much or more on the recipient of behavior as on the agent of behavior. The context can change not only because the agent alters the frequency or intensity of behavior, but also because the recipient receives the behavior differently. If the wife is more accepting of her husband's negativity and does not take it so personally, or if the husband is more understanding of his wife's lack of affection and is not so offended by it, then the context of their relationship and also their sentiment about it will change.

There are three major reasons for the shift in emphasis in IBCT from the agent to the recipient of behavior. First, according to IBCT, there are in every relationship some "unsolvable" problems that the agent is unwilling or unable to change to the level the recipient desires. Improvement in these cases will be mediated by increased acceptance and tolerance. Second, IBCT theory suggests that, paradoxically, increased acceptance in one partner may at times also mediate increased change. In this way, IBCT suggests, at times it may be the pressure for change from one partner that contributes to the maintenance of the undesirable partner behavior. Thus, when the pressure to change is eliminated by increased acceptance or tolerance, change may follow. As partners let go of their efforts to change one another, they become less emotionally reactive; as a result, change becomes more likely. Third, IBCT theory suggests that in most cases the reaction to an offending behavior is as much a problem as the offending behavior itself. In their book on IBCT for couples, Christensen and Jacobson (2000) write that the "crimes of the heart are usually misdemeanors" (p. 273). Garden-variety couple problems usually do not concern major, egregious transgressions, such as violence or infidelity. They concern minor hurts and annoyances that are made more dramatic by the vulnerability with which they are received. Thus, the emphasis upon change in the behavior of the agent should be balanced by an emphasis upon acceptance by the recipient.

IBCT has not only a different focus of change (the recipient vs. the agent of behavior) but also a different strategy of change than TBCT. In TBCT, the mechanism of change is through rule-governed behavior, whereas in IBCT, the primary mechanism of change is through contingency-shaped behavior. This important distinction by Skinner (1966) between rule-governed and contingency-shaped behavior refers to what controls the behavior in question. In "rule-governed behavior," an individual is given a rule to follow and is either reinforced for following it or punished for not following it. Reinforcement depends on the degree to which the behavior parallels the rule. For example, if a member of a couple were to engage in a positive behavior toward his or her partner because the therapist had prescribed the task (i.e., rule) "Do one nice thing for your partner each day," his or her behavior would be shaped by the rule rather than anything in the natural environment. Rule-governed behavior is often, although not always, reinforced arbitrarily. In other words, the conditions under which the individual will be reinforced (i.e., for following the rule) and the reinforcer (e.g., a reciprocal behavior on the part of the partner resulting in therapist praise) are specified in advance; they do not emanate naturally from the experience. In contrast, "contingency-shaped behavior" is determined by the natural consequences of doing the behavior. For example, if something elicits one's feelings of tenderness and he or she does "one nice thing" for the partner, the behavior is shaped not by a rule, but by natural contingencies in the couple's environment. In this case, the behavior is reinforced by the experience itself (e.g., a spontaneous expression of feelings, a sense of doing something nice for the partner) and its consequences (e.g., the partner's genuine surprise and gratitude).

Change that comes about through rule-governed behavior is deliberate change that often involves effort by the participants. Often in couple therapy, the therapist or the partners specify "rules" that they wish to follow, such as going out on a date night once a week. They are reinforced by the therapist and/or each other when they put forth the effort and follow the rule. In contrast, change that comes about through contingency-shaped behavior is "spontaneous change." It happens "naturally" as partners respond to the contingencies of the situation.

In TBCT, change is created deliberately, through attention to rule-governed behavior using the strategies of behavior exchange (BE) and communication/problem-solving training (CPT). In BE, partners specify positive actions that they can take individually and jointly to improve their relationship. In CPT, partners learn the rules of good communication, such as using "I" statements rather than "you" statements, and summarizing and paraphrasing what the other has said. TBCT is founded on the assumption that the rules prescribed or generated by BE and/or CPT generate positive behavior and that this behavior, over time, provides its own reinforcement, thereby maintaining the rules.

The theory of IBCT, however, challenges these assumptions of TBCT and suggests that enduring changes are more likely to result from shifts in the natural contingencies operating in couples' lives than from generation of rule-governed behaviors. Importantly, behavior shaped by rules often "feels" different (i.e., less genuine, less authentic) than contingency-shaped behavior. For instance, a kiss from one's partner upon awakening in the morning, which is generated by a spontaneous feeling of attraction, is often experienced differently than a kiss generated by an intervention prescribed during therapy to "express more physical intimacy to each other."

Not only is rule-governed behavior likely to feel different than contingency-shaped behavior, it is also likely to be interpreted differently. Positive behavior as a result of therapeutic directives or business-like negotiations in therapy is likely to be interpreted less positively than "spontaneously" generated behavior. A partner might wonder whether the other "really meant" a rule-governed behavior or whether it was "really a sign of love" by the other.

Furthermore, many changes that couples cite as goals for therapy are not easily achieved by a focus on rule-governed behavioral changes. Whereas it may be fairly straightforward to address a partner's desire for more help with housework by negotiating new rules for housecleaning, it is much more difficult to address desired emotional changes with rule-governed behavior. For example, if one wants the other to "be more enthusiastic about sex" or to have "more genuine interest in me," it is not more challenging to address these issues with negotiation about rules.

Therefore, IBCT focuses on making changes in the natural contingencies that occur during the couple's life. The therapist becomes a part of the context of the couple's interactions within the session, and the interventions used by the therapist create a different experience for the partners than they have experienced on their own. For instance, rather than teaching partners that they should not blame or criticize one another (a rule), the IBCT therapist models noncritical behavior by validating each partner's perspective. Instead of teaching the partners the value of talking openly about their feelings (another rule), the IBCT therapist tries to create the experience of open disclosure. The therapist may inquire about the feelings of each partner or suggest possible feelings, particularly looking for so-called "soft" feelings, such as hurt, sadness, loneliness, as opposed to anger, hostility, and other "harder" emotions. These disclosures in session might spontaneously lead to greater responsiveness, and the partners may feel a sense of connection with each other. Thus, the therapist has created a reinforcing experience for the couple. He or she has had them *experience* the value of disclosure rather than telling them to do it. In these and other ways discussed in detail below, the IBCT therapist may work to increase the frequency of positive behavior or improve a couple's communication and problem-solving skills; however, the therapist is consistently seeking to generate these shifts by modifying the context of the partners' life rather than by teaching them new rules. Each intervention in IBCT is guided by this emphasis on using the natural contingencies of the partners' life to engage them in a new experience that will shift their behavior both within and outside sessions.

Finally, the IBCT theory of change also suggests that the successful practice of IBCT depends heavily on particular therapeutic clinical skills and attributes, which are reviewed below (see "The Role of the Therapist"). IBCT posits that therapist attributes and the couple–therapist relationship are central to the practice of competent IBCT.

THE STRUCTURE OF IBCT

IBCT is typically provided in an outpatient setting and generally includes one therapist and the couple. Typically, neither other family members nor cotherapists are included, though nothing in the IBCT theory precludes doing so if such inclusions seem warranted by the needs of a particular case.

In our empirical investigations of IBCT, we have used as a format a maximum of twenty-six 50-minute weekly sessions comprising three initial evaluation sessions, a fourth session devoted to feedback about the evaluation, and most of the remaining sessions devoted to intervention, with a final session or two devoted to summation and termination. However, from a conceptual standpoint, the structure and duration of therapy should be individually tailored to the needs of each couple. In general, the 50-minute weekly session format is well suited to many couples, who need the continuity and intensity of this structure. However, it is important to note that other couples may elect to

have less frequent meetings of the same or a longer duration (e.g., 2-hour sessions), due to demands of work or family life.

In IBCT, the duration of therapy and the timing of termination should be discussed collaboratively by the therapist and couple. The therapist should review with the partners their original presenting problems and the goals of each, and should help them to assess the progress they have made. Because IBCT is based on the premise that differences and disagreements are a natural part of a couple's relationship, neither the therapist nor the couple needs to wait until all problems are resolved to decide to terminate treatment. If the partners are able to discuss issues more calmly and find that they have a better understanding of one another's perspectives, and are less distressed by behaviors that formerly disturbed them, therapy has been successful, and it is appropriate to begin discussing termination. Some couples may prefer to employ a gradual fading procedure or return for booster sessions, whereas others may not. In fact, there are no hard-and-fast rules regarding when or how to terminate; as with other aspects of IBCT, we believe that listening carefully to the hopes and feelings of each partner is the best guide. We have found that, on average, couples participate in approximately 15–26 sessions.

The structure of each IBCT session is more flexible and open than is common in TBCT. In IBCT, the therapist and couple develop an agenda based on issues or incidents that are most salient to the couple. This initial agenda can shift if more salient issues or incidents come to mind for the couple. Acceptance-oriented sessions generally focus on four areas: (1) general discussions of the basic differences between the partners and related patterns of interaction, (2) discussions of upcoming events that may trigger conflict or slip-ups, (3) discussions of recent negative incidents, and (4) discussions of a recent positive interaction between the partners. These discussions, whether they focus on positive, negative, or upcoming incidents, reflect issues germane to the formulation. For example, a couple might discuss an incident in which the wife left on a short business trip, if such partings reflect a problematic theme such as closeness and independence in the relationship; however, the couple would not typically focus on a positive parting, such as a warm kiss goodbye, or a negative parting, such as the husband losing his way to the airport, if it did not reflect an ongoing relationship theme. In contrast, change-oriented sessions may be more structured and often include more didactically focused training provided by the therapist, as well as in-session role-play exercises and feedback from the therapist.

THE ROLE OF THE THERAPIST

The IBCT therapist functions in different ways depending on the context of a particular session. Although the IBCT therapist is frequently very active and directive in sessions, the particular form of the therapist's interventions will vary. In this way, being a good IBCT therapist requires comfort with a high degree of flexibility and change. In fact, it has become axiomatic among IBCT therapists that although it is essential to enter each session with a general plan or framework, there is nothing more important than a partner's most recent statement.

There are times, for instance, when the therapist may play the role of teacher or coach during a session, helping a couple to develop or improve skills in communication or problem solving. During these times, the therapist may be more didactic with the couple and rely on specific and structured rules of engagement and communication techniques (Gottman, Markman, Notarius, & Gonso, 1976). The therapist may, for example, instruct the couple to have a conversation during the session using specific communication guidelines, then provide feedback on the partners' performances.

Most often, however, the highest priority for the IBCT therapist is maintaining a focus on the case formulation of the couple (described below). In this sense, being a good and compassionate listener is one of the most important roles of the IBCT therapist. The therapist must be attentive to both verbal and nonverbal communications throughout the sessions and find skillful ways to maintain a focus on the couple's central theme, despite myriad specific issues and complaints that may arise. To maintain a focus on the formulation, the therapist must also take care to do so in a way that expresses genuine understanding and empathy for each partner. Thus, the therapist often acts as a balanced mediator, pointing out to each partner how current problems relate to ongoing themes that cause distress for them both. The therapist as mediator is also a teacher, however. IBCT therapists try to balance change and acceptance techniques. Rather than teaching rules in a didactic fashion (e.g., akin to a classroom teacher giving a lecture), the IBCT therapist tries to provide the

couple with a different experience in the session (e.g., akin to the same classroom teacher choosing instead to take students on a field trip). In general, the role of the IBCT therapist is to take a non-confrontational, validating, and compassionate stance in interactions with the couple (Jacobson & Christensen, 1998).

Another role of the IBCT therapist is to attend to and highlight the *function* of behaviors. Often, this requires that the therapist pay close attention to the function—rather than the content—of both verbal and nonverbal communications. For instance, Beth and Rick's therapist was able to ascertain that Beth's frequent smiling and laughter during the couple's heated confrontations functioned to express her anxiety about conflict, and her fear that Rick wanted to divorce. The therapist's emphasis on the function of Beth's behavior was in marked contrast to the couple's previous arguments over the content of Beth's behavior, which Rick had interpreted as scorn and indifference.

Interestingly, paying attention to the function of behavior frequently requires the IBCT therapist also to play the role of historian with couples. Consider, for instance, the role played by the therapist of Carol and Derek. Carol complains that her partner, Derek, always goes directly to the sofa and reads the newspaper when he comes home from work. She is angry and frustrated, because she would like to have time to interact with him. Derek, on the other hand, believes that he should have time to himself to unwind when he comes home from a very stressful day at work. The therapist recognizes that each partner feels isolated and blamed in this interaction; Derek feels accused of being lazy and disengaged, and Carol feels accused of being needy. The therapist also, however, has remained alert to salient historical information during previous interviews. The therapist may know that Derek's father died of a heart attack at the age of 46 and was a "workaholic," or that Carol's family never discussed issues, and that she had grown up believing her parents were not interested in her.

Using this historical context, the therapist suggested that these histories have occasioned the current behaviors and associated feelings. The therapist then solicited information about how Carol and Derek felt during earlier times and asked if they felt similarly now. Often, this focus will promote softer responses and greater empathy on the part of both partners. Thus, instead of saying, "He never talks to me; he just sits around and reads that damned paper!," Carol might say, "Yeah, when he is reading the paper I feel lonely. It seems like that is what home always has felt like, and I didn't want that to happen in my own home when I became an adult. I just want to feel cared about." Instead of saying, "Why can't she give me a break? I work hard all day and I just want some peace and quiet," Derek might say, "You know, I saw Dad dog tired every single day. He never stopped working, never took time for himself. He gave and gave to everyone, and it killed him. I am so scared that I'll turn into the same thing." The therapist, listening carefully, can then point out the theme of loneliness and isolation that is behind each partner's behaviors. Neither wants to abandon the other or to be abandoned. The therapist—as listener, mediator, and historian—can redirect the conversation in a fashion that allows the couple to talk about feelings, memories, and fears that are often obscured by the typical emphasis on accusation and blame.

Finally, a good IBCT therapist is also skilled at using language in a way that "hits home" (Jacobson & Christensen, 1998). The IBCT therapist uses language as an important intervention tool, because impactful language is one important way to alter a couple's relationship context. The therapists should be alert to ways to incorporate metaphors and terms that hold meaning for the couple and to increase the power of interventions and the likelihood that the couple will integrate the therapeutic ideas into their daily lives.

ASSESSMENT AND TREATMENT PLANNING

A comprehensive and structured assessment process provides the foundation for all future interventions in IBCT. Typically, the assessment phase is structured to involve three to four sessions that include an initial conjoint meeting with the couple, individual sessions with each partner, and a conjoint feedback session in which the results of the assessment are discussed and a plan for treatment is developed. Optimally, the therapist also has each partner complete a battery of questionnaires prior to the first conjoint meeting. Self-report questionnaires provide invaluable information for the therapist and can be easily mailed to the couple prior to the first session. Table 3.1 details questionnaires that we have found to be particularly helpful and each questionnaire's intended usage.

TABLE 3.1. Summary of Recommended Questionnaires

- *Dyadic Adjustment Scale* (Spanier, 1976): a useful global measure of couple satisfaction.
- *Frequency and Acceptability of Partner Behavior Inventory* (Christensen & Jacobson, 1997; Doss & Christensen, 2006): measures both the frequency of problem behaviors and the degree of dissatisfaction partners feel about such behaviors.
- *Marital Status Inventory* (Weiss & Cerreto, 1980): measures the number of specific steps a partner has taken toward divorce or separation.
- *Conflict Tactics Scale* (Straus, 1979): a widely used measure of domestic violence.

Functional Analysis

The foundation of any truly behavioral assessment process is the functional analysis. A clinician examines a problematic behavior and finds the stimuli that have given rise to it. With that information, the clinician can then alter the controlling stimuli and change the problematic behavior. In marriage, the problematic behaviors are negative feelings and evaluations of the relationship that participants often voice to themselves and others (and rate on our measures of relationship satisfaction). In both TBCT and IBCT, a functional analysis seeks to determine the events that give rise to this distress. However, typically in TBCT, assessment focuses on defining specific, discrete, and observable actions or inactions that partners mention as problematic. For example, a client may mention that his or her partner watches too much television. In a sense, assessment in TBCT highlights the "topography" of the behaviors that couples cite as problematic; therefore, the therapist learns a great deal about the size and shape of particular behaviors (e.g., how often and how much time the partner watches television). Unfortunately, as Christensen et al. (1995) suggest, this approach risks eclipsing the "true, controlling variables in marital interaction" (p. 35), with a focus on variables that are, in fact, only derivative of the controlling ones. This risk is particularly salient in couple therapy given that most couples present with a wide array of seemingly disparate complaints.

In contrast, assessment in IBCT aims to highlight the function as opposed to the topography of behavior. Therefore, the therapist seeks to understand the variables that control dissatisfaction, which are more often broad response classes of behavior (or themes, as we discuss below) than derivative variables. This emphasis on broad classes of controlling variables allows the IBCT therapist to see the common thread in diverse complaints and problems. Hence, Eva may complain that Dillon spends too much time watching television, but she may also become angry when he goes hiking with friends. In TBCT, these derivative variables are specified and pinpointed behaviorally as problems for the couple to address. However, in doing the functional analysis and emphasizing broad response classes, the IBCT therapist is able to see the themes of abandonment and responsibility in Eva's complaints. Actions by Dillon that abandon her and leave her shouldering family responsibilities are distressing.

A functional analysis in IBCT emphasizes not only the broad class of behaviors by the "agent" that is a source of dissatisfaction for the recipient but also the reactions of the recipient partner. For example, for Eva, these behaviors by Dillon are reminiscent of her past, when she was often left by her working parents to care for her younger siblings, and rouse similar feelings of abandonment and unfairness in her.

How is a functional analysis conducted? Ideally a therapist conducts a functional analysis by manipulating the conditions that are antecedent or consequent to the target behaviors and observing the behavioral response to such manipulations. Unfortunately, however, couple therapists do not have experimental control over the conditions that control the couple's interactions, so their ability to conduct a functional analysis is limited in a number of ways (Christensen et al., 1995). First, the therapist must rely on the partners' reports of their behavior and his or her observations of their behavior in session. He or she cannot directly observe the conditions surrounding their behavior in the natural environment. Second, people have idiosyncratic learning histories, and diverse stimulus conditions can serve similar functions. For example, Mike might become angry when Ruth gives him the silent treatment, but he might also become angry when Ruth tells him how she feels about his behavior. Thus, two different stimulus conditions, Ruth's silence and her talking, serve the same function of eliciting an angry response in Mike. Third, the therapist cannot directly influence the conditions of the couple's lives. He or she can not experimentally alter conditions to see their causal effect. Because of these limitations, the IBCT therapist is aware that his or her ideas about

the controlling events in couples' lives, developed from observations of their behavior in session and their reports about their behavior in and out of session, must always be held as tentative.

Case Formulation

The primary goal of the functional analysis is the development of a case formulation and a resultant treatment plan. In IBCT, the "formulation" comprises three primary components: the theme, the polarization process, and the mutual trap.

As noted earlier, the "theme" describes categories of conflictual behavior with similar functions. The theme is the broad class of behavior that serves as a basic unifying link among apparently disparate areas. In this way, the theme describes the group of behaviors in which each partner engages that serves a similar overriding function in the relationship. Thus, although the IBCT therapist continues to seek behavioral specificity in the assessment process, this aim is balanced by the need to attend to the *linkages* among problem behaviors. For instance, closeness–distance is one of the most commonly observed themes among couples seeking treatment. Among couples characterized by this theme, one partner seeks greater closeness, while the other seeks greater distance.

Jack and Suzanna, for example, struggled with the theme of closeness and distance throughout their 26 years of marriage. Jack prided himself on the values of autonomy, independence, and a stalwart approach to life. Suzanna, in contrast, valued open communication, connection, and closeness. Although they argued about many specific issues, ranging from what time Jack returned home from work in the evening to Suzanna's frustration with Jack's stoic response to her recent diagnosis of breast cancer, the function of each of their behaviors was consistent. Whether by staying late at work or retreating to his workshop at home, Jack sought greater distance. Whether by planning shared outings or tearful expressions of frustration, Suzanna sought greater closeness. Thus, the basic theme of closeness–distance remained consistent and captured the essential *function* of each of their behaviors.

In addition to the closeness–distance theme, some examples of other common themes in couple therapy include the control and responsibility theme (in which a couple argues about who maintains control and responsibility over particular domains of the relationship), and the artist and scientist theme (in which arguments surround one partner's tendency to value spontaneity and adventure, and the other's need for predictability and goal attainment). It is, however, important to emphasize that this list is not exhaustive; there are countless themes (and variations on themes) among couples. This discussion is intended to provide merely some examples of frequently observed themes among couples, and the ways that such themes can serve to unify a range of seemingly disparate conflicts.

In evaluating the theme for each couple, it is helpful also to assess the vulnerabilities that make this theme so emotionally distressing for partners. What past experiences may have made each partner's behavior in the theme so emotionally potent for the other? For example, with Jack and Suzanna's theme of closeness and distance, perhaps Jack experienced his mother as invasive and smothering and now experiences Suzanna in a similar way. He reacts to Suzanna's attempts at closeness as an effort by her to restrain his freedom. For Suzanna's part, her experience growing up in a large family may have given her the sense that she can never get the attention she needs. She experiences Jack's response to her efforts at closeness as the kind of brush-off that has been painful throughout her life.

The "polarization process" refers to the interaction patterns that are initiated when conflict around the theme occurs. Themes typically involve some expression of difference in a couple. Often, couples who contend with conflicts about their central theme assume that these basic differences are the problem, and that eliminating such differences is the necessary solution. Unfortunately, partners' attempts at eliminating these differences often have the unintended effect of strengthening—or polarizing—the differences even more! Thus, the "polarization process" refers to the ways that partners' efforts to change one another drive them farther apart. As polarization continues, these basic differences become further entrenched and are experienced as intractable and irreconcilable. The "mutual trap" refers to this effect, highlighting the impact of the polarization process on both partners. Both partners feel stuck, discouraged, and hopeless—in a word, trapped.

A good formulation includes a careful description of the theme and the associated vulnerabilities in each partner, the polarization process, and the mutual trap. However, the success of a formulation is not determined by the presence of these elements alone. The value of the formula-

tion is evaluated primarily according to what has been called the "pragmatic truth criterion" (Popper, 1942); that is, does it work? If a formulation "works," it will be a helpful organizing concept for the couple, one that the partners will integrate into their understanding of the relationship, and that will help to diminish blame and criticism and increase their readiness for acceptance and change. In contrast, an unsuccessful formulation fails to serve as such a central organizing concept; couples do not feel understood by the presentation of the formulation and do not integrate it into the basic vocabulary of the relationship. Although all formulations are modified and expanded in an ongoing and iterative fashion throughout the course of treatment, the core of the formulation is developed during the assessment phase of treatment. Both the structure and the content of the assessment phase have been carefully designed to facilitate the development of the formulation.

Guiding Questions

Overall, six primary questions guide the assessment phase and ensure that the therapist gathers information central to the development of the formulation:

1. How distressed is this couple?
2. How committed is this couple to the relationship?
3. What issues divide the partners?
4. Why are these issues such a problem for them?
5. What are the strengths holding them together?
6. What can treatment do to help them?

These questions are explored during both the conjoint interview and the individual interviews, and the information gathered is then summarized during the feedback session. These components of the assessment phase are discussed in turn below.

The First Conjoint Interview

During the first interview, it is important for the therapist to socialize the couple to the treatment model, establish trust, and instill hope. To socialize couples, therapists should explain the structure of the therapy, focusing in particular on the distinction between the assessment and treatment phases of the model. It is important to help couples anticipate the sequence of the upcoming sessions and remind them that treatment goals and an overall agreement regarding therapy will be the focus of the feedback session. Often, carefully explaining the separation of the assessment and treatment phases of IBCT is helpful for couples who have some hesitation about beginning treatment; therefore, the very structure of IBCT helps to honor and respect what is often the very natural ambivalence that couples experience.

The overall goal of the first interview is to achieve a successful balance between focusing on the partners' current presenting problem and on their relationship history. It is important for the therapist to understand what types of problems and conflicts have brought the couple into treatment. Moreover, couples often enter the first session wanting and expecting to talk about their dissatisfactions and disappointments. It is critical that couples leave the first session feeling heard, understood, and supported by the therapist. Therefore, the therapist should ask about the content of the problems, as well as basic interaction processes that occur when conflict arises. In addition, the therapist should be alert for precursors of the present problem in the couple's history (e.g., particular stressors the partners experienced in the past).

At the same time, however, it is important for the therapist to balance attention to these areas with a focus on the couple's history. Probing for information about how the couple behaves when things are going well, obtaining a history of initial attractions, and allowing partners time to talk about the time when their relationship was rewarding is critical for the development of the formulation. Unless the couple never had such a time and/or became partners for reasons other than love and romance, these strategies allow the therapist to begin to set the stage for a different kind of communication between the partners from the very first interview. Moreover, focusing on these areas helps to minimize the risk of increasing the couple's hopelessness, which may occur if the first session focuses exclusively on the presenting problems.

When discussing the relationship history, the therapist should inquire about the partners' early attraction to one another. Important questions may include the following:

"How did you meet?"
"What was your courtship like?"
"What was your relationship like before problems began?"
"What initially attracted you to one another?"

Often, the initial attraction is a central component of the formulation, because partners often find that the qualities that attracted them initially are the very same one that later cause distress and conflict. Partners may be attracted by qualities they themselves do not have, such as when an emotionally stoic person is attracted to an emotionally reactive person, and vice versa. The mesh or synchrony between these complementary qualities may be positive at times, such as when the reactive partner adds color to the relationship and the stoic partner adds stability to it. However, these very qualities can also be disruptive when, for example, the stoic partner finds the emotionally reactive one grating, or the emotionally reactive partner finds the lack of response from the stoic partner frustrating.

To inquire about relationship strengths, the therapist inquires about strengths present in the early phases of the relationship and asks what happens when things are going well. For instance, the therapist may ask,

"What parts of your relationship worked well when you were first together?"
"What parts of your relationship were you proud of?"
"How is the relationship different now during times that you are getting along?"

In addition, the therapist may want to focus on the couple's possible strengths and hopes for the future. It may be helpful to ask the partners how their relationship might be different if their current problems no longer existed.

Finally, we often close the initial conjoint meeting by assigning the first part of the IBCT manual for couples, *Reconcilable Differences* (Christensen & Jacobson, 2000). This reading assignment helps to engage couples in the treatment process and further socializes them to the model. Couples often recognize themselves in the case examples, and the book may help them consider their problems in light of the formulation proposed by the therapist during the upcoming feedback session. In addition, the partners' success at completing this first assignment also provides important information for the therapist about their level of motivation and commitment to therapy.

Individual Interviews

In IBCT, the therapist meets individually with each partner of the couple. Ideally the therapist would meet with each partner for a full 50-minute session. However, there are times when financial constraints or limitations of insurance plans make it difficult for a couple to come for two full-length, individual assessment sessions. Nevertheless, the therapist must stress that at least a split session is important as part of the assessment process. Time with each partner individually is necessary to gather critical information and to begin the process of building a strong alliance with the couple.

Each individual interview begins with an explicit discussion of confidentiality. The therapist explains that his or her confidentiality agreement with the couple differs from such agreements characteristic of individual therapy, in that the therapist has a responsibility to both partners. In general, IBCT therapists explain to each partner, "Unless you tell me otherwise, I will assume that any information you share with me is OK to discuss in our conjoint sessions." Given this, the IBCT therapist agrees to maintain the confidentiality of each partner's private communications to the therapist. If an individual communicates privately some information that is relevant to the current relationship, such as an ongoing affair or a decision to hide money from the partner, the therapist will keep this information confidential from the other. However, the therapist will ask the partner in question to resolve the issue (e.g., end an ongoing affair) or disclose the information to the other partner (e.g., tell the partner about the affair or the hiding of the money). If the individual cannot agree to the aforementioned options, the therapist should indicate that he or she cannot do couple therapy under these circumstances; that person is then left with the responsibility for communicating to the partner that couple therapy will not continue. The therapist should review these confidentiality provisions carefully with each partner at the outset of the individual session.

During the individual interviews, the therapist gathers information about four primary areas: presenting problems and current situation; family-of-origin history; relationship history; and level of commitment. Other special assessment issues, which are discussed in detail in the following section, are also covered during the individual interviews.

In regard to presenting problems, the therapist may begin by referring to the discussion of presenting problems during the conjoint meeting. The Frequency and Acceptability of Partner Behavior Inventory (FAPBI; Christensen & Jacobson, 1997; Doss & Christensen, 2006) is also a very effective method of assessing the major issues in the rela-

tionship from the perspective of each partner. The therapist should also assess the interaction patterns that pertain to these major issues and be alert for polarization processes and/or traps associated with these issues. Discussion of an individual partner's family history should include inquiry about his or her parents' marriage, the parent–child relationship, and the general family atmosphere. In general, the therapist should be alert to possible ways these early relationships may serve as a model for the couple's current problems. The individual interview also provides an important opportunity for the therapist to review each partner's individual relationship history with previous partners. Therapists should be alert to similar patterns or problems in prior relationships and/or ways that earlier relationships may serve as a possible model for the current couple's functioning.

Finally, the therapist assesses each partner's level of commitment to the relationship. Toward this end, it is important to inquire directly about commitment and to assess each partner's understanding of his or her role in the current problems. Often it is helpful to ask partners, "How do you contribute to the problems in your relationship?" and "What are some of the changes that you need to make for your relationship to improve?" Partners' answers to these questions help the therapist to determine the couple's degree of collaboration and commitment.

Feedback Session

The feedback session serves as the link between the assessment and treatment phases of IBCT. During this session, the therapist provides a summary of his or her understanding of the formulation and outlines a plan for treatment. The therapist should remind the couple of the focus of this session at the outset:

"This meeting is our feedback session, during which I will be providing an overview of my understanding of the problems you are facing and the way in which we will work on these problems. My hope is this will be a collaborative process and that you will both also provide feedback to me, correcting, confirming, and/or elaborating what I have to say."

In the best feedback sessions, the therapist solicits the couple's reactions throughout the session and frequently checks to make sure the formulation is meaningful to the couple. If one member of the couple disagrees, the therapist asks for clarification, then incorporates the feedback into the formulation. The therapist should never be defensive about his or her formulation, keeping in mind the centrality of the pragmatic truth criterion for evaluating the success of the formulation. Although the IBCT therapist wants the couple to buy into the formulation, he or she needs to remain flexible, taking into account the partners' understanding of their own problems and presenting the main points of the formulation using the couple's words and ideas.

The structure of the feedback session follows directly from the six primary assessment questions that guide the first three sessions. First, the therapist provides feedback about the couple's level of distress. Towards this end, it may be useful to discuss the couple's scores on relevant questionnaires that assess marital satisfaction or adjustment (e.g., the Dyadic Adjustment Scale [DAS]). Second, the therapist addresses the issue of commitment, again drawing from both the completed questionnaires (e.g., the Marital Status Inventory) and the individual sessions to discuss commitment. In regard to both distress and commitment, the therapist needs to evaluate whether it is more advantageous to emphasize the couple's relative high distress/low commitment to highlight the gravity of the partners' problems ·or their relative satisfaction/high commitment to assuage anxieties about their prognosis. Third, the therapist focuses on the issues that divide the partners, or their basic theme, referring to specific incidents that the partners mentioned in their joint or individual sessions and the specific items they noted on the FAPBI (Christensen & Jacobson, 1997) to present the theme. Fourth, the therapist provides an overview of why these issues create such problems for the couple. He or she discusses the vulnerabilities that make these issues so upsetting and details the polarization process, vilification, and mutual trap that the partners experience as they interact around these issues. Fifth, the therapist stresses the couple's strengths, often focusing on the partners' initial attraction to one another. Finally, the feedback session should include a clear discussion of what treatment can do to help the couple. During this part of the session, the therapist outlines clear treatment goals and a corresponding plan on which both the couple and therapist agree.

Special Assessment Issues in IBCT

It is important to note that the assessment process may also reveal particular clinical issues deserving of special discussion. As a general rule, there are few contraindications to IBCT; however, evidence of battering, an ongoing and undisclosed extramarital affair, and/or significant individual psychopathology (e.g., one of the partners has a psychotic disorder, or a partner is suicidally depressed) may require a referral to another treatment modality. Methods for assessing these areas and making appropriate treatment planning decisions are discussed below.

In general, the individual sessions provide the primary context in which the therapist probes carefully to determine the presence of these issues. In regard to domestic violence, partners should be asked directly about the use of physical, sexual, and emotional abuse tactics. It is often helpful to begin an assessment of domestic violence with general questions about how the couple manages conflict (e.g., "Can you describe a typical argument?" or "What do you and your partner typically do to express anger or frustration?"), followed by questions that assess the consequences of the escalation of conflict (e.g., "Do your arguments ever get out of control?" or "Have you or your partner even become physical during a conflict?"). It is important to use concrete, behaviorally specific terminology at some point during the assessment process (e.g., "Have you or your partner ever hit, shoved, or pushed one another?"), because some partners will not endorse global constructs of "abuse" or "violence" even when specific acts have occurred. It is always important to attend to safety issues, inquiring about the presence of weapons and other relevant risk factors, as well as the possible presence and/or involvement of children during violent episodes. We also strongly recommend the use of self-report questionnaires to assess the presence of violence (e.g., the Conflict Tactics Scale), because research suggests that wives are often more likely to disclose abuse in written, behaviorally specific questionnaires than on general intake questionnaires or during in-person interviews (O'Leary, Vivian, & Malone, 1992). We have couples complete the questionnaires prior to their individual session, so that we can probe for further information about any violence indicated. Finally, it is essential to assess the function of violent tactics, because violence used for the purposes of obtaining or maintaining a position of power and control in a relationship is a particular concern when assessing the appropriateness of couple therapy. If the assessment of violence reveals the presence of battering, we strongly recommend against couple therapy (Holtzworth-Munroe, Meehan, Rehman,

& Marshall, 2002). "Battering" is defined as the use of violence to control, intimidate, or subjugate another human being (Jacobson & Gottman, 1998); our specific, operational criterion for battering is a history of injury and/or fear of violence by a partner, almost always the woman. Given that couple therapy can provoke discussion of volatile topics, couple therapy sessions may increase the risk of battering (Jacobson, Gottman, Gortner, Berns, & Shortt, 1996). Moreover, the conjoint structure of IBCT may communicate to the couple that the responsibility for the violence is shared by both partners. For these reasons, we consider battering to be a clear contraindication of couple therapy. In such cases, we refer the abusive partner to a gender-specific domestic violence treatment program, and the victim to a victim service agency that provides support, safety planning, and legal services, if appropriate. If the assessment of violence, however, indicates the presence of low-level aggression, in which partners do not report injury or fear, IBCT may be indicated. In these cases, therapists should continue to use great caution and care; and as a prerequisite to beginning treatment, insist upon clearly stipulated "no-violence" contracts that specify detailed contingencies if violations occur.

During the individual sessions therapists should also ask partners directly about their involvement in extramarital relationships, including both sexual relationships and significant emotional involvements. In general, IBCT is not conducted with couples in which one partner is engaged in a current and ongoing affair. In such cases, the therapist recommends that the involved partner disclose the affair to the spouse and/or terminate the affair. If the partner agrees to terminate the affair but wants to keep it secret, the therapist arranges to meet periodically with each partner individually. During these individual sessions, the therapist finds out whether the partner's efforts to terminate the affair have been successful. It is often easier to start an affair than to end it. If the involved partner is unwilling to end the affair or to disclose it, the therapist informs him or her that couple therapy cannot be conducted with such an ongoing secret affair. The responsibility for handling the resulting situation is left to the client, who may suggest to his or her partner dissatisfaction with the therapy or therapist. If the unsuspecting partner calls the therapist for an explanation, the IBCT therapist simply tells that person to consult his or her partner about the reasons for ending the therapy. For example, in one case seen by Christensen, a couple sought marital therapy but the wife revealed a longstanding secret affair. She wanted to continue her secret affair but not reveal it to her husband, because the revelation might jeopardize her marriage and family (two children); however, she did want to improve some communication problems with her husband.. After Christensen discussed this issue with her and gave her individual referrals, she ended the treatment. If her husband had called to ask why therapy ended, Christensen would have told him that his wife made the decision and he should seek further information from her. For further discussion of affairs, see Jacobson and Christensen (1998).

Finally, therapists are advised to inquire directly about the presence of significant psychopathology, including current or past experience of mood disorders, substance abuse, and other relevant psychological problems. Therapists should employ standard diagnostic assessment practices, inquiring about major symptom criteria and the course of relevant disorders. In addition, current and/or past treatments should also be reviewed. In general, IBCT is often appropriate to treat couple issues when individual problems are successfully managed in concurrent individual psychological or pharmacological treatment, or when individual problems are closely tied to the problems in the relationship (e.g., depression as a result of marital discord). If there is evidence that a current episode of a disorder is not well managed by an ancillary treatment, therapists may want to consider postponing couple therapy and making a referral, so that an appropriate individual treatment plan can be established.

GOAL SETTING

The major treatment goals in IBCT are to help couples better understand and accept one another as individuals and to develop a collaborative set whereby each partner is willing to make necessary changes to improve the quality of the relationship. The manner in which this overall goal is achieved differs for each couple, depending on the partners' unique presenting problems and history. Specific goals for treatment are determined collaboratively by the therapist and couple, and are explicitly discussed during the feedback session. In general, treatment goals are guided in particular by the formulation developed during the assessment phase. Jacobson and Christensen (1998) recognize the formulation to be so important that they suggest an overarching goal in IBCT is to get couples to see their relationship through the lens provided by the formulation. Through reiterating the formulation as it relates to their daily struggles and joys, the therapist helps the couple process their interactions throughout the treatment. Using this linchpin of treatment, the therapist can then create an atmosphere in which problems are discussed in a fashion that differs from the typical conflict in which the couple has engaged.

Implicit in the goals of understanding, acceptance, and collaboration is the acknowledgment that staying together is not always the right outcome for all couples. It is important for the IBCT therapist to work diligently with couples to improve the quality of their relationship, while remaining neutral with regard to the ultimate outcome of their relationship status. This element of IBCT derives from both philosophical and pragmatic bases. Philosophically, IBCT takes no moral position on divorce. In the context of a particular case, IBCT might help a couple consider the benefits and costs of staying together versus separating, for both the partners and their children. Pragmatically, a strong emphasis on "saving the relationship" may also have iatrogenic effects. Often a strong emphasis on the importance or value of staying together strengthens the demand from one partner that the other change. However, the IBCT theory stipulates that often this very demand maintains and exacerbates the couple's distress. Thus, if Belinda believes she can tolerate Jonathan and stay with him only if he refrains from working excessive overtime and watching ball games on weekends, her desire to stay in the relationship will heighten her sense of needing these changes to happen. However, Belinda's demand for change may spiral into conflict and increase the discord in the relationship rather than allow her to reach the desired goal, a happier marriage. When partners are allowed to interact with one another, without the demand of staying together at all costs, it may be easier for them to begin to understand the motivations and histories behind one another's behaviors, and to become more accepting of those behaviors.

PROCESS, TECHNIQUES, AND STRATEGIES OF IBCT

The interventions used in IBCT fall into three categories: acceptance strategies, tolerance strategies, and change strategies. There are two strategies for promoting acceptance, namely, empathic joining and unified detachment. These strategies attempt to provide partners with a new experience of the issues that divide them; in essence, these strategies aim to help couples turn their problems into vehicles for greater intimacy. In contrast, tolerance strategies allow partners to let go of their efforts to change one another, without aspiring to the somewhat loftier goals of empathic joining and unified detachment. Tolerance is promoted through techniques such as pointing out the positive features of negative behavior, practicing negative behavior in the therapy session, faking negative behavior between sessions, and self-care (Jacobson & Christensen, 1998). Finally, change strategies are used directly to promote changes in partners' behavior and consist largely of behavior exchange (BE) techniques and communication/problem-solving training (CPT) interventions (Gottman et al., 1976; Jacobson & Margolin, 1979).

The principal strategies and techniques of IBCT are described below, followed by a discussion of how these interventions are sequenced throughout a typical course of therapy.

Acceptance through Empathic Joining

One of the two primary techniques to foster acceptance is empathic joining around the problem. When a couple enters therapy, both partners are typically experiencing a great deal of pain. Unfortunately, when they express their pain, they often do so with accusation and blame, which typically exacerbates their marital distress. Thus, the goal of empathic joining is to allow partners to express their pain in a way that does not include accusation. Jacobson and Christensen (1998) proposed the following formula: "Pain plus accusation equals marital discord, pain minus accusation equals acceptance" (p. 104).

Often, the therapist attempts to promote empathic joining by listening to the couple detail particular interactions, then reformulating the problem in light of the theme discussed during the feedback session. For example, a couple that experiences the theme of "the scientist and the artist," wherein one partner, Madeline, is very analytical in her approach to life and the other, Stephanie, is creative and free-spirited, may get into arguments over being on time for appointments. The therapist may say something like,

"As I see it, this argument between the two of you goes right back to the theme that we have discussed before. The two of you deal with life very differently. (*to Madeline*) You are very analytic, as we have said, you are the scientist. You like to have everything set and orderly. This makes complete sense given your upbringing and history. I completely understand that you want to be on time when an appointment is scheduled; you get very frustrated otherwise. I also imagine that you feel embarrassed or humiliated to show up late at events. Is that true? (*Madeline nods.*) However, Stephanie (*turning to partner*), you feel very stifled by such orderliness. What is most important to you is that life be comfortable and fluid. You feel very tied down by deadlines and structure. Having a structure makes you feel controlled, like you are a little kid unable to make up her own mind. (*Stephanie says, "Yes, that is exactly right."*) You aren't late in order to annoy Madeline, and Madeline, you don't push to be on time in order to control Stephanie. You both have very different feelings in this situation. You each feel very vulnerable in these situations in your own way."

Another empathic joining strategy is to encourage soft rather than hard disclosures. "Hard disclosures" often express feelings of anger or resentment and may place the speaker in a dominant position relative to the listener. IBCT assumes that a corresponding "soft" side to most hard disclosures expresses the hurt and vulnerability behind the anger. In therapy, this is often referred to as getting the partner to talk about the "feeling behind the feeling." Using this metaphor, the therapist communicates to the couple that the public expression is not always the full picture of the private experience of each partner. Encouraging soft disclosures is done to soften not only the speaker but also the listener.

For instance, one partner might say, "You never take time to ask me how my day went. You're just concerned with yourself. Well, I'm sick of it." In this statement, anger, resentment, and accusation are resoundingly communicated. To encourage soft disclosure, the therapist might ask the partner what other feelings might also exist with the anger. Or, alternatively, the therapist might suggest a feeling by saying, "I imagine that if I were in your situation I would feel. ... " The partner then is encouraged to disclose the softer feeling. In our example, the partner might say, "I feel like my day doesn't matter to anybody. I spend all of my time taking care of others, and I feel so drained. I feel lonely and unappreciated." The therapist would then turn to the other partner and high-

light the soft disclosure and elicit feedback. The therapist might say, "I wonder if you are surprised that your partner felt lonely during these times?" Ideally, the listener will begin to soften and may respond with a similar soft disclosure, such as "I never meant to make you feel unloved. You know I love you very much, and am sorry that I often get so wrapped up in my own day that I neglect to check in with you."

Another way of finding the soft disclosures is to create a safe environment where couples can talk about their vulnerabilities. In fact, it can sometimes be helpful for the therapist to point out mutual vulnerabilities in a couple. For example, Ellen and Craig had frequent arguments about money and child rearing. The therapist was able to help each of them articulate their vulnerabilities in these areas. Both were very responsible people who wanted to be successful in their endeavors. Ellen took primary responsibility for raising the children; therefore, she was very sensitive to doing a good job in this area. When Craig would take the children out for ice cream without first washing their faces or brushing their hair, Ellen would become irate. He considered this an overreaction. However, Craig was very meticulous about money and wanted to be a good provider for the family. When Ellen spent money that Craig did not anticipate, even if it was just a few dollars, it would lead to an argument. In this situation, Ellen thought Craig was the one who overreacted. The therapist pointed out their mutual vulnerability to being less than successful in their respective roles, and the two of them were able to empathize with the reactions that initially seemed irrational and exaggerated.

We should note a final warning in the use of soft disclosure interventions. When we speak of "soft" and "hard," we are referring to the function of the speech and not the form or content of the speech. For instance, not all apparently soft statements actually soften the emotional reaction of a partner. Imagine a couple whose distress is in response to the wife's depression. If a therapist were to try to get the wife to make a soft disclosure, such as "Sometimes I just feel so sad, like I'm just not good enough," this could lead to an angry response from the husband, who might anticipate such self-deprecating remarks. Although a statement may move the therapist, it might have the opposite effect on a partner. In this case, the proper "soft" disclosure may actually, in form, look harder. The husband may soften if the wife were to say something more assertive, such as "What I really want is to have you tell me that you like how my projects turn out at work, and I'd be happy if you would spend just a few minutes looking over the results with me." Here, there is an expression of the client's need, without accusation, and without the depressive self-debasement.

Therapists must therefore be aware and forewarned not to fall into a trap of accepting statements that appear "soft" as the type of disclosure necessary to actually soften a particular couple. Frequently therapists can be lulled into feeling that they have hit on something good when the speaker begins to cry; however, they must always remember that what is gold in the eyes of the therapist may possibly be tin in the eyes of the client. It is essential that therapists rely on a good functional analysis and the basic formulation to help guide them in selecting the most salient areas to promote soft disclosure.

Acceptance through Unified Detachment

The second principal method for promoting acceptance is unified detachment. Once referred to as seeing the problem as an "it," this strategy aims to help partners develop distance from their conflicts by encouraging an intellectual analysis of the problem. Like empathic joining, unified detachment aims to help couples talk about their problems without accusation and blame; however, unified detachment emphasizes the use of detached and descriptive discussions rather than emotionally laden discussions. Thus, when using unified detachment interventions, the therapist works with the couple to understand the interaction sequences that become triggered and that lead to the couple's sense of frustration and discouragement. The problem is reformulated as a common adversary that the partners must tackle together.

The therapist can promote unified detachment by continually referring back to the major theme in the partners' interactions, their polarization process, and the mutual trap into which they both fall. For instance, when Ray and David tried to resolve conflict about Ray's "flirtatiousness" with other men at social gatherings, the discussions quickly deteriorated. Ray accused David of being "jealous, timid, prudish, and overcontrolling." David accused Ray of being "insensitive, rude, slutty, and shameless." The therapist had earlier defined a theme of "closeness–distance" for Ray and David. In essence, Ray, a fiercely independent man, thrived on doing things his own way. He liked time alone and had been raised as

an only child. David, however, liked frequent interaction. He had grown up with three siblings, had never lived entirely on his own even in adulthood, and was very attracted to sharing time with others. Although the theme of closeness–distance was not readily apparent in the interaction about flirtatiousness, the therapist was able to make a connection, relating Ray's behavior as being consistent with his independence and need to have time to himself, even when the couple was in public; and David's behavior to his desire for closeness with Ray and for a feeling of belonging. The therapist was then able to help David and Ray recognize that they shared a dilemma they could seek to resolve together. This removed the element of blame and allowed them to look at the problem in a more detached manner.

Another way that an IBCT therapist can promote unified detachment is by helping the couple articulate the pattern in a particular conflict. By encouraging partners to take an observer's perspective on the conflict, the therapist can have each identify his or her triggers for emotional reactions, the escalating efforts to get the other to understand, the subsequent distance between partners as they "lick their wounds," and their perhaps unsuccessful efforts to bridge the gap between them. As the partners describe the pattern of interaction between them, they begin to see it in a less emotional, more detached, and, ideally, more unified way.

An IBCT therapist can also promote unified detachment by getting the partners to compare and contrast incidents that occur between them. For example, perhaps José was less disturbed by Maria working last Sunday than he was the previous Sunday, because they had spent such a close time together on Saturday night. If they both see how genuine closeness alleviates the distress of emotional distance, they may be able to better manage their needs for both.

At times, therapists may also choose to bring in a fourth chair and suggest that the partners imagine that the problem is sitting in the chair. This visual and experiential cue may help them remember to think of their problem as an "it," and as something that is external to their relationship. Often, it may also be helpful for the therapist to suggest that they designate a chair for the therapist during conflicts that arise between sessions. They can be instructed to talk to the imaginary therapist about what they would like to say, rather than actually saying such things to each other. The effectiveness of these techniques may vary widely across couples; but if the techniques enable the couple to talk about the problem at a distance, then they are successful.

Tolerance Building

Like acceptance interventions, tolerance interventions aim to help partners let go of fruitless struggles to change one another. Tolerance interventions are used with problems that the therapist believes have little likelihood of serving as a vehicle for greater intimacy for the couple. For these types of problems, the therapist attempts to help the partners build tolerance, so that they will be able to interrupt and/or recover from their conflicts more quickly. However, the therapist may also use tolerance interventions for the problems that were the focus of unified detachment and empathic joining. As illustrated below, the tolerance intervention of enacting negative behavior in the session may be an effective and dramatic way to create unified detachment and empathic joining.

It should be noted, however, that some types of problems are not amenable to acceptance or tolerance interventions. Some situations should neither be accepted nor tolerated, the most obvious of which are domestic violence and battering. No one should be subjected to abuse and danger in his or her own home. Other situations that may be intolerable include substance abuse, extrarelational affairs, or compulsive behaviors, such as gambling, that may jeopardize the well-being of both members of a couple. Thus, tolerance is not promoted as a means of maintaining an intolerable status quo. Individuals are not asked to tolerate all of their partner's bad choices; rather, they are helped to develop tolerance of partner behaviors that are not destructive and are unlikely to change. The four strategies used to promote tolerance are described and illustrated below.

Pointing Out Positive Aspects of Negative Behavior

Pointing out the positive aspects of behaviors that are problematic can be a useful method of increasing tolerance. Therapists are alert to ways that one partner's negative behavior may have positive aspects for the other, currently or in the past. Interestingly, the areas of conflict between partners in the present are often the very same areas that cause them to be attracted in the past. Alternatively, negative behaviors may serve a useful function in the present by helping partners to balance one another and provide greater equilibrium in some area of the relationship. Highlighting these aspects may help partners see the benefits of behaviors that are otherwise experienced as so distressing. It is important to note that the therapist relies on an understanding of the function of the behavior, rather than on concocting a "silver lining" and simply doing a positive reframing of a negative behavior.

Eva and Eric differed significantly in their attitudes towards spending money: Eva was more conservative about spending, whereas Eric was more liberal. Eric liked to buy new technological gadgets every payday, and he had gotten into the pattern of stopping off at a store on his way home, so that Eva would not prevent him from doing so. Eva, however, took money from her paycheck and put it in a savings account to which Eric had no access. Both became irritated by the other's behavior, and this led to many arguments. They had difficulty compromising in this area, because Eric felt that they were living like "paupers" if they did not spend a little money, and Eva feared that they would squander savings for their future if they spent too casually. Both had legitimate reasons for feeling as they did. The therapist chose to promote tolerance by pointing out the ways their behaviors served to balance one another. To do so, she asked each partner what would happen if his or her way of doing things were the only way the couple managed money. Through this intervention, they both were able to acknowledge the importance of the other partner's style. The therapist summarized the balancing function of their behaviors, explaining,

> "If you were both like Eva, you would have very few luxuries and life might seem rather dull, although it would feel stable. If you were both like Eric, you would be a little short-sighted when it comes to handling money and might occasionally have problems paying your bills. So, even though these differences may continue to irk you both, from my perspective, they are necessary to keep you enjoying life in a responsible fashion."

As with all IBCT interventions, the therapist remains nonjudgmental, validating both Eric's and Eva's perspectives. Notice, also, that the therapist does not point out the positive side of the negative behavior, then convey the message, "Great, now you are fixed!" In fact, she says, "These problems may continue to irk you." In other words, IBCT therapists are comfortable with the fact that problems may remain long after therapy is over. The hope, however, is that increasing partners' tolerance of their differences will break them free from the traps created by trying to change one another and allow them to live with a greater sense of satisfaction. It also may make them more open to specific compromises and solutions that might ease the problem.

Practicing Negative Behavior in the Therapy Session

The purpose of this technique is both to desensitize each partner to the other's negative behaviors and to sensitize the offending partner to the impact of his or her behavior on the other. These two objectives apply also to faking the negative behavior at home, which we address next. Asking couples to practice negative behavior in the session also allows the therapist to observe the interaction closely and may lead to either an empathic joining or unified detachment intervention, although this is not always the case.

Daren and Meg were polarized around issues of responsibility and control. They couple struggled significantly with a pattern in which Meg complained frequently, while Daren purposely did the opposite of what Meg requested when he thought she was nagging him. In the session, the therapist asked Meg to complain as much as she could, to really get into complaining. Daren was asked to be obstinate and to disagree with everything Meg said, even if he agreed with her. The first time the therapist tried this exercise, the spouses got into their usual emotional states: Meg got frustrated and felt powerless to influence Daren, who felt attacked and simply counterattacked by being obstinate. The therapist interrupted the sequence and use empathic joining to connect with the immediate emotional impact the exercise had on them. Another time that the therapist tried the exercise, the spouses found it funny. They were unable to get into their usual roles and laughed at what they perceived to be the "silliness" of their pattern. In this way, the exercise helped them achieve some unified detachment from the problem. Thus, the exercise to practice negative behavior in the session not only help partners achieve greater tolerance of the behavior but also may provide a vivid occasion for empathic joining and unified detachment.

Faking Negative Behaviors at Home between Sessions

Partners are instructed to engage in the behavior that has been identified as problematic, but only when they do not feel naturally compelled to do so. In other words, they are to do the behavior when they are not emotionally aroused. In the previous example, Meg was directed to complain at home when she did not feel like complaining; she was given this instruction in front of Daren, who was warned that he would not know when Meg was being real or being fake. Meg was to continue with the behavior for only a few minutes, then inform Daren that it was a "fake." They were then instructed to take a few minutes and debrief the interaction. Partners should tell each other what they observed during the interaction, and the partner who faked the behavior should, in particular, explain what he or she observed the impact of the faked behavior to be.

Partners frequently report that although they have difficulty actually completing this kind of homework, being given the assignment makes them more aware of their behavior. This increased awareness itself serves to decrease the problematic behaviors. Moreover, because the partners choose moments during which they engage in negative behaviors, these behaviors are brought under their voluntary control. This experience helps partners to realize that they have choices about how they want to respond to or interact with one another. Finally, because partners expect to be "faked out," they tend to react less severely to the negative behaviors that formerly annoyed them. In essence, each partner becomes desensitized to the negative behavior through repeated exposure and, as a result, tolerance is promoted.

Promoting Tolerance through Self-Care

Because there are many fixed patterns of behavior that individuals have great difficulty changing, it is often important to help partners learn to engage in self-care. Oftentimes, a partner who uses self-care to address important personal needs or areas of vulnerability is more able to tolerate his or her partner's negative behavior. For instance, Mary's job occasionally requires her to work later than she expects to manage crises that arise. On such days, she may arrive at home 1 or 2 hours later than when she and her partner Mark usually arrive home to make dinner together. Mark often becomes frustrated by Mary's tardiness on these nights, and his sense of frustration, combined with feeling hungry while waiting for her, often leads him to be irate by the time she gets home. It is on these nights that Mary and Mark have some of their most bitter and painful conflicts. Given that the demands of Mary's job seemed unlikely to change in the near future, their therapist worked with Mark to promote self-care during these times. Together, they decided that, on such nights, Mark would give Mary a grace period of 30 minutes after their appointed meeting time, and if she was late, he would go out to dinner at his favorite restaurant with a friend or on his own. This intervention helped Mark to satisfy his own need for a pleasant and relaxing meal. The couple was then able to discuss more calmly and collaboratively their mutual frustration with the demands of Mary's job when she arrived home.

Change Techniques

In addition to the acceptance interventions described earlier, IBCT incorporates some of the change strategies of traditional behavioral couple therapy. We describe these strategies only briefly, because they have been written about extensively (e.g., Jacobson & Margolin, 1979). Then we discuss their integration with the acceptance interventions of IBCT.

Behavior Exchange

The assumption that people are better at changing themselves than at changing others is the underlying principle of BE interventions. When partners each commit to changing their own behavior in such a way as to provide pleasure for the other, both will ultimately be more satisfied. Although BE can be implemented in many different ways, a classic BE exercise is to have each member of a couple write a list of behaviors that each believes would bring pleasure to the other. They are asked to do this at home, independently. Each is asked to write specific, observable and positive behaviors such as "bring home flowers" or "massage his shoulders," rather than negative behaviors such as "stop yelling at her when she forgets to bring in the recycling can." Once each partner has developed a comprehensive list, the lists are read aloud in the session. Then, the other partner indicates the amount of pleasure he/she would derive from the behavior. Eventually, the partners can make requests for additions to the lists. Neither partner

is committed to doing any of the specific behaviors on their list, although they do commit to doing some of them. They may each agree to engage in some of their behaviors from the list during the week or each partner may agree to set aside a "caring day" and do several of the items from their lists on that special day for the other. At the next session, the couple then relates the effects of the caring day to the therapist, who debriefs their experience and encourages them to continue with additional caring days or daily behavior exchanges to increase their mutual reinforcement.

Communication/Problem Solving

Training in both communication and problem solving is a staple of behavioral couple therapy and has been detailed in many articles and books (e.g., Gottman et al., 1976; Jacobson & Margolin, 1979). In general, in IBCT, both communication and problem-solving training are used, though there is often a greater emphasis on communication training interventions, because active listening and expressive training often overlap more readily with efforts to promote acceptance.

Communication exercises involve teaching partners to level with each other about their feelings, to edit out unnecessarily negative comments, and to validate one another. Each partner pays particular attention to the role of speaker or listener. The speaker is to use "I" statements, to be specific about the behaviors of the other that are distressing, and to edit the content of a statement to remove accusation, contempt, overgeneralizations, and the tendency to drag in "everything but the kitchen sink" (Gottman et al., 1976, Gottman, 1994). The listener is to pay careful attention to the other's message, accurately summarize that message to the other's satisfaction, and only then state his or her own message. Specific communication exercises and relevant reading materials are often assigned from *Reconcilable Differences* (Christensen & Jacobson, 2000) and *A Couple's Guide to Communication* (Gottman et al., 1976).

In problem solving, partners are encouraged to take a collaborative approach, to be willing to accept their role in problems, to define the problem clearly, then to consider solutions to the problem. Couples brainstorm solutions, stating as many as possible, without judging or discussing them. Once partners have generated a list of possible solutions, they use the principles they learned in communication training (i.e., validating, leveling, and editing) to discuss each possible solution. They finally decide on a solution and contract with one another to attempt it, specifying a time limit for trying the solution. After partners attempt the solution, they return to discuss and evaluate its success or failure and to modify it appropriately.

When we do CPT in IBCT, we are generally less rule-governed than in TBCT and try to adapt the principles of communication and problem solving to the idiosyncrasies of the particular couple. For example, we might not insist on the communication formula, "I feel X when you do Y in situation Z," but instead encourage spouses to do more of a particular component that is missing. So, if husband rarely mentions a feeling when he complains to his wife, we might encourage this behavior, even if he says it without the obligatory "I feel" (e.g., "I get really frustrated when you do so and so" would be great). Similarly, if a wife tends to make global characterizations, we would help her to specify the particular behaviors that are upsetting. However, we would also respond to her sense that it is not just one or two behaviors but a class of behaviors that are upsetting to her, and that this class of behaviors communicates something to her (e.g., a variety of distancing behaviors communicate a lack of love to her).

Sequencing Guidelines

Because IBCT promotes both acceptance and change in therapy, the therapist moves fluidly between these types of interventions throughout the therapy process. In general, the primary approach is to use more acceptance techniques than change or tolerance techniques (Jacobson & Christensen, 1998). The overall strategy is to start with empathic joining and unified detachment interventions. When couples appear to be stuck in patterns that are particularly resistant to change, the therapist might consider tolerance interventions. Often, acceptance and tolerance interventions may produce as a by-product the very changes that partners entered therapy requesting. Most partners do care about each other and wish to please each other, so when therapy is able to end the struggle for change, the cycle of "persist and resist" that is common in distressed couples, partners may accommodate each other. In these cases, the need for change-oriented techniques may be obviated.

With other couples, the acceptance and tolerance work creates the collaborative spirit required for change-oriented work, and therapy naturally progresses toward communication and problem-solving exercises. In all cases, change

techniques can also be interspersed throughout the therapy, though therapists should be quick to return to acceptance interventions if the emphasis on change appears to exacerbate conflict. IBCT therapists should never try to "force-feed" change strategies to couples at any point in the process of therapy.

Although we recommend these sequencing guidelines for therapists, they are only "rules of thumb." In some cases, for instance, couples may enter treatment with a strong collaborative set, and it may be appropriate to begin with change-oriented interventions. In general, the intervention chosen by a therapist at any time is highly dependent on the context in which a certain interaction is occurring, and fixed rules are difficult to delineate.

MECHANISMS OF CHANGE

As indicated earlier, IBCT theory suggests that improvements in relationship satisfaction and stability come about through changes in behavior, and changes in the emotional reactivity (acceptance) of that behavior. Using data from a large clinical trial of IBCT and TBCT (described below), Doss, Thum, Sevier, Atkins, and Christensen (2005) conducted a detailed examination of the mechanism of change. They found that changes in target behaviors were associated with improvements in satisfaction early in treatment, but that changes in acceptance of those target behaviors were associated with improvements in satisfaction later in treatment. TBCT generated larger changes in behavior than IBCT early, but not later, in treatment. However, IBCT generated larger changes in acceptance throughout treatment. Thus, the study provided important validation for the mechanisms of change in both IBCT and TBCT.

Perhaps all approaches to couple therapy agree that couples typically come in to therapy mired in unpleasant or destructive patterns of interpersonal interaction, such as patterns of mutual attack, attack and defense, attachment and withdrawal, or mutual withdrawal. The goal of therapy is to alter those patterns. One common method of achieving that goal is to alter those patterns directly and deliberately by instructing couples to behave differently (e.g., therapeutic directives, behavioral exchange strategies) or teaching them to behave differently (e.g., by teaching various communication, problem-solving, and social support skills). IBCT is not opposed to direct and deliberate approaches, if they work. However, IBCT suggests that those approaches may not work, or may work only temporarily, because the numerous contextual cues that elicit and maintain the problematic interactions in the natural environment will overwhelm any temporary benefit and momentum from the deliberately changed interactions. Instead of attempting to institute wholesale change in behavior, IBCT suggests instead that features of the problematic interactions themselves can lead to positive alterations in their occurrence. For example, suppressed fears, unspoken thoughts, and unvoiced emotions that occur during the interactions may, when vocalized with the help of a sensitive therapist, lead to important changes in couples' interactions. In the strategy of empathic joining, the therapist facilitates the expression of emotions and thoughts that may alter problematic interaction. Similarly, when IBCT therapists engage in unified detachment interactions by, for example, assisting a couple in a nonjudgmental description of the sequence of their problematic interactions, detailing the triggers that activate each, and the understandable but often dysfunctional reactions that each makes, the couple begins to alter those longstanding interactions. Thus, IBCT therapists often seek solutions to problems within the very problems themselves.

There is some evidence that couples in IBCT become more emotionally expressive and engage in more nonblaming, descriptive discussion. One early study documented that couples treated with TBCT and IBCT demonstrated significant differences in the types of interactional changes observed over the course of treatment (Cordova, Jacobson, & Christensen, 1998). For example, observations of early, middle, and late therapy sessions indicated that IBCT couples expressed more "soft" emotions and more nonblaming descriptions of problems during late stages of therapy than did TBCT couples.

TREATMENT APPLICABILITY AND EMPIRICAL SUPPORT

IBCT has been developed for use with both married or cohabitating couples and same-gender couples, though outcome investigations to date have focused only on married, heterosexual couples. In the latest and largest of these studies, efforts were made to recruit ethnically and racially diverse couples (Latino and African American therapists were

available) from diverse economic backgrounds, although the majority were still middle-class European American couples. Participation was limited to seriously and chronically distressed couples.

Couples Inappropriate for Treatment

In these clinical trials, couples in which there was evidence of battering were excluded. Also, couples in which a partner had a specific, individual psychological disorder that might undermine treatment were excluded: current Axis I disorders of schizophrenia, bipolar disorder, or alcohol/drug abuse or dependence; or current Axis II disorders of borderline, schizotypal, or antisocial personality disorder. Other disorders were allowed. In fact, in the most recent and largest clinical trial (discussed below), over half of the participants met criteria for a past or current DSM disorder. Participants were allowed to be on psychotropic medication as long as they were on a stable dosage and no change in medication during the clinical trial was anticipated. This latter requirement was instituted to ensure that changes as a result of medication were not confounded with changes as a result of couple therapy. The presence of a DSM diagnosis was neither a predictor of initial status nor a response to treatment (Atkins, Berns, George, Doss, Gattis, & Christensen, 2005). However, only 16% of the spouses had a current diagnosis, which may have reduced the likelihood of finding an effect for diagnosis. A quantitative measure of overall mental health was related to initial satisfaction but not to change in satisfaction.

Exclusion of these disorders from the clinical trials was primarily for methodological reasons. People with these kinds of serious disorders often need other, concurrent treatment besides couple therapy, but a requirement of the study was that no other psychotherapy was allowed except couple therapy during the treatment period, so that any improvements (or deterioration) could be attributed to the couple therapy. However, in practice, one might conduct IBCT with a couple, while one or both partners are receiving additional treatment. In fact, important research by O'Farrell and Fals-Stewart (2006; Fals-Stewart & O'Farrell, 2003) has shown that the addition of behavioral couple therapy enhances the effectiveness of treatment for substance use disorders. Therefore, the only couples we would categorically exclude from IBCT would be those in which one partner is a batterer.

Application to Same-Sex Couples

For the most part, same-sex couples present with the same problems as heterosexual couples (Kurdek, 2004). Although stereotypes suggest that same-sex couples cannot maintain stable relationships, especially gay male couples, who are more likely to have agreements about nonmonogamy (Solomon, Rothblum, & Balsam, 2005), such stereotypes are not borne out by the data comparing same-sex couples to heterosexual couples (Kurdek, 2004). However, one area in which same-sex couples may be more vulnerable is in the area of self-acceptance. Mohr and Fassinger (2006) found that individuals whose partners showed higher levels of identity confusion (i.e., difficulty accepting their own sexual orientation) tended to view their relationship more negatively. Individuals who believed they were similar to their partners in comfort or discomfort with a lesbian, gay, or bisexual identity reported higher satisfaction. Alternatively, individuals reporting difference in their partner's level of comfort reported lower ratings of satisfaction. Perceived similarity ratings were inversely associated with each partner's own levels of internalized homonegativity, stigma sensitivity, and identity confusion. Thus, couples with less positive sexual orientation identity may be least likely to experience the benefits of perceived similarity, despite actual similarity, given that individuals who have internalized such negative beliefs do not perceive similarity with their partners. A sensitive IBCT therapist employing empathic joining or unified detachment techniques may help partners in such situations process their disagreements and gain a better understanding for one another and, we hope, greater acceptance of themselves in the long run.

As in any therapy with lesbian, gay, and bisexual clients, IBCT therapists need to be aware of their own biases and gather objective information about working with such clients. Several general texts may help therapists less familiar with working with lesbian, gay, or bisexual clients to gain understanding prior to working with same-sex couples (e.g., Martell, Safren, & Prince, 2004). It is suggested that therapists who cannot practice affirmative therapy with same-sex clients should not work with these couples. There is not a great deal of modification required to the therapy, however, for skilled IBCT therapists who understand some of the issues facing same-sex couples and can affirm such relationships.

Empirical Support

Three empirical studies of IBCT have been conducted. In his dissertation, Wimberly (1998) randomly assigned eight couples to a group format of IBCT and nine couples to a wait-list control group, and found superior results for the IBCT couples. In an early, small-scale clinical trial (Jacobson, Christensen, Prince, Cordova, & Eldridge, 2000), 21 couples were randomly assigned to TBCT or IBCT; results demonstrated that both husbands and wives receiving IBCT reported greater increases in marital satisfaction than those receiving TBCT (as measured by the DAS and the Global Distress Scale [GDS]) at the end of treatment. Moreover, with use of clinical significance criteria, results further suggested that a greater proportion of couples treated with IBCT improved or recovered (80%) compared to couples treated with TBCT (64%).

In a large-scale clinical trial conducted at UCLA and the University of Washington, 134 seriously and chronically distressed couples were randomly assigned to IBCT or TBCT. Treatment comprised a maximum of 26 sessions, typically over a period of 8–9 months. Couples participated in extensive assessments prior to, during, and after treatment, and for 2 years following treatment. Couples in both conditions showed substantial gains during treatment (Christensen et al., 2004) that were largely maintained over the 2-year follow-up period; 69% of IBCT couples and 60% of TBCT couples demonstrated clinically significant improvement at the 2-year follow-up relative to their initial status (Christensen, Atkins, Yi, Baucom, & George, 2006). However, results favored IBCT over TBCT couples (e.g., IBCT couples who stayed together were significantly happier than their TBCT counterparts).

CASE ILLUSTRATION

The following case illustration provides a more detailed example of a typical course of IBCT and some of its primary interventions. First, information that can be gathered in the initial joint interview is provided. Second, the information about each individual that is gathered during the individual interviews is reviewed. Third, the themes, traps, and polarization process presented during the feedback session are described. Finally, because IBCT sessions typically focus on debriefing weekly incidents, several of the key incidents that occurred during this couple's therapy are discussed, and examples of empathic joining, unified detachment, and tolerance techniques used with the couple are illustrated.

Information from the Initial Session

Jennifer and Cole, introduced earlier, came to therapy because they believed themselves to be as stuck as they had been 7 years earlier. During that earlier time, they had considered divorce, entered therapy, and found that couple therapy was very helpful. They had been married for 15 years and had known one another for 19 years. Cole was 53 years old, and Jennifer was 39. They had two small children, a son age 3 and a 3-month-old daughter. Jennifer had worked as an executive assistant, and Cole was an artist. After the birth of their second child, Jennifer was approaching a time when she would need to return to her former job, and Cole was preparing to be the primary parent at home during the day. Cole's art work provided less steady employment and income for the family; however, his experience in the past had been that one good commission could provide enough income for the family to live on for a year, even if he only worked for a few months out of the year. Cole did not want to have to give up his career to settle into a full-time job. He needed the flexibility that he currently had in his schedule to prepare for exhibitions and to solicit commissions. Therefore, during times when his artwork provided little income, Jennifer took primary financial responsibility for the family. Unfortunately, Jennifer now found that rather than return to work, she wanted to be a "stay-at-home mom." The couple began therapy, locked in conflict regarding this issue.

Cole believed that the issues regarding the division of parenting and employment had been debated and resolved prior to the birth of their second child. He was surprised when Jennifer told him that she wanted to stay at home and not return to work. Jennifer said that she had always wanted to be the primary parent, but that it just was not feasible with their financial situation. Cole and Jennifer agreed that this type of exchange typified their disagreements. They would discuss an issue, and Cole would believe that the issue was resolved; however, then Jennifer would mentioned the issue again several months later.

Jennifer and Cole had met when Jennifer was in college. Cole had frequently exhibited artwork in a restaurant where Jennifer worked part-time as a waitress. Jennifer had been impressed, because Cole was very handsome and outspoken. Although she did not think much of exhibiting artwork in a restaurant, she knew that Cole also had pieces on exhibit in reputable local galleries and that he was successful in his career. She liked the fact that he was older, because she had become disillusioned with the apparent irresponsibility of men her own age. Cole had been married before and had been divorced for 3 years prior to meeting Jennifer. He thought she was one of the most beautiful young women he had ever seen. Jennifer's interest in his artwork and her guileless approach to life were very appealing to Cole. He believed Jennifer was someone who would respect and admire him.

The two began dating soon after they met, and she moved into his apartment three months later. Although Cole was not interested in getting married again, Jennifer recalled feeling that she knew he was the man she would eventually marry. They lived together for 4 years prior to getting married. Cole had remained reluctant about getting married and wanted to be able to have a sense of freedom regarding his career. His first marriage had ended over differences about the area of the country they would live in, income, and the lack of stability inherent in Cole's profession. Jennifer had always planned to be married. She had tolerated living together for the first 3½ years, but then had demanded that they legalize their union. Cole did not want to lose her, so he agreed.

Information from the Individual Interview with Jennifer

Jennifer had been raised by working-class parents in a suburban community. Her parents were very protective of her, and her mother had been demanding and controlling when Jennifer was growing up. She would experience very dark moods, in which she harshly criticized Jennifer. Jennifer would cope with her mother's emotional displays by shutting her out. Although her mother was never abusive, she would demand that Jennifer do chores around the house exactly her way, and Jennifer resented the control her mother had over her. Jennifer had wanted to move away for college, but her mother demanded that she stay at home. When Jennifer first met Cole, her parents thought he was too old for her. They were particularly unhappy when Jennifer moved in with him so soon after they met. To Jennifer, this was a way out of her mother's house, although she also had fallen deeply in love with Cole.

Jennifer always worried that Cole did not love her. She wanted to please him and usually complied with his requests or demands. They agreed on most issues, such as politics and religion, and shared many values. Cole, however, had not been as interested in parenting as Jennifer, and she had to work hard over the years to convince him to have children. In fact, it was the issue of children that had brought them to therapy 7 years earlier. At that time, Jennifer had decided she wanted to be a mother and that Cole must either agree to having children or she would leave the marriage. Cole was angry, because he thought that he had made it clear to Jennifer prior to marriage that he did not want children.

The two had many arguments, but the arguments never involved physical aggression or violence. Jennifer did not feel intimidated by Cole, although she did not like it when he became intense and loud. She felt that she could not think fast enough on her feet during those arguments, and that Cole usually got his way. She was tired of the instability of his career and wanted him to get a regular, full-time job so that she could stay home with the new baby. At the same time, Jennifer was very committed to the relationship and interested in doing what she could to make the marriage work. She denied having any extramarital affairs.

Information from the Individual Interview with Cole

Cole corroborated much of Jennifer's story about the early years of the relationship. He had particularly liked the fact that Jennifer seemed open-minded toward new ideas and nontraditional styles of living. Being an artist, he knew that it required flexibility, and he had already seen one relationship ruined because of the difficulty of living an artist's life. However, Cole believed that he needed to sacrifice for his art, and his profession was very important to him. He had agreed to have children with Jennifer provided that they work out a way it would not interfere with his profession. Now that Jennifer wanted to stay home and take care of the baby, Cole felt resentful. Still, he also felt very committed to Jennifer and stated that he was in the marriage "for the long haul." He also denied any domestic violence or extramarital affairs.

Cole was the eldest of two children. His brother had been killed suddenly in a car accident when Cole was in his early 20s. Soon afterward his mother had been hospitalized for a major depressive episode, after which, Cole reported, she was

never the same. He had felt abandoned by both his brother and his mother during the early years of his career. His mother ultimately died by suicide when he was 27, which increased Cole's fears of being left. Cole did not have a history of depression or other psychiatric problems, though he described himself as moody. Prior to the death of his brother and mother, Cole had believed his family was very stable. His mother's psychological difficulties had been a shock to him.

The Feedback Session

Cole and Jennifer had completed several questionnaires prior to beginning therapy. The combination of scores on the DAS (Spanier, 1976) and the FAPBI (Christensen & Jacobson, 1997) showed them to be moderately distressed. Jennifer's score on the DAS indicated that she had significantly greater distress than Cole. Areas of concern for the couple included child rearing, being critical of one another, and finances.

Initially, it appeared that a theme akin to "artist and scientist," with one partner very free-spirited and the other very analytical, applied to Cole and Jennifer. However, upon reflection, it became clear that this was not the case. Though Cole was clearly the artist, Jennifer was also a dreamer. They were simply more artistic or more analytical in different areas of their lives. Instead, the themes of abandonment and control versus responsibility seemed most salient for Jennifer and Cole.

Both were vulnerable to the theme of abandonment because they responded to each other in ways reminiscent of their families of origin. When Cole became critical or animated, Jennifer would become concerned that he was going to leave her. She had felt unloved when her mother was critical, and Cole's criticism also made her feel unloved. Cole, on the other hand, feared that Jennifer would leave if she disagreed with him, or if life became too complicated. He always tried to come up with a solution to everything. When she would apparently agree with his solutions, then tell him months or even years later that she did not agree with him, Cole would feel that his life was changing in a "flash," just as it had when his brother was killed.

They were polarized around issues of managing finances and taking care of the children, because they could not agree on who should be the primary breadwinner. Although Jennifer had been intrigued by Cole's career as a professional artist when they were first together, she had begun to resent it as she experienced the necessary compromises that needed to be made. Cole, who liked the fact that Jennifer had admired and perhaps even idolized him when they were first married, now resented the fact that she did not want to take the primary responsibility for earning money for the family.

They became trapped when they tried to resolve these issues; Cole would try to solve the problem, becoming more and more adamant about the solutions he generated. As he got more "intense," however, Jennifer would stop talking and simply become silent. Cole would interpret her silence as agreement. The discussions would end, and the couple would not address the issues until Jennifer would bring them up again at some point in the future. At this point, Cole would be surprised that an issue he believed to be resolved was again causing distress. He then became more critical of Jennifer, believing that she was "changing on him." Then the pattern would begin again, with Cole taking control and pushing for a solution, and Jennifer becoming silent.

Examples of the Three Primary Techniques Used in IBCT

The three primary techniques of IBCT—empathic joining around a problem, unified detachment, and tolerance—are illustrated with examples from Cole and Jennifer's case.

Empathic Joining around the Problem

At one point in therapy, Jennifer's maternity leave was about to end, and she had contacted her boss to discuss returning to work. Cole and Jennifer had a therapy appointment 2 days before her scheduled return to work. She was very upset about needing to go back to work. Cole was angry with Jennifer for being upset. He, as usual, had believed that the issue of Jennifer returning to work was resolved.

COLE: You know, I just don't understand it. This is always what happens. Jennifer knew she would go to work, we had agreed on this a long time ago.

JENNIFER: I didn't realize it would be so hard to go back. I feel like I have so little time with the baby as it is.

COLE: But that was our agreement—if we had kids, it wouldn't interfere with my art. You know you make more money than I do, and you act as if

my staying at home with the kids isn't work as well.

JENNIFER: (crying) This just makes me very angry.

COLE: (increasing the volume of his voice) Well, that makes two of us who are getting angry.

THERAPIST: (to Cole) You know, this sounds to me like a situation that is similar to others we have talked about in the past, in which you feel like Jennifer is changing her mind on something midstream.

COLE: Exactly, I thought we had settled this.

THERAPIST: (to Jennifer) I suspect that you had settled it, in theory. But I'd imagine now that you find yourself very attached to the baby, and that it is very hard to break away and go back to work.

JENNIFER: It is terribly hard. I feel like I'm only going to see her when she is sleeping, and I want to be able to spend all of my time with her.

COLE: But we agreed . . .

THERAPIST: Hold on a second, Cole. Jennifer, I could be wrong, but it seems like you are not necessarily refusing to go to work, but that you really just need to feel this sadness right now.

The therapist at this point is trying to elicit a softer response from Jennifer, in the hope that this will in turn soften Cole's angry responses.

JENNIFER: Yes, I know that I need to return to work, but I feel terrible about it. I just want Cole to understand that this is hard for me.

COLE: I know it is hard. It always has been hard.

THERAPIST: (to Cole) I want to make sure that you are really hearing what Jennifer is saying. You are getting angry because you think she is changing her mind about returning to work, but in fact she is planning to return to work. She just feels really sad. I'm hearing Jennifer say that she just wants you to sympathize with her sadness, is that right, Jennifer?

JENNIFER: Yes.

THERAPIST: (to Cole) So, do you see that this is not about changing plans, that it is about feelings associated with the plan the two of you have agreed upon?

COLE: I do see that, but what can I do?

THERAPIST: Now, I think that is why you get so angry, because you want to fix this and make Jennifer's feelings go away. To do that, you'd have to take a "straight" job, which would mean sacrificing your art. Jennifer isn't asking you to do that, isn't that right, Jennifer?

JENNIFER: Well, I'd be glad if Cole did take a regular job, but I know he'd ultimately be unhappy. Plus, he couldn't make as much money as I do anyway at this point.

THERAPIST: But you want him to know that this is hard.

JENNIFER: I just want his love and support, and I want him not make me feel like I need to just return to work and be a trouper.

COLE: I do support you, Jennifer. I don't know what I can do to let you know that.

JENNIFER: Just acknowledge that I am making a sacrifice, and that this sacrifice hurts.

COLE: I know this is a very painful sacrifice for you. I want to make you feel better about it and I feel impotent to do anything.

JENNIFER: You don't have to do anything, just be OK about my not being OK about this.

COLE: I can do that.

When using an empathic joining intervention, the therapist does not attempt to encourage the partners to resolve the conflict or to compromise with one another. The task of empathic joining is to help the partners discuss problems in a way that allows them both to feel that they are being heard. In this example, Cole was feeling accused and guilty. The therapist further explored Cole's feelings later in the session. It was important for Cole first to acknowledge that Jennifer's feelings were valid, and that he could feel empathy for her situation. Although this did not resolve the problem, it softened the interaction, so that they could discuss the problem in a kind and understanding way.

Unified Detachment

Cole had an opportunity to make a financial investment; however, he and Jennifer had become polarized around this issue. Jennifer wanted to pay back debts, and Cole wanted to invest, in the hope that he could obtain a good return to help support their children's future. As in many unified detachment interventions, the therapist used empathic joining to help soften the couple around the issue, then pointed out the problem, which was framed as "Cole and Jennifer both want to have a secure

future but disagree how that is best accomplished." When they were able to see the situation as both of them wanting a secure future, they were able to compromise on the investment. Although Cole still made the investment, Jennifer was able to express her concern about their debts and to develop a plan for paying off the debts in a more rapid fashion than they had been doing. Also, Jennifer agreed to become more involved in following the investments, so that she would be aware of what was going on with their money.

Tolerance

One of the primary patterns of distress involved Cole's raising his voice during arguments and coming across like a salesman rattling off reasons for Jennifer to accept his point of view. Jennifer would consequently "shut down" and become silent. The therapist determined that the partners would likely experience great difficulty in breaking this pattern, because it had existed for so long and paralleled many of the patterns present in their families of origin. Thus, the therapist decided that a tolerance exercise could help to desensitize them to this pattern and alleviate some of the difficulty it generated. Therefore, the therapist was not attempting to change the behavior but was instead helping the couple to build tolerance, so that Cole was less distressed when Jennifer became silent, and Jennifer was less distressed when Cole raised his voice or adamantly argued his point of view.

During a discussion, the therapist suggested that the couple demonstrate this behavior.

THERAPIST: Cole, I want to see you get intense in this session. I'd like you to demonstrate this for me here and now. I want to see how you convince, cajole, and sell your perspective.

COLE: Really? As intense as I can be?

THERAPIST: Yes, I want to actually see what happens between the two of you at home. Can you do that?

COLE: I'll try.

THERAPIST: Jennifer, I'd like you to tell me if you think that Cole is showing it here like you see it at home, OK?

JENNIFER: OK.

COLE: Ready?

THERAPIST: Go ahead.

COLE: I think that we should take money out of

our CD and invest it in Harold's venture. I trust Harold, and I wouldn't suggest that we do this if I didn't. (*Speaks rapidly and raises his voice.*) I don't understand why you don't want to do that. It makes complete sense to me.

THERAPIST: (*to Jennifer*) Is this the way Cole is at home?

JENNIFER: Well, not exactly. He gets more demanding, and more demeaning. Also he just fires his points, one after another.

COLE: (*speaking very loudly*) I don't understand how you think I am demanding about this. I think that what I am saying about this investment makes perfect sense. I've looked into other investments. I called about Harold's ideas and I looked into the reputations of the other investors. I don't demean you. I think things out and I come to you with careful decisions. You seem to think that I'd just toss away our family's security . . .

JENNIFER: (*to therapist*) now you're seeing it.

Jennifer was then able to talk about Cole's behavior and her impulse to shut down. She did not shut down in the session, however, and was able to provide feedback to Cole about how his "salesmanship" made her feel. She could identify Cole's exact behaviors that emitted her desire to withdraw. The beginning of tolerance happened in the session. There was great improvement in Jennifer's ability to tell Cole when she felt like shutting down, and to allow the therapist to help her to remain focused and express the impulse aloud. This is a good example of a tolerance exercise in session, but it also highlights the fact that acceptance interventions often overlap. This tolerance exercise also resulted in empathic joining when Cole was better able to understand the impact his behavior had on Jennifer, and to tell her how he felt when she shut down.

The therapist later suggested the following "faking negative behavior" exercise for them to try at home regarding a related behavior. Cole was troubled by their frequent bickering, because he interpreted bickering as indicative of a bad relationship. They often bickered over issues that Cole thought they had resolved, because of the pattern identified earlier—that he would rattle off his opinions and solutions, and Jennifer would withdraw. He would interpret her resignation as resolution, but when she decided to approach the topic again, Cole would be shocked, thinking that

she had shifted positions on him. Jennifer was not as concerned. She thought that bickering was a part of relationships, although she found it to be unpleasant when it occurred. They agreed to try a tolerance assignment about bickering. Jennifer was to bring up a topic that she knew had been resolved. She was only to allow this interaction to continue long enough to see Cole's reaction, then tell him that it was part of the therapy assignment.

Cole was also given a "fake negative" assignment. Jennifer would get annoyed when she sought emotional support from Cole and he responded with solutions. For example, when she would say, "I am really stressed about work," Cole would immediately say, "Well, maybe you should switch to three-quarter time." His faking behavior was to propose a solution when he knew that Jennifer wanted support, maintain his position for a moment and observe her response, then debrief the assignment with her.

Cole and Jennifer never actually followed through with their assignments intentionally, but they reported in the following session that expecting one another to fake the behavior made the behaviors less aversive when they did occur. Moreover, they were able to gain greater awareness of this pattern and to identify it more readily when it did occur. The IBCT therapist places less emphasis than a TBCT therapist on requiring couples to complete the homework. Rather, he or she highlights the shifts that occur through the interventions, regardless of the clients' absolute compliance. The therapist maintains a stance of acceptance but also trusts the shift in context to promote both change and acceptance, even if the couple complies poorly but benefits by becoming more aware and desensitized to behaviors that had previously caused distress.

Case Summary

Jennifer and Cole completed 26 sessions of IBCT. At the termination of therapy, both stated that they were better able to understand each other's positions on a number of issues. Cole felt discouraged that they still bickered as much as they did; however, they had developed greater humor about these ongoing patterns and began jokingly to refer to one another as the "Bickersons." Treatment did not resolve all of their problems. Jennifer still had to go to work full-time when she did not want to. Cole, however, recognized the reality of their situation, empathized with Jennifer, and spontaneously took steps to change. He took a part-time job outside of his profession to help support the family, and was then able to devote only a portion of his time to his art. At the end of therapy, however, both partners felt that they were on the same side and supported each other in areas in which they were both vulnerable.

Throughout therapy, there were frequent discussions of familial patterns that were relevant to current feelings. Both of Jennifer's parents had been very poor in their youth, and they had a very strong work ethic. To them, being in the arts was a luxury. Jennifer realized that she often dismissed Cole's art the same way her parents would have, as not being legitimate labor. Cole recognized that he was always waiting for Jennifer to change suddenly and do something irrational, although she was, in fact an extremely rational and emotionally even person. His expectations related more to the tragedies that had occurred in his family of origin than to Jennifer's behavior. As they began to understand one another's emotional and behavioral repertoires, they were able to feel less isolated from one another during times of disagreement. Jennifer felt more comfortable expressing her opinions and was less likely simply to choose silence in response to Cole. Cole continued to express himself in a fashion that Jennifer considered intense, but he was more solicitous of her input than he had been prior to therapy.

All three of the IBCT interventions were applicable with Jennifer and Cole. They had become polarized over the major theme of responsibility and control, and around the theme of abandonment. Cole softened in his interactions with Jennifer as the empathic joining techniques were used during therapy. They were able to recognize their problem as an "it" that they could work together toward solving when the therapist made unified detachment interventions. Furthermore, there were areas that were unlikely to change, because they involved overlearned, emotion-based, habitual behaviors, such as Cole's rapid-fire intensity when trying to fix problems and Jennifer's tendency to shut down. Tolerance exercises helped to desensitize the partners to these interactions, even though they were unlikely to change. Jennifer and Cole also illustrate how IBCT can be useful with couples when traditional behavioral interventions do not work. When the therapist attempted to have them practice "active listening" during one session, they thought that paraphrasing one another felt impersonal and stated emphatically that they were unlikely to do this at home. By using

empathic joining and helping them articulate the "feelings behind the feelings," the therapist was able to achieve the same goals without teaching a specific skills set of active listening. Natural contingencies were more powerful than artificial reinforcers or rules in maintaining shifts in this couple's behavior.

Objective measures showed improvement for Jennifer, who had been significantly more unhappy in the beginning of treatment. On the DAS and GDS she made reliable improvements that moved into the nondistressed range. Cole verbally acknowledged that therapy had helped tremendously, but this was not reflected in objective measures, which changed very little for him. Long-term follow-up will allow the final analysis of the benefit of therapy for this couple.

SUGGESTIONS FOR FURTHER READING

Treatment Manual

Jacobson, N. S., & Christensen, A. (1998). *Acceptance and change in couple therapy: A therapist's guide to transforming relationships*. New York: Norton.—This is the current treatment manual used the in large clinical trial discussed earlier.

Guide for Couples

Christensen, A., & Jacobson, N. S. (2000). *Reconcilable differences*. New York: Guilford Press.—This self-help book was assigned to couples as they went through treatment.

Research Studies

The following studies describe clinical trials of IBCT: Wimberly (1998); Jacobson et al. (2000); Christensen et al. (2004); and Christensen et al. (2006). A study of predictors of response to treatment can be found in Atkins et al. (2005); a study of the mechanism of change in IBCT can be found in Doss et al. (2005).

REFERENCES

Atkins, D. C., Berns, S. B., George, W., Doss, B., Gattis, K., & Christensen, A. (2005). Prediction of response to treatment in a randomized clinical trial of marital therapy. *Journal of Consulting and Clinical Psychology, 73*, 893–903.

Baucom, D. H., Shoham, V., Meuser, K. T., Daiuto, A. D., & Stickle, T. R. (1998). Empirically supported couple and family interventions for marital distress and adult mental health problems. *Journal of Consulting and Clinical Psychology, 66*, 53–88.

Christensen, A., Atkins, D. C., Berns, S., Wheeler, J., Baucom, D. H., & Simpson, L. E. (2004). Traditional versus integrative behavioral couple therapy for significantly and chronically distressed married couples. *Journal of Consulting and Clinical Psychology*, 72, 176–191.

Christensen, A., Atkins, D. C., Yi, J., Baucom, D. H., & George, W. H. (2006). Couple and individual adjustment for two years following a randomized clinical trial comparing traditional versus integrative behavioral couple therapy. *Journal of Consulting and Clinical Psychology*, 74, 1180–1191.

Christensen, A., & Heavy, C. L. (1999). Interventions for couples. *Annual Review of Psychology*, 50, 165–190.

Christensen, A., & Jacobson, N. S. (1997). *Frequency and Acceptability of Partner Behavior Inventory*. Unpublished questionnaire, University of California at Los Angeles.

Christensen, A., & Jacobson, N. S. (2000). *Reconcilable differences*. New York: Guilford Press.

Christensen, A., Jacobson, N. S., & Babcock, J. C. (1995). Integrative behavioral couple therapy. In N. S. Jacobson & A. S. Gurman (Eds.), *Clinical handbook of couple therapy* (pp. 31–64). New York: Guilford Press.

Cordova, J. V. (2001). Acceptance in behavior therapy: Understanding the process of change. *Behavior Analyst*, 24, 213–226.

Cordova, J. V., Jacobson, N. S., & Christensen, A. (1998). Acceptance versus change interventions in behavioral couples therapy: Impact on couples' in-session communication. *Journal of Marriage and Family Counseling*, 24, 437–455.

Doss, B. D., & Christensen, A. (2006). Acceptance in romantic relationships: The Frequency and Acceptability of Partner Behavior Inventory. *Psychological Assessment*, 18, 289–302.

Doss, B. D., Thum, Y. M., Sevier, M., Atkins, D. C., & Christensen, A. (2005). Improving relationships: Mechanisms of change in couple therapy. *Journal of Consulting and Clinical Psychology*, 73, 624–633.

Fals-Stewart, W., & O'Farrell, T. J. (2003). Behavioral family counseling and naltrexone for male opioid-dependent patients. *Journal of Consulting and Clinical Psychology*, 71, 432–442.

Gottman, J. (1994). *Why marriages succeed or fail . . . and how you can make yours last*. New York: Simon & Schuster.

Gottman, J., Markman, H., Notarius, C., & Gonso, J. (1976). *A couple's guide to communication*. Champaign, IL: Research Press.

Hahlweg, K., & Markman, H. J. (1988). The effectiveness of behavioral marital therapy: Empirical status of behavioral techniques in preventing and alleviating marital distress. *Journal of Consulting and Clinical Psychology*, 56, 440–447.

Holtzworth-Munroe, A., Meehan, J. C., Rehman, U., & Marshall, A. D. (2002). Intimate partner vio-lence: An introduction for couple therapists. In A. S. Gurman & N. S. Jacobson (Eds.), *Clinical handbook of couple therapy* (3rd ed., pp. 441–465). New York: Guilford Press.

Jacobson, N. S. (1984). A component analysis of behavioral marital therapy: The relative effectiveness of behavior exchange and problem solving training. *Journal of Consulting and Clinical Psychology*, 52, 295–305.

Jacobson, N. S., & Addis, M. E. (1993). Research on couples and couple therapy: What do we know? Where are we going? *Journal of Consulting and Clinical Psychology*, 61, 85–93.

Jacobson, N. S., & Christensen, A. (1998). *Acceptance and change in couple therapy: A therapist's guide to transforming relationships*. New York: Norton.

Jacobson, N. S., Christensen, A., Prince, S. E., Cordova, J., & Eldridge, K. (2000). Integrative behavioral couple therapy: An acceptance-based, promising new treatment for couple discord. *Journal of Consulting and Clinical Psychology*, 68, 351–355.

Jacobson, N. S., Follette, W. C., Revenstorf, D., Baucom, D. H., Halhlweg, K., & Margolin, G. (1984). Variability in outcome and clinical significance of behavioral marital therapy: A reanalysis of outcome data. *Journal of Consulting and Clinical Psychology*, 52, 497–504.

Jacobson, N. S., & Gottman, J. M. (1998). *When men batter women: New insights into ending abusive relationships*. New York: Simon & Schuster.

Jacobson, N. S., Gottman, J. M., Gortner, E., Berns, S., & Shortt, J. W. (1996). Psychological factors in the longitudinal course of battering: When do the couples split up? When does the abuse decrease? *Violence and Victims*, 11, 371–392.

Jacobson, N. S., & Margolin, G. (1979). *Marital therapy: Strategies based on social learning and behavior exchange principles*. New York: Brunner/Mazel.

Jacobson, N. S., Schmaling, K. B., & Holtzworth-Munroe, A. (1987). A component analysis of behavioral marital therapy: Two-year follow-up and prediction of relapse. *Journal of Marital and Family Therapy*, 13, 187–195.

Karney, B. R., & Bradbury, T. N. (1995). The longitudinal course of marital quality and stability: A review of theory, method, and research. *Psychological Bulletin*, 118, 3–34.

Kurdek, L. A. (2004). Do gay and lesbian couples really differ from heterosexual married couples? *Journal of Marriage and the Family*, 66(4), 880–900.

Martell, C. R., Safren, S. A., & Prince, S. E. (2004). *Cognitive-behavioral therapies with lesbian, gay, and bisexual clients*. New York: Guilford Press.

Mohr, J. J., & Fassinger, R. E. (2006). Sexual orientation identity and romantic relationship quality in same-sex couples. *Personality and Social Psychology Bulletin*, 32, 1085–1099.

Noller, P., Beach, S., & Osgarby, S. (1997). Cognitive and affective processes in marriage. In W. K. Halford & H. J. Markman (Eds.), *Clinical handbook of mar-*

riage and couples intervention (pp. 43–71). New York: Wiley.

O'Farrell, T. J., & Fals-Stewart, W. (2006). *Behavioral couples therapy for alcoholism and drug abuse*. New York: Guilford Press.

O'Leary, K. D., Vivian, D., & Malone, J. (1992). Assessment of physical aggression against women in marriage: The need for multimodal assessment. *Behavioral Assessment, 14*, 5–14.

Patterson, G. R., & Hops, H. (1972). Coercion, a game for two: Intervention techniques for marital conflict. In R. E. Ulrich & P. Mounjoy (Eds.), *The experimental analysis of social behavior* (pp. 424–440). New York: Appleton.

Skinner, B. F. (1966). An operant analysis of problem solving. In B. Kleinmuntz (Ed.), *Problem solving: Research method teaching* (pp. 225–257). New York: Wiley.

Solomon, S. E., Rothblum, E. D., & Balsam, K. F. (2005). Money, housework, sex, and conflict: Same-sex couples in civil unions, those not in civil unions, and heterosexual married siblings. *Sex Roles, 29*(9/10), 561–575.

Spanier, G. B. (1976). Measuring dyadic adjustment: New scales for assessing the quality of marriage and similar dyads. *Journal of Marriage and the Family, 38*, 15–28.

Straus, M. A. (1979). Measuring intrafamily conflict and violence: The Conflict Tactics Scales. *Journal of Marriage and the Family, 41*, 75–88.

Weiss, R. L., & Cerreto, M. C. (1980). The Marital Status Inventory: Development of a measure of dissolution potential. *American Journal of Family Therapy, 8*(2), 80–85.

Weiss, R. L., & Heyman, R. E. (1997). A clinical-research overview of couples interactions. In W. K. Halford & H. J. Markman (Eds.), *Clinical handbook of marriage and couples intervention*. New York: Wiley.

Wile, D. B. (1988). *After the honeymoon: How conflict can improve your relationship*. New York: Wiley.

Wimberly, J. D. (1998). An outcome study of integrative couples therapy delivered in a group format [Doctoral dissertation, University of Montana, 1997]. *Dissertation Abstracts International: Section B: The Sciences and Engineering, 58*(12-B), 6832.

Humanistic—Existential Approaches

CHAPTER 4

Emotionally Focused Couple Therapy

SUSAN M. JOHNSON

Emotionally focused couple therapy (EFT) is empirically based in a number of ways. First, EFT interventions focus on relational elements that in research have been found to be critical to marital satisfaction and distress. Second, EFT is rooted in attachment theory—an empirically validated theory of adult love. This model also offers a systematic and relatively well-researched change process, and empirical evidence of positive outcomes not only for recovery from marital distress but also relative to variables such as forgiveness of injuries, trust, and partner anxiety and depression. Finally, there is evidence of the stability of treatment effects across time. EFT has led the way in fostering the inclusion of a focus on emotion and attachment in the field of couple therapy. An EFT therapist is a process consultant who supports partners in restructuring and expanding their emotional responses to each other. In so doing, partners restructure and expand their interactional dance and create a more secure bond.

BACKGROUND

EFT is an integration of an experiential/gestalt approach (e.g., Perls, Hefferline, & Goodman, 1951; Rogers, 1951) with an interactional/family systems approach (e.g., Fisch, Weakland, & Segal, 1983). It is a constructivist approach, in that it focuses on the ongoing construction of present experience (particularly experience that is emotionally charged), and a systemic approach, in that it also focuses on the construction of patterns of interaction with intimate others. It is as if Carl Rogers and Ludwig von Bertalanffy (1956), the father of systems theory, sat down to tea to discuss how to help people change their most intimate relationships. Imagine further that, during this discussion, the attachment theorist John Bowlby (1969, 1988) came along to help them understand the nature of those relationships more clearly, and that these three great thinkers then whispered in the ears of two confused but earnest couple therapists at the University of British Columbia, Leslie Greenberg and Susan Johnson. These therapists had been dismayed to find that dealing with the potent, evolving drama of a couple's session was no easy matter, even for therapists who were experienced in treating individuals and families.

When EFT was taking form in the early 1980s, only behavioral therapists offered clearly delineated interventions for distressed relationships and had data concerning treatment outcome. There was also some literature on how helping couples attain insight into their families of origin might change partners' responses to each other. However, neither training couples to problem-solve and to make behavioral exchange contracts nor fostering insight into past relationships seemed to address the potent emotional dramas of couple sessions. After watching numerous tapes of therapy sessions, Johnson and Greenberg began to see patterns in the process of therapy that led to positive changes. They observed both internal changes in how emotions were formulated and regulated, and external changes in interactional sequences. These therapists began to map the steps in the change process and to identify interventions the therapist made that seemed to move this process forward. EFT was born and, even though it was barely out of infancy, began to be empirically tested (Johnson & Greenberg, 1985).

Although the new therapy was a synthesis of systemic and experiential approaches, it was referred to as "emotionally focused" therapy. This was done as an act of defiance and a statement of belief. Although clinicians such as Virginia Satir (1967) were talking about the power of emotion, the prevailing climate in the couple and family therapy field was mistrustful of emotion. As Mahoney (1991) has pointed out, it was seen as part of the problem and generally avoided in couple sessions. If addressed at all, emotion was regarded as a relatively insignificant tag-on to cognition and behavioral change for behavioral therapists. Systems theorists did not address emotion in spite of the fact that there is nothing inherently nonsystemic about recognizing emotion and using it to create change (Johnson, 1998). The name was, therefore, both an attempt to stress a crucial element that was missing from other interventions and a statement about the value and significance of emotions.

Experiential Influences

The experiential perspective has always seen the wisdom in focusing on emotional responses and using them in the process of therapeutic change. In couple therapy emotional signals are the music of the couple's dance, so a focus on emotion in therapy seemed most natural. In this and other ways, EFT shares commonalities with traditional humanistic approaches (Johnson & Boisvert, 2000). EFT adheres to the following basic premises of experiential therapies:

1. The therapeutic alliance is healing in and of itself, and should be as egalitarian as possible.

2. The acceptance and validation of the client's experience is a key element in therapy. In couple therapy, this involves an active commitment to validating each person's experience of the relationship, without marginalizing or invalidating the experience of the other. The safety created by such acceptance then allows each client's innate self-healing and growth tendencies to flourish. This safety is fostered by the authenticity and transparency of the therapist.

3. The essence of the experiential perspective is a belief in the ability of human beings to make creative, healthy choices, if given the opportunity. The therapist helps to articulate the moments when choices are made in the relationship drama and supports clients to formulate new responses. This approach is essentially nonpathologizing. It assumes that we find ways to survive and cope in dire circumstances, when choices are few, but then later find those ways limiting and inadequate for creating fulfilling relationships and lifestyles. For example, in working with a couple in which one partner has been diagnosed with borderline personality disorder, the EFT therapist would view this person's intense, simultaneous need for closeness and fear of depending on others as an understandable adaptation to negative past relationships that can be revised. As Bowlby (1969) suggested, all ways of responding to the world can be adaptive; it is only when those ways become rigid and cannot evolve in response to new contexts that problems arise. It is first necessary, however, to accept where each partner starts from, the nature of his or her experience, and to understand how each has done his or her best to create a positive relationship.

4. Experiential therapies encourage an examination of how inner and outer realities define each other; that is, the inner construction of experience evokes interactional responses that organize the world in a particular way. These patterns of interaction then reflect and, in turn, shape inner experience. Focusing on this ongoing process and helping clients bring order to and coherently engage with these realities in the present is the hallmark of EFT. The EFT therapist moves between helping partners reorganize their inner world and their interactional dance. Humanistic therapists also encourage the integration of affect, cognition, and behavioral responses. They tend to privilege emotions as sources of information about needs, goals, motivation, and meaning.

5. Experiential approaches take the position that we are formed and transformed by our relationships with others. Feminist writers, such as

the Stone Center group (Jordan, Kaplan, Miller, Stiver, & Surrey, 1991) attachment theorists (Mikulincer, 1995), and developmental psychologists (Stern, 2004) also focus on how identity is constantly formulated in interactions with others. By helping partners change the shape of their relationships, the EFT therapist is also helping them reshape their sense of who they are. Couple therapy then becomes a place where partners may revise their sense of self and so become more able to deal with problems such as depression, anxiety, or post-traumatic stress disorder.

6. Experiential approaches attempt to foster new corrective experiences for clients that emerge as part of personal encounters in the here and now of the therapy session. The therapist not only tracks how clients encounter and make sense of the world but also helps them to expand that world.

Systemic Influences

The other half of the EFT synthesis is the contribution from family systems theory (Johnson, 2004a). In systems theory, the focus is on the interaction (feedback loop) that occurs between members of the system (e.g., von Bertalanffy, 1956). As applied to families, the assumption is that symptoms/problems are a consequence of recurring patterns of interaction between family members. Arguably, the hallmark of all family systems therapies is that they attempt to interrupt family members' repetitive cycles of interaction that include problem/symptomatic behavior.

Family systems therapies differ is how they attempt to break these cycles. Thus, for example, the structural family therapist may have clients physically move to help create a boundary (e.g., Minuchin & Fishman, 1982). The strategic family therapist may give a paradoxical directive to bypass resistance in motivating clients to change the cycle of interaction (e.g., Weeks & L'Abate, 1979).

EFT falls within this tradition of family systems therapies, drawing upon systemic techniques, particularly those of Minuchin's structural systemic approach, with its focus on the enactment of "new" patterns of interaction. The unique contribution of EFT is the use of emotion in breaking destructive cycles of interaction. By helping partners identify, express, and restructure their emotional responses at key points in patterned interactions, the EFT therapist helps them to develop new responses to each other and a different "frame" on the nature of their problems. Clients can then begin to take new steps in their dance, to interrupt destructive cycles, such as demand–withdraw, and to initiate more productive ones.

EFT adheres to the following basic premises of family systems theory:

1. Causality is circular, so it cannot be said that action A "caused" action B. For example, the common couple pattern, in which one partner demands interaction while the other tries to withdraw, is a self-perpetuating feedback loop. It is not possible to say whether the "demanding" led to the "withdrawal" or whether the "withdrawal" led to the "demanding."

2. Family systems theory tells us that we must consider behavior in context. This is summed up by the familiar phrase, "the whole is greater than the sum of the parts" (e.g., Watzlawick, Beavin, & Jackson, 1967); that is, to be understood, the behavior of one partner must be considered in the context of the behavior of the other partner.

3. The elements of a system have a predictable and consistent relationship with each other. This is represented by the systems concept of homeostasis (Jackson, 1965), and is manifested in couples by the presence of regular, repeating cycles of interaction.

4. All behavior is assumed to have a communicative aspect (e.g., Watzlawick et al., 1967). What is said between partners, and the manner in which it is communicated, defines the roles of the speaker and the listener. The nature of a relationship, and that of participants, is implicit in every content message and is particularly seen in the way participants talk to each other. Levels of communication may also conflict. "I am sorry—OK?" can communicate dismissal and be heard as commentary on the unreasonable nature of an injured party rather than as a sincere apology.

5. The task of the family systems therapist is to interrupt stuck, repetitive, negative cycles of interaction, so that new patterns can occur. Systems theory, in itself, does not offer direction as to the nature of these new patterns, only that they be more flexible and less constrained. To define such a direction a theory of intimate relatedness is needed.

The Experiential–Systemic Synthesis in EFT

Experiential and systemic approaches to therapy share important commonalities that facilitate integration. Both focus on present experience rather than historical events. Both view people as fluid or "in process" rather than as possessing a rigid core or character that is inevitably resistant to change. The two approaches also bring something to each other. The focus of experiential approaches traditionally is within the person, whereas systemic therapies focus on the interactions between people, to the exclusion of a consideration of the emotional responses and associated meanings that organize such interactions.

To summarize the experiential–systemic synthesis of EFT, there is a focus on both the circular cycles of interaction between people and the core emotional experiences of each partner during the different steps of the cycle. The word "emotion" comes from a Latin word meaning to move. Emotions are identified and expressed as a way to help partners move into new stances in their relationship dance, stances that they then integrate into their sense of self and their definition of their relationship. This results in a new, more satisfying cycle of interaction that does not include the presenting problem and, more than this, promotes secure bonding.

Contributions of Attachment Theory

Since its initial development, the greatest change in EFT has been the growing influence of attachment on EFT's understanding of the nature of close relationships. Although these relationships have always been seen as bonds in EFT, rather than negotiated, quid pro quo bargains (Johnson, 1986), the focus on attachment as a theory of adult, love in recent years has increased and become more explicit (Johnson 2003a, 2004a, 2004b). This has particularly helped us to intervene with depressed and traumatized individuals and their distressed relationships (Johnson, 2004a, 2004c). The research on attachment theory, and the application of this theory to adults and to clinical intervention, has in the last decade exploded and become more directly relevant to the practitioner. This theoretical aspect of EFT is discussed in greater detail in the section "Perspective on Relationship Health."

Recent Developments in the Practice of EFT

As experience with EFT has increased, the therapy has been applied to an increasing range of types of couples, cultural groups, and clinical problems. Although clients were always diverse in terms

of social class, EFT has recently been applied to couples with more varied ethnic backgrounds (e.g., Chinese and Indian clients) and to same-sex couples (Josephson, 2003). Originally used in the treatment of relationship distress, EFT is now being used with clients who have other types of dysfunction, such as anxiety disorders, posttraumatic stress disorder, eating disorders, bipolar and unipolar depression, and traumatic illnesses such as breast cancer and stroke (Johnson, Hunsley, Greenberg, & Schindler, 1999; Johnson, Maddeaux, & Blouin, 1998; MacIntosh & Johnson, in press; Naaman & Johnson, in press).

Although outcome studies demonstrate that recovery rates after a brief course of EFT are very positive, further investigations into the change process in couples whose relationships improve but still remain in the distressed range have taught us about the nature of impasses that block relationship repair. We have recently delineated the concept of attachment injuries as traumatic events that damage the bond between partners and, if not resolved, maintain negative cycles and attachment insecurities; these events occur when one partner fails to respond to the other at a moment of urgent need, such as when a miscarriage is occurring or a medical diagnosis is given (Johnson, Makinen, & Millikin, 2001). A recent outcome study has found that EFT is generally effective in helping couples create forgiveness and reconciliation in their relationship (Makinen & Johnson, 2006). The ongoing study of the change process has been part of the EFT tradition and continues to help to refine EFT interventions.

Also, there has generally been an increase in appreciation within the behavioral sciences of the role emotion plays in individual functioning and health (Salovey, Rothman, Detweiler, & Steward, 2000; Ekman, 2003). Whereas lack of emotional connection to others and isolation in general have been found to impact immune functioning, responses to stress, and cardiovascular functioning (Coan, Schafer, & Davidson, 2006), findings on the link between supportive relationships and physical and emotional resilience have been compelling. The field of psychotherapy has also moved toward more explicit and refined models of emotional processing (Kennedy-Moore & Watson, 1999). Models of catharsis and expulsion have shifted to models of integration and to a view of emotion as a motivational factor in therapy. Systemic therapists have also begun to focus on both the self and emotion in their work (Schwartz & Johnson, 2000). With these developments, along with increasing research evidence supporting efficacy, EFT has become less marginalized and experienced greater respect as an intervention.

Placing EFT in the Context of Contemporary Couple Therapy

Recent developments in the practice, theory, and science of couples and couple therapy are very compatible with EFT (Johnson & Lebow, 2000; Johnson, 2003b), making EFT a relevant and attractive approach to working with couples in today's world. Some of these developments include the following:

1. In a climate of managed care, EFT is a relatively brief treatment (Johnson, 1999). Most research studies have utilized 10–12 therapy sessions, although clinical practice without the supervision offered in research projects, and with couples facing additional problems, may involve more sessions.

2. EFT is consonant with recent research on the nature of couple distress and satisfaction within the developing science of personal relationships. The findings of Gottman and others (Gottman, Coan, Carrere, & Swanson, 1998; Huston, Caughlin, Houts, Smith, & George, 2001) have emphasized the significant role of negative affect in the development of relationship distress, and stress the importance of helping couples find new ways to regulate such affect. Gottman et al. (1998) have recommended that rather than help couples resolve content issues, therapy should help couples develop soothing interactions and focus on how to create a particular kind of emotional engagement in disagreements. This parallels EFT practice, in that EFT focuses on how partners communicate and on general patterns that are repeated across a variety of content areas. The process of change in EFT is also very much one of structuring small steps toward safe emotional engagement, so that partners can soothe, comfort, and reassure each other.

3. There is an increasing focus in couple therapy on issues of diversity. The experiential roots of EFT promote a therapeutic stance of respect for differences and openness to learning from clients what is meaningful for them and how they view intimate relationships. Every couple relationship is seen, then, as a culture unto itself, and the therapist must learn about and adapt interventions to this unique culture to formulate effective interventions. Like narrative approaches, the EFT therapist's stance is then "informed not-knowing" (Shapiro, 1996). However, EFT also assumes that certain universals tend to cut across differences of culture, race, and class; that we are all "children of the same mother." In particular, it assumes that key emotional experiences and attachment needs and behaviors are universal. There are convincing similarities across people in the recognized antecedents, shared meanings, physiological reactions, facial expression of emotions, and actions evoked by emotions (Mesquita & Frijda, 1992). This is particularly true for the eight basic emotions listed by Tomkins (1962): interest/excitement, joy, surprise, distress/anguish, disgust/contempt, anger/rage, shame, and fear/terror. There are, of course, also differences in how central an emotional experience may be to a culture (e.g., shame and guilt seem to be particularly powerful in the Japanese culture). There are also different accepted ways of regulating emotion and display rules in different cultures. However, there is also considerable evidence that attachment needs and responses are universal (van IJzendoorn & Sagi, 1999).

4. EFT parallels feminist approaches to couple therapy in a number of ways. Foremost is that both the EFT attachment perspective on relationships and the work of feminist writers such as Jordan and her colleagues (1991) depathologize dependency. This particularly challenges the Western cultural script for men. EFT interventions have been found to be particularly effective for male partners described as inexpressive by their mates (Johnson & Talitman, 1997). This would seem to reflect the emphasis in EFT on supporting both partners to express underlying feelings, especially fears and attachment needs. A feminist-informed therapy should then examine gender-based constraints, work to increase personal agency, and "develop egalitarian relationships characterized by mutuality, reciprocity, intimacy and interdependency" (Haddock, Schindler Zimmerman, & MacPhee, 2000, p. 165).

5. There has been a move toward integration of interventions across models in the last decade (Lebow, 1997). EFT integrates systemic and experiential perspectives and interventions. It is also consonant with narrative approaches in some respects, particularly in Step 2 of the change process, when the therapist "externalizes" the cycle and frames it as the problem in the couple's relationship (Johnson, 2004a). EFT has also influenced the evolution of other approaches. For example, new versions of behavioral interventions, such as integrative behavioral couple therapy (Koerner &

Jacobson, 1994), share with EFT a focus on both promoting acceptance and compassion, and evoking softer emotional responses.

6. Postmodernism has had considerable impact on the field of couple therapy in the last decade. This perspective promotes a collaborative stance wherein therapists discover with their clients how those couples construct their inner and outer realities. This attitude parallels the perspective that Carl Rogers, one of the key founders of humanistic/experiential approaches, offered to individual therapy (Anderson, 1997). The concern is to not pathologize clients, but to honor and validate their realities. This perspective particularly focuses on how reality becomes shaped by language, culture, and social interactions (Neimeyer, 1993). In terms of perspective, EFT might be thought of as a postmodern therapy. In terms of specific interventions, EFT therapists help clients deconstruct problems and responses by bringing marginalized aspects of reality into focus, probing for the not yet spoken, and integrating elements of a couple's reality that have gone unstoried. They also help couples create integrated narratives about their cycles, problems, and the process of change. On the other hand, EFT does not fit with the more extreme postmodern position that there are no common existential conditions or processes, and that reality is arbitrary and random—a position that has been questioned in the literature (Martin & Sugarman, 2000). This position suggests that problems generally exist only in language and can therefore be "dis-solved" in language; that it is not possible to delineate patterns in how people deal with problems, and that we do not need models of intervention or theory but can simply use metaphors as guides to intervention (Hoffman, 1998). In general, in a postmodern world, couple therapy seems to be turning away from impersonal strategic approaches toward a more collaborative approach to change that recognizes clients as actively creating their experience and their world.

7. Last, but not least, there is increasing pressure for clinicians to be able to document the effectiveness of their interventions. There is now a sizable body of research on EFT outcomes (Johnson et al., 1999). In brief, results indicate that 70–75% of couples see their relationships as no longer distressed at the end of treatment, and these couples appear to be less susceptible to relapse than couples in other approaches. Interventions with families (Johnson et al., 1998) and with partners struggling with depression have also been positive.

PERSPECTIVE ON RELATIONSHIP HEALTH

A model of a healthy relationship is essential for the couple therapist. It allows the therapist to set goals, target key processes, and chart a destination for the couple's journey. Couple therapy has generally lacked an adequate theory of love and relatedness (Johnson & Lebow, 2000; Roberts, 1992). Healthy relationships were seen as rational, negotiated contracts until it became clear that such contracts actually characterized distressed couples (Jacobson, Follette, & McDonald, 1982). Concepts such as "differentiation" and "lack of enmeshment" have also been associated with healthy relationships in other approaches. A healthy relationship, in EFT terms, is a secure attachment bond. Such a bond is characterized by mutual emotional accessibility and responsiveness. This bond creates a safe environment that optimizes partners' ability to regulate their emotions, process information, solve problems, resolve differences, and communicate clearly. In the last 15 years, the research on adult attachment has demonstrated that secure relationships are associated with higher levels of intimacy, trust, and satisfaction (Cassidy & Shaver, 1999; Johnson & Whiffen, 1999).

Bowlby published the first volume of his famous trilogy on attachment in 1969. He believed that seeking and maintaining contact with significant others is a primary motivating principle for human beings that has been "wired in" by evolution. Attachment is an innate survival mechanism. In the first two decades after the publication of that first volume of his trilogy, Bowlby's work was applied mostly to mother and child relationships, despite that fact that he developed his theory as a result of work with delinquent adolescents and bereaved adults. Furthermore, Bowlby believed that attachment needs ran "from the cradle to the grave." He believed in the power of social interactions to organize and define inner and outer realities. Specifically, he believed that a sense of connection with key others offers a safe haven and secure base. Inner and outer worlds then become manageable, allowing individuals to orient toward exploration and learning. Safe attunement and engagement with attachment figures then lead to attunement and engagement with the world and the ability to modulate stress.

More recently, attachment theory has been applied to adult attachment relationships (Hazan & Shaver, 1987; Mikulincer & Goodman, 2006; Rholes & Simpson, 2004). Adult attachment, when compared to attachment between children and caregivers, is more mutual and reciprocal. It is less concrete (e.g., adults need to touch their loved ones less, because they carry them around with them as cognitive representations) and may be sexual in nature. The caregiving and sexual elements of adult relationships were once viewed as separate from attachment. Now, however, they are seen by most theorists as elements of an integrated attachment system. Sexual behavior, for example, connects adult partners, just as holding connects mother and child (Hazan & Zeifman, 1994), and adult attachments are formed almost exclusively with sexual partners.

This perspective depathologizes dependency in adults (Bowlby, 1988) and views the ability to be autonomous and connected as two sides of the same coin, not as two different ends of a continuum. It challenges the North American tradition of rugged individualism and the myth of self-reliance. In Bowlby's view, it is not possible for an infant or an adult to be either too dependent or truly independent. Rather, people may be effectively or ineffectively dependent (Weinfield, Sroufe, Egeland, & Carlson, 1999).

Security in key relationships helps us regulate our emotions, process information effectively, and communicate clearly. With adults, as with children, proximity to an attachment figure is an inborn affect regulation device that "tranquilizes the nervous system" (Schore, 1994, p. 244). If distressing affect is aroused by the relationship itself, the secure person, who has experienced relationship repair, believes disruptions are repairable. When we are securely attached, we can openly acknowledge our distress and turn to others for support in a manner that elicits responsiveness. This enhances our ability to deal with stress and uncertainty. It makes us more resilient in crises. It also makes us less likely to become depressed when relationships are not going well (Davila & Bradbury, 1999). The ability to seek comfort from another appears to be a crucial factor in healing from trauma (van der Kolk, Perry, & Herman, 1991).

Security in relationships is associated with a model of others as dependable and trustworthy, and a model of self as lovable and entitled to care. Such models promote flexible and specific ways to attribute meaning to a partner's behavior (e.g., "He's tired; that's why he's grouchy. It's not that he is trying to hurt me"). They allow people to be curious and open to new evidence, and enable them deal with ambiguity (Mikulincer, 1997). It may be that secure individuals are better able to articulate their tacit assumptions and see these as relative

constructions rather than absolute realities. They are then better able to take a meta-perspective and meta-communicate with their significant others (Kobak & Cole, 1991). Secure individuals tend to be able to consider alternative perspectives, to reflect on themselves (Fonagy & Target, 1997), and to integrate new information about attachment figures. They can reflect on and discuss relationships (Main, Kaplan, & Cassidy, 1985). In general, insecurity acts to constrict and narrow how cognitions and affect are processed and organized, and so constrain key behavioral responses.

Security involves inner realities, cognitive models and ways of regulating emotion, and patterns of interaction. Each reflects and creates the other. Emotional communication is the bridge between inner and outer realities. A secure partner is more able to engage in coherent, open and direct communication that promotes responsiveness in his or her partner, and to disclose and to respond to the partner's disclosures. Confidence in the partner's responsiveness fosters empathy and the ability to see things from the other person's point of view. In conflict situations, such a partner tends to respond with balanced assertiveness, collaborate more, and use rejection and coercion less (Feeney, Noller, & Callan, 1994; Kobak & Hazan, 1991).

Communication behaviors are context-dependent. It is precisely when stress is high and spouses are vulnerable, that less secure partners have difficulty engaging emotionally and responding to each other. Attachment theory suggests that incidents in which partners need comfort and reassurance, and find the other unresponsive, are pivotal in terms of defining a relationship as satisfying and/or distressed (Johnson, 2008).

PERSPECTIVE ON RELATIONSHIP DISTRESS

EFT looks at distress in relationships through the lens of attachment insecurity and separation distress (Johnson, 2004b). When attachment security is threatened, human beings respond in predictable sequences. Typically, anger is the first response. This anger is a protest against the loss of contact with the attachment figure. If such protest does not evoke responsiveness, it can become tinged with despair and coercion, and evolve into a chronic strategy to obtain and maintain the attachment figure's attention. The next step in separation distress is clinging and seeking, which then gives way to depression and despair. Finally, if all else fails, the relationship is grieved and detachment ensues. Separation from attachment figures can be conceptualized as a traumatic stressor that primes automatic fight, flight, and freeze responses. Aggressive responses in relationships have been linked to attachment panic, in which partners regulate their insecurity by becoming controlling and abusive to their partner (Mikulincer, 1998).

The EFT perspective fits well with the literature on the nature of relationship distress, specifically, with the research of Gottman (1994). Furthermore, it offers attachment theory as an explanatory framework for the patterns documented in this observational research. First, both research and attachment theory suggests that the expression and regulation of emotion are key factors in determining the nature and form of close relationships. Absorbing states of negative affect (where everything leads into this state and nothing leads out) characterize distressed relationships (Gottman, 1979). In EFT, we speak of an "alarm being constantly on" in a distressed relationship and the "noise" blocking out other cues. Gottman has demonstrated that he is able to predict accurately from partner's facial expressions which couples are on the road to divorce. Emotional disengagement also predicts divorce better than the number or outcome of conflicts. His research also indicates that anger is not necessarily bad. This is understandable, if expression of anger helps to resolve attachment issues and evoke responsiveness. From an attachment point of view, any response (except an abusive one) is better than none. This perhaps explains why "stonewalling" has been found to be so corrosive in couple relationships. This explicit lack of responsiveness and directly threatens attachment security, thus inducing helplessness and rage.

Second, research suggests that rigid interaction patterns, such as the familiar demand–withdraw pattern, can be poisonous for relationships. Attachment theory would suggest that this is because these patterns maintain attachment insecurity and make safe emotional engagement impossible. Research suggesting that how people fight is more important than what they fight over fits well with the concept that nonverbal, process-level communication is all important. What people are fighting about is the nature of the attachment relationship and what that implies about who they are. So Ann criticizes Roger's parenting skills, and Roger ignores her. In the next moment, Ann is criticizing Roger's tone of voice and how it negates her input into the relationship. In 5 more seconds the

couple is fighting about who is " the saint" and who is "the devil." Anne concludes that Roger is incapable of being close and responsive in their relationship. It is worth noting that the endemic nature of cycles, such as criticize–pursue followed by defend–withdraw, is predictable from attachment theory. There are only a limited number of ways to deal with the frustration of the need for contact with a significant other. One way is to increase attachment behaviors to deal with the anxiety generated by the other's lack of response (and perhaps appear critical in the process). The other's response may then be to avoid and distance him- or herself from the perceived criticism. Both Gottman's research and attachment research suggest that this strategy does not prevent emotional flooding and high levels of emotional arousal. Habitual ways of dealing with attachment issues and engaging with attachment figures may be learned in childhood, but they can be revised or confirmed and made more automatic in adult relationships.

Third, Gottman points out that the skills taught in many communication training formats are not generally apparent in the interactions of satisfied couples. Attachment research suggests that the ability to "unlatch" from negative cycles depends on the level of security in the relationship. Factors such as empathy and self-disclosure, and the ability to meta-communicate, are associated with security. When flooded by attachment fears, it is unlikely that a partner can connect well with his or her cortex and follow rules. However, it may be that more secure couples may use such skills as rituals to deescalate negative cycles. One treatment outcome study (James, 1991) added a skills component to EFT interventions, but this addition did not enhance outcome.

Fourth, both this research and attachment theory stress the importance of "soothing" interactions. Attachment theory suggests that events in which one partner asks for comfort and the other is not able to provide it violate attachment assumptions and disproportionately influence the definition of the relationship (Simpson & Rholes, 1994). In the EFT model, we refer to such events as "attachment injuries" (Johnson, Makinen, & Milligan, 2001). There is evidence that a person who generally takes the "avoider" position in problem discussions may be relatively social in many situations but is particularly likely to withdraw when his or her partner exhibits vulnerability (Simpson, Rholes, & Nelligan, 1992). Attachment theory would also suggest that creation of soothing interactions at such times has the power to redefine close relationships. Research on "softenings" (change events in EFT) suggests that this is true.

It is possible to extrapolate specific links between other research on relationships and the nature of attachment relationships. Attachment is being used as a way of understanding the links between depression and marital distress (Anderson, Beach, & Kaslow, 1999); indeed, Bowlby viewed depression as an inevitable part of separation distress. An explanation of why Gottman found that contempt is so corrosive in couple relationships may be found in the concept that interactions with attachment figures create and maintain our models of self. Contemptuous responses may directly convey feedback as to the unworthiness of the self and so create particular anguish and reactivity in distressed partners.

Research on relationship distress then, along with contributions from attachment research, provides the couple therapist with an emerging science of relationships (Johnson, 2003b, 2008). This can help us as therapists understand and predict clients' responses to each other and to our interventions. It should also help us depathologize them. For example, viewing a client's behavior as a "disorganized attachment strategy" may be more helpful than viewing the client as having "borderline personality disorder." Such a science of relationships should help us formulate goals and target interventions to create lasting change in an efficient manner (Johnson, 2008b).

KEY PRINCIPLES

The key principles of EFT, which have been discussed in detail elsewhere (Johnson, 2004a; Greenberg & Johnson, 1988), can be summarized as follows:

1. A collaborative alliance offers a couple a secure base from which to explore their relationship. The therapist is best seen as a process consultant to the couple's relationship.

2. Emotion is primary in organizing attachment behaviors and how self and other are experienced in intimate relationships. Emotion guides and gives meaning to perception, motivates and cues attachment responses, and when expressed, communicates to others and organizes their response (Johnson, 2005).

The EFT therapist privileges emotional responses and deconstructs reactive, negative emotions, such as anger, by expanding them to include marginalized elements, such as fear and helplessness. The therapist also uses newly formulated and articulated emotions, such as fear and longing or assertive anger, to evoke new steps in the relationship dance. Dealing with and expressing key emotions, then, from the EFT perspective, can be the best, fastest, and sometimes only solution to couple problems. Emotion transforms our world and our responses rapidly and compellingly, and evokes key responses, such as trust and compassion, that are difficult to evoke in other ways.

3. The attachment needs and desires of partners are essentially healthy and adaptive. It is the way such needs are enacted in a context of perceived insecurity that creates problems.

4. Problems are maintained by the ways in which interactions are organized and by the dominant emotional experience of each partner in the relationship. Affect and interaction form a reciprocally determining, self-reinforcing feedback loop. The EFT therapist first has to deescalate negative interactions patterns and the reactive emotions associated with them. The therapist then helps partners shape new cycles of positive interactions in which positive emotions arise and negative emotions can be regulated in a different way.

5. Change occurs not through insight into the past, catharsis, or negotiation, but through new emotional experience in the present context of attachment-salient interactions.

6. In couple therapy, the "client" is the relationship between partners. The attachment perspective on adult love offers a map to the essential elements of such relationships. Problems are viewed in terms of adult insecurity and separation distress. The ultimate goal of therapy is the creation of new cycles of secure bonding that offer an antidote to negative cycles and redefine the nature of the relationship.

The three tasks of EFT, then, are (1) to create a safe, collaborative alliance; (2) to access and expand the emotional responses that guide the couple's interactions; and (3) to restructure those interactions in the direction of accessibility and responsiveness.

THE PROCESS OF CHANGE

The process of change in EFT has been delineated into nine treatment steps. The first four steps involve assessment and the deescalation of problematic interactional cycles. The middle three steps emphasize the creation of specific change events in which interactional positions shift and new bonding events occur. The last two steps of therapy address the consolidation of change and the integration of these changes into the everyday life of the couple. If couples successfully negotiate these steps, they seem to be able both to resolve long-standing conflictual issues and to negotiate practical problems. This may be because such issues are no longer seeped in attachment significance.

The therapist leads the couple through these steps in a spiral fashion, as one step incorporates and leads into the other. In mildly distressed couples, partners usually work quickly through the steps at a parallel rate. In more distressed couples, the more passive or withdrawn partner is usually invited to go through the steps slightly ahead of the other. It is easier to create a new dance when both partners are on the floor and engaged. The increased emotional engagement of this partner also then helps the other, often more critical and active partner, shift to a more trusting stance.

The nine steps of EFT are presented next.

Stage One: Cycle Deescalation

Step 1: Identify the relational conflict issues between the partners.

Step 2: Identify the negative interaction cycle where these issues are expressed.

Step 3: Access the unacknowledged, attachment-oriented emotions underlying the interactional position each partner takes in this cycle.

Step 4: Reframe the problem in terms of the cycle, underlying emotions that accompany it, and attachment needs.

The goal, by the end of Step 4, is for the partners to have a meta-perspective on their interactions. They are framed as unwittingly creating, but also being victimized by, the cycle of interaction that characterizes their relationship. Step 4 is the conclusion of the deescalation phase. The therapist and the couple shape an expanded version of the couple's problems that validates each person's reality and encourages partners to stand together against the common enemy of the cycle. The partners begin to see that they are, in part, "creating their own misery." If they accept the reframe, the changes in behavior they need to make may be obvious. For most couples, however, the assumption is that if therapy stops here, they will not be able to maintain their progress. A new cycle that promotes attachment security must be initiated.

Stage Two: Changing Interactional Positions

Step 5: Promote identification with disowned attachment needs and aspects of self. Such attachment needs may include the need for reassurance and comfort. Aspects of self that are not identified with may include a sense of shame or unworthiness.

Step 6: Promote each partner's acceptance of the other experience. As one partner said to another, " I used to be married to a devil, but now. . . . I don't know who you are."

Step 7: Facilitate the expression of needs and wants to restructure the interaction based on new understandings and create bonding events.

The goal, by the end of Step 7, is to have withdrawn partners reengage in the relationship and actively state the terms of this reengagement; for example, a spouse might state, " I do want to be there for you. I know I zone out. But I can't handle all this criticism. I want us to find another way. I won't stand in front of the tidal wave." The goal also is to have more blaming partners "soften" and ask for their attachment needs to be met from a position of vulnerability. This "softening" has the effect of pulling for empathic responsiveness from a partner. This latter event has been found to be associated with recovery from relationship distress in EFT (Johnson & Greenberg, 1988). When both partners have completed Step 7, a new form of emotional engagement is possible and bonding events can occur. These events are usually fostered by the therapist in the session, but they also occur at home. Partners are then able to confide in and seek comfort from each other, becoming mutually accessible and responsive.

Stage Three: Consolidation and Integration

Step 8: Facilitate the emergence of new solutions to old problems.

Step 9: Consolidate new positions and cycles of attachment behavior.

The goal here is to consolidate new responses and cycles of interaction, for example, by reviewing the accomplishments of the partners in therapy and helping the couple create a coherent narrative of their journey into and out of distress. The therapist also supports the couple to solve concrete problems that have been destructive to the relationship. As stated previously, this is often relatively easy given that dialogues about these problems are no longer infused with overwhelming negative affect and issues of relationship definition.

OVERVIEW OF INTERVENTIONS

The therapist has three primary tasks in EFT that must be properly timed and completed. The first task, creating an alliance, is considered in a later section.

The second task is to facilitate the identification, expression, and restructuring of emotional responses. The therapist focuses upon the "vulnerable" emotions (e.g., fear or anxiety) that play a central role in the couple's cycle of negative interactions. These are usually the most salient emotions in terms of attachment needs and fears. The therapist stays close to the emerging or leading edge of the client's experience and uses humanistic–experiential interventions to expand and reorganize that experience. These include reflection, evocative questions (e.g., "What is it like for you when ... "), validation, heightening (e.g., with repetition and imagery techniques) and empathic interpretation. Such interpretation is always done tentatively and in very small increments. So, a therapist might ask a man whether he might not only be "uncomfortable," as he had stated but also, in fact, quite "upset" by his wife's remarks. When the therapist uses these interventions, reactive responses, such as anger or numbing, tend to evolve into more core primary or "vulnerable" emotions, such as a sense of grief, shame, or fear.

In the third task, the restructuring of interactions, the therapist begins by tracking the negative cycle that constrains and narrows the partners' responses to each other. The therapist uses structural systemic techniques such as reframing and the choreographing new relationship events. Problems are reframed in terms of cycles and of attachment needs and fears. So, the therapist may ask a person to share specific fears with his or her partner, thus creating a new kind of dialogue that fosters secure attachment. These tasks and interventions are outlined in detail elsewhere, together with transcripts of therapy sessions (Johnson, 1999, 2004a).

Timing and delivery of the interventions are as important as the interventions themselves. The process of therapy evolves, with the couple and the therapist attuning to each other, and the thera-

pist matching interventions to each partner's style (Johnson & Whiffen, 1999). Expert EFT therapists, for example, slow down their speech when evoking emotion; use a low, evocative voice; and incorporate simple images to capture people's felt experience. It is as if they emotionally engage with the clients' experience, reflect it, then invite the clients to enter it on the same engaged level. Emotional responses take longer to process, particularly when they are unfamiliar or threatening, and are more easily evoked by concrete images than by more abstract statements (Palmer & Johnson, 2002).

THE ASSESSMENT OF COUPLE FUNCTIONING AND DYSFUNCTION

Although a variety of questionnaires have been used in research on EFT (e.g., the Dyadic Adjustment Scale [DAS; Spanier, 1976]) no instruments are unique to EFT and, clinically, assessment takes place through client interviews. After a period of joining, the partners are asked about what brings them to therapy, and the therapist begins to listen for relational problems experienced by each partner (e.g., "arguments," "poor communication," or "lack of intimacy"). Therapists must be able to identify one or more problems that all parties (including the therapist) can agree to as goals for therapy. It is not uncommon that the partners' complaints may initially seem unrelated. In this case, the therapist see how the complaints are related and "weave" them into a common complaint/goal that both partners accept as encompassing their own concerns.

The therapist then begins to identify the negative cycle of interaction that typifies the couple's complaint. He or she may either observe the cycle actually being played out in the session or begin carefully to "track" the cycle. This is a skill common to most family systems therapists. Briefly, the therapist wants to find out exactly how the cycle begins, who says and does what as the cycle unfolds, and how it concludes. In this assessment phase, the clients may or may not begin to identify spontaneously the emotions underlying their positions in the cycle. The therapist may facilitate this by asking questions (e.g., "What was that like for you?"). At this early stage, expressed emotions tend to be rather "safe" and superficial.

Although EFT is a present-focused therapy, a small amount of relationship history is obtained during the assessment phase. Clients can be asked how they met, what attracted them to each other, and at what point the present problems began to manifest themselves. Life transitions and shifts (e.g., birth of children, retirement, immigration) associated with the beginning of the problem and clients' cultural heritages are particularly noted. A very brief personal history may be elicited, with questions like, "Who held and comforted you when you were small?" The answer to such questions gives the therapist a sense of whether safe attachment is familiar or foreign territory.

The therapist then asks partners about their specific treatment goals and what they hope to gain from therapy. The response to this question tends to be the inverse of the complaints solicited at the beginning of the assessment. Initially, partners were asked what they were unhappy about, but at this point in the assessment they are asked how they would like their relationship to be and are helped to specify particular changes they want to make.

The process of therapy usually evolves, with one or two conjoint sessions followed by one individual session with each spouse. These individual sessions serve to cement the alliance with the therapist, to provide an opportunity for the client to elaborate on perceptions of the other spouse and relationship problems, and to allow the therapist to ask sensitive questions about physical and sexual abuse in past attachment relationships and in the current relationship. If the client discloses information relevant to the relationship that has not been shared with the other spouse, he or she is encouraged to reveal this information in the next couple session. Keeping secrets, particularly secrets about alternative relationships that offer apparent escape from the trials of repairing the marriage, is presented as undermining the objectives of therapy and the client's goals.

A therapy contract is discussed briefly with the partners, who are told that the purpose of therapy is to shift the negative cycle of interaction, so that a new cycle can emerge that fosters a safer and more supportive relationship. Many EFT therapists share an expectation that treatment will in all likelihood be concluded in approximately 8–15 weekly sessions. The number of sessions is not set in this manner if one of the partners shows signs of or has a diagnosis of posttraumatic stress. In this case, the number of sessions is left open to respond to the couple's need for longer treatment or treatment that is coordinated with the demands of other treatment modalities in which the affected partner may be involved.

EFT therapists attempt to be transparent about the process of change, and explain how and why they intervene whenever doing so seems appropriate. So, if a partner wants to renew passion in the relationship, the therapist breaks down the process into intermediate goals, suggesting that the couple will first need to deescalate their negative interactions. Couples are encouraged to view therapists as consultants who can and will be corrected, and who will need the partners' active participation to redefine their relationship. Therapists then can admit mistakes and allow clients to teach them about the unique experience in their relationship.

ABSOLUTE AND RELATIVE CONTRAINDICATIONS

In EFT, the therapist asks partners to allow themselves gradually to be open and therefore vulnerable to each other. The primary contraindication to the use of EFT occurs when the therapist believes that such vulnerability is not safe or advisable. The most obvious situation involves ongoing physical abuse. In this case, partners are referred to specialized domestic violence treatment programs. They are offered EFT only after this therapy is completed and the abused partner no longer feels at risk. It is important that this be used as the criterion for couple therapy readiness rather than the abusive partner's assessment that the behavior is now under control. The goal of treatment, after the assessment, then, is to encourage the abusive spouse to enter treatment and the victimized partner to seek supportive counseling or individual therapy. In general, the field is beginning to address treatment feasibility issues in this area and to systematize assessment in a way that benefits all couple therapists (Bograd & Mederos, 1999). There may be other, more ambiguous situations when the therapist does not feel it is safe to ask one or both partners to make themselves vulnerable (e.g., certain instances of emotional abuse), or when one partner seems intent on harming or demoralizing the other.

Finally, EFT is designed to improve relationships for couples who wish to stay together and have a better relationship. Some partners need the therapist's help first to clarify their needs and goals, before they are ready to work toward this end. This might include a situation in which one or both partners admit to being involved in an extramarital affair and are not sure which relationship they wish to maintain, or one in which partners in a separated couple are not sure whether they want to work toward reconciliation.

PREDICTORS OF SUCCESS

Research on success in EFT (Denton, Burleson, Clark, Rodriguez, & Hobbs, 2000; Johnson & Talitman, 1997) allows therapists to make some specific predictions as to who will benefit most from EFT, and so fit client to treatment. First, the quality of the alliance with the therapist predicts success in EFT. This is to be expected; it is a general finding in research on all forms of psychotherapy that a positive alliance is associated with success. In fact, the quality of the alliance in EFT seems to be a much more powerful and general predictor of treatment success than the initial distress level, which has not been found to be an important predictor of long-term success in EFT. This is an unusual finding, because initial distress level is usually by far the best predictor of long-term success in couple therapy (Whisman & Jacobson, 1990). The EFT therapist, then, does not have to be discouraged by the couple's initial distress level but should take note of the couple's commitment to the therapy process and willingness to connect with the therapist and join in the therapy process. Research indicates that perceived relevance of the tasks of therapy seems to be the most important aspect of the alliance, more central than a positive bond with the therapist or a sense of shared goals. The couple's ability to join with the therapist in a collaborative alliance and to view the tasks of EFT, which focus on issues such as safety, trust, and closeness, as relevant to their goals in couple therapy seems to be crucial. Of course, the therapist's skill in presenting these tasks and in creating an alliance is an element here. Generally, this research suggests that EFT works best for couples who still have an emotional investment in their relationship and are able to view their problems in terms of insecure attachment and conflicts around closeness and distance. The first concern of the EFT therapist must be to form and maintain a strong, supportive alliance with each partner.

A lack of expressiveness or of emotional awareness has not been found to hamper the EFT change process. In fact, EFT seems to be particularly powerful in helping male clients who are described by their partners as "inexpressive." This may be because when such clients are able to discover and express their experience, the results are often compelling, both for them and for their partners. As feminist writers have suggested, it is often positive to challenge typical gender styles and assume that needs are basically the same for both sexes (Knudson-Martin & Mahoney, 1999),

particularly in a safe, validating environment. Traditional relationships, in which the man is oriented to independence and is often unexpressive, while the woman is oriented to affiliation, seem to be responsive to EFT interventions. Some research results suggest that EFT is also more effective with older men (over 35), who may be more responsive to a focus on intimacy and attachment.

There is evidence that the female partner's initial level of trust, specifically, her faith that her partner still cares for her, is a very strong predictor of treatment success in EFT. Women in Western culture have traditionally taken most of the responsibility for maintaining close bonds in families. If the female partner no longer has faith that her partner cares for her, then this may mean that the bond is nonviable and may stifle the emotional investment necessary for change. This parallels evidence that emotional disengagement, rather than factors such as the inability to resolve disagreements, is predictive of long-term marital unhappiness and instability (Gottman, 1994) and of lack of success in couple therapy in general (Jacobson & Addis, 1993). Low levels of this element of trust may then be a bad prognostic indicator for couples engaging in any form of marital therapy. The EFT therapist might then help such a couple to clarify its choices, and the limits of those choices.

The effects of EFT have been found not to be qualified by age, education, income, length of marriage, interpersonal cognitive complexity, or level of religiosity (Denton et al., 2000). In fact, there is some evidence that clients with lower levels of education and cognitive complexity may gain the most from EFT. These findings are significant: People learning about EFT for the first time sometimes assume that it would be most helpful for highly educated, psychologically minded individuals, because it involves the expression of internal feeling states. Available evidence suggests that EFT may actually be of great benefit for people who have fewer personal resources in their lives to draw upon (e.g., cognitive complexity, finances, and education).

ALLIANCE BUILDING AND ENGAGEMENT IN TREATMENT

From the beginning, the EFT therapist validates each partner's construction of his or her emotional experience and places this experience in the context of the negative interaction cycle. This reflection and validation not only focuses the assessment process on affect and interaction, and encourages disclosure but it also begins immediately to forge a strong alliance. A focus on the negative interaction cycle surrounding the problem allows the therapist to frame both partners as victims and to assign responsibility without blame. This aids in creating a secure base and confidence in the process of therapy. The negative interaction cycle in the relationship then becomes the partners' common enemy, and battles about who is "the villain" and who is "the saint" are gradually neutralized.

Assessment and the formation of an alliance are neither precursors nor are they separate from EFT treatment. They are an integral part of active treatment. By the end of the first session, an EFT therapist usually has a clear sense of the typical problem cycle. The therapist might summarize it from one person's perspective as, for example, "I feel alone and enraged, so I pick at you. You feel you will never please me, and you become numb and distant. I then intensify my criticisms. You shut down and avoid me for 2 or 3 days, and then we begin again."

Part of the assessment is to search actively for and validate the strengths of the relationship. So, a therapist asks a husband what is happening for him as his wife weeps. He states in a wooden voice that he has no empathy. The therapist points out that when she is upset about something other than his behavior, he is very empathic, offering a tissue and asking her about her feelings. As therapists observe interactions between partners, they begin to form tentative hypotheses as to key underlying emotions and definitions of self and other that operate at an implicit level in the couple's interactions. As the therapist actively intervenes with the couple, it is possible to assess how open they are and how easy they will be to engage in therapy. From the beginning, the EFT therapist both follows and leads. The therapist is active and directs the partners' disclosures toward attachment-salient interactions, attributions, and emotional responses.

The creation of the alliance in EFT is based on the techniques of humanistic–experiential therapies (Greenberg, Watson, & Lietaer, 1998; Rogers, 1951). The EFT therapist focuses upon empathic attunement, acceptance, and genuineness. Humanistic therapies in general take the stance that the therapist should not hide behind the mask of professionalism, but should attempt to be nondefensive, fully present and authentic. As therapists, we assume that the alliance must always be monitored, and any potential break in this alliance—and there will surely be at least one such

break in a course of therapy—must be attended to and repaired before therapy can continue. The alliance is viewed in attachment terms as a secure base that allows for the exploration and reformulation of emotional experience and engagement in potentially threatening interactions. We begin by taking people as they are. We then try, by the leap of imagination that is empathy (Guerney, 1994), to understand the valid and legitimate reasons for partners' manner of relating to each other and exactly how this maintains their relationship distress. This fits well with the tenets of attachment theory. Bowlby always believed in the perfect reasonableness of apparently "dysfunctional" responses once they were considered in context. He speaks of sympathizing with a grieving widow's sense of "unrealism and unfairness," so that she experiences him as her champion rather than telling her to be more realistic (1979, p. 94). We assume that everyone has to deal with difficult life situations where choices are limited, and that the very ways we find to save our lives in these situations, such as blaming ourselves or numbing out, then narrow our responses in other contexts and create problems. *We tend to frame patterns of interaction and patterns in the processing of inner experience rather than seeing the person as the problem. This facilitates the building and maintenance of the alliance.* In EFT, if therapists find themselves becoming frustrated and blaming or categorizing a client, they are encouraged to disclose that they do not understand a particular aspect of a client's behavior and need the client's help in connecting with his or her experience. The therapist takes a deliberate stance, not only choosing to believe in the client's ability to grow and change but also allowing each client to dictate the goal, pace, and form of this change. So, if the therapist suggests that a partner confide in the spouse rather than the therapist at a particular moment and this partner refuses, the therapist respects this. However, the therapist will then slice the risk thinner by asking the partner to confide to the spouse that it is too difficult to share sensitive material directly with him or her right now. The therapist sets the frame, but the clients paint the picture.

CORE INTERVENTIONS

Once the alliance is established, there are two basic therapeutic tasks in EFT: (1) the exploration and reformulation of emotional experience, and (2) the restructuring of interactions.

Exploring and Reformulating Emotion

The following interventions are used in EFT to address this task:

1. Reflecting emotional experience.
   Example: "Could you help me to understand? I think you're saying that you become so anxious, so "edgy" in these situations that you find yourself wanting to hold on to, to get control over everything, that the feeling of being "edgy" gets so overwhelming, is that it? And then you begin to get very critical with your wife. Am I getting it right?"
   Main functions: Focusing the therapy process; building and maintaining the alliance; clarifying emotional responses underlying interactional positions.
2. Validation.
   Example: "You feel so alarmed that you can't even focus. When we're that afraid, we can't even concentrate, is that it?"
   Main functions: Legitimizing responses and supporting clients to continue to explore how they construct their experience and their interactions; building the alliance.
3. Evocative responding: Expanding, by open questions the stimulus, bodily response, associated desires and meanings or action tendency.
   Examples: "What's happening right now, as you say that?"; "What's that like for you?"; "So when this occurs, some part of you just wants to run, run and hide?"
   Main functions: Expanding elements of experience to facilitate the reorganization of that experience; formulating unclear or marginalized elements of experience and encouraging exploration and engagement.
4. Heightening: Using repetition, images, metaphors, or enactments.
   Examples: "So could you say that again, directly to her, that you do shut her out?"; "It seems like this is so difficult for you, like climbing a cliff, so scary"; "Can you turn to him and tell him? 'It's too hard to ask. It's too hard to ask you to take my hand.'"
   Main functions: Highlighting key experiences that organize responses to the partner and new formulations of experience that will reorganize the interaction.
5. Empathic conjecture or interpretation.
   Example: "You don't believe it's possible that anyone could see this part of you and still accept you, is that right? So you have no choice but to hide?"

Main functions: Clarifying and formulating new meanings, especially regarding interactional positions and definitions of self.

These interventions, together with markers or cues as to when specific interventions are used, and descriptions of the process partners engage in as a result of each intervention are discussed in more detail elsewhere (Johnson, 2004a; Johnson et al., 2005).

Restructuring Interventions

The following interventions are used in EFT to address this task:

1. Tracking, reflecting, and replaying interactions.
   Example: "So what just happened here? It seemed like you turned from your anger for a moment and appealed to him. Is that OK? But Jim, you were paying attention to the anger and stayed behind your barricade, yes?"
   Main functions: Slows down and clarifies steps in the interactional dance; replays key interactional sequences.
2. Reframing in the context of the cycle and attachment processes.
   Example: "You freeze because you feel like you're right on the edge of losing her, yes? You freeze because she matters so much to you, not because you don't care."
   Main functions: Shifts the meaning of specific responses and fosters more positive perceptions of the partner.
3. Restructuring and shaping interactions: Enacting present positions, enacting new behaviors based upon new emotional responses, and choreographing specific change events.
   Examples: "Can you tell him? 'I'm going to shut you out. You don't get to devastate me again'"; "This is the first time you've ever mentioned being ashamed. Could you tell him about that shame?"; "Can you ask him, please? Can you ask him for what you need right now?"
   Main functions: Clarifies and expands negative interaction patterns, creates new kinds of dialogue and new interactional steps/positions, leading to positive cycles of accessibility and responsiveness.

The EFT therapist also uses particular techniques at impasses in the process of change.

IMPASSES IN THERAPY: INTERVENTIONS

It is quite unusual for the EFT therapist to be unable to help a couple create deescalation or to foster greater engagement on the part of a withdrawn spouse. The most common place for the process of change to become mired down is in Stage Two. This is particularly true when a therapist is attempting to shape positive interactions to foster secure bonding and asks a blaming, critical person to begin to take new risks with his or her partner. Often, if the therapist affirms the difficulty of learning to trust, and remains hopeful and engaged in the face of any temporary reoccurrence of distress, then the couple will continue to move forward.

The therapist may also set up an individual session with each partner to explore the impasse and soothe the fears associated with new levels of emotional engagement. The therapist can also reflect the impasse, painting a vivid picture of the couple's journey and its present status and inviting the partners to claim their relationship from the negative cycle. This can be part of a general process of heightening and enacting impasses. When a partner can actively articulate her stuck position in the relationship dance, she feels the constraining effect of this position more acutely. So, by sadly stating to her partner, "I can never let you in. If I do ... ," she begins to challenge this position. The partner often can then respond in reassuring ways that allow her to take small new steps toward trust.

If emotions run very high and interfere with any kind of intervention, the therapist can also offer images and tell archetypal stories that capture the dilemma of the most constrained spouse and his or her partner. In the EFT model, these stories are labeled "disquisitions" (Millikin & Johnson, 2000; Johnson, 2004a). The couple is then able to look from a distance, exploring the story and therefore their own dilemma. This "hands-off" intervention offers the couple a normalizing but clarifying mirror but does not require a response. Instead, it poses a dilemma that presents the couple with a clear set of choices within a narrative framework that is universal and as unthreatening as possible.

As discussed previously, research into the change processes in EFT has examined a particular event that appears to block the renewal of a secure bond. This event we have termed an "attachment injury" (Johnson & Whiffen, 1999). Attachment theorists have pointed out that incidents in which one partner responds, or fails to respond, at times of urgent need seem to influence the quality of an attachment relationship disproportionately (Simpson & Rholes, 1994). Such incidents either shatter or confirm one's assumptions about attachment relationships and the dependability of one's partner. Negative attachment-related events, particularly abandonments and betrayals, often cause seemingly irreparable damage to close relationships. Many partners enter therapy with the goal of not only alleviating general distress but also bringing closure to such events, thereby restoring lost intimacy and trust. During the therapy process, these events, even if they occurred long ago, often reemerge in an alive and intensely emotional manner, much like a traumatic flashback, and overwhelm the injured partner. These incidents, which usually occur in the context of life transitions, loss, physical danger or uncertainty, can be considered "relationship traumas" (Johnson et al., 2001). When the partner then fails to respond in a reparative, reassuring manner, or when the injured spouse cannot accept such reassurance, the injury is compounded. As the partners experience failure in their attempts to move beyond such injuries and repair the bond between them, their despair and alienation deepen. So, a partner's withdrawal from his wife while she suffers a miscarriage, as well as his subsequent unwillingness to discuss this incident, becomes a recurring focus of the couple's dialogue and blocks the development of new, more positive interactions.

Attachment has been called a "theory of trauma" (Atkinson, 1997), in that it emphasizes the extreme emotional adversity of isolation and separation, particularly at times of increased vulnerability. This theoretical framework offers both an explanation of why certain painful events become pivotal in a relationship and an understanding of what the key features of such events will be, how they will impact a particular couple's relationship, and how they can be optimally resolved.

Our present understanding of the process of resolution of these injuries is as follows. First, with the therapist's help, the injured spouse stays in touch with the injury and begins to articulate its impact and it attachment significance. New emotions frequently emerge at this point. Anger evolves into clear expressions of hurt, helplessness, fear, and shame. The connection of the injury to current negative cycles in the relationship becomes clear. For example, a spouse says, "I feel so hopeless. I just smack him to show him he can't pretend I'm not here. He can't just wipe out my hurt like that."

Second, the partner begins to hear and understand the significance of the injurious event and to understand it in attachment terms, as a reflection of his or her importance to the injured spouse, rather than as a reflection of his or her personal inadequacies or insensitivity. This partner then acknowledges the injured partner's pain and suffering, and elaborates on how the event evolved for him or her.

Third, the injured partner then tentatively moves toward a more integrated and complete articulation of the injury, expressing grief at the loss involved in it and fear concerning the specific loss of the attachment bond. This partner allows the other to witness his or her vulnerability. Fourth, the partner becomes more emotionally engaged and acknowledges responsibility for his or her part in the attachment injury and expresses empathy, regret, and/or remorse.

Fifth, the injured spouse then risks asking for the comfort and caring from his or her mate that were unavailable at the time of the injurious event. The mate responds in a caring manner that acts as an antidote to the traumatic experience of the attachment injury.

Sixth, the partners are then able to construct together a new narrative of the event. This narrative is ordered and includes, for the injured spouse, a clear and acceptable sense of how the partner came to respond in such a distressing manner during the event.

Once the attachment injury is resolved, the therapist can more effectively foster the growth of trust, softening events and the beginning of positive cycles of bonding and connection.

MECHANISMS OF CHANGE

Change in EFT is not seen in terms of the attainment of cognitive insight, problem-solving or negotiation skills, or a process of catharsis or ventilation. The EFT therapist walks with each partner to the leading edge of his or her experience and expands this experience to include marginalized or hardly synthesized elements that then give new meaning to this experience. What was figure may now become ground. Once each partner's experience of relatedness takes on new color and form, the partners can move their feet in a different way in the interactional dance. So, "edginess" and irritation expand into anxiety and anguish. The expression of anguish then brings a whole new dimension into an irritated partner's sense of relatedness and his or her dialogue with the mate. Experience becomes reorganized, and the emotional elements in that experience evoke new responses to the partner. So, as the irritated partner becomes more connected with his or her fear and aloneness (rather than contempt for the mate), he or she wants to reach for the mate and ask for comfort. Partners encounter and express their own experience in new ways that then fosters new encounters, new forms of engagement with the other. Experience is reconstructed, and so is the dance between partners.

The research on the process of change in EFT has been summarized elsewhere (Johnson et al., 1999). In general, couples show more depth of experiencing and more affiliative responses in successful sessions. Although deescalation of the negative cycle and reengagement of the withdrawn partner can be readily observed in EFT sessions, the change event that has been demonstrated in research is the softening. A "softening" involves a vulnerable request, by a usually hostile spouse, for reassurance or comfort, or for some other attachment need to be met. When the other, now accessible spouse is able to respond to this request, then both spouses are mutually responsive and bonding interactions can occur. Examples of these events are in the literature on EFT. A brief set of snapshots of the softening partner's progress through such an event follows:

"I just get so tense, you know. Then he seems like the enemy."
"I guess maybe, maybe I am panicked—that's why I get so enraged. What else can you do? He's not there. I can't feel that helpless."
"I can't ask for what I need. I have never been able to do that. I would feel pathetic. He wouldn't like it; he'd cut and run. It would be dreadful." (The partner then invites and reassures.)
"This is scary. I feel pretty small right now. I would really, well, I think (*to the partner*), I need you to hold me, could you, just let me know you care, you see my hurt."

There are many levels of change in a softening. The ones most easily identified follow:

• An expansion of experience that includes accessing attachment fears and the longing for contact and comfort. Emotions tell us what we need.
• An engagement of the partner in a different way. Fear organizes a less angry, more affiliative

stance. The frightened partner has put her emotional needs into words and changed her part of the dance. New emotions prime new responses/actions.

- A new view of the "softening" partner is offered to the spouse. The husband in the previous example sees his wife in a different light, as afraid rather than dangerous, and is pulled toward her by her expressions of vulnerability.
- A new, compelling cycle is initiated. She reaches and he comforts. This new connection offers an antidote to negative interactions and redefines the relationship as a secure bond.
- A bonding event occurs in the session. This bond then allows for open communication, flexible problem solving, and resilient coping with everyday issues. The partners resolve issues and problems and consolidate their ability to manage their life and their relationship (Stage Three of EFT).
- There are shifts in both partners' sense of self. Both can comfort and be comforted. Both are defined as lovable and entitled to care in the interaction, and as able to redefine and repair their relationship.

Research suggests (Bradley & Furrow, 2004) that certain interventions such as evocative responding, are crucial in facilitating the deepening of emotion and so completing these softening events. For a therapist to be able to guide a couple in the direction of such an event and help them shape it, he or she has to be willing to engage emotionally. He or she has to learn to have confidence in the process, the inherent pull of attachment needs and behaviors, and in clients' abilities to reconfigure their emotional realities when they have a secure base in therapy. Even so, not every couple is able to complete a softening. Some couples improve their relationship, reduce the spin of the negative cycle, attain a little more emotional engagement, and decide to stop there. The model suggests that although such improvement is valid and significant, these couples will be more vulnerable to relapse.

TERMINATION

In this phase of treatment, the therapist is less directive and the partners themselves begin the process of consolidating their new interactional positions and finding new solutions to problematic issues in a collaborative way. As therapists we emphasize each partner's shifts in position. For example, we frame a more passive and withdrawn husband as now powerful and able to help his spouse deal with her attachment fears, whereas we frame his spouse as needing his support. We support constructive patterns of interaction and help the couple put together a narrative that captures the change that has occurred in therapy and the nature of the new relationship. We stress the ways the couple has found to exit from the problem cycle and create closeness and safety. Any relapses are also discussed and normalized. If these negative interactions occur, they are shorter, less alarming, and are processed differently, so that they have less impact on the definition of the relationship. The partners' goals for their future together are also discussed, as are any fears around terminating the sessions. At this point, the partners express more confidence in their relationship and are ready to leave therapy. We offer couples the possibility of future booster sessions, but this is placed in the context of future crises triggered by elements outside the relationship, rather than any expectation that they will need such sessions to deal with marital problems per se.

TREATMENT APPLICABILITY

EFT has been used with many different couples facing many different kinds of issues. It was developed in collaboration with clients in agencies, university clinics, private practice and in a hospital clinic in a major city, where partners were struggling with many problems in addition to relationship distress. Many of these hospital clinic couples' relationships were in extreme distress. Some of these partners were in individual therapy, as well as couple therapy, and some were also on medication to reduce the symptoms of anxiety disorders, bipolar depression, posttraumatic stress disorder, or chronic physical illness. The EFT therapist typically links symptoms such as depression to the couple's interactional cycle and attachment security. The therapist focuses on how the emotional realities and negative interactions of the partners create, maintain, or exacerbate such symptoms and how, in turn, symptoms then create, maintain, or exacerbate these realities and interactions. In general, it seems that placing "individual" problems in their relational context enables the couple to find new perspectives on and ways of dealing with such problems. As one client, Doug, remarked, "I am less edgy now that we are more together, but also, if I feel that edginess coming, well, I can go and ask her to touch me, and it makes it more manageable. So I have reduced my meds a bit, and that makes me feel better."

As mentioned previously, EFT is used in clinical practice with couples who are diverse in age, class, background, and sexual orientation. The traditionality of the couple does not appear to impact interventions negatively (Johnson & Talitman, 1997). It seems that it is not the beliefs that partners hold but how rigidly they adhere to such beliefs that can become problematic in therapy. Some beliefs, particularly those that pathologize dependency needs, are challenged in the course of EFT. Women, for example, may be labeled as "sick," "immature," "crazy," or generally "inappropriate" when they express their attachment needs in vivid ways that their partners do not understand. The ambivalence about closeness expressed by women who have been violated in past relationships can also be pathologized by frustrated spouses. In terms of sensitivity to gender issues, EFT appears to fit with the criteria for a gender sensitive intervention defined by Knudson-Martin and Mahoney (1999), in that the model focuses on connection/mutuality and validates both men's and women's need for a sense of secure connectedness that also promotes autonomy. The ability to share power and to trust rather than to control the other coercively is inherent in the creation of a secure adult bond.

EFT is used with gay and lesbian couples, and although special issues are taken into account, these relationships seem to follow the same patterns and reflect the same attachment realities as those of heterosexual relationships. Special topics, such as partners' differing attitudes about coming out and the realities of HIV, arise and have to be dealt with in sessions, but the process of EFT is essentially the same with these couples. We have not found lesbian partners to be particularly "fused" or gay male partners to be "disengaged," and research now suggests that these stereotypes are inaccurate (Green, Bettinger, & Zacks, 1996). An EFT therapist would tend to see the extreme emotional reactivity that might be labeled as evidence of fusion as reflecting attachment insecurity, and the negative relationship dance that maintains that insecurity.

What does the EFT research tell us about how interventions impact couples with different presenting problems? Low sexual desire been found to be difficult to influence significantly in a brief number of sessions (MacPhee, Johnson, & van der

Veer, 1995). This presenting problem seems generally difficult to impact in psychotherapy. However, there is empirical evidence that for other problems that typically go hand in hand with distressed relationships, effects are positive. Depression, the common cold of mental health, seems to be impacted significantly by EFT (Dessaulles, Johnson, & Denton, 2003). Marital discord is the most common life stressor that precedes the onset of depression, and a 25-fold increased risk rate for depression has been reported for those who are unhappily married (Weissman, 1987). Research also demonstrates that EFT works well with couples experiencing chronic family stress and grief, for example, families with chronically ill children (Gordon-Walker, Johnson, Manion, & Clothier, 1997).

Traumatized Partners

EFT has also been used extensively for couples in which one partner has posttraumatic stress disorder (PTSD) resulting from physical illness, violent crime, or childhood sexual abuse (Johnson, 2002, 2004c). EFT appears to be particularly appropriate for traumatized couples, perhaps because it focuses on emotional responses and attachment. PTSD is essentially about the regulation of affective states, and "emotional attachment is the primary protection against feelings of helplessness and meaninglessness" (McFarlane & van der Kolk, 1996, p. 24). As Becker (1973) suggests, a deep sense of belonging results in "the taming of terror," and such taming is a primary goal of any therapy for PTSD.

Trauma increases the need for protective attachments and, at the same time, undermines the ability to trust and, therefore, to build such attachments. If the marital therapist can foster the development of a more secure bond between the partners, then this not only improves the couple relationship but also helps partners to deal with the trauma and mitigate its long-term effects. So a husband might say to his wife, "I want you to be able to feel safe in my arms and to come to that safe place when the ghosts come for you. I can help you fight them off." When his wife is able to reach for him, she simultaneously builds her sense of efficacy ("I can learn to trust again"), her bond with her husband ("Here I can ask for comfort") and her ability to deal with trauma ("I can lean on you. You are my ally when the ghosts come for me").

Trauma survivors have typically received some individual therapy before requesting couple therapy and may be referred by their individual therapist, who recognizes the need to address relationship issues. Indeed, for someone who has experienced a "violation of human connection" (Herman, 1992) such as sexual or physical abuse in his or her family of origin, the specific impact of such trauma manifests itself in relationship issues, and it is in this context that the effects of trauma must be addressed and corrected. When EFT is used with traumatized partners, an additional educational component on trauma, and the effects of trauma on attachment, is added to the usual Stage One interventions. This is often crucial, especially for the trauma survivor's partner, who often has no real understanding of what his spouse is dealing with and cannot be expected to respond empathically.

In general, with these couples, cycles of defense, distance, and distrust are more extreme, and emotional storms and crises must be expected. The therapist has to pace the therapy carefully, containing emotions that the trauma survivor is unable to tolerate. Risks must be sliced thin and support from the therapist must be consistent and reliable. The endpoint of therapy may be different than that with nontraumatized partners; for example, some kinds of sexual contact may never become acceptable for the traumatized spouse. For a survivor of sexual or physical abuse, the spouse is at once the source of and solution to terror (Main & Hesse, 1990). Such partners often swing between extreme needs for closeness and extreme fear of letting anyone close. This ambivalence has to be expected and normalized in therapy. The therapist also has to expect to be tested and, in general, has to monitor the always fragile alliance on a constant basis. The solutions that trauma survivors find to the recurring terror that stalks them are often extremely problematic and include substance abuse, dissociation, and violence against self and others. The Stage One of therapy, then, may also include the formulation of "safety rules" around key stressful moments when trauma cues arise in the relationship (e.g., sexual contact), and general strategies for dealing with fear and shame. Shame is particularly problematic with survivors. Confiding or showing oneself to a valued other is often very difficult. A negative model of self as unworthy, unlovable, deserving of abuse, and even toxic will likely come up especially in key moments of change (see transcript in Johnson & Williams-Keeler, 1998). The first antidote to such shame may be the validation of a therapist; however, the most potent antidote is the support and responsiveness of one's primary attachment figure, one's spouse. The EFT treatment of trauma survivors and their partners is dealt with extensively elsewhere (Johnson, 2002).

The treatment of disorders such as PTSD or even clinical depression can seem intimidating to a couple therapist who is already dealing with the multilayered, complex drama of a distressed relationship. What helps the EFT therapist here is, first, the way the client is conceptualized and the alliance is viewed and, second, the map of close relationships offered by attachment theory. Humanistic theory view clients as active learners who have an intrinsic capacity for growth and self-actualization. The therapist then learns to trust that when clients can be engaged, in contact with, and fully present to their experience—including the neglected emotions, felt meanings, and tacit knowing inherent in that experience—they can be creative, resourceful, and resilient. The clients evolving experience is then a touchstone to which the therapist can return when confused or unsure as to the best road to take at a particular moment in therapy. The therapist can also use his or her own feelings as a compass to decode client's responses and dilemmas.

Depressed Partners

The map offered by attachment theory also facilitates couple therapy with partners dealing with multiple problems as well as relationship distress. Let us take depression as an example. Couple therapy is emerging as a potent intervention for depressed partners who are maritally distressed (Anderson et al., 1999). Couple and family therapy is emerging as the logical treatment of choice in all recent interpersonal approaches to depression (Teichman & Teichman, 1990). Research supports this focus. Spousal support and compassion predicts more rapid recovery from depression (McLeod, Kessler, & Landis, 1992), whereas spousal criticism is related to more frequent relapse (Coiro & Gottesman, 1996).

Attachment theory views depression as an integral part of separation distress that arises after protest and clinging/seeking behaviors have not elicited responsiveness from an attachment figure. Research indicates that the more insecure partners perceive themselves to be and the less close they feel to their spouses, the more relationship distress seems to elicit depressive symptoms (Davila & Bradbury, 1999; Beach, Nelson, & O'Leary, 1988). Depressed individuals describe themselves as anxious and fearful in their attachment relationships (Hammen et al., 1995). Attachment theory also suggests that one's model of self is constantly constructed in interactions with others, so problematic relationships result in a sense of self as unlovable and unworthy. The depression literature has identified the key aspects of depression as (1) unresolved loss and lack of connection with others, and (2) anger directed toward the self in self-criticism, together with a sense of failure and unworthiness. There is also a sense of hopelessness, a sense of the self as having been defeated and disempowered. These aspects of depression—self-criticism and anxious dependency—are often highly intertwined. Many persons who cannot find a way to connect safely with a partner, for example, and are engulfed with loss also despise themselves for needing others and contemptuously label themselves as weak. In experiential models of treatment for depression, clients receive support in finding their voices and using their emotions as a guide to determine their goal, whether it be more secure connectedness with others or a more accepting engagement with self (Greenberg, Watson, & Goldman, 1998).

So when a depressed partner is nagging, seeking reassurance, and trying to control the other's behavior—all behaviors that have been found to characterize depressed partners interactions with their spouses—the therapist views this behavior as attachment protest. This perspective also predicts that depressive symptoms will arise at times of crisis and transition, such as after the birth of a child, when attachment needs become particularly poignant and couples are not able to support each other to create a safe haven and a secure base (Whiffen & Johnson, 1998). An EFT therapist assumes that even if a person enters a relationship with a particular vulnerability to depression or insecurity, new kinds of emotional engagement with one's emotional experience and with one's spouse can break old patterns and create new realities and relationships.

How might the process of change in EFT specifically impact a partner's depression? In the Stage One of therapy, depressive responses are placed in the context of interactional cycles and unmet attachment needs. The partners then become allies against the negative cycle and the effects of this cycle, including the dark cloud of depression. Legitimizing depressive responses as natural and as arising from a sense of deprivation or invalidation in an attachment relationship tends to balance partners' tendency to feel shameful about their struggle with depression. In the Stage Two of therapy, the experience of depression evolves into explicit components, such as grief and longing, which evoke reaching for one's spouse, or anger, which evokes an assertion of needs or shame that can be explored and restructured in the session. The process of therapy directly addresses the sense

of helplessness that many partners feel by offering them an experience of mastery over their own emotional states and their relationship dance. New, positive interactions then offer the depressed partner an antidote to isolation, and feedback from an attachment figure demonstrates the lovable and worthy nature of the self.

For instance, when Mary stepped out of her career and had a baby, she was "dismayed" a year later to find her new life "disappointing" and "lonely." Her physician diagnosed her as clinically depressed and referred her for couple therapy. Whereas she accused her partner David of caring only about his work, he stated that he did not understand what she wanted from him, and that he was working for their future. David had withdrawn more and more and began sleeping downstairs so as not to wake the baby. Mary became more critical of him, and more overwhelmed and depressed. She also felt like a "bad mother" and decided "David doesn't really care about me. I was a fool to marry him." As therapy evolved, Mary began to formulate her sense of abandonment and David, his sense of failure and need to "hide" from his wife. After 10 sessions of EFT, this couple was no longer distressed, as assessed on the Dyadic Adjustment Scale. More specifically, Mary's scores rose from 80 at the beginning to 102 at the end of therapy. Mary's physician independently reported that she was no longer depressed, and the couple displayed new cycles of emotional engagement and responsiveness. These partners experienced themselves as coping with stress more effectively, and at 1-year follow-up these results remained stable. Because a partner's criticism and lack of supportiveness predicts relapse into depression, and secure attachment is a protective factor against stress and depression, we assume that cycles of positive bonding interactions will help prevent a reoccurrence of Mary's depressive symptoms. If we were to take snapshots of key moments in David's reengagement in the relationship and of Mary's move to a softer position, what would these snapshots look like?

David

"I don't want to run away from you. I saw only your anger, not that you needed me."

"I want to support you and be close, but I need some help here. I need some recognition when I try, like when I look after the baby."

"If you are fierce all the time, it makes it hard for me to hold and support you. I feel like I'm a disappointment. So I hide out and work harder at my job."

"I want to feel like I can take care of you and the baby. I want you to trust me a little and help me learn how to do it."

Mary

"I'm afraid that I will start to count on you and off you will go again. I was let down in my first marriage and now in this one too. I'm afraid to hope."

"Maybe I am fierce sometimes. I don't even know that you are hearing me. It's hard for me to admit that I need your support."

"I need to know that I am important to you, and that we can learn to be partners and parents together."

"I want to know that I can lean on you, and that you will put me and the baby first sometimes. I need you to hold me when I get overwhelmed and scared."

Violence in Relationships

Although violence is a contraindication for EFT and for couple therapy in general, couple therapy is considered if violence and/or emotional abuse is relatively infrequent and mild, if the abused partner is not intimidated and desires couple therapy, and if the perpetrator takes responsibility for the abuse. The therapist will then talk to the partners about a set of safety procedures for them to enact if stress becomes too high in the relationship and increases the risk of abusive responses. The position taken by authors such as Goldner (1999), that perpetrators must be morally challenged but not reduced to this singular shameful aspect of their behavior, their abusiveness, fits well with the stance taken in EFT. So, for example, a man who has become obsessed with his wife's weight and frequently becomes contemptuous and controlling is challenged when he minimizes his wife's outrage and hurt at his behavior. However, he is also listened to and supported when he is able to talk about the desperation and attachment panic that precedes his jibes and hostile criticisms. The therapist supports his wife as she expresses her pain and her need to withdraw from him, and facilitates her assertion of limits and insistence on respect from her husband. He is encouraged to touch and confide his sense of helplessness rather than to regulate this emotional state by becoming controlling with his wife.

The couple is helped to identify particular cues and events that prime this partner's insecurities and lead into the initiation of abuse, as well as key responses that prime the beginnings of

trust and positive engagement. Rather than being taught to contain his rage per se, such a client is helped to interact from the level of longing and vulnerability. When he can express his sense of helplessness and lack of control in the relationship, he becomes less volatile and safer for his wife to engage with. It is interesting to note that we do not teach assertiveness in EFT, yet clients, like the wife in this couple, become more assertive. How do we understand this? First, her emotional reality is accepted, validated, and made vivid and tangible. The therapist helps her tell her spouse that she is burnt out with "fighting for her life" and he is becoming "the enemy." Once this client can organize and articulate her hurt and anger, the action impulse inherent in these emotions, which is to protest and insist on her right to protect herself, naturally arises. She is able to tell him that she will not meet his expectations about her physical appearance, and he is able to piece together how he uses her concern about her appearance as a sign that she cares about his approval and still loves him. This couple seemed to illustrate the work of Dutton (1995), which suggests that the abusive behaviors of many partners are directly related to their inability to create a sense of secure attachment and their associated sense of helplessness in their significant relationships. Having discussed the use of EFT with different kinds of couples and problems, let us now look a little more closely at a typical distressed couple going through the therapy process.

BECOMING AN EFT THERAPIST

What are some of the challenges that face the EFT novice therapist? We presume that all couple therapists struggle with integrating the individual and the system, the within and the between dimensions of couple relationships. We also presume that most couple therapists struggle with leading and following their clients. Most couple therapists also struggle to foster not only new behaviors but also new meaning shifts (Sprenkle, Blow, & Dickey, 1999). However, the EFT therapist assumes that emotional engagement with inner experience and with the other partner is necessary to render new responses and new perspectives powerful enough to impact the complex drama of marital distress. The novice therapist has to learn to stay focused on and to trust emotion, even when the client does not (Palmer & Johnson, 2002). My experience has been that clients do not disintegrate or lose control when they access the emotional experience in the safety of the therapy session, but novice therapists may, in their own anxiety, dampen key emotional experiences or avoid them all together. Novice therapists are reassured when given techniques such as grounding to enable them to help clients, for example, trauma survivors, regulate their emotions in therapy (e.g., see Johnson & Williams-Keeler, 1998) on the rare occasions that this becomes necessary. In the same way, novice therapists who are distrustful of attachment needs may find themselves subtly criticizing a partner's fragility. The cultural myths around attachment are that "needy" people have to "grow up," and that indulging their neediness will elicit a never-ending list of demands. On the contrary, it seems that it is when attachment needs and anxieties are denied or invalidated that they become distorted and exaggerated. Supervision or peer support groups that provide a safe base can help such therapists explore their own perspectives on emotional experience, and attachment needs and desires.

The novice therapist also has to learn not to get lost in pragmatic issues and the content of interactions, but to focus instead on the process of interaction and how inner experience evolves in that interaction. The therapist has to stay with the client rather than the model and not try to push partners through steps when they are not ready for them. Sometimes it is when the therapist just stays with the client in his or her inability to move or change that new avenues open up. It is when the frightened client is able explicitly to formulate his fear of commitment, and the therapist stands beside him in that fear, that he is then able to touch and become aware of the small voice telling him that all women will leave him, just as his first love did on the eve of their wedding. As he grieves this hurt and registers the helplessness he still feels with any woman who begins to matter to him, his partner is able to comfort him. He then begins to discover that he can address his fears with his current partner, and they begin to subside. This process differs from that in a previous session, when the novice therapist had pushed the client to list risks he was willing to take and when he would take them, only to find that he became even more withdrawn after the session.

Novice therapists may also have problems at first moving from intrapersonal to interpersonal levels. Therapists can get caught in the vagaries of inner experience and forget to use this experience to foster new steps in the dance. The purpose of expanding emotional experiences in EFT is to shape

new interactions. The therapist then has to move into the "Can you tell him?" mode on a regular basis. Inexperienced therapists may also become caught in supporting one partner at the expense of the other. It is particularly important, for example, when one partner is moving and taking new risks, to validate the other spouse's initial mistrust of this and his or her sense of disorientation and inability to respond immediately to this new risk-taking behavior. Despite all of these factors, recent research (Denton et al., 2000) suggests that novice therapists can be effective using this model.

CASE ILLUSTRATION: "OUT OF THE BLUE"

Trevor and Mandy came to see me because Trevor's individual therapist, who was treating him for depression, told Trevor that he had to work on his marriage. Trevor, a handsome, high-powered executive in his late 40s, with a long history of many brief relationships, had been with Mandy, a rather quiet lawyer who was 10 years his junior, for 5 years. After much initial reluctance on Trevor's part, they had gone to great lengths to conceive a child, who was now 18 months old. The infertility procedures had been hard on them, but they both very much enjoyed being parents to their little son. However, 6 months before coming to see me, Trevor had announced that he was unhappy in the marriage and in love with a colleague, and that he had to leave. Mandy was taken totally by surprise and completely devastated. But Trevor did not leave and after a few weeks the brief affair with his colleague petered out. He then realized that this highly manipulative person was attempting to get his support for her promotion. He expressed shame about the affair in the session, stating that it was completely against his own moral code and had nearly cost him wife, whom he loved, and his family. Mandy constantly pushed her short blonde hair out of her eyes and quietly wept through the entire session, telling me that she was "obsessed" with Trevor's affair and still did not understand why this had happened. She described herself as alternating between surges of rage, relief that her husband was still with her, a desire for constant closeness and constant sex, and a "spacey kind of shut down." As I listened to her, I was reminded of the state of emotional disorganization and seemingly inconsistent responses that have been observed in mothers and children when the mother is experienced as both a source of traumatizing pain and a solution to that pain.

As I asked about their relationship before this incident, Trevor shared that Mandy was the first woman with whom he had ever really felt close. Despite many brief relationships, he had never let himself "count" on anyone until he met Mandy. His parents had both been serious alcoholics, and he had left the family home to live with an uncle at 14 and then gone off to college. He had met Mandy just after his mother's death, which had "thrown him off balance," and had bonded with Mandy when she had helped him with the grieving process. Mandy had grown up in a very strict, religious home in which she was required to be "pretty well perfect" and had been jilted just before marriage by a long -term lover. After this, she had avoided relationships for many years until she met Trevor at an evening class and he had avidly courted her. She had been "amazed" that someone as attractive and confident as Trevor would want to be with her, because she saw herself as a "quiet, very ordinary person." Mandy described their relationship before the affair as "great," although she had been very tired for many months after their son had been born. She had been very "careful" to make sure, though, that she and Trevor still found time for lovemaking. The affair had been a total shock to her. She stated, "I thought we were bullet proof."

Mandy and Trevor were very articulate, empathic and respectful of each other, and committed to their marriage. At first, I could not really see any rigid repetitive interaction cycle in their interactions. The affair was obviously an attachment injury for Mandy, but Trevor assured her any number of times in the first sessions that he was sorry, very sorry, totally sorry. She said she believed him. They commented that they made love almost every day and enjoyed their evenings together after the baby went to sleep. Perhaps this couple did not need a full course of EFT. They just needed a couple of sessions to complete the reconciliation process.

Then I asked Trevor how he understood his apparently sudden and intense involvement with his lover. It must have been an overwhelming impulse. He thought for a moment, then commented that he had considered having the affair long enough to insist that this person go on birth control pills and that she prove to him that she was actively taking them. This did not sound like frenzied passion. He then went on to tell me, "It came out of the blue. I have no idea why I did this. I know I live in my head a lot. I think of lots of reasons why I did this, but really, I don't know

what came over me." Mandy pointedly turned her chair away, and her face became still and mask-like.

We began to talk more about the period of time after the baby was born, before Trevor began to be close with his colleague. Mandy wept and recalled Trevor telling her that she was not responding to his sexual cues, and she had then made sure they made love more often. Trevor agreed that he felt distant and "somehow rejected" during that time, but he could not really explain his feelings. "I would get mad, without even really knowing why I was mad," Trevor continued. "But the minute I got upset, she'd just change the subject or say nothing. There would be this silence. It sucked all the air out of the space between us." And then? "I would feel foolish and go buy her flowers. But then it would happen again. We would make love lots, so why didn't I feel close and desired?"

Mandy bursts into tears here. "Nothing I ever say or do satisfies you. I don't like it when you're mad. I just don't like fighting. I freeze up. How could you love me and do this? I get flashbacks all the time of his talking to that woman on the phone and telling me he is leaving. I can't sleep. Keep thinking about all this. I was suicidal for a good month or two. My first boyfriend left me and then you left me." Trevor comforts her. He says, "I am a bastard. I wrecked havoc here," Then in a quiet voice he adds, "All I know is that the affair felt like an escape. I felt empty and lost in our marriage. I should just be quiet about my feelings." The pattern that had left Mandy and Trevor alienated from each other and tipped both of them into a spiral of insecurity was suddenly apparent to me.

Step 2 of EFT is identifying the negative cycle, so I reflected on the pattern in their story and the moves in the interaction that I saw in front of me. Trevor was unsure of his emotions but felt rejected, disconnected. He tried to talk about this and became frustrated when Mandy moved away. As she shuts down more, he "gives up" on his feelings, becomes confused or tries to act in a conciliatory way. Trevor added that he then "goes analytic and cross-examines her, my motives, us, until I am exhausted." Trevor talked a little here about how Mandy was the first women he had ever "needed" and to whom he really felt committed. He felt "off balance" when these vulnerable feelings would emerge. In past relationships, he had dismissed these feelings and the needs that went with them. With Mandy he could not do this. We began to talk about this pattern, in which the primal code of attachment needs and fear play out and direct the action but remain hidden and a "spiral of separateness" takes over. This pattern could be labeled as demand–withdraw, but Trevor and Mandy have their own idiosyncratic, subtle version. Trevor did not even know what he was fighting about; he just knew he felt somehow empty and rejected. Mandy became more outwardly compliant but more emotionally wary and distant as Trevor became more upset. They both focused on the ball but could not see the game.

Step 3 of EFT is to bring each partner's underlying attachment emotions into this picture. Mandy reminded Trevor of the statements he had made as part of his announcement that he was leaving with his lover. "You said that you were happier single. That you were never happy with our sex life. That you never felt safe with me." Trevor responded, "I was just trying to justify what I was doing." "I didn't know how to talk about the emptiness. But the never feeling safe—that was true." So we talk about the emptiness and lack of safety.

As we unpacked this emotional experience, with interventions such as reflection, evocative questions, and heightening, Trevor first became angry: "I feel like I am responsible for the relationship. I ask for sex, you do it to please me. But I don't feel desired. And if I get upset, I can't find you. You change the subject. You go off—shut down." Then he got sad: "I can't connect, and I can't lean on you, trust you when I need to." He began to understand that when he felt "empty," he had "escaped" into his old strategy for relationships, which was to numb out, detach, and go off with someone new. Mandy said, "I never see your need. You are Mr. Self-Sufficient. You are the perfectionist. I am always afraid of hearing that I am doing it wrong. You don't like the way I clean, the way I dress. I am not passionate enough. I was always terrified of losing you, even before the affair. You judge me." She began to cry. She told him, "I need a shell to deal with the fear. It's like I'm back home trying so hard to be a good little girl and never making it. I just want to die, to disappear." Trevor leaned forward and held her.

Trevor and Mandy moved into deescalation. They were able to integrate their sense of relationships patterns and underlying emotions, and could see these patterns as the problem that prevented them from being open and responsive to each other, and that set up the crisis of the affair. However, they still needed to create new levels of accessibility and responsiveness, and to heal the pain of the affair.

In Stage Two, the more habitually withdrawn partner usually goes one step ahead, so that this person becomes reasonably accessible before the other, more blaming, controlling partner is encouraged to risk asking for his or her attachment needs to be met. Both Trevor and Mandy withdrew at times. Trevor pushed for contact but then, when disappointed, felt "empty," shut down, and pretended for a while that everything was OK before getting openly frustrated again. Mandy was very anxious to please Trevor and to be close to him, but when she picked up negative cues from him, she habitually went into her shell, dismissing his concerns. The therapist then began the Stage Two process by encouraging Mandy to explore her attachment fears and needs more deliberately.

A summary of two the key moments and key interventions in Stage Two of EFT follows:

Step 5. Unpacking and Deepening Mandy's Emotions as Part of Withdrawer Reengagement

Trevor told Mandy how hard it was for him that she insisted he always "stay calm" if he had any issue in the relationship, and then went silent and did not discuss his points. Mandy stayed silent. Then she brought up an intellectual point, and a rather abstract discussion of closeness began. We refocused and began to unpack Mandy's emotions as she listened to Trevor's concern.

THERAPIST: What is happening for you right now, Mandy, as Trevor says this? As he tells you that it is hard for him for always be "calm" and to know how to deal with your silence at those times?

MANDY: I don't know. He's the most important thing to me. I don't know how I feel.

THERAPIST: But what comes up for you is a sense of how important he is. What do you hear him saying ? [Focus on emotional cue.]

MANDY: I hear that he is mad at me. That I am failing here. That is why he had the affair.

THERAPIST: That is what you hear, that you are failing—disappointing him. How do you feel as you say that?—emotionally, in your body? [Focus on somatic sense.]

MANDY: I feel sick. Like I am going to throw up. The other day, when I burnt the muffins we were going to have for breakfast, it was the same. It's worse since the affair, but I think it's always been like this really.

THERAPIST: So what comes up is, he is so important to you, and he is mad, you are failing, you feel sick, and then what do you do with this feeling? [Focus on action tendency.] You go "into your shell"?

MANDY: I just give up. (*Throws her hands in the air and starts to cry.*) I have lost him already.

THERAPIST: And the feeling that comes with that? [It can only be sadness, shame, primal attachment panic.]

MANDY: I am terrified. Terrified. I have nothing to say. I can't say anything. I am not enough. And I shouldn't even feel this way. It's stupid. I shouldn't be so sensitive to his disapproval, especially after all this affair stuff. My mind spins.

THERAPIST: So, in these moments, when you sense that Trevor is in any way disappointed in you, you feel terror. It brings up all your fears that you are not good enough here, and then you feel stupid for even feeling this way. That is unbearable—yes? So you just go still and silent. (*Mandy nods.*) Can you tell him, "I am so afraid that I am not enough for you—so scared."

MANDY: (*Looks at Trevor and then points to the therapist.*) What she said. (*Laughs and then cries.*) Yes. That's right. I am scared, so I go into my shell.

THERAPIST: Trevor, can you hear your wife? What happens to you when she says this?

TREVOR: I feel sad. I am hard on Mandy. I'm demanding. (*Turns to Mandy.*) But when you blow me off like I don't matter, when you just go silent, I can't handle that. I don't want you to be scared of me. Either way it seems like we are stuck. If I get demanding, you go into your shell and shut me out. If I numb out and pretend there is nothing wrong and that I don't need you, that still doesn't work. I guess we are both terrified here.

As Mandy became more engaged and began to articulate her longstanding insecurities, Trevor was also able to explore his emotions. He began to be able to articulate these emotions in statements, such as "I realize now that I cannot tolerate your withdrawal. I feel so alone, so helpless" and "The baby was your big project. Then you were so tired. I couldn't find you." Mandy was more and more able to order and articulate her experience coherently and to demand that they now deal more openly with the trauma of the affair, so that she

could begin to feel safe with Trevor again. Trevor was more able to engage actively in the steps for the forgiveness of attachment injuries now that he had access to his underlying emotions.

Steps in the Forgiveness of Injuries Conversation

The therapist guides Trevor and Mandy through the steps in this conversation, heightening emotional responses and shaping enactments as they go.

Step 1 in this process is where the nub of the injury is outlined, and the traumatic nature of the injury articulated. Step 2 is where Mandy, the injured partner, is able to voice her hurt and its attachment significance. She puts her finger on the core of this experience when she tells him, "The night that I keep going back to is when you said you were leaving, and then you blamed me for the affair. I was literally on the floor, and you announced that it was all my fault, and went off wondering about what your life was going to be like without me. I was irrelevant. How could you love me and do that?"

In Step 3, the injuring partner acknowledges his pain and explains his actions in a coherent way that makes them predictable again to the wounded partner. Trevor no longer says that the affair came "out of the blue." He says,

"I got lost. I didn't know how to talk about my feelings. I didn't know how to ask for comfort. And I felt so helpless. You didn't seem to want me. You were closed off from me; even when we made love it felt like we weren't connected. I got angrier and emptier and more and more numb. The affair was an escape and an attempt to get back to my old life, when I didn't need anyone—didn't need you. When I woke up, I was horrified that I might lose you. Horrified at myself and what I had done. I understand that I broke your heart, and that I even blamed you for my craziness. I decided that you didn't desire me. I turned into a sexual thing."

As Trevor opened up, Mandy could move into Step 4—a coherent, clear statement of her ongoing pain and attachment fears. The therapist supports, reflects, validates, and helps her stay engaged with and order her experience. Mandy tells Trevor, "All my worst fears came true. You were leaving me and it was all because I wasn't enough. I couldn't meet your needs. And then my dismay and my hurt didn't matter at all. I wanted to die then. And now, how do I know if your love is real? All that stuff did come out of the blue for me. Do I really know you? I get into this frantic state."

Trevor now cried with his wife and expressed his shame and his remorse (Step 5). He told Mandy,

"I told myself lies. I focused on the sex. This wasn't about sex. It was about me getting desperate and alone, and not knowing how to reach for you. You are so perfect, so beautiful, and I can see that all my flailing around and making demands freaked you out. I didn't know how to say, 'Let me in. I want to feel cherished'. So I turned away and I hurt you so badly. I don't know if you can ever forgive me. I am ashamed, I feel sick that I did this. I am afraid that you will never trust me again. I squandered our love. Now I want to make you feel safe, make you feel happy."

Mandy could now move into Step 6 and ask for the attachment needs sparked by this relationship trauma to be met. She said,

"I get frantic and spacey, not sure what to trust or believe. Not sure which way is up. I need a ton of reassurance from you. I need to cling to you sometimes. Right now, I just can't get enough caring and holding. And if I get mad, I want you to hear it. I have to know you are right here with me." And Trevor could move into Step 7 of this forgiveness and reconciliation process by responding to his wife's needs and so creating a safe haven for her. He says, "I am so grateful for a second chance. I want to hold and comfort you. I want us to be close. I will never risk losing us again. I am here."

Trevor and Mandy could now stand back and create a clear narrative of their relational problems and attachment injury and how they had healed this injury. They were able to continue to confide, with Trevor discovering and sharing more about his needs for emotional connection and how hard it was for him to admit this need, and Mandy opening up and sharing her fears and asserting her limits in the face of her partner's demands and perfectionistic style. They told me that they had a better relationship than ever before, but that this time, the big change did not come "out of the blue." Now, they knew how they had lost each other, and they knew how to create a sense of safe connection.

EFT AS A MODEL OF INTERVENTION FOR THE NEW MILLENNIUM

One of the clear strengths of the EFT model is that its interventions are clearly delineated, but it still places these interventions in the context of the client's process and responses. It is not an invariant, mechanical set of techniques. It can then address general patterns found across many relationships and the uniqueness of a particular couple's relationship. The need for efficient, brief interventions also requires that interventions be on target. It requires that they reach the heart of the process of relationship repair. EFT formulations and interventions are consonant with recent research on the nature of distress and satisfaction in close relationships, and with the ever-expanding research on the nature of adult love and attachment relationships. In the present climate, it is also particularly pertinent that EFT interventions have been empirically validated and found to be effective with a large majority of distressed couples. Results also seem to indicate that it is relatively stable and resistant to relapse. This model appears, then, to be able to reach different kinds of couples in a brief format and create clinically significant and lasting change.

A recent review of the field (Johnson & Lebow, 2000) points out that the utilization of couple interventions has increased enormously in the last decade, and that couple therapy is used more and more as a resource to augment the mental health of individual partners, particularly those with problems such as depression or PTSD. These two individual problems seem to be particularly associated with distress in close relationships (Whisman, 1999). As a client remarked, "Trying to deal with my depression without addressing my unhappy relationship with my wife is like pushing against both sides of the door. I never get anywhere." For individual changes, once made, to endure, they must also be supported in the client's natural environment (Gurman, 2000). EFT fits well into the emerging picture of couple therapy as a modality that can address and significantly impact "individual" problems that, more and more, are now viewed in their interpersonal context.

EFT also seems to fit with the need for the field of couple therapy to develop conceptual coherence. We need conceptually clear treatment models that not only link back to theories of close relationships but also forward to pragmatic "if this ... then that" interventions. Research into the process of change in this model offers a map of pivotal steps and change events to guide the couple therapist as he or she crafts specific interventions to help partners move toward a more secure bond. One coherent theme that is emerging in the couple and family therapy field is a renewed respect for, and collaboration with, our clients. We learned, and continue to learn, how to do EFT from our clients. To echo Bowlby's (1981) words in the final volume of his attachment trilogy, we must then thank our clients, who have worked so hard to educate us.

SUGGESTIONS FOR FURTHER READING

Johnson, S. (2004). *The practice of emotionally focused marital therapy* (2nd ed.). New York: Brunner/Routledge.

Johnson, S. M. (2002). *Emotionally focused couple therapy with trauma survivors.* New York: Guilford Press.

Johnson, S. M. (2008). *Hold me tight: Seven conversations for a lifetime of love.* New York: Little Brown.

Johnson, S. M., Bradley, B., Furrow, J., Lee, A., Palmer, G., Tilley, D., et al. (2005). *Becoming an emotionally focused couple therapist: The workbook.* New York: Brunner/Routledge.

Karen, R. (1998). *Becoming attached.* New York: Oxford University Press.

REFERENCES

Anderson, H. (1997). *Conversation, language and possibilities.* New York: Basic Books.

Anderson, P., Beach, S., & Kaslow, N. (1999). Marital discord and depression: The potential of attachment theory to guide integrative clinical intervention. In T. Joiner & J. Coyne (Eds.), *The interactional nature of depression* (pp. 271–297). Washington, DC: American Psychological Association Press.

Atkinson, L. (1997). Attachment and psychopathology: From laboratory to clinic. In L. Atkinson & K. J. Zucker (Eds.), *Attachment and psychopathology* (pp. 3–16). New York: Guilford Press.

Beach, S., Nelson, G. M., & O'Leary, K. (1988). Cognitive and marital factors in depression. *Journal of Psychopathology and Behavioral Assessment, 10,* 93–105.

Becker, E. (1973). *The denial of death.* New York: Free Press.

Bograd, M., & Mederos, F. (1999). Battering and couples therapy: Universal screening and selection of treatment modality. *Journal of Marital and Family Therapy, 25,* 291–312.

Bowlby, J. (1969). *Attachment and loss: Vol. I. Attachment.* New York: Basic Books.

Bowlby, J. (1979). *The making and breaking of affectional bonds.* London: Tavistock.

Bowlby, J. (1981). *Attachment and loss: Vol. III. Loss.* New York: Basic Books.

Bowlby, J. (1988). *A secure base.* New York: Basic Books.

Bradley, B., & Furrow, J. (2004). Towards a mini-theory of the blamer softening event. *Journal of Marital and Family Therapy, 30,* 233–246.

Cassidy, J., & Shaver, P. (1999). *Handbook of attachment: Theory, research, and clinical applications.* New York: Guilford Press.

Coan, J., Schafer, H. S., & Davidson, R. J. (2006). Lending a hand: Social regulation of the neural response to threat. *Psychological Science, 17,* 1–8.

Coiro, M., & Gottesman, I. (1996). The diathesis and/or stressor role of EE in affective illness. *Clinical Psychology: Science and Practice, 3,* 310–322.

Davila, J., & Bradbury, T. (1999). *Attachment security in the development of depression and relationship distress.* Paper presented at the 33rd Annual Convention of the Association for the Advancement of Behavior Therapy, Toronto, Canada.

Denton, W. H., Burleson, B. R., Clark, T. E., Rodriguez, C. P., & Hobbs, B. V. (2000). A randomized trial of emotion focused therapy for couples in a training clinic. *Journal of Marital and Family Therapy, 26,* 65–78.

Dessaulles, A., Johnson, S. M., & Denton, W. (2003). The treatment of clinical depression in the context of marital distress. *American Journal of Family Therapy, 31,* 345–353.

Dutton, D. G. (1995). *The batterer: A psychological profile.* New York: Basic Books.

Ekman, P. (2003). *Emotions revealed.* New York: Holt.

Feeney, J. A., Noller, P., & Callan, V. J. (1994). Attachment style, communication and satisfaction in the early years of marriage. In K. Bartholomew & D. Perlman (Eds.), *Advances in personal relationships: Vol. 5. Attachment processes in adulthood* (pp. 269–308). London: Jessica Kingsley.

Fisch, R., Weakland, J. H., & Segal, L. (1983). *The tactics of change: Doing therapy briefly.* San Francisco: Jossey-Bass.

Fonagy, P., & Target, M. (1997). Attachment and reflective function: Their role in self-organization. *Development and Psychopathology, 9,* 679–700.

Goldner, V. (1999). Morality and multiplicity: Perspectives on the treatment of violence in intimate life. *Journal of Marital and Family Therapy, 25,* 325–336.

Gordon-Walker, J., Johnson, S. M., Manion, I., & Clothier, P. (1997). An emotionally focused marital intervention for couples with chronically ill children. *Journal of Consulting and Clinical Psychology, 64,* 1029–1036.

Gottman, J. (1979). *Marital interaction: Experimental investigations.* New York: Academic Press.

Gottman, J. (1994). *What predicts divorce?* Hillsdale, NJ: Erlbaum.

Gottman, J. M., Coan, J., Carrere, S., & Swanson, C. (1998). Predicting marital happiness and stability from newlywed interactions. *Journal of Marriage and the Family, 60,* 5–22.

Green, R. J., Bettinger, M., & Zacks, E. (1996). Are lesbian couples fused and gay male couples disengaged?

In J. Laird & R. J. Green (Eds.), *Lesbians and gays in couples and families* (pp. 185–230). San Francisco: Jossey-Bass.

Greenberg, L., Watson, J. C., & Goldman, R. (1998). Process experiential therapy of depression. In L. Greenberg, J. Watson, & G. Lietaer (Eds.), *Handbook of experiential psychotherapy* (pp. 227–248.) New York: Guilford Press.

Greenberg, L. S., & Johnson, S. M. (1988). *Emotionally focused therapy for couples*. New York: Guilford Press.

Greenberg, L. S., Watson, J. C., & Lietaer, G. (1998). *Handbook of experiential psychotherapy*. New York: Guilford Press.

Guerney, B. (1994). The role of emotion in relationship enhancement marital/family therapy. In S. M. Johnson & L. S. Greenberg (Eds.), *The heart of the matter: Perspectives on emotion in marital therapy* (pp. 124–150). New York: Brunner/Mazel.

Gurman, A. (2000). Brief therapy and family/couple therapy: An essential redundancy. *Clinical Psychology: Science and Practice, 8*, 51–65.

Haddock, S., Schindler Zimmerman, T., & MacPhee, D. (2000). The power equity guide: Attending to gender in family therapy. *Journal of Marital and Family Therapy, 26*, 153–170.

Hammen, C., Burge, D., Daley, S., Davila, J., Paley, B., & Rudolph, K. (1995). Interpersonal attachment cognitions and prediction of symptomatic responses to interpersonal stress. *Journal of Abnormal Psychology, 104*, 436–443.

Hazan, C., & Shaver, P. (1987). Conceptualizing romantic love as an attachment process. *Journal of Personality and Social Psychology, 52*, 511–524.

Hazan, C., & Zeifman, D. (1994). Sex and the psychological tether. In K. Bartholomew & D. Perlman (Eds.), *Attachment processes in adulthood* (pp. 151–180). London: Jessica Kingsley.

Herman, J. (1992). *Trauma and recovery*. New York: Basic Books.

Hoffman, L. (1998). Setting aside the model in family therapy. *Journal of Marital and Family Therapy, 24*, 145–156.

Huston, T. L., Caughlin, J. P., Houts, R. M., Smith, S. E., & George, L. J. (2001). The connubial crucible: Newlywed years as a predictor of marital delight, distress and divorce. *Journal of Personality and Social Psychology, 80*, 237–252.

Jackson, D. D. (1965). The study of the family. *Family Process, 4*, 1–20.

Jacobson, N. S., & Addis, M. E. (1993). Research on couples therapy: What do we know? Where are we going? *Journal of Consulting and Clinical Psychology, 61*, 85–93.

Jacobson, N. S., Follette, W. C., & McDonald, D. (1982). Reactivity to positive and negative behavior in distressed and non-distressed married couples. *Journal of Consulting and Clinical Psychology, 50*, 706–714.

James, P. (1991). Effects of a communication component added to an emotionally focused couples therapy. *Journal of Marital and Family Therapy, 17*, 263–276.

Johnson, S. M. (1986). Bonds or bargains: Relationship paradigms and their significance for marital therapy. *Journal of Marital and Family Therapy, 12*, 259–267.

Johnson, S. M. (1998). Listening to the music: Emotion as a natural part of systems theory [Special issue]. *Journal of Systemic Therapies, 17*, 1–17.

Johnson, S. M. (1999). Emotionally focused couples therapy: Straight to the heart. In J. Donovan (Ed.), *Short term couples therapy* (pp. 11–42). New York: Guilford Press.

Johnson, S. M. (2002). *Emotionally focused couple therapy with trauma survivors: Strengthening attachment bonds*. New York: Guilford Press.

Johnson, S. M. (2003a). Attachment theory: A guide for couples therapy. In S. M. Johnson & V. Whiffen (Eds.), *Attachment processes in couples and families* (pp. 103–123). New York: Guilford Press.

Johnson, S. M. (2003b). The revolution in couples therapy: A practitioner–scientist perspective. *Journal of Marital and Family Therapy, 29*, 365–385.

Johnson, S. M. (2004a). *The practice of emotionally focused marital therapy: Creating connection* (2nd ed.). New York: Brunner/Routledge.

Johnson, S. M. (2004b). Attachment theory as a guide for healing couple relationships. In W. S. Rholes & J. A. Simpson (Eds.), *Adult attachment* (pp. 367–387). New York. Guilford Press.

Johnson, S. M. (2004c). Facing the dragon together: Emotionally focused therapy with trauma survivors. In D. R. Catherall (Ed.), *Handbook of stress, trauma and the family* (pp. 493–510). New York: Brunner/Routledge.

Johnson, S. M. (2005). Emotion and the repair of close relationships. In W. Pinsof & J. Lebow (Eds.), *Family psychology: The art of the science* (pp. 91–113). New York: Oxford University Press.

Johnson, S. (2008a). *Hold me tight: Seven conversations for a lifetime of love*. New York: Little Brown.

Johnson, S. M. (2008b). Attachment and emotionally focused therapy: Perfect partners. In J. Obegi & E. Berant (Eds.), *Clinical applications of adult attachment*. New York: Guilford Press.

Johnson, S. M., & Boisvert, C. (2001). Humanistic couple and family therapy. In D. Kane (Ed.), *Humanistic psychotherapies* (pp. 309–338). Washington, DC: American Psychological Association Press.

Johnson, S. M., Bradley, B., Furrow, J., Lee, A., Palmer, G., Tilley, D., et al. (2005). *Becoming an emotionally focused couple therapist: The workbook*. New York: Brunner/Routledge.

Johnson, S. M., & Greenberg, L. (1985). The differential effects of experiential and problem solving interventions in resolving marital conflict. *Journal of Consulting and Clinical Psychology, 53*, 175–184.

Johnson, S. M., & Greenberg, L. (1988). Relating process to outcome in marital therapy. *Journal of Marital and Family Therapy, 14*, 175–183.

Johnson, S. M., Hunsley, J., Greenberg, L., & Schlinder, D. (1999). Emotionally focused couples therapy: Status and challenges. *Journal of Clinical Psychology: Science and Practice, 6,* 67–79.

Johnson, S. M., & Lebow, J. (2000). The "coming of age" of couple therapy: A decade review. *Journal of Marital and Family Therapy, 26,* 23–38.

Johnson, S. M., Maddeaux, C., & Blouin, J. (1998). Emotionally focused family therapy for bulimia: Changing attachment patterns. *Psychotherapy, 35,* 238–247.

Johnson, S. M., Makinen, M., & Millikin, J. (2001). Attachment injuries in couple relationships: A new perspective on impasses in couple therapy. *Journal of Marital and Family Therapy, 27,* 145–155.

Johnson, S. M., & Talitman, E. (1997). Predictors of success in emotionally focused marital therapy. *Journal of Marital and Family Therapy, 23,* 135–152.

Johnson, S. M., & Whiffen, V. (1999). Made to measure: Adapting emotionally focused couple therapy to partners attachment styles. *Clinical Psychology: Science and Practice, 6,* 366–381.

Johnson, S. M., & Williams Keeler, L. (1998). Creating healing relationships for couples dealing with trauma: The use of emotionally focused marital therapy. *Journal of Marital and Family Therapy, 24,* 227–236.

Jordan, J. V., Kaplan, A. G., Miller, J. B., Stiver, I. P., & Surrey, J. L. (1991). *Women's growth in connection: Writings from the Stone Center.* New York: Guilford Press.

Josephson, G. (2003). Using an attachment-based intervention with same-sex couples. In S. M. Johnson & V. Whiffen (Eds.), *Attachment processes in couple and family therapy* (pp. 300–320). New York: Guilford Press.

Kennedy-Moore, E., & Watson, J. (1999). *Expressing emotion: Myths, realities and therapeutic strategies.* New York: Guilford Press.

Knudson-Martin, C., & Mahoney, A. (1999). Beyond different worlds: A post gender approach to relationship development. *Family Process, 38,* 325–340.

Kobak, R., & Cole, H. (1991). Attachment and meta-monitoring: Implications for autonomy and psychopathology. In D. Cicchetti & S. Toth (Eds.), *Disorders and dysfunctions of the self* (pp. 267–297). Rochester, NY: University of Rochester Press.

Kobak, R., & Hazan, C. (1991). Attachment in marriage: Effects of security and accuracy of working models. *Journal of Personality and Social Psychology, 60,* 861–869.

Koerner, K., & Jacobson, N. (1994). Emotion and behavioral couple therapy. In S. M. Johnson & L. S. Greenberg (Eds.), *The Heart of the matter: Perspectives on emotion in marital therapy* (pp. 207–226). New York: Brunner/Mazel.

Lebow, J. (1997). The integrative revolution in couple and family therapy. *Family Process, 36,* 1–17.

MacIntosh, H. B., & Johnson, S. M. (in press). Emotionally focused therapy for couples and childhood sexual abuse survivors. *Journal of Marital and Family Therapy.*

MacPhee, D. C., Johnson, S. M., & van der Veer, M. C. (1995). Low sexual desire in women: The effects of marital therapy. *Journal of Sex and Marital Therapy, 21,* 159–182.

Mahoney, M. (1991). *Human change processes.* New York: Basic Books.

Main, M., & Hesse, E. (1990). Parent's unresolved traumatic experiences are related to infant disorganized attachment status. In M. Greenberg & D. Cicchetti (Eds.), *Attachment in the preschool years* (pp. 331–349). Chicago: University of Chicago Press.

Main, M., Kaplan, N., & Cassidy, J. (1985). Security in infancy, childhood and adulthood: A move to the level of representation. In I. Bretherton & E. Waters (Eds.), Growing points of attachment theory and research. *Monographs of the Society for Research in Child Development, 50,* 66–104.

Makinen, J., & Johnson, S. (2006). An EFT approach to esolving attachment injuries in couples. *Journal of Consulting and Clinical Psychology, 74,* 1055–1064.

Martin, J., & Sugarman, J. (2000). Between modern and postmodern. *American Psychologist, 55,* 397–406.

McFarlane, A. C., & van der Kolk, B. A. (1996). Trauma and its challenge to society. In B. van der Kolk, A. McFarlane, & L. Weisaeth (Eds.), *Traumatic stress* (pp. 24–46). New York: Guilford Press.

McLeod, J., Kessler, R., & Landis, K. (1992). Speed of recovery from major depressive episodes in a community sample of married men and women. *Journal of Abnormal Psychology, 101,* 277–286.

Mesquita, B., & Frijda, N. (1992). Cultural variations in emotions: A review. *Psychological Bulletin, 112,* 179–204.

Mikulincer, M. (1995). Attachment style and the mental representation of self. *Journal of Personality and Social Psychology, 69,* 1203–1215.

Mikulincer, M. (1997). Adult attachment style and information processing: Individual differences in curiosity and cognitive closure. *Journal of Personality and Social Psychology, 72,* 1217–1230.

Mikulincer, M. (1998). Adult attachment style and individual differences in functional versus dysfunctional experiences of anger. *Journal of Personality and Social Psychology, 74,* 513–524.

Mikulincer, M., & Goodman, G. (Eds.). (2006). *Dynamics of romantic love.* New York: Guilford Press.

Millikin, J., & Johnson, S. M. (2000). Telling tales: Disquisitions in emotionally focused therapy. *Journal of Family Psychotherapy, 11,* 75–79.

Minuchin, S., & Fishman, H. C. (1982). *Techniques of family therapy.* Cambridge, MA: Harvard University Press.

Naaman, S., & Johnson, S. (in press). *Emotionally focused couple therapy with breast cancer survivors and their spouses: An outcome study.*

Neimeyer, R. (1993). An appraisal of constructivist psychotherapies. *Journal of Consulting and Clinical Psychology, 61,* 221–234.

Palmer, G., & Johnson, S. M. (2002). Becoming an emotionally focused couple therapist. *Journal of Couple and Relationship Therapy, 1*, 1–20.

Perls, F., Hefferline, R., & Goodman, P. (1951). *Gestalt therapy*. New York: Dell.

Rholes, S., & Simpson, J. (2004). *Adult attachment*. New York: Guilford Press.

Roberts, T. W. (1992). Sexual attraction and romantic love: Forgotten variables in marital therapy. *Journal of Marital and Family Therapy, 18*, 357–364.

Rogers, C. R. (1951). *Client-centered therapy*. Boston: Houghton Mifflin.

Salovey, P., Rothman, A. J., Detweiler, J. B., & Steward, W. T. (2000). Emotional states and physical health. *American Psychologist, 55*, 110–121.

Satir, V. (1967). *Conjoint family therapy*. Palo Alto, CA: Science and Behavior Books.

Schore, A. (1994). *Affect regulation and the organization of self*. Hillsdale, NJ: Erlbaum.

Schwartz, R., & Johnson, S. M. (2000). Does couple and family therapy have emotional intelligence? *Family Process, 39*, 29–34.

Shapiro, V. (1996). Subjugated knowledge and the working alliance. *In Session: Psychotherapy in Practice, 1*, 9–22.

Simpson, J. A., & Rholes, W. S. (1994). Stress and secure base relationships in adulthood. In K. Bartholomew & D. Perlman (Eds.), *Attachment processes in adulthood* (pp. 181–204). London, Penn: Jessica Kingsley.

Simpson, J. A., Rholes, W. S., & Nelligan, J. S. (1992). Support seeking and support giving within couples in an anxiety provoking situation: The role of attachment styles. *Journal of Personality and Social Psychology, 62*, 434–446.

Spanier, G. B. (1976). Measuring dyadic adjustment: New scales for assessing the quality of marriage and similar dyads. *Journal of Marriage and the Family, 38*, 15–28.

Sprenkle, D., Blow, A., & Dickey, M. H. (1999). Common factors and other non-technique variables in marriage and family therapy. In M. Hubble, B. Duncan, & C. Miller (Eds.), *The heart and soul of change* (pp. 329–359). Washington, DC: American Psychological Association Press.

Stern, D. (2004). *The present moment*. New York: Norton.

Teichman, Y., & Teichman, M. (1990). Interpersonal views of depression: Review and integration. *Family Psychology, 3*, 349–367.

Tomkins, S. (1962). *Affect, imagery and consciousness*. New York: Springer.

van der Kolk, B., Perry, C., & Herman, J. (1991). Childhood origins of self-destructive behavior. *American Journal of Psychiatry, 148*, 1665–1671.

van IJzendoorn, M. H., & Sagi, A. (1999). Cross cultural patterns of attachment: Universal and contextual dimensions. In J. Cassidy & P. Shaver (Eds.), *Handbook of attachment: Theory, research and clinical applications* (pp. 713–734). New York: Guilford Press.

von Bertalanffy, L. (1956). General system theory. *General Systems Yearbook, 1*, 1–10.

Watzlawick, P., Beavin, J., & Jackson, D. (1967). *Pragmatics of human communication*. New York: Norton.

Weeks, G. R., & L'Abate, L. (1979). A compilation of paradoxical methods. *American Journal of Family Therapy, 7*, 61–76.

Weinfield, N. S., Sroufe, L. A., Egeland, B., & Carlson, E. A. (1999). The nature of individual differences in infant–caregiver attachment. In J. Cassidy & P. Shaver (Eds.), *Handbook of attachment: Theory, research, and clinical applications* (pp. 68–88). New York: Guilford Press.

Weissman, M. M. (1987). Advances in psychiatric epidemiology: Rates and risks for major depression. *American Journal of Public Health, 77*, 445–451.

Whiffen, V., & Johnson, S. M. (1998). An attachment theory framework for the treatment of childbearing depression. *Clinical Psychology: Science and Practice, 5*, 478–492.

Whisman, M. (1999). Marital dissatisfaction and psychiatric disorders: Results from the National Comorbidity Survey. *Journal of Abnormal Psychology, 108*, 701–706.

Whisman, M., & Jacobson, N. S. (1990). Power, marital satisfaction and response to marital therapy. *Journal of Family Psychology, 4*, 202–212.

CHAPTER 5

Gottman Method Couple Therapy

JOHN MORDECHAI GOTTMAN
JULIE SCHWARTZ GOTTMAN

BACKGROUND

The Masters and Disasters of Relationships

We believe that couple intervention must be grounded in basic research. When we began this work there were only a handful of studies dedicated to understanding why some couples sustained their marriages, while others did not. Unfortunately, those studies gave no clue as to how to proceed with intervention. For example, Newcomb and Bentler (1980) found that clothes-conscious women were less likely to divorce, but there was no such correlation for men. The correlations, when significant, were small. Imagine, as a humorous aside, a therapy based on these results. The therapist would discuss Martha's wardrobe with her but tell George that it did not matter in his case. Men, it doesn't matter what you wear. Women, go shopping.

So we begin this chapter with a review of the empirical work that underlies our therapeutic methods. This work has been conducted over the last three decades and continues today. Fundamentally descriptive, it arises from the notion that to understand couples, one must follow them for long periods of time to investigate change and stability. We wanted to observe not only distressed relation-

ships but also well-functioning heterosexual and same-sex relationships. Understanding good relationships has helped us define the goals of couple therapy, because we believe that clinicians should rely on reality and not fantasies of what a good relationship is like. Over the past three decades John Gottman and Robert Levenson (1984, 1985, 1988, 1992, 2002) together have conducted most of this basic research.

Levenson and Gottman were surprised by the enormous stability of couples' interaction over time and the data's ability to predict the longitudinal course of relationships. They were able to predict both stability and relationship satisfaction with relatively small samples of observational, self-report, and physiological data. On the basis of these predictions, John and Julie Gottman developed a theory of how relationships function well or fail, and methods to facilitate change in these relationships through psychoeducational, preventive, and therapeutic interventions.

Before describing this theory, we briefly review its empirical basis. More detail is available in previous editions of this volume. In seven nonintervention studies with over 700 couples, Robert Levenson, John Gottman, and their colleagues identified what they later called the "masters" of relationships within representative samples of heterosexual and same-sex couples. Couples were studied across the life course and for as long as 18 years. Observed phases of relationships included everything from the newlywed years through retirement. The "masters of relationships" were those couples who remained stable and relatively happy across time. The "disasters" of relationships were couples who either broke up or stayed unhappily together. With Neil Jacobson and his students (e.g., Jacobson & Gottman, 1998) John Gottman also studied the extreme disaster cases, those couples with both characterological and situational domestic violence. That longitudinal research has spanned the life course. In his own laboratory, Gottman longitudinally studied newlyweds (Gottman, Coan, Carrère, & Swanson, 1998; Driver & Gottman, 2004b; Tabares, Driver, & Gottman, 2004; Gottman, Driver, Yoshimoto, & Rushe, 2002), the transition to parenthood (Shapiro & Gottman, 2000, 2005), and couples with young children (Katz & Gottman, 1993). With Robert Levenson and Laura Carstensen, John Gottman studied two groups: couples in their 40s and couples in their 60s. That study is now in its 19th year (see Levenson, Carstensen, & Gottman, 1993). Couples were followed longitudinally with particular emphasis on major life transitions, such as parenthood, midlife, and retirement. When the couples had children, the Gottman lab studied parent–child interaction and followed infants' or children's emotional, behavioral, social, and intellectual development. Some of these parent–child and child results have been reported in books entitled *Meta-Emotion* (Gottman, Katz, & Hooven, 1996) and *The Heart of Parenting: Raising an Emotionally Intelligent Child* (Gottman & DeClaire, 1996), and Gottman and Gottman's (2007) *And Baby Makes Three*.

A multimethod approach has characterized this research. Couples were videotaped in various contexts of interaction, including a discussion of the events of the day after being apart for at least 8 hours, a conflict discussion, a positive discussion, and 12 consecutive hours with no instructions in a specially designed apartment laboratory (dubbed "The Love Lab" by the media). The collected data ranged from synchronized interactive behavior (coded in various ways) and self-report (interviews and video recall ratings) to physiology (e.g., heart rate, blood velocity, skin conductance; Levenson & Gottman, 1985). Also, Gottman developed, tested, and validated a set of questionnaires that arose from the Gottmans' relationship theory. Data

from these questionnaires were gathered and analyzed. In addition, questions about the history and philosophy of the relationship (the Oral History Interview) were coded with the Buehlman coding system (Buehlman, Gottman, & Katz, 1992). Other data were analyzed with methods that coded emotional interaction during conversation (Gottman's Specific Affect Coding System; Gottman, McCoy, Coan, & Collier, 1996), repair during conflict (Repair Coding; Tabares et al., 2004), everyday interaction in an apartment laboratory (the bids and turning system; Driver & Gottman, 2004a, 2004b), and parent–infant interaction (developed by Shapiro) and parent–child interaction (developed by Kahen, Katz, & Gottman, 1994). The Meta-Emotion Interview (feelings and philosophy about emotions) also generated additional data (Gottman, Katz, et al., 1996; Yoshimoto, 2005). Examples of results of this research may be found in Gottman's *What Predicts Divorce?* (1994), *The Marriage Clinic* (1999), Gottman and Silver's (1999), *The Seven Principles for Making Marriage Work*, and Julie Gottman's edited (2004) *The Marriage Clinic Casebook*.

The accomplishments of this approach included an ability to predict divorce or stability with accuracy, which has now been replicated across four separate longitudinal studies, and an ability to predict eventual relationship satisfaction among newlyweds. These findings on divorce prediction and their replications are based on strong statistical relationships, unlike those typically found in the social sciences (Buehlman et al., 1992; Gottman & Levenson, 1992; Gottman, 1994; Jacobson & Gottman, 1998; Carrère et al., 2000). The researchers have been able to predict the fate of marriages in three measurement domains: interactive behavior, perception (self-report on questionnaires, interviews, and video playback ratings), and physiology. The studies have also yielded: (1) an understanding of how relationships function or fail; (2) an ability to predict newlyweds' adaptations to the transitions of parenthood, midlife, and retirement; and (3) nonlinear dynamic difference and differential equations for mathematical modeling of marital interaction. These equations have produced a theory of how relationships work that integrates the study of affect and power in relationships. The modeling permits one to fit actual equations to observational data over time. The equations estimate couples' "emotional inertias," their "influence functions," and the homeostatic set points to which their interactions are drawn. It is then possible to *simulate* what a couple would be like under new conditions and to conduct experiments to create proximal change. What this means is that the goal of the study is to improve the second of two conversations a couple has, which is a much smaller goal than changing the entire relationship forever. These are specific experiments to change the couple's interaction in very specific ways (e.g., reduce emotional inertia). With many of these experiments one can incrementally build a science of change for couples. These methods are detailed in several articles (e.g., Cook et al., 1995; Gottman, Swanson, & Murray, 1999) and a book entitled *The Mathematics of Marriage* (Gottman, Murray, Swanson, Tyson, & Swanson, 2002; also see Tung, 2006).

The conclusions of this research build on previous research work intervention with couples, yet in some ways they depart dramatically from the past. Here are the central findings:

1. Most relationship conflict is not solvable, but it is "perpetual," based on lasting personality differences between partners; some of that perpetual conflict becomes destructively "gridlocked," but it may also persist in the form of more constructive dialogue.
2. Gridlocked conflict is not about negative affect reciprocity but about its escalation from mild negative affects (e.g., whining) to the more extreme "Four Horsemen of the Apocalypse" (criticism, defensiveness, contempt, and stonewalling).
3. Escalating conflict may characterize couples who divorce early, but a second destructive, emotionally disengaged interaction pattern involves the absence of both negative and positive affect during conflict; this pattern points to the importance of positive affect during conflict.
4. A gentle approach (gentle "startup," accepting influence, and compromise) distinguishes the masters from the disasters of relationships, as do neutral interaction, low levels of physiological arousal, and humor and affection.
5. Physiological soothing versus diffuse physiological arousal (DPA) is predictive of improvement versus deterioration over time in relationships.
6. The basis for a "dialogue" with a perpetual issue lies in dealing with its core existential nature, or the "dreams within conflict."
7. Building general positivity in the relationship (during both conflict and nonconflict contexts) is essential to ensure lasting change,

and this needs to be based upon improving the couple's friendship, intimacy, and building and savoring the positive affect systems (e.g., play, fun, humor, exploration, adventure, romance, passion, good sex).
8. Friendship processes, working via "sentiment overrides," control the effectiveness and thresholds of the repair of problematic interaction (conflict and regrettable incidents).
9. The couple's construction of a "shared meaning system" facilitates stability and happiness.
10. All three systems need to be understood—conflict, friendship/intimacy/positive affect, and shared meaning—and they interact bidirectionally.

The Sound Relationship House Theory

Arranged in hierarchical order are the seven levels of what we have called our "sound relationship house" theory:

1. Build love maps. A love map is a road map of one's partner's inner world, built by asking open-ended questions.
2. Build the fondness and admiration system by expressing affection and respect in small, everyday moments.
3. Turn toward instead of away or against by noticing a partner's bids for emotional connection.
4. Allow positive sentiment override, which means not taking neutral or negative partner actions personally (if processes 1, 2, and 3 are not working, negative sentiment override results, in which even neutral acts are perceived as negative).
5. Take a two-pronged approach toward managing conflict by using a gentle approach in presenting complaints, accepting influence, physiological soothing, and compromise, and by establishing a dialogue with perpetual problems that examines the existential dreams within conflict.
6. Honor one another's life dreams.
7. Build the shared meaning system by establishing formal and informal rituals of connection, supporting one another's life roles, creating shared goals and values, and common views of symbols.

The sound relationship house concepts generally extend to the masters and disasters of gay and lesbian relationships. The sound relationship house theory guides our interventions.

We have conducted several randomized clinical trials of our intervention methods. One study comprised programmatic, 2-day friendship-building and conflict-management psychoeducational workshops (Day 1 only vs. Day 2 only vs. combined Day 1 and Day 2) versus the combined workshop plus nine sessions of couple therapy, all compared to a control group (Ryan & Gottman, in press). Shapiro and Gottman (2005) also studied a prevention program for couples expecting a baby. In the latter study, we found that, compared to a control group, with a 2-day workshop we could reverse the drop in relationship satisfaction experienced by nearly 70% of couples transitioning into parenthood, plus reduce their hostility and mothers' postpartum depression. In the next study we added a support group to the workshop and considerably enhanced the treatment effect (Gottman & Gottman, 2007). Finally, we are now engaged in two 5-year randomized clinical trials, both with lower-income couples: one on situational domestic violence and the other with unmarried couples in poverty expecting a baby.

Based on these findings, rather than offering a checklist of what needs to be changed in ailing relationships, we present our updated theory of how marriages either work or fail, then interventions based on this theory. In our view, a "theory" must provide a "recipe" for therapeutic change, and describes the push–pull causal processes through which relationships work or fail.

THERAPY BASED ON THEORY OF WHAT MAKES RELATIONSHIPS SUCCEED OR FAIL

Overview

We have augmented our theory with the knowledge provided in Jaak Panksepp's superb guide to the unexplored world of both positive and negative affect, his book *Affective Neuroscience* (1998). In it, Panksepp documents seven affect systems that have distinct behavioral and neurophysiological patterns shared by all mammals. Gottman and De-Claire's (2001) book, *The Relationship Cure*, called these systems "emotional command systems" and specifically named them:

1. The Sentry, with the primary affects of fear (being vigilant for danger, and its opposite, the feelings of security and safety.
2. The Nest Builder, with the feelings involved in bonding, security, affection, love, connection and attachment, and the opposite emotions of separation–distress/panic, grief, sadness, and loss.
3. The Explorer, or the seeking system, with primary affects of curiosity and the joy of learning, exploration, and adventure.
4. The Commander-in-Chief, with its primary affects of anger, hostility, rage, dominance, control, and status, and its opposites of submission and helplessness.
5. The Sensualist, with affects involving sensuality, sexuality, and lust.
6. The Jester, with affects related to play, fun, humor, amusement, laughter, and joy.
7. The Energy Czar, which is involved in managing bodily needs concerned with energy, food, warmth, shelter, and so on.

Panksepp found that these seven emotional command systems are the primary colors of affect for mammals. They can operate exclusively but are often recruited in the service of one another. For example, the Explorer may be recruited in the service of finding a sexual partner. Or the Sentry and Nest Builder may be employed along with the Commander-in-Chief to create a potentially ferocious protector of the young. We believe that these systems form the affective underpinnings for sound relationships. In other words, because every individual possesses these systems to varying degrees, they color the relationships between individuals. Through pure forms or blends, they supply interactions with relative affective richness.

These systems plus environmental factors also create an individual's attitudes, values, and feelings about the expression of various emotions, known as "meta-emotion." When individuals enter into relationship with one another, they form unique meta-emotion combinations. In the masters of relationship, partners are often well-matched in meta-emotion, or they have found ways to coexist harmoniously with meta-emotion mismatches. But in couples who experience distress, meta-emotion mismatches have often disrupted the relationship (Gottman, Katz, et al., 1996). Thus, couples often present in therapy with meta-emotion mismatches. According to Gottman and his colleagues, plus Panksepp's work, to help couples deal with meta-emotion mismatches, down-regulating negative conflict is not enough. Positive affect must be created or enhanced as well. The theory-based therapy that we will now present contains both. Intervention processes are organized by therapeutic goal.

Our therapy begins with an assessment of a couple's relationship strengths and challenges that need improvement. Over the course of one conjoint session and two individual sessions, we use interviews. We begin with the partners' narrative of what brings them to the therapy. We then administer our Oral History Interview (questions about the history and philosophy of their relationship and their parents' relationships). We tape a conflict discussion with physiological monitoring, conduct individual sessions, and ask couples to fill out written questionnaires that follow the sound relationship house theory (see below and Gottman, 1999). The information gathered from these sessions and the written materials inform our assessment. In a third session, we present this assessment and discuss the treatment goals engendered by it. Once appropriate goals are agreed upon with the couple, intervention can begin.

We begin each therapeutic session with the concerns and emotions that a couple brings into the therapeutic hour, building the relationship by using these emotions in the context of an empathic and accepting therapeutic alliance. Like Johnson's emotionally focused couple therapy (see Chapter 4, this volume), our therapy is emotion-focused, experiential, and centered in the here and now. But we also provide the couple with explicit "blueprints" we have gleaned from the masters of relationship for down-regulating negative conflict, enhancing positive affect, and creating shared meaning in the relationship. These "blueprints"

provide the therapist and the couple a guide that makes explicit the skills necessary to accomplish therapeutic goals. The therapist makes the therapy process as dyadic as possible, serving as a validating, compassionate emotion coach, and a "translator" of the feelings and needs of each person in the interaction (see Wile, 1993). The therapist also explains and teaches constructive alternatives to the couple's ineffective patterns of interaction.

What Makes Couples' Relationships Successful?

Figure 5.1 is a summary of the five central processes that make relationships successful. All five processes are stated as verbs, because they are goals of our therapeutic recipe. We will describe both the research that underscores these goals and the interventions that help to achieve them. What is our theory as to why some people behave in unfortunate ways that create relationship misery? Our view is that the culprit is entropy. As the Second Law of Thermodynamics suggests, if energy is not supplied to a closed system, it will deteriorate and run down; entropy will increase. Some people prioritize parts of life other than their closest relationships. Without adequate maintenance the best vehicle will fall apart over time. This sad fact is even more true of love relationships. We turn to a consideration of how to do the required maintenance, should we choose to preserve our love.

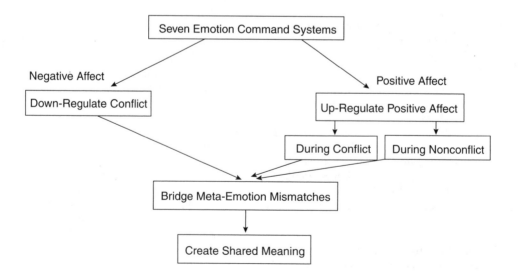

FIGURE 5.1. Flowchart for Gottman method therapy.

Goal 1: Down-Regulate Negative Affect during Conflict

We have found that conflict is inevitable in relationships. It has many prosocial functions, such as culling out interactions that do not work, helping us to know one another as we change, and continually renewing courtship. Therefore, we do not declare war on negative affect, or try to eliminate it. The first consistent finding that emerged from longitudinal studies by Gottman and Levenson is that higher levels and escalation of negative affect predict relationship instability. This was a surprising finding at the time, because many previous writers have targeted negative affect reciprocity as the key symptom of conflictual relationship dysfunction. However, in Gottman and Levenson's research, sequential analysis of the mere reciprocity of negative affect (e.g., anger-to-anger sequences) did not discriminate stable and satisfied couples from their opposite. But the *escalation* of mild negative affect, particularly to one of the Four Horsemen of the Apocalypse (criticism, defensiveness, contempt, and stonewalling), did predict instability and increasing dissatisfaction with the relationship. An added contribution of this research was that physiological arousal of the autonomic nervous system predicted a decline in relationship satisfaction, whereas physiological calm predicted increased relationship satisfaction over a 3-year period. This was true of all systems measured (e.g., heart rate, blood velocity, skin conductance, gross motor movement). In a later, 14-year longitudinal study, escalation of relationship conflict predicted early divorce an average of 5.6 years after the wedding. Taken directly from the research, an example of this escalating negative affect follows:

WIFE: I wish you'd stop laughing. Makes me so mad that I'm late every morning because you won't get up on time.

HUSBAND: (*sad voice tone, avoiding eye contact*) Yeah, I shouldn't laugh. I know what it feels like to be late because of someone else.

WIFE: (*angry*) Oh, do you know what it feels like?

HUSBAND: Yeah, I sort of know what it feels like.

WIFE: (*mocking, contemptuous*) You sort of know what it feels like, you sort of know what it feels like. (*intensely angry*) They why don't you show a little respect for me?

In this short interaction, the husband's laughter appears to mock the wife's anger, which is contemp-

tuous behavior on his part, and she subsequently responds by escalating her anger to mockery and contempt.

Busting Myths about Conflict

We have learned a great deal about conflict in the past four decades. In 1965 Bach published *The Intimate Enemy*, in which he suggested that couples need to express their resentments toward one another, and that great harm can come from suppressing their anger. He believed in a catharsis theory of marriage. He had partners take turns expressing their resentments toward one another, and even had them hit one another with foam-rubber bats called "batakas." At the end of one of his sessions, however, people left even more resentful and angry than before they came for therapy. In her superb book on anger, Tavris (1989) reviewed hundreds of studies indicating that the mere expression of anger leads the angry person (and others) to feel more, not less anger. There is no evidence for a catharsis theory of anger expression. Anger must be guided to become constructive.

What is the alternative to Bach's approach? We have learned that in stable, satisfying relationships people take a gentle approach to conflict. They soften the way they bring up issues. They are influenced by one another (which is easier to do if the issue is presented gently). They emphasize their common ground. There is give and take. They use neutral and positive affect and constructive conflict management and problem solving to down-regulate both their own and their partner's physiological arousal. They reach a compromise. They attempt to repair ruptures early and to accept repair attempts.

Perpetual Unsolvable Conflicts

Our knowledge about conflict itself has also deepened. The focus in many couples' therapies is primarily about "conflict resolution." The therapist sees the goal as helping partners "resolve" their issues and put them away forever. However, we have learned in our research that 69% of couple conflicts are perpetual. They never get resolved. Bring a couple into a lab 4 years later and they are talking about the same issues in very much the same ways, albeit often in different forms. When current and past videotapes are edited together, it looks like no time has passed at all. These conflicts have lasting sources that arise from consistent personality and need differences between partners. In a remarkably insightful book *After the Honeymoon*, Wile (1988) wrote, "Choosing a partner is choosing a set of problems" (p. 12), that problems are a part of any relationship, and that a particular person would have some set of problems no matter who that person married. He wrote:

> Paul married Alice and Alice gets loud at parties and Paul, who is shy, hates that. But if Paul had married Susan, he and Susan would have gotten into a fight before they even got to the party. That's because Paul is always late and Susan hates to be kept waiting. She would feel taken for granted, which she is very sensitive about. Paul would see her complaining about this as her attempt to dominate him, which he is very sensitive about. If Paul had married Gail, they wouldn't have even gone to the party because they would still be upset about an argument they had the day before about Paul's not helping with the housework. To Gail, when Paul does not help she feels abandoned, which she is sensitive about, and to Paul, Gail's complaining is an attempt at domination, which he is sensitive about. The same is true about Alice. If she had married Steve, she would have the opposite problem, because Steve gets drunk at parties and she would get so angry at his drinking that they would get into a fight about it. If she had married Lou, she and Lou would have enjoyed the party but then when they got home the trouble would begin when Lou wanted sex because he always wants sex when he wants to feel closer, but sex is something Alice only wants when she already feels close. (p. 13)

Wile also wrote:

> There is value, when choosing a long-term partner, in realizing that you will inevitably be choosing a particular set of unsolvable problems that you'll be grappling with for the next ten, twenty, or fifty years. (p. 13)

So, we think that it is the case that relationships (without therapy) work to the extent that people have chosen a relationship with a set of perpetual problems with which they can learn to live. Well-functioning relationships establish what we call a "dialogue" regarding these issues. Partners keep revisiting them and talking about them with humor, affection, and some irritability, but without escalating negative affect.

For many couples these perpetual issues seem to arise out of thin air. In hundreds of research interviews about conflict at home, we also found that couples do not necessarily argue about "issues." There may be no topic to the argument. The conflict, as in the following example, appears to be about interaction itself:

WIFE: Stop channel surfing. Just leave it. I want to see this show.

HUSBAND: (*holding the remote*) Let me just see what else is on.

WIFE: No. I might want to watch this show.

HUSBAND: In a minute. There could be a film on.

WIFE: Leave it.

HUSBAND: Fine!

WIFE: That's your problem, the way you just said "Fine"? Why did you say that? We were having a perfectly good time until you said that.

HUSBAND: I said "fine" because, have it your way, you're going to have it your way, anyway.

WIFE: Fine!

On the surface, this fight is about nothing. However, a deeper look suggests that there are hidden agendas based on accepting differences in preferences and personality. In a similar way, conflicts can arise from different ideas about punctuality, affection, power, money, fairness, or emotion itself.

Methods for Accomplishing Goal 1: How to Down-Regulate Negative Affect during Conflict

Here are a number of interventions that can be used to down-regulate negative affect.

STEP 1: REPAIR—PROCESSING FIGHTS AND REGRETTABLE INCIDENTS

Couples come into a therapeutic hour with a combination of successes and hot regrettable incidents (conflict or failing to connect emotionally). These become the focus of therapy. Our analyses of over 900 videotaped conflicts in our laboratory and over 1,000 play-by-play interviews about conflict at home have led us to the conclusion that most of the time most couples fight about what appears to be absolutely nothing (Gottman & Gottman, 2007). Conflicts usually arise from mismatches in perception and need in everyday interaction that very rapidly lead to misunderstanding, hurt feelings, escalation, anger, pouting, sulking, and emotional withdrawal. One or both people say and do things that they later regret. Processing regrettable incidents such as these is an essential part of conflict management. We focus on the emotions and perceptions in these events.

Our "Aftermath of a Fight or Regrettable Incident" format involves both people agreeing that in a regrettable incident there are two subjective realities, both of which are right. Even if we have people view a videotape of their interaction, there will still be two very different subjective realities about the interaction. Processing a fight means being able to talk about it without getting back into it. This may require some physiological soothing. Then the partners process the regrettable incident by (1) taking turns talking about their feelings and needs during the incident, (2) taking turns describing their subjective realities, (3) validating part of their partner's reality, (4) admitting their role in the conflict, and (5) talking about one way to make the conversation better next time. The therapist assists by building acceptance, empathy, and understanding.

Following these five parts of processing, the next step is to understand the fight by mapping what we call "the anatomy" of the fight. This involves identifying the "triggers" for each person that escalated the conflict, and unearthing the original emotional injuries that caused them, usually dating back to childhood (i.e., understanding why these are triggers). These triggers are made public parlance for the couple, whereby partners can experience empathy for one another and soften their response accordingly. Thus, an alliance between the couple can be built from understanding the conflict itself.

Repair will be ineffective, however, if the couple is in a state of "negative sentiment override," in which accumulated resentment renders understanding impossible to achieve. Then, additional work must accompany repair work.

STEP 2: REDUCING THE FOUR HORSEMEN

By heightening partners' awareness of the four best predictors of relationship meltdown, the "Four Horsemen of the Apocalypse" and their antidotes, the therapist can also gentle-down conflict interaction. Sometimes the therapist stops the couple when the Four Horsemen appear and works on their antidotes, but not every time. For some couples, the Four Horsemen are wreaking such havoc on interaction that constantly stopping them could render the couple stone silent. So the therapist uses discretion about when to stop, but always does so when there is verbal contempt (name-calling, direct insults). If it is hard to stop a couple, some simple techniques can be very effective. One method is to ring a soft chime when one of the horsemen appear. A second is to use a kitchen timer to break the interaction into 2-min-

ute segments, with feedback. A third method is to use video playback.

The first horseman, "Criticism," is stating a problem as a deficit in the partner's character. The antidote for criticism is complaining by talking about what one feels ("I" statements, no "you" statements, no blaming) about a specific situation and expressing a positive need. A positive need is a way that one's partner can shine for one. For example, if a man is upset that his partner talked at dinner about her day, a criticism would be "You are so selfish. All you think about is yourself." The antidote or alternative way to express the complaint would be "I'm upset about the conversation at dinner. I need you to ask me about my day." If a partner has trouble voicing needs, the "expressing needs" card deck can help by offering a broad spectrum of needs from which to choose. A gentle form of complaint especially helps when one initially raises a problem.

"Defensiveness," the second horseman, offers a form of self-protection through whining ("innocent victim" stance) or counterattacking ("righteous indignation" stance). The antidote for defensiveness is taking responsibility for even a small part of the problem. For example, if one's partner has said, "I hate you being late. I need you to be on time," a defensive statement would be a counterattack: "You think you're so perfect? When did you last balance the checkbook?" Accepting responsibility would sound like "That's a good point. I do take longer than you'd like." It is also important that the therapist help partners acknowledge responsibility without also feeling criticized by the therapist.

"Contempt," the third horseman, is a statement made from a position of superiority that often includes sarcasm, direct insults, or name-calling, or something more subtle (e.g., correcting someone's grammar when he or she is angry). It is essential that the therapist not empathize with statements of contempt; to do so runs the risk of creating a coalition with abuse. The therapist needs purposely to stop any insults, put-downs, or name-calling, define these as contempt, and tell the couple that contempt is our best predictor of relationship dissolution. The masters of relationships may regularly demonstrate the other three horsemen (at low levels), but they rarely voice contempt. The antidote for contempt is not only the absence of contempt, but also the presence of respect. The therapist must help the couple create a culture of appreciation and admiration, which is not a quick fix. This involves teaching partners how to have a positive habit of mind in which they scan the environment for actions of the other to appreciate and respect. The therapist can begin by having each partner express appreciations for one another either spontaneously or by using our Expressing Appreciations card deck. Over time, couples can learn to see the good in their partners, not the contemptible.

The fourth horseman, "stonewalling," is emotional disengagement from interaction. We observe this in the laboratory in the absence of cues that a listener is tracking the speaker (e.g., head nods, brief vocalizations, facial movement); the listener seems like a stone wall. What predicts stonewalling in heterosexual relationships is being male and having a heart rate over 100 beats a minute. The antidote for stonewalling is self-soothing to reduce one's own physiological arousal and staying emotionally engaged. To decrease stonewalling within sessions we use physiological monitoring (with two pulse oximeters), asking people about their own inner monologue during arousal (in stonewalling this monologue is usually about emotional withdrawal); Gendlin's (1981) method (within a couple session) of focusing, so that people can learn to articulate the nuances of what they are feeling and what their bodies are telling them; relaxation and meditation training within the couple session, actively asking the partners questions; and biofeedback. Another method we use for soothing is to teach the partner to do the soothing. We think this method is far superior to having the therapist do the soothing. The therapist cannot be there in important emotional moments of flooding and stonewalling. In the natural environment, stonewalling might be accompanied by a partner actually leaving the scene of the physiological arousal; this escape serves to condition new triggers signals associated with the arousal (e.g., the partner's voice, the partner's smell, the partner's presence). Teaching the physiologically aroused client to self-soothe in the presence of the partner and teaching the partner to soothe the client has the potential to reverse the escape conditioning that stonewalling offers. Because we think there is so much state-dependent learning, we do not generally teach these methods of self-soothing in an individual session. "State-dependent learning" means that when people learn something in a particular emotional state (e.g., anger), they will have more access to that learning when they are again in the same emotional state. If this is true, and the therapist wants a client to learn to cope with anger, the client needs to be angry in session

and learn to cope with the anger in that moment. So rather than calm people down to make an interpretation, we stay with the emotions of the moment.

STEP 3: RAPOPORT'S BLUEPRINT FOR SPEAKER AND LISTENER

Following Rapoport's work (1960) on international conflict, we need to establish emotional safety for partners by *postponing persuasion* until each person can state the partner's position to that partner's satisfaction. The goal is to make conflict discussions at the outset more gentle. We use an exercise that includes responsibilities for *both* the speaker and the listener. Here is the simple blueprint: Each partner is given a clipboard with paper and pen. The speaker expresses feelings using "I" statements (not "you" statements) about a specific issue and states a positive need, in other words, what he or she does want. This requires a mental transformation. The therapist may need to help convert blaming, "you" statements into feelings about a specific situation and a positive need. Next, the listener needs to be able to state the speaker's feelings and needs to the speaker's satisfaction and, at least to some degree, to validate them. The therapist often needs to aid the listener here. A useful guide for the therapist is the technique of speaking for the client, as described by Wile (1993) in *After the Fight*. We give clients a small, laminated blueprint card that lists speaker and listener roles, so they can also practice at home.

STEP 4: PROBLEM SOLVING, PERSUASION, AND COMPROMISE

Once partners understand each other's positions and feel validated and understood, persuasion can begin. Then, the couple can move toward problem solving and compromise. We use our "two-circle" method to facilitate compromise. The therapist hands each partner a diagram of two concentric circles. Each person is asked to identify a core need in the issue on which he or she *cannot* compromise. These needs are written inside the inner circle. Then each partner writes down aspects of the issue on which he or she has more flexibility. Finally, the partners share what they have written with one another and discuss a compromise, using a series of questions that they are given. The idea is that compromises fail if people give up too much that is crucial to them, so safety is established by first identifying and helping partners identify their core needs and communicating why these needs are so central, then identifying areas of greater flexibility in which there can be movement toward compromise.

STEP 5: BLUEPRINT FOR PERPETUAL, UNSOLVABLE CONFLICT: DREAMS WITHIN CONFLICT

This intervention is for conflicts that are "deal breakers," when to one or both people the very thought of compromise seems like giving up some central part of one's personality that one treasures, and compromise, in essence, feels like giving up one's self. At these times, there is a control struggle in which each person's position is interlaced with deep symbolic meaning and dreams that lie camouflaged beneath the surface. We use a method to unearth these hidden nuggets that again employs a listener–speaker exercise and provides specific questions. Again, safety becomes the focus, because the dreams harbored by each partner are often vulnerable ones. The key, we tell our couples, is that understanding must precede advice or problem solving.

STEP 6: DOWN-REGULATING NEGATIVE AFFECT WITH PHYSIOLOGICAL SOOTHING

One replicated finding in Levenson and Gottman's research is the important role of physiological soothing in down-regulating negative affect. Diffuse physiological activation (DPA), meaning higher heart rate, skin conductance, and blood velocity, characterized relationships that declined versus relationships that increased in marital satisfaction over a 3-year period, when researchers controlled initial levels of satisfaction (Levenson & Gottman, 1983). The difference between groups was substantial; for example, husbands in the group whose relationships improved over time had a preconversation heart rate in the presence of their partners that was 17 beats a minute lower than that of husbands whose relationships declined in satisfaction. These findings suggest that methods for muscle relaxation, deep breathing, meditation, and biofeedback may be helpful in couple therapy. In our offices, in addition to video cameras for replay and discussion within the therapeutic hour, we each have two pulse oximeters that measure the beat-to-beat heart rates and oxygen concentration in each person's blood during a conflict discussion. The oximeters have an alarm we can set that beeps when heart rate exceeds the intrinsic heart rhythm and a person is likely to start secreting adrenaline. This rate is 100 beats a minute in normal people and 80 beats a minute in highly trained athletes. At these rates, the oxygen concentration may also go below 95%. During the session, when the oximeters beep, clients know that they are physiologically aroused, or flooded, and need to calm down before proceeding. They are guided by the therapist to deep-breathe, do muscle relaxation work, or do guided visual imagery to help them in that process. Once their heart rates return to more normal levels, they continue the therapeutic work. This system of biofeedback enables partners at home to begin to sense when they are flooding and need to take a break. Their new sensitivity to body responses enables them to down-regulate escalations that may occur during conflict.

Goal 2: Up-Regulate Positive Affect during Conflict

The Research

In our 14-year longitudinal study, a group of couples emerged who divorced later, an average of 16.2 years after their wedding (Gottman & Levenson, 2002). Looking back at the coding of their Time 1 conflict interaction, the couples did not have very much negative affect or negative affect escalation. What characterized their interaction and discriminated them from couples who remained together or divorced early was the absence of *positive affect during conflict*. Specifically, the 5:1 ratio of positive coded interactions to negative coded interactions characterized stable couples, while a ratio of 0.8:1 positive codes to negative codes characterized unstable couples. The couples who later divorced appeared emotionally disengaged. For example, one couple in the study said the following:

WIFE: In all the years we've been married, seems to me that you don't know very much about me at all (*distressed tone, angry, whining*).

HUSBAND: (*avoiding eye contact, long pause, then in a neutral voice tone*) Yeah, that's pretty much true about the both of us.

In that interaction, the importance of the husband's response can be seen by imagining the alternative response of an engaged husband:

IMAGINED HUSBAND: Oh no, that's a terrible way to feel. No wonder you're upset. Let's talk about that and put an end to your feeling that I don't know you. I want to know you. It's very important to me.

What is surprising about this interaction is that the wife's complaint is actually a bid for connection. What makes it so dramatic is that the husband, instead of responding with alarm, concern, or empathy, responds with sadness and resignation. In observational research, information is only dramatized by actively imagining alternatives.

The Importance of Agreement, or Just Say, "Yes, Dear"

Imagine a salt shaker filled with words and nonverbal actions that communicate all forms of agreement, verbal and nonverbal ways of saying "yes" (e.g., "Yes," "You're right," "Good point," "What are your concerns here?" "You're making total sense," "That's so smart," "OK," "I can agree with some of what you're saying"). Levenson and Gottman (1985) also discovered that during conflict an affectively *neutral* way to present and respond to complaints is also a way of saying "yes"; it is actually positive. Untrained observers tend either to ignore neutral affect during couples' conflict as unimportant or to view it as boring; therefore, they are poor at predicting from videotapes of couple conflict which couples will divorce and which will stay together (Ebling & Levenson, 2003). But now imagine sprinkling the "Yes" salt shaker throughout the conflict interaction over time. That characterizes the interaction of stable, satisfied couples. Now imagine another salt shaker filled with words and nonverbal actions that communicate all forms of disagreement, ways of saying "No" (e.g., "no," "You're wrong," "You're so cold," "You're a total jerk," "What's wrong with you is ... ," "You are the problem," "You never ... ," "You always ... ," "I'm right," "Screw you," "You bitch," "That's ridiculous!," "Let me tell you what your problem is," "You're completely irrational," "I disagree with everything you're saying," "You are so stupid," "Yes, but ... "). Now, imagine sprinkling the "No" salt shaker throughout the conflict interaction. That characterizes the interaction of unstable, dissatisfied couples.

The interaction of the masters of relationships is characterized by some of the words and actions in this "No" salt shaker, just fewer of them, and, in fact, it is counterbalanced by five times more from the "Yes" salt shaker (Gottman, 1994), and effective repair at a lower threshold of negativ-

ity. The masters are particularly low on contempt. However, it would be a mistake for clinicians to declare war on negative affect based on these results. Like predators in an ecology who cull out the weakest of the prey species, negative affect can cull out those parts of interaction that are not working. Negative affect can improve the relationship over time, if it is followed by accepting influence. Anger expressions can reduce unfairness and injustice in the relationship, for example. Negative affect happens in all relationships. However, in good relationships, it is counterbalanced by positive affect and by repair. We have used these facts in therapy to *require* that a negative statement be followed by five positive statements (e.g., thus far unstated appreciations) from that person. One characteristic of the masters of relationship is the threshold and the effectiveness of repair. In a study of newlyweds, Gottman et al. (2002) reported that newlyweds who remained stable 6 years after the wedding had a lower threshold for initiating repair attempts during conflict than newlyweds who divorced. The stable couples did not wait to repair negative affect until it escalated. They repaired before the cumulative negative affect became too negative.

In an apartment laboratory Driver and Gottman (2004a) were able to study the relationship between nonconflict interaction during everyday moments in a 10-minute dinnertime, and both negative affect and positive affect during conflict. Analyzing the more than 600 hours of video generated in the apartment laboratory took nearly a decade. Driver (2006) assessed the response to what her coding system called "bids" for "emotional connection" (verbal and nonverbal attempts to get one's partner's attention, conversation, interest, enthusiasm, humor, affection, playfulness, emotional support, etc.). Driver found, among other things, that couples who stayed together after 6 years had initially (in the first year of marriage) turned toward one another's bids for emotional connection about 86% of the time, whereas couples who later divorced had turned toward their partner's bids only 33% of the time. Furthermore, those couples who turned toward one another's bids at a higher rate had less negative affect and more positive affect during a conflict discussion, particularly more shared humor and affection.

The exciting thing about Driver's work was that when we built the apartment lab, we expected Sidney Jourard's (1966) ideas to be validated, namely, that couples would naturally build intimate connection through self-disclosure conversations, and we would observe these conversations with fairly high frequency, particularly in our newlywed population. In fact, Driver discovered that couples build intimacy in very ordinary moments when partners first bid for the other's attention and, following the partner turning toward them, move up a hierarchy of bids that demand increasingly more emotional connection. Our rough *emotional connection hierarchy* included (1) attention, (2) interest, (3) conversations of various types (from reading the newspaper together to discussing a relative who is having problems), (4) shared humor, (5) affection, and (6) emotional support and empathy. We concluded that self-disclosure interactions were rare, because partners turn away at lower levels of the hierarchy. Driver's (2006) data show that turning away even at low levels of the emotional connection hierarchy can be somewhat devastating, as measured by the probability of rebidding after one's partner has turned away: 0% of the time in less happy newlyweds and 22% of the time in happier newlyweds. Both probabilities were surprisingly low. In these mundane, everyday moments of potential emotional connection, in our view, lie the roots of secure attachment in a relationship.

Driver's (2006) findings are important, because we need to know how a therapist can build a couple's positive affect during conflict. It is clearly not effective simply to tell partners to laugh more the next time they discuss his mother. Furthermore, we claim that it is much more difficult to change a couple's interaction during conflict than to change the mostly neutral interaction of turning toward bids for connection. We also believe that there is a positive feedback effect of turning toward bids: Turning toward leads to more bidding and more turning toward. If this is true, people need not have high standards for turning toward; they can simply start noticing and responding to bids at lower levels of the emotional connection hierarchy. Of course, Driver and Gottman (2004a) only reported correlational data, so we were not sure at that point in the research that changing turning toward could actually increase positive affect during conflict. The randomized clinical trial experiment with Ryan showed that the effect is causal: Turning toward bids and building the friendship in the relationship through increasing the activation of positive affect systems *in nonconflict contexts* build positive affect *during conflict* (Ryan & Gottman, in press). To be fair, Ryan and Gottman changed turning toward bids, as well as two other components of friendship: (1) building

"love maps," that is, knowledge of one another's inner psychological world through asking open-ended questions using our Love Map Card Deck exercises, and (2) expressing fondness and admiration often for small things, which changes a habit of mind from commenting on one's partner's mistakes to catching one's partner doing things right and offering genuine appreciation, being proud of one's partner's accomplishments, and communicating respect. Turning toward bids for emotional connection may simply involve increasing mindfulness of how one's partner expresses needs, combined with a willingness to meet these needs.

In an important study, Robinson and Price (1980) placed two observers in a couples' home, one observing positive acts of husband and the other, positive acts of the wife. Husband and wife were also trained to do the same observations. They found that when the couple was happily married, the couple and the observers were veridical. When the couple was unhappily married, the couple only detected 50% of the positive events the observers noticed. This suggests that even in unhappy relationships there may be a lot of positive affect that either does not get noticed or is not viewed as positive. The therapist's initial task may not be so much to build positive affect as to get people to notice what is already there.

Goal 3: Build Positive Affect during Non-Conflict

The World of Positive Affect: Further Considerations and Comparisons

Turning toward bids for emotional connection opens up an entire world of positive affect that we have yet to fully explore in couple research. The universe of positive affect includes far more than turning toward one's partner's bids or building love maps, or fondness and admiration. There has been a hidden assumption in couple therapy: If we adequately deal with couples' conflicts, a sort of vacuum will be created, and all the positive affects will rush in to fill this void. We suggest that this assumption is wrong. Positive affect systems need to be built separately in therapy. In our research on the effects of the first baby on the couple's relationship, for example, we found that the first couple interactions to vanish are play, fun, exploration, adventure, curiosity, self-disclosing conversations, romance, courtship, female libido, and good sex.

As Seligman (2002) pointed out, psychology and psychiatry have largely thought of mental health as the elimination of symptoms; figuratively, we take the couple system from a score of –200 to 0. The hidden assumption has been that once symptoms are eliminated, health will rush in to fill the vacuum; figuratively, we now take the couple system from a score of 0 to +200. But this may be a fantasy. We may actively need to build methods of going from 0 to 200. In terms of affect, our previous thinking in couple therapy has amounted to attempting to eliminate dysfunctional conflict, in effect taking the couple system from a place of insecurity, anxiety, anger, rage, bitterness, fear, loathing, betrayal, disappointment, and hurt to a peaceful, neutral place, or –200 to 0. An exception is Johnson's emotionally focused couple therapy (EFT), which emphasizes building secure bonds and intimate connection. This intimate connection is about not only healing previous attachment injuries but also creating emotional availability and responsiveness.

However, EFT may have pointed to only the tip of the positive affect iceberg. We suggest that *the savoring* of positive affect in multiple positive affect systems is what builds a wonderful and secure relationship, as well as attachment and security. Therefore, we propose the following hypothesis: Once negative affect is down-regulated, positive outcomes in relationships are a result of being able to savor positive affect. But we need a guide to this world of savoring positive affect. What is "savoring"? We suggest that the secret of savoring comes from an understanding of the two ways infants respond to incoming information and energy. One way infants respond to incoming information and energy is Sokolov's orienting reflex (see Ushakova, 1997). We call it the "Oh, what's this?" response. This is an opening to information and energy that in the infant involves a heart rate reduction, pupil dilation, suspension of sucking and self-soothing behavior, and behavioral stilling. The other way infants respond to incoming information and energy is a defensive response. We call it the "What the hell is this?" response. This is a closing to information and energy that in the infant involves a heart rate increase, pupil constriction, an increase in sucking and self-soothing behavior, and behavioral activation (e.g., pumping the limbs). One part of savoring is an openness to information and energy. The other part of savoring is a heightened awareness of sensual responding, taste, smell, touch, and access to sensual memories. The positive and negative affect systems are related. Just as relaxation is an antidote to anxiety, negative affect eliminates savoring, whereas savoring acts as a powerful antidote to the experience of negative affect.

Rapprochement between Gottman Method Therapy and EFT

Our thinking is compatible with both Johnson's EFT (e.g., Johnson, 2004) and its attachment theory basis. We embrace the EFT focus on emotion; it has guided our work for decades. However, Jaak Panksepp's seven emotional command systems are also critical for creating a complete theory of the role of emotion in couple relationships. Toward explaining this point, we now undertake a brief and friendly critique of attachment theory as a complete basis for couple therapy. We say "friendly," because there is no doubt in our minds that Johnson's EFT is a powerful basis for a couple therapy that recognizes the key role emotion plays in the development and maintenance of intimacy. As the great physicist Isaac Newton said, "If I have seen far, it is because I have stood on the shoulders of giants." Johnson is our giant; the conceptual and empirical contributions of EFT are invaluable. What are the contributions of EFT?

The experiential–emotional basis of EFT has been demonstrated in empirical research as a valid guide for the couple therapist in healing attachment injuries, dealing with trauma, and creating secure bonds. Its contributions to couple therapy are vast, including (1) the focus on emotional reprocessing to heal attachment injuries and (2) the legitimization of dependency in human relationships. Let us consider each contribution in turn. First, in our view the EFT focus on emotional reprocessing of attachment injuries provides the necessary tools for healing deep injuries in secure connections, some of which have their roots in the current relationship and others in childhood family relationships. In EFT language, these injuries are the result of important attachment figures turning away or against bids for emotional connection during times of great need. Second, in our view, the focus on the legitimization of dependency in human relationships corrects the misguided emphasis on what Bowen called "differentiation." To understand the immense importance of Johnson's contribution, let us first understand what Johnson was confronting and correcting: Bowen's concept of differentiation.

The concept of differentiation has two components. As Papero (1995) stated, "differentiation" was envisioned by Bowen as a scale that ranged from 0 to 100; at 0, there was no differentiation, by which Bowen meant that emotion was not controlled by reason; at 100 was full differentiation, by which Bowen meant that reason controlled emotion. Bowen was fond of saying to a couple in therapy, "Don't tell me what you feel, tell me what you think" (Michael Kerr, personal communication, June 28, 2001). Bowen followed a limited view of MacLean's (1990) model of the triune brain; MacLean viewed the brain in evolutionary terms as having reptilian (brainstem), mammalian (limbic), and primate (developed cortical) parts. Bowen chose to view MacLean's triune brain as suggesting that emotions were evolutionarily more primitive, limbic, impulsive, out-of-control, and antithetical to a more cortical highly evolved rationality. This view is outdated by modern neuroscience; research and neurological practice shows that there is an integration of reason and emotion in the prefrontal cortex, as well as bidirectional feedback with limbic areas (LeDoux, 1996; Siegel, 1999). For example, in *Descartes' Error* (1994), Damasio demonstrated that a patient who had a tumor removed from the prefrontal area was no longer able to process emotions and to use intuition, a central emotional component of problem-solving or prioritizing information. The man had lost his job and his marriage. In his initial evaluation of the patient, Damasio discovered that the man could solve puzzles and mazes well. Damasio was puzzled until he scheduled another appointment with the patient, who was able to list times he was available in the following week, but unable to prioritize those times and select a best time for the next appointment. Without emotion and intuition, he was incapable of prioritizing his needs and making fundamental decisions for himself. This demonstrated, in contrast with Bowen's view, that rational thought is fundamentally intuitive and emotional, as well as cognitive, and that during emotional moments people are able to think. The distinctions between reason and emotion are not part of the brain's evolution, structure, or functioning.

An example of the importance of these new facts for therapy is that there may be some evidence of emotional, state-dependent learning (Forgas & Bower, 2001); this implies that, for example, it may be best for clients in therapy to learn about their anger when they are actually angry, because they will then be more able to access what they learned therapeutically the next time they are angry. This view is directly contrary to the idea that we have to make therapeutic interpretations when a client is in a neutral affective state, because that is when he or she is rational and can understand the interpretation.

The second component of Bowen's differentiation was interpersonal. It proposed a developmental theory on the one hand that high levels of interdependence and interconnection in a couple amounted to pathological "enmeshment" and "symbiosis," a kind of biological host–parasite relationship. One the other hand, high levels of independence and the creation of boundaries were viewed by Bowen as highly developed, and the basis of healthy relationships.

Bowlby (1988) and others criticized this view. For example, in his work on the birth of families, the eminent psychiatrist Lewis (1989) suggested that every couple finds its own balance of independence and interdependence. He suggested that it is not helpful to pathologize strong needs for connection, nor is it helpful to pathologize relationships that select greater emotional distance and independence. Lewis suggested that there is no optimal amount of interdependence or independence. Our research findings support the views of Lewis. In our typology of couple relationships, we found that there is also no optimal amount of emotional expression, nor an optimal amount of conflict engagement or avoidance. Raush's classic observational and sequential analytic work (Raush, Barry, Hertel, & Swain, 1974) on the transition to parenthood suggested that both bickering and conflict avoidant (and disinterested in psychological insight) couples were dysfunctional, and that only middle-ground "harmonious" couples were psychologically healthy. However, our typological longitudinal research found that, despite his monumental contributions, Raush was wrong on this point. So long as partners are matched on the amount of conflict they desire or wish to avoid, the amount of emotional expression and exploration they wish, and the amount of intimacy, passion, and interdependence or independence they desire, everything is fine. Their relationships turn out to be happy and stable, and their children are also fine on measures of cognitive and affective child outcome. Problems occur when there are mismatches between partners, and these mismatches create central, perpetual issues for the relationship.

As the foundation for her research and therapy, Johnson used attachment theory, which has demonstrated that a developmental theory of increasing independence in close relationships is entirely misleading. Johnson understood that attachment theory correctly normalized dependency in close relationships.

In addition, research has demonstrated that relationships are all about being emotionally connected, and that the amount of connection and emotion is a matter of personal choice and comfort. Both low and high levels of emotional connection have their own risks and benefits; neither choice is perfect. In our work (Gottman, 1994), as long as the ratio of positivity to negativity during conflict is 5:1, all relationships (passionate, validating, and conflict-avoidant) are stable. However, when the ratio of positivity to negativity during conflict falls to 0.8:1, all of these relationships are unstable. Bowlby's theory (1988) has also been supported by basic research on attachment in nonhuman primates (e.g., see Blum, 2002). Harlow's groundbreaking research showed that love in baby rhesus monkeys is based on secure attachment, comfort, nurturance, emotional availability and responsiveness, touch, affection, and contact. It is not based on a surrogate providing milk delivered by a nipple, no matter how readily available the nipple is. Johnson understood this, too, and based EFT on the need for secure attachment, not the alleged need for differentiation.

The implications of this work are dramatic for the couple therapist. Rather than differentiation being the therapist's royal road to intimacy, the royal road is emotional availability and responsiveness. Instead of fostering a process of controlling emotion with reason in clients, couple therapy needs to focus on the integration of emotion and thinking, the understanding of emotional connection, couples' negative cycles, and the dynamics of emotional connection, turning away or against, and the dynamics of attachment betrayal. EFT has shown us the pathway. Yet we maintain that there is still more distance to go along this road, and Panksepp's work provides us with the road map we need.

The Limits of Attachment Theory

Only two of Panksepp's seven emotional command systems are central to attachment theory, the Sentry and the Nest Builder. It was Bowlby's contention that once an infant was safe and securely attached, it would naturally explore and play, occasionally returning to the mother's secure presence for comfort. The research of Ainsworth, Blehar, Waters, and Wall (1978) and Campos, Frankel, and Camras (2004) supported these contentions for mothers and infants. Johnson has written that adult attachment differs from the parent–child system in that it is far more reciprocal and also sexual. We agree with her,

but we also believe that were Bowlby alive today, he would agree with Panksepp that each of the seven emotional command systems can and often do operate independently and are also essential to ensure healthy adult couple relationships.

This idea of including all seven emotional command systems (and not just two) is critical for couple therapists. It suggests that a secure attachment does not necessarily result in well-matched partners in the emotional command system for lust, romance, passion, sex and intimacy (the Sensualist), nor for play and fun (the Jester), nor for exploration and adventure (the Explorer), nor for balancing energy inputs and expenditures (the Energy Czar), nor for managing power and anger (the Commander-in-Chief). Although Bowlby may have suggested that all these emotional command systems will work well by themselves once there is secure attachment, we disagree. It is our contention that every emotional command system needs the special attention of the couple therapist. For example, the entire world of positive affect (the Sensualist, the Jester, the Explorer, and the Energy Czar) needs to be built intentionally, and the therapist cannot assume that these command systems are activated, function well, or are matched across partners once conflict is managed or attachment is secure.

In addition, we agree with Darwin (1873) that all the emotions are functional and serve adaptive values. For example, as Darwin pointed out, the disgust facial expressions close the nostrils against potentially noxious odors. In fact, contempt and disgust might have been the basis for the evolution of morality. Anger and rage can be in the service of justice, or the establishment of specialization, leadership, and fair and equitable dominance relationships in couples (research has shown that a dominance structure is neither bad nor good). Sadness and grief are the opposite sides of the coin of attachment and connection. Because the emotional command systems, when paired with negative affects, are also quite capable of operating independently, it is not the case that "behind" anger and rage there is necessarily a primary emotion, such as fear. Johnson (2004) suggested that anger is often a natural reaction to an unavailable attachment figure. We agree. However, many contexts (e.g., a frustrated goal; Ortony, Clore, & Collins, 1988) also generate anger. Anger can be just anger; it need not be related to the attachment system. We especially draw attention to anger here as a way to dramatize the need for the therapist to consider *all* of Panksepp's emotional command systems. The therapist needs to be able to understand all the affects and not assume that any need is necessarily hierarchically related to insecurity; in other words, none should be dismissed. The expression and understanding of pure anger (unblended with fear), for example, can be the basis for greater understanding, fairness, emotional connection, and bonding for partners.

In summary, we believe that attachment theory deals with only two out of seven of Panksepp's emotional command systems. We agree with Johnson that the couple therapist needs to be an emotion expert. However, that therapeutic expertise must be based on awareness of all seven emotional command systems.

Methods for Accomplishing Goals II and III: How to Up-Regulate Positive Affect during Both Conflict and Non-Conflict Contexts

Our blueprint for building friendship and intimacy, and up-regulating positive affect has four steps.

STEP 1: EMOTIONAL CONNECTION DURING EVERYDAY MOMENTS

The action components of building emotional connection during everyday moments follows:

1. *Build love maps*, which are road maps of one's partner's inner psychological world, formed by showing active interest and asking open-ended questions. We use a Love Map Card Deck.

2. *Build a culture of appreciation and respect* by catching one's partner doing something right and thanking him or her; this involves cultivating a positive habit of mind in which one partner scans the environment for things to appreciate and to respect in the other, and employs politeness and consideration. Robinson and Price (1980), using both independent observers and partners observing one another at home, reported that partners in happily married couples noticed almost all the positive behaviors of their partner, whereas unhappily married partners noticed only half of the positive behaviors of their partner. The fundamental process they identified is mindfulness of positivity. This is an important point because rather than thinking he or she needs to build positivity, the therapist can assume a lot of it is already there but unnoticed. The therapist's job, then, is to increase couples' awareness of and expression of positivity.

3. *Turn toward bids* involve building an emotional bank account by becoming mindful of the

way one's partner asks for what he or she needs, and responding positively to those needs. Bids are verbal or nonverbal requests for connection along a hierarchy of intimate interactions, beginning with getting the partner's attention, then showing active interest, having conversations, giving affection, sharing humor, and offering empathy and emotional support. This is based on the work of Driver (Driver & Gottman, 2004a). People who are unsuccessful at bidding and receiving a response at a lower level on this hierarchy will not make bids that are higher up, with increasing potential for intimacy. Recall that the probability of rebidding after one's partner has turned away is always fairly low. People seem to crumple a bit when their partners turn away from a bid for emotional connection. It is our belief (as yet untested) that one's partner's turning away *leads* to less bidding. In a 10-minute dinnertime segment, Driver found that bid scores ranged from 2 to 100. Tabares et al. (2004) also found a significant relationship between turning toward bids and the quality of repair during conflict. Turning toward bids is discussed in Gottman and DeClaire's (2001) *The Relationship Cure*.

4. *Emotion coaching* is about periodically taking one's partner's emotional temperature by asking a question, such as "How are you? Talk to me," and being able to engage in an emotionally satisfying conversation.

5. *Increase and savor positive affect.* Robinson and Price (1980) were partly right. A lot of positivity goes unnoticed in ailing relationships. But they were also wrong. There is a huge deficit in positive affect in ailing relationships. The final part of building friendship and intimacy is to build positive affect. We maintain that each positive affect system requires effort and prioritization of time. This involves the therapist helping the couple to increase the Panksepp positive affect systems, such as play, comfort, humor, laughter, interest, amusement, curiosity, learning, fun, exploration, and adventure. Dealing effectively with conflict or adding insight into negative patterns, or creating bonding by healing attachment injuries, will not enhance these positive affect systems. They are separate emotional command systems (see Gottman & DeClaire, 2001) that will not flourish by themselves, unless the therapist prioritizes them.

It is not enough for the couple and therapist to plan events that are likely to generate more positive affects, because it is equally important to work on *savoring* positive affect. That is difficult for many clients, and problems in this area have a history that is worth exploring. We go so far as to claim that attachment security is about partners savoring positive affective experiences that they have shared. This process of savoring is important for events that are in memory as well. It is like periodically lifting out of one's memory a many-faceted jewel, each face of which contains a lovely and loving memory of how the partner or the relationship has enriched one's life. In this way positive events become more and more precious and indicative of what a wonderful relationship the partners have built. This is an active way that people naturally work on their cost–benefit view of the relationship.

STEP 2: DAILY STRESS-REDUCING CONVERSATION

Jacobson, Schmalling, and Holtzworth-Munroe (1987) discovered that one of the secrets to maintaining gains in couple therapy over 2 years was for partners together to cope actively with stress outside the relationship and to buffer the relationship from these stresses. Such couples actively engaged in stress-reduction. This finding was even more fascinating because stress management was not a component of the therapy. Instead, the couples who maintained gains thought of this themselves. The work has been extended in Switzerland by the work of Bodenmann, Pihet, and Kayser (2006). In our therapy we suggest that couples engage daily in a 20-minute stress-reducing conversation, and we help couples with guidelines for this conversation. Our motto, taken from the groundbreaking work of Ginott (1965) is "Understanding must precede advice."

STEP 3: BUILD AFFECTION, GOOD SEX, ROMANCE, AND PASSION

In our research on the transition to parenthood (see Gottman & Gottman, 2007) we studied couples 3 years after the arrival of a baby. We asked them about their sex life and found factors that differentiated between couples whose sex life was going well in their view and those whose sex life was not going very well. The partners whose sex life was going well tended to (1) continue courtship and most important, they occasionally let the partner know occasionally that he or she was sexually desirable to them; (2) give compliments, surprise gifts, poems, or daily messages that said, "You are special to me"; (3) express nonsexual physical and verbal affection often; (4) have an agreed-upon ritual for initiating and refusing sex;

(5) have an agreed-upon way to talk about sex—often talking only about what was erotic or a "turn on"; (6) have moments of cuddling that turned into sensual touch and massage, much like Masters and Johnson's nondemand pleasuring, and taking in sensual experience; and (7) make it a priority to engage in a wide variety of sexual activities. For example, they had "quickies" as well as gourmet sex without having a long list of prerequisites for having sex. They said, "Yes, OK," a lot when their partners initiated sex, even if they were not totally in the mood; they accepted masturbation (together or separately); they continued oral sex; and they explored and accepted one another's sexual fantasies. To help couples work on their sexual relationship, we have developed a card deck for affection, romance, and good sex that we call the "Salsa Deck."

STEP 4: PROCESS FAILED BIDS FOR EMOTIONAL CONNECTION

Just as the conflict blueprint has a method for processing fights and regrettable incidents, the friendship blueprint has a method for processing failed bids for emotional connection. These are moments when one partner turns away or against a bid for connection, or turns toward a bid unenthusiastically. Most of the time when couples come into a therapy hour (or, in our case, 80-minute sessions) in one of two negative states: There has been either a fight or a regrettable incident, or failed bids for connection, or both. We use a very similar, but not identical, blueprint for processing a failed bid for connection.

Goal 4: Bridge Meta-Emotion Mismatches

People have emotional reactions to being emotional. In a series of investigations we examined "meta-emotions," or how people feel about feelings. With the Meta-Emotion Interview we studied people's history with specific emotions, their feelings about having these emotions and seeing them in others, and also their general philosophy about emotional expression and exploration. Gottman, Katz, et al. (1996) focused on the parent–child relationship. Nahm (2006) extended the parent–child work to the cross-cultural context, comparing Korean American and European American families. Yoshimoto (2005) focused on meta-emotion in couple relationships. The results were quite complex. For example, people can have negative meta-emotions about anger, but not about sadness. The enormous specificity makes the Meta-Emotion Interview a rich tool for the therapist.

In attachment theory there are two major insecure attachment classifications: avoidant and anxious–preoccupied. The avoidantly attached person has suppressed his or her negative affects and has little access to what he or she is feeling or needs. In Main's Adult Attachment Interview (see Cassidy & Shaver, 1999), the avoidantly attached person has few memories of childhood and gives a glowing, positive account of it. Avoidant insecure attachment is created by an unavailable attachment figure. The anxious–preoccupied insecurely attached person, however, is unable to give a coherent story of childhood, gives a disorganized account of childhood trauma, is filled with negative affects about attachment figures, and is still absorbed by issues in the relationship with the attachment figure. A couple in which one person is avoidant and the other is anxious–preoccupied will be characterized by pursuer–distancer patterns of conflict and attempts to form connection during moments of heightened attachment need. To some extent these descriptions are pathologized male (avoidant type) and female (anxious–preoccupied type) stereotypes, similar to those in prior eras, when narcissistic–borderline or earlier hysterical–obsessive–compulsive descriptions prevailed.

We suggest that meta-emotion provides a much richer descriptive language of mismatches than these two broad classifications of attachment insecurity and, as a result, the clinician has more tools for assessment and intervention. People have complex needs and relationships illustrated by each of Panksepp's seven emotional command systems and their associated emotions. For example, some people have a troubled history with the emotion anger but not sadness. One of our clients had been traumatized by his parents' anger during arguments he observed as a child. As a result, he had a great deal of trouble with his wife's anger. Some people have similar difficulties with sadness but not anger. One woman we interviewed said that in observing her bullied and depressed mother, she and her sisters had made a pact when they were children never to feel sad, but if in a sad situation, to be angry instead. So she had a great deal of difficulty when her son became sad. At those times, she said she went out for a run and let her husband deal with her son's sadness. However, she used her anger effectively to become a crusader for many important causes. There are many cultural variations

in how people are supposed to feel about specific emotions or about emotional expression in general. One of our therapists in Norway talked about the informal cultural rule in Norway known as the "Yante Law," in which it is considered shameful to be proud of one's accomplishments. The attitude comes from Aksel Sandemose's (1933) novel *A Refugee Crosses His Tracks*. There are ten rules in the Law of Yante:

1. Do not think that *you* are special.
2. Do not think that you are of the same standing as *us*.
3. Do not think that you are smarter than *us*.
4. Do not fancy yourself as being better than *us*.
5. Do not think that you know more than *us*.
6. Do not think that you are more important than *us*.
7. Do not think that *you* are good at anything.
8. Do not laugh at *us*.
9. Do not think that anyone cares about *you*.
10. Do not think that you can teach *us* anything.

Parents who express pride when their child accomplishes something are considered bad parents under the Yante Law, because they may be leading their child to be boastful and feel better than other people. People in many Asian cultures have shame about having needs; being dependent or "needy" is seen as shameful (Nahm, 2007). British and Scottish cultures have trouble with touch and affection (Montague, 1971).

Jourard (1966) observed how often people touched one another in an hour in public restaurants in London, Paris, Mexico City, and Gainesville, Florida. The average was 0 in London, 115 in Paris, 185 in Mexico City, and 2 in Gainesville, Florida. Field (2001) later corroborated some of Jourard's findings. Obviously, meta-emotions regarding touch vary tremendously from culture to culture.

Despite the enormous complexity of meta-emotion we observed in our research, people could be divided into two broad categories: emotion dismissing/out of control, and emotion coaching. Emotion-dismissing people believed that they could decide which emotion they would have through a force of will, a Norman Vincent Peale "power of positive thinking" view. They believed in action rather than introspection, and used expressions such as "Suck it up and get on with life" or "Roll with the punches." Emotion-dismissing people generally had a poorly developed lexicon for the different emotions and often did not really know or care to investigate what they were feeling. They tended to view not having needs as a strength, and having needs as being "needy" and weak. They tended to view introspection about negative feelings as a waste of time or even as toxic. They considered emotional expression a loss of control, and tended to use explosion metaphors for anger, mental illness metaphors for sadness, and weakness or cowardice metaphors for fear. They were impatient with their children's negative affect and tended to view it as a failure of their own parenting. When they taught their children something new, they waited for their children to make a mistake, then became critical, directive, and even more critical and intrusive if the child's performance worsened. Emotion-dismissing people emphasized action over introspection in any situation and tended to suppress their own needs and feelings in any situation in favor of getting things done. These people were effective at compartmentalizing and suppressing emotion.

A subdivision of this category that resembles the anxious–preoccupied insecure attachment classification: the emotion-out-of-control group. In our research, emotion-out-of-control people often expressed disapproval with respect to specific negative affects and tended to be anxiously preoccupied with these affects in their past and current relationships. For example, some people were disapproving of and preoccupied with anger; they tended to see anger as aggression and disrespect, and their disapproval was triggered by the partner's anger. They also felt that their own anger was out of control. Many such people avoided conflict but also had intense blowups in which they screamed and raged at their partner. Some people were disapproving of and preoccupied with sadness. These people were not effective at compartmentalizing and suppressing emotion. On the contrary, they felt out of control and labeled themselves as overly emotional.

In contrast, emotion-coaching people believe that emotions are a guide for how to proceed through life. To such people, anger meant that one had a blocked goal, fear meant that one's world was unsafe, and sadness meant that something was missing in one's life. They did not think they could or should decide which emotion they would have. They viewed emotions like a GPS (global positioning system) for action. They believed in introspection, and understanding emotions as a prelude for action, and believed in validating their children's emotions even when they misbehaved. Their philosophy was that all feelings and wishes

are acceptable, but not all behavior is acceptable. They set strong limits on misbehavior and gave their children choices. Emotion-coaching people generally had a good lexicon for the different emotions, noticed mild forms of emotion, and believed that their children's expressions of emotion were an opportunity for intimacy or teaching. They tended to view having needs and knowing what one needs as strengths, and to view introspection about negative feelings as productive and emotional expression as positive, within limits. They were patient with their children's negative affect and thought of it as healthy, even if their children were disappointed or sad, and believed they should respond with empathy and validation of their children's feelings before problem solving or giving advice. When teaching their children something new, they waited for their children to do something right, offering genuine praise and enthusiasm before giving advice or direction. Emotion-coaching people emphasized introspection over action and tended to explore their own needs and feelings in any situation rather than getting things done.

Obviously, most people, as well as most couples, arrive at some balance of emotion-dismissing/out-of-control and emotion-coaching behavior. Often they work on defining that balance through dialogue about a perpetual issue. For example, let us say parents are discussing their child's tension about doing math. Empathy and support are important in helping the child deal with this fear; but at some point the child will have to learn to do math, plus developing math competence should help to mitigate this fear. The parents might arrive at a balance by deciding on the use of both emotion coaching and a more dismissing attitude of simply getting on with it.

In contrast, for some couples, a meta-emotion mismatch like this can be a source of great conflict. Rather than dialogue regarding their mismatch and the resultant actions to be taken, the partners might end up in a state of "gridlock." To continue with the child's math fear example, if the parents were gridlocked whenever they discussed the child's math fear, each might feel that the other disrespected his or her perspective. Gottman, Katz, et al. (1996) reported that an untreated meta-emotion discrepancy between married parents predicted divorce with 80% accuracy.

Similar to classifications of insecure attachment in attachment theory, our clinical experience is that a meta-emotion mismatch (a coaching person combined with a dismissing person, or a coaching person coupled with an out-of-control person) predicts a pattern of turning away from bids, or what has been called the "pursuer–distancer" or the "demand–withdraw" pattern. Driver (2006) found that turning away from bids tends to lead to escalating conflict. Turning against bids tends to lead to emotional withdrawal. These two predictions from non-conflict to conflict contexts are a bit counterintuitive; one might usually predict from a trait model that turning away in non-conflict contexts would be consistent with emotional withdrawal during conflict, whereas the more hostile turning against in non-conflict contexts would lead to escalation during conflict. However, we found the opposite. Wile's (1993) observation that a great deal of conflict is about the conversation the couple never had helps us understand our results. The reaction to turning away during non-conflict contexts, as Johnson (2004) pointed out, is anger. Turning away has created an unavailable and unresponsive partner. The reaction to one's partner turning against bids in non-conflict is fear, as if the partner is saying that even in non-conflict situations a bid for connection will be met with threatening irritability. The effect shuts down the bidding partner and creates conflict avoidance and emotional withdrawal. Turning against bids create a scary, disapproving, and rejecting partner. The result is emptiness and loneliness.

Over time, without clinical intervention, we therefore suggest that meta-emotion mismatch can lead to loneliness and to secrets in the relationship, largely in the interest of avoiding more conflict. The late Shirley Glass and Jean Staeheli (2003) described this pattern in their book, *Not Just Friends*, as the basis for emotional and sexual extramarital affairs. They used as an example of a couple who had recently had a baby and, as is typical (see Gottman & Gottman, 2007), wound up avoiding one another and feeling lonely.

One day the husband has a great conversation with a female colleague at work. He talks about how lonely he has become in his marriage and his colleague sympathizes with him. They laugh a lot and, unlike his wife, his colleague is very interested in what he has to say. He drives home and thinks he should talk to his wife and say, "I'm worried because we haven't talked like that for a long time, and that worries me." But he thinks, well, nothing untoward has really happened with this female colleague, and there might be an ensuing fight with his wife, so he decides not to bring it up. Then he has a secret. His colleague has a "window" into his marriage, and the man has created a "wall" between his wife and his relationship with

his colleague. Slowly over time, he gives himself permission to cross boundaries into forbidden intimacy, and an emotional or sexual affair develops.

Johnson's seminal EFT work highlights the attachment injuries created by one partner turning away from another in a time of great need. Many of the examples she gives reveal to us a meta-emotion discrepancy in which the partner who turns away is dismissing and the partner who is abandoned is emotion coaching. EFT provides a systematic method for healing these attachment injuries and creating a secure relationship bond.

If both partners are emotion-coaching individuals, we predict that they will turn toward bids at a high rate and have higher levels of emotional expression and intimacy. These are the "volatile" couples described by Gottman (1994). They are better described as "passionate." If they have a 5:1 ratio of positive to negative affect during conflict, their relationships will be stable and happy, though they may also have a high need for repair.

Yoshimoto (2005) extended meta-emotion research to couple relationship and found that coaching, particularly by husbands, was related to reduced negative affect during conflict and higher levels of marital satisfaction.

Attachment theory has also focused on two main insecure forms of attachment, avoidant and anxious–preoccupied attachment. The avoidant person is cut off from his or her feelings and seems to resemble our emotion-dismissing meta-emotion, while the anxious–preoccupied attachment seems to resemble our out-of-control and overwhelmed meta-emotion. Yoshimoto's thesis shows that the broader view of meta-emotion mismatches can lead to precise clinical interventions. The interventions begin with the Meta-Emotion Interview, which asks about each partner's history of specific emotions (especially emotions that are problematic in the couple's interaction; e.g., anger), what it was like when others expressed that emotion toward him or her, and when he or she has felt that emotion. It is very enlightening for partners to hear each other's answers to these questions. In another specific intervention we have trained partners in the art of intimate conversation. They practice taking turns as speaker or listener. The speaker expresses a need and the listener either asks emotion-focused questions (e.g., "What is the full story of that event?"), or makes statements of interest, understanding, and compassion. To reduce defensiveness, the need must be stated as a "positive need," in which one asks for something that the partner can do to shine for one, instead of a negative need, which is what the partner must stop doing.

Methods for Accomplishing Goal 4: Bridge Meta-Emotion Mismatches with Emotion Coaching

The world of different emotional experiences and needs is the source of either emotional connection or alienation. In our experience, alienation often involves one person making a bid for emotional connection and the other person either not being aware of the bid or not knowing what to do. No one seems to escape hurt and injury within a relationship. Johnson's EFT has shown us how to reprocess these injuries in light of old childhood injuries and to create bonding where, in the past, there has been anger or sadness about the emotional unavailability or lack or responsiveness of one partner in a time of high attachment need.

In addition to this focus on times of "not being there," we now know that there are continual opportunities on a daily basis for healing through positive emotional connection and bids. We build awareness of these bids, and of typical styles and personal histories of turning away or against. We use the Meta-Emotion Interview to build awareness between partners of their different attitudes, histories, and experiences with expressing and experiencing specific emotions, and their different attitudes toward emotion, introspection, seeking self-insight, self-disclosure, exploration of feelings, and their emotion lexicon. Gendlin (1981) explored some of these aspects of emotion in his work on "focusing," which helps people creatively give the right words and phrases to bodily experiences of emotion.

In this part of our therapy we create mechanisms that allow people to connect during times of emotional need. Emotion coaching is about viewing emotional moments as opportunities for intimacy, asking questions about feelings, putting words to emotional experience, and understanding and validating the partner's emotions before problem-solving. A similar blueprint is used in the stress-reducing conversation. Using these skills and awareness during these moments of need, emotion coaching becomes a source of connection rather than alienation. In some ways this puts the emotion-focused skills of the therapist in the couple's skills repertoire. We teach people how to make their bids and needs explicit (sometimes using the Expressing Needs Card Deck), and

how to engage in the art of intimate conversation. We teach them how to ask open-ended questions (using the Open-ended Questions Card Deck, and the Emotion Coaching Questions Card Deck), and how to make statements that express interest and empathy (Emotion Coaching Statements Card Deck).

REPAIR AND META-EMOTION MISMATCH

It is easy to prove mathematically that repair must be the *sine qua non* of good relationships. If we estimate, generously, that a person in a good relationship is emotionally available to his or her partner 50% of the time (probability = .5), then, assuming these are independent events, the joint probability that both will be emotionally available to one another at the same time is ($.5 \times .5 = .25$) 25%. Therefore, we can expect that in a good relationship, partners will be unavailable or mismatched 75% of the time. Some of these times hurt feelings may accompany the mismatch in emotional availability. The 50% figure is probably a gross overestimation of how much a person in a good relationship is emotionally available to his or her partner.

This brief thought experiment is consistent with Tronick and Gianino's (1986) research on face-to-face mother–infant interaction, considered by many to be the best possible type of relationship in the world. They actually found that mothers and 3-month-old babies in face-to-face play were mismatched 70% of the time, and that the mothers who repaired interactions were the ones who had securely attached babies at 1 year of age. So we suggest that repair is likely to be an important part of adult relationships as well. Therapists should expect clients to make mistakes in the process of communication on a regular basis and need help to make repair processes more effective.

If both partners are emotion-coaching individuals, they turn toward bids at a high rate and have high levels of emotional expression and intimacy. They will also have a high need for effective repair. They will be the volatile, or passionate, conflict-engaging couples described by Gottman (1994) in *What Predicts Divorce?* If both partners are emotion-dismissing individuals, then they will bid at a lower rate and subsequently turn toward one another less often. They may also have low levels of emotional expression and intimacy, and as a result, a lower need for effective repair. They are the conflict-avoiding couples described by Gottman (1994). Raush, Barry, Hertel, and

Swain (1974) suggested that both bickering and conflict-avoiding couples are both dysfunctional. Our research suggests, on the contrary, that these conflict-avoiding couples, contrary to the assumption of Raush, can be stable and happy if their ratio of positive to negative conflict is 5:1; the same is true for the passionate couples who are both emotion coaching (Raush's bickering couples), and validating (Raush's harmonious couples).

Goal 5: Create and Nurture a Shared Meaning System

The final part of Figure 5.1 is the creation of a shared meaning system. All couples build a shared meaning system either intentionally or unintentionally. This is a very important system for creating connection and positive affect. We are a symbol-generating, storytelling species engaged in a search for meaning. Frankl (1959) based his psychotherapy on the human existential search for meaning and purpose, and suggested that psychopathology emerges from an existential vacuum. His idea was that people's emotions help direct this search for meaning. Frankl rejected Maslow's hierarchy of needs (1968), suggesting instead that spirituality, kindness, generosity, creativity, art, science, and beauty can and do emerge from suffering, even when people face terminal illness. He first observed this phenomenon in the German concentration camps of World War II. Frankl observed that in the darkest moments of intense suffering people fashion meaning, community, and spiritual connection.

The couple's shared meaning system puts Frankl's work in the relationship context. We observed the importance of the shared meaning system at several levels of our analysis of couple relationships. The search for shared meaning and a shared story emerged from Buehlman et al.'s (1992) coding of our Oral History Interview. We also observed the importance of Frankl's work in our analysis of partners' repetitive conflicts in which "hidden agendas" are the symbolic meaning of each person's positions. We now know that comprise is impossible in these conflicts, unless what we call the "dreams within conflict" are addressed (i.e., the stories and wishes behind each person's intractable position). These positions are compromise "deal breakers." The very thought of compromise to both persons feels like giving up the core of who they are and what they most respect about themselves and their life journeys.

The "dreams within conflict" intervention reveals the tip of the iceberg of the shared meaning system. First, in gridlocked perpetual conflict with hidden agendas, partners need to talk about the story behind their positions, their dreams and wishes, why they are so central to each person, and what their life dreams are on the issue, then to find a way to honor these dreams and adapt to the perpetual dialogue surrounding these recurring conflicts. Master couples discuss the meaning of their positions with one another. Over the years they reveal the dreams within their positions and talk about them.

Second, at a deeper level of analysis of couple relationships, we also find evidence of the importance of Frankl's ideas. In our interviews we find that master couples intentionally build a shared story of their relationships and a sense of purpose and shared meaning in which their own individual existential struggles become merged, in part, into a system of shared meaning.

People create this shared meaning system in several ways:

1. *They build rituals of connection.* First they create shared meaning simply in the way they move through time together, establish priorities, and build rituals of connection. A "ritual of connection" is a way of turning toward one another that each person can count on. There are *formal* and *informal* rituals of connection. For example, dinnertime can include a ritual of everyone talking about their day. Fiese and Parke (2002) studied dinnertimes in people's primary families and in their current families. People always had stories about wonderful dinner rituals and nightmare meals. Doherty (1997) reported that most American families do not eat dinner together regularly, and half of those who do have the television on during dinner (which wipes out conversation). There are many areas of informal connection, including weekends; rituals of parting and reunion; what happens when one person gets sick, or succeeds or fails at work; and sexual initiation and refusal, to name a few. Formal rituals include a yearly holiday cycle and what each holiday should mean and why. What should Christmas mean? Or Ramadan, Passover, or Kwanza? What shared beliefs are represented and celebrated in this holiday cycle? Other rites of passage are formal rituals of connection, such as birthdays, anniversaries, confirmations, graduations, weddings, and funerals. Most families take photographs and keep albums

of noble and not-so-noble ancestors and relatives. Many families have pictures of these ancestors on their walls and tell stories of their families' legacies. They create a culture of values by giving meaning to the past and this legacy of values is passed down to the children.

2. *They create shared meaning through supporting life's roles.* Couples create meaning by honoring the roles they play in life. Work careers, their roles as father, mother, son, daughter, sister, brother, friend, philanthropist, leader, and so on, display the variety of roles we all play in life. How do families honor and support these roles? Do people feel appreciated and joined in these roles? Do they complement one another's roles?

3. *They create shared meaning through shared life goals.* Partners also create meaning in the goals they set for their family and for themselves. They make plans, problem-solve around these plans, build a home and manage a life together, distribute labor and work together as a team, and express their values as a family. They gather around them a set of friends. They give and receive from their community. They grieve losses together and celebrate successes with their friends and relatives. They sometimes create community, ethical orientation, or spiritual connections and religious or other community affiliations emanating from these shared values. They create a life mission and culture as part of their legacy. They create things together as part of this process. They raise children, they perform music, they write or appear in plays and musicals. They travel and explore together, and learn together. They celebrate their triumphs and strivings, and suffer together when they are in pain. And even in desperate pain, they still create meaning together. Or, couples may fail to do all these things intentionally.

There is a story about Alfred Nobel, the inventor of dynamite, who became wealthy from this invention. When his brother died, the leading newspaper in Stockholm made a mistake. They thought Alfred Nobel had died, and they printed his obituary. He was horrified to read it in the morning paper. It said that he was the most destructive man in all of Europe. He had caused more people to die than any other man in Europe. Horrified by people's view of him, Nobel turned his attention to doing good. He created the Nobel Prize for peace, and for medicine and other sciences—the prize for which he is now remembered. He had a chance to influence the world for good rather than harm. When partners intentionally fail to create a shared meaning system, they have closed a door to enormous sources of positive affect with one another, and in life.

Methods for Accomplishing Goal 5: Create and Nurture the Shared Meaning System

There are two steps in building the couple's shared meaning system.

STEP 1: CREATE SHARED MEANING BY MAKING RITUALS OF EMOTIONAL CONNECTION INTENTIONAL

The therapist works to make intentional the aspects of the couple's shared meaning system and culture that have hitherto remained implicit or undeveloped. We believe that every couple's relationship is a cross-cultural experience. Partners come from very different families even if they are part of the same ethnic, racial, religious, national, and cultural group. When they unite, they form a new culture together, in the sense that almost anything they do together repeatedly has the potential of having some meaning.

The first aspect of building the shared meaning system is to nurture the feeling of building something valuable together. One way is to help partners create meaningful *rituals of emotional connection* (both formal and informal), by answering specifics questions (e.g., "What should moving through time together mean?"). Informal rituals of connection involve discussing things, such as "What should happen when one person gets sick" and "What should dinnertime be like at our house?" We have a card deck for these informal rituals. Defined, formal rituals of connection surround events such as birthdays, rites of passage (confirmations, graduations, bar and bat mitzvahs, weddings, funerals), and, very importantly, the couple's yearly holiday cycle and its meanings.

STEP 2: CREATE SHARED MEANINGS BY MAKING GOALS AND VALUES INTENTIONAL

What is made intentional here is partners talking about their shared goals, missions, and legacy. Couples often have scrapbooks and photograph albums that contain memorabilia and photographs of noble ancestors, and important places and events in their past. These pictures can be a catalyst for these discussions. Also partners talk about how they can support each other's central life roles (e.g., mom, dad, son, daughter, brother, sister, friend, worker, leader) and central symbols (e.g., "What is a home?" or "What does love mean?"). Parts of these conversations involve talking about what is sacred to each partner, and what spiritual, moral, or ethical connections they wish to honor in their family. Through these methods, partners are helped to weave together a system of meaning that enriches them both.

Practical Considerations

Gottman method couple therapy is generally not a time-limited program. For couples seeking relationship enhancement, it averages 5–10 sessions; for distressed couples, 15–20 sessions; for couples with serious comorbidities or a recent extramarital affair, it averages 25–50 sessions. For minor domestic violence (not characterological) we are pilot-testing an approach that comprises 21 two-hour sessions of couples group therapy, with a structured social skills curriculum. Termination is handled in our therapy by talking to the clients in the first session about phasing out the therapist toward the end of therapy and following couples for 2 years after termination. We discuss our "dental model" of follow-up. Couples can return on an as-needed basis for a checkup and some repair. The two most common errors our beginning therapists make are as follows:

1. Not understanding the immediate experiential and affective nature of the therapy; and trying to follow a prescribed recipe instead of staying with the moment and the couple's affect, that is, ignoring what the couple brings into a session and being inattentive to process. An example of trying to follow a recipe is that some beginning therapists may think they must work on conflict for the first five sessions, when the couple may not need that.
2. Not understanding the existential nature of the deepest conflicts, for example, trying to apply the "dreams within conflict" intervention to people's overall life dreams rather than to their position on a specific issue.

We work with individual therapists and often recommend medication as an adjunct to our therapy, provided that there is a flow of information between the individual and the couple therapist. However, in our couple work we are often doing individual therapy in a couple context. None of us seems to escape childhood without some scars that last forever, and these scars manifest themselves in the anatomy of every regrettable incident we experience. As William Faulkner (1984) said in *Requiem for a Nun*, "The past is never dead. In fact, it's not even past" (p. 103). Effective repair requires insight into the stories of these lasting injuries and how they are revealed in our interactions. Couple therapy in Gottman method is contraindicated when there is an ongoing extramarital affair and when there is characterological (as opposed to situational) domestic violence.

Resistance to Change

When we encounter resistance to change, we viewed it in several ways. Resistance may appear as distrust of the therapist or therapy process based on old attachment injuries; there may also be fear or discomfort with the experience of intimacy. In these cases, the therapist has to work with the resistant partner's fear using empathy, taking care to not pressure that partner to change, but understanding that partner's need to stay in place and voicing his or her feelings without blame or judgment, creating an extremely safe environment, so that the desire for greater connection can grow. Resistance also appears as a systematic distortion of one of the fundamental processes of the sound relationship house. Let us consider a few of these processes. Most people enjoy discovering more about their partners and being known, and enjoy being appreciated and enhancing fondness and admiration. Most people want to make their own needs known and to discover and meet their partners' needs. In these cases, the therapist helps to make these processes easier and to establish them as pillars of the relationship. However, some people have trouble engaging in these processes. For example, people with low self-esteem may have trouble being admired by their partner. Some people may have trouble with having needs, or with knowing how they feel. They are then revealing to the therapist the ways in which they are stuck in this relationship. There is a story and a history behind this resistance. Such clients are telling the therapist to go deeper into this part of their lives. We work with people's internal working model of relationships around the very process with which they have trouble. The therapist asks him- or herself: What is their story? Can that story be rewritten in this relationship? In this view, resistance is seen by the therapist as "hitting paydirt." It is exactly where the therapy needs to go, and the sound relationship house points the way.

Minimal Conditions for Being in a Long-Term Relationship

Unlike individual therapy, when two people appear in a therapist's office, there is not necessarily a relationship there to work on. A relationship is a contract of mutual nurturance. The wedding vows allude to these minimal conditions in the marriage contract. Clearly, not everyone should be in a long-term relationships. For some people, it may be better advice for them to have short-term liaisons with people that minimize obligation and responsibility. In the follow-up we have done in our clinical practice, one of the most common issues is when the fundamental beliefs necessary for a long-term relationship are missing. We identify six minimal beliefs as necessary: (1) a belief that commitment is necessary for a long-term relationship to succeed; (2) an agreement of romantic and sexual exclusivity; (3) an agreement that there will be no secrets, deceptions, or betrayals; (4) an agreement of fairness and care (e.g., when a person is sick, he or she will be cared for); (5) an agreement to treat one another with respect and affection; and (6) an agreement in principle to try to meet one another's wants and needs.

CONCLUSION

Our basic research, our theory, and our therapy remain a work in progress. We aim to integrate various approaches to couples—analytic, behavioral, existential, emotionally focused, narrative, and systems—into a theory we find elegant, parsimonious, mathematical, and eminently testable. We aim to improve our ideas over time with both empirical research and clinical experience. We aim to bridge both worlds respectfully. It is our goal to honor those thinkers on whose work we build. It is our goal to generate questions that will stimulate research. It is also our goal to be prescriptive and practical, and to develop tools that will be useful for clinicians.

Couples are endlessly complex. They teach us something new every day, through both our research and clinical work. We also are always learning from others like ourselves, who are fascinated by the turnings of relationships. Thus, we never claim that the methods we have described are the *sine qua non* of couple intervention. Our work is constantly informed by the mistakes we make, the misunderstandings we commit, and the questions we ask. We are deeply grateful to our research subjects and our clients for their generosity in sharing their worlds with us, and to our clients, for their patience.

SUGGESTIONS FOR FURTHER READING

Gottman, J. M. (1999). *The marriage clinic*. New York: Norton.

Gottman, J. M., & DeClaire, J. (1996). *The heart of parenting*. New York: Simon & Schuster.

Gottman, J. M., & DeClaire, J. (2001). *The relationship cure*. New York: Simon & Schuster.

Gottman, J. M., & Gottman, J. S. (2007). *And baby makes three*. New York: Crown.

Gottman, J. M., & Silver, N. (1999). *The seven principles for making marriage work*. New York: Crown.

Gottman, J. S. (Ed.). (2002). *The marriage clinic casebook*. New York: Norton.

REFERENCES

Ainsworth, M. S., Blehar, M. C., Waters, E., & Wall, S. (1978). *Patterns of attachment*. Oxford, UK: Erlbaum.

Bach, G. (1965). *The intimate enemy*. New York: Basic Books.

Blum, D. (2002). *Love at goon park: Harry Harlow and the science of affection*. New York: Berkeley.

Bodenmann, G., Pihet, S., & Kayser, K. (2006). The relationship between dyadic coping and marital quality: A 2-year longitudinal study. *Journal of Family Psychology, 20*, 485–493.

Bowlby, J. (1988). *A secure base*. London: Routledge.

Buehlman, K., Gottman, J. M., & Katz, L. (1992). How a couple views their past predicts their future: Predicting divorce from an Oral History Interview. *Journal of Family Psychology, 5*, 295–318.

Campos, J. J., Frankel, C. B., & Camras, L. (2004). On the nature of emotion regulation. *Child Development, 75*(2), 377–394

Carrère, S., Buehlman, K. T., Coan, J. A., Gottman, J. M., Coan, J. A., & Ruckstuhl, L. (2000). Predicting marital stability and divorce in newlywed couples. *Journal of Family Psychology, 14*, 1–17.

Cassidy, J., & Shaver, P. R. (1999). *Handbook of attachment*. New York: Guilford Press.

Cook, J., Tyson, R., White, J., Rushe, R., Gottman, J., & Murray, J. (1995). The mathematics of marital conflict: Qualitative dynamic mathematical modeling of marital interaction. *Journal of Family Psychology, 9*, 110–130.

Damasio, A. (1994). *Descartes' error*. New York: Putnam.

Darwin, C. (1873). *The expression of emotions in man and animals*. New York: BiblioBazaar.

Doherty, W. (1997). *The intentional family*. Reading, MA: Perseus Books.

Driver, J. L. (2007). Observations of newlywed interactions in conflict and in everyday life. *Dissertation*

Abstracts International: Section B: The Sciences and Engineering, 67(9-B), 5441.

Driver, J. L., & Gottman, J. M. (2004a). *Turning toward versus turning away: A coding system of daily interactions.* In P. K. Kerig & D. H. Baucom (Eds.), *Couple observational coding systems* (pp. 209–225). Hillsdale, NJ: Erlbaum.

Driver, J. L., & Gottman, J. M. (2004b). Daily marital interactions and positive affect during marital conflict among newlywed couples. *Family Process, 43*(3), 301–314.

Ebling, R., & Levenson, R. W. (2003). Who are the marital experts? *Journal of Marriage and the Family, 65,* 130–142.

Faulkner, W. (1984). *William Faulkner: Novels 1942–1954: Go Down, Moses/Intruder in the Dust/Requiem for a Nun/A Fable.* New York: Library of America: Penguin/Putnam.

Field, T. (2001). *Touch.* New York: Bradford Books.

Fiese, B. H., & Parke, R. D. (2002). Introduction to the special section on family routines and rituals. *Journal of Family Psychology, 16,* 379–380.

Forgas, J., & Bower, G. H. (2001). Mood and social memory. In P. W. Gerrod (Ed.), *Emotions in social psychology* (pp. 204–215). New York: Psychology Press.

Frankl, V. E. (1959). *Man's search for meaning.* Boston: Beacon Press.

Gendlin, E. (1981). *Focusing.* New York: Bantam.

Ginott, H. G. (1965). *Between parent and child.* New York: Three Rivers Press.

Glass, S., & Staeheli, J. C. (2003). *Not just friends.* New York: Free Press.

Gottman, J. M. (1994). *What predicts divorce?* Hillsdale, NJ: Erlbaum.

Gottman, J. M. (1999). *The marriage clinic.* New York: Norton.

Gottman, J. M., Coan, J., Carrère, S., & Swanson, C., (1998). Predicting marital happiness and stability from newlywed interactions. *Journal of Marriage and the Family, 60,* 5–22.

Gottman, J. M., & DeClaire, J. (1996). *The heart of parenting: Raising an emotionally intelligent child.* New York: Simon & Schuster.

Gottman, J. M., & DeClaire, J. (2001). *The relationship cure.* New York: Simon & Schuster.

Gottman, J. M., Driver, J., Yoshimoto, D., & Rushe, R. (2002). Approaches to the study of power in violent and nonviolent marriages, and in gay male and lesbian cohabiting relationships. In P. Noller & J. A. Feeney (Eds.), *Understanding marriage: Developments in the study of couple interaction* (pp. 323–347). Cambridge, UK: Cambridge University Press.

Gottman, J. M., & Gottman, J. S. (2007). *And baby makes three.* New York: Crown.

Gottman, J. M., Katz, L., & Hooven, C. (1996). *Meta-emotion.* Hillsdale, NJ: Erlbaum.

Gottman, J. M., & Levenson, R. (1984). Why marriages fail: Affective and physiological patterns in marital interaction. In J. Masters (Ed.), *Boundary areas in so-cial and developmental psychology* (pp. 110–136). New York: Academic Press.

Gottman, J. M., & Levenson, R. W. (1985). A valid procedure for obtaining self-report of affect in marital interaction. *Journal of Consulting and Clinical Psychology, 53,* 151–160.

Gottman, J. M., & Levenson, R. W. (1988). The social psychophysiology of marriage. In P. Noller & M. A. Fitzpatrick (Eds.), *Perspectives on marital interaction* (pp. 182–200). Clevedon, UK: Multilingual Matters.

Gottman, J. M., & Levenson, R. W. (1992). Marital processes predictive of later dissolution: Behavior, physiology, and health. *Journal of Personality and Social Psychology, 63,* 221–233.

Gottman, J. M., & Levenson, R. W. (2002). A two-factor model for predicting when a couple will divorce: Exploratory analyses using 14-year longitudinal data. *Family Process, 41,* 83–96.

Gottman, J. M., McCoy, K., Coan, J., & Collier, H. (1996). The Specific Affect Coding System (SPAFF). In J. M. Gottman (Ed.), *What predicts divorce: The measures.* Hillsdale, NJ: Erlbaum.

Gottman, J. M., Murray, J., Swanson, C., Tyson, R., & Swanson, K. (2002). *The mathematics of marriage: Dynamic nonlinear models.* Cambridge, MA: MIT Press.

Gottman, J. M., & Silver, N. (1999). *The seven principles for making marriage work.* New York: Crown.

Gottman, J. M., Swanson, C., & Murray, J. (1999). The mathematics of marital conflict: Dynamic mathematical nonlinear modeling of newlywed marital interaction. *Journal of Family Psychology, 13*(1), 3–19.

Gottman, J. S. (Ed.). (2004). *The marriage clinic casebook.* New York: Norton.

Greenberg, L. S., & Johnson, S. M. (1988). *Emotionally focused therapy for couples.* New York: Guilford Press.

Jacobson, N. S., & Gottman, J. M. (1998). *When men batter women.* New York: Simon & Schuster.

Jacobson, N. S., Schmaling, K., & Holtzworth-Munroe, A. (1987). Component analysis of behavioral marital therapy: 2-year follow-up and prediction of relapse. *Journal of Marital and Family Therapy, 13,* 187–195.

Johnson S. M. (2004). *The practice of emotionally focused couple therapy* (2nd ed.). New York: Brunner/Routledge.

Johnson, S. M., Bradley, B., Furrow, J., Lee, A., Palmer, G., Tilley, D., et al. (2005). *Becoming an emotionally focused couple therapist.* New York: Brunner/Routledge.

Jourard, S. M. (1966). *The transparent self.* New York: Van Nostrand Reinhold.

Kahen, V., Katz, L. F., & Gottman, J. M. (1994). Linkages between parent–child interaction and conversations of friends. *Social Development, 3,* 238–254.

Katz, L. F., & Gottman, J. M. (1993). Patterns of marital conflict predict children's internalizing and externalizing behaviors. *Developmental Psychology, 29,* 940–950.

LeDoux, J. (1996). *The emotional brain.* New York: Simon & Schuster.

Levenson, R. W., Carstensen, L. L., & Gottman, J. M. (1993). Long-term marriage: Age, gender and satisfaction. *Psychology and Aging, 8,* 301–313.

Levenson, R. W., & Gottman, J. M. (1983). Marital interaction: Physiological linkage and affective exchange. *Journal of Personality and Social Psychology, 45,* 587–597.

Levenson, R. W., & Gottman, J. M. (1985). Physiological and affective predictors of change in relationship satisfaction. *Journal of Personality and Social Psychology, 49,* 85–94.

Lewis, J. M. (1989). *The birth of the family.* New York: Brunner Mazel.

MacLean, P. (1990). *The triune brain in evolution.* New York: Plenum Press.

Main, M., Goldberg, S., Muir, R., & Kerr, J. (Eds.). (1995). *Recent studies in attachment.* Hillsdale, NJ: Analytic Press.

Maslow, A. H. (1968). *Toward a psychology of being* (2nd ed.). New York: Van Nostrand.

Montague, A. (1971). *Touching.* New York: Harper & Row.

Nahm, E. Y. (2007). A cross-cultural comparison of Korean American and European American parental meta-emotion philosophy and its relationship to parent–child interaction. *Dissertation Abstracts International: Section B: The Sciences and Engineering, 67*(7-B), 4136.

Newcomb, M. D., & Bentler, P. M. (1980). Assessment of personality and demographic aspects of cohabitation and marital success. *Journal of Personality Assessment, 44,* 11–24.

Ortony, A., Clore, G., & Collins, A. (1988). *The cognitive structure of emotions.* New York: Cambridge University Press.

Panksepp, J. (1998). *Affective neuroscience: The foundations of human and animal emotions.* New York: Oxford University Press.

Papero, D. V. (1995). Bowen family systems and marriage. In N. S. Jacobson & A. S. Gurman (Eds.), *Clinical handbook of couple therapy* (pp. 11–30). New York: Guilford Press.

Rapoport, A. L. (1965). *Fights, games, and debates.* Ann Arbor: University of Michigan Press.

Rausch, H. L., Barry, W. A., Hertel, R. K., & Swain, M. A. (1974). *Communication conflict and marriage.* Oxford, UK: Jossey-Bass.

Robinson, E. A., & Price, M. G. (1980). Pleasurable behavior in marital interaction: An observational study. *Journal of Consulting and Clinical Psychology, 48,* 117–118.

Ryan, K., & Gottman, J. M. (in press). Evaluation of five psycho-educational interventions for distressed couples. *Journal of Marital and Family Therapy.*

Sandemose, A. (1933). *A refugee crosses his tracks.* Copenhagen: Boker in Boker.

Seligman, M. E. P. (2002). Positive psychology, positive prevention, and positive therapy. In C. R. Snyder & S. J. Lopez (Eds.), *Handbook of positive psychology* (pp. 3–9). New York: Oxford University Press.

Shapiro, A. F., & Gottman, J. M. (2005). Effects on marriage of a psycho-communicative–educational intervention with couples undergoing the transition to parenthood, evaluation at 1-year post intervention. *Journal of Family Communication, 5,* 1–24.

Shapiro, A. F., Gottman, J. M., & Carrère, S. (2000). The baby and the marriage: Identifying factors that buffer against decline in marital satisfaction after the first baby arrives. *Journal of Family Psychology, 14,* 59–70.

Siegel, D. (1999). *The developing mind.* New York: Guilford Press.

Tabares, A. A., Driver, J. L., & Gottman, J. M. (2004). Repair attempts observational coding system: Measuring de-escalation of negative affect during marital conflict. In P. K. Kerig & D. H. Baucom (Eds.), *Couple observational coding systems* (pp. 227–241). Hillsdale, NJ: Erlbaum.

Tavris, C. (1989). *Anger: The misunderstood emotion.* New York: Simon & Schuster.

Tronick, E. Z., & Gianino, P. (1986). Interactive mismatch and repair: Challenges to the coping infant. *Zero to Three, 6,* 1–6.

Tung, K. K. (2006). *Topics in mathematical modeling.* Lecture Notes available on the University of Washington website at *http://press.princeton.edu/titles/8446.html.*

Ushakova, J. N. (1997). Russian psychology. *European Psychologist, 2,* 97–101.

Von Bertalanffy, L. (1968). *General system theory.* New York: Braziller.

Wile, D. B. (1988). *After the honeymoon.* New York: Wiley.

Wile, D. B. (1993). *After the fight.* New York: Guilford Press.

Yoshimoto, D. K. (2005). Marital meta-emotion: Emotion coaching and dyadic interaction. *Dissertation Abstracts International: Section B: The Sciences and Engineering, 66*(6-B), 3448.

Psychodynamic and Transgenerational Approaches

CHAPTER 6

Object Relations Couple Therapy

JILL SAVEGE SCHARFF
DAVID E. SCHARFF

BACKGROUND

Object relations couple therapy (D. Scharff & Scharff, 1987) was developed from psychoanalytic object relations theory that had been applied to family therapy and modified by ideas from group therapy, then integrated with behavioral approaches in sex therapy, and illuminated by systems theory and, more recently, chaos theory. So it is not surprising that object relations couple therapy has some features in common with the two other major models, behavioral and systems approaches (Gurman, 1978), even though these are arrived at from different theoretical viewpoints. This technical flexibility has been welcomed by Gurman and Jacobson (1986) as a sign of willingness to learn from other models and join the common ground of therapeutic efficacy. Given that all the major models deal with thoughts, feelings, and behavior, and the interactions among the mind, the body, the significant other, and the environment, what distinguishes the object relations approach? Derived from both a psychoanalytic object relations model of the mind of the individual and group analytic theory, it relates to the couple as a small group of two and as two individuals, and moves easily between their shared external and internal real-

ity. This focus on the interaction of the dynamic unconscious in the interpersonal situation of being a couple is the main point of difference from other major models.

Before describing object relations couple therapy in depth, we look at some early psychoanalytic applications to understanding and treating families and couples. Before object relations theory entered the mainstream of American psychoanalysis, psychoanalytic theory had an impact on couple therapy through its influence on the early family therapists. Ackerman, Bowen, Cooklin, Lidz, Minuchin, Selvini Palazzoli, Stierlin, Shapiro, Watzlawick, Wynne, Zilbach, and Zinner are graduates of analytic training programs. Andolfi, Byng-Hall, and Jackson had analytic training. Framo and Paul acknowledged being influenced by analytic theory, and Skynner was a group analyst. Working in the 1960s and 1970s with Haley, Bateson, and Weakland, the communications and systems family theorists at the Mental Research Institute, Satir and its directors, Jackson and Riskin, both of whom had analytic training, along with Watzlawick, formerly a Jungian training analyst, integrated psychoanalytic understanding with systems models and preserved a concern for the individual, as well as for the family life group. Sullivan's (1953) interpersonal psychiatry offered a relational view that was kept out of the mainstream of psychoanalysis but succeeded in influencing Ryckoff and Wynne (Ryckoff, Day, & Wynne, 1959; Wynne, 1965), who, however, were mainly interested in families, not couples. According to Bodin (1981), whereas Sullivan's (1953) theory of etiology and psychotherapy influenced Jackson, the Chicago Institute of Psychoanalysis influenced Satir's training at the Chicago School of Social Work and led to her interest in corrective emotional experience and the importance of self-concept and self-esteem.

Skynner (1976) applied Freud's (1905) concept of fixation and regression in the psychosexual stages to family functioning. Shapiro (1979) and Zinner (Zinner & Shapiro, 1972) showed how families that are more in tune with the attitudes of an earlier developmental stage are unable to proceed to the developmental tasks of adolescence. Although all of these writers addressed the subject of marriage, they tended not to emphasize developmental regression and fixation in couple dynamics. Bowen (1978) noted that spouses tend to operate at a similar level of differentiation, by which he meant that each spouse was the same distance along the developmental path toward personal integrity, with a capacity for tolerating anxiety, appreciating self and otherness, and taking responsibility for one's own being and destiny (Friedman, 1991). Zilbach (1988), influenced by Erickson (1950), applied a developmental perspective to the family life cycle and described how changes in family needs appropriate to changing developmental stages alter the parents' functioning as a couple, but marriage was not her primary focus. Though equally rare, the developmental perspective on marriage can be quite revealing. Sager (1971; Sager et al., 1976), who noted that intrapsychic factors determine transactional aspects of a couple relationship, found that conflict dynamics specific to the marriage contract must be interpreted in terms of the spouses' unconscious wishes and aims.

By the late 1950s, partners were seen together by the same therapist, an approach that Mittelmann (1994, 1998) had used but for which no name was invented until the term conjoint couple therapy was coined by Jackson and Weakland (1961). Greene (1970) and collaborating cotherapists used individual, concurrent, and conjoint psychoanalytic therapy sessions in a combination that, though flexible, had to adhere to a predictable sequence (Hollender, 1971; Zinner, 1989). Some object relational and self psychological ana-

lysts persevered to understand the effects of complementary neuroses of the marriage partners on mate selection and in married life. Kohut's (1971, 1977, 1982) self psychological theory of narcissistic character pathology, and Kernberg's (1975) theory of ego splits and alternating ego states in borderline pathology have been applied to the couple relationship by Lansky (1986), Kernberg (1991), and Solomon (1989).

OBJECT RELATIONS THEORY APPLIED TO COUPLE THERAPY

Basic Object Relations Terminology and Models

Object relations psychoanalytic theory is the one brand of psychoanalysis that also illuminates family dynamics (D. Scharff & Scharff, 1987, 1991; J. Scharff, 1989). An individual psychology drawn from study of the relationship between patient and therapist, *object relations theory holds that the motivating factor in growth and development of the human infant is the need to be in a relationship with a mothering person, not the discharge of energy from some instinct.* Impulses and driven activity are now seen not as primary elemental forces but as desperate attempts to relate or as breakdown products of failed relationships. According to Sutherland (1980), object relations theory is an amalgam of the work of British Independent group analysts Balint (1968), Fairbairn (1952), Guntrip (1961, 1969), and Winnicott (1951/1958, 1958/1975, 1965, 1971), and of Klein (1948, 1957) and her followers. Of those, Fairbairn gave the most systematic challenge to Freudian theory. His schema of the endopsychic situation (Fairbairn, 1963) was picked up by Dicks (1967), who applied it to his work with spouses. In Britain, Bannister and Pincus (1965), Clulow (1985), Dare (1986), Main (1966), Pincus (1960), and Skynner (1976), and in the United States, Framo (1970/1982), Martin (1976), Meissner (1978), Nadelson (1978), D. Scharff and Scharff (1987, 1991), Willi (1984), and Zinner (1976, 1988), all acknowledge the influence of Dicks' (1967) work on the psychoanalytic model of couple interaction. In his study of unconsummated marriages, Friedman (1962) integrated Dicks's (1967) concepts with those of Balint (1968). Bergmann (1990) applied Dicks's formulation to his study of love. McCormack (1989), who applied Winnicott's concept of the holding environment to the borderline–schizoid marriage, Finkelstein (1987), Slipp (1984), and Stewart,

Peters, Marsh, and Peters (1975) all advocated an object relations approach to the theory of couple therapy.

Before we describe Dicks's model of couple dynamics, we need to summarize Fairbairn's (1944/1952, 1952, 1954) theory of the individual, then extend it to the relational context. In Fairbairn's view, the infant is not the inchoate conglomerate of drives that Freud described. The infant is born with a whole self, through which it executes behaviors that secure the necessary relatedness. Infant research (Stern, 1985) has now corroborated this view of the infant as competent. The infant is looking for attachment, not discharge. As the infant relates to the mother (or mothering person), attachment develops. Out of the vicissitudes of this experience, psychic structure is built. The experience—even with a reasonably good mother who responds well to her infant's regulatory cycles (Brazelton, 1982; Brazelton & Als, 1979)—is always somewhat disappointing in that needs cannot be met before they cause discomfort, unlike the situation in the womb. When the frustration is intolerable, the infant perceives the mother as rejecting. To cope with the pain, the infant takes in ("introjects") the experience of the mother as a rejecting object and rejects that image inside the self by "splitting" it off from the image of the ideal mother and pushing it out of consciousness ("repressing" it). This is called the "rejected object." It is further split into its "need exciting" and "need rejecting" aspects, associated with feelings of longing and rage, respectively. The part of the self that related to this aspect of the mother is also split off from the original whole self and is repressed along with the relevant, unbearable feelings. Now the personality comprises (1) a "central self," attached with feelings of satisfaction and security to an "ideal internal object"; (2) a "craving self," longingly but unsatisfyingly attached to an "exciting internal object"; and (3) a "rejecting self," angrily attached to a "rejecting internal object."

Fairbairn's terminology for the unconscious parts of self and object were "libidinal ego and exciting object" and "antilibidinal ego and rejecting object," but these terms have been discarded in favor of the "exciting" and "rejecting" parts of the self and objects, respectively. The exciting part of the self is sometimes called "the craving self," as suggested by Ogden (1982). Along with the relevant affects, these comprise two repressed, unconsciously operating systems of self in relation to object, called "internal object relationships." Fairbairn's genius was to recognize that the reject-ing object relationship system further suppressed the exciting object relationship system. Now, we have a view of the personality in which subsystems of the object relationship are in dynamic interaction with each other. Dicks's genius was to see how two personalities in a marriage united not only at the level of conscious choice, compatibility, and sexual attraction but also at the unconscious level, where they experienced an extraordinary fit of which they were unaware. Glimmers of lost parts of the self are seen in the spouse, and this excites the hope that, through marriage, unacceptable parts of the self can be expressed vicariously.

Dicks noted that the fit between partners, their "unconscious complementarity," leads to the formation of a "joint personality" (1967, p. 69). When two people fall in love, they connect at conscious and unconscious levels. Whether they remain in love is determined by the aptness of fit at the unconscious level. Dicks noted three major systems that support their bond: shared cultural values, shared individual values, and unconscious fit. Given the rapid mixing of cultures in today's global economy, shared cultural values are less common, so the role of the couple's unconscious fit is greater than ever before. In the healthy marriage, this unconscious complementarity allows for derepression of the repressed parts of one's object relations, so one can refind lost parts of the self in relation to the spouse. In the unhealthy marriage, the fit cements previous repression, because undoing of the defenses would also undo the spouse's similar defensive armature that the marriage is supposed to consolidate rather than threaten. Now, we have a model of two minds united in marriage, their boundaries changing and their internal economies in flux, for better or worse.

To account for unconscious communication between partners, Dicks turned to projective identification (Klein, 1946) as the crucial bridging concept between the intrapsychic and the interpersonal. "Projective identification" is a mental process that is used to defend against anxiety during the earliest months of life. Like Freud, Klein remained true to instinct theory. Segal (1964) and Heimann (1973) gave clear accounts of Klein's ideas. Klein thought that the infant had to defend against harm from the aggression of the death instinct by splitting it off from the self and deflecting it by projecting aggressively tinged parts of the self into the maternal object, especially her breast. Boundaries between self and object being unformed, the infant sees those parts of the self as if they were parts of the object. Now the infant fears attack from the breast as an aggressive object. Klein called this stage of personality development, the "paranoid–schizoid position." Under the influence of the life instinct, the infant also projects loving parts of itself into the breast and experiences it as a loving object. Aspects of the breast, sorted in primitive fashion into all-good or all-bad, are identified with and taken into the infant through "introjective identification" (Klein, 1946). According to Klein, psychic structure forms through repeated cycles of projective and introjective identification. Maturation over the course of the first half-year of life enables the infant to leave behind primitive splitting between good and bad, and to develop an appreciation of a whole object that is felt to be both good and bad. The infant becomes capable of tolerating ambivalence, recognizing the destructive effect of its aggression, feeling concern for the object, and making reparation for damage done to it. When this is accomplished, the infant has achieved the "depressive position."

At this early age, according to Klein, the infant already has a concept of the parents as a couple involved in mutually gratifying intercourse, perceived as a feeding experience at first and later as a genital relationship from which the child is excluded. This image forms the basis for another aspect of the child's psychic structure, namely, the "internal couple" (J. S. Scharff, 1992). Understanding the functioning of this part of the therapist's personality is particularly important in couple therapy, where it is stirred by interaction with the patient couple. Couple therapy may founder or be avoided by the therapist who cannot face the pain of exclusion by or frightening fusion with the couple.

The paranoid–schizoid and depressive positions remain active throughout the life cycle as potential locations along a continuum from pathology to health. Projective identification is retained as a mental process of unconscious communication that functions along a continuum from defense to mature empathy. It is difficult to describe exactly how the processes of projective and introjective identification actually take place. We can become aware of them from their effect upon us as therapists (and hopefully also in our domestic life as spouses). Each is usually experienced as a feeling that is alien or unexplainable, perhaps a feeling of excitement or of numbness. It could be a sudden idea, a fantasy, a sense of in-touchness, or fear, such as a fear of going mad. Fantasies can be communicated by tone of voice, gesture, changes in blood flow to the skin, or in other overt macro- or micro-behaviors. But other times the experience is not detectable with present methods. To some, this may sound a bit mystical, but others are willing to accept the occurrence of projective and introjective identification on the basis of their own experience of complexity, ambiguity, and awe in relationships.

Marriage, like infancy, offers a relationship of devotion, commitment, intimacy, and physicality. It fosters regression and offers the partners a durable setting in which to explore the self and the other. Repressed parts of the self seek expression directly in relation to an accepting spouse, or indirectly through uninhibited aspects of the spouse. There is a mutual attempt to heal and to make reparation to the object refound in the spouse through projective identification, then to find through introjective identification a new, more integrated self. The dynamic relation between parts of the self described by Fairbairn can now be conceptualized as occurring between the conscious and unconscious subsystems of two personalities united in marriage. Figure 6.1 illustrates this process diagrammatically.

The Steps of Projective and Introjective Identification in a Couple

Figure 6.1 summarizes the mutuality of the processes. They have been described as a series of interlocking steps (D. Scharff & Scharff, 1991; J. S. Scharff, 1992). To describe them more fully, we have to begin at some point along the chain of reciprocity. We start from the original projection of a partner we will call "the wife."

- *Projection.* The wife expels a part of herself that is denied (or overvalued) and sees her spouse as if he were imbued with these qualities, whether he is or not. He will certainly be imbued with some of them, accounting for the attraction that his wife felt for him. In other words the projection may or may not fit. If it does, the spouse has a *valency* (Bion, 1961) for responding to the projection.
- *Projective identification.* The husband may or may not identify with the projection. If he does, he may do so passively, under the influence of his wife's capacity to induce in him a state of mind corresponding to her own, even if it feels foreign to him, or actively, by the force of his valency compelling him to be identified that way. He tends to identify either with the projected part of the wife's self ("concordant identification") or with the object ("complementary identification") that applies

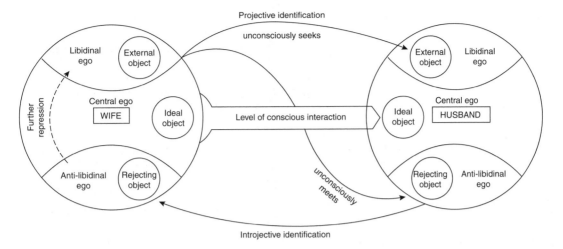

FIGURE 6.1. Projective and introjective identification. Adapted from D. E. Scharff (1982). Copyright 1982 by David E. Scharff. Adapted by permission of Taylor & Francis.

to that part of herself (Racker, 1968). Although the husband inevitably has been chosen because of his psychological valencies and physical (including sexual) characteristics that resonate with parts of the wife's self and object, he also has his own personality and body that are different from those of his wife and her external objects on whom her internal objects are based. In this gap between the original and the new object lies the healing potential of these bilateral processes. The husband as a new object transforms his wife's view of herself and her objects through accepting the projection, temporarily identifying with it, modifying it, and returning it in a detoxified form through a mental process of *containment*, analogous to the mother's way of bearing the pain of her infant's distress and misperceptions of her (Bion, 1962). Now, through *introjective identification* the wife takes in this modified version of herself and assimilates her view of herself to it. She grows in her capacity to distinguish self and other. If her husband is not willing or able to offer her the containment that she needs, and instead returns her projections either unaltered or exaggerated, growth is blocked.

• *Mutual projective and introjective identificatory processes.* The wife is simultaneously receiving projections from her husband and returning them to him. Together, they are containing and modifying each other's internal versions of self and object. Mutual projective and introjective processes govern mate selection, falling in love, the quality of the sexual relationship, the level of intimacy, and the nature of the marriage in general and its

effect on the partners' development as adults (D. Scharff, 1982; D. Scharff & Scharff, 1991). In a mutual process, husband and wife connect according to unconscious complementarity of object relations. Similarly, couple and therapist relate through the reciprocal actions of transference and countertransference.

How is unconscious complementarity of object relations different from the familiar term "collusion" (Willi, 1982)? We think that "collusion" is another way of describing the same process, at least in those writings where collusion refers to an unconscious dynamic between a couple. We tend to avoid the term "collusion," because it seems to judge and blame the husband and wife, as if they were intentionally colluding to thwart each other, their families, and therapists. Nevertheless, mutual projective and introjective identificatory processes cement the couple in an unconscious collusive attempt to avoid anxiety.

Couple dysfunction occurs when more distress than can be tolerated upsets the balance in the mutual projective identificatory system. This happens when some of the following conditions apply: (1) Projective and introjective identificatory processes are not mutually gratifying; (2) containment of the spouse's projections is not possible; (3) cementing of the object relations set happens instead of its modification; (4) unarousing projective identification of the genital zone cannot be modified by sexual experience; (5) aspects of the love object have to be split off and experienced in a less threatening situation, leading to triangulation involving a child, hobby, work, friend, parent, or lover.

The following snapshot, taken from a vignette of a couple described later in the chapter, illustrates the way the balance in a couple may shift and lead to breakup.

Michelle and Lenny were drawn to each other by mutual projective and introjective identificatory processes. She saw in him a solid, loving, thoughtful, and successful man who treated her well, and whom her hatefulness could not destroy, whereas he was proud to be her stable base, and in return enjoyed her vivacity and outrageous disregard of his sensibilities, loving her in spite of herself and treating her like a queen. Lenny treated Michelle as special, the way his mother had treated him, and as her mother had treated her, and her brother even more so. Michelle treated Lenny as she had felt treated: He was special to her, as she was to her mother, but not as wonderful as the other person, namely, a man like her brother. The problem arose when Lenny could not contain Michelle's projective identification of him as her brother because he was not as exciting, not as aggressive, and not as enviable. Michelle could not contain his projective identification of her as his adored self, because she was so hateful and destroyed by envy. Michelle longed for Lenny to be more aggressive, but the more she pestered him to be so, the less space she gave to his initiative, and the more she became like a repressed, nagging image of his mother, whom he preferred to think of as adoring. Lenny had helped Michelle with her fear of sex, and so she had been able to modify her unarousing projective identification of the genital zone due to her envy of her brother's genitalia and preferred status, but not sufficiently to reinvest her vagina as a gratifying organ of pleasure and bonding for the couple. No actual triangulation had occurred, but in fantasy Michelle kept herself attached to the hope of a better man who would fulfil all her expectations of virility. She wished to break up, but could not. Against his own wishes, but facing the reality of the destructiveness of their attachment, Lenny decided to break up, because the balance of the re-creation of projective and introjective identificatory processes had shifted from the gratifying into the intolerable range, and hope of their modification was lost.

THE PROCESS OF OBJECT RELATIONS COUPLE THERAPY

The Structure of Therapy

The couple therapy session may be of any predetermined length, from 45 minutes to 1½ hours, and may occur weekly or twice weekly for as long as necessary, with 2 years being the average duration

of treatment. Although object relations couple therapy is a long-term method for in-depth work, the same approach can be applied by those at work in managed care situations. In such a limited time frame, we would offer as much understanding as we could of the couple's defensive system, without feeling under pressure to produce quick changes. We admit the limits of what we can offer rather than delude ourselves, the families, and their health care planners into thinking that the minimum is all that is necessary, just because it is all that we are authorized to provide.

Family therapists of various orientations share a common goal in seeking to improve technique, so that more families can be helped more economically. Fewer sessions can be quite effective in crises and in families with short-term goals. When families see that their presenting symptom is part of a broader dysfunction, some of them make it a financial priority to work for more fundamental change in the family system and in their internal object relations. These are the families for whom short-term, focused methods provide a window of opportunity through which to move on to in-depth family therapy with plenty of time to do the work.

Both in brief therapy and in long-term therapy formats, beginnings and endings of the sessions are important. Anxiety is often most accessible at these times of separation and reunion. The object relations couple therapist is attentive to boundary phenomena, because they illuminate the interior of the couple relationship. Other than having a beginning, a middle, and an end, the object relations couple therapy session has no structure imposed upon it, because the therapist does not direct how the couple will use the session. Instead, we follow the couple's lead and comment on how their use of the session reflects their way of dealing with other times, tasks, authorities, and intimate situations.

The main ingredient of the approach is the working space provided by the therapeutic relationship. Training, supervision, peer discussion, and personal therapy ensure that the therapist maximizes the availability of the therapeutic self and calibrates it for use as an effective therapeutic instrument.

The Role of the Therapist

The working alliance is fostered mainly by the therapist's capacity for tolerating anxiety. The therapist is neither aloof nor gratifying, but is willing to be accommodating, to share knowledge when that will be helpful, and to negotiate a way of working that meets the couple's needs without compromising the therapist's integrity. Some couples may need more support or advice than others (including behavioral sex therapy for some), yet the principle of remaining fundamentally nondirective at the unconscious level still applies. That is to say, when the couple responds to some parenting advice or resists an assignment in sex therapy, for example, the therapist waits for associations to the spouses' reactions, including any dreams and fantasies, through which to trace the unconscious thread and its relation to the transference. The general attitude is one of not doing too much so as to let themes emerge in their own form and time. Once the shape of the couple's experience declares itself, the therapist takes hold of it, interacts, shares the experience, and puts words on it. Reaching into the couple's unconscious life in this way gives the couple the feeling of being understood and "held" psychologically in the treatment situation. This fosters the working alliance and sustains the couple and the therapist through times when the relationship to the therapist inevitably bears the brunt of the couple's distress.

The therapist aims to become an object that the couple can use—and abuse, if necessary. She becomes a transitional object that their relationship encompasses and uses, as a child uses a toy or a pet to deflect yet express feelings about self, sibling, or parent. In the quality of their relationship to her, she can discover and reveal to the partners the defenses and anxieties that confound their relationship. The therapist is not a traditional blank screen analyst, impassively awaiting the onslaught from the id. The object relations couple therapist is personable yet not seductive, and she remains neutral as to how the couple chooses to use therapy. She will follow rather than lead. She is both supportive and confrontational when communicating to the partners her experience of the use they have made of her. She uses her own presence and feelings, yet she is somewhat distant, in that she does not allow her mood to dominate the session. She does not share information from her personal life, but she may share a fantasy or a feeling that occurs to her in association to the couple's material. Her therapeutic stance changes little over the course of the therapy, but the way that she interacts with the partners will change as couple and therapist become progressively more

able to give up defensive patterns, to tolerate shared anxiety, and to engage in a collaborative relationship. In the following section on technique, we return to a more detailed examination of the use of the therapist's self.

The most usual error is that of doing too much. The therapist gets anxious about being worthwhile and takes action to dispel the uneasy, helpless feeling. She may end a session early, start late, forget an appointment, make a slip, lose a couple's check, or call partners by the wrong names. She may speak too much, cut off the flow of communication, or retreat into a withholding silence. She may substitute asking questions for realizing how little she knows or how frustrated she has been by a withholding couple. All of these happenings are to be expected as part of the work of allowing herself to be affected. Instead of calling them errors, we can call them deviations from which we can recover as soon as we subject them to process and review.

Another common error is to deviate from the neutral position: Now, the therapist is siding with the husband; now, she takes the wife's point of view. Object relations couple therapists agree that a neutral position is important and that partiality to either spouse is an error. But we disagree about the need to avoid it. Dare (1986) advises scrupulous fairness to spouses and absolute symmetry in the seating arrangements. We share his ideal of fairness as an intention, but we leave room for error. Rather than rigidly guarding against them, we prefer to work with deviations and jealousies that arise, and to understand their source in difficulties with triangles in the family of origin.

Assessment and Treatment Planning

Setting the Frame

Thinking about a frame (Langs, 1976; Zinner, 1989) within which to establish a reliable space for work begins in the first moment of the consultation. The frame may be established at the beginning or may emerge according to need as the consultation proceeds. The frame includes the number and length of sessions, the setting of the fee, the therapist's management of the beginning and end of sessions, and the establishment of the way of working. Usually about five sessions are needed before we are ready with a formulation and recommendation. This allows for one or two couple sessions, one or more individual sessions for each spouse as indicated, and a couple session in which formulations and recommendations about treatment are given. The couple's reactions to the frame and any attempts to bend it are explored in terms of the couple's transference to the therapist's attempts to provide a safe therapeutic space. This exploration is undertaken both to secure the frame against unconscious forces tending to distort it and to discover the nature of the flaws in the couple's holding capacity.

Creating Psychological Space for Understanding

The therapist creates psychological space for understanding (Box, 1981) by containing the couple's anxieties as they begin the consultation. As object relations couple therapists we do this through dealing with the couple relationship rather than the individuals who comprise it, and the way we listen, allow feelings to be expressed, experience those feelings in relation to ourselves, and interpret our experience. The couple identifies with our containing function and develops the capacity to create space in which to arrive at understanding.

Listening to the Unconscious

We listen in a relaxed way that is attentive yet not closely focused. We try to be free of the need to get information and to make sense of things, so we do not take a formal history. We wait until the salient facts emerge at moments of affective intensity. We listen not to the individuals alone but to the communication from the couple as a system in relation to us. We listen to not only the conscious communication but also the unconscious communication. We do this by following the themes emerging from the verbal associations, by noting the meaning of silences, by integrating our observation of nonverbal language with words and silence, and by working with fantasy and dream material. We also attend to the unconscious communication expressed in the physical aspects of sexual functioning. As we listen, we let our senses be impinged on. We hold the experience inside. Then we allow meaning to emerge from within.

Following the Affect

We are interested in moments of emotion, because these provide access to the unconscious areas from which the feeling has emerged. These mo-

ments bring us a living history of relationships in the families of origin that is more immediate and useful than a formally obtained social history or genogram. Some psychoanalytic couple therapists, however, such as Dare (1986), do recommend the use of the genogram.

Transference and Countertransference

Creating the space, listening, and following the affect come together in the "countertransference" (Freud, 1910b), namely, our feelings about the couple and the individual spouses in response to the couple's "transference" (Freud, 1917), namely, partners' feelings about us as new editions of figures from their family histories. At times, our countertransference remains unconscious in a way that supports our being in tune with the couple and doing our work. At other times, it obtrudes as a feeling of discomfort, a fantasy, or a dream, and we can take hold of it and get to work on what it means.

Interpretation of Defense

We point out the couple's recurring pattern of interactions that serve a defensive purpose. Then, speaking from our own emotional experience of joining in unconscious communication with the couple, we interpret the couple's pattern of defenses. Only when we can point out the partners' pattern and the way in which we have been involved in it can we work out what they and we have been defending ourselves against.

Confronting Basic Anxiety

Finally, we work with the basic anxieties that have seemed too intolerable to bear in consciousness. When they are named, faced, and adapted to, the partners can proceed to the next developmental phase of their life cycle. During assessment, we are content to identify some aspect of the basic anxiety revealed in the defensive patterns that we have pointed out, without any attempt at thorough exploration.

Couples who are not ready for couple therapy and who have not responded to interpretations of their resistance to it are given a choice of psychoanalytically oriented separate or concurrent marital, family, and individual therapies, with or without necessary or preferred adjunctive treatment or referral for behavioral or communications-based therapy as either an alternative or preliminary treatment. Given a free choice, partners can then sometimes move in the direction of the therapist's original emphasis on the couple relationship, but if not, their right to begin therapy as they see fit must be respected and accommodated. If they choose to work with the therapist, then by mutual agreement, couple and therapist settle upon the treatment plan. Then the policy of sticking to the plan is explained and discussed: unless future experience dictates a shift, no change in the arrangements is undertaken except after thorough discussion and mutual agreement. So the frame is secure but flexible.

Then we outline other policies, such as fees, vacations, and billing practice. Our billing practice is to bill at the end of the month and to have the couple's check by the 10th of the month. We do this because it helps us to keep in mind the moment when the bill was rendered and to focus on how the couple is dealing with the financial aspects of the commitment. We sell our time not by item of service but by long-term commitment, so we expect the couple to attend as planned. If they have to be absent, we are willing to reschedule within the week, but if that is not possible then we hold them responsible for the time. Unlike our work with families in which we see the family with a member absent, in couple therapy we do not work unless both members of the couple are present. Suddenly doing individual therapy with one spouse poses a threat to the therapist's neutrality and capacity to help the couple. Of course, in keeping with the flexible frame, individual sessions can be scheduled by plan and by mutual agreement, but not as filler for absences from therapy.

Goal Setting

Goals are not closely specified, because we find this to be restricting. We do not tailor our approach to the removal of a symptom, because we value the symptom as a beacon that leads us through the layers of defense and anxiety from which it stems. In any case, goals tend to change over time as the partners are freed to experience the potential of their relationship. So we prefer a somewhat openended formulation of a couple's aims for treatment. We are content with a general statement of the wish to change behavior, to become more accommodating, to improve communication and understanding, and to function better as a couple. In technical terms, our therapeutic goals are as listed in Table 6.1.

TABLE 6.1. The Goals of Object Relations Couple Therapy

- To recognize and rework the couple's mutual projective and introjective identifications.
- To improve the couple's contextual holding capacity so that the partners can provide for each other's needs for attachment and autonomy, and developmental progression.
- To recover the centered holding relationship that allows for unconscious communication between the spouses, shown in their capacity for empathy, intimacy, and sexuality.
- To promote individuation of the spouses and differentiation of needs including the need for individual therapy or psychoanalysis.
- To return the couple with confidence to the tasks of the current developmental stage in the couple's life cycle.

The Move from Assessment to Treatment

At the moment of moving from assessment to treatment, the couple is given the choice of accepting the frame or accepting referral to another therapist whose conditions seem preferable. Here is an example from such a session.

Mr. and Mrs. Melville had both had previous individual therapies and now wanted to work with me (Jill Scharff) in couple therapy. He was a successful organizational consultant who loved his work; enjoyed food, sports, and sex; and felt great about himself except in his marriage, where he felt unloved. She was a good homemaker, mother of three little ones, and ran a small business selling jewelry from her home. She felt exhausted, unaccomplished, and uninterested in sex. Both tended to overspend, so short-term cash flow problems created financial stress in addition to their couple tension.

I told them my fee and my billing policy. They had no problem agreeing to the amount of my fee and my payment schedule. But charging for mixed sessions was another matter. Mr. Melville did not want to be charged, because he was a punctual person, and because his business travel was out of his control. Mrs. Melville was concerned that her vacation would have to be tied to mine, but since our vacation periods happened to overlap, she was not concerned.

I said, "I see that you react differently to my policy. You, Mr. Melville, feel that since you are a good, responsible person, you do not deserve to be charged, which to you feels like a punishment and a rejection of your worth. You, Mrs. Melville, feel afraid of being trapped in the relationship with me. I assume these feelings also come up between you as you deal with the consequences of the marriage commitment."

Mrs. Melville rushed to concur. She said that she felt so trapped in marriage. She was terrified of feeling financially and emotionally destitute as she had at the time of her divorce. She felt she could lose herself. She thought that her husband felt punished by her need for space and for her own charge account. Mr. Melville agreed that he felt that way. Unlike her first husband, he insisted on sharing his inheritance with her, even though all her money went directly to her children. He had already recovered financially from his divorce, he had been generous with his former wife, and he was not worried about risking all in marriage again. He had no idea how frightened she was.

In their transference reactions to the frame, the Melvilles revealed their fundamental problems. His self-worth was tied to his earning capacity rather than to being loved, because the former was more dependable than the latter. His willingness to provide for his wife could not assuage her sense of insecurity, because it emphasized his independence from her and defended against love. How could anyone so apparently confident ever understand her terror of dependency and her fears of annihilation? How could someone so generous be married to someone to whom it meant so little? The answer must lie in their mutual projection of the good, abundant, nourishing, energetic breast into him (as, it turned out, both had experienced their fathers) and the shrivelled, nonreplenishing breast, depleted by their neediness into her (an image that derived from their shared views of their mothers). As the therapist expecting to be paid, Dr. Scharff was a replenishing breast to which they had to contribute in partnership, an expectation that threatened them in ways unique to each individual in reflection of the object relations set.

Some couples come already seeking couple therapy. Others have to be shown that that is the approach most likely to help them, rather than the individual therapy that one of the partners had requested. In that case an individual problem has to be redefined as a symptom of the relationship. We do not suppose, however, that couple therapy is always best, or that every couple is ready for it. We find it best to start where the spouses are, and to recommend the form of treatment that they will accept and follow through on, including referral for adjunctive medication or behavioral treatment, where indicated, or for individual psychoanalysis when that is an appropriate, definitive choice, not a defense against couple therapy.

Process and Technical Aspects of Object Relations Couple Therapy

As object relations couple therapists we observe the couple relationship primarily, through noticing the way the couple deals with us, but we are also interested in how the partners interact with each other. We are concerned with not only the conscious aspects of their bond but also the internal object relations operating through mutual projective identificatory processes in the partners' unconscious minds.

In keeping with this focus, our technique employs nondirective listening for the emergence of unconscious themes, following the affect, analyzing dream, and fantasy material and associations offered by both members of the couple, and exploring the family history of each partner as it relates to the current couple relationship. We point out patterns of interaction that tend to recur and look for unconscious forces that drive the repetition. Gradually we become familiar with the defensive aspects of these repeating cycles. We do this over and over, covering the same ground and making inroads into defended territory, which we find particularly accessible at times when the couple's transference has stirred a countertransference response through which we can appreciate the couple's vulnerability. As the partners' trust builds, we can help them figure out and face the nameless anxiety behind the defense. Our help comes in the form of interpretations of resistance, defense, and conflict, conceptualized as operating through unconscious object relation systems that support and subvert the marriage. These interpretations are imparted after being metabolized in the countertransference. Interpretation may lead to insight that produces change in the unconscious object relations of the couple, or it may lead to increased resistance to the unconscious conflict. Progression and regression succeed each other in cycles as we work through the defensive structures of the marriage to the point that these no longer interfere with the partners' capacity for working together as life partners, loving each other, integrating good and bad, and building a relationship of intimacy

---

TABLE 6.2. The Tasks of Object Relations Couple Therapy

1. Setting the frame
2. Maintaining a neutral position of involved impartiality
3. Creating a psychological space
4. Use of the therapist's self: Negative capability
5. Transference and countertransference
6. Interpretation of defense, anxiety, fantasy, and inner object relations: The "because" clause
7. Working with dreams
8. Working through
9. Termination

---

and sexuality that is free to develop through the developmental life cycle of the marriage.

What does all this mean in practice? Our technique can be explored through its components, as summarized in Table 6.2.

Setting the Frame

Our first priority is to hold to a frame for therapy that we established during the assessment interviews (Langs, 1976). This frame offers "a secure and consistent environment in which highly sensitive, private feelings and fantasies can be expressed and explored without the threat of actualizing the feared consequences" (Zinner, 1989, p. 321). The partners try to bend the frame so that unconscious wishes can be gratified, but their efforts are frustrated by the therapist, who holds firm. The ensuing conflict brings into the treatment the issues that have been dividing the marriage.

Listening to the Unconscious

At the conscious level we listen to what the partners are saying, which partner is saying what, in what order, and with what affect. We try to listen just as carefully to the silence and to the nonverbal communications in the form of gestures. Yet this careful listening is not as consciously attentive as our description sounds so far. Instead, we experience a drifting state of mind, at one level interacting, maybe even asking a question and hearing the answer, at another level not listening for anything in particular. Freud (1912) described this as "evenly-suspended attention," the therapist turning "his own unconscious like a receptive organ toward the transmitting unconscious of the patient" (pp. 112–115). Through experience, supervision, peer consultation, ongoing process, and review of our work in sessions, therapy, and self-analysis, we develop an understanding of our own unconscious so that we can separate our own from the patients' material. We tune in our calibrated, unconscious receiving apparatus at the deepest level of communication to the unconscious signals from the couple, coming through to us as a theme that emerges from the flow of associations and silences, amplified by dream and fantasy, and resonating in us as countertransference experience from which we can share in and reconstruct the couple's unconscious object relations. When we give the couple our reconstruction in the form of an interpretation, we can check out its validity by evaluating the ensuing associative flow.

Holding the Neutral Position

We maintain a position of neutrality, with no preference for one spouse or the other, for one type of object relationship versus another, for lifestyle choices, or treatment outcome. Our attention hovers evenly between the intrapsychic dimensions of each spouse, their interpersonal process, and their interaction with us. While we obviously value marriage as an institution, we do not have a bias about continuation of a couple's marriage or divorce. We are invested in our work with the couple and in the possibility of growth and development, but we do not want to invest in the couple's achievement. We want to hold a position described as one of "involved impartiality" (Stierlin, 1977). Any deviations from that occur in directions that are quite unique to each couple. From reviewing the specific pull exerted upon us, we learn about the couple's unconscious object relationships.

Creating the Psychological Space

This willingness to work with one's experience demonstrates an attitude of valuing process and review. It offers the couple a model for self-examination and personal sharing, and creates the psychological space into which the couple can move and there develop its potential for growth. We offer a therapeutic environment in which the couple can experience its relationship in relation to the therapist. Our therapeutic stance derives from our integration of the concepts of container–contained (Bion, 1962) and the holding environment (Winnicott, 1960). The relationship to the therapist creates a transitional space in which the couple can portray and reflect upon its current way of functioning, learn about and modify its projective identificatory system, and invent new ways of being. Through clinical experience, training and supervision, and intensive personal psychotherapy or psychoanalysis, the therapist develops a "holding capacity," the capacity to bear the anxiety of the emergence of unconscious material and affect through containment and to modify it through internal processing of projective identifications. The therapist contributes this capacity to the transitional space that is thereby transformed into an expanded psychological space for understanding. The couple then takes in this space and finds within the couple relationship the capacity to deal with current and future anxiety. Once this happens, the actual therapeutic relationship can be terminated, because the therapeutic function has been internalized.

The Use of the Self

Clearly, the use of the therapist's self is central to our technique. Some of this can be learned from reading (Jacobs, 1991; J. S. Scharff, 1992), but mainly we must develop an openness to learning from experience, nurtured in training and supervision. For fullest use of the self in the clinical setting, we need to have had the personal experience of understanding our own family history and object relations in psychoanalysis or intensive psychotherapy, including couple and family therapy, even in the rare instance when this has not been necessary for a satisfactory personal life. This gives the therapist the necessary base of self-knowledge to calibrate the self as a diagnostic and therapeutic instrument. Its continued refinement is a lifelong task, accomplished mainly through process and review in the clinical situation, discussion with colleagues, and teaching and writing.

Developing Negative Capability

Once the therapist's self is cleared for use as a receiving apparatus and as a space that can be filled with the experience of the couple, the therapist is able to know, without seeking to know actively, about the couple's unconscious. Striving to find out distorts the field of observation. Instead we recommend a nondirective, unfocused, receptive attitude best described as "negative capability," a term invented by the poet Keats to describe Shakespeare's capacity as a poet for "being in uncertainties, mysteries, doubts, without any irritable reaching after fact and reason" (Murray, 1955, p. 261). Bion (1970), expanding on Keats's term, urged the therapist to be without memory or desire, that is, to abandon the need to know and to impose meaning. Negative capability, however, is an ideal state, and we do not advocate striving for it. Instead, negative capability is a state to sink into, best achieved by not doing too much and allowing understanding to come from inside our experience. In their anxiety to be understood and cared about, some couples react with frustration to the therapist's apparent lack of directiveness, activity, and omniscience. As long as their reactions are recognized and interpreted, these couples usually come to value the deeper level of understanding that is promoted by the therapist's inhibition of surface engagement activity. Some couples will not be able to tolerate the initial frustration or the ensuing depth of intimacy offered by the analytic therapist and will do better with a therapist who relates in a more obviously supportive way, and who does not intend to offer an in-depth, growth experience.

Working with Transference and Countertransference

Negative capability fosters our capacity to respond to the couple's transference, namely the partners' shared feelings about the therapist. The transference gives rise to ideas, feelings, or behavior in the therapist, namely, countertransference. As Heimann (1950) pointed out, "The analyst's countertransference is an instrument of research into the patient's unconscious" (p. 81). The analyst must value and study this countertransference, because "the emotions roused in him are often nearer to the heart of the matter than his reasoning" (p. 82). This elaboration of countertransference stresses an understanding of the normal countertransference and its deviations (Money-Kyrle, 1956) rather than emphasizing the pathology of the therapist's responses.

In studying our reactions to unconscious material in psychoanalysis, psychotherapy, and couple and family therapy, we have found that our countertransference experiences tend to cluster in relation to two kinds of transferences: the contextual and the focused transferences (Scharff & Scharff, 1987).

"Contextual countertransference" refers to the therapist's reaction to the patient's contextual transference, namely, the patient's response to the therapeutic environment, shown in attitudes about the frame of treatment, unconscious resistance in general, specific conscious feelings, and behavior toward the therapist as an object for providing a holding situation.

"Focused countertransference" occurs in response to the focused transference, namely, feelings the patient transfers to the therapist as an object for intimate relating. Usually the contextual transference–countertransference predominates in the opening and closing phases of individual treatment and throughout family therapy. In couple therapy, there is often rapid oscillation between the contextual and focused countertransference, as the following vignette from an opening session with Jill Scharff shows:

Mrs. Rhonda Clark, a tall, angular woman with a short, burgundy-colored, spiked hairdo, stormed ahead of her husband, Dr. Clark, a short, round-faced, gentle-looking man. She wore high-style black leather pants and a studded jacket, which she threw on the couch. He meekly laid down his own sheepskin coat and looked expectantly at her through his traditional, rimmed glasses, which unexpectedly, however, were bright purple. She was emitting hostility but no words.

I asked if they were waiting for me to start. He said that she almost didn't come today.

I said, "How come? You, Mrs. Clark, were the one who called me and made the arrangements."

Mrs. Clark explained that was just mad today at him, the big shot, Mr. Doctor God, who, she told me angrily, was indeed no god. Turning back to me, she told me of his berating and belittling her in front of his office staff. Dr. Clark agreed that he had been rude, because he was annoyed by being pestered at the office, where she caused upset among the staff. All he wanted was to be in a happy situation with a decent sex life and no ruckus. His friends recommended divorce, but he wanted to work it out for the sake of their four children.

Mrs. Clark responded that she did not feel like being sexual with a man who was so rude about her.

At first I felt ashamed that my sympathies were with the doctor, who was calm and reasonable, and not asking much. But I knew from experience that this was not an opinion; it was just a temporary reaction, not just to her but to them as a couple. For some reason as this couple crossed the boundary into the therapy space, Mrs. Clark became dominating, interruptive, and crude. But as she was being thrust forward, his feelings were hiding behind her anxious and aggressive front.

I said to Dr. Clark, "Is Mrs. Clark the only one who is anxious or do you have questions, too?"

Dr. Clark replied that he was not anxious, but that he did have questions. He wanted to interview me about where I went to school.

This is one question that must always be answered. Without commenting on the denigrating, aggressive tone in his question, I told Dr. Clark my professional background. He was glad to learn that I had graduated from medical school in 1967. He had thought that I was a psychologist (which he would not like) and that I seemed too young. So he felt relieved that I had been practicing as a board certified psychiatrist for 15 years. I was temporarily protected from his denigration by the fact of my sharing his medical background, a feature about me that he and his wife overvalued.

I said that I was glad to hear of his concerns, because until then it had appeared as though Mrs. Clark was the one who had all the feelings about therapy being no use. I told them that I had the impression that she expressed her anxiety by getting angry, but that he expressed his anxiety through her. Now, usefully, he was admitting to it. Both of them, for their own reasons and in their individual ways, were anxious about therapy and about their marriage.

In my countertransference, I experienced a deviation from involved impartiality (Stierlin, 1977) and realized that Mrs. Clark was expressing a focused transference toward me as the doctor (the same profession as her husband), and that this was a cover for the couple's

shared contextual transference of distrust in the context of treatment. My task was to address the contextual transference with them so that, as a couple, Dr. and Mrs. Clark could modify their reluctance to begin treatment.

This example serves to illustrate another idea that is helpful in work with our reactions to focused transferences, namely, Racker's (1968) concept of concordant and complementary transference.

Racker described countertransference as a fundamental condition of receiving the patient's projections and tolerating them inside himself as projective identifications. His reception of the projections was unconscious, out of his awareness until he subjected his experience to process and review. In Racker's view, countertransference is a fundamental means of understanding the patient's internal world, a view that object relations couple therapists share. Racker went further to point out that the therapist might identify with parts of either the patient's self or objects. Identification with the patient's self he called "concordant identification." Identification with the object was called "complementary identification." As couple therapists, we can now think of our therapeutic task as the reception and clarification of the couple's projections, followed by analysis of the interpersonal conditions under which these occur.

In the session with the Clarks, Mrs. Clark experienced me as a contemptuous and rejecting object, like the object that she projected into her husband, and she evoked in me an unwelcome state of mind in which I felt contempt for her. My countertransference was one of complementary identification to her object. Dr. Clark experienced me as a denigrated object, like the one he projected into his wife, then switched to seeing me as a part of himself, the wise physician. To him, my countertransference was one of concordant identification with part of his self. I did not experience an identification with his object, perhaps because my identity as a physician protected me from it, but more likely because I was tuning in to an internal process in which Dr. Clark used his ideal object to repress his rejected object, which he split and projected more readily into Mrs. Clark than into me at this stage of the assessment.

Interpreting Defense and Anxiety about Intimacy

The next example from Jill Scharff comes from the midphase of couple therapy with Aaron and Phyllis.

Aaron and Phyllis had had a fulfilling marriage for 10 years—until Aaron's 16-year-old daughter Susie came to live with them. Phyllis had raised their shared family without much criticism from Aaron, and without challenge from their very young son and daughter. She felt supported by Aaron in her role as an efficient mother who ran a smooth household. She felt loved by him and by her dependent children. Her self-esteem was good, because she was a much better mother than her own mother had been.

But when Susie came to stay, trouble began. Phyllis had firm ideas on what was appropriate for Susie and, in contrast, Aaron was extremely permissive. So Phyllis became the target for Susie's animosity. Aaron saw no need for limits and, indeed, saw no problem between Phyllis and Susie. Phyllis became increasingly angry at Aaron. He bore the situation stoically, only occasionally confronting the problem. Then, he would tell Phyllis that she was being small-minded and awful, because she was acting out her jealousy, and he felt that this was making her stepchild miserable. Phyllis was angered by that attack on her self-esteem and never did recover from it.

They saw a family counselor, who verified the 16 year-old's need for limits, supported Phyllis's views, and worked to get Aaron's cooperation. Aaron turned around and in a short time his daughter was behaving well and Phyllis could enjoy her. To this day, 10 years later, Phyllis enjoys visits from her.

This seemed to have been a spectacular therapeutic success. I asked Aaron how he conceptualized the amazing turnabout. He said that once the therapist had made the situation clear to him, he simply told his daughter to do what Phyllis said or she would be out of the house. But Phyllis's anger at Aaron's ignoring her pleas until then was still there. Although she continued to enjoy sex with Aaron, Phyllis walked out emotionally for several years, in equal retribution for the years in which she felt Aaron had walked out on her. The family counselor had treated the family symptom and its effect on the couple with a useful prescription that removed the symptom, but she did it so rapidly that the underlying problem in the marriage was not recognized. The use of the focus upon a problem child as a defense against problems of intimacy had not been addressed, so the issue came up again in their second treatment opportunity.

The force of Aaron's ultimatum about complying or leaving the house suggested to me that he had lived by the same rule himself for the preceding 10 years. Then, however, he began to challenge Phyllis's rule by expressing his alternative way of coping with children—with predictable results. Now, the same old problem they had had with Susie was surfacing with their shared older daughter, who was now 15. Because no work had been done on their differences, they had not developed a shared method of child rearing. Now that Aaron was challenging Phyllis, they fought about the right way to do everything, but nowhere as painfully as over the care of their children.

Phyllis went on to give an example, however, that concerned not the problem daughter but their 11-year-old son. He had asked to go on a date, and Phyllis had promptly told him that this was inappropriate because he was too young. Aaron had immediately intervened to offer a ride, and Phyllis told me that she had felt undermined. Aaron said that he had spoken up because he felt that she was being unhelpful to their son's social development. I said that I could see how either position could be defended, but the problem was that they had not discussed things to arrive at a shared position that addressed their anxiety about their 11-year-old's burgeoning social independence.

Phyllis was furious at me for a whole day. She thought that I had been unaccommodating and controlling. But to my surprise, and to her credit, she said that she had had to laugh when it struck her that it was not what I was doing to annoy her, but what *she* was bringing to the session. She could have made the interpretation herself.

I realized that Phyllis was seeing me in the transference as Aaron saw her, and I was speculating on the origin of this projective identification and admiring her insight, when suddenly Phyllis returned to her argument and pointed out how anyone who could let a child date at the age of 11 could just as well let them be murdered and cut into pieces. I felt ridiculed for suggesting that they could consider their son's request together. I felt put down, as if I had not a clue about an 11-year-old's social development. I felt I was being small-minded, getting into the fight with them about a child, when we knew they had come for help not with child rearing but with their marriage. I thought that dating, meaning independence and intimacy, was equated with severe damage and loss.

Perhaps Phyllis felt that she needed her son close to her and could not yet face being cut off from him. Perhaps Aaron, while wishing to facilitate their son's date, was offering to drive to stay close to him, too, or possibly to stay close to the issue of intimacy vicariously. I also wondered if dating signaled sexuality causing loss, but that was probably not the case, because sexuality for Phyllis and Aaron was relatively free of conflict. So I concluded that the loss referred to sexuality being cut off from intimacy in the rest of the relationship.

I stuck to my point. I said, "I'm not really talking about whether or not an 11-year-old should date. I'm taking you to task about the effect of sticking to alternative positions and not talking about them together."

Here I was confronting their defense of using a child to portray their conflict about intimacy. Aaron agreed that intimacy was a problem, even though sex was not. He said that he felt cramped in every part of his life, because he felt that Phyllis was so vulnerable. Phyllis was more concerned with how much they argued. Conflict was killing them and smashing up their marriage, and she was tired of it. She did not want to leave again, as she had had to do to get away from her mother, a dreadful, intrusive person. Phyllis got out by being perfect, an overachiever. Having struggled so hard not to be evil like her mother, Phyllis felt threatened when Aaron said she was small-minded and evil. She did not want to be anything like the mother she disliked so much.

Now, I understood that my countertransference response of feeling small and no good reflected a complementary identification with Phyllis's internal maternal object and, at the same time, a concordant identification with the most repressed part of Phyllis's self. Using the explanation that Phyllis had worked out, I was able to make an interpretation that integrated her words and my countertransference.

I said to Phyllis, "Now, we can see that you retreated from Aaron because you wished to keep your relationship together as the harmonious marriage it used to be and occasionally is when you have enjoyable sex. You were trying to protect yourself and him from your becoming as horrible as the angry, intrusive mother spoiling the relationship, or else facing the calamity of having to leave the marriage to leave that part of you behind."

This interpretation illustrates the use of "the because clause" (Ezriel, 1952). Ezriel noted that transference contained three aspects: (1) a required relationship that defended against (2) an avoided relationship, both of which were preferable to (3) a calamity. We have found it useful in couple therapy to follow his interpretive model, because it brings the avoided relationship into focus as both anxiety and defense.

Aaron had not yet told me enough about himself to let me complete the picture. It was clear that Phyllis was still using projection and overfunctioning within the marriage to keep herself above being horrible. And Aaron, feeling cramped like the children, was finding her control just as horrible. When he suppressed his angry or critical feelings, as he did most of the time except in irrational fights, he also suppressed his warm, affectionate feelings except when he and Phyllis had sex.

In this example, the sexually exciting object relationship was the required relationship being used to repress the avoided rejecting object constellation. Aaron's conscious suppression felt withholding to Phyllis, who longed for feedback and emotional involvement. Aaron's eventual outbursts against her led Phyllis to relentless pursuit of his attention, approval, and affection. The emergence of the avoided relationship unleashed the energy of the exciting object constellation, because it was no longer needed for repression. When Phyllis failed to get what she hoped for from Aaron, she then suppressed her longings and withdrew. Now the rejecting object system was repressing the exciting one. But when this happened, Phyllis appeared to Aaron to be pouting, and he withdrew. The cycle continued, with their needs for intimacy defended against and frustrated by their mutual projective identifications.

As we read this case account, we could see this pattern, but we would have to wait for more object relations information from Aaron to clarify his contribution. We cannot always achieve the same depth or specificity in interpretation, but "the because clause" is still useful to stimulate an inquiring attitude in which we can ask the family to join as we move toward understanding.

Working with Fantasy and Inner Object Relations

Instead of taking a genogram to evaluate couples and to tell them their relationship to their families of origin, we prefer to wait for a living history of inner objects to emerge through our attention to object relations history at affectively charged moments in therapy.

Dr. and Mrs. Clark had been working with me (Jill Scharff) for a year. I had worked on Arthur's passivity, his inability to earn Rhonda's admiration of him as a successful, ambitious, caring man, and his need to denigrate Rhonda by comparing her to the nurses at the office. I worked on her tirades and her outrageous behavior that alienated Arthur, his office staff, and his family and left her feeling contemptible. Their sex life had improved because he was less demanding and she was less likely to balk and cause a fight. Their tenacious defensive system, in which she was assigned the blame and was the repository for the rage, greed, ambition, and badness in the couple, had not yet yielded to interpretation, although Rhonda was no longer on such a short fuse. I could see improvement in the diminution in the volume and frequency of her reactions, and in the degree of his contempt, but the basic pattern stayed in place until Arthur felt safe enough to tell Rhonda and me the full extent of his sadistic and murderous fantasies against women who had abandoned him. Catharsis played a part in securing some relief for him, but the major therapeutic effect came from work done in the countertransference on the way he was treating the two actual women in the room with him, his wife and me, as he told his fantasies about other women.

As he concluded, Arthur said that he was terrified that people would think that he would act out his fantasies, which, he assumed I would understand, he had never done and would not do in real sex.

I felt extremely uncomfortable. If I acknowledged that I was familiar with such a fear, I felt I would be siding with him in assuming that his wife was ignorant. His wife was hurt that he thought I would understand, as if she would not. Rhonda felt that neither I nor she, nor Arthur for that matter, could be sure, because he seemed afraid that it could happen.

I said, "There is no evidence that Arthur will act out the fantasies in their murderous form. But there is evidence that he's scared they'll get out of hand. We also have evidence right here that you do sadistic things to each other in this relationship, not physically, but emotionally."

Rhonda got it immediately. She said that she knew that as well as I did. She was grateful to Arthur for sharing his fantasies, because she felt so relieved that he was taking responsibility instead of blaming her for all that was wrong between them. Arthur maintained that he had always told her about his sadistic fantasies, but Rhonda pointed out that he had never gone into it in detail. She had felt that the fantasies were exciting at first, but now she knew that they were out of hand.

I said, "To some extent the threatening part of the fantasy is arousing to both of you. But by the end of it, Arthur, you are terrified of losing control, and Rhonda, you are frightened for your life."

Rhonda felt that understanding this was a breakthrough.

I was inclined to agree with Rhonda's evaluation. The longer Arthur kept the fantasy to himself, the more it seemed to be the real him. He was terrified of being found out, his secret hidden inside yet demanding to be heard. Furthermore, it was heard through projection into Rhonda, who identified with it: Her rages and aggression against Arthur gave expression to that attacking, chopping up part of him, for which she had a valency. Meanwhile, he contained for her the greater calamity of the wish for death, a wish and fear that stemmed from early loss of an envied and hated older brother.

Working with Dreams

An important part of the therapeutic process with couples is the analysis of the interpersonal–intrapsychic continuum expressed in dreams. Individual partners often report dreams during the course of treatment, and sometimes both of them have dreams that are found to overlap. Split-off aspects of shared unconscious object relations and linkages within the couple system of mutual projections and multiple unconscious communications are manifested in the couple's dreams. So, dreams communicate to the therapist the couple's unconscious object relations, and the couple can then be made conscious of them.

Dreams reveal underlying psychic conflict, repressed affects, shifts from one developmental level to another, attempts to master anxiety and to control affective flooding, longings, hurts or failures in development, transferences to the therapist or the partner, and refinding lost objects. The

dream remains the dreamer's own production, a reflection of his or her own internal object relations, but then the couple's free association and their analysis of the dream with the therapist's help turns the dream into an opportunity to explore the couple's intrapsychic–interpersonal narrative. Describing the dream, associating freely to the dream, and eliciting the partners' responses in couple therapy delivers the individual unconscious into the couple arena, where it becomes clear that the individual dream is dreamed and shared on behalf of the couple.

DISCOVERING THE INTERPERSONAL MEANING OF A DREAM

Dreams play an important role in therapy with couples, allowing access to the internal world of the partners at the same time that they give metaphors for their interaction. We treat any dream reported in the course of couple therapy as a joint product of the marriage, illustrating something about the joint marital personality, the two partners in interaction, individual and shared unconscious fantasy, and the transference. Split-off and repressed aspects of individual and shared unconscious organization, conscious and unconscious links, and multidirectional unconscious communication are all potential factors in the reporting of a dream. We can see the links to repressed affects: underlying conflict; shifts in developmental levels; attempts to master anxiety, to control overwhelming emotion, longings, and hurts; failures in development; and the refinding of repressed lost objects.

REPORTING OF DREAMS IN COUPLES

When first hearing a dream in couple therapy, we proceed in the following way. We first ask the partner who reports the dream what comes to mind about the dream; and only then do we listen to the other partner's associations. After that, we ask for partners' reactions to each other's thoughts about the dream. In this way, we learn how they know each other and gain access to their unconscious fantasies. We track the shifting affect that accompanies the unfolding of fantasy material. When we have been working with a couple for some time, we continue to respect the individual creativity of the dreamer, but we may respond sooner with our own associations as part of the co-construction of the dream analysis (as shown in the example that follows). In active dialogue with the couple around a dream, we get a living sample of the partners' interplay around depth issues: This lets us understand them better as individuals and as a couple. We see and interact with the joint marital personality. As the couple relates to the therapist while dealing with dream material, we note the transference and analyze our countertransference responses. From inside our own experience with the couple we can arrive at deeper understanding of the communication of the dream, and use the dream to help us understand their conflict.

DREAM WORK WITH A COUPLE IN SEX THERAPY

Lucien and Rachel are in their late 40s and have been married for 10 years. They were referred to me (David Scharff) because theirs had been a sexless marriage for several years. Sex therapy progressed slowly, because Lucien was phobic at every step, avoiding exercises, finding reasons to delay, and blaming Rachel for pressuring him, which she did despite the fact that this drove him away. Slowly he became able to tolerate sexual interaction. Three months before these dreams, Lucien and Rachel had managed pleasurable intercourse for the first time in years, and Lucien admitted he found it exciting, but he continued to tell Rachel that she should not pressure him by wanting to schedule intimate times together. Although sex therapy was technically successful, the couple still did not have sex outside of situations structured by therapy. There continued to be a barrier in the approach phase of every encounter, so weekly couple therapy continued.

• *A dream that shows direct transference in relationship to the dreamer's fears about himself and the persecuting object.* Lucien reported a dream. "In my dream, I'm an observer. There is a man with salt-and-pepper hair holding a bundle the size of a watermelon. I see it's a dead baby in a towel, but there's no blood. I conclude that there had been an evisceration. This man asks me to understand that the baby has no internal organs, and that something has just happened." Lucien said the baby's lack of internal organs referred to one of his business deals that a partner was threatening to eviscerate.

I said, "Well, it seems to me that another of your babies is our project here to restore your sexual life."

Ignoring me, Lucien said, "Well there was a sense of emotional detachment: looking at a horror scene without shrieking. It reminds me of my perennial dream as a child, seeing an axe man and not being disturbed. But there's no connection to here."

Rachel said, "The dream sounded like a nightmare. I thought perhaps it was you as the baby."

I asked about the man with salt-and-pepper hair, feeling that image referred to me. Lucien said, "He had

an oval face with shortish, gray hair with just a little black, late 50s, with a dark complexion." He turned to Rachel, "You never met Uncle Frank, my aunt's boyfriend, who was like a mobster from *The Sopranos.*"

I said, "Perhaps it referred to me—a salt-and-pepper-haired physician holding your baby."

Lucien said that he was not trying to let things slip away, and he was not sure about the resemblance to me. So I now asked about Frank, his aunt's boyfriend.

Lucien said, "My aunt has come to be known as the 'black widow' because she's had a husband and several boyfriends who have died, including Frank, whom I was fond of. At 73, my aunt's not necessarily finished. ... She is the horror show at family Christmas. She's not fit for society. She has money, which she uses strategically to attract men."

I said, "Well, there's the theme of a lethal woman who attracts men. Here you're afraid of Rachel's control of you, just as you feared getting too close to your intrusive mother."

Lucien said, "My mother has much more power over me than my aunt."

I now summarized, "I think the dead baby is the sexual project here and the association to your "black widow aunt" has to do with the risk you feel. Rachel thought the baby might also be you. I see a picture of the salt-and-pepper-haired man as me, but also partly as an image of you and your future. The man is heavyset, as if you had kept gaining weight, his hair gray with remnants of black, holding the baby that was this project, and emotionally detached from the horror that you have killed it. This is a way of telling yourself about the horror of what you might be doing right now, while acting as though you had no part in it. At the same time you are afraid of me for exposing you to this deadly situation. You cut yourself off from those fears and put them into Rachel, whom you get mad at because she expresses the anxiety that you both have."

The dream leads by association to the threatening maternal object imposed on the wife, and Lucien's distancing attachment to Rachel in fear of her intrusiveness. She feels his fear more acutely than he does consciously, then anxiously clings to him, and in the process frightens him further. He cuts off affect to maintain inner controls, but the anxiety comes back to him anyway in the form of a disowned and almost unnamed dread that comes back from his wife. As the cycle repeats, his automatic sense of dread (perhaps amygdala-directed) creates his withdrawal, which interacts with the anxiety about abandonment that Rachel brings from her own history. Together they construct a shared marital personality characterized by intrusion and retreat. This conjoint mental constellation is lived out in a sexual disjunction. The emotional pattern makes a detour through a bodily pattern, which makes recognition of emotion even harder. The couple's joint pattern is also expressed in relation to the therapist, who, struck by the horror in the dream and by the absence of feeling in Lucien over this nightmare, feels acutely the murder of the therapy project.

• *Work when the dreams elaborate on previous intervention.* In the next session, Lucien brought another dream. "This time you *were* in it. It takes place here in your office. The furniture and décor were different. You were sitting where you are. I spoke first, then I moved off the couch and Rachel moved onto it and spoke. It was the tail end of the session, and Rachel only got to speak a couple of minutes. Most of the dream took place after the session. Rachel gets her coat on and leaves. I linger in your vestibule though, unlike this office, the vestibule had two levels with a double staircase. Rachel slipped out down the staircase, while I went up the other stairs, landing in front of your house. (My office is next to my house.) I opened the door and realized it was the door to an armoire, a 5- or 6-foot-tall, pretty armoire decorated in gilt. It was not your front door, so I closed it. To the right of the furniture, a 12- to 14-year-old girl stood admiring an iron sculpture of a young girl like herself. I played with the furniture, she looked at the sculpture of the girl, and you and your wife entered the vestibule. I admired the furniture and your wife accepted the compliment, and then showed me a spot the size of a postage stamp on the lower right-hand corner where the gilt had been rubbed off. She took gilt from the other side and repaired it magically. It was like a magic armoire. You entered and said, 'Did you see the summer intern who walked on and off the stage?' You reminded me that Rachel was waiting for me to go and I scurried off." Then he added, "Oh, yes, I forgot: Your wife told me the furniture is 'Clemenceau.' I asked if that was a politician. She giggled and said it was an art term I wasn't familiar with."

In the work on this dream, Lucien thought the word "Clemenceau" referred to his love of France, his parents' homeland, the place to which his first therapist had retired, and a place to which he himself imagined returning. He thought the armoire represented the process of therapy, and with its magical quality, it healed itself. I noticed I had drawn on my wife's magical quality to heal his gilt ("guilt") miraculously. That image of a woman contrasted with his intrusive "black widow" aunt and mother; therefore, the collaboration of my wife and me provided a contrast to the destructive internal couples both of them had. The "armoire" seemed to be a pun, a magical chest, a pun for love (*amour*) and for defensive armor. Rachel agreed, saying that the right words would be "armor" and "guilt." (As in the dream, Rachel said only a few words in the session).

Lucien ended the session: "I think of the two of you as priests in a healing sense, keepers of the image. In that way it's completely different than my mother, who was a destructive force of nature. She captured too much of me. And my father just stood by passively. You and your wife are restorative kinds of earth mothers."

The French word *amour* led me to the idea that love could be repaired by getting beyond his usual armor and into his arms, repairing the gold of his unloved internal situation, removing his guilt, and readying him

for a return to Rachel. Instead of having to take the stairs up from the vestibule to live in my house, something happens that readies him for going down and out to her. In attachment terms, Lucien had taken a step toward an earned secure attachment that let him be less distancing. In neuroscience terms, he became less guilty and was therefore less reactive, less amygdala driven, more supported in the right orbitofrontal cortex exchange to maintain contact with a regulating internal mother.

Lucien's transference fantasy now refers to an idealized internal couple who cares for his armoire/armor, as he imagines an idealized mother in a couple relationship with me. A new internal object is forming that will help Lucien see himself as a man in a couple relationship.

• *Reciprocal dreaming as the couple refinds new internal objects through the transference.* In the couple session that followed, Lucien reported that he had managed to initiate sex, which had gone well. It happened on Sunday, after Rachel had had a nightmare on Saturday night and woke up screaming.

Rachel reported the dream that had awoken her: "We were in Paris, my favorite place in the world, looking for ice cream (We'd gone on a hunt for ice cream that day). We were looking for an ice-cream shop and got separated by crowds. When I saw Lucien again he was on the Pont Neuf bridge, happily carrying a thin, young French woman who was feeding him his favorite flavor, bad-for-you ice cream. I started yelling at him that he'd been lying, and that some other woman did make a difference."

Rachel talked about how she had been blaming herself for Lucien's lack of desire, and that this dream was a way of not blaming herself. He was carrying this woman just as she would like him now to carry the project about their sexual life. Lucien asked whether the French woman could be his mother. This seemed a stretch, because his mother is obese. But she had been thin when he was young, and in Rachel's mind the woman is attractive and seductive. "Perhaps yes, a thinner version of your mother," Rachel said.

The search for ice cream is the residue from the couple's day together, which kicks off the story that powerfully depicts their individual internal struggles, the problem in their couple relationship, and their reaction to my intervention of the previous week. Rachel depicts Lucien carrying the bad mother who poisons him with bad-for-you ice cream in Paris, the place she and he would most like to be. This Lucien–mother couple represent Rachel's own persecutory internal couple invading her space, and the ice cream connects with her "scream" at the outrage of the invasion. Her dream represents her screaming response to Lucien's need for distance (the armor mentioned in the previous session) and reveals her anxious, clinging attachment. When Lucien distances himself from her, she fills the inner void with this persecutory picture and feels betrayed by him in her most highly valued place (geography here substituting for emotional space).

This dream was also a reaction to those Lucien had reported previously, so we went back to those dreams and worked again with their shared reaction. Lucien's involvement with the invasive mother had led him to create an idealized couple and healing mother, but to Rachel his flight had seemed like a seduction by the feeding mother. Rachel's dream reminded Lucien of the slim mother of his childhood, and now we could talk about the two younger women in his dream. Lucien remembered that the young woman and my wife appeared when he was opening the door to look for something. He remembered that he was searching for guidance in the dream. Lucien talked about how, in the dream, he was searching for guidance, and then my wife showed him how to fix a scratch. I said that he was searching for a more complex woman in Rachel than he had been able to allow himself to know about, because of many things in the way. Rachel's dream shows that she shares his fear of what he'll find inside—inside himself, inside her, and inside the armoire/armor/amour. Rachel's nightmare belongs to both of them.

Thanks to training and personal psychoanalysis the therapist (David Scharff) has developed an expanded range of internal couples, from the intrusive, destructive woman–helpless man couple to the collaborative, creative, healing couple. These internal couples resonate with the couples that he is treating and become available to further the work. It helps him to experience the nightmare with them and to move beyond it. In association to his more flexible, strange attractor system, the fixed system of the couple relationship that is dominated by fear and reactivity, breaks up into fear and chaos, and then reorganizes (J. S. Scharff & Scharff, 2005; D. Scharff & Scharff, 2006). As Lucien opens himself to the possibility of new internal objects, Rachel and Lucien slowly become less reactive to the fear of the destructive "black widow"–dominated couple and see the glimpse of a gilded couple with powers to deal with guilt constructively. That is to say, they move toward an earned security together, to possibilities of better coregulation of affect, and toward the creative coconstruction of new emotional patterns.

Working Through Late in the Midphase

We return now to the Clarks who were in treatment with Jill Scharff.

Following Dr. Clark's revelation of his sadistic fantasies, the Clarks had a session in which Rhonda talked of her continued sense of gratitude that her husband had shared his fantasies with her. Although she felt unusually tentative about responding to him sexually, she felt

close to him and committed to working things out. For the first time, she felt an equal level of commitment from him. Summer was approaching, and Rhonda was taking the children to visit her family in Maine for a month as usual. Until now, Rhonda had viewed her annual summer trip as a chance to get away from Arthur's criticism of her and demand for sex. For the first time, she felt sad that they would have to spend the summer apart.

The sharing of the fantasy had been a healing experience. The couple could now move beyond a level of functioning characteristic of the paranoid–schizoid position, toward the depressive position in which there is concern for the object whose loss can be appreciated.

In a session following their vacation, Rhonda reported that she had got so much from the last session; it had kept her thinking and working for 4 weeks. Even when Arthur expressed no affection during his phone call to her in Maine, when he did not even say he missed her, she felt hurt but not outraged as before. She realized that in some way he just was not there.

I suggested that Arthur had been unaware of feeling angry that Rhonda had left him alone for a few weeks, and had dealt with it by killing her off.

Rhonda said she had managed not to take it personally. Even though Arthur continued to belittle her, she no longer felt like a little person, and she was glad to have changed.

Arthur's revelation of his murderous fantasies released Rhonda's capacity for growth, confirming that the silent operation of the unconscious projective identification expressed in the fantasy had been cutting her down and killing off her adult capacities.

Working Through

As we peel away layers of repression, we experience more resistance. Sometimes, it feels as though the further we go, the more we fall behind. The couple is suffering from a defensive system of object relationships that are mutually gratifying in an infantile way inside the couple system. Until more mature forms of gratification are found within the system, it is going to resist efforts at change. "Working through" is the term Freud (1914a) gave to the therapeutic effort to keep working away at this resistance and conflict. Sessions in this phase can feel plodding, laborious, repetitive, and uninspired. Resolution comes piecemeal, until one day the work is almost done.

Curative Factors and Mechanisms of Change

Object relations couple therapy creates a therapeutic environment in which the couple's pattern of defenses can be displayed, recognized, and analyzed until the underlying anxieties can be named, experienced, and worked through together. In the language of psychoanalysis, one might say, the couple develops insight, after which change becomes possible. In the language of object relations couple therapy, we conceptualize the process as one of improving the couple's capacity for containment of projections. Spouses learn to modify each other's projections, to distinguish them from aspects of the self, then take back their projections. The wife is then free to perceive her husband accurately, as a separate person whom she chooses to love for himself, rather than for the gratification he had afforded to repressed parts of herself. Through this process, reinforced by the joy of more mature loving, the wife refinds herself and becomes both more loving and more lovable. Doing the same work for himself, her husband grows in the same direction. Sometimes, however, their improved capacities for autonomy and mature love will take them in directions opposite to marriage to each other. Saving the marriage is not the primary goal. Ideally, freeing the marriage from the grip of its obligatory projective and introjective identification processes is the goal of treatment. In practice, something short of the ideal may be all that the partners need to be on their way again. More realistically, the goal of treatment is to enable the projective identification cycle to function at the depressive rather than the paranoid–schizoid end of the continuum more often than before therapy (Ravenscroft, 1991).

This is accomplished through a number of techniques. These are not the familiar techniques of communications-trained or behavioral couple therapists. The techniques of object relations couple therapy comprise a series of attitudes toward the couple and the therapeutic process, as we described in the section on the process of couple therapy. This type of therapy is not for every couple, and it is not for every therapist. It is for the couple that values complexity and subscribes to long-term goals of growth and development. It is for the therapist who can listen and respond without jumping to action, who has a capacity for waiting, holding anxiety, following the affect, tolerating a variety of feelings and impulses that arise in response to particular couples, reflecting and processing experience, and generally maintaining a non-action-oriented, nonimpulsive position. Some therapists have this naturally; others learn it in their own analysis, or therapy, and in seminars and supervision.

Common Obstacles to Successful Treatment of a Marriage

Obstacles to treatment include secrets withheld from spouse or therapist; an ongoing affair that dilutes commitment to the marriage; severe intrapsychic illness in one spouse; financial strain from paying for treatment; severe acting out in the session in the form of violence or nonattendance; and the intrusion of the therapist's personal problems into the therapeutic space, unchecked by training or personal therapy. Unresolved countertransference can lead to premature termination (Dickes & Strauss, 1979).

If we can assume an adequate therapist, then the main obstacle to treatment is a lack of psychological mindedness in the couple. Despite a therapist's best effort, the spouses do not want to deal in frightening areas of unconscious experience. They will do better with a more focused, short-term, symptom-oriented approach. But it is better to discover this from experience than to assume it from a single diagnostic session. Every couple deserves a chance for in-depth work. Some will take to the waters and others will not.

Treatment Applicability and Limitations

Object relations couple therapy is indicated for couples who are interested in understanding and growth. It is not for couples whose thinking style is concrete. The capacity to think psychologically does not correlate with low intelligence or social disadvantage. So object relations couple therapy is not contraindicated in couples from lower social classes, some of whom will be capable of in-depth work. D. Scharff and Scharff (1991) have described its usefulness for developmental crises; grief and mourning (Paul, 1967); communication problems; lack of intimacy, including sexuality (D. Scharff, 1982), unwelcome affairs and secrets (D. Scharff, 1978), remarriage (Wallerstein & Blakeslee, 1989), paraphilia, homosexual conflict, unwanted pregnancy, infertility; and apparently individual symptomatology that predates the marriage. It is not good for couples who require support and direction, financial assistance, and budgetary planning. Alone, it is not sufficient for couples in which one partner has an addiction to alcohol or drugs that requires peer group abstinence support, addiction counseling, or rehabilitation. It cannot produce major character change, although it produces enough change that a person comes to view his or her character as a modifiable quality.

Managed care considers object relations therapy a luxury. Even though therapists who work in managed care are constrained to work in a brief format with specific, limited goals, they help couples more by applying psychoanalytic couple therapy theory to their conceptualization of the problem and giving couples a full understanding of what their relationship can aim for and how to approach that goal, than by using the time to get rid of a few symptoms.

Integration with Other Interventions

Object relations couple therapy integrates well with other psychoanalytic interventions with which it may be combined sequentially or concurrently. It is fully compatible with individual object relations therapy because of the common theory base. Particularly in the case of object relations couple therapy, the theory is compatible both with individual therapy and with couple, group, or family therapy because the theory refers to endopsychic systems that are expressed in the interpersonal dimension. The therapist can integrate a structural or strategic approach with in-depth object relations understanding of defensive patterns (Slipp, 1988).

When a patient in psychoanalysis needs couple therapy, object relations couple therapy is the treatment of choice because of compatibility between the underlying theories. Then, the patient will not be told to quit analysis, as has happened, in favor of a short-term intervention that, however helpful, will not effect major character change for which analysis has been recommended. Sometimes, individual problems cannot be managed with couple therapy alone, but this should not be concluded too early. Individual referral is not resorted to readily, because it tends to load the couple problem in the individual arena, but when the couple can correctly recognize and meet individual needs, referral for one of the spouses may be helpful to the treatment process and to the marriage. Object relations couple therapy can then be combined with other treatment for the individual spouse such as medication, addiction rehabilitation, phobia desensitization programs, or psychoanalysis. When psychoanalysis is required, the couple therapist may become anxious that the greater intensity of individual treatment will devalue the couple therapy. That is not at all inevitable. When it occurs, it does so because one therapist is being idealized, while the other is being denigrated due to a splitting of the transference that will need to

be addressed. This risk to couple therapy is more likely to be a major problem if the couple therapist secretly admires psychoanalysis and puts down his or her own work. It is helpful for the concurrent treatments if both therapists are comfortable communicating with each other, but some analysts will not collaborate, because they are dedicated to preserving the boundaries of the psychoanalysis for good reason and will not betray the patient's confidentiality. Perhaps the greater betrayal lies in not confronting the acting out of split transference.

Object relations couple therapy may be combined with a family session with children, who may say helpful things about which the grown-ups are unaware. Sessions for one spouse with parents and/or siblings may be added, then the couple reviews that partner's experience and its implications for their marriage (Framo, 1981). A couple may also be treated in a couples' group, either as an adjunct to the couple therapy or as a primary treatment method (Framo, 1973). Object relations couple therapy can be combined serially or concurrently with behavioral sex therapy (Levay & Kagle, 1978; Lief, 1989; D. Scharff, 1982; D. Scharff & Scharff, 1991). The sex research of Masters and Johnson (1966, 1970) and Kaplan (1974) vastly improved couple therapists' understanding of sexuality. Kaplan linked an analytic approach with sex therapy methodology. She showed how blockade in the progression through the behavioral steps requires psychoanalytic interpretation to help clients get over underlying anxieties. She described hypoactive sexual desire (1977, 1979) as a spectrum of disorders usually relating to psychodynamic issues that require psychoanalysis or psychoanalytic therapy, sometimes in conjunction with medication (1987). The object relations couple therapist may apply this knowledge within the usual frame of therapy or switch to a specific sex therapy format, if qualified to do so. We may prefer to refer the couple to a colleague temporarily or concurrently, to free us from the strain of holding to the nondirective attitude at the unconscious level during directive behavioral formats or if the couple needs a therapist who is more experienced and qualified in specific sex therapy or behavioral methods. Object relations couple therapists who work regularly in nonanalytic modes combine them without compromising the integrity of their analytic stance, by recognizing and working with the couple's transference to their directiveness in the nonanalytic role. Systems-oriented or structurally trained couple therapists can integrate the analytic stance into their current way of working by attending to the

impact of therapist personality and directive behavior on the partners' attitudes toward them. The
object relations perspective gives more access to
the use of the therapist's psyche (Aponte & Van-
Deusen, 1981) and provides the systems therapist
with greater understanding of the system through
patterns that the therapist will find re-created in
relation to him- or herself (Van Trommel, 1984,
1985).

An illustration of the link between internal
object relations, psychosexual stages of development, and sexual symptomatology is provided
in the following vignette from an initial couple
therapy evaluation, with David and Jill Scharff as
cotherapists:

Michelle and Lenny had a hateful attachment. Although diametrically opposite in character and family background, they had been together for 4 years, but
Michelle, an outgoing social activist, had been unable
to marry quiet, conservative Lenny because he seemed
so passive. A nice, attractive man from an upper-class
family, successful in business, and loyal to her, Lenny
had many appealing qualities. He treated Michelle well,
he adored her, but she hated his steadfeastness. He just
could not meet her expectations. Her ideal man would
be like her amazingly energetic, confident, and admira-
ble brother. Unlike steady Lenny, Michelle was bubbling
with energy. So, why was she still with Lenny? Lenny
was a kind, loyal boyfriend, but Michelle criticized him
for being boring to her, and she put him down relentlessly. He seemed immune to criticism and maintained
his steady love for her.

The therapists felt uncomfortable with this frustrating relationship and David Scharff, who is normally
rather energetic, almost fell asleep to avoid the pain of
being with Michelle and Lenny. His countertransference
response led David and Jill to see the underlying sadness
in the couple's relationship and to experience the void
they would have to face if their destructive bantering
were to stop. Lenny's void came from the lack of a father when he was growing up. Michelle's came from her
perception of herself as a girl whose brother had more
than she did.

Unlike the way she felt about boring old Lenny, Michelle felt special. So why did she hate herself? Her mother had felt that Michelle's brother was a special child,
and this had given him the immense confidence that Michelle was missing. Michelle explained that because of
this, a part of her constantly found holes in herself.

To an analyst, these words speak of penis envy
from the phallic stage of development. Usually, we address this issue in the broader terms of envy of the man's
world. But in this case, both aspects of Michelle's envy
were close to consciousness. And Lenny was not far behind her in the extent of his envy of Michelle's brother.
Lenny wished he could be like him.

It turned out that, in bed, Lenny was a confident
sexual partner who had shown great sensitivity to Michelle's vaginismus. He helped her to tolerate intercourse and find sexual release with him. He found her
beautiful whether she was fat or thin. For Michelle, who
hated her body, on the one hand, although Lenny's ado-
ration was gratifying, it was also contemptible, because
sex was difficult for her. On the other hand, Michelle
was grateful for his patience, his sexual restraint, and his
comfort with sex. Nevertheless, penetration by a powerful phallus was frightening to her.

Jill said, "It's sad for you that you can't take sexual
pleasure from the penis, because you see it as a source of
envied and threatening power."

Michelle agreed that she hated it, adding that
this was because it seemed like a way of controlling a
woman.

Applying Freudian theory, we can say that, as a
child, Michelle had thought that boys like her brother
did not feel the emptiness and longing that she felt in
relation to her rejecting mother, because they each had
the penis that she was missing, whereas her vagina felt
like an empty hole. In her adulthood, the penis continued to be threatening, because it could enter that painful
hole. Michelle now directed the childhood hatred for
the penis toward the man in her adult sexual relationship. The better Lenny did with her sexually, the more
Michelle had to attack him enviously. Lenny, though
sexually competent, had some inhibition against being
assertive generally and sexually, and he used Michelle as
a phallic front for himself, so that he could avoid castra-
tion anxiety.

In object relations terms, each partner was using
Michelle as a manic defense against emptiness and
sadness. Each was using Lenny as a depository for the
schizoid defense against emptiness. Painful longing was
projected into Michelle's vagina, for which she had a
psychophysiological valency. In therapy they would
need to take back these projective identifications of
each other and develop a holding capacity for bearing
their shared anxieties.

Common Significant Clinical Issues

Working with the Difficult Couple

There are many varieties of difficult couples. "Difficulty" depends partly on the degree of fixity and
severity of the partners' unconscious complementarity and pathology, and partly on their fit with
the object relations set of their therapist. Difficult
couples may transfer from previous therapists in
whom they were disappointed. A common trap
is to suppose that the new therapist will be better
than the previous therapist. Sometimes, treatment
does go better, usually because of the couple's projection of negative objects into the former thera-

pist. Unless the therapist can address that issue, the couple may seem better but will not have developed the capacity to integrate good and bad objects. The turning point in treatment of the difficult couple often comes when the therapist is able to experience fully in the countertransference the hopelessness and despair that underlies the couple's defense of being difficult (D. Scharff & Scharff, 1991). Sometimes the couple cannot use the assessment process to develop sufficient trust in the therapist to make a commitment to therapy. The disappointment that the therapist feels in failing to make an alliance activates guilt about not being able to repair the damage of the therapist's internal parental couple (J. S. Scharff, 1992).

Managing Resistance and Noncompliance

At worst, the couple may remain too resistant to engage in couple therapy. Nevertheless, one of the spouses may be willing to have individual therapy. It is important to start where the couple is. Change in one partner may effect change in the system, so that couple therapy may be possible later. Before arriving at that conclusion, however, psychoanalytic couple therapists try to be understanding of the reasons for the resistance. We do not try to seduce the couple into making a commitment or promise symptomatic relief. We do not remove the resistance by paradoxical prescription. We analyze the resistance with the aim of freeing the partners from the inhibition imposed by their defenses against intervention, and giving them control over their decision about treatment.

Sometimes, a couple makes the commitment but cannot keep it when anxieties surface. They may miss appointments, forget or refuse to pay the bill, or substitute a single partner for the couple. The therapist discusses all these attempts to bend the frame, in the hope that making conscious the unconscious reluctance will help the couple to confront the therapist about the treatment process and the therapist's style. But therapists do not agree to work without pay, both because they cannot allow their worth and earning potential to be attacked in that way, and because it produces unconscious guilt in the couple. Our policy is that we do not see a spouse alone to fill a session from which the other spouse is missing. On the other hand, each of us has at times done so when the situation seemed to call for it. Policies differ among psychoanalytic couple therapists, as they do among therapists of other backgrounds, but the important thing is to establish a policy and a way of working, and hold to it as a standard from which to negotiate, experiment, and learn.

Working with the Couple When There Is an Affair

Greene (1970) warned that premature discussion of the affair can disrupt the marriage, and Martin (1976) agreed that the mate should not always be told the secret. D. Scharff (1978) advocated revelation of the secret in every case but has since modified the rigidity of his view (D. Scharff & Scharff, 1991). Revelation puts couple and therapist in position to learn from the affair and to understand the meaning of the secret in developmental terms (Gross, 1951), the significance of the affair (Strean, 1976, 1979), and the attraction of the lover for the spouse. Only when the affair is known can the therapist work with the couple's expression of disappointment, envy, rage, love, and sadness. In the affair (as in a fantasy) lies important information about repressed object relations that cannot be expressed and contained within the marriage. It is worth remembering that the affair is an attempt to maintain the marriage, even while threatening its existence.

The revelation of extramarital affairs constitutes one of the frequent reasons for referral to couple therapy. Perhaps even more often, an evaluation will uncover undisclosed affairs in the current life of one of the partners or in their history. When the affair has been disclosed, our stance is to explore the meaning of the affair to each of the partners and to the marriage (or partnership). Is the attitude of the partner who has had the affair one of remorse, dismissiveness as to its importance, self-righteousness? And does the offended spouse feel that he or she has done nothing to justify the affair? Or does the spouse understand something about an erosion of the bond in the marriage that had a role in setting up the affair? For instance, one woman who had lost interest in sex early in the marriage had over several years become quite contemptuous of her husband. She felt her attitude had no importance in triggering a sense of desperation in her husband that preceded his affair with one of her friends, and when they began couple therapy, she was interested only in getting the therapist to condemn him. Not surprisingly, this couple moved toward divorce.

In contrast, in the case of a couple in treatment for the crisis following the wife's one-night stand, the husband recognized that the infidelity was connected to the fact that he had withdrawn from sex with his wife following the birth of their son, and that this had left her feeling lonely and bereft. This couple was in a much better position to examine the origins of strain in the marriage, brought on by the arrival of the son, the husband's unconscious jealousy, and his feeling of exclusion from his wife's concern and affection. The origins of this strain could be traced to his feeling pushed aside by his mother in favor both of his father and his younger brother. At the same time, his wife turned toward their new baby boy and away from him in identification with the baby, to repair in fantasy a history of neglect by her own mother. Over the years, the partners' shared feeling of being overlooked had ripened into a sense of mutual neglect in the intimate relationship with loss of sexual desire. Without the renewal of the bond supplied by sexuality, the marriage was in a state of unspoken vulnerability until the wife acted out the shared sense of disconnection and desperation in her brief affair. The partners used therapy to explore their shared loneliness, individual vulnerabilities, and the persisting sense of concern for each other to reconstruct their marriage with a strengthened sense of commitment despite the mutual hurt.

There are many patterns of affairs, from the brief, one-night stand of the wife mentioned earlier to those lasting many years, constituting a parallel (usually secret) marriage. Sometimes these affairs are accepted implicitly and to mutual advantage by partners who feel locked in a loveless marriage they prefer to preserve. But more often, they constitute a secret ground into which issues from the marriage are projected and, therefore, not dealt with directly.

The secrecy of an affair is central to its dynamic meaning. The spouse who is having the affair is often aware that keeping the affair quiet has to do with avoiding the reaction to its revelation, but he or she does not usually realize that the secrecy serves to avoid issues that cannot be addressed prior to the need for the affair. Frequently, the partner with the secret affair claims that he or she cannot tell, because it would hurt the spouse too much. We take the position that this kind of protection is almost always a form of disguised self-protection, and that its meaning needs to be explored. Most often, such secrets come to the therapist's attention in individual interviews that are part of an initial evaluation. When this occurs, the therapist works with the partner with the secret to

understand the unconscious meaning, and the way the secret often controls the unknowing spouse. Respecting individual confidentiality, the therapist does not have the right to reveal such secrets, and takes some time to show the partner who is having the affair its effect and its cost to help him or her confront what lies behind the fear of being found out and to work toward revelation so as to offer the possibility of rebuilding the marriage on a firmer footing. Maintaining such a secret corrupts the integrity of the marriage and of the therapist's ability to be open and honest with the partners. So, if the partner refuses full disclosure, the therapist must decide whether effective further work is at all possible, and may at times have to be willing to resign from the treatment.

A different situation exists when the therapist becomes suspicious of an affair because of hints and hunches. For instance, the husband may be absent for periods for which he cannot or will not account, or a wife discovers multiple phone calls and credit card charges while the husband is traveling with a female business partner. In this case, one can say openly to the couple that it certainly looks as though there is an affair, and speculate as to either the dynamics that might have led to it or to the appearance of the situation. We as therapists are empowered to do this, because we comment on whatever we feel is important, and because, in this case, we are not betraying any secrets. This tends to push the couple to consider the distancing of emotions, resentment, and their unconscious roots.

In one case of loss of sexual interest by the wife, both husband and wife revealed to the therapist that there had been affairs during their marriage. The wife's two affairs had been in the distant past, and the husband had had inklings of both affairs. The husband's affair was recent and with a close friend of the wife. The therapist worked with each of them toward revelation, to which they reluctantly agreed. Although they almost split up, the work that followed dealt with the mutual resentment that was crucial to understanding their sexual decline and emotional distance, and led, not without difficulty, to a much stronger marriage and a return of sexual life.

Handling Acute Couple Distress

The prompt offer of a consultation appointment is usually enough to contain an acute situation. In more extreme cases, a suicidal or psychotic spouse may require medication or hospitalization, whereas a violent one may necessitate temporary separation. When distress is acute, and there is no time to deal with an emergency, it is better to refer the case to someone who has time than to make the couple wait for an appointment. During the delay, a couple problem may be redefined as an individual illness, and the advantage of the healing potential of the crisis in the system is lost. If the therapist does take the referral, a longer appointment time than usual is required to allow the partners enough time to express their distress and the therapist to develop the necessary holding capacity. The therapist needs time to contain the partners' anxiety, offer them a therapeutic relationship on which they can count, and demonstrate the possibility of understanding their overwhelming emotion. Another appointment time within the week is scheduled before the couple leaves the session.

Working with a History of Trauma

Partners experience any overwhelming recent trauma in terms of any previous trauma. They may try to dissociate from it by splitting off their awareness of the traumatic experience and sequestering it in traumatic nuclei inside the marriage. An apparently satisfactory marital relationship may cover these traumatic nuclei or gaps. In that case, the couple therapist may get access to the dissociated material by analyzing his or her own feelings of discomfort or by examining gaps in the treatment process. When the material inside the nuclei is too toxic to be managed, affect explosions or absences of affect and motivation may bring the couple into treatment, as in the following case:

Tony and Theresa had been happy together in their marriage and now had three children, with the eldest adopted from Theresa's first marriage. Tony and Theresa both worked to support the family and shared household chores. A sudden fulminating infection in Tony's right arm could not be treated medically, and he had to have his shoulder and arm amputated to save his life. An easygoing, cheerful man, Tony bounded right back at first, then depression hit as he realized the enormity of his loss. He refused rehabilitation work and prosthetic fittings. He sat around at home while his wife went out and did his work as well as her own. Then when she came home, he complained about her being away. They were arguing an unusual amount, their oldest daughter avoided coming home, the middle child was doing badly in school, and the youngest one seemed simply sad.

After telling the therapist about the trauma relieved their stress somewhat, it was possible to reveal the trauma base against which their marriage had been organized. Both Tony and Theresa had been physically abused by their parents, and both had taken the role of the child who will get hit to protect the others. When they got married, each promised to respect the other. There would never be any violence in their relationship. When tempers flared, they punched the wall instead. The bricks absorbed their anger and in so doing built a wall between them and their feelings. Now Tony had lost his punching arm, and without it, he did not know how to express his rage and grief.

The couple therapist (David Scharff) noted considerable improvement in Tony and Theresa's capacity to acknowledge anger, but he was puzzled by their new pattern of skipping sessions. Their silences and his own discomfort led him to guess that they were creating a gap to cover over another traumatic nucleus. Perhaps another recent trauma lay beneath the loss of Tony's arm. Since they had already told him about their problems with anger, he asked if they might be avoiding discussion of some other feeling, perhaps in relation to their sexual life. Theresa replied that since she had had a hysterectomy some years earlier, she had suffered from recurrent vaginal infections. Previously the couple had enjoyed a vigorous sexual life; now sex had become less frequent. Theresa admitted that she avoided sex because it was painful for her, a secret that she had kept from Tony until that moment.

Prior to the loss of Tony's arm, the couple had lost the use of Theresa's vagina as an accepting, sexually responsive organ. They lost one body part that stood for the control of aggression (Tony's arm) and another that stood for their loving connectedness (Theresa's well-functioning vagina), both vital to the maintenance of their commitment to each other. Work with the couple would have to focus on mourning their losses, then finding gratifying ways to express love and anger.

In couples whose current sexual interaction is traumatic, compulsively enacted, or phobically avoided, we as therapists inquire about earlier sexual experience, including unwanted sexual experience in the family of origin. We help couples that tend to invoke abusive behavior in one spouse by showing that this is a way of repeating the abuse instead of remembering it. Other couples need to see that their successful efforts to avoid repetition of abuse require a high degree of close control that is less successful for them, because it inhibits not only the marital relationship but also the next generation. We try to put words to experience. We help couples to develop a narrative of the abuse history to share with their family as an alternative to the reenactment of trauma and the defenses against it.

Termination

The couple has had some rehearsal for termination when ending each time-limited session and facing breaks in treatment due to illness, business commitments, or vacations. We as therapists work with the couple's habitual way of dealing with separations in preparation for the final parting. Our criteria for judging when that will be are in Table 6.3.

These goals that provide the criteria for terminating are really only markers of progress. Couples decide for themselves what their goals are and whether they have been met. Sometimes they coincide with the therapist's idea of completion and sometimes not. We as therapists have to let ourselves become redundant and to tolerate being discarded. As we mourn with the couple the loss of the therapy relationship (and in some cases the loss of the marriage), we rework all the earlier losses. The couple now relives issues from earlier phases of the treatment with greater capacity for recovery from regression. Separating from the therapeutic relationship, therapist and couple demonstrate their respective capacities for acknowledging experience, dealing with loss, understanding defensive regressions, and mastering anxiety. As the couple terminates, now able to get on with life and love without us, the therapist partners take their leave of the real couple and at the same time resolve another piece of the ambivalent attachment to their internal couples. Such a thorough experience of termination seasons the therapist and prepares him or her to be of use to the next couple.

TABLE 6.3. Criteria for Termination

- The couple has internalized the therapeutic space and now has a reasonably secure holding capacity.
- Unconscious projective identifications have been recognized, owned, and taken back by each spouse.
- The capacity to work together as life partners is restored.
- Relating intimately and sexually is mutually gratifying.
- The couple can envision its future development, and the partners can provide a vital holding environment for their family.
- The couple can differentiate among and meet the needs of each partner.
- Alternatively, the partners recognize the failure of their choice, understand the unconscious object relations incompatibility, and separate with some grief work done, and with a capacity to continue individually to mourn the loss of the marriage.

SUGGESTIONS FOR FURTHER READING

Case Report

Scharff, J. S., & de Varela, Y. (2000). Object relations therapy. In F. M. Dattilio & L. J. Bevilacqua (Eds.), *Comparative treatments for relationship dysfunction* (pp. 81–101). New York: Springer.—A demonstration of the object relations approach in the case of a conflict-avoidant couple with a nagging mother–fretful child dynamic, no sexual relationship, and a diminished social network, a couple in which one partner has a history of depression, substance abuse, attention deficit disorder, and sexual abuse, and the other has depression over surgical loss of fertility.

Research

Scharff, J. S., & Scharff, D. E. (1998). Clinical relevance of research: Object relations testing, neural development, and attachment theory. In *Object relations individual therapy* (pp. 117–151). Northvale, NJ: Aronson.—A summary of the research relevant to object relations therapy.

Reference Books

Scharff, D. E., & Scharff, J. S. (1991). *Object relations couple therapy*. Northvale, NJ: Aronson.—A comprehensive guide to doing object relations couple therapy to help couples achieve emotional and sexual intimacy, in which the therapists focus on transference and countertransference to arrive at interpretation of the projective and introjective processes that mar the couple relationship.

Scharff, J. S., & Scharff, D. E. (2005). *The primer of object relations* (2nd ed.). Northvale, NJ: Aronson.—Clear answers to beginners' questions about object relations expanded to include simple explanations of complex ideas from neuroscience, attachment theory, chaos theory, and trauma theory, all of which are being integrated into contemporary object relations theory.

REFERENCES

Aponte, H. J., & VanDeusen, J. M. (1981). Structural family therapy. In A. Gurman & D. Kniskern (Eds.), *Handbook of family therapy* (pp. 310–360). New York: Brunner/Mazel.

Balint, M. (1968). *The basic fault: Therapeutic aspects of regression*. London: Tavistock.

Bannister, K., & Pincus, L. (1965). *Shared phantasy in couple problems: Therapy in a four-person relationship*. London: Tavistock Institute of Human Relations.

Bergman, M. (1990, November). *Love and hate in the life of a couple*. Paper presented at the Washington School of Psychiatry Conference on Romantic Love, Washington, DC.

Bion, W. R. (1961). *Experiences in groups*. London: Tavistock.

Bion, W. R. (1962). *Learning from experience*. London: Heinemann.

Bion, W. R. (1970). *Attention and interpretation*. London: Tavistock.

Bodin, A. M. (1981). The interactional view: Family therapy approaches of the Mental Research Institute. In A. S. Gurman & D. P. Kniskern (Eds.), *Handbook of family therapy* (pp. 267–309). New York: Brunner/Mazel.

Bowen, M. (1978). *Family therapy in clinical practice*. New York: Jason Aronson.

Box, S. (1981). Introduction: Space for thinking in families. In S. Box, B. Copley, J. Magagna, & E. Moustaki (Eds.), *Psychotherapy with families* (pp. 1–8). London: Routledge & Kegan Paul.

Brazelton, T. B. (1982). Joint regulation of neonate–parent behavior. In E. Tronick (Ed.), *Social interchange in infancy* (pp. 7–22). Baltimore: University Park Press.

Brazelton, T. B., & Als, H. (1979). Four early stages in the development of mother–infant interaction. *Psychoanalytic Study of the Child*, *34*, 349–369.

Clulow, C. (1985). *Couple therapy: An inside view*. Aberdeen, Scotland: Aberdeen University Press.

Dare, C. (1986). Psychoanalytic couple therapy. In N. S. Jacobson & A. S. Gurman (Eds.), *Clinical handbook of couple therapy* (pp. 13–28). New York: Guilford Press.

Dickes, R., & Strauss, D. (1979). Countertransference as a factor in premature termination of apparently successful cases. *Journal of Sex and Couple Therapy*, *5*, 22–27.

Dicks, H. V. (1967). *Marital tensions: Clinical studies towards a psycho-analytic theory of interaction*. London: Routledge & Kegan Paul.

Erickson, E. H. (1950). *Childhood and society*. New York: Norton.

Ezriel, H. (1952). Notes on psychoanalytic group therapy: II. Interpretation and research. *Psychiatry*, *15*, 119–126.

Fairbairn, W. R. D. (1944). Endopsychic structure considered in terms of object relationships. *International Journal of Psycho-Analysis*, *25*(1 and 2). Reprinted in *Psychoanalytic studies of the personality* (pp. 82–135). London: Routledge & Kegan Paul.

Fairbairn, W. R. D. (1952). *Psychoanalytic studies of the personality*. London: Routledge & Kegan Paul.

Fairbairn, W. R. D. (1954). Observations on the nature of hysterical states. *British Journal of Medical Psychology*, *27*, 105–125.

Fairbairn, W. R. D. (1963). Synopsis of an object relations theory of the personality. *International Journal of Psycho-Analysis*, *44*, 224–225.

Finkelstein, L. (1987). Toward an object relations approach in psychoanalytic couple therapy. *Journal of Couple and Family Therapy*, *13*, 287–298.

Framo, J. L. (1973). Marriage therapy in a couples' group. *Seminars in Psychiatry*, *5*, 207–217.

Framo, J. L. (1981). The integration of couple therapy with sessions with family of origin. In A. S. Gurman & D. P. Kniskern (Eds.), *Handbook of family therapy* (pp. 133–158). New York: Brunner/Mazel.

Framo, J. L. (1982). Symptoms from a family transactional viewpoint. In *Explorations in couple and family therapy: Selected papers of James L. Framo* (pp. 11–57). New York: Springer. (Original work published in 1970)

Frank, J. (1989). Who are you and what have you done with my wife? In J. S. Scharff (Ed.), *Foundations of object relations family therapy* (pp. 155–173). Northvale, NJ: Jason Aronson.

Freud, S. (1905). Three essays on the theory of sexuality. *Standard Edition*, *7*, 135–243.

Freud, S. (1910). The future prospects of psycho-analytic therapy. *Standard Edition*, *11*, 141–151.

Freud, S. (1912). Recommendations to physicians practicing psychoanalysis. *Standard Edition*, *12*, 111–120.

Freud, S. (1914a). Remembering, repeating, and working through. *Standard Edition*, *12*, 147–156.

Friedman, E. H. (1991). Bowen theory and therapy. In A. Gurman & D. Kniskern (Eds.), *Handbook of family therapy* (Vol. 2, pp. 134–170). New York: Brunner/Mazel.

Friedman, L. (1962). *Virgin wives: A study of unconsummated marriages*. London: Tavistock.

Greene, B. L. (1970). *A clinical approach to couple problems*. Springfield, IL: Thomas.

Gross, A. (1951). The secret. *Bulletin of the Menninger Clinic*, *15*, 37–44.

Guntrip, H. (1961). *Personality structure and human interaction: The developing synthesis of psychodynamic theory*. London: Hogarth Press and the Institute of Psycho-Analysis.

Guntrip, H. (1969). *Schizoid phenomena, object relations and the self*. New York: International Universities Press.

Gurman, A. S. (1978). Contemporary couple therapies: A critique and analysis of psychoanalytic, behavioral and system approaches. In T. J. Paolino & B. S. McCrady (Eds.), *Marriage and couple therapy* (pp. 455–566). New York: Brunner/Mazel.

Gurman, A. S., & Jacobson, N. S. (1986). Couple therapy: From technique to theory, back again, and beyond. In N. S. Jacobson & A. S. Gurman (Eds.), *Clinical handbook of couple therapy* (pp. 1–9). New York: Guilford Press.

Heimann, P. (1950). On counter-transference. *International Journal of Psycho-Analysis*, *31*, 81–84.

Heimann, P. (1973). Certain functions of introjection and projection in early infancy. In M. Klein, P. Heimann, S. Isaacs, & J. Riviere (Eds.), *Developments in psycho-analysis* (pp. 122–168). London: Hogarth Press and the Institute of Psycho-Analysis.

Hollender, M. H. (1971). Selection of therapy for couple problems. In J. H. Masserman (Ed.), *Current psychiatric therapies* (Vol. 11, pp. 119–128). New York: Grune & Stratton.

Jackson, D. D., & Weakland, J. H. (1961). Conjoint family therapy. *Psychiatry, 24,* 30–45.

Jacobs, T. J. (1991). *The use of the self.* Madison, CT: International Universities Press.

Kaplan, H. S. (1974). *The new sex therapy: Active treatment of sexual dysfunctions.* New York: Brunner/Mazel.

Kaplan, H. S. (1977). Hypoactive sexual desire. *Journal of Sex and Couple Therapy, 3,* 3–9.

Kaplan, H. S. (1979). *Disorders of sexual desire and other new concepts and techniques in sex therapy.* New York: Brunner/Mazel.

Kaplan, H. S. (1987). *Sexual aversion, sexual phobias, and panic disorder.* New York: Brunner/Mazel.

Kernberg, O. F. (1975). *Borderline conditions and pathological narcissism.* New York: Jason Aronson.

Kernberg, O. F. (1991). Aggression and love in the relationship of the couple. *Journal of the American Psychoanalytic Association, 39,* 45–70.

Klein, M. (1946). Notes on some schizoid mechanisms. *International Journal of Psycho-Analysis, 27,* 99–100.

Klein, M. (1948). *Contributions to psycho-analysis, 1921–1945.* London: Hogarth Press.

Klein, M. (1957). *Envy and gratitude.* London: Tavistock.

Kohut H. (1971). *The analysis of the self.* New York: International Universities Press.

Kohut, H. (1977). *The restoration of the self.* New York: International Universities Press.

Kohut, H. (1982). Introspection, empathy, and the semi-circle of mental health. *International Journal of Psycho-Analysis, 63,* 395–407.

Langs, R. (1976). *The therapeutic interaction: Vol. II. A critical overview and synthesis.* New York: Jason Aronson.

Lansky, M. (1986). Couple therapy for narcissistic disorders. In N. S. Jacobson & A. S. Gurman (Eds.), *Clinical handbook of couple therapy* (pp. 557–574). New York: Guilford Press.

Levay, A. N., & Kagle, A. (1978). Recent advances in sex therapy: Integration with the dynamic therapies. *Psychiatric Quarterly, 50,* 5–16.

Lief, H. F. (1989). *Integrating sex therapy with couple therapy.* Paper presented at the 47th Annual Conference of the American Association of Marriage and Family Therapy, San Francisco, CA.

Main, T. (1966). Mutual projection in a marriage. *Comprehensive Psychiatry, 7,* 432–449.

Martin, P. A. (1976). *A couple therapy manual.* New York: Brunner/Mazel.

Masters, W. H., & Johnson, V. E. (1966). *Human sexual response.* Boston: Little, Brown.

Masters, W. H., & Johnson, V. E. (1970). *Human sexual inadequacy.* Boston: Little, Brown.

McCormack, C. (1989). The borderline–schizoid marriage. *Journal of Couple and Family Therapy, 15,* 299–309.

Meissner, W. W. (1978). The conceptualization of marriage and couple dynamics from a psychoanalytic perspective. In T. J. Paolino & B. S. McCrady (Eds.), *Marriage and couple therapy* (pp. 25–28). New York: Brunner/Mazel.

Mittelmann, B. (1944). Complementary neurotic reactions in intimate relationships. *Psychoanalytic Quarterly, 13,* 479–491.

Mittelmann, B. (1948). The concurrent analysis of married couples. *Psychoanalytic Quarterly, 17,* 182–197.

Money-Kyrle, R. (1956). Normal countertransference and some of its deviations. *International Journal of Psycho-Analysis, 37,* 360–366.

Murray, J. M. (1955). *Keats.* New York: Noonday Press.

Nadelson, C. C. (1978). Couple therapy from a psychoanalytic perspective. In T. J. Paolino & B. S. McCrady (Eds.), *Marriage and couple therapy* (pp. 101–164). New York: Brunner/Mazel.

Oberndorf, P. (1938). Psychoanalysis of married couples. *Psychoanalytic Review, 25,* 453–475.

Ogden, T. H. (1982). *Projective identification and psychotherapeutic technique.* New York: Jason Aronson.

Paul, N. (1967). The role of mourning and empathy in conjoint couple therapy. In G. Zuk & I. Boszormeny-Nagy (Eds.), *Family therapy and disturbed families* (pp. 186–205). Palo Alto, CA: Science and Behavior Books.

Pincus, L. (Ed.). (1960). *Marriage: Studies in emotional conflict and growth.* London: Methuen.

Racker, H. (1968). *Transference and countertransference.* New York: International Universities Press.

Ravenscroft, K. (1991, March). *Changes in projective identification during treatment.* Paper presented at the Washington School of Psychiatry Object Relations Couple and Family Therapy Training Program Conference, Bethesda, MD.

Ryckoff, I., Day, J., & Wynne, L. (1959). Maintenance of stereotyped roles in the families of schizophrenics. *Archives of General Psychiatry, 1,* 93–98.

Sager, C. J. (1976). *Marriage contracts and couple therapy: Hidden forces in intimate relationships.* New York: Brunner/Mazel.

Sager, C. J., Kaplan, H. S., Gundlach, R. H., Kremer, M., Lenz, R., & Royce, J. R. (1971). The marriage contract. *Family Process, 10,* 311–326.

Scharff, D. (1978). Truth and consequences in sex and couple therapy: The revelation of secrets in the therapeutic setting. *Journal of Sex and Marital Therapy, 4,* 35–49.

Scharff, D. (1982). *The sexual relationship: An object relations view of sex and the family.* Boston/London: Routledge & Kegan Paul.

Scharff, D., & Scharff, J. S. (1987). *Object relations family therapy.* Northvale, NJ: Jason Aronson.

Scharff, D., & Scharff, J. S. (1991). *Object relations couple therapy.* Northvale, NJ: Jason Aronson.

Scharff, D., & Scharff, J. (Eds.). (2006). *New paradigms in treating relationships.* Lanham, MD: Jason Aronson.

Scharff, J. S. (Ed.). (1989). *Foundations of object relations family therapy.* Northvale, NJ: Jason Aronson.

Scharff, J. S. (1992). *Projective and introjective identification and the use of the therapist's self.* Northvale, NJ: Jason Aronson.

Scharff, J. S., & Scharff, D. E. (2005). *The primer of object relations* (2nd ed.). Lanham, MD: Jason Aronson.

Segal, H. (1964). *Introduction to the work of Melanie Klein*. London: Heinemann.

Shapiro, R. L. (1979). Family dynamics and object relations theory: An analytic, group-interpretive approach to family therapy. In J. S. Scharff (Ed.), *Foundations of object relations family therapy* (pp. 225–245). Northvale, NJ: Jason Aronson.

Skynner, A. C. R. (1976). *Systems of family and couple psychotherapy*. New York: Brunner/Mazel.

Slipp, S. (1984). *Object relations: A dynamic bridge between individual and family treatment*. New York: Jason Aronson.

Slipp, S. (1988). *Theory and practice of object relations family therapy*. Northvale, NJ: Jason Aronson.

Solomon, M. (1989). *Narcissism and intimacy*. New York: Norton.

Stern, D. (1985). *The interpersonal world of the infant: A view from psychoanalysis and developmental psychology*. New York: Basic Books.

Stern, D. (2004). *The present moment in psychotherapy and everyday life*. New York: Norton.

Stewart, R. H., Peters, T. C., Marsh, S., & Peters, M. J. (1975). An object relations approach to psychotherapy with married couples, families and children. *Family Process, 14*, 161–178.

Stierlin, H. (1977). *Psychoanalysis and family therapy*. New York: Jason Aronson.

Strean, H. S. (1976). The extra-marital affair: A psychoanalytic view. *Psychoanalytic Review, 63*, 101–113.

Strean, H. S. (1979). *The extramarital affair*. New York: Free Press.

Sutherland, J. (1980). The British object relations theorists: Balint, Winnicott, Fairbairn, Guntrip. *Journal of the American Psychoanalytic Association, 28*, 829–860.

Sullivan, H. S. (1953). *The interpersonal theory of psychiatry*. New York: Norton.

Van Trommel, M. J. (1984). A consultation method addressing the therapist–family system. *Family Process, 23*, 469–480.

Van Trommel, M. J. (1985, October). *Getting to the heart of the matter with the Milan method*. Presented at the annual meeting of the American Association of Marriage and Family Therapy, New York.

Wallerstein, J. S., & Blakeslee, S. (1989). *Second chances*. New York: Ticknor & Fields.

Willi, J. (1982). *Couples in collusion*. Claremont, CA: Hunter House.

Willi, J. (1984). *Dynamics of couples therapy*. New York: Jason Aronson.

Winnicott, D. W. (1958). Transitional objects and transitional phenomena. In *Collected papers: Through paediatrics to psycho-analysis*. London: Tavistock. (Original work published in 1951)

Winnicott, D. W. (1958). *Collected papers: Through paediatrics to psycho-analysis*. London: Tavistock.

Winnicott, D. W. (1960). The theory of the parent–infant relationship. *International Journal of Psycho-Analysis, 41*, 585–595.

Winnicott, D. W. (1965). *The maturational processes and the facilitating environment*. London: Hogarth Press.

Winnicott, D. W. (1971). *Playing and reality*. London: Tavistock.

Wynne, L. (1965). Some indications and contraindications for exploratory family therapy. In I. Boszormenyi-Nagy & J. Framo (Eds.), *Intensive family therapy* (pp. 289–322). New York: Harper & Row.

Zilbach, J. (1988). The family life cycle: A framework for understanding children in family therapy. In L. Combrinck-Graham (Ed.), *Children in family contexts* (pp. 46–66). New York: Guilford Press.

Zinner, J. (1976). The implications of projective identification for couple interaction. In H. Grunebaum & J. Christ (Eds.), *Contemporary marriage: Structure, dynamics, and therapy* (pp. 293–308). Boston: Little, Brown.

Zinner, J. (1988, March). *Projective identification is a key to resolving couple conflict*. Paper presented at the Washington School of Psychiatry Psychoanalytic Family and Couple Therapy Conference, Bethesda, MD.

Zinner, J. (1989). The use of concurrent therapies: Therapeutic strategy or reenactment. In J. S. Scharff (Ed.), *Foundations of object relations family therapy* (pp. 321–333). New York: Jason Aronson.

Zinner, J., & Shapiro, R. (1972). Projective identification as a mode of perception and behavior in families of adolescents. *International Journal of Psycho-Analysis, 53*, 523–530.

CHAPTER 7

Transgenerational Couple Therapy

Laura Roberto-Forman

Transgenerational (TG) therapies were pioneered in the 1950s. As a group of methods, one could say that their development has reached only its early adulthood, having experienced a consolidation of work in the 1990s (Roberto, 1991, 1992; Roberto-Forman, 1998, 2002). This chapter reviews major current TG theories, relevant research and applications, and current techniques in view of what TG therapies offer for couple treatment.[1] Couple therapists of every persuasion use at least some TG tools, although these tools often are not formally recognized as "transgenerational." In fact, Carl Whitaker (1982) once referred to the central tenets of TG theory as "universals." For example, one prestigious training institute's most recent training brochure offers a "coaching group" (defined later in this chapter) for examining the therapist's position in his or her own family of origin. As a second example, a survey reveals that in the flagship marital and family therapy journal *Family Process*, between its inception in 1962 and March 2007, the terms "transgenerational," "intergenerational," and "multigenerational" were cited in 388 articles. In yet another example, most therapists and health care professionals routinely assess and refer to family-of-origin issues when treating

partners, if only to create a genogram, or to take a medical or sexual history. Until the late 1970s, this was not standard practice. However, although TG ideas permeate most marital therapy, TG therapies are often not explicitly acknowledged as a school of thought.

Transgenerational family process is, as I discuss later, a series of unfolding relational dynamics that evolve over the course of 20–40 years or more, such as in the concept "adult child of an alcoholic" (ACoA). This term encapsulates a self-definition, identity, set of roles and implicit family mandates, and behavioral repertoires that develop over the course of a child's life up to age 18 and beyond. Similarly, the concept of the "memorial candle" (Vardi, 1990) describes the strong mutual bond between the parent survivor of genocide and a chosen child. A small but growing number of qualitative research papers look at the connection between family-of-origin problems (e.g., alcoholism) and later relationship issues in couples, yet this research is not commonly pulled together under the umbrella of "TG." This chapter aims to address that deficit, pulling together, comparing, and combining different TG perspectives on couple therapy to demonstrate several points:

1. TG theory and TG therapy provide a powerful, nonhierarchical approach to framing and voicing problems, and understanding and working with couples in distress.
2. TG therapy moves beyond immediate symptom reduction to increase marital resilience and prevent future symptoms through the facilitation and development of intimacy, mutual problem solving, and satisfaction in couples.
3. Expansion of previous work identifies common bridging concepts among several historical TG schools, working toward a unitary, powerful TG model.
4. TG can inform a new generation of health professionals, who personally may not have studied with the departed founders of TG models or their earlier proponents, about central tenets and practices that can inform their research, theory, and practice with couples.

BACKGROUND

The major schools of TG theory and therapy over the past five decades include natural systems (Bowen) theory, symbolic–experiential (Whitaker) theory, contextual (relational ethics, Boszormenyi-Nagy) theory, and some aspects of object relations theory (Roberto, 1992; Scharff & Bagnini, 2002; Scharff & Scharff, 1987; Slipp, 1984; Wachtel & Wachtel, 1985). Although object relations marital and family therapy (MFT) in particular has been more in vogue since the 1980s, all of these models are widely used by MFTs to explain problems and inform treatment of couples. Current object relations theory has become more systemic, striving to address relational problems, even though its interview style focuses on affective, intrapsychic experience. Certain kinds of object relations interventions, such as holding, interpreting, eliciting unconscious material, fostering integration of painful memories, and working through in the present, have all been modified for use with couples in conjoint therapy. Because object relations theory includes family-of-origin material to understand marital behavior, some of its tenets are included in this discussion (also see Scharff & Scharff, Chapter 6, this volume). Although none of these major theories has been explicitly named transgenerational, they can be grouped together as theories that draw on intergenerational (long-term, slow to change) family processes to explain couples' problems.

TG models have been extended to examine specific spousal, family, and larger systems problems: personal authority in marriage and family (Williamson, 1981, 1982a, 1982b); family-of-origin consults (Framo, 1976); sexual dysfunction (Hof & Berman, 1989; Scharff, 1989; Schnarch, 1997); unconscious marital contracts (Sager, 1976); unresolved loss (Litvak-Hirsch & Bar-On, 2006; Paul, 1967); gender/power conflicts (Goodrich, 1991; Walters, Carter, Papp, & Silverstein, 1988); domestic violence work (Jory, 1998); late-life reconciliation (Hargrave, 1994; Hargrave & Anderson, 1992); and multicultural marriages (McGoldrick, 1989; McGoldrick, Pearce, & Giordano, 1982). A number of authors have sought specifically to apply feminist theory to TG couple therapy (Carter & McGoldrick, 1989; Knudson-Martin, 1994; Roberto, 1992; Walters et al., 1988). Their ideas have informed and enriched all of the methods presented in this chapter.

The TG therapies formulated in the last half of the 20th century reflected their time, in that they stemmed from individual models of human development, normality, and dysfunction. The work of early theorists aimed to observe, describe, and restructure the context of individual problems by looking "one level up" at the structure of the family of origin surrounding, supporting, and maintaining the views, values, cultural, religious, and personal identity, options, mandates, and subjective interpretations of people in therapy. As we will see, the transition involved in moving "one level up" meant that many TG techniques were formed to allow a client in individual psychotherapy to reflect on family-of-origin contexts without the entire family being in the room—or even the spouse. Over the last 50 years, TG techniques have evolved to include family members in the psychotherapy process.

I share the hopefulness of Johnson and Lebow (2000), who stated in their decade review of couple therapy that "we are, perhaps, beginning to build a generic base for couple intervention that is less constrained by differences in language" (p. 33). However, over the last 50 years, each of these four theories has been disseminated in different postgraduate training institutes, different publications, and even different professional organizations and conferences. For example, during Murray Bowen's years at Georgetown University, his family systems training program held its own conferences and symposia, and published its own archives. Although Bowen served as a President of the American Family Therapy Academy (AFTA), neither he nor Carl Whitaker (the founder of symbolic–experiential therapy) presented at AFTA's prestigious annual conference or other family therapy conferences (Ivan Boszormenyi-Nagy alone did so). Thus, the history of these four methods developed within separate groups of writers and institutes at the expense of developing common vocabularies. Furthermore, each of the four models is also based on the work of a highly charismatic male founder and his trainees: Natural systems theory is based heavily on Murray Bowen's work; symbolic–experiential theory, on that of Carl Whitaker; contextual therapy, on the work of Ivan Boszormenyi-Nagy; and object relations therapy on the work of D. W. Winnicott. Even though TG work is now in its fourth professional "generation" (assuming that a younger generation of trained professionals moves toward the leading center of a science every 20 years), literature bringing together common concepts and compatible interventions among the four models is still quite sparse.

Natural Systems Theory

Natural systems theory (Bowen) developed out of research observations of the interactions in families with a schizophrenic member. While at the National Institutes of Health from 1954 to 1959, Bowen sought to describe dysfunctional cycles of behavior between the parents and the psychotic patient (Bowen, 1972/1985b). At that time, he was looking for a relational basis for the striking lack of personal boundaries and autonomy of patients with psychotic disorders. He was especially interested in the possible role of family-of-origin enmeshment (and a related problem of "cutoff") in the eventual emergence of schizophrenia over generations of a family's life. Bowen subscribed to the diathesis–stress model of psychosis, which holds that illnesses do not necessarily emerge unless a person is stressed and cannot mobilize self-observation and self-regulation skills.

Early clinical researchers looked only at connections between inpatients and their mothers. Later, Bowen began to look at the role of the father and the quality of parental marriage as well. Bowen's team observed that in parent–child relationships situations with very highly involved–low interpersonal boundaries ("enmeshment" or "fusion"), emotional tensions increase to the point that a "triangle" (inclusion of a third person) evolves. The team began to look for evidence of fusion and triangulation in families whenever a psychiatric patient experienced frequent relapses. Bowen also predicted that if certain patterns of fusion are present in a marriage or family, then modifying these patterns in family therapy will lead to improvement in psychotic symptoms and improved individual resilience ("differentiation").

After 1967, Bowen developed and experimented with methods to diffuse family enmeshment, to increase individual differences and self-focus, and to promote give and take in family-of-origin relationships (a direction later continued by Williamson [1981] in his theory of "personal authority"). Bowen became increasingly interested in the connection between fusion and differentiation, and, in one famous appearance, even reported audaciously at a national medical conference on his own personal experiences increasing differentiation with his family of origin (Anonymous, 1972). This first reported use of self in the history of marital and family therapy had a powerful effect on both Bowen, who believed that experiential learning is potent for professional, as well as psychotherapeutic, growth, and on the audience, whose members saw a new modality for training in front of their eyes. Through this personal family-of-origin work, Bowen redefined differentiation—which had been viewed as an internal developmental phenomenon—as a function of family tolerance for individual differences and self-expression. He posited that once set during rearing, differentiation of self is very difficult to increase later in life. This concept has tremendous implications for therapists working with issues of partner selection and maturity in couple therapy.

A training institute was opened at Georgetown University in Washington, D.C. Bowen began to use assignments and family-of-origin visits as training tools with his own psychiatry residents as a way to teach his model and to address professional growth (Bowen, 1974). He observed that trainees who completed family-of-origin assignments seemed to possess more clinical effectiveness than those trainees who did not. By 1971, he concluded that work focused on creating one-on-one, well-delineated relationships with one's parents essentially raised one's own level of differentiation, increasing a therapist's ability to function in marriage, parenting, and practice of therapy. Trainees were encouraged to present their own families of origin in classes and conferences, and to enter psychotherapy with their spouses to look at how stagnant, unresolved family dilemmas colored their marriages and views of themselves. Although graduate training institutes are no longer encouraged to allow dual relationships in training, family of origin presentations and experiential learning are still highly utilized in advanced therapy externships and supervision.

Like his contemporaries, Bowen used the genogram, an old medical tool for charting family history—but with a twist. He and his trainees mapped symptom-bearers in relation to their extended families, then looked for intense relationships and triangles that might be helping to maintain clients' distress. Students such as Fogarty (1978) and Guerin (1976) applied the concept of triangles to problems of individual despair (emptiness), disconnection, and emotional distancing, and began to examine specifically the effect of distancing on marriage. The technique of "coaching" was developed to allow adult individuals and couples to disengage from family triangles, control distress ("reactivity"), and create one-on-one relationships with parents and key family members. Bowen also saw marital counseling as a way to prevent enmeshment problems from emerging between parents and their children.

Eventually, the natural systems group at Georgetown created a "think tank" to generalize these findings on the nature of enmeshment and triangulation in larger systems. Students applied the concepts of poor differentiation, fusion, and "undifferentiated ego mass," triangles, and "projection" (of unresolved issues) to less impaired families, workplace "families," social groups, and the training of clinicians. This expansion has included consultation in many types of workplaces. For example, Friedman (1985), an ordained rabbi, created a training model for clergy to apply to church/synagogue relations. Throughout the 1980s and 1990s, groups for clergy were run under his direction to examine the minister's/rabbi's relationship with congregational members and boards. The natural systems model works seamlessly with genogram study, because it focuses on recursive, repetitive, chronic cycling of symptoms between marital partners, parents, grandparents, and children. After Bowen's death, one of his principal students, Michael Kerr, took over direction of their institute. The influence of this model of family functioning has also helped to shape the curriculum at a number of important training institutes, including programs such as the Multicultural Training Institute at Rutgers University in New Jersey.

Symbolic–Experiential Therapy

Carl Whitaker also began working in the 1940s with adults hospitalized with psychotic symptoms. Trained as a psychoanalytic child psychiatrist, a contemporary of Murray Bowen, Lyman Wynne, Gregory Bateson, Ivan Boszormenyi-Nagy, Virginia Satir, and Nathan Ackerman, he also worked in public and Veterans Administration hospitals. Consistent with the predominant androcentric model in the 1940s, his emphasis was initially on parental (especially maternal) dysfunction as a contributor to relapse. However, he also consulted at the Oak Ridge atomic research facility during World War II, where he counseled scientists and war veterans showing severe stress reactions to the classified project. This experience gave Whitaker a sense of how personal disintegration can be a reaction to intolerable breakdowns of societal order, and everyday ethics and norms—what Whitaker (1982, p. 36) later called "being driven [as opposed to being] crazy." He later emphasized that one goal of therapy is to allow individuals to believe more in themselves and their potential, and to externalize the forces that lead us to view ourselves as different and marginalized. Externalization has become a central feature of some narrative therapies.

As a faculty member in the Department of Psychiatry at Emory University in the 1950s, Whitaker continued to shift from a psychoanalytic, internal conflict model of mental illness to an interactional, systemic model. The symbolic–experiential school of TG therapy thus echoes the same bridging ideas linking individual symptoms to larger family dysfunction as does natural systems theory. Unlike later methods, which are more problem-, present-, and solution-focused, TG models were created to provide a relational view of lifetime vulnerability and to explain why emotional breakdown occurs in one family member rather than others. Because he was a child psychiatrist (Neill & Kniskern, 1982; Whitaker & Ryan, 1989), Whitaker continued to feel that nonverbal affective experiences are an important avenue to self-awareness and resilience. This view distinguished him from peers, such as Bowen, who were viewing the same dysfunctional patterns in troubled families but emphasized intervention on the verbal and cognitive level to treat them (Roberto, 1991, 1992).

In addition, working with vulnerable clients such as children, worried parents, and trauma-related cases at the Oak Ridge facility, Whitaker came to believe that couple and family therapy require a high level of emotional safety and therapist transparency. Whitaker referred to this as "use of self": the ability to respond personally to the needs and concerns of clients in therapy. In symbolic–experiential therapy, the role of the therapist is unique: He or she shows multilateral caring rather than neutrality (Roberto, 1992). It is a proximal, emotionally focused, personal therapy rather than an abstract, coaching, educational therapy. As we will see, this view of the therapist's role overlaps the view held by Boszormenyi-Nagy in contextual therapy.

Finally, in a "third period" of work at Emory University, Whitaker began using a cotherapist and including the family of origin in therapy sessions. Like Bowen, he also began to make his residency training groups more systemic, having them do family-of-origin presentations in class. These ideas were picked up by other systemic therapies and elaborated into observing and reflecting teams, including family-of-origin consults in couple therapy (Framo, 1976) and in-session consultation with multiple therapists. The Emory faculty formed a process group and generated the Sea Island Conference of 1955—the first family process conference.

After Whitaker went to the University of Wisconsin Psychiatry Department, until the mid-1980s, he and colleague David Keith trained residents using live and videotaped interviews of extended families to teach marital and family therapy. Symbolic–experiential techniques remain heavily rooted in this collegial context of peer supervision, personal family-of-origin work, and use of self in therapy. To the other TG models of therapy it added heart, warmth, and therapist–client connectivity.

Contextual Therapy

Beginning around 1965, Ivan Boszormenyi-Nagy and colleagues focused on the concept that unresolved relationship problems over the course of several generations create, or "feed forward," into later emotional symptoms. He viewed families as possessing an implicit, invisible network of felt loyalties between parents and children, and believed that these bonds of attachment and loyalty constitute a separate dimension of relationship—an "ethical" dimension. By adding the concept of "relational ethics" (Boszormenyi-Nagy & Krasner, 1986; Boszormenyi-Nagy, Grunebaum, & Ulrich,

1991), contextual theory adds a layer of family experience to therapy that is not addressed by other TG models (Roberto, 1992).

In 1957, Boszormenyi-Nagy founded and directed the Department of Family Psychiatry at Eastern Pennsylvania Psychiatric Institute in Philadelphia. Like the workplaces of his peers, it contained both research programs and a clinical service, until state funding ended in 1980. His early family observation was, like that of his contemporaries, based on intensive care of inpatients with schizophrenia and their families (Boszormenyi-Nagy, 1962, 1965, 1972; Boszormenyi-Nagy & Spark, 1973). The Institute sponsored several of the earliest family therapy conferences in the 1960s, and Boszormenyi-Nagy was a founder of AFTA, formed in 1977.

Contextual theory draws on the ideas of European object relations writers such as Fairbairn (1952) and existentialist, experience-based theorists such as Buber. These ideas were brought to the United States by Sullivan (1953), Fromm-Reichmann (1950), Searles (1960), and others in the Chestnut Lodge group. One of the dominant interests for therapists at that time was *trustworthiness*—especially how a therapist's trustworthiness affects a client's ability to tolerate and manage psychotic symptoms. In the late 1950s and 1960s, Boszormenyi-Nagy made his theoretical shift to systems thinking and began to apply it in his medical setting. At that same time, cybernetic theory was also being developed. It was difficult to stimulate dialogue and attention to the idea of relational ethics—*loyalty binds, entitlement, merit, trust,* and *mutuality*—with cybernetic theory in vogue (Boszormenyi-Nagy & Ulrich, 1981). Contextual theory focuses on implicit emotional communication and types of bonding between people, so it has a poor "fit" with purely behavioral, problem-focused thinking. Rather, contextual theory explains how the quality of long-term family relationships affects intimate behavior that people bring to marriage and to parenting two to three generations later.

Object Relations Theory

In the history of marital and family theory, the influence of psychoanalytic theory is enormous. This was especially the case in the work of Norman Paul (1967) and James Framo (1976, 1981), whose techniques are reviewed here. Virginia Satir (1983), a TG therapist, was trained in analytic theory, as were Jackson, Wynne, Bowen, Whi-taker, Boszormenyi-Nagy, Minuchin, Palazzoli, and Stierlin—many of the originators of current marital and family techniques (Jackson & Lederer, 1968; Minuchin, Montalvo, Guerney, Rosman, & Schumer, 1967; Satir, 1983; Stierlin, 1981; Palaz-zoli, 1974; Wynne, 1965). In the United States, psychoanalytic theory existed mainly as Freudian theory through the 1950s. In Europe, however, an-alytic theory was modified between the late 1950s and the 1970s to become a theory of how self is created from intimate relationships. Object rela-tions theory was a revolutionary departure from Freud's wish-defense theory of the mind.

Object relations theory is based on a Euro-pean view of self-in-relation—how a young indi-vidual adapts to the encircling environment of the parent(s). Through adaptation to the loved other, the young person's deeply held wishes, beliefs, and emotional responses arise in the context of family responses and initiations (Roberto, 1992). Some object relations theorists devoted their life's work to how family systems shape the individual's experi-ence of self. That body of work uses the linear view that the parent shapes the child's experience—in a unilateral fashion (Bowlby, 1969, 1973; Fraiberg & Fraiberg, 1980; Mahler, Pine, & Bergman, 1975). Initially, the theory focused mostly on individual behavior and self-concept (Fairbairn, 1952; Klein, 1957; Winnicott, 1965). Fairbairn focused on how internal views of the "ideal object [other]" evolved from interaction between baby and mother, and how painful and disappointing events are taken in ("introjected") and then repressed or buried to preserve this ideal. Klein extended the idea of re-pression to propose that repressed experiences stay buried to avoid emotional pain but emerge as pro-jections onto important caretakers. Dicks, in an early application to couple work (1963), looked at how projection colors marriage. He posited that although a trusting marriage gives us the oppor-tunity to revisit and come to terms with painful, repressed experiences, frequently the repression–projection cycle is repeated instead.

Object relations theory has been applied in many settings in Europe, the Americas, Aus-tralia, and Canada, and has suffused most MFT theories in use now. Ideas about the place of the unconscious or unintegrated experience, ego, or self-definition, and internal experiences, such as introjection, projection, and attribution, are part of the bedrock in our understanding of psychologi-cal development.

WHAT WE HAVE LEARNED FROM RESEARCH

A number of associations have been identified be-tween family-of-origin relationships and courtship/marriage behavior in sons and daughters. A review of the literature shows that the family of origin has been shown to pass on a number of marital pat-terns. Preferred values (VanLear, 1992), patterns of coping with stress in marriage and with children (Juni, 1992), adjustment in and readiness for mar-riage (Campbell, Masters, & Johnson, 1998; Haws & Mallinckrodt, 1998), and age at marriage and/or pregnancy (Manlove, 1997; Thornton, 1991) are transgenerationally linked. Illness and resilience patterns (Abrams, 1999; Jankowski, Leitenberg, Henning, & Coffey, 1999; Wallerstein, 1996), ability to hold a "double vision" of marriage and to resolve conflict (Wallerstein, 1996), and intimacy (Prest, Benson, & Protinsky, 1998) are also trans-generationally linked.

These intergenerational patterns provide the blueprints and patterns of connection that will evolve later in every couple. Yet, when couples are interviewed to clarify the structure of their mar-riage and patterns of interaction, therapists often do not explore how the couple may be replaying lessons learned in their families of origin. I discuss this issue as it applies to the most current empirical models of marital dysfunction.

Research on Couples in Distress

Gottman (1998; Gottman & Gottman, Chapter 5, this volume) identified seven complex patterns of marital interaction that distinguish between satisfied and unsatisfied couples: greater reciproc-ity of negative affect; lower ratios of positive to negative behaviors; high levels of criticism, defen-siveness, contempt, and stonewalling (the "four horsemen"); and negative and lasting attributions about the partner. The researchers also identi-fied a frequent pattern that they called the "wife demand–husband withdraw" cycle. They con-cluded that positive affect and persuasion work better to preserve stability in marriage: Positive affect buffers conflicts, prevents negative attribu-tions (attributing bad motives for the partner's behavior), and protects against pathologizing one another.

These findings are extremely germane to TG theory. For example, the Gottman team likened the function of stable marriages to a bank account in which each partner's positive contributions compensate for negative feelings during conflicts. This finding parallels a central tenet of contextual therapy, which holds that the level of trust built up over time colors and influences people's ability to negotiate and reconcile. The initial fund of trust in a marriage also partly reflects each spouse's history in previous love relationships, as well as needs and abilities each has brought out of his or her family of origin. But Gottman's research to date in looking at his couples' transactions does not include concepts from TG theory.

Two-generational research studies help to explain the factors that lead to and maintain the skewed interactions of unhappy couples. Goodrow and Lim (1997) described a pattern of high reactivity and defensiveness in an engaged couple and the relevant behavior patterns transmitted from their respective parents. Larson and Thayne (1998) showed that fusion and triangulation in subjects' families are related to negative opinions and feelings about marriage. In Nelson and Wampler's (2000) study of 96 couples in counseling, in which one or both partners reported childhood abuse (physical or sexual), the partner who reported abuse functioned especially poorly, and the trauma affected the other partner as well. The authors concluded that "a person may experience secondary trauma issues resulting from identification with the trauma victim" (p. 180). One wonders to what extent the negative attributes discussed by Gottman's team could reflect such mediating family-of-origin problems and their serious marital consequences.

Interestingly, Gottman and Levenson (1999a, 1999b) stated that in their samples, couple interaction is remarkably durable over a 4-year period. These patterns probably "become part of the fabric of a couple's life and [are] resistant to change" (Lebow, 1999, p. 169). Couples also present with the same issues after a 4-year period in their samples. Therefore, the viability of a marriage must depend not so much on whether issues are resolved, or what issues are resolved, but on *how partners engage each other*. *Degree* of engagement about marital issues is crucial. We can speculate that when transactions between spouses are so remarkably stable over time, then it is probable that we are viewing patterns that are "trait" rather than "situational" behaviors (i.e., they reflect fundamental underlying perceptions and characteristics that each spouse brings to the marriage).

I conclude that families of origin pass on preferred values; styles of intimate relating, meanings and beliefs about difference, tolerance and acceptance, fairness, and mutuality; and other intrinsic aspects of family life. Their children then go into marriage with expectations, needs, and dreams colored by these formative experiences. Marriages either develop characteristics of safety, mutual regard, and hope or are compromised by the past. It seems imperative, given these findings, that couple therapy provide powerful ways to identify and to change the modes of attachment by which partners relate to one another. These emotional processes, so deeply ingrained and colored by one's birth family, are beautifully addressed and described by the TG model. In fact, it is the TG model's *pièce de résistance*.

THE HEALTHY PARTNERSHIP

Formulated as they were in European American societies, most TG theories hold that healthy marriage begins with a love bond in which the partners have chosen each other. It is certain that the deep psychological bond of love allows the couple to form an emotional boundary around the twosome that is preeminent and different from other connections—more intense, focused, and intimate. Although a love bond turns the partners' focus toward one another, the boundary around them must be somewhat permeable for a healthy partnership. The loyalty between partners in a marriage of choice is typically stronger than the loyalty to family-of-origin or other relationships.

Falling in love as a basis for marriage is a 20th-century European and American concept. However, the love bond may be of increasing importance in marriage historically. As women and girls are allowed greater access to education and paid work, the economic factors sustaining marriage become less crucial, and marital commitment becomes increasingly more choice-based. Yet it is important to understand the TG forces of culture and religion that have shaped marital structure—even the concept of marriage as a twosome—rather than committing the "beta bias" (Hare-Mustin, 1987) of assuming that all marriages are alike regardless of ethnicity. And in many communities and countries (e.g., in observant Islamic and Orthodox Jewish families), marriage (or at least the meeting of prospective mates) is arranged by a trusted elder. Ethnicity, religion, and class are so fundamental and crucial in defining the concept of a "marital dyad" that I discuss them in a separate section of this chapter.

Empathy and Mutuality

There is a flow of empathy or understanding in a healthy marriage—a shared framework in which each partner's behaviors and intentions are for the mutual good of the couple. It is difficult for partners to build empathy unless each member has an imaginative sense of the other's experience. Empathy partly comes from dialogues in which each partner confides the personal meanings he or she derives from the marriage, personal beliefs, and responses to past events that have been significant and formative. Empathy is also to some extent a developmental ability that requires an internal sense of well-being and the wish to be considerate and generous with others. In dysfunctional families of origin, painful or traumatic events and disasters can destroy any empathic connection and turn members aside into self-absorption, hatred, or mistrust (Boszormenyi-Nagy's "destructive entitlement").

There is no term for the shared emotional "flow" that occurs in satisfied couples. This flow is referred to as "give and take" in contextual theory (Boszormenyi-Nagy & Krasner, 1986), as a sense of "we"-ness (Whitaker & Keith, 1981, p. 192) in symbolic–experiential theory, and as reciprocity in behavioral theory. I prefer the term "mutuality," which implies that there is a back-and-forth affective quality: "One extends oneself out to the other and is also receptive. ... There is openness to influence, emotional availability. ... There is both receptivity and active initiative toward the other" (Jordan, 1991, p. 82). This interconnectedness sustains a couple during times of conflict, because partners rely on their fundamental attachment. Trust evolves from the reciprocity: If one goes to one's partner, the partner then responds with concern.

Mutuality and marital *quid pro quo* involve agreeing to clear rules. Rules are unique to each couple and allow partners to carry out their responsibilities and commitments as a team. In healthy couples, the agreements and requests are not oriented so much toward "doing" as toward "supporting"; trading car repair for housecleaning is not mutuality. It is the sense of bilateral agreement *behind* the responsibilities that constitutes mutuality. When empathy and consideration are flowing back and forth, each partner has a feeling of being understood. Attachment theory considers this quality to be central in producing emotional security in couples (Silverstein, Buxbaum Bass, Tuttle, Knudson-Martin, & Huenergardt, 2006).

There is a dimension of imagination in healthy couples: Partners can share fantasies, hopes, and expectations together. In secure marriages, emotional energies are freed up to anticipate the future-connectedness that transcends today and adds depth that may not be apparent to the casual observer. Partners have mutual curiosity about each other. It is a good sign when couples come together to marital therapy because one or both partners want to increase marital satisfaction. When a spouse refuses to participate in the emotional work of therapy despite an available and caring therapist, the ensuing distance will likely harm the marriage. The death of hope and imagination is a primary sign of eventual marital dissolution.

Differentiation, Commitment, and Marital Choice

"Differentiation" is the ability to experience difference, the self as separate although in relation to everyone else. Many definitions have been offered to conceptualize differentiation and what comprises "enough" or "good" differentiation. Bowen was foremost among writers trying to define and explain differentiation, not only psychologically, but also biologically and sociologically (1966/1985a).

Well-functioning couples are able to change their dynamics over time as shifts in family and social network produce "reality stresses of life" (Bowen, 1966/1985a, p. 171). The partners' familiar ways of interrelating have to adapt to the inevitable triangles that form through other commitments, such as children, friends, family, and work (Whitaker & Keith, 1981). Relationships and connections "outside" the dyad are accepted and encouraged between healthy spouses. When each partner has a differentiated sense of self (self-identity), he or she can be resilient in the face of change. Without self-awareness, partners revert to emotionally volatile, reactive modes of responding, and cannot tolerate stress well. Bowen speculated that "the highest level of differentiation that is possible for a family is the highest level that any family member can attain and maintain against the emotional opposition of the family unit in which [s]he lives" (Bowen, 1966/1985a, p. 175). Bowen believed that the capacity for differentiation becomes gradually more and more "set" over generations, with a downward drift into what Bowen termed "undifferentiated ego mass," or family fusion. Certainly this is seen in families with a multigenerational history of violence, incest, addiction, or neglect.

Differentiation includes the ability to discern one's internal emotions and thoughts, to identify them as separate from others' emotions, and to maintain one's own observations and judgment—one's own "voice." Differentiation includes personal goals and direction, self-knowledge, self-guidance, and self-soothing. It allows personal problem solving and self-correction. Since the 1980s, when science began to study female, as well as male, development, our view of differentiation has been modified to acknowledge that self-knowledge always occurs in the context of significant, long-term, intimate relationships—"self-in-relation" rather than "self" (Boszormenyi-Nagy & Ulrich, 1981; Fishbane, 1999; Knudson-Martin, 1994). Differentiation is a prerequisite to a healthy marriage because when one can be emotionally self-sufficient, then "dependency on each other is voluntary" (Framo, 1981, p. 139). Neither partner feels burdened from constantly having to be in the "helper" role, a situation that Bowen referred to as "losing self," popularly known as codependency.

TG models view differentiation as a cornerstone of people's ability to enter into long-term commitments and live together. We have only to look at marriages in which one or both spouses have poor differentiation to see how even trivial and unimportant disagreements lead to defensiveness, recrimination and blaming, self-centeredness; and discrediting the partner.

Individual differentiation probably influences how we select our partners. Although many other models of couple therapy do not examine issues of marital choice, TG models provide a framework to understand variations in commitment, marital readiness, and choosing one's partner. The reason for this is that TG models do not view young marrieds as individuals, but as members of two families who have been launched (to a lesser or greater degree), and are expected to form their own relationships.

Intimacy and Healthy Attachment

Attachment is the metaphor used to explain the supportive properties of committed relationships (Johnson & Lebow, 2000). However, attachment has to develop hand in hand with individual self-awareness. Maturana (personal communication, March, 1986), a research biologist, remarked that from the point of view of environmental biology, love is "the intention to coexist." Attachment and adaptation evolve in the context of two different people who have decided to share their lives. Research and clinical study in the areas of emotional, traumatic, and developmental disorders have also shown that there is a neurobiological element in the ability to attach to loved ones (Siegel, 2006). The ability to regulate and integrate emotion, to engage, and to respond are neurological activities. Secure (consistent, empathic) attachment and attunement to others require a healthy mind that has not been traumatized. Abuse, neglect, and disaster survivors have difficulty with secure attachment.

Marriage requires a significant amount of "accommodation" (Jory, Anderson, & Greer, 1997), or tolerance. Individual differences demand that partners accept each other's limits, in spite of whatever expectations each carried into the relationship. Accommodation is part of the "relational ethics" of caring and fairness. It involves following through on requests and expressed needs instead of questioning or criticizing each other's vulnerabilities. Accommodation does not occur unless partners are able to show fairness; in families where pathological hurt has occurred, fairness can be erased or distorted. For example, in the situation of the *revolving slate* (Boszormenyi-Nagy & Krasner, 1986), people whose families have harmed or wronged them tend to feel entitled or that they are "owed" compensation in their own families later. If there is not a reasonable amount of accommodation in the marriage, neither partner feels cared for or safe.

Marital intimacy also "requires a keen sense of self-identity and self-differentiation. … In contrast to distancing, the feelings *inside* a person and *between* people are critically important in developing closeness" (Fogarty, 1978, p. 70). To a large extent, people's capacity for intimate relating also includes willingness to examine their own internalized beliefs about love, fulfillment, caring, and mutuality (Jory et al., 1997; Schnarch, 1997). It is this self-examination that clarifies their values and expectations regarding closeness, reciprocity, sexual intimacy, and nurturance, so that they can evaluate marriage and identify desired changes.

Self-examination is the direct experience of the inner self, subjectivity, and "going deep" into one's core assumptions and expectations of the social world. It is not possible to share this kind of spiritual and emotional subjectivity with a spouse, unless one is first willing to explore and reflect on personal experiences. When scrutinized, internalized beliefs and memories of love relationships draw heavily on family-of-origin experiences.

Schnarch (1997) points out that intimacy is thus a "two-pronged" process of both examining the self and expressing one's self to the partner. Partners who are capable of self-validation rather than approval seeking are better able to contribute to their marriage. This view of intimacy reflects the natural systems concept that chronic anxiety (e.g., approval seeking) is a relational obstacle.

Defining "Good" Communication

The prevailing view of couple communication is that "good" communication provides active listening, openness, and empathy toward one's partner's views. However, in this "open" process, the connection between partners is *not* necessarily "good." There are many forms of "open" but troubled communication as well: spilling of anxiety (venting), expressions of self-doubt, unresolved issues, and projections carried from other relationships. In contrast, "good" communication is dialogue with personal accountability and is relevant to the partner who is listening. Concerns expressed must be resolvable, the stress level has to be controlled, emotions must be contained to some degree, and the spouse must have room to respond. A good dialogue occurs between two people who are reflecting on an issue from different vantage points in which each has some understanding and emotional equilibrium.

This view, called "self-validated" (Schnarch, 1997) communication, creates gender-specific tasks for couples in therapy. Women are socialized to move toward the partner, trying to clarify their feelings through connection with others (Jordan, Kaplan, Miller, Stiver, & Surrey, 1991). As Knudson-Martin and Mahoney (1999) point out, women may feel pressure to "seek relationship and connection," sometimes compromising or suppressing parts of themselves that appear different (p. 331). Men, pressured by gender expectations that they should "protect their independence" (p. 331), hide parts of themselves that would foster connection. In couple therapy, therapists tend to follow this gender bias and call on the female partner to open the dialogue. It is assumed that this will help the male partner learn to disclose himself. Gender-stereotypical behavior—women pursuing while men detach—leads to the burnout (hers) and disengagement (his) that ends marriages (Johnson & Lebow, 2000). Ideally, good communication involves investment of each partner's true, not hidden, self (Scheel et al., 2000). The

woman does not aim to be the "sole keeper" of the connection and can formulate thoughts that are different, and the man is willing to risk emotional contact and can express thoughts that connect.

THE DYSFUNCTIONAL PARTNERSHIP

As I have mentioned elsewhere (Roberto, 1992), "structural" (connectivity vs. distance, hierarchy vs. equality, conflict vs. cooperation) symptoms reflect problems in a couple's emotional "process." Structural symptoms are transactions that can be marked on a genogram. They may look like boundary problems, in which the marital dyad is distant, "locked" (fused or enmeshed) together in dependency and/or fighting about it, or pseudomutual (a social relationship with no attachment). The marriage may be too open to intrusions from others, or so closed that a spouse is punished for any outside connection. The partners may have triangled in a third party. Or there may be extreme complementarity (codependent–addict or caretaker–patient marriages); extreme symmetry (two partners with similar symptoms); and "tilts," where there is an imbalance of power or equity (e.g., the "dollhouse" or "one-up–one-down" marriage).

In contrast to structural symptoms, the underlying process problems do not show on any genogram. "Process problems" include unworkable types of bonding that produce stress and emotional pain. There may be unrealistic or destructive expectations, such as contempt, disrespect and ridicule, narcissism, or exploitiveness. One or both partners may have problems with idealization and perfectionism. Or there may be indifference, sexism, or prejudice. Process problems easily escape discussion in marital therapy, because they are implicit in thought, difficult to verbalize, and painful to admit.

Delegation and Negative Attributions

"Delegation" is the transmission of unresolved family stress onto a child, which is internalized (Boszormenyi-Nagy & Krasner, 1986; Stierlin, Levi, & Savard, 1973). The child experiences "obligation," learning that his or her personal wishes are less significant than family needs. As the offspring tries to carry out the expectations delegated to him or her, choices become narrower, and the obligations become a heavy burden. The sense of burden is usually not in conscious awareness and is instead expressed in the marriage. Paul (1967) commented on how "losses and associated sense of deprivation lead to deposit of such affects as sorrow ... guilt ... bitterness, despair, and regret" (p. 189).

There can be "displaced exploitation," such as expecting the spouse to share the sense of obligation also—especially with family of origin. These are the situations in which a husband dines with a parent several times a week and expects his wife to participate. Or a wife expects to take in an irresponsible sibling to live with the couple indefinitely. When a delegated child lacks empathy for him- or herself, by extension he or she lacks consideration for the spouse.

Projection has been well discussed in the object relations literature—in fact, it is part of the oldest literature on couple problems (e.g., Jackson & Lederer, 1968). Dynamically, the bond with a parent is idealized in childhood, and painful events are often distorted by children to maintain that idealization. As a young person splits off negative or problematic characteristics of the parents or elder siblings, these perceptions are suppressed to maintain the loving connection (Fairbairn, 1952). Clinicians are familiar with the problem of an adult child of abusive parents, who refuses to admit that the parents were abusive and instead overreacts when the spouse raises his or her voice or makes the slightest dissatisfied comment. When the spouse then protests, the negative reaction seems to validate those projections (Roberto, 1992). This is one of the central problems of abusive relationships: The violent or abusive partner, who him- or herself was once harmed, has difficulty believing that the other cares, because the parents did not show caring. There can also be "mutual attribution" (Dicks, 1963), in which each spouse perceives the other as similar to hurtful persons in the past.

What we cannot accept in ourselves, we deny—and then despise it in our significant other. In the phenomenon of "projective identification," the spouse is viewed (erroneously) as having certain attitudes or reactions with which we ourselves struggle but will not admit. For example, a wife may feel critical toward her husband's devotion to his work, viewing him as too job-oriented; at the same time, she pushes herself and everyone around her toward her own goals for success. It is not hard to understand how these long-standing, disowned perceptions come to cloud the deep and primary attachment of a marriage. Because this is not a conscious or deliberate act, it is to some degree inevitable.

Through understanding the dynamics of suppression and projection, we can recognize Gottman's discovery in the marriage lab of negative attributions as an example of projective behavior. As he and his colleagues noted, this problem spells the end of marital viability. There can be no trust in a marriage if there is not hope that it will comfort and give support, and attributions are self-fulfilling prophecies that do not allow healing to take place.

Fusion and Distancing Patterns

Fusion

Natural systems therapists coined the term "fusion" to describe the "glue" that makes some couples too attached. In fused marriages, one partner tends to show greater passivity under stress than the other, and appears dependent on the other while seeming to give in or adapt. Bowen's (1966/1985a, 1972/1985b) group believed that the overly adaptive partner loses a sense of competence, while the underadaptive partner seems to gain it. Over time, the partners merge into a tightly locked unit, with little overt conflict. Bowen's theory holds that the "competent" spouse is protected from stress in this way—at the expense of the "incompetent" spouse (Roberto, 1992). One or both partners finally form emotional symptoms—usually the overly adaptive spouse (Bowen, 1966/1985a; 1972/1985b; Kerr, 1981, 1985). The "competent" spouse, who is gaining functional "self" from the other, may be completely unaware of the pressures on the "incompetent" spouse. The conflict that drives them into therapy comes when neither spouse will further accommodate the other in the fusion, or when the one who formerly gave up self cannot function very well anymore.

In the natural systems view of fusion, the "locking" together of partners is seen as a response to chronic anxiety or "unresolved emotional attachments" to a dysfunctional family of origin (Bowen, 1974). Family members are drawn into intense and anxiety-ridden positions with each other. The anxiety level in the family results in a lack of focus on self and overfocusing on others. "Family projection process," a related concept, describes how particular children become enmeshed in a triangle with the parents, then fail to develop ("differentiate") a focus on self. In an interesting empirical study of fusion and family projection, alcoholics who were children of alcoholics and their nondrinking spouses showed similar scores on a codependency measure. They also reported similar levels of dysfunction in their families of origin. Participants endorsed items on a family systems questionnaire indicating low individuation, high anxiety, low transgenerational intimacy, and low spousal intimacy (Prest et al., 1998).

Unconscious Marital Contracts

Object relations theory maintains that when an adult has not addressed important developmental needs before leaving home, they are played out in mate selection. This has been called an "unconscious marital contract" (Sager, 1976). In those areas in which we feel inadequate, we project that need and are then attracted to others who appear correspondingly stronger. For example, a woman who believes that she is not competent to make decisions may seek out a spouse who seems more decisive. Of course, she then experiences frustration when he is decisive because in reality she can make workable decisions and only assumed that his were preferable. A man who sees himself as abandoned and vulnerable may choose a partner who appears self-confident enough to protect him. Attraction is extremely powerful between incomplete or suppressed parts of ourselves and the image we form of another who appears more complete. It is very difficult to form a dispassionate perspective on this unconscious agenda until well into a marriage, when the spouse show human frailty and fails to fulfill the wishes and desperately desired missing qualities.

Transitions and life challenges bring a feeling of emptiness and confusion. The tension that accompanies emptiness challenges our sense of competence, and adults turn to their marriage anticipating support. What people expect from each other creates anticipation and demands, disappointment, hurt and anger. The expectations, which always come from past experience outside the marriage, stress the relationship (Fogarty, 1978). Each partner must be able to tolerate disappointments and understand his or her own dissatisfaction. In the process, "one should not expect any more from husband or wife than he would expect from any man or woman outside the family" (p. 83). These startling remarks go against the instinctive sense of intimacy as togetherness.

One extreme form of unconscious contract is the self-fulfilling prophecy, in which a partner is so greatly distressed by fears or anxieties in the marriage that he or she actually makes them come to pass. For example, a man whose mother left him in childhood may be so riddled with fear that his wife will leave him, or be unfaithful, that he pushes her away with his doubts and suspicions. Pathological jealousy, pathological guilt, and destructive entitlement (Boszormenyi-Nagy & Krasner, 1986) are examples of self-fulfilling prophecy.

Marital Violence as Fusion

Marital violence is probably the premier symptom of marital fusion. Goldner (1998) commented particularly on the "compelling, automatic projection process that has come to possess the [abusively connected] couple" (p. 277, my brackets). In battered spouse syndrome, batterers retain a sense of control and personal meaning. Because the batterer frightens his or her spouse into agreement, the victimized spouse progressively loses any sense of self apart from trying to contain and look out for the next episode of violence. Both partners are reluctant even to seek help without the other—a complex situation that forces therapists into interviewing them together, despite the danger in the home. The victimized partner, who spends energy adapting to the demands of the violent, poorly controlled partner, ceases to be self-protective over time. Instead, he or she becomes protective of the batterer.

Exploring family histories of abusive spouses has clarified some confusing aspects of violence—for example, why there is TG transmission. The concept of "destructive entitlement," discussed later in this chapter, describes the exploitive behavior of abusers as a reaction to family-of-origin abuse: if one's parent was not accountable for hurting the family, then why should one be accountable to one's spouse now? Denial and minimization, used to cope with the violent family of origin, leads to lack of accountability in one's own marriage later. Imitation is the purest form of fusion.

To unpack any of these underlying issues in the marital fusion, "careful deconstruction of each individual's personal biography is a necessary preamble for the morally crucial discussion of personal responsibility and agency" (Goldner, 1998, p. 277). Jory, using intimate justice theory, also points out that to treat violence, there must be an examination of internalized family experiences. One major clinical intervention involves "exploring experiences with empowerment, disempowerment and the abuses of power in the family of origin" (Jory & Anderson, 1999, p. 350).

Triangles

Fusion is expressed not only in "locking together" but also in the reactive conflict and backing away that ensues. In many couples, periods of dependency explode into anger and pushing apart. The marriage is unstable and shifts back and forth between two poles of coming together and backing away. Couples react to these extremes by pulling in a third person, who moderates the closeness and distance by being available to one or both partners. This person becomes a "boundary keeper," who stabilizes the shifting marriage (Byng-Hall, 1980, p. 355), much as a goalie guards a goalpost and keeps the ball in play. The partners then continues their back-and-forth shifting, approaching and then backing away, but without extremes. Common triangles include affairs, job entanglements, or forming a family or child "confidante." However, once the triangle has become persistent, one or both spouses begin to have loyalty binds, and it is difficult to focus attention on the marriage. In many couples, emotional triangles may affect the very future of the relationship. Extramarital affairs are a dramatic example.

Children are often the most common third parties in a cross-generation triangle called a "coalition." The couple becomes child-focused or creates a "three-way marriage" (Palazzoli, 1974). The couple maintains stability for decades of child rearing, with one or both partners relying on a son or daughter for support. When the son or daughter becomes more separate from the parent(s), often after individual therapy, these marriages destabilize (e.g., see Braverman's 1981 study). That child's increased independence, even later in life, creates a significant loss for the parent(s). The subsequent emotional distance is not balanced by a strong marriage tie.

The other most common third party is an in-law, usually a mother-in-law. One or both of the spouses remains highly interconnected with the mother, who maintains an active part in the couple's relationship, occupies time, aids in decision making, and furnishes support. However, theories about the harm caused by this cross-generational triangle combine a Western concern about the primacy of the married pair and the misogynist idea that female interdependency is a problem. The concept of cross-generational triangles as dysfunctional is culturally linked to Western individualist societies (Falicov, 1998). In collectivist cultures, such as Asian, East Indian, Mediterranean, and Latino societies, the weight of the parent–child bond is equal to that of the marital bond and may actually be more enduring and important. Empathy and receptiveness between a parent and a child are expected, and differentiation from the family of origin is not expected or tolerated.

Entitlement and Revolving Slates

Any discussion of attributions, projection, and mutual projection leads into discussion of "entitlement," which is the expectation that because one has sacrificed for others, one deserved acknowledgment and consideration back (Boszormenyi-Nagy & Spark, 1973; Boszormenyi-Nagy & Ulrich, 1981). "Destructive entitlement" is the belief that one is being denied acknowledgment or consideration. Healthy feelings of entitlement begin in formative years, when a young person is given the care and attention that is part of normal family development. In dysfunctional families, unmet needs for care and acknowledgment are carried forward into adult love relationships and marriage as negative feelings of entitlement. In a painful and unfair "revolving slate," the position of "giver" is passed on to the spouse. Meanwhile, the partner who feels destructive entitlement feels justified in making demands and expecting care from his or her mate, because it should be his or her turn to benefit.

People caught in a revolving slate of unrequited caring with their family of origin, play out this unresolved problem with a spouse. I believe that many repeating marital patterns seen on a genogram are the result of the revolving slate phenomenon. For example, the neglected son of a busy father may expect that his spouse will let his own life revolve around him. On the marital genogram, we see a "dotted line" of distancing between the "entitled" man and his father, and the same "dotted line" between the two husbands now. Whitaker, joking about problems of the revolving slate, commented that marriages are "really just two scapegoats sent out by two families to reproduce each other. … The battle is which one it will be" (cited in Neill & Kniskern, 1982, p. 368). Destructive entitlement in marriage is most clearly seen in codependent marriages. Somehow, one partner's needs and perceptions are valued as more important, and the other partner's needs and perceptions are overlooked by both of them. If the situation is not rectified, the children in that household are at risk to play out this revolving slate of "who gets and who gives." In marital therapy, pointing out this risk can be a powerful motivator for a codependent spouse in setting limits and learning not to make so many sacrifices.

Distancing and Cutoff

Chronic fusion can produce a distant marriage. For example, in the distancer–pursuer pattern, one partner tries to speak for, approach, or draw out the other's concerns, and usually misreads them. An overexpressive spouse pursues an underexpressive spouse. In turn, the underexpressive partner acts without expressing his or her thoughts or feelings, leaving the "mind-reader" to follow along completely mystified and usually approaching again for some explanation. The more nonexpressive one partner is, the harder the other one works, and the couple becomes trapped in this pattern, with one as the "rock" and the other as the "emotional wreck."

Significant tension underlies the distancer–pursuer pattern. The tension is related to each partner's deeply held beliefs about how to gain security and love, desire for validation from the other, fears of the dangers of conflict, and expectations about who must do the work in a relationship. These beliefs and tensions are internalized from previous relationships, including experiences with the family of origin. Distancers want to see themselves as self-sufficient, and carry an idealized and depersonalized view of marriage that tends to break down under stress. Pursuers see themselves as dependent, and believe that their hope for a viable marriage comes from carrying both partners' dissatisfactions so they can unilaterally "patch up" areas of conflict. It is also possible to have a symmetrical distancer–pursuer pattern in which each spouse dances toward the other, then away, like the characters Scarlett O'Hara and Rhett Butler in the book *Gone with the Wind*.

The extreme of distancing is cutoff. Central features of cutoff include minimization or denial of attachment, as if the relationship never existed, acting completely self-sufficient, and even physically running away. The cutoff is not subjectively seen as a problem, but as a justified feeling that "I have to get away from this." At the receiving end, the partner who is cutting off seems to have great self-determination, strength, and more self-esteem than the partner who is left behind. In reality, it reflects severe deficits in the ability to tolerate frustration, to preserve hope in the face of crisis, and to maintain connection under stress.

Religion, Culture, and Class

Feminist-informed theories of culture and the family have provided powerful larger-system explanations for marital dysfunction. Feminist theory focuses on the ways that male-centered culture rules how husbands and wives differently approach marital conflict, problem solving, intimacy, managing stress, self-empowerment, sexuality, financial and emotional power distribution, and even defining what constitutes a problem or a marital crisis. Each TG model in its original form, built in the 1950s and 1960s, neglected to examine biases of male-centered culture (beta bias). "Beta bias" here would be the assumption that gender differences are unimportant, thus placing them outside the scope of discussion (Hare-Mustin, 1987). Symbolic–experiential theory does point out the importance of addressing gender inequities in marital therapy, either by moving couples toward egalitarianism, or acknowledging justice issues for women, such as the need for autonomy in family life. Yet there has been little focus on gender inequities in marriage. For example, feminist theorists would argue that entitlement is gendered—that in marriage, the needs of the husband tend to be valued as more worthy than the wife's needs. Slipp (1994) has pointed out that because male children are pushed away from nurturance in their socialization, they carry a certain amount of destructive entitlement into marriage. If, in this transitional society, fathers were to pick up nurturance functions for their sons, there would not be a deficit for their sons to carry into marriage. In the past decade, feminist theory has focused more on larger-system problems, analyzing social and political movements that color the expectations of men and women in marriage. The implication for marital therapy is that the therapist must take a position about the larger system that refuses to ignore gender inequity, or else the therapist will *be in* the position of beta bias. As Goldner (1995) put it, "Given that we are born into a symbolic and material world that is *already* gendered ... it is impossible to overstate its effects on mind and culture. ... We cannot 'see through' gender to the person 'inside,' since gender and self have co-evolved throughout the developmental process" (p. 46). Even if a couple is not aware of or complaining about inequities in their marriage or families of origin, the culturally competent marital therapist must address the impact of cultural stereotypes on the couple's functioning.

Therapists must carefully look at what is normative for a family's cultural group when evaluating structural or process symptoms. Marital problems can reflect and even be mediated or have their meaning changed by cultural issues. Culture affects how a family defines its members, and where the boundaries exist within a family or a multicultural marriage (McGoldrick, 1989). For example, not every nuclear family is defined as persons who live in the home. In a Roman Catholic family, parents, godparents, and the spouses of sons and daughters are all seen as part of the nuclear family. In an African American household, neighbors and church fellows may be part of the spousal support system. In a religiously observant family, if a relative is a minister, he or she may be treated as a member of the nuclear family during times of crisis.

In East Indian, Asian, and Southeast Asian families, the in-laws are central to a couple's loyalties. Traditional Chinese and Japanese families are similar in their emphasis on filial loyalty, and family structure derives from Buddhist and Confucian ideals emphasizing patriarchy and the extended family (Tamura & Lau, 1999). In these families, the emphasized relationship is between mother and child (especially a son), not husband and wife. In extreme contrast, Caucasian Eurocentric Christian families (e.g., British families) expect the married pair to be split off from other family members when it comes to personal problems and concerns; parents and in-laws are peripheral (Tamura & Lau, 1999). The structure of a family and the boundary (if there is one) around the couple are defined by at least three to four generations of family tradition and ethnicity.

Generational and gender hierarchies are culturally linked. The idea I just expressed—that couples should move toward egalitarianism to the extent that their relational symptoms reflect gender inequities—is a Western concept. The individualist societies of the West locate the couple as a unit of leadership in the family, so symmetrical interactions are considered ideal (Falicov, 1989). The "united front" of two parents making decisions about children stems from the view of couple as a unit of leadership. In extended-family societies, leadership is vertical across generations, with lifelong authority given to elders. For example, Mexican American couples defer to the parents throughout married life, until the parents are gone; hence, there is no stage of "personal authority" in one's own married home (Williamson, 1981, 1982a, 1982b). Because of centuries of male-dominated economics and law, authority extends through fathers to husbands to brothers to sons.

Emotional process is also cultured. For example, the concepts of entitlement (what is owed to us by our spouse and family), destructive entitlement, and attendant problems such as the revolving slate, cannot be used in the same way across cultures. For example, the current generation of Korean American young adults has risen to educational and financial advantages through the personal sacrifice and hard work of their parents. They carry a tremendous sense of obligation to respond by choosing work and marriage that will please their parents. In Japanese families, individual happiness is considered less important, and happiness is considered to be linked to achieving the well-being of the whole group; excessive demands by any one member would disturb *ki*, or harmony (Tamura & Lau, 1999).

Conflict and communication are culturally linked. In extended-family societies, where large-group harmony must be preserved due to proximity and involvement, indirect and implicit communication is preferred. Rather than being able to assert oneself and make "I"-focused statements in the Bowenian mode, the couple relies on careful listening to read wishes underlying each other's much more compact comments. Or, an ally is temporarily triangled in to represent the interests of one spouse; for example, a wife may confide in a sister-in-law, who tells her mother, who tells her son (the husband) of the wife's concerns.

Political movements create legacies that are expressed in marriage. Young couples now are the third generation after the American Depression, and it is no accident that many of them are driven by the job market and financial ambition. Some middle-aged adults whose parents were refugees during World War II have seen their parents sue for international reparation. This historic set of events will create for some people a shift in social identity from "second- or third-generation American" to a more long-term, healing, self-respectful view of family history. We can also expect to see changes in the social class and privilege experienced by families of reparation, who, once impoverished refugees, are able to attain financial privilege two generations later.

ASSESSMENT OF COUPLES

Procedures for TG assessment of couples are not well articulated. Several well-researched tests of family functioning are available that use a circumplex model to assesses families regarding distribution of power, intimacy and cohesion, autonomy and other important factors. These tools have been underutilized, reflecting the predominant thinking that the frame for couple work can be completely constructed within the married dyad, instead of being viewed as an extension of larger-family problems. Thus, despite the wealth of information about family impact on later adult functioning, couple therapy is too often cordoned off as a modality separate from family therapy. In contrast, TG therapists "punctuate" the problems experienced within a couple by looking at their place in the three-generation grid of their two families during assessment.

It is also important for the therapist to understand what effects flow outward from changes within a couple, to their families of origin. The two families, connected as they are to each spouse in dyads and triangles, will be changed if the couple changes. In fact, this is one of the tenets of natural systems therapy. The two families will probably experience these shifts as uncomfortable and unfamiliar, and will have their own responses. For example, families with low differentiation tend to "pull" harder when boundaries are moved, and the pressure to move boundaries back will challenge the couple. These responses need to be predicted, planned for, and considered in couple work (Roberto, 1992).

Genograms

Assessment usually takes place in the first one to three meetings with both spouses present. Partners are not divided up for individual interviews, unless there are issues of safety and well-being to be assessed (e.g., partner violence). The major tool for identifying problem patterns is the family genogram. Genograms have been adapted in various ways for clinical use. Dynamic markings have been well developed (Guerin & Pendagast, 1976), so that dyad and TG patterns can be easily shown (see Figure 7.1).

These markings are used to make certain couple interventions, such as pointing out repeated problem patterns in bonding; generations of symptoms, such as alcoholism and codependency; or complementarity of behaviors. Initially, however, genograms guide the clinician to address problem-maintaining issues in either or both families of origin, and to plan realistically regarding long-term family change. The time-line genogram (Friedman, Rohrbaugh, & Krakauer, 1988) plots important family-of-origin events clearly in their time frames.

Genograms have also been adapted for clinicians treating specific types of couple problems, such as sexual dysfunction, family illness patterns, spiritual and religious histories, medical and genetic disorders that could affect planning of children, and even providing self-study for medical

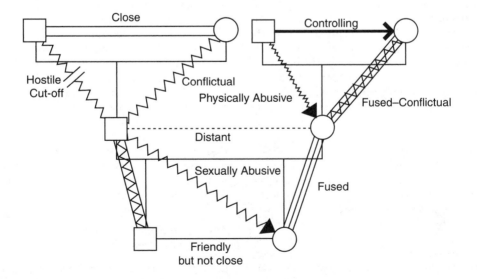

FIGURE 7.1. Relationship lines on a genogram. From McGoldrick, Shellenberger, and Gerson (1999, p. 30). Copyright 1999 by W. W. Norton & Co., Inc. Reprinted by permission.

students and their spouses. Assessment includes looking at historical patterns of work, religion, and even political affiliation. For example, a husband whose family has always been religious, with himself being the exception, will probably mean that there is tension between the husband and his spouse, and his family of origin, and this tension probably contributes to the couple's presenting problem. It is common to find people whose parents, grandparents, uncles or aunts, and even in-laws have all been physicians, businessmen, or military officers.

Whereas in other schools of couple therapy, genogram information is used to look mainly at family structure, the TG therapist is looking for multigenerational patterns (e.g., Wachtel, 1982). Sometimes patterns of relationship repeat themselves over generations without varying—spousal abuse, poor health, depression or anxiety, underachievement, abandonment and neglect, drug addiction. These patterns feed forward into marriage problems, such as distancing, fusion, chronic mistrust, communication problems, or triangling in third parties.

Finally, the clinician looks for critical incidents (e.g., natural disasters), lived trauma or violence ("common shock," e.g., war; Weingarten, 2004), and immigration/resettlement and other social upheavals that have created or challenged family coping and resilience.

The clinician uses a couple's first one or two sessions to identify key figures in each family of origin, formative events in each family's past, and the history of the marriage. Dynamic markings are made to indicate proximity and distance with key family members and within the dyad, presence of fusion or cutoff that may be affecting the boundary around the marriage, and any repetitive patterns found in more than one generation. For example, the younger partner in a couple may show a pattern of always deferring decisions to her spouse, and in her parents' marriage, her mother may also defer decisions to her father.

The couple is asked for their own narrative about the problem, and how each spouse perceives its origin, meaning, and sequence. This technique is not different from other systemic, even ahistorical therapies. However, TG therapists interview and observe couples with a "wide-angle lens" (Roberto, 1992) to inquire and track three-generational patterns of culture, marital and family structure, and beliefs about marriage. The TG therapist who asks a wife her theory of why and how she chose her partner is not looking to explain why they met, but rather for a theory that explains the needs, wishes, and drives present in that wife for many years before she courted her partner.

Spouses are asked to describe whether and how key family members have reacted to their problem to clarify whether triangles exist and need to be addressed. For example, in the classic "mother-in-law" triangle, the husband acts distant from his wife, who turns to her mother for advice, following which the husband distances more. Of course, assessment is not the same process as therapy, and not all triangles are targeted for change. However, creating a "macro" view of key participants in a couple's problems helps ensure that a clinician creates workable goals of change by understanding the forces around the couple's relationship. During therapy, participants are also more aware of potential extended-family reactions to marital changes.

Clinicians using genograms for couple assessment must be culturally competent regarding normative family structures. The dynamic markings for genograms as they currently exist are culture-blind and can imply that some relationships are pathological, when in a particular cultural group they are normative. For example, in Islamic families, the mother, mother-in-law, and other female relatives are an important support to the wife. In a hierarchical family, religion and culture are governed by men. Class also intersects with what TG therapists consider "normal" family dynamics. In poor families, young women bear children young fathers are not able to provide resources, and relatives may become central to their lives as helpers, such as child care providers. Poor families are more likely to experience chronic stress, fragmentation, unemployment, illness and addiction, violence, obstacles to education, difficulty planning children, and broad lack of access to health care. Unless the genogram contains information about class, cultural, religious, and historical differences that intersect with couple dynamics, the clinician runs the risk of pathologizing couples instead of understanding their needs and the TG meaning of their symptoms.

Assessing Relational Quality: The Clinical Interview

Each partner is interviewed regarding his or her subjective experience of the presenting problem, as well as the habitual ways the partners interact around it. TG therapies do not bypass central complaints. Rather, they use identified problems to expand the field of inquiry into the "macro" context of the couple's long-term connection with each other and with the past (Roberto, 1991). The object is to begin framing the family-of-origin context immediately, so that one can return to this frame repeatedly while addressing the couple's problem.

TG therapies utilize classical circular interviewing to identify unique differences in each partner's views. The binocular picture prized by systemic therapists emerges easily in initial assessment. Each spouse attaches personal meanings to events in the marriage, and these personal meanings must be brought into the dialogue. For example, a man may personally feel that he has deliberately tried to depend more on his lover to show his trust, whereas his lover believes that his increased dependence is only a temporary reaction to stress. *The individual meanings attached to the couple's experiences are used as the dynamic core of couple therapy to highlight each partner's emotional needs and the family inheritance behind them.* When the differences cause confusion or conflict, the couple is helped to frame them in ways that are protective of the marriage.

Timing of symptoms is very important to TG therapies. Once each partner's view of the problems is elicited, the clinician works to construct a hypothesis that accounts for their emergence at the present time. Most marital dysfunction involves repeated impasses, not isolated or short-term stressors. The clinician must have a theory about when and why those impasses reached runaway proportions. Many long-term emotional patterns combine with life stressors to "blow up" a marriage: unrealistic expectations, feelings of entitlement or frustrated wishes, low supportiveness or empathy, lack of self-expression and warmth, legacies of abuse, and maltreatment or losses that color partners' ability to extend trust or be trustworthy.

It is important to address the distribution of power—power to name problems, power to make decisions and to problem-solve, power to make requests or claims on one's spouse. Currently, there are no dynamic markings to depict power relationships on a genogram, nor have we a precise language to describe power. Assessing the distribution of power in a marriage is as important as assessing its affective and functional quality. Although some clients maintain that they do not mind an unequal balance of power, too often they avoid the issue,

because power affects privilege and resources in a relationship. For example, it may be easier for a woman to claim she has lost sexual desire because she is depressed than to admit she is dissatisfied with her mate. Money and sex are good illustrations of how a couple manages power: Are the decisions democratic, unilateral, obtained under pressure, hidden, or avoided completely?

To be "emotionally intelligent" (Schwartz & Johnson, 2000), beginning interviews must also include assessment of affect. Affective factors include the degree of security and trust in the marital bond; presence of negative attributions and/or disrespect (two of Gottman and colleagues' "Four Horsemen of the Apocalypse"), significant reactivity that might stem from fusion, dissatisfaction, and the desire for change (particularly when shown by the more accommodating partner); and emotions that might be biologically significant (related to mood and physical health). Affective tone gives important clinical information: The words "My partner asked me to come" mean one thing when said with concern, and another thing entirely when said in a manner that is flat and disengaged.

Only recently have marriage therapists understood the importance of a positive affective bond to the survival of a marriage. Each school of TG therapy tends to emphasize certain domains of information from the clinical interview, with object relations and symbolic–experiential therapists more focused on assessment of affect. As Wachtel has noted, "Such a focus enables the therapist to learn more about what the client values than he could disclose consciously" (1982, p. 340). Marital therapies need to explore and describe different types of affective bonding more clearly. For example, there are vast differences among the kinds of intensity found in a couple fused together by (1) anxiety and dependency, (2) addictive behavior, and (3) a traumatic bond through mutual abandonment or survival of loss. More work is necessary on a typology of attachment.

At the end of the assessment phase, the clinician should have a clear genogram, a description of the presenting problem from each partner's position in the marriage, a theory explaining the differences in their ideas and responses to the problem, information regarding long-term contributing factors in the families of origin, and an idea about what the partners wish to change. These ideas are fed back to the couple in the goal-setting phase of therapy. The therapist must do the following:

- Articulate mutual values and goals underlying the partners' views of commitment, including an understanding of cultural underpinnings of those values.
- Articulate any differences or conflicts between spouses' closely held beliefs and family legacies.
- Describe the position of each spouse in his or her family of origin regarding important family issues and experiences.
- Predict how these positions will shift if the partners solve their problem.
- Ally with each spouse in a way that creates a basis of trust for doing couples work and initiating change.

SETTING TREATMENT GOALS

TG couple work seeks to achieve greater relationship competence, enhance self-knowledge and self-esteem, increase partners' confidence that they can solve their own problems, and help the dyad support important individual and mutual developmental tasks (Roberto, 1992). The TG therapist recommends a relational therapy even when the problem appears individually based. Even though the general public is better informed about the value of spouse-assisted counseling for severe emotional disorders (e.g., mood and thought disorders), coming to therapy together can be daunting. And, often the serious concerns seem to be one's own burden. A common example of this is sexual dysfunction: Many clients assume that they will explore and resolve physical and emotional symptoms about sexuality individually with a therapist, then take home what they have learned. In reality, both partners have to communicate about their sexual needs. Whitaker referred to two decision points in planning MFT: the "battle for structure" and the "battle for initiative" (Napier & Whitaker, 1978). The term "battle for structure" is a somewhat adversarial way to describe how the therapist and clients agree to include the relationship as the unit of change rather than one of the partners alone.

There are two types of goals. I have made the distinction previously between mediating goals and ultimate goals in systemic work (Roberto, 1991, p. 454). In intermediate-length therapy, unlike brief, symptom-focused therapy, clinician and client couple can take the time to evolve an ongoing, deep personal bond. In this therapeutic triangle, "mediating goals" of therapy include (1) expanding the presenting problem into a TG frame, (2) activating and holding "positive anxiety" about change (Whitaker & Ryan, 1989), (3) encouraging a multilateral perspective of problems, (4) creating a boundary around the partners and their relationship work, and (5) creating a shared meaning about the origin and nature of the problem. By agreeing to ongoing work, a couple in TG therapy also creates time to investigate and understand formative family-of-origin experiences. This mediating goal that may at first seem irrelevant to the current problem becomes clearer. For example, a man with a chronically alcoholic parent is unable consistently to set limits on his involvement in his spouse's drinking. He may be asked to explore whether he believes that recovery is possible without his help, considering the fact that his own parent never sought help.

Like other types of couple therapies, TG therapies hold that ultimate goals of change are created by couple and therapist together. These can vary widely: greater autonomy; decrease in fights and tension; greater intimacy, including sexual intimacy, support of career, work, and personal development; greater self-esteem and effectiveness; commitment; empathy and nurturance; and a decision whether or not to have children. It has been noted that ultimate goals are sometimes difficult to articulate clearly (Whitaker & Keith, 1981): A couple may know only that they "aren't getting along," "aren't close anymore," or "don't have sex." Discussion of crucial family experiences and legacies helps partners to make sense of the painful issues playing out between them.

Problem-focused couple therapy addresses one problem or a prioritized list of clearly delineated problems. However, this means another course of therapy in the future, if there are other problems (Watzlawick, 1984). TG marital therapy aims to go beyond symptoms to increase a couple's relationship competence. The therapy must strengthen trustworthiness, consideration, understanding and speaking up for personal beliefs and needs, tolerance for differences, mutual respect, nurturance, and identification. I call this goal "restoration."

In the TG therapy model, because the course of therapy is intermediate-term, sessions are often held less often—typically every 2 weeks—so that partners can integrate a larger perspective, contact family-of-origin members and hold visits, and have time to focus on self. Therapy may extend from 3–12 months in length; therefore, whereas brief therapy may conclude after 3–10 sessions, TG therapies may take from 10 to 24 sessions. However, unlike most couple therapies that adjourn during holidays, TG therapies are more likely to hold family-of-origin consults (see comments later in this chapter) over 2 to 3 consecutive days while family members are in town. Such meetings are usually 2 to 2-½ hours in length to allow for a meaningful dialogue about past events and important, unresolved family issues.

ROLE OF THE THERAPIST

The Therapeutic Alliance

A strong, compassionate, "partial" (in contextual therapy terms) alliance is pivotal in this type of couple work. *Partiality replaces neutrality.* A TG focus opens up the therapy conversation to emotionally laden issues in a way that requires a high degree of trust in the therapist. Spouses discussing stories of abandonment, illness, conflict and betrayal, abuse, loss, and stressful family loyalties are looking at a dimension of experience that feels far more vulnerable than that in problem- or solution-based talk. The therapist is a participant from inside the therapeutic triad, helping to create and protect a safe environment to expand symptoms into their deeper relational context. If neutrality means that no member, after a session, can tell whose side the therapist is on, then partiality means that, after a session, each member knows that the therapist is on his or her side. Systemic neutrality, the position of therapists holding circular interviews, does not build the partial, concerned alliance necessary.

The strength of partiality provides "anesthesia for the operation," as Whitaker called it. It is only when the therapist can offer an affective connection that spouses in therapy feel empowered to work on their affective connection. Finally, as Napier commented (1983), it is a mark of our commitment to a caring and humane society that therapists offer kindness and compassion rather than the distant "expert" stance, to the clients who entrust to them their love relationships.

Use of Self: Therapeutic Transparency

Part of exercising partiality means that the TG therapist has to be actively engaged and personally responsive, which calls for a certain amount of transparency (Roberto, 1992). In the early symbolic–experiential literature, "use of self" meant "transparency." The clinician shares fragments of experience, personal reflections, and teaching stories (Roberto, 1991) to deepen, expand, or enter into a dialogue in a way that is intimate but also

instructive. As Framo wrote, it is important "that the therapist convey in some form that he has experienced pain and loss, shame, guilt, and disappointment, as well as the exhilaration and joys of living. ... It is just as unwise to support the fantasy of the therapist's life as ideal as it is to overburden clients with one's own problems" (1981, p. 147).

Use of self connotes the possibility of change for therapy couples, because the therapist is communicating thoughts and actions regarding events in and out of the therapy session that may differ from those of the spouses. The therapist's comments include a high degree of disclosure, but they are selected deliberately and thoughtfully. Issues shared with a couple must be resolved issues to be useful, so it is best not to share information that is anxiety-provoking or confusing to the therapist. Ideally, they are well-digested thoughts that while mirroring or paralleling a couple's dilemmas hold a view that leads to a solution. The therapist's self-disclosure does not have to be a lived experience, but can be a metaphor, an idea, an echo of the clients' thoughts, a reflection, a wish, or an imaginative vision.

A RELATIONSHIP IN STAGES

TG therapies unfold in stages as a couple's framework moves from the particular (events at home) to the larger system (their families of origin), and from the here and now (recurring conflicts) to the longer term (beliefs about marriage, themselves, and their union). The structure moves from high to low, the therapist moves from a central position toward the periphery, interventions move from directive to nondirective, and use of self increases (Roberto, 1991). This is not as true of Bowen therapy, but even in natural systems therapy, as clients go home to visit their families and work on diffusing triangles, the ensuing debriefings and insights probably change a therapist's role toward less directiveness.

In early-stage work, the "battles for structure and initiative" take place as the therapist recommends couple sessions and creates a setting in which partners focus on their relationship. During this time, partners are encouraged to begin self-study of their marriage, genograms are made, family histories are taken, and the marriage is examined from each partner's standpoint. The mid-phase of couple work aims to reorganize partners' understanding of key problems in a newly expanded, relational, context. Use of self communicates that the clinician understands the complexity of intimate relating, the difficulty of accepting and changing oneself, and the flux between intimacy and autonomy. Each partner becomes more clearly defined: self in relation to the other.

Late-stage couple work calls for less therapist coaching. At this point, the partners can observe themselves responding to one another without the therapist's help. They are usually reporting progress in areas of intimacy, disclosure, self-knowledge, and mutuality, and can identify and discuss flashpoints as they push themselves and each other toward change. Partners create innovative ways of supporting their own and the other's needs and requests—often in ways that the therapist could not have predicted. They are a flexible system that generates its own solutions, and the clinician serves more as a sounding board.

PROCESS AND TECHNICAL ASPECTS

Creating a Transgenerational Frame

Earlier, I explained genogramming as an assessment tool. It is also a teaching tool in early therapy (Roberto, 1992; Wachtel, 1982). When shared with the couple, it is a technique of change, because it adds to partners' sense of "where they are each coming from." The mutual self-disclosure and willingness to expose vital and often unprocessed information also has a healing quality. Creating the genogram stimulates therapist and clients to think about extended family issues, and contributes to forming connections between events in the marriage and the legacies that came before.

Genograms enable family members to develop a metaperspective together about their history. Gaining perspective helps to calm intensity and may help to diffuse a crisis atmosphere in couple work when there are "hot" conflicts, such as affairs, religious differences, parenting problems, or extreme complementarity. Where there is a power imbalance in the relationship, genogramming "levels the playing field," so that both partners must look at both strengths and challenges in their past lives. Finally, mapping the family of origin can increase a feeling of confidence that symptoms are not random but are instead responses to ongoing family issues. Therefore, it is one core technique.

Tracking Problem Cycles

If one asks where a TG clinician's focus is during a therapy session, the answer would be the same as

that for other clinicians. Dysfunctional, reactive, "stuck," conflictual, disengaged, or ineffective responses and the cycles around those responses are always the target of couple work. The therapist watches to see which spouse names the problems and which one defers, elicits their individual theories about underlying tension and differences, and observes how they handle the differences. For example, if their symptom is distance and coldness, the therapist notes what happens when one spouse tries to attract attention, and whether one or both spouses try to engage each other, and how this is done. Their structural characteristics—distance, fusion, disengagement or cutoff, conflict or pseudomutuality—are noted.

Tracking Antecedents: Trailing

A TG therapist tracks presenting problems with an eye toward antecedent events in the couple's life and the partners' own lives with their families of origin. It is like watching a "trailing cursor" on a computer mouse, looking to see where it has come from and where it is going. I call this "trailing." Trailing antecedents uses a time frame of up to two, or even three, generations.

Trailing inquiries do not replace discussion of alternative ways partners can approach relationship problems. Rather, a trailing question acknowledges another dimension of a client's experience. Trailing keeps partners located on their TG map. The experience of trailing back from complaints to antecedents makes people feel that they are "getting to the root of things." The spouse gets a sense that there is an entire family and its members' histories behind a loved one's behavior, and it makes more sense. Sparring decreases, and context and mutual understanding increase. For example, a woman who hears in session that her partner was criticized by his family for leaving school may understand more clearly that his low support for her recent promotion does not reflect lack of caring, but an unresolved conflict about being seen as equally worthy.

Family-of-Origin Consults

There are few tools so clarifying to a couple therapist as a family-of-origin consult. When a marital partner sits in to witness a meeting between the spouse and the spouse's parents and/or siblings, that clarity is even more powerful. Framo produced a body of work (1976, 1981) on his experiences in meeting families of couples in counseling. It reflects the orientation that " ... When ... adults are able to go back to deal directly with their parents and brothers and sisters about the previously avoided issues that have existed between them, an opportunity exists for reconstructive changes to come about in their marital relationship" (1981, p. 134). It is important to note that consults are rarely requested by the couple. They are a tool initiated by the therapist in midphase couple work.

Family-of-origin consults can usually occur only once or twice during couple therapy because of distance and cost. They can be scheduled in 2-hour segments on 2 consecutive days, although they have also been organized for entire extended families for up to a week (Whitaker, personal communication, October, 1979). Meetings are not structured with therapeutic tasks, but are organized around making intergenerational connections visible, explicit, and available for discussion.

Couples in therapy experience extreme anxiety about bringing parents in, and the idea should be "seeded" for at least a month prior to the meeting. There are usually many reservations that need to be worked through regarding whether the parents (and siblings, if possible) should attend. In itself, experiencing this anxiety and struggling to come to terms with it directly challenges a client's illusion that the spouse is causing all of his or her distress. One family of origin is brought in at a time. Whereas some TG therapists do not include the spouse (Framo, 1976, 1981), others believe that observing can greatly aid clarity and understanding in the marriage (Roberto, 1992). When attending, the spouse is invited to sit in without participating, because unresolved family issues are easily displaced onto a son- or daughter-in-law.

Family consults are arranged by the partner who is preparing for the visit. The invitation can be framed as: an invitation to parents to help move therapy forward by giving the family's viewpoint or to help clarify important family issues while their son or daughter is in therapy. Family members are told that they will not be made into clients by the therapist; rather, they are there to give the therapist important history. TG therapists agree on the crucial importance of respecting the generational boundary and do not demote parents in the eyes of their grown children. While awaiting the visit, the husband or wife in therapy is asked to reflect on personal concerns and issues in the marriage that may be connected to previous experiences with the family. These key experiences become part of the material for the interviews.

Siblings are sometimes reluctant to attend a consult. When this occurs, it is most probably because the client in marital therapy has formed an ambivalent relationship with that sibling, or because that sibling is even more distressed by the family than the client. It is important to expend all means to bring about sibling participation. Later, the bond formed by this visit may become a powerful means of support for the client, one that may have been absent since childhood, and create an alliance that meets needs the client once expected in the marriage.

At the consult, the client is asked to describe for the family the problems that brought him or her to couple counseling. Because this is a midphase technique, the client usually explains his or her subjective difficulties coping with stresses in their marriage. The family is encouraged to discuss what they know of their child's difficulties and to ask questions, so that the focus is firmly placed on their child. Every consult is unique in its emotionality, pace of discussion, degree of openness and disclosure, participation, and historical perspective (Framo, 1981). Some families need 2 days just to acknowledge that their son or daughter might be having relationship problems and that family issues might be involved. Others begin with a request for help from a parent that opens the way immediately for a deep and sincere discussion. The meeting can be audiotaped or videotaped, and there should be an agreement that all family members who wish to may receive a copy, including absent members.

Although couples do not explicitly connect changes in their families of origin to progress in their marriage, consults add depth to their understanding of the relational problems they have brought into their commitment. There is less other-focus, more self-observation and investment in change, and greater self-respect after a consult is held. This is true even though the consult itself may be painful or complicated. Seemingly little movement creates a very different view of self, and of self-in-relationship.

Enhancing Personal Authority

"Personal authority" in the family system (Williamson, 1981, 1982a, 1982b) is defined as the ability to discern and use one's own opinions and judgment, to choose whether or not to express oneself, to hold a metaperspective on relationships, to take responsibility for one's actions and beliefs, to choose whether and when to be close to someone, and to treat elders as peers. Williamson's work on personal authority hinges on the idea that many marital impasses reflect intergenerational intimidation and failure to develop an adult relationship with self (1981). This theory holds that, by midlife, there is a normative life-cycle transition that involves ending the hierarchy with one's parents and moving toward an adult–adult connection.

An unrecognized power issue, the investment of lifetime authority in parents, produces a tilt in the family's distribution of power that limits the personal sense of choice. The term "intimidation" refers to the reluctance we feel about challenging parents, family history, and the values with which we were reared (Roberto, 1992). Williamson suggests that in middle adulthood, the generational hierarchy of the first half of our lives has to be terminated, leaving in its place an egalitarian, mutual, give-and-take relationship. Otherwise, that hierarchy creates pressures via old legacies (unresolved issues) and delegations (unlived and transferred expectations; see Stierlin, 1981; Stierlin et al., 1973). It is an enormous challenge to "leave home" in the sense of seeing and relating to parents as peers instead of authority figures (Williamson, 1981).

A husband in his early 60s developed a psychotic depression with suicidal thoughts; left his wife, children, and grandchildren; and began living with a young woman he met in a shop, several years after his own father disinherited him and died, following which his mother refused to oppose the will and give him a share of the inheritance.

Couples commonly come for counseling in response to one or both spouses' exploitation of their marriage to conform to stagnant family relationships (e.g., expecting a partner to help care for a frail parent but refusing to give care oneself). Williamson's belief is that couples must give up their expectation of getting approval, and their image of the parents as dispensers of approval.

The technique for creating and enhancing personal authority is a coaching technique, in which the client begins to seek more information about the parent as an aging individual and to mourn the end of the parent's protection (or the wish for it). The client examines his or her lifelong perceptions of the parents, exploring these images and how they arose (Williamson, 1982a). Meetings focus on the relationship with each parent and the changes that need to occur to move the relationships forward into the here and now. The client works to express him- or herself clearly and

to ask important family questions. There is usually at least one visit home, in which the client talks one-on-one with each parent, then with both parents about their early life and experiences with love relationships. The object is for the client to see the parents as real people.

When the client is no longer reluctant to discuss parent–child issues, a family-of-origin consult is held to propose changes and to discuss them. As with any other family consult, the partner ideally should attend; he or she will have the opportunity to view significant issues that he or she previously has only heard about secondhand. It may be the first time that a woman's depression, or a man's distancing, is completely visible in the context in which it originally formed. It may be the focal point at which a client finally lets go of blaming the mate for marital problems. As Paul (1967) pointed out, facing loss has profound potential to unlock personal resources for solving problems in marriage and personal life.

CURATIVE FACTORS

Historically, couple and family therapy has never been comfortable with emotions. The models that dominated their early development (structural and strategic) were aimed primarily at changing behavior patterns and, through reframing, the cognitions that maintained them. Increasingly, due to advances in neurobiology and attachment theory, emotionality is being viewed as the underpinning of adaptive behavior and a positive organizing force in human functioning (Damasio, 1994; Johnson & Greenberg, 1994). TG therapies, with the exception of Bowen techniques, acknowledge and utilize the emotions that arise through bonding, and use them as motivators for change.

When clients listen to their own subjective responses in a dialogue with each other, reflections, emotions, beliefs, and recollected behavior are integrated (Schwarz & Johnson, 2000). If emotions carry constructive messages, as research indicates, adding them to therapeutic dialogue helps each partner "get the message." Anger can be seen as a demand for change; sadness, as loss; pleasure, as the hope and joy of connection. Conversation that includes personal responses helps to evoke in clients the respect and acceptance that couple therapists desire—it increases intimacy.

There are gender differences in expression of affect that need to be considered. Women may tend to value expression of emotion because it is normally suppressed. When women in families are marginalized from the executive unit, they are expected to accept the decisions of others and not show "negativity." Therefore, in trust relationships, women seek openly to admit the opinions and concerns that they are expected to suppress daily. From this point of view, it is important to encourage this avenue to intimacy for women and to teach men to respect and value their wives' wish to engage them in honest conversation.

In addition to integrating affect into therapy, TG therapies consider contextual and experiential learning as curative. The encounter between partners and the clinician, who participates, as well as conducts, the sessions, increases their awareness of alternative ways to solve problems. Therapist transparency has unique qualities that model disclosure and self-acceptance rather than justification and defensiveness. The processes of genogram work, and family-of-origin visits and consults, create metaperspectives on recurring problems. Like the "connect the dots" puzzle in which the solution is a single line leading *outside* the group of dots, a TG perspective allows couples to rework their marital connection in ways that are "outside" their previous cycling repertoires.

Negative Therapeutic Reactions

Freud (1937/1964) first coined the term "negative therapeutic reaction" (p. 243), referring to intense negative emotions that spike after discussing material with a therapist. Couples frequently experience negative effects during and after meetings that focus on painful subjects. In my experience, the stress of couple work exceeds the stress of family therapy, in which clients can perceive responsibility for change as shared among parents and children. For some clients there is great anxiety related to verbalizing intentions or reactions that have never been voiced in their marriage, especially in Western societies, where marriage is a voluntary contract and our rates of separation and divorce are high. Other clients find the intensity of the process overwhelming—for example, an overaccomodating spouse who "smoothes over" conflicts, or a rigid, walled-off spouse who is unaccustomed to integrating emotional information. What appears matter-of-fact or easily voiced to a clinician may be extremely difficult for clients to acknowledge.

Some couples feel shamed by the disclosure of marital problems. For example, in a European American Protestant couple, discussing sexual problems is experienced as too intimate and as evidence of personal inadequacy. A Jewish couple that prides itself on family accomplishments may feel shame after discussing job problems or destructive behavior, such as spousal abuse or addiction. A Japanese pair may feel they have "lost face" after voicing complaints about each other or their extended family. Cultural competence requires that the clinician understand his or her role in relation to families that are culturally different. Attending to partiality includes asking couples for their consent to discuss specific issues, and for feedback about their willingness to disclose each subject.

Court-mandated marital therapy is complicated by the fact that the therapist is a representative of social control. The therapist in this situation must work hard to hold the boundary between legitimate community concerns (e.g., personal or public safety) and legitimate couple concerns. These couples benefit from transparency, which enables the therapist to express the wish to help partners strengthen the relationship and protect themselves and each other of further intervention from legal or community agencies. Maintaining a TG framework for couple work does not preclude use of safety contracts, setting the terms and limits of outpatient therapy (e.g., procedures for emergency calls), creating a safe home through setting of rules, and other basic security needs. These techniques add to the client's view that the therapist cares about his or her welfare.

Applicability of Transgenerational Methods

Whitaker commented that, when interviewing a couple whose cultural legacy is different from one's own, it is best to use a cotherapist with the same heritage as the couple. The decline in use of cotherapy and treatment teams outside training institutes is related to insurance industry restrictions on therapy benefits. In the 1990s, standards of practice moved toward *every* clinician establishing and exercising a personal knowledge base, to the degree possible, for understanding and attending to cultural differences. To date, this awareness has not extended to religious differences. Couple and family work has tended to split off religious discussion to the clergy or self-identified pastoral counselors, and this schism can be seen clearly in the histories of the two major North American family associations (the American Association for Marital and Family Therapy and AFTA). In the field as a whole, spirituality has been relegated to the margins as a therapeutic resource and as a cultural identity issue. The TG clinician needs carefully to ascertain whether a couple has cultural or spiritual needs that are more effectively served by a clinician who has the same cultural heritage or religious community.

It is commonly thought that relational, dynamic therapies require intellectual or academic achievement and self-observation or insight. In fact, some of the TG theories, as well as foster care and community mental health agencies and therapeutic schools, were created from hospital-based work in large metropolitan areas comprising a spectrum of cultures, social classes, and religions. For example, symbolic–experiential theory was developed at Emory University in Atlanta, Georgia, and University of Wisconsin in Madison. The clinics at University of Wisconsin, located in the capital, serve families that include rural Lutheran families of Swedish descent, farming families, urban families, survivalist and cultist families living in remote rural areas, Czech families that historically migrated to its industrial cities for jobs, health care professionals, poor families, and clients with chronic schizophrenia and addiction.

TG therapies have a unique capacity to address gender-based problems common in Western marriage. For men, the opportunity to explore the relationship with their parents is precious. It is extraordinarily moving to see a man who has been withdrawn and unresponsive begin to examine his relationship with his parents and realize that in pushing away his wife, he has pushed away the most important and intimate relationship of his adult life. For women, whose focus may be on connection to the exclusion of their internal experience, family-of origin work creates a venue to reexamine their own needs and wishes.

There are complexities with therapy for couples from Middle Eastern, Indian and Pakistani, and Asian and Southeast Asian families. Cultural groups that ascribe power to parents and previous generations are sensitive to any intervention that may appear to lay blame on family elders. The marriage may actually be at the behest of the parents. In some societies, as mentioned earlier, couples are not viewed as a unit of two at all, on any rung of the family hierarchy. Power here is not really defined by generations of family, but rather from outside, as a reflection of religious traditions that venerate authority and duty, as well as societal mores. There are profound implications in these differences for couples' awareness and commitment to their connection as dyads. They must be treated in therapy as a segment of their family

and their religious community, or therapy may fail. Interactionally based and ahistorical therapies are likely to ask clients to "put the marriage first," or to "make a boundary around the marriage." We believe that, if properly applied, TG therapy is *uniquely* relevant for these families, because one's place in one's family is respected contextually.

CASE ILLUSTRATION

Karen and Keith, two previously divorced professionals in their 40s, requested couple therapy 3 years into their courtship. Although they considered themselves a committed couple and spent much time together and with their respective families (visits with parents and children), they did not live together. Both stated in the initial interview that they were troubled by a number of relationship problems. Keith, a musician and band leader, felt that he did not get as much of Karen's attention as he would like when he was off work during the day, and there was constant bickering, in which Karen insistently took his words and acts as personal insults and malicious slights. He could not seem to please her. Karen, the director of a nonprofit agency, worried that Keith refused all social invitations, showed little warmth to her children, and exhibited a lack of social experience and refinement that she attributed to his blue-collar background. The result of these tensions was a pattern of being overly careful (pseudomutuality) when approaching each other, marked by a lack of spontaneity and rapidly decreasing sex, combined with anger in Karen and depression in Keith.

Both had become distressed enough that they feared they would never be able to live together without the relationship deteriorating. In fact, Karen had received an exciting job offer from a larger nonprofit in the nearby capital, and wondered if she should take it.

Both partners also said that they had been miserable in their first marriages, and that their spouses had left them. Because of the chronicity of their relationship problems and the severity of the current discord, the first four sessions were devoted to exploring family-of-origin and relationship history up to the present day. A session was devoted to gathering family-of-origin and previous marital history from each partner, with the other present to observe. In genograms created for each spouse, they were asked to think about and choose the dynamic markings that described each significant relationship.

Keith saw himself as the "different," more artistic member of his hardworking New England family, the product of a closely bonded couple that married out of high school and had high expectations for him and his brothers. The youngest child, Keith described his father as a no-nonsense tradesman for whom wealth was the most important goal for his sons, and his mother as concerned mainly for his father's happiness and her sons' achievements. His father had died suddenly of heart failure; Keith had not had time to say goodbye to him. He spoke to his mother only twice a year—before the Jewish High Holy Days and around her birthday—and described his relationships with both parents as distantly polite. Keith had two older brothers living close to their mother's home. Both were professionals: a high-stakes lawyer in a fast-track litigation practice, and a physician. He did not feel respected by either of them.

His first marriage was to the high school sweetheart with whom he grew up with and who, he assumed, would give him the affection and acceptance he craved. Keith gradually felt alienated, because she had more career advancement and made more money than he, and did not seem to show appreciation. This relationship was described as originally quite close, but eventually distant–conflictual. His ex-wife had asked for a divorce in their 30s, seemingly as soon as their daughter Krista graduated from high school. His ex-wife confirmed all of his feelings that he was unvalued when she sued for, and got, most of their marital assets, their home, and even their pets. He saw Krista as disrespectful and superficial, feeling that she had looked down on him as a breadwinner and was too materialistic, and he usually felt depressed when he and Karen saw her on holidays. Keith lived in a small, undecorated, uncomfortable apartment furnished with his business equipment, and he did not socialize.

Karen, in contrast, described her childhood as magical. She and her younger brother had been good friends, and their popular parents—older, academic people—had kept the house full of visiting colleagues, friends, and neighbors. All the adults seemed to dote on the two children. She believed that she had never faced adversity. She had expected to and had done well at college and "fell into" her nonprofit job through her father's connections, without having to stress over a job search. She described her relationship with her parents as "quite close" and spoke to them often. They were a bit perplexed by her choice of Keith as a partner. Her current relationship with her brother, a his-

tory professor, was more uneasy—although they had always gotten along, they seemed to exchange only good news on the phone now and she felt a confusing lack of desire to be more disclosive.

In Karen's first marriage, she was shattered to discover that her husband had conducted a secret affair after falling in love with someone he met at work. Although she had tried to stay after the discovery to save the marriage, he later told her that he felt the relationship had been a mistake and that his lover "needed him more than she ever had." To her added horror, their son Kevin had elected to live with his father after the couple finally divorced, and she felt he sided with father and stepmother whenever she confronted him about his choice, which was often.

It was difficult for Karen and Keith to give their histories in front of each other, and at one point Keith asked if they could give history separately. He seemed to want more response from the female therapist, and said that his concern was "looking bad" in front of Karen and her family, whom he angrily dubbed "The Perfects." Because there did not seem to be dangerous (e.g., abuse-related) history, he was asked to work with Karen in the room. The couple was given the framework that hearing each other's challenges and needs would help them to understand each other in a different way. They were also encouraged to consider that although, after 3 years, it might seem that they knew each other inside and out, each was attributing motives to the other that were probably inaccurate and counterproductive. Intrigued and challenged, they began to work together.

The fifth session was used to assess the partners' goals for their work. They asked for (1) help to find some way of relating to each other instead of disconnecting with disinterest and boredom; (2) help in discussing Karen's job offer; and (3) help in constructing a social life as a couple with their families, children, and friends. The therapist noted that the process of four sessions devoted to family-of-origin and marital history had already opened a window into both spouses' pain, disappointments, and underlying needs and wishes for themselves and their family life.

Mediating goals of TG therapy call for expanding the focus of therapy to its larger family-of-origin context rather than pathologizing the couple relationship. Therefore, in the sixth through 10th sessions (the "midphase"), the couple was asked to consider what legacies (unresolved family-of-origin patterns) they had carried with them into their first marriages and into this courtship. Karen began to focus on the familiar, gratifying, attention that her parents had garnered for themselves and their children, and admitted that it had left her intolerant of disagreements, disconnected when not catered to, and easily frustrated. With active input provided by Keith and the therapist, she recognized her pattern of playing out her sense of learned entitlement with both Keith and Kevin, and their reactions of hurt and withdrawal. The therapist worked with Karen to examine specifically how her pattern of responding during conflicts was to privilege her own feelings, to assume that the other was inadequate, and to make demands that belittled and disempowered her loved ones.

Keith became aware that he avoided taking risks and held on to people and things that made him feel successful and secure, because he had not felt secure as a young person. Underlying competitiveness and resentment of the successes of others, which had emerged especially with women, caused him to withhold love and to pull back from supporting Karen and Krista. This meant that the affection he sought was withheld as the women pulled back from him in turn, which made them appear uncaring even as he blamed them for the problem. He was asked to look at how he undermined Karen when they fought, hitting "below the belt" with spiteful and rejecting yet indirect remarks that he told himself were simply giving his opinion.

In the 11th through 15th sessions, Karen and Keith were given assignments to reconnect with parents and siblings in a way that reflected their growing understanding of their roles in their families/marriage. During this process, each partner was asked to (1) accompany the other to an upcoming family function as an "anchor" in the present, (2) schedule couple time alone during the visits and stay together at night in a separate hotel, (3) debrief with each other privately when they experienced distress, rather than expecting the other to fit in and avoid family issues.

Karen was given the following tasks: (1) to focus on how Keith or Kevin were perceiving and feeling incidents at home, rather than on her own feelings; (2) to reframe her parents' legacy as handicapping (rather than preparing her) for adult intimacy; and (3) to begin speaking with her parents and brother about personal problems and ask about family problems that had not been discussed. Karen particularly decided to tell her parents about the pain she experienced when her first marriage ended. She admitted to them that

she felt she had contributed to the breakup by seeing herself and the past as perfect. She asked her parents to see her as a real person and to acknowledge that she had been raised in a somewhat self-congratulatory, self-righteous manner. Her parents responded by opening up the life experiences that had driven each of them to seek constant approval and entertainment, while neglecting personal time with their children. She and Keith made a trip to visit her brother and his wife and children, where Karen spoke with him about their childhood years and gathered her brother's memories of important family events that had previously been ignored and whitewashed. For example, he disclosed that their father had been briefly married some years before marrying their mother, and that he had left his young ex-wife and their baby because he did not find her supportive enough.

Keith was assigned to (1) tell Karen clearly and firmly what he expected and needed from her as his mate; (2) share his views with his mother and brothers regarding his talent, commitment, and success in music; (3) spend several visits alone with Krista, in which he allowed her to choose their activity and introduce him to her friends. He began calling his family and shared with his mother how he had internalized a sense that he must earn well, and that being a musician was self-indulgent and unimportant. He admitted that this had made him angry at his brothers and ex-wife, even though he was working in the profession he believed he had chosen. He and Karen attended a nephew's graduation with his brothers, and spent time talking about his father's reserve and difficulty getting his affection.

As both partners faced and challenged the sources of their perceptions and family legacies, they saw each other in a more hopeful, more respectful, less suspect light. They expressed feeling closer, more loving and sexual, and began to consider living together in Karen's home. Karen spoke with her son, admitting her own problems and apologizing for personalizing his boyhood choice. She told him how much she loved and respected him, and he in turn began to call and to visit more often.

Toward the end of the fourth month of couple work, Keith's daughter became engaged. His ex-wife contacted him about a lavish wedding shower that she and her family were planning and for which they would pay. Keith had to face the fact that he could not contribute much money. With Karen's loving support, he was able to think through realistically and with dignity how he wished to contribute, and decided instead on a satisfying personal gift that he checked out with his grateful daughter. He now felt dignified, respect-worthy and content, able to handle Karen in an assertive but warm manner, and the couple felt ready to terminate therapy and continue their life together.

NOTE

1. This chapter refers to committed couples, irrespective of sexual orientation, as spouses.

SUGGESTIONS FOR FURTHER READING

Roberto, L. G. (1992). *Transgenerational therapies.* New York: Guilford Press.

Roberto, L. G. (1998). Transgenerational family therapy. In F. M. Datillio (Ed.), *Case studies in couple and family therapy* (pp. 257–277). New York: Guilford Press.

Whitaker, C. A., & Ryan, M. C. (1989). *Midnight musings of a family therapist.* New York: Norton.

REFERENCES

Abrams, M. S. (1999). Intergenerational transmission of trauma: Recent contributions from the literature of family systems approaches to treatment. *American Journal of Psychotherapy, 53,* 225–231.

Anonymous. (1972). On the differentiation of self. In J. Framo (Ed.), *Family interaction: A dialogue between family researchers and family therapists* (pp. 111–173). New York: Springer.

Boszormenyi-Nagy, I. (1962). The concept of schizophrenia from the point of view of family treatment. *Family Process, 1,* 103–113.

Boszormenyi-Nagy, I. (1965). A theory of relationships: Experience and transaction. In I. Boszormenyi-Nagy & J. L. Framo (Eds.), *Intensive family therapy: Theoretical and practical aspects* (pp. 33–86). New York: Hoeber.

Boszormenyi-Nagy, I. (1972). Loyalty implications of the transference model in psychotherapy. *Archives of General Psychiatry, 27,* 374–380.

Boszormenyi-Nagy, I., Grunebaum, J., & Ulrich, D. (1991). Contextual family therapy. In A. S. Gurman & D. P. Kniskern (Eds.), *Handbook of family therapy* (Vol. 2, pp. 200–238). New York: Brunner/Mazel.

Boszormenyi-Nagy, I., & Krasner, B. (1986). *Between give and take: A clinical guide to contextual therapy.* New York: Brunner/Mazel.

Boszormenyi-Nagy, I., & Spark, G. (1973). *Invisible loyalties.* Hagerstown, MD: Harper & Row.

Boszormenyi-Nagy, I., & Ulrich, D. N. (1981). Contextual family therapy. In A. S. Gurman & D. P. Kniskern (Eds.), *Handbook of family therapy* (pp. 159–186). New York: Brunner/Mazel.

Bowen, M. (1974). Toward the differentiation of self in one's own family of origin. In F. Andres & J. Lorio (Eds.), *Georgetown Family Symposia* (Vol. 1). Washington, DC: Georgetown Medical Center.

Bowen, M. (1985a). The use of family theory in clinical practice. In M. Bowen (Ed.), *Family therapy in clinical practice* (3rd ed., pp. 147–181). Northvale, NJ: Aronson. (Original work published 1966)

Bowen, M. (1985b). On the differentiation of self. In M. Bowen (Ed.), *Family therapy in clinical practice* (3rd ed., pp. 467–528). Northvale, NJ: Aronson. (Original work published anonymously 1972)

Bowlby, J. (1969). *Attachment and loss: Vol. 1. Attachment.* New York: Basic Books.

Bowlby, J. (1973). *Attachment and loss: Vol. 2. Separation: Anxiety and anger.* New York: Basic Books.

Braverman, S. (1981). Family of origin: The view from the parents' side. *Family Process, 20,* 431–437.

Brown-Standridge, M. D., & Floyd, C. W. (2000). Healing bittersweet legacies: Revisiting contextual family therapy for grandparents raising grandchildren in crisis. *Journal of Marital and Family Therapy, 26,* 185–197.

Byng-Hall, J. J. (1980). The symptom bearer as marital distance regulator: Clinical implications. *Family Process, 19,* 355–365.

Campbell, J. L., Masters, M. A., & Johnson, M. E. (1998). Relationship of parental alcoholism to family-of-origin functioning and current marital satisfaction. *Journal of Addictions and Offender Counseling, 19,* 7–14.

Carter, B., & McGoldrick, M. (Eds.). (1989). *The changing family life cycle: A framework for family therapy* (2nd ed.). Boston: Allyn & Bacon.

Damasio, A. R. (1994). *Descartes' error: Emotion, reason and the human brain.* New York: Putnam.

Dicks, H. V. (1963). Object relations theory and marital status. *British Journal of Medical Psychology, 36,* 125–129.

Dicks, H. V. (1967). *Marital tensions.* New York: Basic Books.

Fairbairn, W. R. D. (1952). *An object-relations theory of the personality.* New York: Basic Books.

Falicov, C. J. (1998). The cultural meaning of family triangles. In M. McGoldrick (Ed.), *Re-visioning family therapy: Race, culture and gender in clinical practice* (pp. 37–49). New York: Guilford Press.

Fishbane, M. D. (1999). Honor thy mother and thy father: Intergenerational spirituality and Jewish tradition. In F. Walsh (Ed.), *Spiritual resources in family therapy* (pp. 136–156). New York: Guilford Press.

Fogarty, T. F. (1978). On emptiness and closeness. In E. Pendagast (Ed.), *The best of the family* (pp. 70–90). New Rochelle, NY: Center for Family Learning.

Fraiberg, S. (Ed.), & Fraiberg, L. (Collaborator). (1980). *Clinical studies in infant mental health.* New York: Basic Books.

Framo, J. (1976). Family of origin as a therapeutic resource to couples therapy: You can and should go home again. *Family Process, 15,* 193–210.

Framo, J. (1981). The integration of marital therapy with sessions with family of origin. In A. S. Gurman & D. P. Kniskern (Eds.), *Handbook of family therapy* (pp. 133–158). New York: Brunner/Mazel.

Freud, S. (1964). Analysis terminable and interminable. *Standard Edition, 23,* 216–253. (Original work published 1937)

Friedman, E. H. (1985). *Generation to generation: Family process in church and synagogue.* New York: Guilford Press.

Friedman, H., Rohrbaugh, M., & Krakauer, S. (1988). The time-line genogram: Highlighting temporal aspects of family relationships. *Family Process, 27,* 293–303.

Fromm-Reichmann, F. (1950). *Principles of intensive psychotherapy.* Chicago: University of Chicago Press.

Goldner, V. (1995). Boys will be men: A response to Terry Real's paper. Copublished simultaneously in *Journal of Feminist Family Therapy, 7,* 45–48, and in K. Weingarten (Ed.), *Cultural resistance: Challenging beliefs about men, women and therapy* (pp. 45–48). New York: Haworth.

Goldner, V. (1998). The treatment of violence and victimization in intimate relationships. *Family Process, 37,* 263–286.

Goodrich, T. J. (Ed.). (1991). *Women and power: Perspectives for family therapy.* New York: Norton.

Goodrich, T. J., Rampage, C., Ellman, B., & Halstead, K. (1988). *Feminist family therapy: A casebook.* New York: Norton.

Goodrow, K. K., & Lim, M. (1997). Bowenian theory in application: A case study of a couple intending to marry. *Journal of Family Psychotherapy, 8,* 33–42.

Gottman, J. M. (1998). *What predicts divorce.* Hillsdale, NJ: Erlbaum.

Gottman, J. M., & Levenson, R. W. (1999a). What predicts change in marital interaction over time?: A study of alternative models. *Family Process, 38,* 143–158.

Gottman, J. M., & Levenson, R. W. (1999b). How stable is marital interaction over time? *Family Process, 38,* 159–165.

Guerin, P. J. (Ed.). (1976). *Family therapy: Theory and practice.* New York: Gardner.

Guerin, P. J., Jr., & Pendagast, E. G. (1976). Evaluation of family system and genogram. In P. J. Guerin, Jr. (Ed.), *Family therapy: Theory and practice* (pp. 450–464). New York: Gardner.

Hare-Mustin, R. T. (1987). The problem of gender in family therapy theory. *Family Process, 26,* 15–33.

Hargrave, T. D. (1994). *Families and forgiveness: Healing wounds in the intergenerational family.* New York: Brunner/Mazel.

Hargrave, T. D., & Anderson, W. T. (1992). *Finishing well: Ageing and reparation in the intergenerational family.* New York: Brunner/Mazel.

Haws, W. A., & Mallinckrodt, B. (1998). Separation–individuation from family of origin and marital adjustment of recently married couples. *American Journal of Family Therapy, 26,* 293–306.

Hof, L., & Berman, E. M. (1989). The sexual genogram: Assessing family-of-origin factors in the treatment of sexual dysfunction. In D. Kantor & B. F. Okun (Eds.), *Intimate environments: Sex, intimacy, and gender in families* (pp. 292–321). New York: Guilford Press.

Jackson, D., & Lederer, W. (1968). *The mirages of marriage.* New York: Norton.

Jankowski, M. K., Leitenberg, H., Henning, K., & Coffey, P. (1999). Intergenerational transmission of dating aggression as a function of witnessing only same sex parents vs. opposite sex parents vs. both parents as perpetrators of domestic violence. *Journal of Family Violence, 14,* 267–279.

Johnson, S., & Lebow, J. (2000). The "coming of age" of couple therapy: A decade review. *Journal of Marital and Family Therapy, 26,* 23–38.

Johnson, S. M., & Greenberg, L. S. (1994). *The heart of the matter: Perspectives on emotion in marital therapy.* New York: Brunner/Mazel.

Jordan, J. V. (1991). The meaning of mutuality. In J. V. Jordan, A. G. Kaplan, J. B. Miller, I. P. Stiver, & J. L. Surrey (Eds.), *Women's growth in connection: Writings from the Stone Center* (pp. 81–96). New York: Guilford Press.

Jordan, J. V., Kaplan, A. G., Miller, J. B., Stiver, I. P., & Surrey, J. L. (Eds.). (1991). *Women's growth in connection: Writings from the Stone Center.* New York: Guilford Press.

Jory, B. (1998). The intimate justice question. In L. Hecker & S. Deacon (Eds.), *The therapist's notebook* (pp. 215–220). New York: Haworth Press.

Jory, B., & Anderson, D. (1999). Intimate justice II: Fostering mutuality, reciprocity, and accommodation in therapy for psychological abuse. *Journal of Marital and Family Therapy, 25,* 349–364.

Jory, B., Anderson, D., & Greer, C. (1997). Intimate justice: Confronting issues of accountability, respect, and freedom in treatment for abuse and violence. *Journal of Marital and Family Therapy, 23,* 399–419.

Juni, S. (1992). Family dyadic patterns in defenses and object relations. *Contemporary Family Therapy: An International Journal, 14,* 259–268.

Kerr, M. E. (1981). Family systems theory and therapy. In A. S. Gurman & D. P. Kniskern (Eds.), *Handbook of family therapy* (pp. 226–264). New York: Brunner/Mazel.

Kerr, M. E. (1985). Obstacles to differentiation of self. In A. S. Gurman (Ed.), *Casebook of marital therapy* (pp. 111–154). New York: Guilford Press.

Klein, M. (1957). *Envy and gratitude.* New York: Basic Books.

Knudson-Martin, C. (1994). The female voice: Applications to Bowen's family systems theory. *Journal of Marital and Family Therapy, 20,* 35–46.

Knudson-Martin, C., & Mahoney, A. R. (1999). Beyond different worlds: A "postgender" approach to relational development. *Family Process, 38,* 325–340.

Larson, J. H., & Thayne, T. R. (1998). Marital attitudes and personal readiness for marriage of young adult children on alcoholics. *Alcoholism Quarterly, 16*, 59–73.

Lebow, J. L. (1999). Building a science of couple relationships: Comments on two articles by Gottman and Levenson. *Family Process, 38*, 167–173.

Litvak-Hirsch, T., & Bar-On, D. (2006). To rebuild lives: A longitudinal study of the influences of the Holocaust on relationships among three generations of women in one family. *Family Process, 45*, 465–483.

Mahler, M., Pine, F., & Bergman, A. (1975). *The psychological birth of the human infant: Symbiosis and individuation.* New York: Basic Books.

Manlove, J. (1997). Early motherhood in an intergenerational perspective: The experiences of a British cohort. *Journal of Marriage and the Family, 59*, 263–279.

McGoldrick, M. (1989). Ethnicity and the family life cycle. In B. Carter & M. McGoldrick (Eds.), *The changing family life cycle: A framework for family therapy* (pp. 70–91). Boston: Allyn & Bacon.

McGoldrick, M. (1995). *You can go home again: Reconnecting with your family.* New York: Norton.

McGoldrick, M., Anderson, C. M., & Walsh, F. (Eds.). (1989). *Women in families.* New York: Norton

McGoldrick, M., Pearce, J. K., & Giordano, J. (Eds.). (1982). *Ethnicity and family therapy.* New York: Guilford Press.

McGoldrick, M., Shellenberger, S., & Gerson, R. (1999). *Genograms: Assessment and intervention* (2nd ed.). New York: Norton.

Minuchin, S., Montalvo, B., Guerney, B. G., Rosman, B. L., & Schumer, F. (1967). *Families of the slums: An exploration of their structure and treatment.* New York: Basic Books.

Napier, A. Y. (1983). *Coming of age: Reflections on the journey.* General session presented at the 41st Annual Meeting of the American Association for Marriage and Family Therapy, Washington, DC.

Napier, A. Y., & Whitaker, C. A. (1978). *The family crucible.* New York: Harper & Row.

Neill, J. R., & Kniskern, D. P. (Eds.). (1982). *From psyche to system: The evolving therapy of Carl Whitaker.* New York: Guilford Press.

Nelson, B. S., & Wampler, K. S. (2000). Systemic effects of trauma in clinic couples: An exploratory study of secondary trauma resulting from childhood abuse. *Journal of Marital and Family Therapy, 26*, 171–184.

Palazzoli, M. S. (1974). *Self-starvation: From the intrapsychic to the transpersonal approach to anorexia nervosa.* London: Human Context Books.

Paul, N. L. (1967). The role of mourning and empathy in conjoint marital therapy. In G. H. Zuk & I. Boszormenyi-Nagy (Eds.), *Family therapy and disturbed families* (pp. 186–205). Palo Alto, CA: Science and Behavior Books.

Prest, L. A., Benson, M. J., & Protinsky, H. O. (1998). Family of origin and current relationship influences on codependency. *Family Process, 37*, 513–528.

Roberto, L. G. (1991). Symbolic–experiential family therapy. In A. S. Gurman & D. P. Kniskern (Eds.), *Handbook of family therapy* (Vol. II, pp. 444–476). New York: Brunner/Mazel.

Roberto, L. G. (1992). *Transgenerational therapies.* New York: Guilford Press.

Roberto, L. G. (1998). Transgenerational family therapy. In F. M. Datillio (Eds.), *Case studies in couple and family therapy: Systemic and cognitive perspectives* (pp. 257–277). New York: Guilford Press.

Roberto-Forman, L. (2002). Transgenerational marital therapy. In A. S. Gurman & N. S. Jacobson (Eds.), *Clinical handbook of couple therapy* (pp. 118–147). New York: Guilford Press.

Sager, C. J. (1976). *Marriage contracts and couple therapy.* New York: Brunner/Mazel.

Satir, V. (1983). *Conjoint family therapy* (3rd ed.). Palo Alto, CA: Science and Behavior Books.

Scharff, D. E. (1989). Family therapy and sexual development: An object relations approach. In D. Kantor & B. F. Okun (Eds.), *Intimate environments: Sex, intimacy, and gender in families* (pp. 1–27). New York: Guilford Press.

Scharff, D. E., & Bagnini, C. (2002). Object relations couple therapy. In A. S. Gurman & N. S. Jacobson (Eds.), *Clinical handbook of couple therapy* (pp. 59–85). New York: Guilford Press.

Scharff, D. E., & Scharff, J. S. (1987). *Object relations family therapy.* Northvale, NJ: Aronson.

Scheel, M. J., Forsythe, N., Kristjansson, S., Pranata, H., Packard, T., & Packard, K. (2000). Marital enrichment: Linking research to practice. *The Family Psychologist, 16*, 6–10.

Schnarch, D. (1997). *Passionate marriage: Love, sex, and intimacy in emotionally committed relationships.* New York: Holt.

Schwartz, R. C., & Johnson, S. M. (2000). Commentary: Does couple and family therapy have emotional intelligence? *Family Process, 39*, 29–33.

Searles, H. F. (1960). *The nonhuman environment in normal development and in schizophrenia.* New York: International Universities Press.

Siegel, D. (2006, June). *Brain, culture, and development.* Lecture presented to the annual meeting of the American Family Therapy Academy, Chicago, IL.

Silverstein, R., Buxbaum Bass, L., Tuttle, A., Knudson-Martin, C., & Huenergardt, D. (2006). What does it mean to be relational?: A framework for assessment and practice. *Family Process, 45*, 391–405.

Slipp, S. (1984). *Object relations: A dynamic bridge between individual and family treatment.* New York: Aronson.

Slipp, S. (1994). *Object relations and gender development.* Paper presented to 16th Annual Meetings of American Family Therapy Academy, Santa Fe, NM.

Stierlin, H. (1981). *Separating parents and adolescents* (2nd ed.). New York: Aronson.

Stierlin, H., Levi, L., & Savard, R. (1973). Centrifugal versus centripetal separation in adolescence: Two patterns and some of their implications. In S. Feinstein & P. Giovacchini (Eds.), *Annals of American Society of Adolescent Psychiatry* (Vol. 2, pp. 211–239). New York: Basic Books.

Sullivan, H. S. (1953). *The interpersonal theory of psychiatry.* New York: Norton.

Tamura, T., & Lau, A. (1999). Connectedness versus separateness: Applicability of family therapy to Japanese families. *Family Process, 31,* 319–340.

Thornton, A. (1991). Influence of the marital history of parents on the marital and cohabitational experiences of children. *American Journal of Sociology, 96,* 868–894.

VanLear, C. A. (1972). Marital communication across the generations: Learning and rebellion, continuity and change. *Journal of Social and Personal Relationships, 9,* 103–123.

Vardi, D. (1990). *Nerot zikaron* [Memorial candles]. Jerusalem: Keter.

Wachtel, E. F. (1982). The family psyche over three generations: The genogram revisited. *Journal of Marital and Family Therapy, 8,* 335–343.

Wachtel, E. F., & Wachtel, P. L. (1985). *Family dynamics in individual psychotherapy: A guide to clinical strategies.* New York: Guilford Press.

Wallerstein, J. S. (1996). The psychological tasks of marriage II. *American Journal of Orthopsychiatry, 66,* 217–227.

Walters, M., Carter, B., Papp, P., & Silverstein, O. (1988). *The invisible web: Gender patterns in family relationships.* New York: Guilford Press.

Watzlawick, P. (1984). *The problems of change, the change of problems.* Invited seminar, Eastern Virginia Family Therapy Institute, Norfolk, VA.

Weingarten, K. (2004). *Common shock: Witnessing violence every day.* New York: Signet.

Whitaker, C. A. (1982). Gatherings. In J. R. Neill & D. P. Kniskern (Eds.), *From psyche to system: The evolving therapy of Carl Whitaker* (pp. 365–375). New York: Guilford Press.

Whitaker, C. A., & Keith, D. V. (1981). Symbolic–experiential family therapy. In A. S. Gurman & D. P. Kniskern (Eds.), *Handbook of family therapy* (Vol. 1, pp. 187–224). New York: Brunner/Mazel.

Whitaker, C. A., & Ryan, M. C. (1989). *Midnight musings of a family therapist.* New York: Norton.

Williamson, D. (1981). Personal authority via termination of the intergenerational hierarchical boundary: A "new" stage in the family life cycle. *Journal of Marital and Family Therapy, 7,* 441–452.

Williamson, D. (1982a). Personal authority in family experience via termination of the intergenerational hierarchical boundary: Part II. The consultation process and the therapeutic method. *Journal of Marital and Family Therapy, 8,* 23–37.

Williamson, D. (1982b). Personal authority in family experience via termination of the intergenerational hierarchical boundary: Part III. Personal authority defined, and the power of play in the change process. *Journal of Marital and Family Therapy, 8,* 309–323.

Winnicott, D. W. (1965). *The maturational processes and the facilitating environment.* New York: International Universities Press.

Wynne, L. (1965). Some indications and contraindications for exploratory family therapy. In I. Boszormenyi-Nagy & J. Framo (Eds.), *Intensive family therapy: Theoretical and practical aspects* (pp. 289–322). New York: Harper & Row.

Social Constructionist Approaches

CHAPTER 8

Narrative Couple Therapy

JILL FREEDMAN
GENE COMBS

BACKGROUND OF THE APPROACH

Narrative therapy, as we (Freedman & Combs, 1996, 2002) think of it, is a growing body of ideas and practices (e.g., Brown & Augusta-Scott, 2007; Freeman, Epston, & Lobovits, 1997; Monk, Winslade, Crocket, & Epston, 1997; Morgan 2000; Payne, 2000/2006; White, 2007; Zimmerman & Dickerson 1996) that stems from the work of Michael White and David Epston (1990, 1992). Michael White's early published work (e.g., 1986) was based on ideas from the work of Gregory Bateson (1972), which gave it some theoretical overlap with strategic and cybernetic approaches to therapy. David Epston (1989, 1998), who had encountered the narrative metaphor in studying anthropology, and Cheryl White, "who had enthusiasm for this analogy from her readings in feminism" (White & Epston, 1990, p. xvi), encouraged Michael White to use the "story analogy"—the notion that meaning is constituted through the stories we tell and hear concerning our lives. Their advice proved fruitful, so much so that since the early 1990s *narrative* has been the central organizing metaphor for this approach to therapy.

Therapists who began to use the narrative metaphor in the manner of White and Epston experienced quite a large shift in their worldview.

Instead of trying to solve problems, we began to focus collaboratively on enriching the narratives of people's lives. We work to bring forth and develop "thick descriptions" (Geertz, 1978; Ryle, 1971/1990) or rich, meaningful, multistranded stories of those aspects of people's life narratives that lie outside the influence of problems. Through these alternative stories, people can live out new identities, new possibilities for relationship, and new futures.

In therapy organized by the narrative metaphor, we work to help people find new meaning in their lives by experiencing, telling, and retelling stories of as-yet-unstoried aspects of their lives. Imagine that each of the dots below represents a life experience:

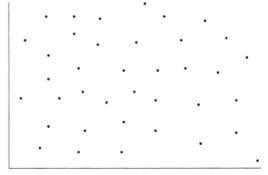

When people consult with a therapist, they are usually caught up in a rather thin story that focuses on only a few of their many life experiences:

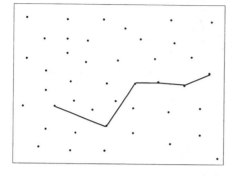

.As therapists, our first job is to listen to this story and orient to it as one of many possible stories. Listening with that attitude helps us notice when people make implicit or explicit reference to events that would not be predicted by the plot of the problematic story. The circled dot below represents such an event.

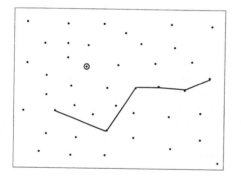

We can then ask questions that invite people to step into those events, and to tell us (and themselves) about the events and the meaning of the events, developing them into memorable and vivid stories, as represented by the new story line in the next picture.

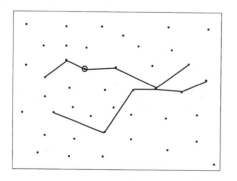

Over time, this process leads to the development of multiple story lines with rich and complex meanings that speak of multiple possibilities for people's lives:

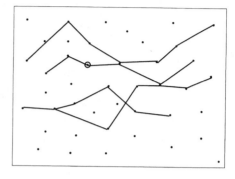

This process does not take away problematic stories, but problematic stories often have a different meaning when they are only one strand of a multistranded story.

This work is more complex than a brief description of the narrative metaphor might suggest. One factor that adds to the complexity is the interplay between culture and stories. In any given culture, some stories have the support of the powers that be, and others do not. Certain stories are much more a part of the taken-for-granted fabric of day-to-day reality than are others. We are born into the dominant stories of our local culture, and they shape our perceptions of what is possible from the day of our birth. However, people do not usually think of the stories they are born into as stories. They think of them as "reality."

Poststructuralism, especially as it is expressed in the late work of Michel Foucault (1980, 1985), has been an important influence on how narrative therapists work with the stories that circulate in our local cultures. Foucault, a French intellectual, studied, among other things, the various ways that Western society has categorized some people as normal and others as not normal. He examined madness (1965), illness (1975), criminality (1977), and sexuality (1985) as concepts around which we have "othered" people by declaring them to be insane, sick, criminal, or perverted. He described how we have separated people, oppressed them, or enrolled them in self-policing on the basis of such distinctions.

To Foucault, people have power in a society in direct proportion to their ability to participate in the various discourses that shape that society. Scholars like Foucault use the word "discourses" to refer to the ongoing political–historical–

institutional conversations within a society that constitute our notions of what is true and what is possible. Foucault showed how the people whose voices dominate the discussion about what constitutes madness, for example, can separate the people *they* see as mad from "polite society," sequestering them in madhouses, where their voices cannot reverberate within the avenues of power.

Foucault argued that there is an inseparable link between knowledge and power. Because the discourses of a society determine which bits of knowledge are held to be true, right, or proper in that society, those who most powerfully influence the discourse control knowledge. At the same time, the dominant knowledge of a given milieu determines who will be able to occupy its powerful positions. We see the discourses of power that Foucault studied as historical, cultural stories—grand narratives that have shaped (and been shaped by) the distribution of power in society.

We all know that society is not necessarily benign, fair, or just. Feminist critics of family therapy (e.g., Avis, 1985; Carter, Papp, Silverstein, & Walters, 1984; Goldner, 1985a, 1985b; Hare-Mustin, 1978; Laird, 1989; Taggart, 1985) have reminded us how, even when we try not to, we see certain possibilities as desirable and are blind to other possibilities. Laird (1989, p. 430) writes, "Sociocultural narratives ... construct the contextual realms of possibility from which individuals and families can select the ingredients and forms for their own narratives." Some people have easier access to a wider range of sociocultural narratives than others. Laird (1989, p. 431) draws our attention to the politics of storymaking when she writes, "Clearly there are both obvious and subtle differences in the power individuals and particular interest groups possess to ensure that particular narratives will prevail in family, group, and national life. Not all stories are equal."

In our experience, some people think that when we emphasize stories and reauthoring, we are acting from a belief that one story is as good as another, and that "nothing is real." We do believe that the stories that shape the meaning of life events are socially constructed, but we do not believe that meaning is trivial, or that meaning is easy to change. Socially constructed narratives have real effects. For example, the myth that "welfare mothers" are engaged in a mini-industry in which they get richer and richer as they make more and more babies has had real effects on already underserved women and children. It has provided a rationalization that has allowed those in power to

cut funds even further. The widely circulated stories in which inner-city males are only interested in drugs, sex, and killing each other support the perverse glorification of certain kinds of misogyny and violence. At the same time, they have served as a rationale for giving up on social policies that might offer inner-city males a real chance at a different way of making it in the world. More pertinent to this chapter is the current struggle over stories of marriage—for instance, the politics of whether same-sex couples can legally be storied as partners in a marriage.

Foucault was especially interested in how the "truth claims" carried in the "grand abstractions" of certain forms of empirical science constitute a discourse that dehumanizes and objectifies many people. He was interested in finding and circulating marginalized discourses—stories that exist, but are not widely circulated or powerfully endorsed—that might undermine the excessive power of the reductionistic scientific discourse. Foucault (1980, pp. 80–84) wrote of the "amazing efficacy of discontinuous, particular, and local criticism" in bringing about a "return of knowledge" or "an insurrection of subjugated knowledges."

Following Foucault (1980), we believe that even in the most marginalized and disempowered of lives, there is always lived experience that lies outside the dominant stories. Narrative therapists have developed ways of thinking and working that bring forth the "discontinuous, particular, and local" (p. 80) stories of couples and other social groups, so that people can inhabit and lay claim to the many possibilities for their lives that lie beyond the pale of dominant narratives.

When we use the narrative metaphor and the lens of poststructuralism to orient our work as therapists, we cultivate an intense curiosity about each new couple we meet. We cherish each couple's stories. We work to invite partners to celebrate their differences and to develop and live out narratives that they prefer around the particularities of their lives. This valuing of the meaning people make of their own experience over the meaning experts make of that experience has been referred to as the "interpretive turn" (Bruner, 1986). It leads us to decenter our meanings and to conduct ourselves not as experts, but as interested collaborators—perhaps with an anthropological or biographical or field researcher's bent—who are skilled at asking questions to bring forth the knowledge and experience carried in the particular stories of the couples with whom we work.

We work to help people notice the influence of restrictive cultural stories in their lives, and to expand and enrich their own life narratives. We strive to find ways to spread the news of triumphs; to circulate stories of accomplishment, fulfillment, and meaningful struggle in order to keep them alive and growing. We believe that these alternative stories of nonstandard lives keep our culture growing and flowing.

THE HEALTHY/WELL-FUNCTIONING VERSUS PATHOLOGICAL/DYSFUNCTIONAL COUPLE/MARRIAGE

"Healthy," well-functioning," "pathological," and "dysfunctional" are not descriptions we generally use. Such terms suggest preset normative scales of the sort that, following Foucault, we want to invite people to avoid. As narrative therapists, one of our principal intentions is to subvert the dominant practice in our society of measuring ourselves, our relationships, and others by standardized norms. For us, two-dimensional normative scales (healthy–ill, gifted–impaired, etc.) invite therapists and the couples who consult with them into thin descriptions—pallid, reductionist accounts—of their multistoried lives. These two-dimensional scales pervade contemporary Western culture, and each of them coexists with a prescriptive story about the right or healthy or successful way to live or to have a relationship. None of us can measure up to the demands of all these norms. When we use them, we are inevitably too fat or too thin, too driven or too passive, too caring or not caring enough. Our relationships are too rigid or too enmeshed, too focused on sex or not sexy enough, too hot or too cold. Even when we do measure up, it is within the dictates of a thin, two-dimensional story.

This does not mean that we are opposed to health or that we approve of dysfunction; it just means that we are cautious about terminology, especially terminology that supports dominant norms. We do make ongoing assessments of the effects of our work with couples. We want people to like the stories they are living out together. We want those stories to support meanings and actions that do not harm or impair other people. Every relationship can be expressed and experienced through a great variety of narratives; many "true" stories may be told about any experience. We take the stories that are currently shaping a relationship and seek to facilitate a collaborative reauthoring process in which more suitable stories can be expressed and experienced.

Because we do not consider the partners in a couple to have essential, relatively fixed, core identities with predictable, stable characteristics, we do not look for fixed or predictable qualities such as "health" or "dysfunctionality" within them. Keeping in mind the interpretive turn, we are interested in people's own evaluations of what is problematic and what is preferred. We want to hear their stories of how the problems they name affect their lives and relationships. This does not mean that we think "anything goes." We are full participants in the process of therapy, and we inevitably bring our own opinions and hard-won lived experience (and biases) along with us. For example, we are opposed to (among other things) abuse, coercion, and cruelty. When one of these problems appears to have invaded a relationship, we consider it our responsibility to ask questions that invite couple members to consider the effects of that problem on their life, their partners' life, and their relationship, and to consider the stand they want to take in relation to it.

We seek to create an interactional space in which people can take responsibility for addressing and ameliorating the effects of problems. To us, this means that we must avoid lecturing or imposing rules from a position of moral superiority. Instead, we want to invite people to bring their "best selves" into a consideration of the problems that diminish their relationship and an exploration of how they might choose ways of living that diminish the effect of the problems on their relationship.

Rather than looking for pathology or flawed functioning within couples, we work to develop awareness of problematic discourses and offer couples the opportunity to describe and evaluate the effects of those discourses on their relationship. To illustrate, let us discuss a conversation our team had with Pat and Bill. Pat complained that Bill always walked ahead of her, and at malls always led them into the stores he wanted to shop in, not the ones she would prefer. When Pat noticed this pattern, she wondered whether it meant that she was a slow person or that Bill did not care about her and her preferences. Bill thought all it meant was that he was a fast walker. As we asked questions to explore the cultural stories that shaped their way of walking, it seemed to all of us that gender socialization had supported Bill in unthinkingly setting the pace and Pat in unthinkingly following along, even though it made her feel like a "little girl" or a "puppy dog." Our conversation allowed Pat and Bill to separate themselves from the problem, notice the effects it had on their lives, and consider what they would prefer for their relationship.

We have worked with couples in which corporate values have played the largest role in creating problems, keeping one member of the couple unavailable and inattentive to what was most important to both him- or herself and to the relationship. We have also worked with couples in which differences in social class contributed to problematic power relations and bred fear and doubt in the relationship. In both instances, the stories about discourses that negatively influenced their relationship, and their preferred directions in life, emerged in collaborative conversation with a couple. Our desires in each instance were for the couple to have the last word as to what was preferred, and for the choices to be made within a multidimensional domain, not against a two-dimensional yardstick.

THE PRACTICE OF COUPLE THERAPY
The Structure of the Therapy Process

Although we take an active role in structuring the therapy, we ask couples to collaborate with us so that the process will fit their circumstances.

Length, Frequency, and Number of Meetings

We negotiate the time of each next meeting as we go along, one session at a time. At the end of meetings with couples, we ask whether the conversation has been useful. If it has, we ask how. Then we ask whether the couple would like to meet again and if so, when.

We ask couples to make these decisions each time, so that they are at least as active as we are in evaluating what schedule would be most useful. Sometimes, such as when partners are in the middle of intense conversations, they want to return very soon. More often, because they have been hearing each other in new ways and making new distinctions, they are interested in allowing some time between sessions so they can find out what difference these new experiences will make in their lives. We listen as they negotiate with each other about how long their explorations might take. Occasionally, because they are not sure how much time would be useful, partners decide to telephone us for the next appointment. If we have an opinion, we offer it—

especially when the couple seems undecided—but we are careful not to impose it.

We generally meet with couples for 60 minutes at a time, but we have negotiated longer meeting times when we all agreed that more time would be useful and affordable.

How long therapy lasts is highly variable and is determined by each couple. Some couples come to consult about a single, clearly defined problem; therapy in such circumstances may require only a very few meetings. Other couples become involved in developing very rich, detailed stories of their lives together, and find therapy a continuing help in the process. Their therapy may go on for several years. Most are somewhere in between.

Focusing on New Directions in Life

Sometimes it seems that simply sitting down for a meeting with a therapist invites people to reimmerse themselves in their most problematic stories. Because of this, we try from the first to invite people to explore, describe, and experience new directions in life that are already unfolding—new distinctions, positions they have taken about their relationship to problems, and new stories. Sometimes we read our notes from the previous session aloud and ask a question such as, "Can you tell us about new developments that relate to what we were talking about last time?" Sometimes we begin by wondering whether there have been important thoughts or events that connect to possibilities identified in our previous conversation.

Another way we structure therapy is through thinking about how to keep stories alive and growing between conversations. We use letters, documents, videotapes, and the like to document and circulate alternative stories. For example, after a therapy interview we may write a letter posing questions that invite the partners to develop an alternative story even further than they had in the interview, or we may send a document noting the stands they have taken in regard to a problem. We think that reading such a document between therapy meetings, and the conversations that may follow such a reading, can contribute to keeping a story alive and growing.

Medication

We are not opposed to the responsible, thoughtful use of medications when people find them helpful. Ideas about medication are so pervasive in contemporary culture that the people who come to us often raise the issue before we think about it. Even so, medications are rarely a primary focus of couple therapy. If it seems that either or both partners struggle with problems that are so pervasive and intrusive that medication might be called for, then we suggest that they consult a psychiatrist, and we will work with him or her as a colleague. If something about one partner's medication or the condition for which it is being prescribed proves to be problematic or divisive for a couple, we address it in the same manner that we address other problems—asking each partner to describe the problem and its effects, considering discourses that might be shaping or supporting the problem, identifying unique outcomes (those events that stand outside of and would not be predicted by the problem story) concerning the problem, and developing the stories of those unique outcomes.

The Role of the Therapist

David Epston (1999, pp. 141–142) writes,

> I chose to orient myself around the co-research metaphor both because of its beguiling familiarity and because it radically departed from conventional clinical practice. It brought together the very respectable notion of research with the rather odd idea of the coproduction of knowledge by sufferers and therapist. … This has led, and continually leads, to practices to discover a "knowing" in such a fashion that all parties to it could make good use of it. Such knowledges are fiercely and unashamedly pragmatic.

We join Epston in thinking of our work as coresearch.

White (2000) describes a therapist's role in this work as decentered but influential. We participate, not as enforcers of professional knowledge, not as authorities on what constitutes a normal or healthy relationship, but as people with skills in facilitating a coresearch project.

We ask questions to help expose gaps or contradictions in the problematic stories that bring couples to therapy, and to open space for and describe alternatives. We work to keep the conversation focused and relevant. We facilitate people's ongoing evaluation of the process by asking how the conversation is going for them and responding to their answers. At times, we reflect and offer alternative directions for our conversations.

We work to create a collaborative context. We situate our ideas in our own experience and make our intentions transparent. We encourage couples to ask questions about our questions and

comments. When therapy goes well (and sometimes even when it does not) we all change. We acknowledge to couples how our work and lives are enriched through meeting with them.

Although we avoid the position of making professional, "expert" assessments, we acknowledge that the role of therapist/interviewer is a powerful one. Each question we ask directs attention to a particular domain and away from many others. We want people to make meaning of their own experience, but our questions inevitably shape the inquiry. For this reason, we situate our questions; that is, we describe where they come from and our intentions in asking them so that people can evaluate our bias and decide how to relate to it. We believe that people are in a better position to interpret, make meaning of, and evaluate their own experience than outsiders are, even outsiders trained to help.

When we participate as coresearchers, we have more questions than answers. The following are some of the questions we (Freedman & Combs, 2000) have found it useful to ask ourselves in order to keep a coresearcher perspective:

- Whose voice is being privileged in this relationship? What is the effect of that on the relationship and on the process of therapy?
- Is anyone showing signs of being closed down, not able to fully enter into the work? If so, what power relations/discourses are contributing to the closing down?
- What are we doing to foster collaboration? Among whom? What is the effect of that collaboration?
- Is this relationship opening up or closing down the experience of "agency" (of being an active agent of change in one's own behalf)?
- Does this relationship take into account other relevant people, communities, and cultures? Are we considering how the ripples of this relationship affect other relationships?
- Are we asking whether and how the work is useful, and modifying it according to the answers we hear?

Assessment and Treatment Planning

In therapeutic conversations, we think about "generating experience" rather than "gathering information." In a rather literal way, we believe that we are making ourselves and each other up as we go along. This is a poststructuralist idea. We do not assume that a couple has a particular interactional or relational structure that we can assess. We do not think of people or relationships as having stable, quantifiable identities or "typical" characteristics, so we do not try to discover or gather information about such characteristics. Instead, we think of people's lives as being multistoried, and we believe that each new telling of a story generates new possibilities for making meaning and taking action.

Because we do not subscribe to normative ideas of what constitutes a healthy couple relationship, any assessments we might make are ad hoc and tentative. Instead of assessing, we are interested in hearing detailed, context-specific narratives. As we ask questions to bring forth their stories, we encourage those with whom we work to evaluate problems and their relationship to problems, as well as the therapy itself.

We ask questions that invite the partners in a couple to:

- Evaluate their current situation.
- Name the problems involved.
- Evaluate their relationship to those problems.
- Take a stand in regard to them.
- Tell more satisfying stories of their relationship.
- Evaluate the usefulness of the alternative stories.

We want to know whether the alternative stories speak to people of a more satisfying identity as a couple. In telling the new stories and reflecting on them, partners collaborate with us in an ongoing evaluation of their new expressions of themselves and their relationship.

Here are some questions we might ask in inviting people's evaluation of their situation and of their therapy experience:

- What name would you give the problem?
- What is it like to experience the problem?
- What effect does the problem have on your life?
- What effect does the problem have on your relationship with each other?
- What has it talked you into about your partner? What impact has that had?
- What effect does the problem have on other relationships?
- How does the problem alter your relationship with yourself?
- Is this what you want for your relationship? Why or why not?
- Is this what you want for yourself? Why or why not?

- Are we talking about what you want to be talking about?
- Is this conversation useful?
- How is it useful?

In telling and living out the strands of alternative stories, the partners in a couple evaluate many aspects of their lives: their private thoughts, feelings, hopes and fears, their dyadic interactions, the contributions of each partner's culture of origin to the couple and to the individual partners, their interrelationship with local institutions and traditions, and more.

Although we bend over backwards to avoid "expert," categorical, reductionist assessment, it would be misleading to imply that we make no assessments of any kind. One kind of assessment that we make has to do with which parts of a couple's story might be shaped by discourses that are invisible to the partners. We ask questions that invite people to unmask the operations of such discourses, and that offer them an opportunity to decide where they stand and how they would like their relationship to be in the face of such discourses.

We think it is important for people to evaluate the power relations in which they participate. This leads us to ask questions that invite them to consider the effects of discourses of gender, ethnicity, heterosexual dominance, class, corporate culture, patriarchy, age, or other sociocultural factors on their relationship. We try to have thoughtful, interactive conversations in which each question is responsive to the previous answer. It is difficult to capture the mood and tone of such inquiries in a series of hypothetical questions. We would not ask these questions in the beginning of a conversation. They would follow a detailed telling of a particular experience. We might initiate such a conversation with questions similar to those that follow:

- Martha, you have just said that fear of humiliation keeps you from wanting to go to social events with Brian. You described his failure to introduce you to people he knows and his talking over you when you try to join in. Is that right?
- Brian, what is it like to hear your actions being described that way? Does it fit with how you like to think of yourself?
- What or who do you think might have introduced you to this way of acting?
- Your father and uncles undoubtedly did not make up this way of being. Where do you think they might have learned it?

- Martha, I've noticed that all of these examples are of men. Do you think that is a coincidence?
- Do you think it is a way of acting only to women, or do you see it with children as well?
- What should we call this way of acting?
- Brian, what do you think it might be like to be a woman or child who experiences discounting?
- Is this what you would want women and children to experience from you? Why not? What would you rather have them know about you?
- You have already said, Martha, that this discounting keeps you from wanting to socialize with Brian. Are there other ways it affects your relationship?
- Is this what you want for your relationship? What would you prefer?
- We've been talking about a strand of our culture in which women and children are invisible or are considered to be property. It is clear, Brian, that this does not fit with your thinking, although you have gotten pulled into some ways of acting that go with it. What name would you give to the ways of acting that you prefer?
- Martha, do you think you've been pulled into some of the actions that go with these ideas as well?
- What would you name them?
- What has that been like for you?
- What has it been like for the relationship, do you think? How would you prefer your relationship to be?

Because we think that "self," "identity," "personhood," and the like are experiences that emerge and are always changing *in relationship*, we do not know exactly which "self" will be answering when we ask a person to draw a distinction or to evaluate the effect of an action. To make this transparent, we might ask, "Is that the problem speaking?" or "Whose values are guiding you in saying that, gay culture's or straight culture's?"

In exposing discourses that support problems, couples can separate from the ways of being that are supported by those discourses, and identify and recognize preferred perceptions, attitudes, and actions. Although we do not think of strengths or resources as fixed commodities, and we do not administer questionnaires to inventory them, we are very interested to hear the stories of relationships and events that help people to have a sense of choice, agency, purpose, and accomplishment in their lives, both as individuals and as partners in a couple.

Goal Setting

Our general goal in therapy is to collaborate with people in living out, moment-by-moment, choice-by-choice, life stories that they prefer, that are more just, and that make their worlds more satisfying. We are more interested in opening up possibilities than in closing them down. This makes us wary of "goal setting" as it is usually defined and practiced. We think that unless they are very tentatively set and rigorously updated, goals can set single, specific trajectories for people's lives. This can all too easily close down possibilities. The narrative metaphor biases us toward thinking about possibilities that unfold in living out a story, rather than about goals, which are usually set in advance and pursued more or less singlemindedly. Instead of goals, we tend to speak of "projects" or "directions in life."

The process of identifying projects is fluid, shifting as new distinctions are made and as alternative stories unfold. Problems can be thought of as plots, and projects as counterplots. Partners in a couple may name joint projects for the relationship, individual projects, or both. For some couples, the collaborative negotiation of shared or complementary directions in life can be a very significant—sometimes even inspirational—part of the therapy.

Process and Technical Aspects of Couple Therapy

Listening

When we meet people for the first time, we want to understand the meaning of their stories for *them*. This means turning our backs on "expert" filters: not listening for chief complaints; not "gathering" the pertinent-to-us-as-experts bits of diagnostic information interspersed in their stories; not hearing their anecdotes as matrices within which resources are embedded; not listening for surface hints about what the core problem "really" is; and not comparing the selves that people portray in their stories to normative standards.

In the beginning, we ask about nonproblematic aspects of the lives of each partner and of their relationship. We are interested in getting to know the members of a couple as people and in making sure that the problem does not trick us into mistaking "them" for "it." Unless people insist on moving quickly into talking about problems, we spend a while listening to stories about their preferences and pleasures. At some point in this process, people do usually begin to spontaneously tell problem-tinged stories.

As we listen to their stories of the problem, we try to put ourselves in people's shoes. We do not assume that we understand the meaning their experience holds for them. We listen and ask. Connecting with people's experience from their perspective orients us to the specific realities that shape, and are shaped by, their personal narratives. This sort of understanding requires that we listen with focused attention, patience, and curiosity while building a relationship of mutual respect and trust.

Deconstructive Listening

When we listen "deconstructively" to people's stories, our listening is guided by the belief that those stories have many possible meanings. The meaning that we as listeners make, more often than not, is at least a little different from the meaning that the speaker has intended. We seek to capitalize on this by valuing the gaps we notice in our understanding and asking people to fill in details, or by listening for ambiguities in meaning, then asking people about those ambiguities.

As people tell their stories, we interrupt at intervals to reflect our sense of what they are saying and to ask whether the meaning we are making fits with their intended meaning. Even though we intend to understand people's realities from something very close to their point of view, their realities inevitably begin to shift, at least a little, as they expand their narrative in response to our retellings and questions. Our very presence makes their world different. Throughout this process, we listen with thoughtfulness about what new constructions are emerging. We wonder aloud whether they are useful or desirable. We strive to co-create a process in which people experience choice rather than "settled certainties" (Bruner, 1986) with regard to the realities that they inhabit.

Deconstructive Questioning

White (1991) defines "deconstruction" actively and politically:

> According to my rather loose definition, deconstruction has to do with procedures that subvert taken-for-granted realities and practices: those so-called "truths" that are split off from the conditions and the context of their production; those disembodied ways of speaking that hide their biases and prejudices; and

> those familiar practices of self and of relationship that are subjugating of person's lives. (p. 27)

The medical model and other discourses of modern power can lead people to a sense of themselves as "docile bodies" (Foucault, 1977), subject to knowledge and procedures in which they have no active voice. Subjugating stories of gender, race, class, age, sexual orientation, and religion (to name a few) are so prevalent and entrenched in our culture that we can get caught up in them without realizing it.

We believe it is our responsibility as therapists to cultivate a growing awareness of the dominant (and dominating) stories in our society and to develop ways of examining the effects of those stories collaboratively when we sense them at work in the lives and relationships of the people who consult with us.

Hare-Mustin (1994, p. 22) has used the metaphor of a "mirrored room" to talk about how the only ideas that can come up in therapy are the ideas that the people involved bring into the therapy room: "The therapy room is like a room lined with mirrors. It reflects back only what is voiced within it. ... If the therapist and family are unaware of marginalized discourses, such as those associated with members of subordinate gender, race, and class groups, those discourses remain outside the mirrored room." This notion implies that therapists must continually reflect on the discourses that shape our perceptions of what is possible, both for ourselves and for the people we work with. Such reflection puts us in the position to ask deconstructive questions—questions whose aim is to examine problems in detail and expose discourses that support them.

Our language ("discourses," "deconstructive questions") can make this whole process sound quite heady and cumbersome. In practice, we strive to keep all that to ourselves. We seek to ask small questions that ask people, one small step at a time, to reflect, in their own language and metaphors, on the taken-for-granted, unquestioned values, beliefs, and customs that shape their daily experience, and to evaluate whether those ways of living suit them.

Externalizing Conversations

White (1987, 1988, 1989; see also Epston, 1993) has introduced the idea that the person is not the problem; the problem is the problem. The narrative practice of "externalizing" puts this idea into action. Just listening with the belief that problems are separate from people has a powerful deconstructive effect. It biases us to interact differently than we would if we saw people as intrinsically problematic. It creates a different receiving context for people's stories, one in which their stories almost always become less restrictive.

We can expose dominant discourses by asking "externalizing questions" about contextual influences on the problem. What "feeds" the problem? What "starves" it? Who benefits from it? In what settings might the problematic attitude be useful? Which people would proudly advocate for the problem? What groups of people would definitely be opposed to it and its intentions? Questions such as these invite people to consider how the entire context of their lives affects the problem and vice versa.

As problems are externalized, it becomes established that, rather than *being* the problem, the person or couple has a *relationship* with the problem. Members of a couple have the opportunity to describe their relationships with problems in a variety of ways. One of the consequences of an externalizing conversation is that it becomes clear that both partners have relationships with the problems they name.

In externalizing conversations, we are particularly interested to hear descriptions of the effects of problems. We ask about the effects of a problem on both members of a couple—on their lives and their relationships. This helps keep the identity of the problem separate from either partner. It mobilizes the members of the couple to join together in opposing the effects of the problem. This is particularly helpful when the problem has kept them apart. People can stop thinking about themselves or their relationships as inherently problematic and, instead, consider how they want to revise their relationships with problems.

Naming the Problem and the Project

Naming a problem can open a way for examining the problem and thinking differently about it. It can be poetic and compelling. We recently saw a young heterosexual couple. The man described the problem as waking him in the middle of the night with a gun to his head. When we asked him to name the problem (which he had called "anxiety attacks"), he named it "the thief" because it was trying to steal his sleep. His partner, who had been scornful of the fear and difficulty in sleeping

until this point, could easily relate to the terror of a burglary in the dark of night. She began to appreciate her partner's bravery in facing it alone. She suggested that he wake her so that she could help.

As we ask people to evaluate their relationship to problems, they often tell us what they would prefer to have in their lives in place of the problems. We are especially interested in hearing about preferred directions in life. We listen for words in people's descriptions that might serve as good names for their preferred directions. We ask questions that invite them to identify the directions and name them as projects. These questions can be quite direct. For example, let us say a couple has named "blaming" as a problem, and that through answering our deconstructive questions the partners have realized that they are living under the influence of the idea that each partner in a couple should intuitively "know" what the other wants. In answering still more questions, they have described how this idea leads to blaming and has each of them feeling that something is wrong with the relationship. In this conversation, they are recounting an incident in which they could have gotten caught up in blaming, but did not. Julie tells how she finished a major project at work, let Fran know it was finally done, and described a way she would like to celebrate. Fran did not arrange the dinner Julie would have liked that night, and did not even come home until late in the evening. In the past, "blaming" would have convinced Julie that Fran did not really care about the relationship. This time, Julie was able to escape "blaming," to ask Fran what went into her actions and believe Fran's answer. In such an instance, we might ask Julie whether asking about Fran's perspective instead of assuming she knew it reflected a preferred direction in life—one that blaming could have kept her from seeing. If Julie agreed, we could ask whether this direction represented a project in which the couple was interested. If they *were* interested, we could ask what name they would give the project.

Sometimes partners share the same problems and projects. Sometimes a problem and/or project concerns one partner but not the other. Even when partners do not describe or experience the same problems and projects, witnessing each other's stories, and hearing the problems and projects that shape them, can lead to new understandings and choices.

As people name problems and projects, we keep track of them. The explicit and direct discussion of projects and how they contrast with problems can be a vital part of therapy. Such discussion brings forth and thickens the counterplots to problematic stories. It heightens the meaning that is made of particular experiences. Without an identified counterplot, experiences that lie outside the problem story may go unnoticed or seem trivial. With a counterplot, people can perceive shape and meaning in their nonproblematic experiences. For example, once the partners in a couple have agreed on "listening more with our hopes and less with our fears" as a shared project, any conversation they have can be plotted into the narrative of how hopes and fears influence their listening. Until such a project is explicitly discussed and agreed upon, conversations could be given many different meanings or no meaning at all.

We keep projects present in the therapy through short names or phrases such as "growing intimacy," "having a voice," "standing against violence." These names often shift as the therapy progresses, and it is the therapist's job to keep up with the couple's changes in language and conceptualization. We seek personal, evocative, and poetic names for problems and projects (Epston, 2000, 2006). Throughout therapy, we ask questions that invite people to shape their perceptions, thoughts, feelings, and actions into stories according to the plots and counterplots they identify as meaningful for their lives.

Unique Outcomes

A "unique outcome," as noted earlier, is any event that would not have been predicted in light of a problem-saturated story. It may be a plan, action, feeling, statement, desire, dream, thought, belief, ability, or commitment (Morgan, 2000). Unique outcomes constitute openings that, through questions and reflective discussion, can be developed into new stories.

Sometimes couples offer unique outcomes quite directly. For example, someone in describing a problem may say, "It's not always like that. Sometimes ... " and go on to describe a unique outcome. It is not unusual as therapy progresses and as couples become involved in the reauthoring process, for them to save up new unique outcomes to tell their therapist. At other times, unique outcomes are so buried in people's descriptions of their problematic stories that it is important to listen very carefully not to miss them. For example, if one partner says, "It would have been OK if he

hadn't ... " and then proceeds to tell a problematic story, if we are listening closely, we can be curious about the "It would have been OK" part, just as we would be curious about the answers to direct unique outcome questions.

Sometimes we might notice events that, given the problematic story, we would not have predicted: Partners who believe they have communication difficulties might eloquently and clearly describe a problem in a way that suits them both, or one partner might show up on time to meet the other for therapy, even though the problematic story is one of irresponsibility.

Most often, as we listen deconstructively and ask couples about the effects of problems on their lives and relationships, we begin to get glimpses of events that lie outside the problem story. If we do not hear of actions that speak of nonproblematic intentions, commitments, or values, we can inquire more directly about their existence. When we are working with an externalized problem, a straightforward way of looking for a unique outcome is to ask about the influence of one or both partners on the life of the problem; that is, we ask questions such as "Has there ever been a time when [the problem] tried to get the upper hand, but you were able to resist its influence?" or "Have you ever been able to escape [the problem] for even a few minutes?" or "Is this problem *always* with you?" When questions of this sort follow a detailed inquiry into the effects of the problem on the person or couple, people can usually find instances in which they were able to avoid the problem's influence. Each such instance is a potential beginning for an alternative life narrative.

The Absent but Implicit

Michael White (2000) describes how it can be useful to listen for purposes, values, hopes, commitments, and the like, that are "absent but implicit" in people's narratives. He draws on the writings of Bateson (1980) and Derrida (1978), which illustrate how we draw distinctions by contrasting one experience with another. No experience has a set meaning that exists independent of other experiences, and one way we make meaning is through operations in which we say (or think, or sense) "This is different from. ... " If we listen closely, using what White has called "double listening," we can hear implications of the experiences that are being drawn on to make a distinction concerning our present experience. These "implied" experiences are a rich source of alternative stories. When we hear problematic stories, we particularly listen for implications about what might be treasured.

For example, in an early therapy conversation, June names the problem as "betrayal," and describes how it is leaving her in grave doubt about continuing her relationship with Larry. When they married, Larry had promised they would live in Cincinnati, where June had family and friends. After 2 years of marriage, June had agreed, with considerable reluctance, to move to Washington, D.C. for Larry's career. A year later, she agreed to move to Chicago. Although June did not like relocating, her sister and her sister's family lived in the area, and this helped her accept the change. After a year and a half in Chicago, Larry lost his job. In a tearful conversation, he agreed to seek only a new job that would let them stay put. This had become even more important to June, because their two children had cousins close by. Larry and June came to therapy when June discovered e-mails that made it clear Larry was looking into jobs all over the country. At several points, she referred to this as a betrayal.

Following the principle of double listening, we began to wonder what experience allowed June to draw distinctions about betrayal. We thought it might be trust, so we asked June whether trust was something that she treasured. She began to weep, saying, "Without trust, I cannot go on." We asked questions that invited her to tell stories about the history of her relationship with trust. Some of the stories she told concerned her marriage with Larry. These stories let to an inquiry about what she contributed to trust and what Larry had contributed. It was important for June to recognize that Larry had contributed substantially in some contexts to the growth of trust in their relationship. Larry witnessed this whole conversation, and that helped him see his career moves in a different light. Rather than feeling like he was being blamed for betrayal, even though he was doing his best to support the family, he could recognize other implications in June's story of trust and its importance. In the therapy, we began to focus on stories of trust and connection. These conversations opened up different possibilities than those that focused on where June and Larry should live. As they continued these conversations outside of therapy, the couple decided that trust and connection could grow and flourish either in Chicago or in Cincinnati, but noplace else. When Larry related this conversation to us, it was with an expression of joy and commitment.

Listening for the absent but implicit helped us find stories and meanings we might never have found if we had continued to focus on betrayal.

Developing Stories from Unique Outcomes

When we find a possible unique outcome—either an overt one, or one that is absent but implicit—that seems relevant and interesting to one or both partners, we ask questions that invite them to develop it into an alternative story. We do not have a formula to follow in this process, but we do keep in mind that stories involve events organized by plot through time in particular contexts, and that they usually include more than one person. A big part of the reason new stories make a difference in people's lives is that a performance of meaning occurs when they tell them to other people. As people tell their stories, others who are present witness them. The telling, witnessing, and retelling make up a ritual of sorts, in which new meanings can be enacted, discussed, and brought into being. We facilitate this process by asking questions to develop an experientially vivid story that is rich in detail.

White (White & Epston, 1990), following Bruner (1986), speaks of the "dual landscapes" of *action* and *consciousness* (or, in his more recent work, *identity*). He suggests the stories that constitute people's lives unfold in both those landscapes, and that it can be helpful for therapists to inquire about both. Let us look first at the landscape of action.

The landscape of action includes *detail* in *multiple modalities* involving the viewpoints of *multiple characters* in a particular *scene* or *setting*. It also includes the action itself. What happened, in what sequence, involving which characters?

Taking the very simple example of Jack and Lisa, who at an initial therapy appointment say that their relationship had been deteriorating for years and that this is the first time they have sought out therapy, we might wonder whether simply deciding and following through to come to therapy is a unique outcome. The following are some questions we might ask:

- Who actually made the suggestion that you come to therapy?
- What was the look on Jack's face when you suggested it? Did the look change as you talked more?
- Jack, what did you think when Lisa first made the suggestion? How did that change for you as you talked?

- Were there conversations or interactions between the two of you that prompted you to bring this up, Lisa? Was there something Jack said?
- Jack, do you remember that? What were you thinking that got you to say that?
- Who would be most pleased that you have taken this step? What would they say about it?

In the landscape of action, we are interested in bringing forth people's "agentive self"; that is, we ask questions with an eye toward enhancing those aspects of the emerging story that support "personal agency" (Adams-Westcott, Dafforn, & Sterne, 1993). The very act of reauthoring requires and demonstrates personal agency, and most people experience that in this work. One way we make personal agency apparent is by asking, in a variety of ways, how people have accomplished what they have. In the preceding example we might ask the following questions for this purpose:

- Given the hopelessness you described, Lisa, what did you draw on in deciding to do something in the face of it?
- Were you preparing somehow to take this step? What went into that preparation?
- Jack, do you think that Lisa knew that you would be willing to come? How did you get past the hopelessness to agree on doing something so foreign?

We think about the *shape* of a story as it comes forth: What happened before the unique outcome? How smoothly did things unfold? Were there false starts involved? To what did this particular episode lead? In this regard, we are especially interested to know whether there is a turning point, a place where the story changes for the good. Although "turning point" is not a fitting metaphor for everyone in every situation, when it does fit, it distinguishes a significant event that we can plot in time. We believe it is useful to focus special attention on this sort of event, bringing forth even more shape and detail, perhaps even treating it as a story within a story.

No matter how vivid a story is in the landscape of action, if it is to have *meaning*, it must also be developed in the landscape of identity. By "the landscape of identity," we refer to that imaginary territory in which people plot the meanings, desires, intentions, beliefs, commitments, motivations, values, and the like, that relate to their experience in the landscape of action. In other words, in the landscape of identity, people reflect on the implications of experiences storied in the landscape of action.

To explore the landscape of identity, we ask what we (Freedman & Combs, 1993) call "meaning questions," which are questions that invite people to step back from the landscape of action and reflect on the wishes, motivations, values, beliefs, learning, implications, and so forth that lead to and flow from the actions they have recounted. For example, we may ask:

- "What do you think it says about your relationship that you agreed to come together to therapy?"
- "Does it characterize the way the two of you do things to have secret hope in the face of hopelessness?"

In coauthoring stories, we move between the landscape of action and the landscape of identity, weaving the two back and forth, again and again.

Time: Developing a "History of the Present" and Extending the Story into the Future

Once we have identified a preferred event and developed a bit of its story, we want to link that event to other preferred events across time, so that their meanings survive and the events and their meanings can thicken a person's or couple's narrative in preferred ways. Therefore, once a preferred event is identified and storied, we ask questions to link it to other past events, and to develop the story of those events. Here are some examples of questions that might identify such events:

- When you think back, what events that you might be building on reflect other times when you could have been pulled apart, but that you came together as a couple?
- If we were to interview friends who have known you throughout your relationship, who might have predicted that the two of you would have been able to accomplish this? What memories might they share with us that would have led them to predict this?

We can also ask how the emerging new story influences a person's ideas about the future. As people free more and more of their past from the grip of problem-dominated stories, they are able to envision, expect, and plan toward futures they like better. We might ask:

- We have just been talking about an accomplishment and several events in the past that paved the way for this accomplishment. If you think of these events as creating a kind of direction in your lives, what do you think will be the next step?
- You have learned some things about each other that have changed your view of each other and of the relationship. If you keep this new view in your hearts, how do you think the future might be different?

Telling and Witnessing

There is a rhythmic alternation between telling and witnessing that characterizes narrative work. We set up a structure early in our work with couples that runs through most of our subsequent conversations. We ask one member of the couple to tell his or her story, while the other listens from a witnessing position. Once a story has been told, we ask the partner in the witnessing position to reflect on what he or she has heard. After the teller reflects on the reflections, we invite the partner in the witnessing position to now relate a story from his or her own experience.

We initiate this process by making eye contact and speaking primarily with one person at a time, asking the other to comment only after we have had enough conversation to bring forth and develop a meaningful bit of story with the first person. Sometimes we need to be more explicit, saying something like, "What I would like to do is speak with you, Rubin, for a while, as you, Ellen, listen. After a bit I'll turn to you, Ellen, and ask what thoughts you have been having as you listened to Rubin. Then we'll switch and you, Rubin, will be in the listening position while Ellen and I have a conversation. Would that be OK?"

Stories need listeners as well as tellers. It is through the interpersonal, societal practice of telling and retelling that stories take on enough substance to change people's lives. When we ask one partner to witness the other's story, we hope that he or she will hear it in a new way. We find that it is important to be thoughtful about what kind of attitude or position is helpful for witnessing in each particular instance. For example, with a certain person we might say, "Would you be willing, as I talk with Vernon, to listen as you would to a friend? With friends, sometimes you can suspend your own point of view and listen just to understand. Would that be all right?"

With another person, or at a different point in the therapy, we might choose very different language. We want to assist people in listening from a vantage point in which they can hear things that are new and worthy of appreciation in their partner's stories. Especially in the beginning of therapy, when the influence of entrenched problems is strong, this takes great care. It helps to know a variety of positions from which to invite people to listen. The following list is not exhaustive, but we hope it illustrates some of the positions for witnessing that we have found useful:

- Ask the person to imagine a particular person or team of people by his or her side, who will help to create and maintain a position of security (or calm, or curiosity—whatever might be a useful attitude).
- Ask the person to identify a context (meditation class, watching his or her daughter perform, listening to an inspirational speaker, coaching a valued student) in which he or she uses skills, abilities, or perceptions that might be helpful in this context. Invite the person to listen from within that imagined context.
- Use the vantage point of a version of self that is attending to "what is important," rather than "being right." Begin by talking with the witness about hopes, values, and wishes for the relationship. Invite the witness to hold these close as he or she listens to what the partner is saying.
- Listen the way a particular other (friend, mentor, role model, etc.) might listen.
- Listen from the vantage point of "the relationship."
- Together, construct an antianger (or antihurt, or antipessimism, etc.) position. Invite the person to tell stories that illustrate that antianger position. Ask enough questions to assist the person in becoming experientially involved in the antianger position. Then ask the person to witness from that place.
- If you have one, use the one-way mirror to physically create a space for appreciative, reflective listening.
- Use videotape or live, closed-circuit video, so that the partner watches the video from a separate location. This can be especially useful when conflict is so pronounced that it prevents partners from having the space to speak.

After the first partner has told a bit of story and the other has listened from an appropriate position, we invite the witnessing partner to give voice to what he or she witnesses. We might ask general questions, such as the following:

- What was it like to hear what Brad was saying?
- What thoughts were you having while Linda was talking?

However, we often find it useful to ask questions that more directly invite people to respond to unique outcomes and preferred directions, rather than leaving the field for response wide open. The following are examples of this sort of question:

- Were you surprised when Raoul described you as taking the time to let others know you care?
- What did it mean to you to hear Chantal say how important the relationship is to her?

We then make space for the original teller to respond to her partner's reflections: we ask story development questions as they seem appropriate. We use this format to facilitate not only witnessing of each partner's versions of events but also deconstruction of the meaning of those events.

We use the alternation of telling and witnessing in other ways as well. Sometimes a couple describes something and the therapist reflects. Although we most often work separately, many people know us to be partners in marriage and in parenthood, as well as in our work. Heterosexual couples, particularly, sometimes ask us to work with them as a cotherapy team. In those instances, one of us takes the role of interviewer and the other reflects. Sometimes we include an outsider witness group (White, 1997) as part of the structure.

Relational Identity

When partners begin describing problems in therapy, it is not unusual for each to describe the problem as if it were inside the other and to give it a very stable description such as, "He is a cold and judgmental person." This kind of description, and the perception on which it is based, coaches blame, regret, resentment, and hopelessness. If we can resist the influence of discourses that support essential identities and think instead about identities as being multistoried and fluid, we are much more free to notice difference in our partners, our relationships, and ourselves, and to notice what contributes to those differences.

We treat identity as a project (Combs & Freedman, 1999). The discourses of popular psychology more often treat identity as a given and

as fixed: They talk about finding one's "true self" as if it were a preexisting treasure just waiting to be dug up; they invite us to categorize ourselves on the basis of 10-point checklists. The focus is much more on who we *are* than on who we are *becoming*, and it is definitely on who we are as individuals. It takes vigilance and the support of others to resist these discourses and approach identity as a project that we undertake in interaction with others.

We have previously described (Freedman & Combs, 2004) a man who had this to say about his marriage that had just ended: "I don't know what happened. I married my baseball card and it still didn't work out!! What more could I have done?" When we asked what he meant by his "baseball card," he said, "You know. Baseball card. It's got a picture and a list of facts about the player. I married my baseball card. She looked perfect, her stats were perfect, but somehow we never had anything to say to each other." Perhaps this is an extreme example, but it illustrates how we conspire together to treat each other as fixed commodities. In narrative therapy, we look for ways to deconstruct this kind of characterization and invite people to consider how together they can help each other enact new ways of being—new identities that partake of new possibilities.

Thinking about identity as something that develops in relationship has led us to wonder aloud with people what difference it would make if, instead of asking, "Does my partner have these qualities?" they asked, "Who do I get to be when I'm with my partner?" or "Am I liking myself better as I spend more time with my partner?"

These have been very useful questions. In answering them, people often recognize that although they may be with someone who has all the "qualities" they are looking for, they do not much like themselves when they are with that person. We have also worked with couples for whom the change of focus from "Does this person measure up to who I think my partner should be?" to "Who do I get to be when I am with this person?" has produced joyous results that are wonderful to behold. This shift in focus often helps people let go of the idea of changing their partners, and work instead on building ways to witness and appreciate each other.

We developed the following exercise to give people an opportunity to practice relational identity questioning in workshops we teach on couple therapy. We include it here to give readers the same opportunity. It can be done alone, but readers may find doing it with a partner even more educational.

EXERCISE: RELATIONAL IDENTITY QUESTIONING

This exercise is for two people. In each pair, one person interviews the other following the suggestions below, then partners switch roles, so that the person who was being interviewed now takes on the interviewer role.

Pick a significant relationship with another person. This does not have to be a couple relationship. It could be a friendship, a mentoring relationship, or some other kind of relationship with one other person that has been important to you.

Consider the following questions:

- In this relationship, have you become (in some way) different than you once were? Is this difference valuable to you? Focusing particularly on the difference, how would you describe the "you" that you have come to know in this relationship?
- What about the relationship facilitates this difference?
- Is this difference related to something that you stand for or value? If so, can you name or say something about the thing for which you stand?
- How does your partner (or friend, etc.) contribute to your becoming this way or knowing yourself in this way, or being able to take this position?
- What experiences might he or she relate if I asked your partner (or friends, etc.) about times that he or she really appreciated this new and different you? Is there a particular time you could tell me about in some detail? How do experiences like these contribute to his or her life?
- What has it been like to be appreciated for this new expression of your self? Has it made this version of your self grow or shrink, or has it changed it in some other way?
- Are there things about this new version of your identity that your partner (or friend, etc.) hasn't yet appreciated that you wish he or she would appreciate more? What difference might it make to you if you experienced that appreciation?
- What might have been lost to you, your partner, and the relationship if you hadn't become the person you have just been describing?
- If you imagine that your partner (or friend, or mentor, etc.) listened to all that you have just been saying from an open, receptive position, what do you think that would have been like for him or her? What might he or she have most appreciated about what you have said?

Outsider Witness Groups

In our discussion of telling and witnessing, we outlined possible witnessing structures: one partner reflecting on the other's story, the therapist reflecting, and an outsider witness group reflecting. In this section, we describe how we set up and use outsider witness groups.

At times, particularly as part of training or consultation, outsider witness groups are composed of therapists. At other times, in response to our raising the possibility, couples agree to our inviting another couple (whose members have insider experience in dealing with a particular problem) to serve as an outsider witness group. Or, the couple may invite other people who are important in their lives to join in as outsider witnesses.

For example, if we are working with a couple that is struggling with infertility, with the couple's permission, we might ask other couples who have been through infertility struggles to join the group. When we have an outsider witness group we structure it in a very particular way that includes four parts (Cohen, Combs, DeLaurenti, DeLaurenti, Freedman, Larimer, & Shulman, 1998; White, 1995, 1997, 2005).

In the first part, the therapist interviews the couple while the outsider witness group observes the interview from behind a one-way mirror (or at a bit of a distance). In the second part, the group switches places with the couple and the therapist. The couple and therapist listen as members of the group have a conversation, raising questions and commenting about what they have watched. In the third part, the couple and therapist switch back to their original places, and the couple responds to the reflections as the group observes. In the fourth part, everyone meets together for the purpose of deconstructing the interview or making it transparent. The therapist and outsider witness group members respond to questions about their purposes, questions, and the directions they pursued in the interview.

In the second part of the interview, if an outsider witness group with little experience is reflecting, the therapist may ask questions that draw out team members, keeping the focus on what moved them and on possible preferred directions that emerged during the interview. We ask team members to situate their reflections in their own experience, to acknowledge the trust couples have shown in opening their lives to the presence of others, and to comment on the difference that being part of the conversation makes to their own lives.

Documenting and Circulating New Stories

Because we believe the new stories that emerge in therapy become transformative as they are enacted outside of the therapy room, we are interested in documenting and circulating the new stories (White & Epston, 1990). We take notes in therapy that document new stories as they develop. We often refer back to these notes and read them aloud. When couples take stands or achieve new things, or reach turning points, we might create a document or certificate together that formalizes this newly distinguished event in their story. We often make videotapes for their personal use in which couples reflect on how far they have come. We may make tapes or documents about what they have learned that, with their permission, can be viewed by others facing similar problems (White & Epston, 1990). Through this kind of exchange, couples can band together with others in virtual leagues.

We sometimes write letters between therapy meetings. In these letters, we reflect on unique outcomes and ask questions that we did not ask in the therapy conversation. We hope that this will thicken and extend the knowledge that had begun to emerge there. We sometimes generate formal documents that list important elements of new narratives (Freedman & Combs, 1997). To encourage the circulation of this knowledge, we invite couples to share these documents with other people in their lives.

Curative Factors in Couple Therapy/ Mechanisms of Change

We approach therapy as an experiential process through which people reclaim, relive, and make meaning of stories that add new substance and new possibilities to their lives. In our work with couples, therapy is also a process in which partners witness each other fleshing out their stories of alternative events. The mechanism of change in narrative therapy is the telling, retelling, witnessing, and living out of multistoried lives.

People's life narratives are condensations and abstractions: They contain only a small portion of the events and circumstances of their lives. Of the countless events that occur each day, only a few are storied and given meaning. When couples come to therapy, their accounts of their relationships are generally problematic and limited. This has to do, at least in part, with larger cultural stories or discourses that support particular sets of stories and meanings and not others. We think that people's

experience of the meaning of their lives and relationships changes through changes in their life narratives. As people's narratives change, what they do and perceive change as well. We facilitate this process by asking questions to highlight unstoried events and to encourage meaning making around those events, then we tie the meaning to memorable actions and contexts.

We recently had an experience with someone in therapy that illustrates the way lives change when narratives change. Rhonda, a 42-year-old woman, had been sued for legal malpractice some 15 years previously. Although the suit was settled out of court, there was considerable publicity and scandal. After that lawsuit, Rhonda first experienced devastation. As time passed, she felt numb. Her life was on hold. Although she did not find her relationship with Greg to be satisfying, she stayed in it. She stayed in her job. Life went on, but she did not. She missed her childbearing years.

After 13 years, Rhonda started therapy and began to reclaim her life. She began to consider her career and whether she would like to interview for other jobs. She ended the relationship with Greg and became involved in what she described as the best relationship of her life—with Jeff.

One day Jeff said, "I can't believe you stayed in that relationship with Greg for so long. Why did you do it?" Rhonda said that she did not know, and they became involved in talking about other things. Two days later, Jeff apologized profusely to Rhonda, saying that he had been really thoughtless in asking that question about Greg. He had somehow forgotten about the whole lawsuit and how it had put her life on hold. Rhonda burst into gales of laughter and told him that she had forgotten too!

She, of course, knew that it had happened, but it was no longer the central story of her life. Other stories had been told, retold, witnessed, documented, and—more importantly—reexperienced. The thicker version of Rhonda's narrative supported new actions and possibilities: a new relationship, new ways of thinking about work, and many smaller changes. The way Rhonda experienced her life had changed through restorying events. Her immersion in the alternative stories supported new relationships and other possibilities.

Another way to describe our ideas about change is to say that in successful therapy new meanings are performed. "Performance of meaning" is a concept that narrative therapists have borrowed from poststructural anthropology, particularly from the work of Myerhoff (1982, 1986), who gave numerous examples of how meaning instead of being an innate quality, arises through performance. Unless a story is told and retold (circulated, written down, acted out, sung, etc.), it has no lasting meaning. In the light of this notion, the new strands of story that emerge in response to our questions must be circulated and put into action before they can become meaningful.

When Jeff apologized to Rhonda for his memory lapse, he was performing meaning around the lapse. When Rhonda realized that she, too, had lost track of those 13 painful years, she added another layer of meaning to Jeff's. Rhonda's retelling of the incident in therapy was a big performance of meaning, and in that performance her new, joyous relationship with Jeff became appreciably more real and memorable.

We believe that change occurs through the performance of meaning that takes place in waves of telling and retelling such as these.

Treatment Applicability and Empirical Support

We have found that the narrative approach has general applicability. Although the length, intensity, and specific outcome vary from problem to problem and from context to context, the approach is as effective for couples seeking premarital counseling as it is for couples struggling to reclaim their relationship from violence and abuse, or for couples in which one partner has been diagnosed with a serious mental illness.

That said, our experience is that some couples prefer a different kind of therapy relationship than what we offer. Some people are seeking instruction or expert advice. Others are more interested in exploring their past histories to find out why they are in particular situations. We regularly ask people how the therapy is going for them, and we are open and willing to refer couples if they are seeking a different kind of therapy relationship.

We find that most couples coming to therapy are concerned less with how the therapy relationship is structured than with whether their relationship improves. Because popular notions of therapy include descriptions such as "getting to the root of the problem" or "improving communication skills," they may initially use words that seem to indicate a preference for a different kind of therapy relationship. With further conversation, we have found that most couples are simply interested in improving their relationships, and we find narra-

tive therapy very useful and effective for that purpose.

If a member of a couple wonders if medication might be helpful, or requests a formal assessment of a particular problem, we talk about it and, if the partner chooses, we make a referral to someone who might collaboratively facilitate a decision about medication, diagnosis, and so forth. We do not consider medication or testing a part of narrative therapy, but we support people in exploring whatever kind of approach they think might be helpful.

We are not opposed to the thoughtful and informed use of drugs, testing, DSM-IV labeling, and so forth; we just do not consider them to be a part of narrative therapy.

For us, the most important aspect of narrative therapy is the worldview. We do not often think of people in terms of the traditional, expert, individual diagnoses that underpin most "legitimate" research. We do not believe that we possess expert knowledge about what would be most helpful to each new couple we meet. Instead, we focus on the insider knowledge that people have acquired through struggling with particular problems in particular contexts. The skills and values we have cultivated to become good narrative therapists make it difficult for us to stand outside of our work and assess it by conventional empirical criteria. Our most common form of research is coresearch (Epston, 1999), in which we ask the people we are sitting with in an ongoing way whether the therapy is helpful, and what in particular is helpful about it. The documentation, compilation, and circulation of coresearch builds up a body of insider knowledge that shapes our work as it continues to evolve (see Maisel, Epston, & Borden [2004] for a vivid illustration of the existence and usefulness of large archives of insider knowledge).

Researchers who are interested in narrative approaches tend to do qualitative rather than quantitative studies. None of the published qualitative studies that we could find (Besa, 1994; Kogan & Gale, 1997; Etchison & Kleist, 2000; Seltzer & Seltzer, 2004; O'Connor, Davis, Meakes, Pickering, & Schuman, 2004; France & Uhlin, 2006) directly addresses couple therapy, but the studies are all supportive of narrative therapy as an effective treatment modality in which clients improve and therapists do what they say they do.

A recent article in *The New York Times* (Carey, 2007) summarizes psychological research concerning narrative and the formation of identity and meaning. In a concluding paragraph, it says:

Taken together, these findings suggest a kind of give and take between life stories and individual memories, between the larger screenplay and the individual scenes. The way people replay and recast memories, day by day, deepens and reshapes their larger life story. And as it evolves, that larger story in turn colors the interpretation of the scenes.

CASE ILLUSTRATION

Pauline and Rick came to consult me (Jill Freedman) about a year after they married. Pauline was 35 years old, and Rick was 51. I began by asking each of them to tell me a little bit about themselves that had nothing to do with the problem that brought them to see me. Because I had spoken briefly with Pauline on the phone when she called to request therapy, I began with Rick.

Rick described himself as a freelance writer and novelist. He had been in Chicago for almost 3 years and in that time had published a number of stories in local papers, but the work of most importance to him was the novel he was writing. Before moving to Chicago, he had traveled in Europe for many years. For fun, he enjoyed not only listening to music, watching television, and reading fiction, but also his work writing. This novel, his second, it meant a great deal to him, as did seeing his craft improve.

Pauline described herself as a fiction writer. She had recently published a short story in a very prestigious magazine. She taught writing in a local master of fine arts (MFA) program. She enjoyed going out with friends to restaurants, clubs, and movies, talking on the phone, and reading. She had grown up in Chicago. While Pauline was in college, her family had moved to the West Coast. She joined them after earning her MFA degree, but had decided 5 years ago to move back to Chicago because her closest friends were still here.

I asked if they could tell me something about their relationship that had nothing to do with the problem. They looked at each other, then Rick said, "We enjoy grocery shopping together. We are good at finding things that will please each other. I indulge Pauline by cooking real meals. She buys extravagant things I appreciate but wouldn't think of buying, like good wine and dark chocolate." Pauline smiled and said, "I love shopping together."

I asked if there were things they would like to ask me before we talked about the problem. They declined to ask any questions at that time, but preferred to begin describing why they had come to see me. They had accepted a joint faculty position in the English department of a university in a different city for the fall. Part of the reason they were consulting me in November was to feel confident about their move the following summer, in anticipation of this new career step. What they described as "fighting" seemed to stand in the way of confidence in their relationship.

As I began speaking with them one at a time to understand and unpack their experience of fighting, it seemed to me that the fighting demonstrated itself. Pauline and Rick punctuated the conversation with interruptions, primarily in the form of loud and lengthy denials and corrections. My reassurance that I understood that their descriptions were different and that each would get a chance to speak had little impact, so I stopped the conversation and instead asked Rick who in his life had listened to him with the most interest and openness. Rick quickly chose Sven, the person to whom he reported to when he worked for a time as a literary critic for a small newspaper in Sweden. Rick said that he had had work experiences in which people did not care what he wrote or vehemently disagreed, or thought his work was great, but Sven, despite his different views, always seemed to be open and interested. In conversation with him, Rick sometimes put ideas into words for the first time and expanded on his original assignments.

I asked Rick if a particular experience came to mind that illustrated this experience with Sven.

Rick looked a bit confused, and Pauline asked what this had to do with their relationship.

I explained that if I hosted the same conversations they had at home, it probably would not be very helpful. Instead, I wanted to look for alternative perspectives, both for listening and for telling. With Pauline's permission to explore this alternative listening position with Rick (so that there might be more room for her experience), I asked Rick if it would be agreeable to explore the possibility of listening from Sven's perspective. He was not sure, but was willing to proceed in thinking about Sven and their relationship.

Rick told a story of going to a club with Sven to listen to jazz. While they were waiting for the music to begin, they talked about a book that Rick was reviewing. As he critiqued the book, Sven asked questions that drew Rick out and helped him crystallize what he wanted to say. Later in the evening, Rick was surprised to discover that Sven did not particularly like the author or have an interest in the book. However, he was interested in bringing Rick's perspective to readers, and although he did not share it, he said that he respected it and even found it compelling. This was startling to Rick, who had not usually been compelled by things with which he did not agree.

I wondered what skills and ideas Sven brought to these kinds of conversations that allowed him to listen the way he did. Rick thought that it must have had to do with believing that there are different ways of looking at things, and that one can like people without agreeing with them. Also, he thought that Sven must somehow have kept in mind a bigger picture, so that he could disagree without losing track of other points of agreement and the working relationship.

I asked Rick if he would be willing to listen to Pauline the way Sven might listen, with the belief that there are different ways of looking at things and that one can like people without agreeing with them. Also, I asked whether he could keep in mind a bigger picture, and think about the relationship rather than only the specific thing that Pauline said at a particular moment.

Rick agreed to try, and I reminded him by repeating key phrases at certain points, when I thought he might be losing track of this position.

As Rick listened, Pauline described the fighting. Pauline said that she wanted to get close to Rick, but whenever she tried to talk, he shut her out and ignored her. Rick met her attempts to talk with irritation, annoyance, anger, and defensiveness. Then, she said, they were into bullying.

I was very alert to the word "bullying," because it implies a power difference. It can signal abuse occurring in a relationship. I paid careful attention to nonverbal cues—voice tone, facial expression, looking or not looking toward each other, and so on—as I asked how the bullying expressed itself. "It is a two-way process," Pauline exclaimed. "Sometimes when I want to be close and Rick won't pay any attention to me, I find myself unloading a barrage of criticism and exploding in anger. At other times he's criticizing everything, and then he goes out or into the other room and won't talk, and I feel even more angry."

In this early conversation, I was interested in engaging in an externalizing conversation with Pauline, so that we could think about their relationships with some of these problems, such as fighting and anger. I summarized: "So when the anger takes over, it makes itself known through criticism. This affects each of you in different ways. It seems to you that it affects Rick by getting

him to withdraw. This withdrawal in turn makes you feel shut out and ignored, is that right?"

Pauline agreed and said that they had different styles. Rick wanted more space, and she wanted to talk and feel understood.

This description provided quite a contrast. What she had earlier described as being shut out and ignored, Pauline was now describing as a difference in style and wanting more space. I asked which was more on the side of anger: to describe what Rick did in these situations as wanting more space, or to describe it as shutting out and ignoring? Pauline answered, "Shutting out and ignoring. But it still feels that way. It is hard to understand why he doesn't want to talk about things, and why he wants so much time alone!"

I asked if she had taken a step away from anger in renaming Rick's actions as "wanting more space." She nodded, then said that she supposed she had. I wondered, in taking this step away from anger, what was Pauline stepping toward? She said that it was a step toward understanding, but that understanding was not easy to hold on to, because she did not have experiences of wanting to move away instead of talk. It would help her if Rick could either stay more present or explain more about how taking time alone was not a move away from her.

I then turned to Rick and asked him what it had been like to listen in the way Sven listens, to hear Pauline describe the problem, holding the belief that there are different ways of looking at things and that you can like people without agreeing with them, also keeping in mind a bigger picture in thinking about the relationship rather than only the specific things Pauline said at a particular moment.

He said it had been interesting. I asked him, in keeping in mind a bigger picture, how what he had been thinking about differed from what Pauline was describing.

"I was thinking that we are ultimately good at compromising," he said, and with a little encouragement, he went on to describe a memory that had to do with a hiking trip they had taken in Colorado. It was their first trip together and they discovered early on that they had different ideas about luxury and roughing it, sleeping late and getting an early start, and eating in nice restaurants and having picnics, but eventually they both compromised and had a great time.

We only had a little bit of time left, and I was curious about several things, so I asked Pauline and Rick what they would prefer to talk about. I said, "At the beginning of our conversation, Pauline, you described wanting to get close to Rick, so I wondered if closeness was something you really valued and I wanted to hear more about that. I am also quite taken with this memory about compromising. We could talk more about that, or if you think it is important to say something else about the problem that brought you, we could fill in some of those gaps. Maybe Rick could describe more of his hopes and intentions in wanting more space. What do you think would be most important to talk about?"

"I think in general it is probably more important to talk about compromising, but I would feel better if I could add some about the problem and then maybe next time we will be in a better position to talk about solutions," Rick said. Pauline nodded her assent.

When Rick began talking about his experience of the problem, Pauline interrupted with disagreements and corrections. After several quick and unsuccessful attempts to establish a listening position for Pauline, I apologized for being in a hurry. I explained that we took the time to find a specific listening position for Rick that seemed to help him experience what Pauline was saying in a different way, and I made a mistake in not insisting we take the same time to establish a listening position for Pauline. I suggested that we could do that next time and added that I hoped my mistake did not obscure some of the new ideas that had been voiced in the conversation. I summarized some of those ideas. Then I reassured Rick that we could begin the next time hearing whatever he thought was important to say about the problem. I asked if we could end with each of them saying what stood out in our first conversation.

Rick said that getting back in touch with their history of compromise made him feel hopeful. Pauline said that what stood out to her was feeling heard and having the space to complete her thoughts.

Session 2

I began the second interview by reading my notes aloud from the first meeting, then wondering if we could proceed with Rick's description of the problem. When they agreed, I said to Pauline that I was interested in establishing a position from which she could usefully listen. "Who in your experience do you feel really listens to you? It could be someone in your current experience or from your past."

Pauline named a teacher from the MFA program she had attended. "When we workshopped something with Fran," she said, "it was like time stopped. The room was silent except for what you read aloud, and you could just feel her attention. I always heard myself in a different way when she was listening." In unpacking her ideas about Fran's listening skills, Pauline named letting go of everything except what is being spoken—thinking of nothing else—and the belief that what she said in response would ultimately make things better. Pauline agreed to listen from "Fran's listening position," letting go of everything except what was being spoken and believing that her response would ultimately make things better.

I then turned to Rick and asked what he would like to say about the problem as Pauline listened from Fran's position.

"Last time we were here," Rick said, "I was thinking about compromise, but what stayed with me more was Pauline saying that we have different styles. Pauline always wants to be talking and hanging out with people. I need some time alone. I think that need is misunderstood. And I get angry when she sees me as unfriendly or disagreeable, or not wanting to talk, just because I need space."

I drew Rick out more about his experience. He said that he had been 50 years old when he married. He had spent many years traveling on his own. He had learned to keep his own counsel and work things out through personal reflection. Time alone was a comfort and perhaps, at this point, a necessity. Part of the anger he experienced was being labeled as unsociable and unfriendly. He thought that he was plenty skilled socially, but that his way of working out problems was a solitary one. He did not think that was a bad thing, but he feared that Pauline did.

I asked Pauline, listening from the position of letting go of everything except what was being spoken and believing that her response would ultimately make things better, what she understood about Rick's experience of feeling misunderstood.

Pauline said that maybe she had had the idea that they were both the same, so that when she saw Rick do something, for her it meant what it would mean if she had done it, but that maybe it really did not mean that. "To me it was all about Rick not wanting to be close, but I am willing to consider that it may not mean that at all. In fact, since we met, I have been trying to believe that. It is hard because we are so different."

I asked Rick what it was like to hear Pauline's idea about misunderstanding. "It's great. I think she understands," he said. "I just don't want to be labeled the bad guy, the unfriendly guy, or even the mean guy. I'm not."

One thing that stood out to me, also mentioned in the first interview, had to do with this idea of wanting to be close. When I asked if that was something she treasured, Pauline said that it was.

I continued, "I don't want to impose this idea, but I was wondering, when you talked about not wanting to be labeled unfriendly or even mean, Rick, if those perceptions stand in the way of closeness?"

Rick agreed that they did, and that he, too, valued closeness.

I asked whether it might be important to talk about a history of treasuring closeness. The couple spent the rest of the interview telling stories of closeness: reading aloud to each other, hiking together, conversations over wine, candlelit dinners.

I asked whether the conversation was helpful. Both agreed that it was—that it had put them back in touch with the importance of their connection.

Session 3

I began the third interview reading the notes from the previous meeting, then asked whether there were further developments that had to do with connection. With a large sigh Pauline said, "Disconnection is more like it."

"She didn't understand at all," Rick said. Pauline said that she did, and the two began arguing. I interrupted and asked whether anger and misunderstanding had taken over their relationship again. They agreed that it had. I asked if it would be OK to record the effects of the anger on their life and relationship. They agreed and together we composed the following notes: The anger leads to fighting. This fighting tears Rick up and makes him want space, as an alternative to fighting. Although space works for Rick, often it is problematic, because the fighting makes Pauline want to settle things through conversation.

When she promotes the idea of talking, Rick feels cornered. Then Pauline feels that she is not heard. When Rick takes space instead of talking, the anger convinces Pauline that he does not want closeness. This misunderstanding makes both Rick and Pauline feel that they are not on the same side. Once they feel they are on different sides the stage is set for bullying, belittling, criticism, irrita-

tion, patronization, annoyance, and defensiveness. Eventually, hopelessness takes over, and Rick and Pauline lose track of their capabilities of talking rationally, their belief in each other's intelligence, and what the relationship means to each of them. Neither of them wants this anger, misunderstanding, or hopelessness. They would prefer to be more in touch with their connection.

I asked what set the stage for anger (e.g., "If I were anger, how would I know I could take over your relationship at one particular time, but not at another time?"). Pauline said that it had to do with unfairness. When I asked her to talk more about the unfairness, Pauline said that she always has to fit with Rick, not the other way around. I asked whether she thought more women had to fit with men or if men had to fit with women and Rick interrupted loudly,

> "Look! Yes, I am a white male and I am older, but Pauline has made it. She has published in very competitive, well-regarded places. In our apartment she has the office with a door and I have to work in the dining room. People are calling about her work, not mine. She has all this time and I am doing review after review, just to make a little money, and barely getting to my novel. She got the university job and included me as one of the conditions. Everyone there knows it. What do you think it was like for me going to parties where everyone knows Pauline's work, knowing she was watching to see if I was being friendly instead of sitting by myself?"

I summarized how unfairness and power differences set the stage for anger, and how those differences were complicated by different amounts of recognition and status and different amounts of privileges because of gender. In the face of those differences, I wondered about the compromises they had mentioned in an earlier meeting and a statement that Pauline made in this one. When they spoke about their capabilities of talking rationally, their belief in each other's intelligence, and what the relationship meant to each of them, Pauline had said, "When we get along, we really get along well." I reminded her of that statement and asked what happens to the unfairness in those moments of really getting along well.

She did not answer so I asked whether it would be helpful to talk about a time when they really got along well. Then, together we could think about whether they were creating the relationship the way they wanted it or whether the unfairness was structuring the relationship.

Pauline said that for her a particular time had come to mind immediately, but she did not think that Rick would agree that it was a time when they got along really well. Several weeks earlier, Pauline had given a reading at a bookstore. After signing copies she was mingling with the attendees and could not find Rick. Eventually she found him sitting alone in a corner, immersed in a book. When they got home, they had a fight. Pauline said that Rick did not care about her friends. It was an opportunity to be together as a couple and he was sulking. Rick said that he was having a fine time. He had talked to everyone, then found a book he had wanted to explore for some time. He did not see how that was being unsupportive. The argument escalated and Rick walked out of the apartment. He was walking down the alley when Pauline yelled from the back stoop that he come back right then or not at all. "There was this awful look on his face," she reported, "and he froze. But then he came back. He walked up the stairs, enfolded me in his arms and kissed me. Later that night we were in bed, with jazz playing, and he toasted my book with champagne."

I asked for more details of this memory—the words of the toast, the look on Rick's face, the music that was playing. Then I asked Pauline what it meant to her to have this time. She began to weep and said that it was much more important than the signing. It meant that she could be successful as a writer without sacrificing their relationship.

"So the unfairness threatens to take away your relationship, is that right? But you have held on to it in spite of that?"

They agreed.

"I don't think that either of you invented the kind of gender socialization that has women fitting with men, instead of the other way around, or that creates expectations that in a heterosexual relationship the man should have the more obvious markers of what our society calls success. I don't think either of you invented that, but it does seem that these ideas are playing havoc with your relationship, doesn't it?"

They agreed.

I wondered aloud what happened in that moment when Rick froze, then turned around and came back.

"I realized I wanted the relationship, even though I felt humiliated and misunderstood. I

want the relationship. When Pauline described it, she didn't say that I showed her that I was hurt. But I think I did. Then she softened, and it was just the two of us together."

I said that I wished we had more time to contrast what the power differences and the closeness pulled them toward, but we only had time to name what stood out from our conversation.

Each partner talked about the importance of feeling that the other understood something about his or her experience. Because they were both writers, I wondered whether there was something they might write about this. I was not sure what. The idea was only tentative and very vague.

Session 4

At the beginning of the fourth interview I asked Pauline and Rick if they would like me to read the notes from the previous meeting. They declined and reported that they had had a wonderful couple of weeks since seeing me. Pauline told a number of stories about a visit of some friends from her MFA program, and how wonderful Rick had been. She saw him in a different light—as gracious and friendly and wanting to fit with her life.

Two things about the meaning Pauline made of this set of experiences particularly interested me. One had to do with Rick fitting with her life. I reminded her how she previously had described feeling that she had to fit with his life, and now she was saying he wanted to fit with hers. She nodded and said how important and healing it was to see this effort. The second thing I noticed had to do with Rick's identity and the new description of it. Given her description, I wondered whether Pauline had noticed things about Rick or about their relationship that she had not seen before. She said that it was more like getting back in touch with things she had lost track of, and she told several stories about earlier times in their relationship when Rick had worked to fit with her life, and had been a wonderful friend and partner as they mingled with larger groups of people. She could now envision a future of shared friendships and finding their place as a couple in their new work. Rick agreed, and said that he had believed that all along, and that it was a tremendous relief to feel joined by Pauline. He had learned that she could understand his wanting time alone, if he let her know beforehand and made sure it was not at times that Pauline wanted him to join with her friends.

Session 5

Rick started the fifth interview saying that when they had left the time before, they had wondered whether they had solved their problems and did not need to come back, but they had had one of those awful fights just a few days later. They were not scheduled to see me for almost 2 weeks. Rick was getting ready to go out, just to get away.

"Usually in those situations I don't want to listen to anything Pauline says, because it is nothing but blame and it just makes things worse. I was putting on my jacket to go and she said, 'I have an idea. We never did that writing that Jill mentioned.' So we decided to do it. Each of us wrote a description of what had just happened from the other's point of view. It was quite amazing how accurate we were. Neither of us would have predicted that."

I was interested in reading these descriptions, but the couple had not brought them to the meeting. Instead, I asked what each partner most appreciated that the other understood, what it meant to have that understanding, and what the implications were for their relationship. We also talked about how they had moved from fighting to new levels of understanding on their own.

From my notes of this meeting I made the following document:

Important New Understandings

Rick and Pauline understand some things about each other and their relationship that are important for them to remember:

1. Rick is interested in being part of Pauline's social life. When he takes time for himself, it is not because he is unfriendly or distant. It is because time alone, as well as time together, is important for him.
2. Pauline is most comfortable talking about difficulties. When she talks more and more, she is not trying to promote only her view. She is trying to promote talking. When Rick puts into words why he doesn't want to talk and when he will be willing to talk, Pauline can wait for the conversation.
3. Rick is proud of the success and recognition that Pauline's work has brought her. He also finds that success and recognition difficult, because he would like to have it for his work. Both of these sets of experiences are real and do not cancel each other out. He would like for Pauline to keep in mind that even when he withdraws from her success, he is proud of her.
4. Pauline and Rick recognize that they have been able to find joy, comfort, and compromise in their relationship in spite of their different ways of handling problems, their different levels of "success," and their age difference. They believe that this has to do with love, as well as a delightful closeness and connection that is special to their relationship. It is important to their relationship that they always remember the closeness and connection of special times when the two of them are alone.

Session 6

I sent the document to them between meetings. We began the sixth meeting by reading it and considering whether the couple would like to change anything. Rick and Pauline were happy to leave the document as it was, and they gave examples of how the understandings had made a difference in several situations between meetings. An example that stood out for both of them had occurred the weekend before the interview. Pauline's old friend whom Rick had only met briefly at their wedding, came for a weekend visit. On Sunday morning, Rick told Pauline that he liked Blythe, had enjoyed spending time with the two of them, and that he wanted to sit in a coffee shop and read *The New York Times* all morning on his own. Pauline agreed. That morning was an example of understanding for both Pauline and Rick, and contrasted with similar situations in their past. What Rick contributed was an understanding that it helped Pauline to hear his reason for taking time alone, so that she did not attribute other meaning to those intentions. What Pauline contributed was an understanding that Rick's desire for time alone did not mean bad things about him, her, or the relationship. She had a great morning with her friend Blythe, and the three of them enjoyed the afternoon together. Having this experience behind them left the couple optimistic about blending their styles and being a couple together in the world, not just when they were alone.

Session 7

In the seventh meeting, Rick and Pauline stated that their relationship now seemed free of the anger that had been so disruptive in their past. Pauline wondered whether Rick needed individual therapy now that their relationship was on better footing. Rick agreed. I wondered whether it would be useful to talk a bit about the problem with which Rick struggled.

Rick said, "I'm depressed." I asked a number of questions to try to unpack and get an experience-near description of what he was calling "depression." He described feelings of hopelessness, particularly in relationship to his writing. These feelings were keeping him from writing and caused him to see himself as a failure. At the height of these feelings, he was convinced that there was no point taking on the new job in the fall, because everyone at the university would know that he was a fraud.

JILL: How are these feelings of hopelessness affecting your relationship with Pauline?

RICK: It's terrible. They make me doubt whether I can live up to what she wants me to be. In fact, at times I think I would be better off with someone doing completely different work.

JILL: How would that make a difference?

RICK: There wouldn't be these expectations that I could publish, teach, or even be a writer. Then I could just be free to do what I do.

JILL: So, I am beginning to wonder if what we are talking about here could be difficulty with expectations?

RICK: (*Nods.*)

JILL: Pauline, if you think about what is going on as being difficulty with expectations …

PAULINE: This is ridiculous! It is not my expectations that Rick can write and publish. He has! And not only that, I don't care. That is not what is important to me.

JILL: What is important to you about Rick?

PAULINE: His values. That he cares about things. He thinks independently and says what he thinks. I care that we are close and that he wants to share my life.

JILL: And all of that can happen without the writing?

PAULINE: Absolutely.

RICK: Hold on! I wanted to write before I met Pauline. I have always wanted to write and I did write. But living with a writer who publishes and has readings and wins awards puts it on a whole different plane.

JILL: All right. So, are you saying that a tactic that hopelessness uses to get a hold of you is showing you comparisons?

RICK: Umm, I do make comparisons.

JILL: I'm just wondering, if I were hopelessness and I wanted to take over your experience, how would I get those comparisons going? Would I show you images or say something to you?

RICK: You wouldn't have to do anything. I live with a very successful writer.

JILL: OK. But sometimes hopelessness takes over and other times it doesn't. It seems like it might have to do with comparisons. Does hopelessness say to you, "You'll never write as well as Pauline, or … "?

RICK: What happens, I think, is that her editor calls or she gets 50 e-mails about a review, or she gets asked to speak at something, and I want all that for her. I think it is fantastic, but my agent doesn't return my calls.

JILL: So, OK. If I were going to be hopelessness, would I say, "All these people are calling *her* and *my* agent won't even call me back?"

RICK: Yeah. That would be a good start.

PAULINE: But I can't help it that I get these calls. I don't want them.

JILL: Let's keep in mind that Rick is proud of your work and recognition. It is hopelessness that is inciting this problem, through comparisons, not your writing or how many people notice it. In fact, I am beginning to wonder if it is the comparisons that are the problem and hopelessness is one of its effects.

RICK: I think it comes to the same thing.

PAULINE: Yeah.

JILL: What do you think sets the ground for these comparisons?

RICK: All the calls and honors.

JILL: Yeah, but …

RICK: And that we are in the same field.

JILL: Well, yeah …

RICK: Also that I am older and the man.

JILL: What is it about being older and the man that feeds into this?

RICK: You know. The man as the wage earner and life isn't infinite. There is a finite amount of time to accomplish anything. So I have had more time and I am more programmed for success and still, she's the one who got it.

JILL: So that's what hopelessness and comparisons tell you?

RICK: Yeah.

JILL: Hopelessness and comparisons support the idea that the man is the wage earner and the older one is supposed to be successful first?

RICK: Yeah.

JILL: There are so many pieces of this to talk about, I don't know where to start. Let's come back to the part about being the man and being older. Let's talk a little bit about success. Can you define "success"?

RICK: Well, I guess "success" is accomplishing what you want to.

JILL: (*paging through my notes and looking at early ones*) The first time we met, you said that you had written a novel, and you were at work on another one. How many people do you suppose set out to write novels and never finish them?

RICK: Many.

JILL: Yeah, but you completed one and are working on another. You accomplished what you wanted to. Are you successful?

PAULINE: I think so.

RICK: I think so, too, sometimes, and sometimes I don't.

JILL: Would it be fair to say that hopelessness and comparisons convince you at times that you aren't?

RICK: Yeah.

JILL: So what backs up their arguments? I mean, how have they at times recruited you into believing that you aren't successful?

RICK: You know, I think it has to do with the whole community around here. Before I met Pauline, when I told people I wrote a novel and I had an agent, they were totally impressed. Of course, I wanted to publish, but I was leading the writer's life and that was what was important. Now everyone we know leads a writer's life. It is assumed. You either make it or you don't.

I went on to ask about the impact of this idea of success on Rick and on the relationship. It turned out that this idea of success led to feelings of hopelessness, failure, and competition. It came between Rick and Pauline, making Rick wish he were in a relationship with someone who was not so "successful." It also encouraged guilt and at times got Pauline to hide, minimize, or not enjoy her success. This drove Pauline and Rick further apart and made Rick feel infantilized. None of

these things was what either partner wanted. We also talked about how, if Rick had been the one to publish a novel, some of these things might plague Pauline, but undoubtedly not to the same degree, because she is a woman.

I asked whether they wanted this idea of success to be in charge of their relationship or whether they wanted to be in charge. Both Rick and Pauline were committed to being in charge of the relationship.

I wondered whether what they thought of as "depression" had to do with this idea of success taking over their relationship. They agreed that it did.

I then began to ask about times when their own ideas of success were more in the forefront than cultural ideas of what success meant, and they were more in charge of their lives. We were out of time, so after making a few notes about memories to come back to the next time, the meeting ended.

Session 8

After the seventh interview, I called a couple with whom I had previously worked and asked if it would be all right with them if I shared a document we had made with a couple I was currently seeing. I began the eighth meeting by reading my notes from the time before, then asking Rick and Pauline whether they would be interested in hearing a document made by another couple made who had faced similar difficulties. They were interested, so I read the following document to them:

Joy and Frank's Position on Worry

1. Worry creates an experience of being trapped in an ongoing problem. This is not useful, because it encourages Frank and Joy to give up instead of creatively pursuing new possibilities.
2. Worry makes Joy think about sabotaging her own career. This does not fit with the value both Joy and Frank give to doing their best.
3. Worry is making room for the public evaluation of success to take over Frank and Joy's private life. This brings shame to Frank for not succeeding by public standards and leads him to withdraw. Then, Joy feels abandoned. Joy and Frank would prefer to act as partners.
4. Worry promotes the idea that Frank is dragging Joy down with pessimism. This idea keeps Frank from sharing how he is feeling with Joy. This lack of sharing contributes to a growing distance be-

tween them. Both Joy and Frank prefer closeness and sharing of feelings to distance.

5. Worry is eating away at future dreams. Frank and Joy want to reclaim a shared vision of a meaningful and joyful future.

6. Joy and Frank are committed to not letting the worry come between them and to taking back their present, as well as their future.

Pauline and Rick felt a sense of being joined by Frank and Joy through their willingness to share their document. They found this solidarity to be quite moving. They realized that, as a couple they had never talked about this problem with friends or family. It was a tremendous relief to find that another couple struggled and did something about a similar problem. They noted how Frank and Joy preferred intimacy, as they did. This led to a discussion of the experiences they had had since we last met, in which closeness dominated their relationship rather than the "idea of success." One of the stories they told about these times involved playing pool with a couple of Rick's old friends. These friends were not part of the literary world, and Pauline's identity to them was as "a person, a pool player, Rick's partner, and a funny lady." Although it was important for Pauline to keep her identity as a writer, it was good to see that this was not the only way for her to see herself, to be in the relationship, and to be known to others. Pauline supposed that if they had children, there would be contexts in which her identity was "mother." Because they did not have children, they should perhaps be more purposeful in allowing room for identities that had nothing to do with the imbalance created by a focus on "ideas of success."

Session 9

The ninth interview focused on developing and letting stories of Rick and Pauline being in charge of their relationship, rather than other writers' ideas of success take over their relationship. I had made notes in the previous interview about a couple of events in which Pauline and Rick had taken charge. We talked briefly about these memories, but they were much more interested in telling me about a new development. They had signed up as volunteers in a political campaign. Though they shared a political vision and had previously talked about being more politically active, they had never followed through on this idea, because they thought they should devote as much time as possible to writing. After our previous meet-

ing, they had revisited this idea and agreed that if they were to escape the published writers' ideas of success, they needed friends who were not writers and interests that would expand their world. They had spent the previous weekend canvassing for an upcoming primary. To immerse Rick and Pauline in the telling of "being in charge of their relationship" stories, I asked about details of the weekend. I also asked what they appreciated about themselves, each other, and the relationship that the comparisons and the old ideas of success had obscured.

When I asked for his reflections on this conversation, Rick said that he enjoyed listening to Pauline talk. He remembered that her way with language was interesting not only in written form but also in conversation. He reappreciated her enthusiasm, focus, and dedication. Pauline said she appreciated Rick's quiet ability to join in, the solidity he brought to an endeavor, the feeling of safety she had being with him. They both appreciated the fun they could have as a couple and the enjoyment of meeting others together. They liked being part of a mission that was a long shot and were willing to give it their all, just because it was a way of standing for what they both wanted in the world.

I wondered what it was like for each of them to hear the way the other saw him or her. Rick liked Pauline's description. He had not thought about his ability to provide a feeling of safety, but he appreciated it and liked thinking about himself as offering solidity. Pauline was enthusiastic about Rick appreciating her language, because that created more room in their relationship for conversation. When she saw herself through his description, she felt compelled to continue with the enthusiasm, focus, and dedication to the political causes they were embracing. They were committed to continuing and to making new connections in this world as a couple.

Session 10

The tenth interview focused on more stories of Rick and Pauline expanding their relationship to new communities and commitments. Rick described the parity people who were not writers saw in their work. "To them, we are both just writers. They've never heard of either of us. It seems about the same to them that a review of mine was published in the *Tribune* and a story of hers was accepted by *The New Yorker*."

I asked how the perception of these new friends made a difference when they were back with their writer friends. "The world looks bigger," Pauline said. "I know that what happens in this election is more important than my latest story. I think that neither of us gets caught up in other people's critiques or ideas." Rick agreed.

They had not set out to spend time outside of their apartment, but through our conversation, they decided it was important to be in the world, outside of their own space.

Session 11

The eleventh interview was our last. In looking back, several things stood out for Rick and Pauline. The fighting was different. It was less frequent and less intense. The turning point had been the argument in which Rick had left, Pauline had called after him, and he had returned. Although we had never talked about it in therapy, since that time, when fighting began, they had committed to saying, "This argument is not about whether we should stay together. I love you." They were rigorously saying these words at the beginning of every argument, and the statement dramatically changed the arguments, which never again obscured all the wonderful things about their relationship. Pauline said that once they started saying these words to each other, they assumed good motives. This made a huge difference.

They had continued their political involvement and also had learned from it the importance of spending time together that was not work time. This reminded me of the grocery shopping they had mentioned in our first meeting. They realized that what they called "friendship time" made the other time less urgent. If they did something fun together on the weekend, there was more good will between them. Their differences in how much time they wanted alone were not a problem. I asked what each of them contributed to this. For Pauline, it was no longer attributing negative intentions. For Rick it was patience and taking care to say more of his thoughts out loud.

We also reviewed their experience of themselves in the relationship. Rick said that when they started therapy, he had felt like a bad guy. Now, he appreciated the strength Pauline saw in him, and his growing patience. The different levels of "success" were not easy for him, but by keeping in mind a larger context, he could see himself as successful. Pauline said she felt loved. She saw herself as lovable through Rick's eyes. Before, she had seen herself as hysterical. Lovable was much better.

I wondered how it would make a difference to bring these new experiences of themselves and the relationship with them to their new job. They thought they would be more secure in themselves and in the relationship than they otherwise might have been. They also thought that it would be very important to establish themselves as a couple outside of the academic community from the start. They were going to go house hunting in a few weeks. They decided also to spend some time trying to discover other communities that would appreciate them the way they had grown to appreciate themselves.

The following October, I got a card from Pauline and Rick. They reported that they were doing great. They loved their house, and Rick had connected with neighbors around gardening. They were politically active and had new friends, many of whom were not writers. They wrote that they both enjoyed teaching and did not have time to notice whether the rest of the faculty saw them the way they saw themselves or not!

SUGGESTIONS FOR FURTHER READING

Freedman, J., & Combs, G. (2002). *Narrative therapy with couples . . . and a whole lot more: A collection of papers, essays, and exercises*, Adelaide, Australia: Dulwich Centre Publications.

Hare-Mustin, R. (1994). Discourses in the mirrored room: A postmodern analysis of therapy. *Family Process, 33*, 19–35.

Percy, I. (2007). Composing our lives together: Narrative therapy with couples. In E. Shaw & J. Crawley (Eds.), *Couple therapy in Australia: Issues emerging from practice* (pp. 139–158). Melbourne: PsychOz.

White, M. (2004). Narrative practice, couple therapy, and conflict dissolution. In M. White (Ed.), *Narrative practice and exotic lives: Resurrecting diversity in everyday life* (pp. 1–41). Adelaide, Australia: Dulwich Centre Publications.

REFERENCES

Adams-Westcott, J., Dafforn, T., & Sterne, P. (1993). Escaping victim life stories and co-constructing personal agency. In S. Gilligan & R. Price (Eds.), *Therapeutic conversations* (pp. 258–271). New York: Norton.

Avis, J. M. (1985). The politics of functional family therapy: A feminist critique. *Journal of Marital and Family Therapy, 11*, 127–138.

Bateson, G. (1972). *Steps to an ecology of mind.* New York: Ballantine.

Bateson, G. (1980). *Mind and nature—A necessary unity*. New York: Bantam Books.

Besa, D. (1994). Evaluating narrative family therapy using single-system research designs. *Research on Social Work Practice*, 4(3), 309–326.

Brown, C., & Augusta-Scott, T. (2007). *Narrative therapy: Making meaning, making lives*. Thousand Oaks, CA: Sage.

Bruner, J. (1986). *Actual minds/possible worlds*. Cambridge, MA: Harvard University Press.

Carey, B. (2007, May 22). This is your life (and how you tell it). *The New York Times*. Available at *www.NYTimes.com/2007/05/22/HEALTH/PSYCHOLOGY/22NAR.HTML*.

Carter, E., Papp, P., Silverstein, O., & Walters, M. (1984). *Mothers and sons, fathers and daughters* [Monograph Series 2(1)]. Washington, DC: Women's Project in Family Therapy.

Cohen, S. M., Combs, G., DeLaurenti, B., DeLaurenti, P., Freedman, J., Larimer, D., & Shulman, D. (1998). Minimizing hierarchy in therapeutic relationships: A reflecting team approach. In M. Hoyt (Ed.), *Handbook of constructive therapies: Innovative approaches from leading practitioners* (pp. 276–293). San Francisco: Jossey-Bass.

Combs, G., & Freedman, J. (1999). Developing relationships, performing identities. In *Narrative therapy and community work: A conference collection* (pp. 27–32). Adelaide, Australia: Dulwich Centre Publications.

Derrida, J. (1978). *Writing and difference*. Chicago: University of Chicago Press.

Epston, D. (1989). *Collected works*. Adelaide, Australia: Dulwich Centre Publications.

Epston, D. (1993). Internalizing discourses versus externalizing discourses. In S. Gilligan & R. Price (Eds.), *Therapeutic conversations* (pp. 161–177). New York: Norton.

Epston, D. (1998). *Catching up with David Epston: A collection of narrative practice-based papers published between 1991 and 1996*. Adelaide, Australia: Dulwich Centre Publications.

Epston, D. (1999). Co-research: The making of an alternative knowledge. In *Narrative therapy and community work: A conference collection* (pp. 137–157). Adelaide, Australia: Dulwich Centre Publications.

Epston, D. (2000, May 11–12). *Crafting questions for narrative practice*. A two-day workshop at Evanston Family Therapy Center, Evanston, IL.

Epston, D. (2006, March 2–3). *Two-day intensive course in narrative therapy*. A workshop at Evanston Family Therapy Center, Evanston, IL.

Etchison, M., & Kleist, D. (2000). Review of narrative therapy: Research and utility. *Family Journal*, 8, 61–66.

Foucault, M. (1965). *Madness and civilization: A history of insanity in the age of reason* (R. Howard, trans.). New York: Random House.

Foucault, M. (1975). *The birth of the clinic: An archeology of medical perception* (A. M. Sheridan Smith, trans.). New York: Random House.

Foucault, M. (1977). *Discipline and punish: The birth of the prison* (A. Sheridan, trans.). New York: Pantheon Books.

Foucault, M. (1980). *Power/knowledge: Selected interviews and other writings, 1972–1977* (C. Gordon, Ed.). New York: Pantheon Books.

Foucault, M. (1985). *The history of sexuality: Vol. 2. The use of pleasure* (R. Hurley, trans.). New York: Pantheon Books.

France, C., & Uhlin, B. (2006). Narrative as an outcome domain in psychosis. *Psychology and Psychotherapy: Theory, Research and Practice*, 1(79), 53–68.

Freedman, J., & Combs, G. (1993). Invitations to new stories: Using questions to explore alternative possibilities. In S. Gilligan & R. Price (Eds.), *Therapeutic conversations* (pp. 291–303). New York: Norton.

Freedman, J., & Combs, G. (1996). *Narrative therapy: The social construction of preferred realities*. New York: Norton.

Freedman, J., & Combs, G. (1997). Lists. In C. Smith & D. Nylund (Eds.), *Narrative therapies with children and adolescents* (pp. 147–161). New York: Guilford Press.

Freedman, J., & Combs, G. (2000). Therapy relationships that open possibilities for us all. *Dulwich Centre Journal*, 1–2, 17–20.

Freedman, J., & Combs, G. (2002). *Narrative therapy with couples . . . and a whole lot more: A collection of papers, essays, and exercises*. Adelaide, Australia: Dulwich Centre Publications.

Freedman, J., & Combs, G. (2004). Relational identity in narrative work with couples. In S. Madigan (Ed.), *Therapy from the outside in* (pp. 30–40). Vancouver: Yaletown Family Therapy.

Freeman, J., Epston, D., & Lobovits, D. (1997). *Playful approaches to serious problems: Narrative therapy with children and families*. New York: Norton.

Geertz, C. (1978). *The interpretation of cultures*. New York: Basic Books.

Goldner, V. (1985a). Feminism and family therapy. *Family Process*, 24, 31–47.

Goldner, V. (1985b). Warning: Family therapy may be dangerous to your health. *Family Therapy Networker*, 9, 19–23.

Hare-Mustin, R. (1978). A feminist approach to family therapy. *Family Process*, 17, 181–194.

Hare-Mustin, R. (1994). Discourses in the mirrored room: A postmodern analysis of therapy. *Family Process*, 33, 19–35.

Kogan, S., & Gale, J. (1997). Decentering therapy: Textual analysis of a narrative therapy session. *Family Process*, 36, 101–126.

Laird, J. (1989). Women and stories: Restorying women's self-constructions. In M. McGoldrick, C. Anderson, & F. Walsh (Eds.), *Women in families: A framework for family therapy* (pp. 427–450). New York: Norton.

Maisel, R., Epston, D., & Borden, A. (2004). *Biting the hand that starves you: Inspiring resistance to anorexia/bulimia*. New York: Norton.

Monk, G., Winslade, J., Croket, K., & Epston, D. (Eds.). (1997). *Narrative therapy in practice: The archaeology of hope*. San Francisco: Jossey-Bass.

Morgan, A. (2000). *What is narrative therapy?: An easy-to-read introduction*. Adelaide, Australia: Dulwich Centre Publications.

Myerhoff, B. (1982). Life history among the elderly: Performance, visibility, and remembering. In J. Ruby (Ed.), *A crack in the mirror: Reflexive perspectives in anthropology* (pp. 99–117). Philadelphia: University of Pennsylvania Press.

Myerhoff, B. (1986). Life not death in Venice: Its second life. In V. Turner & E. Bruner (Eds.), *The anthropology of experience* (pp. 261–285). Chicago: University of Illinois Press.

O'Connor, T., Davis, A., Meakes, E., Pickering, R., & Schuman, M. (2004). Narrative therapy using a reflecting team: An ethnographic study of therapists' experiences. *Contemporary Family Therapy: An International Journal, 26*(1), 23–40.

Payne, M. (2006). *Narrative therapy: An introduction for counselors*. London: Sage. (Original work published 2000)

Ryle, G. (1990). *Collected papers: Critical essays and collected essays 1929–68*. Bristol, UK: Thoemmes Press. (Original work published 1971)

Seltzer, M., & Seltzer, W. (2004). Co-texting, chronotope and ritual: A Bakhtinian framing of talk in therapy. *Journal of Family Therapy, 26*(4), 358–383.

White, M. (1986). Negative explanation, restraint and double description: A template for family therapy. *Family Process, 25*, 169–184.

White, M. (1987, Spring). Family therapy and schizophrenia: Addressing the "in-the-corner" lifestyle. *Dulwich Centre Newsletter*, pp. 14–21.

White, M. (1988, Summer). The externalizing of the problem and the re-authoring of lives and relationships. *Dulwich Centre Newsletter*, pp. 3–20.

White, M. (1989). *Selected papers*. Adelaide, Australia: Dulwich Centre Publications.

White, M. (1991). Deconstruction and therapy. *Dulwich Centre Newsletter, 3*, 21–40.

White, M. (1995). Reflecting teamwork as definitional ceremony. In *Reauthoring lives: Interviews and essays* (pp. 172–198). Adelaide, Australia: Dulwich Centre Publications.

White, M. (1997). *Narratives of therapists' lives*. Adelaide, Australia: Dulwich Centre Publications.

White, M. (2000). *Reflections on narrative practice: Essays and interviews*. Adelaide, Australia: Dulwich Centre Publications.

White, M. (2005). Outsider–witness responses. In *Michael White workshop notes*. Published September 21, 2005, on *www.dulwichcentre.com.au*.

White, M. (2007). *Maps of narrative therapy*. New York: Norton.

White, M., & Epston, D. (1990). *Narrative means to therapeutic ends*. New York: Norton.

White, M., & Epston, D. (1992). *Experience, contradiction, narrative, and imagination*. Adelaide, Australia: Dulwich Centre Publications.

Zimmerman, J., & Dickerson, V. (1996). *If problems talked: Narrative therapy in action*. New York: Guilford Press.

CHAPTER 9

Solution-Focused Couple Therapy

MICHAEL F. HOYT

When you play songs, you can bring back people's memories of when they fell in love. That's where the power is.
——JOHNNY MERCER (SONGWRITER OF "MOON RIVER" AND OTHER BALLADS, QUOTED IN BERENDT, 1994, P. 90)

Suppose that one night, while you were asleep, there was a miracle and this problem was solved. How would you know? What would be different?
——STEVE DE SHAZER (1988, P. 10)

Solution-focused brief therapy (SFBT) is an intervention approach developed by Steve de Shazer (1982, 1985, 1988, 1991a, 1994a; de Shazer et al., 2006) and Insoo Kim Berg (1994a; Berg & Dolan, 2001; Berg & Kelly, 2000; Berg & Miller, 1992; Berg & Reuss, 1997; DeJong & Berg, 1997; Miller & Berg, 1995), with additional valuable explications from a number of contributors (e.g., Bonjean, 1997, 2003; Dolan, 1991; George, Iveson, & Ratner, 1999, 2006; Lethem, 1994; Metcalf, 2004; Miller, Hubble, & Duncan, 1996; Nelson, 2005; Nelson & Thomas, 2007; O'Connell & Palmer, 2003; O'Hanlon & Weiner-Davis, 1989; Simon & Nelson, 2007; Tohn & Oshlag, 1996a; Walter & Peller, 1992, 2000; Weiner-Davis, 1992). Although there is a theory-based, teachable model with specific techniques—the topic of this chapter—it is important to recognize that the essence of solution-focused therapy is an overarching worldview, a way of thinking and being, not a set of clinical operations (see Lipchik, 1994).[1] As the name implies, the focus is on *solutions*, on *what works for clients*. It is a "post-structural revision" (de Shazer & Berg, 1992; also see de Shazer, 1993a)—a non-normative, constructivist view

that emphasizes the use of language in the social construction of reality (see Hoyt, 1994a, 1996a, 1998, 2000, 2004; McNamee & Gergen, 1992; G. Miller, 1997). It appreciates the power of the subjective and operates with the assumption that clients have the competency and creativity, sometimes with skillful facilitation, to shift perspectives in ways that will open new options for experience and interaction. Solution-focused therapy respects clients' own resources and is directed toward *building solutions* rather than increasing insight into putative maladaptive psychological mechanisms. It is optimistic, collaborative, future-oriented, versatile, user-friendly, and often effective.

BACKGROUND OF THE APPROACH

Solution-focused therapy was developed in the late 1970s and 1980s by Steve de Shazer and his colleagues at the Brief Family Therapy Center (BFTC) in Milwaukee, Wisconsin.[2] de Shazer had been influenced by the work of the pioneering Mental Research Institute (MRI) group in Palo Alto, California (Watzlawick, Weakland,

& Fisch, 1974; Fisch, Weakland, & Segal, 1982; Shoham & Rohrbaugh, 2002), which in turn was influenced by the work of the renowned psychiatrist–psychologist–hypnotherapist Milton Erickson—especially Erickson's ideas about strategic intervention and the fuller utilization of clients' submerged competencies.[3] As indicated by the title of their keynote book, *Change: Principles of Problem Formation and Problem Resolution* (Watzlawick et al., 1974), the MRI group had focused on how clients create and resolve problems, including how efforts to solve a problem sometimes actually perpetuate the problem. de Shazer and his Milwaukee-based group took a somewhat different view, focusing instead on those times ("exceptions") when the presenting problem was not present, as expressed in the title of their signal counterpaper, "Brief Therapy: Focused Solution Development" (de Shazer et al., 1986):

> The task of brief therapy is to help clients do something different, by changing their interactive behavior and/or their interpretation of behavior and situations so that a solution (a resolution of their complaint) can be achieved. (p. 208)

DeJong and Berg (1997, p. 13) describe a watershed moment in their book *Interviewing for Solutions*:

> de Shazer first hit upon the idea that there is not a necessary connection between problem and solution in 1982, when working with a particular family (Hopwood & de Shazer, 1994). As usual, de Shazer and his colleagues asked, "What brings you in?" In response, family members kept interrupting one another until, by the end of the session, they had listed 27 different problems. Since none of the 27 were clearly defined, de Shazer and his colleagues were unable to design an intervention. Still, wishing to encourage the family members to focus on something different from their problems, de Shazer and his colleagues told them to pay careful attention to "what is happening in your lives that you want to continue to have happen." When the family returned, two weeks later, they said that things were going very well and they felt their problems were solved. According to the assumptions of the problem-solving approach, the family should not have improved so dramatically, because the practitioner had not yet been able to isolate and assess the patterns and nature of the problems. Their experience with such cases led de Shazer and his colleagues towards a solution focus in place of a problem focus. They and many others. ... have been continuing to work out the implications of this shift ever since.

The two groups, BFTC and MRI, have complementary approaches (Weakland & Fisch, 1992), both eschewing obfuscating theory in favor of "minimalistic," pragmatic, outcome-oriented approaches. As Shoham, Rohrbaugh, and Patterson (1995, p. 143, emphasis in original) explain in their review in the second edition of the *Clinical Handbook of Couple Therapy*:

> The hallmark of these models is conceptual and technical parsimony. The aim of therapy is simply to resolve the presenting complaint as quickly and efficiently as possible so that clients can get on with life: Goals such as promoting personal growth, working through underlying emotional issues, or teaching couples better problem-solving and communication skills are not emphasized. Both therapies offer minimal theory, focusing narrowly on the presenting complaint and relevant solutions, and both are nonnormative in that neither attempts to specify what constitutes a normal or dysfunctional marriage. Both pay close attention not only to what clients *do* but also to how they *view* the problem, themselves, and each other; in fact, both therapies assume that the "reality" of problems and change is constructed more than discovered. Both therapies also attach considerable importance to clients' "customership" for change and to the possibility that therapy itself may play a role in maintaining (rather than resolving) problems. Finally, in contrast to most other treatments for couples, therapists following the MRI and Milwaukee models often see the partners individually, even when the focus of intervention is a complaint about the marriage itself.

The most fundamental difference between problem- and solution-focused therapy concerns the emphasis each gives to the concept of "solution": While the MRI approach aims to interdict existing solutions that maintain the problem and to promote "less of the same," the Milwaukee model seeks to identify exceptions to the problem and develop new solutions that work.

NON-NORMATIVE (IDIOMORPHIC) ASSESSMENT

Solution-focused therapists meet clients where they are (oftentimes beginning a session by asking, "What brings you in?" or "What are you hoping to accomplish coming here?") and avoid traditional diagnostic categories and preconceived notions of what may be healthy/unhealthy or functional/ dysfunctional for a particular couple, individual, or family. Although general guidelines can be described, every case is considered to be unique. The therapist attempts to "keep it simple" by "taking the patient seriously" (de Shazer and Weakland, cited in Hoyt, 1994b), accepting the clients' version of what is—and is not—a problem. Primacy is given to clients' experiences, goals, ideas, values, motivations, and worldviews, which are respectfully accepted as valid and real. While some discussion of the past allows clients a sense of being heard and acknowledged, and provides an opportunity for exploring clients' ideas about what would be helpful (their theories of change) and a reconnaissance of past successes and exceptions to the problem, the thrust of the solution-focused session is present- to future-oriented.

The therapist needs to have skills to join and work with persons of varying diversities to help them develop solutions that fit *their* frames of reference. The solution-focused approach is client-centered and transcultural, in that it truly respects the "local knowledge" (individual, familial, social) of those who seek therapy; "cultural diversity" is honored in that the emphasis is genuinely on learning *from* clients, not just *about* them. The approach tends to be apolitical, however, and sociocultural topics such as ethnicity, class, race, and gender roles are not usually discussed explicitly unless clients make them the focus of conversation.

Initially, the solution-focused approach emerged in an inductive manner, from studying what clients and therapists did that preceded clients declaring that their problems were "solved." It was noticed that problems were described as "solved" (or "resolved," "dissolved," or simply "no longer problems") when clients began to engage in new and different perceptions and behaviors vis-à-vis the presenting difficulty (Hoyt & Berg, 2000). This recognition led to de Shazer's "basic rules" of solution-focused therapy:

- If it ain't broke, don't fix it.
- Once you know what works, do more of it.
- If it doesn't work, don't do it again; do something different. (quoted in Hoyt, 1996b, p. 68)

As previously noted, at times *solutions* may not even seem to have a direct connection to *problems*—development of a solution often involves a reformulation or different construction, such that the former position loses its relevance or simply "dis-solves." The client–couple has "moved on," and what was once a problem is "no longer an issue."

GOAL SETTING

It's the *clients'* therapy (and life). The solution-focused therapist is on the lookout for the *clients'* notions of what would constitute a viable solution or success. As de Shazer (1991a, p. 112, emphasis in original) has written:

> Early in their conversations, therapists and clients address the question, "How do we know when to stop meeting like this?" Both clinical experience and research indicate that workable goals tend to have the following general characteristics. They are:
>
> 1. small rather than large;
> 2. salient to clients;
> 3. described in specific, concrete behavioral terms;
> 4. achievable within the practical contexts of clients' lives;
> 5. perceived by the clients as involving their "hard work";
> 6. described as the "start of something" and not as the "end of something";
> 7. treated as involving new behavior(s) rather than the absence or cessation of existing behavior(s).
>
> Thus goals are depictions of what will be *present*, what will be happening in the clients' lives when the complaint is absent, when the pain that brought them to therapy is absent and they therefore no longer depict life in problematic terms.

de Shazer (p. 113) goes on to suggest using his well-known future-oriented "Miracle Question" to elicit goals within an interpersonal framework:

> Suppose that one night there is a miracle and while you are sleeping the problem that brought you into therapy is solved: How would you know? What would be different? (de Shazer, 1988, p. 5)
> What will you notice the next morning that will tell you that there has been a miracle? What will your spouse notice?[4]

How (and where) we look helps to determine what we see (Hoyt, 2000). In *Words Were Originally Magic*, de Shazer (1994a, p. 10) elaborates the relevance of this for therapists working with couples:

> What we talk about and how we talk about it makes a difference (to the client). Thus reframing a "marital problem" into an "individual problem" or an "individual problem" into a "marital problem" makes a difference both in how we talk about things and where we look for solutions.

Solution building in SFBT begins with clients' descriptions of how they want their lives to be different; it can be understood as beginning with the end of the story rather than the beginning of the problems (Berg & Dolan, 2001, p. 5). "Goaling" is an on-going, dynamic process, open to renegotiation, often more a process of identifying and moving toward possibilities than locking in fixed behavioral targets (Walter & Peller, 2000). Partners also may have different ideas, of course, about what constitutes the problem and what would constitute the solution; this provides the opportunity for a both/and (not an either/or) negotiation:

> HOYT: What about the situation of the so-called "multiproblem family"? […]
>
> DE SHAZER: […] We think about them as "multigoal families." […] First of all, if you ask the miracle question early enough in the session, you oftentimes avoid that difficulty—having all these multiple goals. Sometimes.
>
> HOYT: Who do you ask the miracle question of?
>
> DE SHAZER: Everybody.
>
> HOYT: And if everyone gives a different answer?
>
> DE SHAZER: That's reasonable.
>
> HOYT: Then you have competing goals.
>
> DE SHAZER: That's normal and reasonable. Then you say "Okay, 10 stands for this package—everything you've been talking about, those kinds of things. Whatever it will take for you guys each individually and collectively to recognize that a miracle has happened, that's 10. Where are we today?" We get different estimates where each of them are. Then we sort of work on getting everybody's number on the scale and ignore, if you will, the fact that their version of 10 is probably different, because it's always going to be different with more than one person. And even with one person, he's going to have more than one goal, and they may conflict with each other anyway. […] Our studies indicate that most people—most families stop with 7 being good enough, and that 6 months later they will have frequently moved up to 8, but that is almost the outer limit. Very few people make 10. Those that do make 10 usually end up going into the teens as well—"overachievers." (Hoyt, 1996b, pp. 70–71, emphasis in original)

Eve Lipchik, a former member of the BFTC group, reminds us of the importance, when working with couples and families, of forming and maintaining a relationship with all the attending members:

> A technique that helps me stay centered is not to listen to one person talk too long without asking the other for their view of what they heard. Frequent switching and checking between clients is a way of communicating that I am equally interested in what all of them have to say. I have been told by clients after treatment that what they think helped them the most was that I never took sides. They said that while they disagreed bitterly with each other, they trusted their relationship with me, and my acceptance of all views motivated them to give consideration to the perspectives of other family members. (Lipchik, 1997, p. 163; also see Ziegler & Hiller's [2001, pp. 39–53] discussion about active neutrality.)

Friedman and Lipchik (1999, p. 325) elaborate and note the utility of using a solution-focused approach:

> Differing perceptions between partners requires great sensitivity in acknowledging often strongly held yet divergent points of view while maintaining a working alliance with each member of the couple. In addition, faced with sometimes volatile and emotionally charged communications and affects, the couple therapist must manage high levels of reactivity in ways that offer the couple a path out of its members' problem-saturated reality. To meet these challenges, the time-effective, solution-focused therapist acts as a facilitator of the therapeutic conversation in ways that open space for the couple to move toward a preferred future. Working from a perspective of competencies and strengths, we take a nonpathologizing approach that respects the clients' goals and utilizes the clients' own resources and "expert knowledges" in reaching these goals. (Friedman, 1997; Lipchik, 1993)

THE STRUCTURE OF THE (COUPLE) THERAPY PROCESS

Although therapy with a couple may present some particular challenges—such as each member vying for the therapist's attention and trying to get the therapist on his or her side, or the partners presenting differing and sometimes seemingly contradictory histories and goals—the basic structure and therapeutic processes of solution-focused intervention are much the same whoever attends the session:

> Is marital therapy somehow different from family therapy? If so, what is the difference? And if there is a difference, does this difference make a difference?
>
>   Since our practice and the practice of the Brief Family Therapy Center (BFTC) involve seeing individuals (people who live alone, half a marital pair, or one member of a larger family group), couples (mar-

ried and unmarried, heterosexual and homosexual pairs), and family groups (two or more people, representing at least two generations or parents without the troublesome child), we found that the distinction between marital therapy and family therapy does not apply. A problem is a problem; the number of people (and their relationship to one another) whom the therapist sees to help solve the problem does not seem a useful distinction. This, of course, presupposes a strong belief in the systemic concept of wholism: If you change one element in a system, or the relationship between that element and another element, the system as a whole will be affected [....]

The only criterion that seems to make a potential difference is that in "marital therapy" the relationship treated is that between two people of the same generation, whereas in family therapy the relationship of concern is often or usually between people of different generations. But does this affect the nature of the problems encountered or the nature of the solutions or the patterns of intervention–response?

A quick check of case records accumulated over the years at BFTC and some research we have been doing indicated that the nature of problems, the nature of solutions, and the patterns of intervention–response do not differ along the lines implied by this distinction. In fact, the process of therapy seems relatively constant across situations. The kinds of intervention messages used appear over and over, and the patterns of response appear over and over. *Marital therapy, individual therapy,* and *family therapy* do not seem to be separate classes of brief therapy. (de Shazer & Berg, 1985, pp. 97–98, emphasis in original)

On initial phone contact, the caller may be invited to bring to the session whomever is involved. "A part is not apart" (de Shazer & Berg, 1985; also see Weiner-Davis, 1995, 1998), however, and it is recognized that working with only one of the partners present can still have powerful effects upon all concerned.

Usually there is one therapist, who sits across from the clients. In some clinics and training situations, a team may observe (with the clients' informed consent) and consult from behind a one-way mirror, but in common practice most solution-focused therapists work successfully without this "stimulating but not necessary" (de Shazer, 1985, p. 18) arrangement.

Solution-focused therapy is typically time-unlimited (no preset session maximum), and session appointments are made one at a time—the implication being that one may be enough. A course of therapy generally lasts 1–10 sessions, sometimes longer, and clients can return on an intermittent or as-needed basis (Hoyt, 1995, 2000). Sessions

may be scheduled as frequently or infrequently as clients and therapists desire and find convenient and useful—often a week to a few weeks apart. A couple wanting another appointment in 1 week might be complimented for "wanting to get right to it," while a couple wanting to wait a month might be complimented for "wanting time to see some progress" before returning.

In 1991, de Shazer (1991a) reported the average number of sessions per case as 4.7; in 1996, he indicated (in Hoyt, 1996b) that the average had dropped to 3. Using an approach based on the BFTC model, single-session therapies were demonstrated to be successful in a wide variety of cases (see Talmon, 1990, 1993; Rosenbaum, Hoyt, & Talmon, 1990; Hoyt, 1994c). Other research results are reviewed in McKeel (1996), DeJong and Hopwood (1996), Zimmerman, Prest, and Wetzel (1997), Gingerich and Eisengart (2000), and Macdonald (2003).

THE ROLE OF THE THERAPIST

The solution-focused therapist serves essentially as a consultant, interviewing purposefully (Lipchik & de Shazer, 1986; Lipchik, 1987; Weakland, 1993; Weiner-Davis, 1993) to "influence the clients' view of the problem in a manner that leads to solution" (Berg & Miller, 1992, p. 70). The therapist functions as "guardian of the conversation" (to borrow an apt phrase from Wile, 2002, p. 300), endeavoring to help the couple build a solution—rather than getting bogged down in "problem talk"—by asking questions (discussed at length below) and carefully punctuating responses to highlight a positive reality facilitative of clients' goals. Clients usually respond directly to the therapist, as well as talking with one another.

The interview process is designed to assist clients in achieving new perceptions and meanings. It is directive in that it deliberately encourages clients to look at things differently, but it does not supply answers. Rather, it provides a context for clients to focus on "what's right" and other possible ways of being "right," rather than on complaints of "what's wrong." A problem arises and a couple seeks therapy when the partners view their situation in such a way that they do not have access to what is needed to achieve what they consider reasonable satisfaction. By directing clients away from the problem-saturated narrative (story) that has embroiled them, the therapist attempts to create a context for the clients to develop their own, more useful ways of looking and responding.

The solution-focused therapist serves as a skillful facilitator, assisting clients to better utilize their own (perhaps overlooked) strengths and competencies, with a recognition that how clients conceive their situation—the way they "story" their lives—will either empower them or cut them off from existing resources: "Our attention is focused primarily in the here and now, and even more importantly, on the future, since the future provides a blank canvas on which the couple can paint a picture of the pair's wishes and hopes" (Friedman & Lipchik, 1999, pp. 325–326). The solution-focused therapist assumes a posture of "not knowing" (Anderson & Goolishian, 1992; Hoyt & Berg, 2000), allowing the clients to be "experts," rather than the therapist telling the clients what is "really" wrong and how to fix it.

The therapist–couple alliance is evolving and dynamic. In his now-classic paper, "The Death of Resistance," de Shazer (1984) noted that traditional theories of resistance were tantamount to pitting the therapist against the client in a fight that the therapist had to win in order for the client to be successful. In contradistinction, de Shazer suggested shifting the focus of therapeutic activity to the study of how people *do* change. As de Shazer and Berg (1985, p. 98) explain:

In our view, the therapist needs to set the stage for the "cooperating" of client and therapist. The therapist needs to assume that the client is also interested in cooperating and, consequently, to build the therapeutic stance on the assumption that changing is inevitable, rather than difficult, as many models built on the concept of resistance assume. Of course, the particular way of cooperating can differ from session to session with the same client. (de Shazer, 1982)

From this perspective, clients could be seen as having unique ways of *cooperating with* rather than resisting the therapist in their mutual efforts to bring about desired changes (see Hoyt & Miller, 2000). Although therapists may know that they are helpers—or at least think they are—clients may not be ready for the kind of help the therapists want to offer. Imposition tends to produce opposition (Hoyt, 2000). Appreciating and working *with* clients' sense of their situation—including their theories, language, motivations, goals, and stages of change (Berg & Miller, 1992; Duncan, Hubble,

& Miller, 1997; Duncan et al., 1998)—maintains therapist–client cooperation and vitiates the concept of *resistance*.

Solution-focused therapists (see Berg, 1989) conceptualize three types of therapist–client relationships, which can (and do) alternate within sessions: *customer, complaint,* and *visitor.* As Shoham et al. (1995, p. 153, emphasis added) explain:

Here the distinction between customer, complainant, and visitor-type relationships offers guidelines for therapeutic cooperation or "fit" (de Shazer, 1988; Berg & Miller, 1992). If the relationship involves a *visitor* with whom the therapist cannot define a clear complaint or goal, cooperation involves nothing more than sympathy, politeness, and compliments for whatever the clients are successfully doing (with no tasks or requests for change). In a *complainant* relationship, where clients present a complaint but appear unwilling to take action or want someone else to change, the therapist cooperates by accepting their views, giving compliments, and sometimes prescribing observational tasks (e.g., to notice exceptions to the complaint pattern). Finally, with *customers* who want to do something about a complaint, the principle of fit allows the therapist to be more direct in guiding them toward solutions. . . .
    Both de Shazer (1988) and Berg and Miller (1992) emphasize that the customer–complainant–visitor categories represent dynamic, changing attributes of the therapist–client relationship, not static characteristics of the clients themselves. Visitors and complainants can become customers and vice versa. In fact, one of the main reasons to cooperate with clients in this way is to increase possibilities for customership.

Even if a couple has not been mandated to treatment by the legal system, one partner may, in fact, be under mandate if he or she has come only under the insistence or threat of the other. With clients who are not there voluntarily, it is especially important to develop goals that appeal to each client (see Friedman, 1993a; Rosenberg, 2000; Tohn & Oshlag, 1996b). "What would it take to get your partner off your back?" may not sound very elegant, but for some clients it may be a more engaging and effective starting place than "How would you like to improve your marriage?" or "Let's look at ways you and your partner can enhance your relationship."

As Hoyt and Miller (2000) have written, therapists may also find it helpful in advancing therapist–client "fit" and cooperation to recognize where the client–couple may be in terms of "stages of change." In Prochaska's (1999) "transtheoretical model," for example, change unfolds over a series of six stages of motivational readiness. Some differential intervention strategies are suggested if one combines Prochaska's stages-of-change model with some ideas from solution-focused and strategic therapy (de Shazer, 1985, 1988; Miller, Hubble, & Duncan, 1996), as discussed at length by Miller et al. (1997, pp. 88–104; see especially Hoyt & Miller, 2000):

> *Precontemplation*: Suggest that the client "think about it" and provide information and education;
> *Contemplation*: Encourage thinking, recommend an observation task in which the client is asked to notice something (such as what happens to make things better or worse), and join with the client's lack of commitment to action with a "Go slow!" directive;
> *Preparation*: Offer treatment options, invite the client to choose from viable alternatives;
> *Action*: Amplify what works—get details of success and reinforce;
> *Maintenance*: Support success, predict setbacks, make contingency plans for relapse prevention;
> *Termination*: Wish well, say goodbye, leave an open door for possible return as needed.

As discussed in the next section, the solution-focused therapist maintains activity to keep the couple moving toward solution rather than engaging in extended blame talk and escalation of negative affect (see Table 9.1).

TECHNIQUES OF SOLUTION-FOCUSED COUPLE THERAPY: TOOLS FOR COLLABORATIVE PRACTICE

> We hesitate to use the words techniques or interventions because those words often connote an idea that the therapist does something to the client. The [solution-focused] approach focuses on collaborative conversations between clients and therapists rather than therapists' doing something to clients. We recognize, however, that therapists in the [solution-focused] approach are trained, supervised, and experienced in particular kinds of conversations—ones that build solutions rather than exploring problems. Therefore, there obviously are certain things that [solution-focused brief] therapists do. We call these practices or tools. (Simon & Nelson, 2007, p. 12, emphasis in original)

Whereas support and encouragement may be given and specific skills are sometimes taught, the hallmark of solution-focused therapy is the use of questions to invite clients to organize and focus their attention, energy, and understanding in one way— toward a richly detailed description of a solution picture—rather than toward another. Questions are asked and selected responses are explored and elaborated to direct clients' toward the realization of their desired outcomes. The therapist functions like a special kind of mirror that can become convex or concave and swivel this way or that. Rather than providing a "flat mirror" that simply "reflects and clarifies," the solution-focused therapist purposely and differentially expands and contracts

TABLE 9.1. Solution-Building Vocabulary

In	Out	In	Out
Respect	Judge	Forward	Backward
Empower	Fix	Future	Past
Nurture	Control	Collaborate	Manipulate
Facilitate	Treat	Options	Conflicts
Augment	Reduce	Partner	Expert
Invite	Insist	Horizontal	Hierarchical
Appreciate	Diagnose	Possibility	Limitation
Hope	Fear	Growth	Cure
Latent	Missing	Access	Defense
Assets	Defects	Utilize	Resist
Strength	Weakness	Create	Repair
Health	Pathology	Exception	Rule
Not Yet	Never	Difference	Sameness
Expand	Shrink	Solution	Problem

Note. From Hoyt (1994d, p. 4). Copyright 1994 by The Guilford Press. Reprinted by permission.

the reflected image, so to speak—opening parts of the story and closing others, making "space" for discourses that support the realization of clients' goals (Hoyt, 2000). As discussed in the following sections, highlighting and amplifying clients' past successes and their agency in bringing about preferred outcomes help empower couples to construct more self-fulfilling realities.

A Guide for the Perplexed

In his book *Clues: Investigating Solutions in Brief Therapy*, de Shazer (1988, p. 86; also see Walter & Peller, 1992) offers a schematic map or "family tree" of solution-focused interviews, as seen in Figure 9.1.

The Structure of Therapy Sessions

de Shazer and Berg (1997, p. 123) have also outlined the formal characteristics of a "classic" SFBT session:

> Characteristic features of SFBT include:
> (1) At some point in the first interview, the therapist will ask the "Miracle Question."
> (2) At least once during the first interview and at subsequent ones, the client will be asked to rate something on a scale of "0 > 10" or "1 > 10."
> (3) At some point during the interview, the therapist will take a break.
> (4) After this intermission, the therapist will give the client some compliments which will sometimes (frequently) be followed by a suggestion or homework task (frequently called an "experiment").

Following this outline, we will first discuss a variety of questions typically asked in solution-focused couple therapy, providing numerous examples. We will then discuss the use of a short break or intermission during the session; and will then consider the postbreak portion of the session, including the use of directives or "homework" assignments.

Sessions, which usually last 50–60 minutes, typically begin with a brief period of socializing and joining. As expressed in the title of the book by Ben Furman and Tapani Ahola (1992), *Solution Talk: Hosting Therapeutic Conversations*, the solution-focused therapist attends to creating ("hosting") a comfortable, collaborative therapeutic situation.

Various types of questions may then be asked. The following sampler provides typical solution-focused therapy questions, many of which have been drawn (with some paraphrasings) from Ziegler (2000; also see Ziegler & Hiller, 2001), with additional sources, including Berg and de Shazer (1993), Berg and Miller (1992), DeJong and Berg (1997), de Shazer (1985, 1988, 1991a, 1994a), George et al. (2006), Hoyt and Miller (2000), S. Miller (1994), O'Hanlon & Weiner-Davis (1989), Walter and Peller (1992, 2000), and Weiner-Davis (1992).

A Sampler of Solution-Focused Therapy Questions

Before the Session: Eliciting Presession Change

It is useful to recognize that the roots of change exist before the first session. On first contact, usually when there is a phone call requesting an appointment, the solution-focused therapist may make a request that helps direct clients' attention toward *exceptions* to the problem, times when the presenting complaint isn't present (de Shazer, 1984; de Shazer & Molnar, 1984):

> Between now and next time we meet, I would like you to observe, so that you can describe to me next time, what happens in your [*pick one:* family, life, marriage, relationship] that you want to continue to have happen. (see de Shazer, 1985, p. 137)

This "Skeleton Key Question" (a generic "key" that can fit any lock) helps shift perspective: it implies (presupposes) that something positive is happening that could observed and recruits the clients' cooperation. Discussing at the session what was noticed (*Eliciting Pre-Session Change*) can help to consolidate and amplify useful new awarenesses (see Adams, Piercy, & Jurich, 1991; Weiner-Davis, de Shazer, & Gingerich, 1987).

Initial In-Session Questions

These questions are intended to build rapport, make space for partners' views and theories, and establish a team (therapist–couple alliance) framework.

- What brings you here today?
- How can I be helpful to the two of you?
- What changes have either of you noticed since you first made the call to set up this appointment?

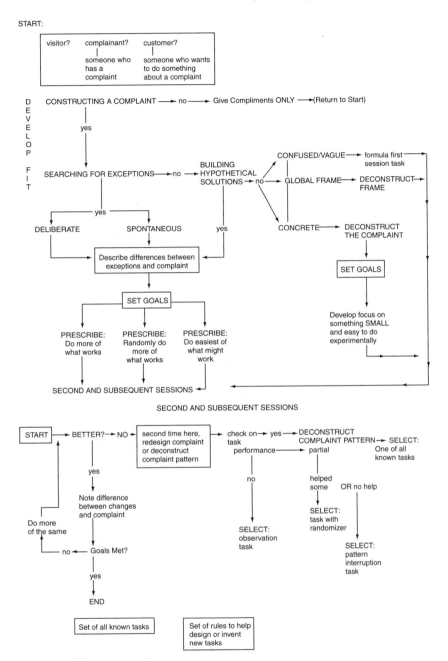

FIGURE 9.1. The central map. From de Shazer (1988, p. 86). Copyright 1987 by Steve de Shazer. Reprinted by permission of W.W. Norton & Co., Inc.

- How do you see the situation—what's your understanding (theory) of what would be helpful?
- What needs to happen here so that when you leave you will think, "It was good that we went to see (the therapist)?
- What can I do that would help you two work better together at getting beyond these troubles and turning your relationship around?

Goal-Building Questions

These questions are intended to identify, in operational (achievable and observable) terms, what the clients' desire from therapy.

- *Miracle question*: Suppose when you go home tonight and go to sleep a miracle happens and the problems that brought you here are solved. But, because you are asleep, you don't know this miracle has happened. So tomorrow, when you wake up and go through your day you notice things are different between you but you don't know the miracle happened. What will be the first things you notice that are different? What will you notice your partner doing differently that will tell you something has changed? What will your partner notice you doing differently?
- *From general to specific*: How will the two of you know you have solved the problems that bring you here (or have reached your goals)? How will things be different? What specifically will tell you that you have solved your problem or reached these goals? What will be the first signs (smallest steps) that will tell you that you two are moving in that direction? What else?
- *Getting specific details—painting the picture*: What will tell you that you are on track? What else? What will that look like? What else will be different? When you are on track, what will you notice, what will be different to give you the confidence that you two will keep heading in that direction even after we stop meeting?
- *Ends and means*: How will it make a difference to you when these changes have happened? How will they change the way you feel about your partner and your relationship?
- *Relationship/outside perception questions*: When your partner is being more the way you want him/her to be, what will (s)he see you doing differently that will tell him/her that his/her changes are having a meaningful effect on you? What will your partner notice different about you when ... ? How do you suppose this will make a difference to him/her? What will tell him/her that you are on track to solving your marital problems? What will your children notice is different? Friends? Other family members?

Exceptions Questions

These questions are intended to identify times when the presenting problem has not been present. A hallmark of solution-focused therapy, they seek a kernel or "germ" that can be expanded into an alternative view that elevates awareness of clients' abilities to make a positive difference, and opens the gateway to a new couple story, one not saturated or dominated by problems. The search is for "symptoms of solutions" (S. Miller, 1992).

- When in the past might the problem have happened but didn't (or was less intense or more manageable)?
- When have you managed not to____?
- What is different about those times when the problem does not happen?
- When (in the recent past) have you experienced some of the things that you say make a difference (tell you that you're heading in the right direction)?
- When have you noticed that the two of you do better with this problem?
- How have you let your partner know when he/she does something that makes a positive difference to you?

Agency (Efficacy) Questions

These questions are intended to call attention to clients' self-efficacy, that is, their abilities to make a difference in the desired direction (see Ziegler & Hiller, 2001).

- How did you do that?
- How did you get that to happen?
- What was each of you doing differently when you were doing better (or when there wasn't a problem, or when the exception happened)?
- How did each of you decide to do that?
- What would you say you (your partner) need to do to get that to happen more?
- What needs to happen first?
- What would your partner say you could do that would encourage him (or her) to do more of the things you think he (or she) could do to make a difference? Would you agree, even though it might be hard to do it or go first?

- What do you know about (your past, your self, your partner, your situation, other people) that tells you that this could happen for you (that you can make it together)?

Coping (Endurance) Questions

These questions are intended both to acknowledge the difficulty and painfulness of some situations and also highlight the clients' contributions to their resiliency.

- How have the two of you managed to cope (survive, endure, keep going)?
- Given the terrible situation, how bad the (pick one: arguing, grief, worrying, lack of communication, etc.) has been how come things aren't worse (how have you managed to avoid it getting even worse)?
- What have you been doing to fight off the (pick one: arguing, grief, etc.)?
- How did you know that would help?
- If you hadn't been through this experience personally, would you have ever thought you had the strength to survive?

Scaling Questions

These questions are typically asked "to make numbers talk" (Berg & de Shazer, 1993, pp. 9–10):

Our scales are used to "measure" the client's own perception, to motivate and encourage, and to elucidate the goals and anything else that is important to the individual client. [...] Scaling questions are used to discuss the individual client's perspective, the client's view of others, and the client's impressions of others' view of him or her. (pp. 9–10)

They go on to elaborate:

Scales allow both therapist and client to use the way language works naturally by agreeing upon terms (i.e., numbers) and a concept (a scale where 10 stands for the goal and zero stands for the absence of progress toward that goal) that is obviously multiple and flexible. Since neither therapist nor client can be absolutely certain what the other means by the use of a particular word or concept, scaling questions allow them to jointly construct a way of talking about things that are hard to describe, including progress toward the client's goal(s). ... Here the scales give us a way to creatively misunderstand by using numbers to describe the indescribable and yet have some confidence that we, as therapists, are doing the job the client hired us to do. (p. 19)

It is important to recognize that the positive direction and valence of a scale helps shift discourse toward a solution (not problem) focus. For example, asking partners to rate themselves along the dimensions of how hopeful or motivated they are or how much progress has been made evokes a very different mind-set than asking how hopeless or unmotivated or how stuck they are. Thinking about where one might be rated along positively worded dimensions *is* much more hopeful, motivating, and likely to stir progress than the latter questions, which are not merely statistical inversions of solutions but entirely different constructions. Once clients give ratings, their responses are respectfully accepted and the question then shifts to "What will it take to move from a 3 to a 4 [or from a 6 to a 7, etc.]?"

- *Hope:* On a scale from 1 to 10, with 1 being *absolutely no hope* and 10 being *complete confidence*, what number would you give your current level of hope? What will tell you that your score has gone up one level? What number will be high enough to warrant your working hard to try and change things?
- *Motivation:* On a scale from 1 to 10, with 1 being *no motivation* and 10 being *a willingness to go to any lengths to solve your problems*, what number would you give your current level of motivation? What will cause that score to go up one level?
- *Progress:* On a scale of 1 to 10, where 10 is *the day after the miracle*, and 1 is *when this situation was at its worst*, where would you say things are today? On a scale from 1 to 10, with 1 being when *the problems were just before you made the call* and 10 being the *problems solved and a thing of the past*, what number would you give your current level of progress (where you're at now)? What will tell you that you have moved up one level? What number will tell you that you have made enough progress in solving this problem so that you can consider it solved?

Self–Other Perception/Meaning Questions

These relationship questions are asked to bring forth and highlight competencies, positive qualities, strengths, and successes, and to weave them into the interpersonal context (see Ziegler & Hiller, 2001).

- What does this say about you as a couple?
- What else would you want your partner to know (or have him/her notice) that would tell him/

her how much you (care or love him/her, are working hard, want the relationship to improve, etc.)?

- As you continue to see yourselves this way, how do you imagine things continuing to change for the better? How do you suppose letting your partner know you see these positive changes in him or her will contribute to the two of you turning your relationship around (continuing to make progress)? How does your partner telling you that he/she notices and appreciates how you are changing affect you in your efforts to keep working for positive change?
- How will this (does this) make a difference that you want to see continue?

Timing of Interventions

The purpose of solution-focused therapy is to help clients build a solution they find acceptable. If the client-couple is making progress that is adequate and satisfying to them, it is important to keep in mind the principle *"If It Works, Don't Fix It."* In these instances, it is helpful to "cheerlead rather than mislead" (Hoyt & Miller, 2000, p. 222)—that is, elicit details of the partners' success, offer encouragement, highlight their role (instrumentality) in bringing it about—and not push.

If the couple gets stuck (or more likely, *when*—because they probably would not be in the therapist's office if they didn't need assistance getting unstuck), the solution-focused therapist earns his or her fee by recognizing how they are getting bogged down in "problem talk," then intervening appropriately to redirect them toward "solution talk." Thus, as discussed earlier, the therapist needs to discern what type of therapist–client collaborative relationship (customer, complainant, visitor) is active and proceed accordingly. A couple may be stuck because of not having a sense of an achievable goal, or because one or both parties do not feel competent to make a positive difference. Good intentions need to be translated into specific actions. They may be ready to proceed as customers but not know what particular steps to take (or not recognize what steps have worked for them in the past).

The solution-focused therapist intervenes, interrupting "problem talk" before it escalates into demoralizing bickering, cycles of blaming and defending, accusations, and unhappy crescendos. Instead, the therapist reminds the couple of what they want and asks questions to redirect attention toward their role in achieving past, present and,

most important, future solutions. The "Miracle Question" captures clients' imaginations and shifts the tone and flow of the conversation (see Nau & Shilts, 2000; Metcalf, 2004). Exceptions, coping, and agency questions evoke resources; relationship questions highlight cooperation and the bond between the partners.

Scaling questions, which can be used at any point during the session, are particularly helpful when complaints (or progress) are vague or nonspecific, such as when couples refer to topics such as "communication":

> [A] couple's perception of how well they communicate with each other varies for each of them from time to time. With 10 standing for communicating as well as is possible for a specific couple to communicate, their joint progress and their different perceptions are simply depicted through their ratings. We frequently ask each partner to guess the other's rating, which again simply depicts progress and differences in perception as well as implying that such differences are both normal and expectable. The question is not "Who is right?" but "What does the one giving the higher rating see that the other one does not?" Thus, no matter how vaguely and nonspecifically the clients describe their situation, scales can be used to develop a useful way for therapist and clients to talk together about constructing solutions. (Berg & de Shazer, 1993, pp. 22–23)

Session Break: A Pause to Reflect and Plan

Although many solution-oriented therapists may not take a formal break during a session, in its "pure" or "classic" form a solution-focused therapy session is characterized by the therapist taking a short (typically 5–10 minute) break or intermission about 30–45 minutes into the session. (The therapist will typically have prepared the clients for this at the beginning of the interview, when he or she indicates the structure of the session and gets the clients' permission to have a team, if available, observe the session.) When the time comes ("Let's take a short break so that I can talk with my colleagues"), the clients may be asked to sit in the interview room while the therapist goes next door to consult with a team of observers, or the clients may be asked to take a brief recess in the waiting room while the therapist talks with colleagues. Even if there are no colleagues observing, the therapist can use the break to organize his or her thoughts, to reflect upon what has occurred, and to plan a message (feedback and possible homework task) to be presented to the couple when the session is resumed.

The couple can also be asked to think about what task or postsession activity might be useful for them. Building on the solution-focused idea that it is the client who is "heroic" (Miller & Duncan, 2000) and whose therapeutic contributions should be kept foremost, Sharry, Madden, Darmody, and Miller (2001) describe an interesting variant in which the session break can be used in a more collaborative or client-directed fashion. They suggest this expectation can be established in the way the therapist describes the purpose of the consultation break:

> We're nearing the end of the session and I'd like to take a five-minute break. This is to give you time to think and reflect about what we have discussed; to pick out any important ideas that came up, or to make any decisions or plans. You might also like to think about whether this session has been useful and how you would like us to be further involved, if that would be helpful. While you're thinking, I will consult with my team for their thoughts. We will think together about what you said. When we get back together, I'll be interested to hear what stood out for you today. I'll also share the team's thoughts with you. Together, then, we can put something together that will be helpful. (pp. 71–72)

This puts the emphasis clearly on the clients' thinking, reflecting, and planning. Clients are encouraged to participate in the evaluation of the session and the decision about further work. There is no "automatic" assumption that more sessions will be needed or desired, and it is the clients rather than the therapist who have primacy in making decisions about the length of treatment. As Sharry et al. (2001, pp. 74–75) write:

> Clients as well as the therapist team are encouraged to use the break as an opportunity to reflect on the session, generate their own conclusions and even assign themselves a homework task. ... It helps clients build on their own strengths and resources, recognizing their central role in any therapeutic change. ... The responsibility for successful therapy is shared between therapist and client.

Resuming and Concluding the Session: Feedback and Tasks

When the therapist returns or brings the couple back into the room after taking a break, the session resumes. If one endeavors to utilize an especially collaborative or client-directed session

break, as Sharry et al. (2001) suggest, it will be important that the therapist "first seeks the views and thoughts of the clients in evaluating the session and constructing a plan of action" (p. 74). The break "punctuates" the session, and clients are usually keen to hear what the therapist has to say after studying the situation and perhaps consulting with other therapists. Hence, although primacy is given to the clients' ideas, the moment also may be ripe for the therapist to introduce a suggestion or a reframing (Erickson & Rossi, 1979; de Shazer, 1985). Feedback and "homework" tasks, which flow from the preceding conversation, can be designed collaboratively to promote goal attainment by reflecting and reinforcing client competencies and any emerging "solution talk." The therapist works to amplify whatever the clients are doing in the direction they want to go. DeJong and Berg (1997, p. 107) distinguish solution building from problem solving:

> End-of-session feedback in solution building is not the same thing as intervention in the problem-solving approach. In the latter case, the practitioner uses assessment information about the nature and severity of client problems to decide on what actions would best benefit the client. The practitioner then takes those actions or encourages the client to do so. These actions—the interventions—are thought to produce the positive changes for the client. ...
>
> In solution-building, by contrast, we do not regard session-ending feedback as any more important than any other component of the process. Instead. [...] we think that solutions are built by clients through the hard work of applying their strengths in the direction of goals that they value. Clients, not practitioners, are the primary agents of change. In the course of the interview, clients disclose information about themselves and their circumstances; session-ending feedback merely organizes and highlights the aspects of that information that might be useful to clients as they strive to build solutions.

Compliments, a Bridging Statement, and the Task

In classic solution-focused therapy, there are typically three components to what the therapist says after the session break: *compliments*; which acknowledge and validate the clients' point of view, affirming what is important to them, their successes and strengths; a *bridging statement* that links compliments to the suggestion or directive that is to be offered; and the *task or directive* itself, often involving performance of an "experiment" or "homework."

[Compliments] are statements from the therapist and/or team about what the client has said that is useful, effective, good, or fun. This helps to promote client–therapist fit and thus cooperation on the task at hand.

With some frequency, the compliments (in the first session) will include statements about the difficulty of achieving the chosen goal and some statements, based on the exceptions, about the progress toward the goal and the general viability of the goal. In later sessions, the main focus of the compliments will often be on the progress toward the goal. (de Shazer, 1988, pp. 96–97)

The use of compliments, acknowledgment and validation, and a bridging statement near the end of a solution-focused couple therapy session is illustrated in these comments excerpted from a report by Hoyt and Berg (2000, pp. 160–161; also see Berg, 1994b):

THERAPIST [INSOO BERG]: I really have to tell you that I think your calling to set up this appointment was really good timing. It sounds like you both are very concerned about what's not happening between the two of you, and you want to do something about that. And I am very impressed, Bill, that you responded to Leslie's initiating this meeting and your willingness to take time from your very busy schedule and obviously this relationship is very important to you. ... And that's why you are here, to do something about this. Both of you really care about this relationship a great deal. But both in a very different way. ... [*She goes on to describe each partner's stated values.*] So there's no question in my mind that both of you care about each other in a very different way. And that gets misunderstood. And I think that both of you need both ways. ... And so I think that you two have a very good start because you're already thinking about right now as well as the future. So the next task for the two of you is to figure out how to fit your concerns together. [*bridging statement*] I don't think it's either your way or your way. It's the blending of the two. In order to do that, both of you have to work together to strike this balance. And I really like the way that you want to get started on this. You have lots of ideas of how to get started on that ...

In this case, the therapist recognized that each member of the couple was in a complainant position, that is, felt aggrieved but not (yet) instrumental to make a difference. Thus, she suggested an *observation task*, one designed to shape viewing (and thus, affect subsequent interaction) by having each partner notice what the other person was doing that was positive:

THERAPIST: So what I would like to suggest to you between now and the next time we get together, is for each of you to keep track of what the other person is doing. For you [to the wife] to keep track of what Bill does, and for you [to the husband] to keep track of what Leslie does to make things a little bit better for the marriage. And it's important for you not to discuss it, but just keep track of them. And when we come back together we will discuss this more, the details of them. But I want you to sort of observe, file it away, and then when we get together we'll talk about it. OK? (Hoyt & Berg, 2000, p. 161; also see Berg, 1994b)

Having each partner notice the positive helped to shift the basis of their interaction from a problem-saturated to a more solution-saturated worldview. Seeing one's partner in a positive light makes one more likely to respond in kind; this may help produce a "virtuous" instead of a "vicious" cycle (see Wender, 1968). Had the partners been in more of a "customer" position, the therapist might have more directly offered them specific suggestions or guidance on how to improve their interaction (as complainants, they would not have felt able to use this information); had they been in the position of "visitors," disavowing any problem or interest in a remedy, the therapist might have simply paid them courteous compliments and invited them to return (as complainants, however, this would not have resulted in their feeling that their complaints had been acknowledged and taken seriously).

de Shazer (1985) provides a decision tree and some suggestions to therapists for how to respond to clients' responses to tasks in the best way for promoting cooperation (thus, solutions). "Fit" is enhanced by attending to the basic solution-focused principles of "Once you know what works, do more of it" and "If it doesn't work, don't do it again; do something different." de Shazer (1988, pp. 97–99, emphasis in original) also provides some general guidelines for designing tasks:

(1) Note what sort of things the clients do that is good, useful, and effective.
(2) Note *differences* between what happens when any exceptions occur and what happens when the complaint happens. Promote the former.
(3) When possible, extract step-by-step descriptions of any exceptions.
   (a) Find out what is working, and/or
   (b) find out what has worked, and/or
   (c) find out what might work, then
   (d) prescribe the easiest.

If some aspects of the exception (or of the complaint) are sort of random, then

  (e) include something arbitrary or make allowances for randomness in the task.

(4) When necessary, *extract* step-by-step descriptions of the complaint.

(5) Note *differences* between any hypothetical solutions and the complaint.

(6) Imagine a *solved* version of the problematic situation by:

  (a) making *exceptions* to the rule,
  (b) changing the *location* of the complaint pattern,
  (c) changing who is *involved* in the complaint pattern,
  (d) changing the *order of the steps* involved,
  (e) adding a *new element* or step to the complaint pattern,
  (f) increasing the *duration* of the pattern,
  (g) introducing *arbitrary* starting and stopping,
  (h) increasing the *frequency* of the pattern,
  (i) changing the *modality* of the problematic behavior.

(7) Decide what will fit for the complainant/customer, i.e., which task, based on which variable (a through i) will make sense to the particular client. Which one will the complainant most likely accept? Which one will the customer most likely perform? For instance: If a couple has a joint complaint, give them a joint, cooperative task. If only one member of a couple presents the complaint like a customer, give the "customer" a task that involves doing something and the other person an observation task.

de Shazer (1994a, 1994b; also see his remarks in Hoyt, 1996b, pp. 61–63) also cautions the therapist to keep it simple and not get caught up in overly clever, complicated strategizing that might have the untoward effects of both disempowering the client and overburdening the therapist.

Lipchik (1997, p. 170) also describes the importance of attending to cooperative "fit" and maintaining a colloborative set throughout the closing portion of the session:

I believe the summation message has an important function in creating a different reality for clients. I now structure this message to reflect what I believe I understand about the clients' reality ("What I heard you say today is … "); my perspective on what I heard ("My response is … "), which includes positives, reinforcements of what the clients are doing that they experience as helpful, normalizing statements and sometimes some information; and a suggestion

about what they might think about, or do until the next session. I present "the task" as a choice, not an assignment. Then I ask the client[s] for a short response. This gives clients an opportunity to correct anything I reflected on or responded to that they do not agree with before leaving the session. I find this format more fitting a collaborative relationship than my former, more "expert" way of structuring the messages.

Common Messages

In their excellent text, *Interviewing for Solutions*, DeJong and Berg (1997, p. 121) provide a number of guidelines for giving feedback and identify various basic statements—called "common messages"—for recurring situations: [W]here you decide to point a client will depend on your assessment of: (1) the type of relationship in which your client stands to your services; (2) the degree to which the client has developed well-formed goals; and (3) the presence or absence of random and deliberate exceptions related to what your client wants.

DeJong and Berg (1997, pp. 120–133, with some paraphrasings here) describe typical common messages for different situations (it is important to remember that *compliments* and *bridging statements* would precede these):

CLIENTS IN A VISITOR RELATIONSHIP

• "We are very impressed that you are here today even though this is not your idea. You certainly had the option of taking the easy way out by not coming. … I agree with you that you should be left alone. But you also realize that doing what you are told will help you get these people out of your life and you will be left alone sooner. Therefore, I would like to meet with you again to figure out further what will be good for you to do. So let's meet next week at the same time."

CLIENTS IN A COMPLAINANT RELATIONSHIP

• *No exceptions and no goal:* "Between now and the next time that we meet, pay attention to what's happening in your life that tells you that this problem can be solved."

• *Exceptions but no goals:* "Between now and the next time we meet, pay attention to those times that are better, so that you can describe them to me in detail. Try to notice what is different about them and how they happen. Who does what to make them happen?"

• *If the clients attribute the exceptions entirely to the other person's actions:* "Pay attention for those times when your partner (relationship) is more the way you want. Besides paying attention to what's different about those times, pay attention to—so you can describe it to me next time—what he/she might notice you doing that helps him/her/the two of you to be more ____. Keep track of those things and come back and tell me what's better."

• *If the clients view the problem as existing outside of themselves but are able to identify random exceptions:* "I agree with you; there clearly seems to be days your partner (relationship) is more _____ and days when he/she/it isn't. So between now and the next time that we meet, I suggest the following: Each night before you go to bed, predict whether or not tomorrow will be a day when _____ or not. Then, at the end of the day, before you make your prediction for the next day, think about whether or not your prediction came true. Account for any differences between your prediction and the way the day went and keep track of your observations so that you can come back and tell me about them."

CLIENTS IN A CUSTOMER RELATIONSHIP

• *A clear miracle picture but no exceptions:* "Pick one day over the next week and, without telling anyone, pretend that the miracle has happened. And, as you live that day, pay attention to what's different around your house, so that you can tell me about it when we meet next time."

• *High motivation but no well-formed goals:* "I am very impressed with how hard you have worked on your problem and how clearly you can describe to me the things you have tried so far to make things better. I can understand why you would be discouraged and frustrated right now. ... Because this is such a stubborn problem, I suggest that between now and the next time we meet, when the problem happens, you do something different—no matter how strange or weird or off-the-wall what you do might seem. The only important thing is that, whatever you decide to do, you need to do something different."

• *Well-formed goals and deliberate exceptions:* "I am impressed how much you want to make things go better between you and your partner, and

that there are already times this is happening (give examples). I agree that these are the things you have to do to have the kind of relationship that you want. So, between now and when we meet again, I suggest that you continue to do what works. Also, pay attention to what else you might be doing—but haven't noticed yet—that makes things better, and come back and tell me about it."

OTHER USEFUL MESSAGES

• *The overcoming-the-urge task:* "Pay attention for those times when the two of you overcome the urge to (argue, return to the old problem, not look for positives in what the other is saying, etc.). Pay attention to what's different about those times—especially to what you are doing to overcome the urge."

• *Addressing competing views of the solution (without taking sides):* "I am impressed by how much both of you want to improve your relationship. I am also impressed by what different ideas the two of you have about how to do this—I can see that, coming from your different perspectives (backgrounds, families, etc.), you have learned different ways to do things. ... I (or, the team) am (are) split on which way to go: Both of you have strong ideas. Therefore, I (we) suggest that each morning, right after you get up, you flip a coin. Heads means that day you improve things the way (Person A) suggests, and the other person goes along; and tails means you improve things the way (Person B) suggests, and the other person goes along. And also—on those days when each of you is not busy being in charge—pay careful attention to what the other does that is useful, and how you help with that, so that you can report it to me (us) when we meet again."

In her bestselling self-help guide, *Divorce Busting: A Revolutionary and Rapid Program for Staying Together,* Michele Weiner-Davis (1992), another former BFTC group member, draws on many solution-focused ideas. Under the heading (pp. 124–125) "Why Focusing on What Works—Works," she provides and discusses four answers:

1. Exceptions Shrink Problems
2. Exceptions Demonstrate that People Are Changeable
3. Exceptions Supply Solutions
4. Focusing on Strengths Strengthens.

Weiner-Davis (1992, pp. 127–140) then provides (with extended discussion and numerous practical suggestions for application) the following nine guidelines to help readers "analyze what works in your marriage and give you information you need to get your marriage back on track":

1. Notice What Is Different About the Times the Two of You Are Getting Along
2. If You Are Having Trouble Identifying Current Exceptions, Recall What You and Your Spouse Were Doing Differently in Years Past that Made Your Marriage More Satisfying
3. You Don't Have to Like It, You Just Have to Do It
4. Focus on What's Doable or Possible
5. A Problem that Recurs Doesn't Necessarily Require a New Solution
6. Pay Attention to How Your Conflicts End
7. If There Are No Exceptions, Identify the Best of the Worst
8. Notice What's Different About the Times the Problem Occurs but Something Constructive Comes from It
9. Notice What's Different About the Times the Problem Situation Occurs but Doesn't Bother You

In *Rewriting Love Stories: Brief Marital Therapy*, Patricia Hudson and Bill O'Hanlon (1991; also see O'Hanlon & Hudson, 1994) also highlight many solution-focused/solution-oriented ideas, including the importance of moving from blame to collaboration, changing the couple's way of "viewing" and "doing" their situation, the use of task assignments, the value of humor, and the power of commitments and consequences. More recently, in their *Brief Couples Therapy Homework Planner*, Gary Schultheis, Bill O'Hanlon, and Steffanie O'Hanlon (1999, p. 1) write:

We use homework assignments for many reasons, including that homework:

• Introduces change to the situation
• Encourages a spirit of experimentation
• Encourages clients to take an active part in therapy
• Evokes resources
• Highlights and allows follow-through on something that happened in the session
• Encourages the client to put more attention on an issue
• Encourages the client to take the next step before the next session
• Enhances the client's search for solutions.

They go on (p. 6):

We want to, at the very least, create some sense that the situation is not hopeless. That means we quickly move into making changes. So, in addition to validating, we immediately set about helping the couple make changes in three areas around the problem:

1. What are they paying attention to in the problem situation and how are they interpreting it? (*Changing the Viewing*)
2. How are they typically interacting with one another, including patterns of how each of them act during the problem situation and how they talk with one another or others about the problem? We are searching for repeating patterns and helping couples change those problem patterns. (*Changing the Doing*)
3. What circumstances surround the problem? That is, what are the family backgrounds and patterns, the cultural backgrounds and patterns, the racial backgrounds and gender training and experiences that are contributing to the problem? In what locations do the couple's problems usually happen? (*Changing the Context*)

In each of these change areas, we have two tasks:

1. Recognizing and interrupting typical problem patterns
2. Seeking, highlighting and encouraging solution patterns.

Drawing upon solution-based (as well as other) ideas, they then provide many ready-to-use between-session assignments. When thoughtfully selected, proffered, and explained to couples, these user-friendly "homework" tasks can help couples develop skills for healthier relationships.

Subsequent Sessions

When a couple returns for a second (or subsequent) session, the solution-focused therapist endeavors to co-create a comfortable, cooperative situation; then inquires about progress, seeking detailed descriptions of any movement toward the couple's desired outcome (solution) and their roles in attaining it; and then assists the couple to look forward to how they will take their next pro-solution steps. This process is nicely summarized (with some examples of opening questions) in the acronym *EARS* (Berg, 1994c; DeJong & Berg, 1997):

E (elicit): "What's better?" or "What worked for you two?" or "What happened that you liked?"

A (amplify): "Tell me more" or "Who/what/where/when/how?" or "Walk me through how the two of you did that"

R (reinforce): "Wow!" or "That sounds great!" or "What part did you especially enjoy?"

S (start again): "And what else is better?" or "So, what do you think the next step might be?" or "How can you keep this going?" or "On a scale of 1 to 10, you say your progress (relationship, communication, love life, etc.) is now at a 5—what would a 6 look like?"

Recalling the marital therapy case (from Hoyt & Berg, 2000) I referred to earlier, consider these excerpts from the therapist's remarks at the beginning of the next session:

> THERAPIST [INSOO BERG]: It's been about 2 weeks since you were here the last time. What's been better for the two of you?. ... No kidding! Really? Wow! How'd you manage to do that? ... No kidding? ... Wow! That must have been hard. ... You did, really—without the kids? Some intimate time. ... You were willing to do that, this time—wonderful! ... Would you agree, was that fun for you, too? ... Wow! That must have taken quite a bit of coordination to pull it off, with 4 people's schedules. ... Huh-huh. ... That's good! ... Right! ... What did Leslie do to make things a little easier for you to do that? ... Huh-huh. ... Great! ... Before we get to that, let me ask you: What did Bill do that was helpful? ... Wow! Yes! It seems like that was very important to you—what does that mean to you? ... Is that one of the things he did? Anything else you noticed to make things better? ... Huh-huh. ... What about for you—what did Leslie do to make things better? What else? Say some more about that. ... Really! ... How hopeful are you now, on a scale of 1 to 10, that this marriage will make it? A 9? And you? ... This is a big change, isn't it? What would it take for you to stay on this track? ... What needs to happen for the two of you to feel you are moving in the right direction? ... So, how do you solve it—what's the next step for the two of you? [from Berg, 1994b]

If, even after careful inquiry, there has been a lack of discernable progress (including not doing homework that was discussed), *coping questions* ("How did you keep things from getting worse?") may be appropriate. The solution-focused therapist may also recognize "no progress" feedback as an opportunity to repair a possible mismatch. The

therapist may have misgauged the clients' stage of readiness or the type of therapist–client relationship pattern (see Hoyt & Miller, 2000). Blaming the client is not useful in building cooperation and solutions. In such instances, questions such as the following may be helpful:

- What's your idea about what would be useful? What do you think the next step should be?
- Are we working on what you want to work on? How is this going for you?
- I seem to have missed something you said. What can I do to be more helpful to you now?

Common Technical Errors and Criticisms

Solution-focused brief therapists focus on solutions. Many traditional therapists, however, are trained and oriented toward problems and pathologies. In addition to highlighting negativities, therapists (solution-focused and otherwise) can engender opposition by trying to take clients where they don't want to go:

> DE SHAZER: Well, if I were to use the word *resistance*—I wouldn't, but if I were—it would translate in my vocabulary as *therapist error*. That would mean to me that the therapist wasn't listening, and therefore he told the client to do something the client didn't want to do. That means he wasn't listening during the interview. Most of our stuff is based on the fact of something they told us about, that they did such and such and it worked in some situation, so it's just a matter of transferring that from situation A to situation B. So there's nothing new. Most of our interventions are nothing new for them [...].
>
> HOYT: I think another advantage, then, to a solution-focused approach is that it doesn't stimulate noncompliance because there's nothing they have to noncomply with. It makes it more user-friendly for both the therapist and for the client. It's less likely to drive clients away.
>
> DE SHAZER: Less likely. What I see sometimes is the amateurs, so to speak—the beginners, who somehow think more is better and, therefore, they give this endless stream of compliments and bore the client silly with them and, therefore, the client stops taking them seriously. That's one thing I see happen with beginners, in particular: There's just too damn many compliments, and that will drive the client away.
>
> HOYT: [...] How do we separate the idea of "influence" from "brainwashing," to call it that? That we're influencing but not imposing our values, manipulating them?
>
> DE SHAZER: There's that line, all right. Clients hire

us to influence them; that's why they come. The more you are using their stuff, the less danger you are in of moving into brainwashing. The more you are putting in your stuff, the closer you're getting to brainwashing. That's pretty clear to me. Those are the two ends of it, perhaps. I'm not sure if it is a continuum, but there certainly in a line in between. And, frankly, I see many, many of the psychotherapy models as being closer to brainwashing than to anything else.

HOYT: I think the respectful ethic is that it's truly informed consent. We're identifying what their goals are and helping them meet their goals, rather than imposing our agenda.

DE SHAZER: Right. You know, we have a saying around here [BFTC]—there used to be a sign made by somebody on the team (probably Gale Miller): "If the therapist's goals and the client's goals are different, the therapist is wrong." (Hoyt, 1996b, pp. 63–65, emphasis in original)

The approach should not be "model driven" or "technique driven" at the expense of the therapist–client relationship (see Lipchik, 1997, 2002; Miller & Duncan, 2000). Several commentators (e.g., Efran & Schenker, 1993; O'Hanlon, 1998) have suggested, however, that solution-focused therapy can be applied in a heavy-handed, formulaic manner that results in clients feeling "solution forced" (Nylund & Corsiglia, 1994) and "rushed to be brief" (Lipchik, 1994), and that embraced solutions may serve to perpetuate problem patterns (Fraser, 1998). de Shazer (in Hoyt, 1994b, p. 39) has made his view clear:

I know what I don't want, and that's for anybody to develop some sort of rigid orthodoxies. I'm afraid of that. I'm always afraid of that. For me, it's a big point of concern. That there's a right way to do this and that. And to see my descriptions—and they've done this to me; I've probably done this to myself—to see my descriptions as prescriptions.

Critics have also suggested that emotion may be downplayed or ignored, and that recurring complaints and important social issues (e.g., oppression of women, domestic violence) will not be recognized unless clients explicitly raise them. When done skillfully, clients in solution-focused therapy do not feel "forced" or "rushed," but assisted to go where they want to go.

We do not believe solution-focused brief therapy encourages practitioners to force solutions on clients. However, because the approach is usually presented with a heavy emphasis on the idea that solution talk, not problem talk, leads to solutions, it is easy for those learning this approach to prevent clients from talking about their concerns and troubles. We have never heard or read anything in the solution-focused brief therapy literature that suggests clients should be forced to talk only about positive things. Watching de Shazer and Berg on videotapes, we have always noted their respectful attitudes and their skillful ways of "leading from behind." (Ziegler & Hiller, 2001, p. 222)

Emotion is not avoided, but it is also not sought or elicited as a therapeutic "royal road" or as an end in itself (see King, 1998; G. Miller & de Shazer, 1998, 2000). As Eve Lipchik (2002, p. 64) has written in her book *Beyond Technique in Solution-Focused Therapy: Working with Emotions and the Therapeutic Relationship*:

Solution-focused therapists have traditionally guided clients toward behavioral descriptions of their goals so they can track progress better, even though most clients describe their complaints in terms of feelings. The therapist's response does not have to be in either a behavioral direction or an emotional one. We can cooperate with clients and use their feeling words in conversation without sacrificing the benefit of more concrete signs of progress (Turnell & Lipchik, 1999).

The solution-focused therapist is present as a real, genuinely concerned person (see Hoyt, 2001b) but does not engage in unneeded (by the client) personal self-disclosure. Therapists resist the temptation to be clever or to explore unnecessary topics, although they do respond appropriately to situations of obvious abuse, and various solution-focused methods have been described (see Johnson & Goldman, 1996; Lipchik & Kubicki, 1996; Tucker, Stith, Howell, McCollum, & Rosen, 2000; Ziegler & Hiller, 2002) for such situations.

Termination

Solution-focused (couple) therapy stops when the clients are satisfied that their goal or goal(s) have been adequately met or achieved, a situation that can be identified by their response to these questions:

- "How can we know when to stop meeting like this?" (de Shazer, 1991a, pp. 120–131)
- "What needs to be different in your life as a result of coming here for you to say that meeting with me was worthwhile?" or "What number

[scaling progress] do you need to be in order not to come and talk with me anymore?" (DeJong & Berg, 1997, pp. 148–149)

In her book, *Family Based Services: A Solution-Focused Approach*, Berg (1994a) elaborates some criteria and methods for ending therapy, including goal achievement, designating a limited number of sessions, no movement in a case, and leaving things open-ended in response to outside restrictions. She writes:

> If you wait until *all* the client's problems are solved, you will never end treatment. … What is important to keep in mind is that "empowering" clients means equipping them with the tools to solve their own problems as far as possible. When they can't do it on their own, they need to know when to ask for help and where to go for help. Termination can occur when you are confident that the client will know when and where to go to seek help, and *not* when you are confident that he [she or they] will never have problems. (Berg, 1994a, p. 163, emphasis in original)

The solution-focused therapist endeavors to become obsolete and thus end therapy as soon as possible. The object is to get the client out of therapy and actively and productively involved in living his or her life (Dolan, 1985). The approach is characterized more by an attitude than by a particular length: "As few sessions as possible, not even one more than is necessary" is the way de Shazer (1991b, p. x) has put it. Hence, the approach is "minimalistic" in two related senses: (1) theoretical elegance, staying close to the clients' goals without introducing unnecessary and potentially distracting topics; and (2) short-term, using the minimum of necessary sessions. When a couple feels ready and able to carry on without therapy—which includes having some strategies to manage future conflicts (see Carlson, 2000)—it is time for termination. Sometimes termination completes a process; other times a couple has gotten "unstuck" and back "on track" (Walter & Peller, 1994; Hoyt, 2000), and the partners carry on without the presence of a therapist. de Shazer made a remark at the end of a published conversation that might serve as good advice for therapists considering when to terminate treatment:

HOYT: How shall we close?

DE SHAZER: Wittgenstein [1980, p. 77e] has some tremendous advice for all authors: "Anything your reader can do for himself, leave to him." (in Hoyt, 1996b, p. 81)

Although "no more than needed" is a guiding desideratum, it is important to make sure that clients' problems have been "heard" and addressed:

> I have occasionally worked with clients who describe their experience with their past solution-focused professional as he or she having been too positive and not providing opportunity for talking about things that really bothered them. Positive reinforcement alone can initially lead to clients feeling better about their situation and themselves. However, as they begin to feel better and talk more about their complaints, the specific goals may shift, and unless the collaborating professional is aware of this, the collaboration may be ended prematurely. When it appears that goals have been reached, it is important for the collaborating professional to become very curious about how clients have been experiencing the sessions, and what they think has been useful or not useful. "What else would you have wanted me to ask you, or talk about?" could prevent premature termination. (Lipchik, 1997, p. 167)

In keeping with the idea of intermittent or episodic therapy (see Cummings & Sayama, 1995; Hoyt, 1995, 2000), it is also important to leave the door open for possible return. Termination should be structured in such a way that a subsequent decision for more treatment will be seen by clients as an opportunity for further growth rather than an indicator of failure.

Opening the Lens: Some Useful Ideas and Techniques for Solution-Focused Therapists from Other Models

A number of writers have suggested ways to integrate ideas and methods from seemingly related orientations into the solution-focused approach. However, although psychotherapy integration or borrowing techniques from different models is a laudatory endeavor if it better equips the therapist to assist clients, it is not without its perils. Neimeyer (1998, p. 62) warns about the "indiscriminate gallimaufry of deconstructive rules deriving from incompatible metatheories" that might result, for example, if a therapist switches from eliciting, affirming, and celebrating a client's emerging self-awareness to suddenly challenging its logical or empirical basis. Although one can explore with clients their intentions or even carefully offer another possible way of construing a situation ("Could that be a way he/she tries to show concern?"), solution-focused therapists are wary of the concept of therapist-provided "insight," because it implies that there is a "right" or "true" psychological reality underlying clients' awareness, and elevates the therapist to the role of The Expert able to interpret what is "real" and what is not:

HOYT: What I'm getting from what you're saying is it's best to accept that what the patient is communicating about is accurate. And it's our job to figure out what it's accurate about.

WEAKLAND: That's an interesting way of putting it, rather than converting them.

DE SHAZER: I'm not even sure about the last part ... just, "it's accurate."

HOYT: It's accurate.

DE SHAZER: Yeah. It's accurate. And that's all there is.

HOYT: But if we're going to be of service to them, not just to take them seriously and listen, what do we add beyond listening?

DE SHAZER: The seriously. Taking them seriously. See, I think a lot of people listen, but they don't take them seriously. (in Hoyt, 1994b, p. 30)

Shoham et al. (1995, p. 156; also see Fraser, 1998) note that there would even seem to be core contradictions between MRI problem-focused brief therapy and BFTC solution-focused brief therapy models:

This is no easy task, because despite similarities, there are also many ways in which specific tactics and the general therapeutic stance prescribed by the two models can be quite incompatible (e.g., investigating complaints vs. exceptions to complaints, offering optimism and encouragement vs. pessimism and restraint).

Saggese and Foley (2000, p. 59), however, note that "The SFBT [solution-focused brief therapy] and PFBT [problem-focused brief therapy] models are prime candidates for integration because they share a number of basic assumptions about both the nature and resolution of human problems." They go on to suggest ways of integrating the different pathways the two models use when seeking to resolve problems.

In practice, most clinicians influenced by solution-focused therapy do borrow from various models (e.g., see Cade & O'Hanlon, 1993; Eron & Lund, 1996; Fish, 1997; Friedman, 1997; Hoyt, 1995, 2000; Jordan & Quinn, 1994; O'Hanlon & Weiner-Davis, 1989; Quick, 1996), and such "technical integration" (Lazarus, 1995) can be consistent with the solution-focused metamessage *Do what works*. All therapists, however, more or less think they "do what works" (why else would

they do what they do?), so it seems reasonable to establish more specific criteria for what may be consistent with the spirit and intentions of solution-focused intervention. In their thoughtful review, Beyebach and Morejon (1999) refer to Michael Hjerth's (1995) idea that solution-focused therapy can be distinguished along the dimensions of its *philosophy* (or basic premises and assumptions), *use of language*, and *techniques*, and then go on to write:

Provisionally, we would like to describe Solution-Focused Therapy as an approach that includes as its *premises* the beliefs that clients have resources, that change is constant, that in therapy a small change is enough (as long as it is noticed), and that therefore there is no need to understand a problem in order to solve it. The *language* used in Solution-Focused Therapy is usually possibility and future-oriented, with the aim of creating cooperation and putting the client in control of the change process. This language creates a *stance* of cooperation on the part of the therapist, who tries to agree with her clients and is always alert to their use of language and to their changing goals during the process of therapy. This stance includes also an attempt to stay "behind" the clients, to carefully listen to them and to avoid pushing them in the therapist's direction. The therapist does not lecture to the clients or tell them what to do, but tries to help them figure out on their own what course of action to follow. Common, but not necessary *techniques* include goal-talk, exception-talk, and scaling questions, all of which could be described as solution-talk as opposed to problem-talk (de Shazer, 1994a). (Beyebach & Morejon, 1999, p. 29, emphasis in original)

In his book, *Time-Effective Psychotherapy: Maximizing Outcomes in an Era of Minimized Resources*, Steven Friedman (1997, p. 234; also see Friedman & Lipchik, 1999) draws heavily from solution-focused therapy as he outlines five major processes that define a time-effective, competency-based approach:

1. *Connection*: Listening, affirming, and acknowledging each partner's story while joining with both around a set of mutually agreed-upon goals;
2. *Curiosity*: Opening space for a discussion of multiple perspectives while attending to the couple's resources;
3. *Collaboration*: Working together with both members [of] the couple in the direction of *their* preferred futures. Highlighting successes ("exceptions") and generating hope;
4. *Co-Construction of Solution Ideas*: (a)introducing novel ideas that emerge from the clinical conversations; (b)defining action steps ("homework");

5. *Closure:* Giving compliments; celebrating and applauding change; offering each partner an opportunity to acknowledge and comment on changes in the other; offering future availability.

Lipchik (2002, pp. 14–21) also describes a series of solution-focused assumptions:

1. Every client is unique.
2. Clients have the inherent strength and resources to help themselves.
3. Nothing is all negative.
4. There is no such thing as resistance.
5. You cannot change clients; they can only change themselves.
6. Solution-focused therapy goes slowly.
7. There is no cause and effect.
8. Solutions do not necessarily have anything to do with the problem.
9. Emotions are part of every problem and every solution.
10. Change is constant and inevitable; a small change can lead to bigger changes.
11. One can't change the past so one should concentrate on the future.

Looking through these "lenses," various competency-based, collaborative, and future-oriented ideas and interventions borrowed from strategic, narrative, and systemic frameworks can be integrated into solution-focused work. I cite a few here from my clinical experience and that of Shoham et al. (1995), Beyebach and Morejon (1999), Ziegler and Hiller (2001), and others referenced earlier:

• *Motivational interviewing* (W. Miller & Rollnick, 1991; Cordova, Warren, & Gee, 2001). Clients' goals are clarified and their motivation for change is enhanced by exploring with them their reactions to their current experience and their reasons for seeking therapy (e.g., "How is what you've been doing working for you?" and "Is that a positive or a negative for you?"). If clients are dissatisfied, sometimes I find it helpful simply to quote the old saying, "If you don't change directions, you'll wind up where you're heading!"[5] Although solution-focused therapists favor solution-talk rather than problem-talk, hearing some of a couple's woes allows the clients to feel heard and understood. We do not want to get stuck or bogged down, but they are going to tell us anyway, and talking about problems can also be used as a starting point to identify times the problems are not present.
• *Appreciative inquiry.* Although appreciative inquiry (AI) developed within an organiza-tional and business management rather than clinical context, this "positive psychology" approach draws upon social constructionist principles, involving

in a central way, the art and practice of asking questions that strengthen a system's capacity to apprehend, anticipate, and heighten positive potential. It centrally involves the mobilization of inquiry through the crafting of the "unconditional positive question." … In AI the arduous task of intervention gives way to the speed of imagination and innovation; instead of negation, criticism, and spiraling diagnosis, there is discovery, dream, and design. … AI seeks, fundamentally, to build constructive union … and the massive entirety of what people talk about as past and present capacities: achievements, assets, unexplored potentials, innovations, strengths, elevated thoughts, opportunities, benchmarks, high point moments, lived values, traditions, strategic competencies, stories, expressions of wisdom, insights into the deeper corporate spirit or soul—and visions of valued and possible futures. […] It assumes that every living system has many untapped and rich and inspiring accounts of the positive. (Cooperrider & Whitney, 1999; also see http://appreciativeinquiry. cwru.edu)

• *Externalization and relative influence questioning* (White, 1989; White & Epston, 1990; Zimmerman & Dickerson, 1993; Roth & Epston, 1996; also see de Shazer, 1993b). These well-known narrative therapy methods place the "problem" outside the person/couple and identify both times the problem entraps them and times they are able to withstand or control the "problem." Times the couple successfully influences the "problem" may be thought of as "exceptions" (and "coping") within the solution-focused framework, providing a basis for solution development. As Michael White (in Winslade & Monk, 1999, p. 42) notes, these "unique outcomes" (to use the narrative therapy term) or "exceptions" (solution focus) may be nascent and manifest themselves as actions, intentions to act, moments when the effects of the problem do not seem so strong, areas of life that remain unaffected by the problem, special abilities or knowledge about how to overcome the problem, or problem-free responses from others that can be learned from vicariously. As I have suggested elsewhere (Hoyt, 2000, p. 44), seeking a "history of the present recovery" may be more salutary than the conventional psychiatric "history of the present complaint"; rather than (or in addition to) the usual genogram (replete with divorces, suicides, and cutoffs), what useful information might a client and therapist gain from constructing a "solution-focused genogram"?

• *"Go slow" messages and predicting setbacks.* Particularly with couples that have experienced a lot of difficulties and are hesitant to make changes, it may be helpful to compliment them on taking a cautious approach and to remind them that although the course ahead may not be smooth, their thoughtful, determined efforts will yield overall progress. Instead of looking at setbacks as failures, slips and relapses can be reframed as reminders that the couple is still improving and needs to remain vigilant about their process (see Berg, 1994a; Norum, 2000). It is also important for therapists, even those who describe themselves as "brief" therapists, to recognize that change sometimes is slow and that they may need patience to allow couples the time and space to make and consolidate hard-earned gains.

• *Role playing (especially in-session rehearsals of possible "solution" behavior).* Suggesting to one or both members of a couple that they "pretend" or act "as if" a miracle has occurred or the problem is solved allows them a glimpse of a problem-free future; having them "try it on" makes it more "real" and more likely that they will see themselves differently and continue the pro-solution enactment (for a good example drawn from narrative couple therapy, see Roth & Chasin, 1994).

• *Kindness, humor, faith, respect, and love.* These often assumed or taken-for-granted qualities provide the soil in which various techniques may take root. Solution-focused therapists operate from a deep, abiding belief that people, if treated right, are competent and capable. We are in search of *their* solutions and, while not always, I generally have found that the harder I listen, the smarter the client gets—often in ways that I would not have expected or imagined. This belief allows the solution-focused therapist "to look for the light instead of cursing the darkness," which is sometimes no mean feat when unhappy couples occupy our offices.

• *Evoking a positive his/herstory.* Asking about good times and happy memories helps people restore a positive sense of themselves, their partner, and their relationship. In his self-help book, *Why Marriages Succeed or Fail . . . and How You Can Make Yours Last*, couple researcher John Gottman (1994, pp. 224–227) recommends "finding the glory in your marital story" and provides questions to help couples focus on early favorable

impressions of one another, identify ways they have overcome problems and made successful transitions, and highlight positive aspects of their marriage.

• *Giving information, education and advice, and building skills.* This is a particularly "slippery slope," since we don't want to interfere with a couple's own solution development. The "prime directive" of solution-focused therapy—that clients' goals and resources be respected—encourages collaboration and purposeful intervention but does not encourage a "strategic" ploy of the therapist using techniques to manipulate or "do" something to the clients, even if it is intended for their own good. However, while respecting clients' capacities and adhering to Erickson's idea (1980, p. 540—see Note 3) that we may not know what is best, I find that particularly when we are in a therapist–couple *customer* relationship, couples often benefit from and appreciate receiving information about ways they may be able to improve their communication, their problem solving, their sex lives, their parenting, and so on. "Insistence produces resistance" (Hoyt, 2004), so invitation, not imposition, is paramount ("Would you be interested in . . . " rather than "You ought to . . . "), but not providing new ideas and perspectives when asked and appropriate may unnecessarily constrain clients to working *only* with what they already have—a restriction that can result in their attempted solution becoming a more-of-the-same repetition of the problem (see Fraser, 1998). There is nothing in the theory or technique of solution-focused therapy that would contravene, say, addressing a client's depression or lack of relationship skills, especially if doing so would be likely to help him or her toward their therapy goal. Similarly, adjunctive psychopharmacology may sometimes support clients' self-empowerment by relieving suffering and allowing them to participate better by "restoring restorying" capacities (Hoyt, 2000, p. 74).

Examination of various effective brief therapies, including solution-focused intervention with couples, suggests that they all share certain basic characteristics (Budman, Hoyt, & Friedman, 1992):

• Rapid and positive alliance.
• Focus on specific, achievable goals.
• Clear definition of client and therapist responsibilities and activities.
• Emphasis on client strengths and competen-

cies with an expectation of change ("After the miracle ... when things are better").

- Assistance for the clients to move toward new perceptions and behaviors.
- Here-and-now (and next) orientation.
- Time sensitivity, making the most of each session with the possibility of intermittent return as needed.

THEORETICAL UNDERSTANDINGS (CURATIVE FACTORS/MECHANISMS OF CHANGE)

Not invisible but unnoticed, Watson. You did not know where to look, and so you missed all that was important.
— SHERLOCK HOLMES (Arthur Conan Doyle; quoted in Kendrick, 2000, p. 68)

In an interview on "Solution Building and Language Games" that I conducted with de Shazer, he explained:

Our whole model is based on this. That the people come in, and if you ask then right, they will tell you about when the problem doesn't happen and, therefore, you can increase the frequency of its not happening. It's very simple. Now, don't get confused— simple does not mean easy. It's a very simple idea. (Hoyt, 1996b, p. 79)

As George et al. (2006, p. 34) have written in *BRIEFER: A Solution-Focused Manual*, "Steve de Shazer was adamant that solution-focused brief therapy is not a theory. Rather, he stated, it is a description of a way of talking with clients." Simon and Nelson (2007, p. 7) elaborate:

The Solution-Focused Brief Practice approach is, above all, an approach, a stance, a perspective. It is not a Theory of how people develop, how people change, or how therapy should be conducted. One could say, we suppose, that "one theory" (note the small *t*) is that a solution-focused approach in therapy helps clients to make the changes they wish to make because they focus on what they want rather than on what they do not want. That is as far as the approach goes, in terms of theory, however.

Solution-focused therapy does not conceive of the therapeutic endeavor in terms of "curative factors" (which would imply a medical model of "disease" and "cure"). Rather, solution-focused therapy emphasizes the human, interactional achievement of meaning making. How we look influences what we see, and what we see influences what we do—around and around. Changes in perception lead to changes in behavior (and vice versa). This happens through language: "As the client[s] and therapist talk more and more about the solution they want to construct together, they come to believe in the truth or reality of what they are talking about. This is the way language works, naturally" (Berg & de Shazer, 1993, p. 9).

Clients in solution-focused therapy are assisted to develop new awarenesses—not "insights" of buried pains and sorrows, but of underappreciated, overlooked, perhaps forgotten hopes, skills and resources. The focus is on enhancing what I call "*solution sight*": "This process of solution development can be summed up as helping an unrecognized difference become a difference that makes a difference" (de Shazer, 1988, p. 10).[6]

In his book *Becoming Miracle Workers: Language and Meaning in Brief Therapy*, Gale Miller (1997, p. 183) elaborates:

Solution-focused therapists ... use their questions to construct mutually satisfactory conversations with clients. The questions are not designed to elicit information about worlds outside ongoing therapy conversations, but to elicit information in building new stories about clients' lives. Within solution-focused brief therapy discourse, then, all questions are constructive. They are designed to define goals and to construct solutions that solution-focused therapists assume are already present in clients' lives.

As noted at the beginning of this chapter, solution-focused therapy is a "post-structural re-vision" (de Shazer & Berg, 1992; also see Riikonen & Smith, 1997); it is an antipathologizing, utilitarian view that emphasizes the use of language (or "conversation") in the social construction of reality. Insoo Berg and Yvonne Dolan (2001, p. 1) put it very nicely in their compendium, *Tales of Solutions: A Collection of Hope-Inspiring Stories*:

If we had to define the SFBT approach in one sentence without talking about philosophy or techniques, we would describe it as "the pragmatics of hope and respect." Rather than focusing on deficits, SFBT therapists view clients as competent and in possession of resources. SFBT therapists do not attempt to educate or "enlighten" clients; instead, they prefer to view clients as having positive rather than negative intentions. Completely accepting of the client's view, the SFBT therapist uses the client's perceptions as valuable resources to help create the change the client desires.

How we make sense of our worlds—the stories we tell ourselves and each other—does much to determine what we experience, our actions, and our destinies. When clients need a better story, they often come to therapy.

As I have described in *Some Stories Are Better than Others*:

What makes some stories better than others? Ultimately, of course, the answer must come from each individual freely, lest we impose our own values or beliefs. In general terms, stories involve a plot in which characters have experiences and employ imagination to resolve problems over time. ... From this perspective, therapy can be understood as the purposeful development of a more functional story; "better" stories are those that bring more of what is desired and less of what is not desired ...

Aesthetics, effects, and ethics are all important. We like stories that are well told; that are vivid and eloquent; that involve the generation and resolution of some tension; that see the protagonist[s] emerge successfully, perhaps even triumphantly. A "good" story does more than merely relate "facts"; a "good" story invigorates. (Hoyt, 2000, pp. 19–22)

Some of the implications of "storying" for therapy with couples are elaborated by Phillip Ziegler and Tobey Hiller (2001, p. 6; also see Atwood, 1993, 1997; Sternberg, 1998) in their book *Recreating Partnership: A Solution-Oriented, Colloborative Approach to Couples Therapy*:

It is a central tenet of our work that all couples live together, interact, and view each other and their relationship through the lenses of certain narratives—narratives that are either relationship supportive or destructive. These stories, some personal and private, others co-authored and shared by the partners, explain and give meaning to past events, shape each partner's perceptions of ongoing encounters and support their expectations about the future. Whatever their specific content, however long they have been influencing the partners' perceptions and interactions, certain stories, in the case of distressed couples, have woven themselves together into narratives destructive to the relationship—these constructs we call the bad story narrative. These bad stories have led to an ongoing and regenerating perception and experience of events on the part of the couple that result in an increasing loss of a sense of partnership. The couple no longer views itself as a team through good times and bad, a unit working together for the common good. People in this situation are becoming less and less able to draw upon what we call a couple's shared good story narrative. This is a co-authored story running both into the past and into the future which, in distinction to the effects of the bad story narrative, keeps good will and feelings of love alive even during times of trouble and struggle. This good story is, in general, one in which a couple views itself as uniquely lucky to be together, with a past pleasing to dwell on and a future full of hope and promise. Attention to the function of the good story/bad story narratives in couples' lives is very important in the therapeutic endeavor.

The solution-focused approach was developed inductively, by noticing what happened that preceded clients declaring their problems solved, and it is a tenet of solution-focused therapy that it is not necessary to know *why* (or even *how*) something works in order to be effective:

For an intervention to successfully *fit*, it is not necessary to have detailed knowledge of the complaint. It is not necessary even to be able to construct with any rigor how the trouble is maintained in order to prompt solution. ... Any really different behavior in a problematic situation can be enough to prompt solution and give the client the satisfaction he seeks from therapy. (de Shazer, 1985, p. 7; emphasis in original)

Still, it is interesting to speculate, and a good theory (like a good story) may point the way to something useful. Solution-focused couple therapy endeavors to help clients construct self-fulfilling ("good story") realities (Hoyt & Berg, 2000), that is, views of themselves, their partner, and their relationship that will bring the couple more of what they want. Solution-focused therapists attend to working *with* clients to identify and amplify client goals and client perceptions of their abilities to achieve those goals. Entire stories need not be rewritten ("reauthored"), however, since clients can often "take the ball and run" once they are "unstuck."

Clients are conceived as cooperative and competent, and behavior change is seen to flow naturally from changes in the partners' views and viewpoints. Stories and narratives transform and clients cooperate (with the therapist and each other) and move forward more readily when they are assisted to develop solutions that embrace their preferred views of self and other (Eron & Lund, 1996; Sluzki, 1998). As Gottman (1994) has noted, marriages are most likely to fail not when there is conflict, but when there is a lack of conflict resolution—specifically, when there is a lack of "reparative gestures," or when one (or both) partners frequently ignore the other's attempts to repair whatever hurts have happened when conflicts have occurred. Gottman and Silver (1999, pp. 63–64) also highlight the importance of what they term a "fondness and admiration system," with the therapist needing to help the couple "unearth those positive feelings even more and put them to work to save their marriage." By focusing on solutions and exceptions to the problem, solution-focused therapy emphasizes these repairs and positive elements, and avoids iatrogenesis.[7]

Solution-focused therapy is prospective, not retrospective. There is usually a "future focus," with the therapist helping clients to break out of their painful, reiterating traps by drawing attention toward what the clients will be doing differently when they have achieved a desired outcome or solution (Gustafson, 2005). Questions are designed to evoke a self-fulfilling map of the future (Penn, 1985; Tomm, 1987). The language presupposes change ("After the miracle … ") and excites positive expectations (Battino, 2006), with the focus on what *will* be different when the solution is achieved.

> Traditional therapies are backward looking. Therapists ask for recountings of the past, why did you feel that way, who did what to whom, what precipitated the current condition, and the like. In effect, therapies that search for origins, trajectories, structures, and dynamics create the reality of the past. It is this reality that may come to dominate the conversational space of therapy. In contrast, a constructionist consciousness invites a focus on future realities—visions of a livable world, positive possibilities, and viable outcomes. It is this creation of a positive vision that provides direction and hope. Solution-focused therapy … and its replacement of problem-oriented discourse with solution talk, is an obvious case in point. (Gergen, 2006, pp. 173–174)

Indeed, the language of SFBT is sometimes hypnotic, collapsing time, conflating present with future. As a picture of a positive future develops (or a positive past is reevoked), the couple begins to see themselves differently, and they respond to what they see. They begin living in the solution, not the problem. Once this "virtuous cycle" gets going, the couple is "unstuck" and moving toward where they want to go.

TREATMENT APPLICABILITY

There is nothing inherent to solution-focused therapy that would preclude working with any particular problem or group. Indeed, the strong emphasis on identifying and working with clients' own goals, motivations, language, and theories of change makes the approach widely applicable. Solution-focused therapy considers each person, each couple, and each case as unique and potentially cooperative. As George et al. (1999, pp. 22–23, emphasis in original) write in *Problem to Solution*:

> Like de Shazer, in recent years we have adopted the assumption that *all* clients are motivated for *something*. What we assume is that if, under any circumstances, a client has agreed to speak with us then they are doing so for a good reason, and one connected with our professional role. If we believe otherwise then we are acting on an assumption about the client which is potentially offensive: that they do things without a good reason. Not a good start to what should be a working relationship!

Clients who are too psychiatrically impaired to participate in talking therapy would not be expected to do well in solution-focused therapy or any other approach. Clients with so-called "chronic and persistent severe psychiatric illness" may find benefit, however, in that solution-focused therapy works in the here and now and toward achievable goals, rather than getting bogged down by long psychiatric histories (see Kreider, 1998; Rowen & O'Hanlon, 1999; Simon & Nelson, 2007). Mandated clients—who usually arrive as visitors or complainants—can be productively engaged if a goal can be identified that appeals to them. Situations involving severe sociopathy and/or domestic violence may require partners to be seen separately until safety can be assured (see Johnson & Goldman, 1996; Lipchik & Kubicki, 1996; Lee, Sebold, & Uken, 2003; Ziegler & Hiller, 2002).

CASE ILLUSTRATION[8]

> Hey, Dad—that's good! Instead of letting them fight, she's getting them to talk about ways they could be happier!
> —ALEXANDER HOYT (then age 7), after watching a videotape of Insoo Berg (1994b) working with a couple (quoted in Hoyt & Berg, 2000, p. 337)

Jane and John, a married couple in their mid-30s, had initially consulted a child psychologist with concerns about their 3½-year-old son, Jimmy, who had been acting disruptively in his preschool day care. The child therapist had determined that Jimmy did not seem to have any neurological problem, but he did have a challenging temperament and was in need of more consistent parenting. She was able to help the couple with parenting skills but noted that they often became critical and argumentative toward one another, so she referred them for couple therapy. The wife, Jane, told the child therapist that she thought this was a good idea, "because John is so difficult to work with"; but John was less than enthusiastic. Still, concerned about their son and wanting to get along better with his wife, he reluctantly accepted the referral.

Due to restraints of space, I can only sketch and summarize a few of the interactions that characterized the "solution-focused" nature of the work with this particular couple. It is important to keep in mind that much (including tone, timing, and nonverbal communication) cannot be conveyed through a written presentation. This is especially relevant because *how* we respond to clients, the twinkle in our eye and what part of their narrative gets us to lean forward and ask questions, is what helps write the song.

Presession Phone Contact

I initially spoke with John on the phone. He called and left his name and number, and I called him back at the end of my clinical day. He told me about their son and the referral, then added: "You should probably know that I'm not comfortable with shrinks. I've seen other therapists before, by myself and with Jane. They always make a big deal about the way I grew up, that my Mom was crazy and my Dad was abusive and drank a lot."

"Has that been helpful?"

"No, but therapists always make a big deal about it and Jane always wants to blame everything I do on that."

"Well, everybody's got a past. But you're an adult now. So, what do you want to get out of therapy?"

There was a pause. "Well, I'd like Jane and me to get along better without fighting so much. Sometimes I do screw up, and I should tell her about my feelings more, but she makes such a big deal about it that we always wind up arguing."

"So, you'd like to deal with things without so much arguing?"

"Yes."

"OK. Would you be willing to do something before we meet? Just notice those times, even if they're not too often yet, when you and Jane do OK, and come and tell me what she and you do differently in those moments that work out without the two of you fighting. OK?"

He agreed to do so, and we set an appointment time for a week hence. Before we hung up, I added, "If Jane asks you what I said, please tell her that I asked for both of you to notice the times that go OK so that you can describe them to me when we meet. It may give us some clues to what helps and what you both need to do more of."

From Session 1

A week later, they were in the waiting room. When we got into my office and sat down, I welcomed them and reiterated my (pretreatment) assignment:

"So, what did you notice in the last week that you would like to see continue to happen?"

Jane looked at John, then at me, then replied: "Did John tell you about the problem he has telling the truth? He usually doesn't tell me his feelings, and sometimes he lies, even about little things, even when it doesn't make any sense. Like, I'll ask him where he went and he'll tell me he went to the supermarket, even if he really went to the gas station. I just don't get it."

"What would you like to be different?"

"I'd like to know why he doesn't tell me the truth."

"And how would that be helpful?"

"Maybe then he would stop doing the stuff he does."

"And how would your lives be different then?"

"And then I wouldn't get so mad, and we could get along better."

"So you'd like to not get mad, and to get along better?"

"Well, yeah."

"And what would you be doing when you're all getting along better?"

Jane looked puzzled. "What do you mean?"

"Well, let me ask you kind of a funny question: Suppose sometime after our meeting today, a miracle happens—and you and John somehow begin to get along better. If someone looked at the two of you, your son or maybe someone else, what would they see going on?"

"A miracle?"

"Well, figuratively speaking. Maybe it would be better simply to say that after you and John change some of what you're doing, what will that look like?"

"John would be doing what he said he was going to do, and he wouldn't get so defensive if I asked him questions."

"And what would you be doing?"

"When?"

"When he's talking and you're not arguing."

"I wouldn't get mad so easily. We'd probably be laughing more, getting along the way we used to."

"And then what?"

"We'd have more fun, and our son Jimmy probably wouldn't be so freaked out."

"When was the last time that happened, even a little bit, that you and John talked without getting into an argument, the way you used to?"

"Well, the other night, but—"

I interrupted. "How'd you do that?"

"I'm not sure, but I think I just decided to listen and not react even if I thought he wasn't telling me the whole truth."

I turned to John. "And what did you do to make it go better?"

He smiled. "I started to say something that wasn't completely, shall we say, accurate—then I caught myself, before Jane got mad, and made sure I wasn't saying anything wrong."

"Wow! How'd you do that?"

"I just did it. I'm not stupid, or crazy. I can tell the truth when I want to—if she'd give me a chance."

I smiled. "I'm sure you can, if you decide to."

Jane then asked if I had spoken with the child psychologist. I said that I had gotten her message that I might be getting a call from a couple, but I had not heard any details. Jane explained that they had seen Dr. Silver because of worries about their child, and that after a few sessions she had recommended couple therapy to improve their communication. Then she added: "Did John tell you that we've seen other shrinks before? Do you really think that you can help us?"

"Well, I think I can—but that will ultimately be up to the two of you. But I have to tell you, I'm really not a *shrink*. I used to be, but I decided that I'd rather be an *expander*.[9]

John leaned forward and listened intently.

"I like to take people at their word, and try to help people go in the directions they want to go, and not try to bust them or 'shrink' them. So, if you and John are interested in that, I can probably help."

"How does that work?" Jane asked.

"Well, most people have heard of a vicious cycle, you know, where one bad thing leads to another, right?"

She nodded.

"Well, there is also a virtuous cycle, where one good thing leads to another, for example, you trust John, he steps up and does the right thing, so you trust him more, so he does the right thing more, and things build up in a positive way, back and forth. Sometimes things can get better pretty quickly if both people work together."

"Hmm."

"I also think that when couples are having trouble and come to see me, they are often acting more like adversaries than friends. Their story is more like 'Jane *versus* John' than 'Jane *and* John.' So my job is really to help them remember ways they could work together as a team, as partners. Sometimes they already know what they need to do and I just need to remind them, and sometimes they also want to learn some new ways of handling things."

We then discussed how they had met (they had worked for the same computer software company), and I spent much of the remaining time eliciting details of their courtship and happy times together. Numerous questions expanded those "exceptions." As they began to see one another more beneficently, slowly shifting figure and ground, moving from problem to solution, I commented: "It sounds like you both have lots of ideas about how to make things better."

At the end of the session I asked if they would be willing to do "some happiness homework." They agreed, and I suggested: "Between now and our next appointment, and maybe even longer, I'd like each of you to notice what the other person does to make things better—but don't tell the person what you've noticed. Just store it in your head and tell me about it next time we meet. OK?" They agreed, and we made an appointment for 1 week later.

From Session 2

"So, how's the state of the union? What's better?"

John smiled. "After our session last week, we sat in the car in the parking lot and really talked."

"OK."

"And we didn't really get into any big fights all week."

"Really? Wow! How'd you both do that?" I looked at John, then at Jane.

"Well, it's true what John is saying, but ... "—she looked hard at John—"why couldn't you do that earlier?"

I could see defeat being snatched from the jaws of victory, so I interrupted: "Remember teamwork? I think a better question might be, 'How could you do that some more, and *what* can I do to help it happen?'"

"Yeah, give me a chance. I know I made mistakes before, but I'm trying."

John went on to describe several instances in the past week where he had been helpful and truthful. I listened and asked a few questions to keep the discussion positive and headed toward where they wanted to go.

One of their stressors was financial. They had purchased a home 2 years earlier, at what in retrospect now seemed to have been the peak of a real-estate boom. They were having trouble keeping up with payments, and had decided to sell the house, but had not yet found any buyers willing to pay the price they were asking. The pressure was taking a toll. In addition to worrying about whether the house would ever sell, they were strapped for cash and unable to afford some of the activities that they might otherwise have used for relaxation and renewal—such as getting a babysitter and having a night out, or taking a vacation. We explored ways they could do something together, as a couple, and John suggested talking with some friends they knew from their son's daycare to see if they would be interested in trading babysitting.

"In a few minutes, we're going to make another appointment, if you'd like, then stop for today. Before we do that, however, I'd like to ask you each a question—OK?"

They both nodded.

"So, on a scale of 1 to 10, where 1 is things are totally hopeless, and 10 is total bliss—where would you each say you are? John?"

"I'd say a 6—we're talking and I'm hopeful."

I considered asking for details, but wanted to keep Jane engaged, so I turned to her.

"And you, Jane?"

"A 4, maybe a 5."

"OK. And let me ask, for each of you: What would it take to bump it up one notch? So for you, John, what would it take to get from a 6 to a 7?"

"I need to keep doing what I'm doing, and Jane needs to trust me and give me a chance."

"Do you have ideas how to do that?"

John smiled. "Sure."

"OK, and for you, Jane: What would move it up for you from a 4 or 5 to maybe a 5 or 6?"

"Well, I'm not sure I'm ready for that."

"OK—sorry, I didn't mean to be pushy. But, then, let me ask you this: What would it take to keep things from going the other way, toward a 3 or a 2?"

"We just need to keep talking and not arguing. I'm sorry, I'm not trying to be difficult. I do think things are getting better."

"You do?"

"Of course, and I appreciate all that John has been doing."

"Does he know that?"

"Well, maybe I haven't said it in so many words. I know I need to give him more credit than I do."

"Do you have ideas of how you could do that?"

She looked at John. "I know you're trying, honey. I love you, and I appreciate how you've been making lots of efforts, like when you helped me with Jimmy, and when you told me what was bothering you the other night."

The session was almost over. I complimented them on their hard work ("You've both come up with some very good ideas"), then asked: "So, when should we meet again? A week or two, or aybe a little longer? What do you think?"

They looked at one another, then Jane spoke. "Well, we've got a lot going on, dealing with the house, and Jimmy's preschool, and stuff. How about 3 weeks, or a month?" John nodded agreement.

"OK," I said. "I really like the way you want to have some time to work on this. I know it's not going to be all perfect, and you've got a lot of other stuff going on, but it will be interesting to hear what each of you does over the next couple of weeks to keep it going in the right direction and not in the wrong direction."

From Session 3

"Hey, it's been almost a month. So, what's better?"

Jane smiled. "Lots!"

"How so?"

She described two situations in which John had come to her and directly said "I'm upset" rather than avoiding her.

"Is that a positive for you?" I asked.

"Are you kidding? That's what I've been wanting all along."

John looked at me and smiled.

"How'd you do that?" I asked.

"I just knew I had to if we were going to be happy—and it really helped that she didn't yell at me or bring up stuff from other times when I had screwed up. I appreciate that."

I turned toward Jane. "Did you know how much that meant to him?" I asked.

"Yeah, and it was great that he didn't try to switch the topic or bring up crap about my family."

I looked back at John. "I thought you knew where you really wanted to go."

He grinned, then reached over and took Jane's hand.

We spent some time talking about ways they had been cooperating—sharing chores around the house, the evening out they finally had after making the babysitting arrangement with friends, a discussion they had had with their realtor about the house, coparenting little Jimmy. We also discussed a couple of what I referred to as "normal inevitable glitches"—those "temporary times" when things get tense. But even in discussing those instances— maybe especially then—I emphasized the ways they avoided making things worse and how they eventually got back "on track." I remarked, "You know yourselves and each other better than I ever could. What do *you* think would work for the two of you?"

The session was almost over, and generally they seemed to be doing quite well.

"So," I asked, "let me ask another one of those scaling questions. In terms of progress, 1 to 10, where would you say you are?"

"A 7 or 8," said Jane.

"How about you, John?"

"Definitely an 8—I think we're doing well."

"So, what do you think about another appointment?" I asked

They glanced at one another, then John took the lead. "Jane and I talked about it, and we decided that we're doing OK now. So I don't think we need to make an appointment right now."

"OK. But will you give a call if you decide you'd like one?"

"Sure."

"In fact, let me ask you this: Sometime down the road, maybe in a few weeks, or shorter or longer, when something happens that's especially good for 'John *and* Jane', will you give me a call and let me know? It sounds like you're doing fine and know what you need to do to keep it going, but sometimes it's good for us therapists to hear good news about how people can get unstuck and make things go the way they want them to."

Jane and John laughed. "Sure. We'll let you know—the pleasure will be ours!"

Follow-Up

About 2 months, later, my voicemail light was flashing when I came into my office one morning. I sat down, then listened to this verbatim message:

"Hi, Dr. Hoyt. This is John, of 'Jane *and* John.' I'm just calling to leave you a message, as we promised. . . . Things are going really well, and Jane, actually Jane *and* I, are doing really really well.

"We ended up pulling our house off the market, and that helped out a lot—some unexpected bonuses and raises that both us got really helped out in that department. Jimmy is mellowing out a little bit, and he is doing incredibly well at school.

"And, I mean, even the bumps in the road aren't all that big . . . and everything is going fantastic. So, I wanted to thank you, and hopefully you won't be seeing us again, just hearing from us. But even if you see us, I think things from here on out are going to be pretty good. So, maybe I'll call you back and leave you another message in the future.

"And again, we have absolutely nothing but positive memories from going to see you. It was really great. I don't have a lot of, well, I have some suspects of authority and people in your position, but you gave me an incredible amount of confidence in your field and just in doctors in general. And so, yeah, I just wanted to thank you again. Sorry for the long message—and goodbye!"

About 3 weeks later, there was another message, this time from Jane:

"Hi. This is Jane. I know that John called you a couple of weeks ago. I thought it was too early for him to call, but last night we had a little argument and we really handled things differently. He didn't try to lie when he had made a mistake, and I didn't get all pissed off the way I used to. We were both a little angry, but we talked about it. I remembered when we talked with you about being 'Jane *and* John,' not 'Jane *versus* John.' Anyway, you asked us to call to let you know when something went the way we want it to, so I'm calling. Thanks!!!"

CODA

When the night has been too lonely and the road has been
  too long
And you think that love is only for the lucky and the
  strong
Just remember in the winter far beneath the bitter snows
Lies the seed that with the sun's love, in the spring,
  becomes the rose.
                    —AMANDA MCBROOM (1979, from "The Rose")

Solution-focused therapy is a constructivist, collaborative, competency-based, future-oriented approach. The basic premise is deceptively simple: *Increase what works; decrease what doesn't work.* What are the "exceptions" to the problem? What are patients doing differently at those times when they are not anxious or depressed or quarrelling? What has worked before? What strengths can the patients apply? What would be a useful solution? How to construct it?

Behind these apparently simple questions is a profound paradigmatic shift: Competencies, not dysfunctions, are the focus; the quest is to access latent capacities, not latent conflicts. The orientation is toward the future, with the guiding belief that with skillful facilitation, people usually have within themselves the resources necessary to achieve their goals. Without obviating the idea of a physical universe, solution-focused therapy operates from the radical assumption that clients' experience of psychological problems is part and parcel of their language-based social construction of reality (see Hoyt & Ziegler, 2004). As I heard my *haiku* muse whisper (Hoyt, 2000, p. 47):

> Focusing language
> On solutions, not problems
> Miracles happen.

Therapeutic intervention, therefore, is construed as a process of assisting clients to play better "language games" (Wittgenstein, 1958). Although new information and relationship skills training may be provided—if they support the clients' worldview and movement toward their desired goals—solution-focused therapists primarily endeavor to help clients envision and realize solutions by assiduously calling attention to clients' strengths, resources, past successes, and ways of looking.

As therapists we are actively involved—whether we realize it or not—in helping clients construe a different way of looking at themselves, their partners, their situations, and their interactions.

How we look influences what we see, and what we see influences what we do—and around and around the process goes, recursively. Even if one is unaware of it, one cannot *not* have an epistemology (Bateson, 1972, 1979). We choose what we use:

> Dear Reader,
>   Suppose tonight, while you're sleeping, a miracle happens! You're asleep, of course, and you don't immediately know it has happened. But tomorrow, while seeing couples in your office, you begin to notice some things about your clients you haven't noticed or thought much about before. You can still see all the things that your training has allowed you to see, but as you look, you begin to see some previously overlooked qualities: perhaps a love or a hope or a dream that somehow manages to survive, maybe some almost forgotten skill or ability, possibly a quirky interest or sense of humor, something. What might you see? What does the couple see that you don't? What does the couple think would help? What might happen if that could be used therapeutically? What difference might it make?

ACKNOWLEDGMENTS

Thanks to the anonymous couple described in the case illustration; to Guilford Publications for permission to use quotations from two published interviews (Hoyt, 1994b, 1996b) with Steve de Shazer as well as the material in Table 9.1 from Hoyt (1994a) and excerpts from Hoyt and Berg (1998); to W. W. Norton and Company for permission to reprint excerpts and Figure 9.1 from de Shazer (1985, 1988, 1991a); to Phillip Ziegler for permission to adapt handout materials from Ziegler (2000); and to Alfred Publishing Company for permission to use the excerpt from the Amanda McBroom song, "The Rose." I am grateful to Phillip Ziegler and Tobey Hiller, Harvey Ratner, Thorana Nelson, and editor Alan Gurman for their helpful comments regarding earlier drafts of this chapter. The work contained herein is dedicated to my wife, Jennifer Lillard.

NOTES

1. As Simon and Nelson (2007, p. 2) note, "The original solution-focused work was centered on therapy. Today, solution-focused ideas are used in a variety of contexts including social services, corrections, and even business. Steve de Shazer suggested the concept of solution-focused brief practice. Therefore, we use the acronym SFBP." However, since this chapter focuses on clinical applications, we shall retain the more conventional term *solution-focused brief therapy* (and its acronym, *SFBT*).
2. Although the pressures of managed care for greater efficiency and cost containment (see Hoyt, 1995,

2000, 2001a) have contributed to the increased popularity of solution-focused and other time-sensitive approaches, de Shazer (quoted in Short, 1997, p. 18, emphasis in original) has made his position clear: "We are not a response to managed care. We've been doing brief therapy for 30 years. We developed this a long time before managed care was even somebody's bad idea."

3. Erickson wrote: "Patients have problems because their conscious programming has too severely limited their capacities. The solution is to help them break through the limitations of their conscious attitudes to free their unconscious potential for problem solving" (Erickson, Rossi, & Rossi, 1976, p. 18) and "The fullest possible utilization of the functional capacities and abilities and the experiential and acquisitional learnings of the patient ... should take precedence over the teaching of new ways in living which are developed from the therapist's possibly incomplete understanding of what may be right and serviceable to the individual concerned" (Erickson, 1980, p. 540).

4. In their book *The Miracle Method*, Scott Miller and Insoo Berg (1995, p. 37, emphasis in original) recount the origins of the "miracle question," which has come to be a signature characteristic of solution-focused therapy:

> "A woman called us [in 1984] for an appointment, demanding that she be seen that day because it was an emergency. She began sobbing as she told the receptionist how her husband's drinking was out of control and that he had even been violent toward her. As [the client] entered the therapist's office and began to sit down, she said, "My problem is so serious that it would take a *miracle* to solve it!" ... The therapist simply followed the client's lead, and said, "Well ... suppose one happened?" Immediately, the client began to describe what she wanted to be different about the situation that was troubling her. As she described what she wanted in more detail, a smile began to creep into her face and the tone of her voice became more hopeful. ... As she stood to leave the office, she told the therapist that she was feeling "much better." ... The following week she returned and reported that she had turned that feeling into some small but significant changes in her life and her marriage."

5. "More of the same" does not make a change. Even a small pattern deviation can get things moving, as Bill O'Hanlon (1999) suggests in the title of his book, *Do One Thing Different*. In a chapter on "solution-oriented relationships," O'Hanlon discusses "Nine Methods for Resolving Relationship Crises":

1. Change Your Usual Conflict Patterns or Style
2. Do a 180: Change Your Usual Pursuer–Distancer Pattern
3. Catch Your Partner Doing Something Right
4. Unpack Vague, Blaming, and Loaded Words; Instead, Use Action Talk
5. Change Your Complaints into "Action Requests"
6. Make a Specific Plan for Change
7. Focus on How You (Not Your Partner) Can Change, and Take Responsibility for Making That Change
8. Blow Your Partner's Stereotype of You
9. Compassionate Listening. (pp. 157–162)

6. Hence the title of de Shazer's book *Putting Difference to Work* (1991a).

7. Also see Glasser and Glasser (2000, p. 15) regarding the importance of avoiding the "Seven Deadly Habits" of criticizing, blaming, complaining, nagging, threatening, punishing, and bribing. For a more tongue-in-cheek view that uses satire and absurdity to emphasize the value of solution language, see Greenberg and O'Malley (1983), *How to Avoid Love and Marriage*.

8. Additional case examples of couple therapy based on solution-focused or solution-oriented principles can be found in Berg (1994b), Beyebach and Morejon (1999), de Shazer (1982, 1985, 1991a, 1994a), de Shazer and Berg (1985), Friedman (1992, 1993b, 1996, 1997), Friedman and Lipchik (1999), Gale and Newfield (1992), George et al. (1999), Hoyt (2002), Hoyt and Berg (2000), Hudson and O'Hanlon (1991), Iveson (2003), Metcalf (2004), Nelson and Kelly (2001), Norum (2000), O'Hanlon and Hudson (1994), Johnson and Goldman (1996); Lethem (1994), Lipchik (2002), Lipchik and Kubicki (1996), Nunnally (1993), Quick (1996), Walter and Peller (1988), Weiner-Davis (1992), Ziegler (1998), and Ziegler and Hiller (2001, 2002, 2007).

9. See Hoyt (1995), especially Chapter 13, "'Patient' or 'Client': What's in a Name?," and Chapter 14, "'Shrink' or 'Expander': An Issue in Forming a Therapeutic Alliance."

SUGGESTIONS FOR FURTHER READING

Berg, I. K., & Dolan, Y. D. (2001). *Tales of solutions: A collection of hope-inspiring stories.* New York: Norton.

DeJong, P., & Berg, I. K. (1997). *Interviewing for solutions.* Pacific Grove, CA: Brooks/Cole.

de Shazer, S. (1985). *Keys to solution in brief therapy.* New York: Norton.

Hoyt, M. F. (2000). *Some stories are better than others: Doing what works in brief therapy and managed care.* Philadelphia: Brunner/Mazel.

Ziegler, P. B., & Hiller, T. (2001). *Recreating partnership: A solution-oriented, collaborative approach to couples therapy.* New York: Norton.

REFERENCES

Adams, J. F., Piercy, F. P., & Jurich, J. A. (1991). Effects of solution-focused therapy's "formula first session task" on compliance and outcome in family therapy. *Journal of Marital and Family Therapy, 17,* 277–290.

Anderson, H., & Goolishian, H. A. (1992). The client is the expert: A not-knowing approach to therapy. In

S. McNamee & K. Bergen (Eds.), *Therapy as social construction* (pp. 25–39). Newbury Park, CA: Sage.

Atwood, J. D. (1993). Social constructionist couple therapy. *Family Journal, 1*, 116–130.

Atwood, J. D. (1997). Social construction theory and therapy. In J. D. Atwood (Ed.), *Challenging family therapy situations: Perspectives in social construction* (pp. 1–40). New York: Springer.

Bateson, G. (1972). *Steps to an ecology of mind.* New York: Ballantine.

Bateson, G. (1979). *Mind and nature: A necessary unity.* New York: Dutton.

Battino, R. (2006). *Expectation: The very brief therapy book.* Norwalk, CT: Crown House.

Berendt, J. (1994). *Midnight in the garden of good and evil.* New York: Random House.

Berg, I. K. (1989). Of visitors, complainants, and customers. *Family Therapy Networker, 13*(1), 27.

Berg, I. K. (1994a). *Family-based services: A solution-focused approach.* New York: Norton.

Berg, I. K. (1994b). *Irreconcilable differences: A solution-focused approach to marital therapy* [Videotape]. New York: Norton.

Berg, I. K. (1994c). *So what else is better? Solutions for substance abuse* [Videotape]. Milwaukee, WI: Brief Family Therapy Center.

Berg, I. K., & de Shazer, S. (1993). Making numbers talk: Language in therapy. In S. Friedman (Ed.), *The new language of change: Constructive collaboration in psychotherapy* (pp. 5–24). New York: Guilford Press.

Berg, I. K., & Dolan, Y. D. (2001). *Tales of solutions: A collection of hope-inspiring stories.* New York: Norton.

Berg, I. K., & Kelly, S. (2000). *Building solutions in child protective services.* New York: Norton.

Berg, I. K., & Miller, S. D. (1992). *Working with the problem drinker: A solution-focused approach.* New York: Norton.

Berg, I. K., & Reuss, N. H. (1997). *Solutions step by step: A substance abuse treatment manual.* New York: Norton.

Beyebach, M., & Morejon, A. R. (1999). Some thoughts on integration in solution-focused therapy. *Journal of Systemic Therapies, 18*(1), 24–42.

Bonjean, M. J. (1997). Solution-focused brief therapy with aging families. In T. D. Hargrave & S. M. Hanna (Eds.), *The aging family: New visions in theory, practice, and reality* (pp. 81–100). New York: Brunner/Mazel.

Bonjean, M. J. (2003). Solution-focused therapy: Elders enhancing exceptions. In J. L. Ronch & J. Goldfield (Eds.), *Mental wellness in aging: Strengths-based approaches* (pp. 201–234). Baltimore: Health Professions Press.

Budman, S. H., Hoyt, M. F., & Friedman, S. (Eds.). (1992). *The first session in brief therapy.* New York: Guilford Press.

Cade, B., & O'Hanlon, W. H. (1993). *A brief guide to brief therapy.* New York: Norton.

Carlson, J. (2000). How to prevent relapse: Treatment strategies for long-term change. *Family Therapy Networker, 24*(5), 23, 84.

Cooperrider, D. L., & Whitney, D. (1999). Appreciative inquiry: A positive revolution in change. In P. Holman & T. Devane (Eds.), *The change handbook* (pp. 245–263). San Francisco: Berrett-Koehler.

Cordova, J. V., Warren, L. Z., & Gee, C. B. (2001). Motivational interviewing as an intervention for at-risk couples. *Journal of Marital and Family Therapy, 27*(3), 315–326.

Cummings, N. A., & Sayama, M. (1995). *Focused psychotherapy: A casebook of brief, intermittent psychotherapy throughout the life cycle.* New York: Brunner/Mazel.

DeJong, P., & Berg, I. K. (1997). *Interviewing for solutions.* Pacific Grove, CA: Brooks/Cole.

DeJong, P., & Hopwood, L. E. (1996). Outcome research on treatment conducted at the Brief Family Therapy Center, 1992–1993. In S. D. Miller, M. A. Hubble, & B. L. Duncan (Eds.), *Handbook of solution-focused brief therapy* (pp. 272–298). San Francisco: Jossey-Bass.

de Shazer, S. (1982). *Patterns of brief family therapy.* New York: Guilford Press.

de Shazer, S. (1984). The death of resistance. *Family Process, 23,* 79–93.

de Shazer, S. (1985). *Keys to solution in brief therapy.* New York: Norton.

de Shazer, S. (1988). *Clues: Investigating solutions in brief therapy.* New York: Norton.

de Shazer, S. (1991a). *Putting difference to work.* New York: Norton.

de Shazer, S. (1991b). Foreword. In Y. M. Dolan (Ed.), *Resolving sexual abuse: Solution-focused therapy and Ericksonian hypnosis for adult survivors* (pp. ix–x). New York: Norton.

de Shazer, S. (1993a). Creative misunderstanding: There is no escape from language. In S. G. Gilligan & R. Price (Eds.), *Therapeutic conversations* (pp. 81–90). New York: Norton.

de Shazer, S. (1993b). Commentary: de Shazer and White: Vive la difference. In S. G. Gilligan & R. Price (Eds.), *Therapeutic conversations* (pp. 112–120). New York: Norton.

de Shazer, S. (1994a). *Words were originally magic.* New York: Norton.

de Shazer, S. (1994b). Essential, non-essential: *Vive la différence.* In J. K. Zeig (Ed.), *Ericksonian methods: The essence of the story* (pp. 240–253). New York: Brunner-Mazel.

de Shazer, S., & Berg, I. K. (1985). A part is not apart: Working with only one of the partners present. In A. S. Gurman (Ed.), *Casebook of marital therapy* (pp. 97–110). New York: Guilford Press.

de Shazer, S., & Berg, I. K. (1992). Doing therapy: A post-structural re-vision. *Journal of Marital and Family Therapy, 18,* 71–81.

de Shazer, S., & Berg, I. K. (1997). "What works?": Remarks on research aspects of solution-focused brief therapy. *Journal of Family Therapy, 19,* 121–124.

de Shazer, S., Berg, I. K., Lipchik, E., Nunnally, E., Molnar, A., Gingerich, W., et al. (1986). Brief therapy: Focused solution development. *Family Process, 25,* 207–227.

de Shazer, S., Dolan, Y., Korman, H., Trepper, T., Mac-Collum, E., & Berg, I. K. (2006). *More than miracles: The state of the art of solution-focused therapy.* New York: Haworth.

de Shazer, S., & Molnar, A. (1984). Four useful interventions in brief family therapy. *Journal of Marital and Family Therapy, 10*(3), 297–304.

Dolan, Y. M. (1985). *A path with a heart: Ericksonian utilization with resistant and chronic clients.* New York: Brunner/Mazel.

Dolan, Y. M. (1991). *Resolving sexual abuse: Solution-focused therapy and Ericksonian hypnosis for adult survivors.* New York: Norton.

Duncan, B. L., Hubble, M. A., & Miller, S. D. (1997). *Psychotherapy with "impossible" cases: The efficient treatment of therapy veterans.* New York: Norton.

Duncan, B. L., Hubble, M. A., Miller, S. D., & Coleman, S. T. (1998). Escaping from the last world of impossibility: Honoring clients' language, motivation, and theories of change. In M. F. Hoyt (Ed.), *The handbook of constructive therapies* (pp. 293–313). San Francisco: Jossey-Bass.

Efran, J. S., & Schenker, M. D. (1993). A potpourri of solutions: How new and different is solution-focused therapy? *Family Therapy Networker, 17,* 71–74.

Erickson, M. H. (1980). *Collected papers* (Vol. 1). New York: Irvington.

Erickson, M. H., & Rossi, E. L. (1979). *Hypnotherapy: An exploratory casebook.* New York: Irvington.

Erickson, M. H., Rossi, E. L., & Rossi, S. I. (1976). *Hypnotic realities: The induction of clinical hypnosis and forms of indirect suggestion.* New York: Irvington.

Eron, J. B., & Lund, T. W. (1996). *Narrative solutions in brief therapy.* New York: Guilford Press.

Fisch, R., Weakland, J. H., & Segal, L. (1982). *The tactics of change: Doing therapy briefly.* San Francisco: Jossey-Bass.

Fish, J. M. (1997). Paradox for complainants: Strategic thoughts about solution-focused therapy. *Journal of Systemic Therapies, 16*(5), 266–273.

Fraser, J. S. (1998). Solution-focused therapy—As a problem. In W. Ray & S. de Shazer (Eds.), *Evolving brief therapies: Essays in honor of John Weakland* (pp. 178–194). Iowa City: Geist & Russell.

Friedman, S. (1992). Constructing solutions (stories) in brief family therapy. In S. H. Budman, M. F. Hoyt, & S. Friedman (Eds.), *The first session in brief therapy* (pp. 282–305). New York: Guilford Press.

Friedman, S. (1993a). Does the miracle question always create miracles? *Journal of Systemic Therapies, 12*(1), 71–74.

Friedman, S. (1993b). Possibility therapy with couples: Constructing time-effective solutions. *Journal of Family Psychotherapy, 4*(4), 35–52.

Friedman, S. (1996). Couples therapy: Changing conversations. In H. Rosen & K. T. Kuehlwein (Eds.), *Constructing realities: Meaning-making perspectives for psychotherapists* (pp. 413–453). San Francisco: Jossey-Bass.

Friedman, S. (1997). *Time-effective psychotherapy: Maximizing outcomes in an era of minimized resources.* Boston: Allyn & Bacon.

Friedman, S., & Lipchik, E. (1999). A time-effective, solution-focused approach to couple therapy. In J. M. Donovan (Ed.), *Short-term couple therapy* (pp. 325–359). New York: Guilford Press.

Furman, B., & Ahola, T. (1992). *Solution talk: Hosting therapeutic conversations.* New York: Norton.

Gale, J., & Newfield, N. (1992). A conversation analysis of a solution-focused marital therapy session. *Journal of Marital and Family Therapy, 18*(2), 153–165.

George, E., Iveson, C., & Ratner, H. (1999). *Problem to solution: Brief therapy with individuals and families* (rev. ed.) London: Brief Therapy Press.

George, E., Iveson, C., & Ratner, H. (2006). *BRIEFER: A solution-focused manual.* London: Brief Therapy Press.

Gergen, K. J. (2006). *Therapeutic realities: Collaboration, oppression and relational flow.* Chagrin Falls, OH: Taos Institute Publications.

Gingerich, W., & Eisengart, S. (2000). Solution-focused brief therapy: A review of the outcome research. *Family Process, 39,* 477–498.

Glasser, W., & Glasser, C. (2000). *Getting together and staying together: Solving the mystery of marriage.* New York: HarperCollins.

Gottman, J. M. (1994). *Why marriages succeed or fail . . . And how you can make yours last.* New York: Fireside/Simon & Schuster.

Gottman, J. M., & Silver, N. (1999). *The seven principles for making marriage work.* New York: Three Rivers Press/Random House.

Greenberg, D., & O'Malley, S. (1983). *How to avoid love and marriage.* New York: Freundlich Books/Schribner.

Gustafson, J. P. (2005). *Very brief psychotherapy.* New York: Routledge.

Hjerth, M. (1995, February). *New developments in solution-focused therapy.* Workshop presented in Salamanca, Spain.

Hopwood, L., & de Shazer, S. (1994). From here to there and who knows where: The continuing evolution of solution-focused brief therapy. In M. Elkaim (Ed.), *Family therapies: The principal approaches* (pp. 555–576). Paris: Editions de Seuil.

Hoyt, M. F. (Ed.). (1994a). *Constructive therapies.* New York: Guilford Press.

Hoyt, M. F. (1994b). On the importance of keeping it simple and taking the patient seriously: A conversation with Steve de Shazer and John Weakland. In *Constructive therapies* (pp. 11–40). New York: Guilford Press.

Hoyt, M. F. (1994c). Single session solutions. In *Constructive therapies* (pp. 40–159). New York: Guilford Press.

Hoyt, M. F. (1994d). Introduction: Competency-based future-oriented therapy. In *Constructive therapies* (pp. 1–10). New York: Guilford Press.

Hoyt, M. F. (1995). *Brief therapy and managed care: Read-*

ings for contemporary practice. San Francisco: Jossey-Bass.

Hoyt, M. F. (Ed.). (1996a). *Constructive therapies* (Vol. 2). New York: Guilford Press.

Hoyt, M. F. (1996b). Solution building and language games: A conversation with Steve de Shazer (and some after words with Insoo Kim Berg). In *Constructive therapies* (Vol. 2, pp. 60–86). New York: Guilford Press.

Hoyt, M. F. (Ed.). (1998). *The handbook of constructive therapies.* San Francisco: Jossey-Bass.

Hoyt, M. F. (2000). *Some stories are better than others: Doing what works in brief therapy and managed care.* Philadelphia: Brunner/Mazel.

Hoyt, M. F. (2001a). Getting unstuck: The squeaky wheel—Don't let managed care shortchange your clients. *Family Therapy Networker, 25*(1), 19–20.

Hoyt, M. F. (2001b). Connection: The double-edged gift of presence. *Journal of Clinical Psychology/In Session: Psychotherapy in Practice, 57*(8), 1–8.

Hoyt, M. F. (2002). Solution-focused couple therapy. In A. S. Gurman & N. S. Jacobson (Eds.), *Clinical handbook of couple therapy* (3rd ed., pp. 335–369). New York: Guilford Press.

Hoyt, M. F. (2004). *The present is a gift: Mo' better stories from the world of brief therapy.* New York: iUniverse Publishers.

Hoyt, M. F., & Berg, I. K. (2000). Solution-focused couple therapy: Helping clients construct self-fulfilling realities. In M. F. Hoyt, *Some stories are better than others* (pp. 143–166). Philadelphia: Burnner-Mazel.

Hoyt, M. F., & Miller, S. D. (2000). Stage-appropriate change-oriented brief therapy strategies. In M. F. Hoyt, *Some stories are better than others* (pp. 207–235). Philadelphia: Brunner-Mazel.

Hoyt, M. F., & Ziegler, P. (2004). The pros and cons of postmodernism in psychotherapy: Stepping back from the abyss. In M. F. Hoyt, *The present is a gift* (pp. 132–181). New York: iUniverse Publishers.

Hudson, P., & O'Hanlon, W. H. (1991). *Rewriting love stories: Brief marital therapy.* New York: Norton.

Iveson, C. (2003). Solution-focused couples therapy. In B. O'Connell & S. Palmer (Eds.), *Handbook of solution-focused therapy* (pp. 61–73). London: Sage.

Johnson, C. E., & Goldman, J. (1996). Taking safety home: A solution-focused approach with domestic violence. In M. F. Hoyt (Ed.), *Constructive therapies* (Vol. 2, pp. 184–196). New York: Guilford Press.

Jordan, K., & Quinn, W. H. (1994). Session two outcome of the formula first session task in problem- and solution-focused approaches. *Journal of Family Therapy, 22,* 3–16.

Kendrick, S. (2000, January–February). Zen in the art of Sherlock Holmes. *Utne Reader, 97,* 65–69.

King, E. (1998). Role of affect and emotional context in solution-focused therapy. *Journal of Systemic Therapies, 17*(2), 51–64.

Kreider, J. W. (1998). Solution-focused ideas for briefer therapy with longer-term clients. In M. F. Hoyt (Ed.),

The handbook of constructive therapies (pp. 341–357). San Francisco: Jossey-Bass.

Lazarus, A. A. (1995). Different types of eclecticism and integration: Let's be aware of the dangers. *Journal of Psychotherapy Integration, 5,* 27–39.

Lee, M. Y., Sebold, J., & Uken, A. (2003). *Accountability for solutions: Domestic violence solution-focused treatment with offenders.* New York: Oxford University Press.

Lethem, J. (1994). *Moved to tears, moved to action: Solution focused brief therapy with women and children.* London: Brief Therapy Press.

Lipchik, E. (Ed.). (1987). *Interviewing.* Rockville, MD: Aspen.

Lipchik, E. (1993). "Both/and" solutions. In S. Friedman (Ed.), *The new language of change: Constructive collaboration in psychotherapy* (pp. 25–49). New York: Guilford Press.

Lipchik, E. (1994). The rush to be brief. *Family Therapy Networker, 18*(2), 34–39.

Lipchik, E. (1997). My story about solution-focused brief therapist/client relationships. *Journal of Systemic Therapies, 16*(2), 159–172.

Lipchik, E. (2002). *Beyond technique in solution-focused therapy: Working with emotions and the therapeutic relationship.* New York: Guilford Press.

Lipchik, E., & de Shazer, S. (1986). The purposeful interview. *Journal of Strategic and Systemic Therapies, 5,* 88–89.

Lipchik, E., & Kubicki, A. D. (1996). Solution-focused domestic violence views: Bridges toward a new reality in couples therapy. In S. D. Miller, M. A. Hubble, & B. L. Duncan (Eds.), *Handbook of solution-focused brief therapy* (pp. 65–98). San Francisco: Jossey-Bass.

Macdonald, A. J. (2003). Research in solution-focused brief therapy. In B. O'Connell & S. Palmer (Eds.), *Handbook of solution-focused therapy* (pp. 12–24). London: Sage.

McBroom, A. (1979). The rose. Song on Bette Midler album, *The rose.* New York: Atlantic Records/Warner Communications Group.

McKeel, A. J. (1996). A clinician's guide to research on solution-focused brief therapy. In S. D. Miller, M. A. Hubble, & B. L. Duncan (Eds.), *Handbook of solution-focused brief therapy* (pp. 251–271). San Francisco: Jossey-Bass.

McNamee, S., & Gergen, K. J. (Eds.). (1992). *Therapy as social construction.* London: Sage.

Metcalf, L. (2004). *The miracle question: Answer it and change your life.* Norwalk, CT: Crown House.

Miller, G. (1997). *Becoming miracle workers: Language and meaning in brief therapy.* Hawthorne, NY: Aldine de Gruyter.

Miller, G., & de Shazer, S. (1998). Have you heard the latest about … ?: Solution-focused therapy as a rumor. *Family Process, 37,* 363–378.

Miller, G., & de Shazer, S. (2000). Emotions in solution-focused therapy: A re-examination. *Family Process, 39*(1), 5–23.

Miller, S. D. (1992). The symptoms of solution. *Journal of Strategic and Systemic Therapies*, *11*, 1–11.

Miller, S. D. (1994). Some questions (not answers) for the brief treatment of people with drug and alcohol problems. In M. F. Hoyt (Ed.), *Constructive therapies* (pp. 92–110). New York: Guilford Press.

Miller, S. D., & Berg, I. K. (1995). *The miracle method*. New York: Norton.

Miller, S. D., & Duncan, B. L. (2000). Paradigm lost: From model-driven to client-directed, outcome-informed clinical work. *Journal of Systemic Therapies*, *19*(1), 20–34.

Miller, S. D., Duncan, B. L., & Hubble, M. A. (1997). *Escape from Babel: Toward a unifying language for psychotherapy practice*. New York: Norton.

Miller, S. D., Hubble, M. A., & Duncan, B. L. (Eds.). (1996). *Handbook of solution-focused brief therapy*. San Francisco: Jossey-Bass.

Miller, W. R., & Rollnick, S. (1991). *Motivational interviewing: Preparing people to change addictive behavior*. New York: Guilford Press.

Nau, D. S., & Shilts, L. (2000). When to use the miracle question: Clues from a qualitative study of four SFBT practitioners. *Journal of Systemic Therapies*, *19*(1), 129–135.

Neimeyer, R. A. (1998). Cognitive therapy and the narrative trend: A bridge too far? *Journal of Cognitive Psychotherapy*, *12*, 57–65.

Nelson, T. S. (Ed.). (2005). *Education and training in solution-focused brief therapy*. New York: Haworth Press.

Nelson, T. S., & Kelly, L. (2001). Solution-focused couples group. *Journal of Systemic Therapies*, *20*(4), 47–66.

Nelson, T. S., & Thomas, F. N. (Eds.). (2007). *Handbook of solution-focused brief therapy: Clinical applications*. New York: Haworth Press.

Norum, D. (2000). The family has the solution. *Journal of Systemic Therapies*, *19*(1), 3–15.

Nunnally, E. (1993). Solution-focused therapy. In R. A. Wells & V. J. Giannetti (Eds.), *Casebook of the brief psychotherapies* (pp. 271–286). New York: Plenum Press.

Nylund, D., & Corsiglia, V. (1994). Becoming solution-focused forced in brief therapy: Remembering something important we already knew. *Journal of Systemic Therapies*, *13*(5), 5–12.

O'Connell, B., & Palmer, S. (Eds.). (2003). *Handbook of solution-focused therapy*. London: Sage.

O'Hanlon, W. H. (1998). Possibility therapy: An inclusive, collaborative, solution-based model of psychotherapy. In M. F. Hoyt (Ed.), *The handbook of constructive therapies* (pp. 137–158). San Francisco: Jossey-Bass.

O'Hanlon, W. H. (1999). *Do one thing different: And other uncommonly sensible solutions to life's persistent problems*. New York: Morrow.

O'Hanlon, W. H., & Hudson, P. (1994). Coauthoring a love story: Solution-oriented marital therapy. In M. F. Hoyt (Ed.), *Constructive therapies* (pp. 160–188). New York: Guilford Press.

O'Hanlon, W. H., & Weiner-Davis, M. (1989). *In search of solutions: A new direction in psychotherapy*. New York: Norton.

Penn, P. (1985). Feed-forward: Future questions, future maps. *Family Process*, *24*, 289–310.

Prochaska, J. O. (1999). How do people change and how can we change to help many more people? In M. A. Hubble, B. L. Duncan, & S. D. Miller (Eds.), *The heart and soul of change: What works in therapy* (pp. 227–255). Washington, DC: American Psychological Association.

Quick, E. K. (1996). *Doing what works in brief therapy: A strategic solution-focused approach*. San Diego: Academic Press.

Riikonen, E., & Smith, G. M. (1997). *Re-imagining therapy: Living conversations and relational knowing*. London: Sage.

Rosenbaum, R., Hoyt, M. F., & Talmon, M. (1990). The challenge of single-session therapies: Creating pivotal moments. In R. A. Wells & V. J. Giannetti (Eds.), *Handbook of the brief psychotherapies* (pp. 165–189). New York: Plenum Press.

Rosenberg, B. (2000). Mandated clients and solution focused therapy: "It's not my miracle." *Journal of Systemic Therapies*, *19*(1), 90–99.

Roth, S., & Chasin, R. (1994). Entering one another's worlds of meaning and imagination: Dramatic enactment and narrative couple therapy. In M. F. Hoyt (Ed.), *Constructive therapies* (pp. 189–216). New York: Guilford Press.

Roth, S., & Epston, D. (1996). Consulting the problem about the problematic relationship: An exercise for experiencing a relationship with an externalized problem. In M. F. Hoyt (Ed.), *Constructive therapies* (Vol. 2, pp. 148–162). New York: Guilford Press.

Rowen, T., & O'Hanlon, W. H. (1999). *Solution-oriented therapy for chronic and severe mental illness*. New York: Wiley.

Saggese, M. L., & Foley, F. W. (2000). From problems or solutions to problems and solutions: Integrating the MRI and solution-focused models of brief therapy. *Journal of Systemic Therapies*, *19*(1), 59–73.

Schultheis, G. M., O'Hanlon, W. H., & O'Hanlon, S. (1998). *Brief couples therapy homework planner*. New York: Wiley.

Sharry, J., Madden, B., Darmody, M., & Miller, S. D. (2001). Giving our clients the break: Applications of client-directed, outcome-informed clinical work. *Journal of Systemic Therapies*, *20*(3), 68–76.

Shoham, V., Rohrbaugh, M., & Patterson, J. (1995). Problem- and solution-focused couple therapies: The MRI and Milwaukee models. In N. S. Jacobson & A. S. Gurman (Eds.), *Clinical handbook of couple therapy* (2nd ed., pp. 142–163). New York: Guilford Press.

Shoham, V., & Rohrbaugh, M. J. (2002). Brief strategic couple therapy. In A. S. Gurman & N. S. Jacobson (Eds.), *Clinical handbook of couple therapy* (3rd ed., pp. 5–25). New York: Guilford Press.

Short, D. (1997). Interview: Steve de Shazer and Insoo Kim Berg. *Milton H. Erickson Foundation Newsletter*, *17*(1), 18–20.

Simon, J. K., & Nelson, T. S. (2007). *I am more than my label: Solution-focused brief practice with long-term users of mental health services.* New York: Haworth Press.

Sluzki, C. E. (1998). Strange attractors and the transformation of narratives in family therapy. In M. F. Hoyt (Ed.), *The handbook of constructive therapies* (pp. 159–179). San Francisco: Jossey-Bass.

Sternberg, R. J. (1998). *Love is a story: A new theory of relationships.* New York: Oxford University Press.

Talmon, M. (1990). *Single session therapy: Maximizing the effect of the first (and often only) therapeutic encounter.* San Francisco: Jossey-Bass.

Talmon, M. (1993). *Single session solutions.* Reading, MA: Addison-Wesley.

Tohn, S. L., & Oshlag, J. A. (1996a). *Crossing the bridge: Integrating solution-focused therapy into clinical practice.* Natick, MA: Solutions Press.

Tohn, S. L., & Oshlag, J. A. (1996b). Cooperating with the uncooperative. In S. D. Miller, M. A. Hubble, & B. L. Duncan (Eds.), *Handbook of solution-focused brief therapy* (pp. 152–183). San Francisco: Jossey-Bass.

Tomm, K. (1987). Interventive interviewing: I. Strategizing as a fourth guideline for the therapist. *Family Process, 26,* 3–13.

Tucker, N. L., Stith, S. M., Howell, L. W., McCollum, E. E., & Rosen, K. H. (2000). Meta-dialogues in domestic violence-focused couples treatment. *Journal of Systemic Therapies, 19*(4), 56–72.

Turnell, A., & Lipchik, E. (1999). The role of empathy in brief therapy: The overlooked but vital context. *Australian and New Zealand Journal of Family Therapy, 20*(4), 177–182.

Walter, J. L., & Peller, J. E. (1988). Going beyond the attempted solution: A couple's meta-solution. *Family Therapy Case Studies, 3*(1), 41–45.

Walter, J. L., & Peller, J. E. (1992). *Becoming solution-focused in brief therapy.* New York: Brunner/Mazel.

Walter, J. L., & Peller, J. E. (1994). "On track" in solution-focused brief therapy. In M. F. Hoyt (Ed.), *Constructive therapies* (pp. 111–125). New York: Guilford Press.

Walter, J. L., & Peller, J. E. (2000). *Recreating brief therapy: Preferences and possibilities.* New York: Norton.

Watzlawick, P., Weakland, J. H., & Fisch, R. (1974). *Change: Principles of problem formation and problem resolution.* New York: Norton.

Weakland, J. H. (1993). Conversation—But what kind? In S. G. Gilligan & R. Price (Eds.), *Therapeutic conversations* (pp. 136–145). New York: Norton.

Weakland, J. H., & Fisch, R. (1992). Brief therapy—MRI style. In S. H. Budman, M. F. Hoyt, & S. Friedman (Eds.), *The first session in brief therapy* (pp. 306–323). New York: Guilford Press.

Weiner-Davis, M. (1992). *Divorce-busting: A revolutionary and rapid program for staying together.* New York: Simon & Schuster/Fireside.

Weiner-Davis, M. (1993). Pro-constructed realities. In S. G. Gilligan & R. Price (Eds.), *Therapeutic conversations* (pp. 149–157). New York: Norton.

Weiner-Davis, M. (1995). *Change your life and everyone in it.* New York: Fireside/Simon & Schuster.

Weiner-Davis, M. (1998). *A woman's guide to changing her man.* New York: Golden Books.

Weiner-Davis, M., de Shazer, S., & Gingerich, W. J. (1987). Using pretreatment change to construct a therapeutic solution: An exploratory study. *Journal of Marital and Family Therapy, 13,* 359–363.

Wender, P. (1968). Vicious and virtuous circles: The role of deviation amplifying feedback in the origin and perpetuation of behavior. *Psychiatry, 31,* 309–324.

White, M. (1989). The externalizing of the problem and the re-authoring of lives and relationships. In M. White (Ed.), *Selected papers* (pp. 5–28). Adelaide, Australia: Dulwich Centre Publications.

White, M., & Epston, D. (1990). *Narrative means to therapeutic ends.* New York: Norton.

Wile, D. B. (2002). Collaborative couple therapy. In A. S. Gurman & N. S. Jacobson (Eds.), *Clinical handbook of couple therapy* (3rd ed., pp. 281–307). New York: Guilford Press.

Winslade, J., & Monk, G. (1999). *Narrative counseling in schools: Powerful and brief.* Thousand Oaks, CA: Corwin Press.

Wittgenstein, L. (1958). *Philosophical investigations* (3rd ed.). New York: Macmillan.

Wittgenstein, L. (1980). *Culture and value* (P. Winch, Trans.). Chicago: University of Chicago Press.

Ziegler, P. B. (1998). Solution-focused therapy for the not-so-brief clinician. *Journal of Collaborative Therapies, 6*(1), 22–25.

Ziegler, P. B. (2000, April 8). *Recreating partnership: A solution-focused, competency-based approach to couples therapy.* Workshop sponsored by John F. Kennedy University, Orinda, CA.

Ziegler, P. B., & Hiller, T. (2001). *Recreating partnership: A solution-oriented, collaborative approach to couples therapy.* New York: Norton.

Ziegler, P. B., & Hiller, T. (2002). Good story/bad story: Collaborating with violent couples. *Psychotherapy Networker, 26*(2), 63–68.

Ziegler, P. B., & Hiller, T. (2007). Solution-focused therapy with couples. In T. S. Nelson & F. N. Thomas (Eds.), *Handbook of solution-focused brief therapy: Clinical applications* (pp. 91–115). New York: Haworth Press.

Zimmerman, J. L., & Dickerson, V. C. (1993). Separating couples from restraining patterns and the relationship discourses that support them. *Journal of Marital and Family Therapy, 19*(4), 403–413.

Zimmerman, T. S., Prest, L. A., & Wetzel, B. E. (1997). Solution-focused couples therapy groups: An empirical study. *Journal of Family Therapy, 19*(2), 125–144.

Systemic Approaches

CHAPTER 10

Brief Strategic Couple Therapy

Varda Shoham
Michael J. Rohrbaugh
Audrey A. Cleary

In this chapter we describe applications and extensions to couples of the "brief problem-focused therapy" developed over 25 years ago by Richard Fisch, John Weakland, Paul Watzlawick, and their colleagues at the Mental Research Institute (MRI) in Palo Alto (Weakland, Fisch, Watzlawick, & Bodin, 1974; Weakland & Fisch, 1992; Watzlawick, Weakland, & Fisch, 1974; Fisch, Weakland, & Segal, 1982). This parsimonious therapy approach is based on identifying and interrupting *ironic processes* that occur when repeated attempts to solve a problem keep the problem going or make it worse. Although Fisch, Weakland, and associates did not themselves use the term "ironic process," it captures well their central assertion that problems persist as a function of people's well-intentioned attempts to solve them, and that focused interruption of these solution efforts is sufficient to resolve most problems.[1]

The hallmark of this approach, sometimes referred to as the Palo Alto or the MRI model, is conceptual and technical parsimony. The aim of therapy is simply to resolve the presenting complaint as quickly and efficiently as possible, so clients can get on with life: Goals such as promoting personal growth, working through underlying emotional issues, or teaching couples

better problem-solving and communication skills are not emphasized. Theory is minimal and non-normative, guiding therapists to focus narrowly on the presenting complaint and relevant solutions, with no attempt to specify what constitutes a normal or dysfunctional marriage. Because the "reality" of problems and change is constructed more than discovered, the therapist attends not only to what clients *do* but also to how they *view* the problem, themselves, and each other. Especially relevant is clients' "customership" for change and the possibility that therapy itself may play a role in maintaining (rather than resolving) problems. Finally, in contrast to most other treatments for couples, therapists working in this tradition often see the partners individually, even when the focus of intervention is a complaint about the marriage itself.

This model is sometimes called "strategic" because the therapist intervenes to interrupt ironic processes deliberately, on the basis of a case-specific plan that sometimes includes counterintuitive suggestions (e.g., to "go slow" or engage in behavior a couple wants to eliminate). Calling this approach "strategic therapy" alone, however, risks confusing it with a related but substantially different approach to treating couples and families developed by Jay Haley (who coined the term "strategic therapy"; 1980, 1987) and his associate Cloé Madanes (1981, 1991).[2] More importantly, the "strategic" label gives undue emphasis to intervention style and detracts attention from the more fundamental principle of ironic problem maintenance on which this brief therapy is based.

Our chapter deals primarily with applications of this brief problem-focused therapy to *couple* complaints, but this is a somewhat arbitrary delimitation. As a general model of problem resolution, this therapy approaches couple problems in essentially the same way it does other complaints. Furthermore, because practitioners of this therapy are inevitably concerned with social interaction, they often focus on marital interaction when working with "individual" problems—for example, depression (Watzlawick & Coyne, 1976; Coyne, 1986a), anxiety (Rohrbaugh & Shean, 1988), and addictions (Fisch, 1986; Rohrbaugh, Shoham, Spungen, & Steinglass, 1995; Rohrbaugh, Shoham, et al., 2001; Shoham, Rohrbaugh, Trost, & Muramoto, 2006)—and for tactical reasons they may avoid calling this "couple therapy" in dealings with the clients. This and the predilection of therapists to treat couple problems nonconjointly (by seeing individuals), make it difficult to distinguish between what is and is not "couple" therapy.

BACKGROUND

Couple therapy based on interrupting ironic processes is a pragmatic embodiment of an "interactional view" (Watzlawick & Weakland, 1978) that explains behavior—especially problem behavior—in terms of what happens between people rather than within them. The interactional view grew from attempts by members of Bateson's research group (which included Weakland, Haley, and MRI founder Don D. Jackson) to apply ideas from cybernetics and systems theory to the study of communication. After the Bateson project ended, Watzlawick, Beavin, and Jackson (1967) brought many of these ideas together in *Pragmatics of Human Communication*. Around the same time, Fisch, Weakland, Watzlawick, and others formed the Brief Therapy Center at MRI to study ways of doing therapy briefly. Their endeavors were also influenced by the "uncommon" therapeutic techniques of Arizona psychiatrist Milton Erickson, whom Haley and Weakland visited many times during the Bateson project (Haley, 1967). In retrospect, it is striking how discordant this early

work on brief therapy was with the psychodynamic *zeitgeist* of the late 1960s and early 1970s, when therapies were rarely designed with brevity in mind. Even today, as Gurman (2001) points out, most brief therapies represent abbreviated versions of longer therapies—and most family therapies are brief by default. In its commitment to parsimony, the Palo Alto group was probably the first to develop a family-oriented therapy that was brief by design.

Since 1966, the MRI's Brief Therapy Center has followed a consistent format in treating over 500 cases. Under Fisch's leadership, the staff meets weekly as a team to treat unselected cases, representing a broad range of clinical problems, for a maximum of 10 sessions. One member of the team serves as a primary therapist, while the others consult from behind a one-way mirror. After treatment (at roughly 3 and 12 months following termination), another team member conducts a telephone follow-up interview with the client(s) to evaluate change in the original presenting problem and to determine whether clients have developed additional problems or sought further treatment elsewhere. The center's pattern of practice has remained remarkably consistent, with the three core members (Fisch, Weakland, and Watzlawick) all participating regularly, until Weakland's death in 1995.[3]

From the work of the Palo Alto Brief Therapy Center emerged a model of therapy that focuses on observable interaction in the present, makes no assumptions about normality or pathology, and remains as close as possible to practice. The first formal statement of this model appeared in a 1974 *Family Process* paper by Weakland et al., "Brief Therapy: Focused Problem Resolution." At about the same time, Watzlawick et al. (1974) also published *Change: Principles of Problem Formation and Problem Resolution*, a more theoretical work that distinguished between first- and second-order change, and provided many illustrations of ironic processes. Eight years later, Fisch et al. (1982) offered *The Tactics of Change: Doing Therapy Briefly*, essentially a how-to-treatment manual that remains the most comprehensive and explicit statement to date of the Brief Therapy Center's clinical method. In 1992, Weakland and Fisch presented a concise description of the model in a book chapter, and most recently Fisch and Schlanger (1999) have provided another concise outline of the model, along with illustrative clinical material, in *Brief Therapy with Intimidating Cases: Changing the Unchangeable*. Although these sources do not deal with marital therapy per se, couple complaints figure prominently in the clinical principles and examples. Other applications to couples, especially when one of the partners is depressed, can be found in the work of former MRI affiliate James Coyne (1986a, 1986b, 1988). Coyne's work highlights the significance of the interview in strategic marital therapy, particularly how the therapist works to (re)frame the couple's definition of the problem in a way that sets the stage for later interventions.[4]

In addition to the ironic process model's historical connection to the "strategic family therapy" of Haley (1980, 1987) and Madanes (1981), we should mention its sometimes confusing connection to the "solution-focused therapy" (Berg & Miller, 1992; de Shazer, 1991; de Shazer et al., 1986). Inspired by the Palo Alto group, de Shazer et al. initially took Weakland et al.'s (1974) "focused problem resolution" as a starting point for a complementary form of brief therapy emphasizing "focused solution development." Subsequently, however, solution-focused therapy has undergone progressive revision (de Shazer, 1991; Miller & de Shazer, 2000) and now has a substantially different emphasis than the parent model (for a detailed comparison, see Shoham, Rohrbaugh, & Patterson, 1995). One of the main points of disconnection is that de Shazer et al. (1986) tried to avoid characterizing their therapy as "strategic," preferring instead to describe it as collaborative, co-constructivist, and (by implication) not so manipulative. This (re)characterization aligns solution-focused therapy with the narrative, postmodern tradition that rejects the model of therapist-as-expert-strategist in favor of therapist-as-collaborative-partner (Nichols & Schwartz, 2000). We suspect that this distinction may be more semantic than substantive. In any case, calling one's therapy "strategic" is today probably not a very strategic thing to do.

Although research at the MRI has been mainly qualitative, it is noteworthy that the original description of brief, problem-focused therapy by Weakland et al. (1974) included tentative 1-year outcome percentages for the first 97 cases seen at the Brief Therapy Center. In 1992, in collaboration with the Brief Therapy Center's staff member Karin Schlanger, we updated the archival tabulation of outcomes for cases seen through 1991 and attempted to identify correlates of success (Rohrbaugh, Shoham, & Schlanger, 1992). For 285 cases with interpretable follow-up data, problem resolution rates of 44, 24, and 32% for success,

partial success, and failure, respectively, were very similar to the figures reported by Weakland et al. (1974) more than 15 years earlier. Thus, at least two-thirds of the cases reportedly improved, and the average length of therapy was six sessions. To investigate correlates of outcome more closely, we identified subgroups of "clear success" cases (n = 39) and "clear failure" cases (n = 33) for which 1-year follow-up data were complete and unambiguous. Then, after coding clinical, demographic, and treatment variables from each case folder, we compared the success and failure groups and found surprisingly few predictors of outcome. Interestingly, however, it appears that about 40% of the cases seen over the years at the Brief Therapy Center have involved some form of marital or couple complaint, and we touch on some findings from the archive study in sections to follow.

A NON-NORMATIVE VIEW OF COUPLE FUNCTIONING

Based primarily on interrupting ironic processes, this approach to couple therapy makes no assumptions about healthy or pathological functioning. In this sense, the theory is non-normative and complaint-based: In fact, if no one registers a complaint, there is no problem (Fisch & Schlanger, 1999). At the relationship level, this means that patterns such as quiet detachment or volatile engagement might be dysfunctional for some couples but adaptive for others. What matters is the extent to which interaction patterns based on attempted solutions keep a complaint going or make it worse—and the topography of relevant problem–solution loops can vary widely from couple to couple.

At the heart of brief problem-focused therapy are two interlocking assumptions about problems and change:

> Regardless of their origins and etiology—if, indeed, these can ever be reliably determined—the problems people bring to psychotherapists persist only if they are maintained by ongoing current behavior of the client and others with whom he interacts. Correspondingly, if such problem-maintaining behavior is appropriately changed or eliminated, the problem will be resolved or vanish, regardless of its nature, or origin, or duration. (Weakland et al., 1974, p. 144)

These assumptions imply that how a problem persists is much more relevant to therapy than how the problem originated, and that problem persistence depends mainly on social interaction, with the behavior of one person both stimulated and shaped by the response of others (Weakland & Fisch, 1992). Moreover—and this is the central observation of the Palo Alto group—the continuation of a problem revolves precisely around what people currently and persistently do (or do not do) to control, prevent, or eliminate their complaint; that is, how people go about trying to solve a problem usually plays a crucial role in perpetuating it.

A problem, then, consists of a vicious cycle involving a positive feedback loop between some behavior someone considers undesirable (the complaint) and some other behavior(s) intended to modify or eliminate it (the attempted solution). Given that problems persist because of people's current attempts to solve them, therapy need consist only of identifying and deliberately interdicting these well-intentioned yet ironic "solutions," thereby breaking the vicious cycles (positive feedback loops) that maintain the impasse. If these solutions can be interrupted, even in a small way, then virtuous cycles may develop, in which less of the solution leads to less of the problem, leading to less of the solution, and so on (Fisch et al., 1982).

Such an ironic feedback loop can be seen in the following passage from *Pragmatics of Human Communication* (Watzlawick et al., 1967), which highlights the familiar demand–withdraw cycle common to many marital complaints:

> Suppose a couple have a marital problem to which he contributes passive withdrawal while her 50% is nagging and criticism. In explaining their frustrations, the husband will state that withdrawal is his only *defense against* her nagging, while she will label this explanation gross and willful distortion of what "really" happens in their marriage: namely, that she is critical of him *because* of his passivity. Stripped of all ephemeral and fortuitous elements, their fights consist in a monotonous exchange of the messages, "I will withdraw because you nag" and "I nag because you withdraw." (p. 56)

Watzlawick et al. (1974) elaborate a similar pattern in *Change*:

> In marriage therapy, one can frequently see both spouses engaging in behaviors which they individually consider the most appropriate reaction to something wrong that the other is doing. That is, in the eyes of each of them the particular corrective behavior of the other is seen as that behavior which needs correction. For instance, a wife may have the impression that her husband is not open enough for her to know where she stands with him, what is going on

in his head, what he is doing when he is away from home, etc. Quite naturally, she will therefore attempt to get the needed information by asking him questions, watching his behavior, and checking on him in a variety of other ways. If he considers her behavior as too intrusive, he is likely to withhold from her information which in and by itself would be quite harmless and irrelevant to disclose—"just to teach her that she need not know everything." Far from making her back down, this attempted solution not only does not bring about the desired change in her behavior but provides further fuel for her worries and her distrust— "if he does not even talk to me about these little things, there *must* be something the matter." The less information he gives her, the more persistently she will seek it, and the more she seeks it, the less he will give her. By the time they see a psychiatrist, it will be tempting to diagnose her behavior as pathological jealousy—provided that no attention is paid to their pattern of interaction and their attempted solutions, which *are* the problem. (pp. 35–36)

The "solutions" of demand and withdrawal in these examples make perfectly good sense to the participants, yet their interactional consequences serve only to confirm each partner's unsatisfactory "reality." How such a cycle began is likely to remain obscure, and what causes what is a matter of more or less arbitrary punctuation: From our perspective, the problem-maintaining system of interaction is its own explanation.

THE PRACTICE
OF BRIEF STRATEGIC COUPLE THERAPY
The Structure of Therapy

The basic template for brief therapy based on interrupting ironic processes can be summarized as follows: (1) Define the complaint in specific behavioral terms; (2) set minimum goals for change; (3) investigate solutions to the complaint; (4) formulate ironic problem–solution loops (how "more of the same" solution leads to more of the complaint, etc.); (5) specify what "less of the same" will look like in particular situations; (6) understand clients' preferred views of themselves, the problem, and each other; (7) use these views to frame suggestions for less-of-the-same solution behavior; and (8) nurture and solidify incipient change (Rohrbaugh & Shoham, 2001). Sessions are not necessarily scheduled on a weekly basis, but allocated in a manner intended to maximize the likelihood that change will be durable. Thus, when the treatment setting formally imposes a session limit (e.g., both the MRI's Brief Therapy Center and our own clinic limit treatment to 10 sessions), the meetings may be spread over months or even a year. A typical pattern is for the first few sessions to be at regular (weekly) intervals and for later meetings to be less frequent once change begins to take hold. Therapy ends when the treatment goals have been attained and change seems reasonably stable. Termination usually occurs without celebration or fanfare, and sometimes clients retain "sessions in the bank," if they are apprehensive about discontinuing contact.

Although two (co)therapists are rarely in the room together, practitioners of this approach usually prefer to work as a team. At the Brief Therapy Center and in most of our own work, a primary therapist sees the clients, with other team members observing (and participating) from behind a one-way mirror. Team members typically phone in suggestions to the therapist during the session, and the therapist sometimes leaves the room to consult briefly with the team. A typical time for such a meeting is late in the session, when the team can help the therapist plan the particulars of a homework assignment or framing intervention.

The team format also opens the possibility of clients' having contact with more than one therapist. As if to downplay the sanctity of "therapeutic relationship factors," the Palo Alto group historically has had no reservations about one therapist substituting for another who could not be present—and in fact, about 25% of cases in the first 3 years of the brief therapy project did see more than one therapist, but this proportion fell to 11% in the early 1970s, and to under 5% by the late 1980s (Rohrbaugh et al., 1992). In our own manual-guided treatments for couples who face drinking or smoking problems in one or both members, we routinely hold brief individual meetings with the partners in the second session and, whenever possible, use different members of the team to do this (Rohrbaugh et al., 1995, 2001).

As a treatment for couples, this approach differs from most others in that the therapist is willing, and sometimes prefers, to see one or both partners individually. The choice of individual versus conjoint sessions is based on three main considerations: customership, maneuverability, and adequate assessment. First, a brief strategic therapist would rather address a marital complaint by seeing a motivated partner alone than by struggling to engage a partner who is not a "customer" for change. In theory, this practice should not decrease the possibility of successful outcome, since the interactional systems view assumes that prob-

lem resolution can follow from a change by any participant in the relevant interactional system (Hoebel, 1976; Weakland & Fisch, 1992). A second reason to see partners separately, even when both are customers, is to preserve maneuverability. If the partners have sharply different views of their situation, for example, separate sessions give the therapist more flexibility in accepting each viewpoint and framing suggestions one way for her and another way for him. The split format also helps the therapist avoid being drawn into the position of referee or possible ally. The goal, however, remains to promote change in what happens between the partners.

A third reason for interviewing spouses separately is to facilitate assessment. Some couples relentlessly enact their arguments and conflicts in the therapy room, whereas others lapse into silence and withdrawal. As Coyne (1988) points out, seeing such patterns at least once is useful, but their repetition can easily handicap the therapist's efforts to track important problem–solution loops that occur outside the therapy session. Strategic therapists often make a point of seeing the partners alone at least once to inquire about their commitment to the relationship; if either is pessimistic, the therapist may request a moratorium on separation, long enough to give treatment a chance to make a difference. In no case, however, does the therapist express more commitment to saving the marriage or to the likely success of therapy than does the client being interviewed (Coyne, 1988). Individual sessions are also used to assess the possibility of spousal abuse or intimidation (Rohrbaugh et al., 1995). This assessment is especially important in cases where there is domestic violence but the abused partner is too intimidated to introduce this violence as a complaint in the conjoint interview.

In our study of the Brief Therapy Center's archives (Rohrbaugh et al., 1992), cases with marital or couple complaints were more likely to be successful when at least two people (the two partners) participated in treatment. This finding would not seem to fit well with the MRI view that marital complaints can be treated effectively by intervening through one partner. On the other hand, we did not evaluate the potentially confounding role of customership in these cases, or the possibility that the absent partners were as uncommitted to the relationship as they apparently were to therapy. In any case, the Center's own data do little to undermine Gurman, Kniskern, and Pinsof's (1986) empirical generalization: "When both spouses are involved in therapy conjointly for marital prob-lems, there is a greater chance of positive outcome than when only one spouse is treated" (p. 572).

A related historical footnote from the ar-chives project bears on the question of brevity it-self: In the mid-1970s, the Brief Therapy Center undertook an experiment to test the feasibility of shortening treatment to 5 sessions and, for nearly a year, randomly assigned new cases to either a 5-ses-sion limit (n = 13) or the usual 10-session limit (n = 14). It turned out that cases treated with the 5-session limit fared substantially *worse* than the "control" cases ($p < .01$)—and when this pattern became clear clinically, the group abandoned this experiment. Thus, although the MRI group found that most problems could be resolved in fewer than 10 sessions, they surmised that attempting to enforce further brevity could itself become a problem-maintaining solution.

Role of the Therapist

The essential role of the therapist, as explained earlier, is to persuade at least one participant in the couple (or most relevant interactional system) to do "less of the same" solution that keeps the com-plaint going. This essential role does not require educating clients, helping them resolve emotional issues, or even working with both members of a couple. It does, however, require that the therapist "work with the customer" and "preserve maneu-verability." The "customership principle" means simply that the therapist works with the person or persons most concerned about the problem (the "sweater" or "sweaters"). Thus a therapist treat-ing a marital complaint would not require or even encourage the participation of a reluctant spouse, especially if this is what the principal complain-ant has been doing. To "preserve maneuverability" means that the therapist aims to maximize pos-sibilities for therapeutic influence, which in this model is his or her main responsibility. In *The Tactics of Change*, Fisch et al. (1982) make plain the importance of control: "The therapist, to put it bluntly, needs to maintain his own options while limiting those of the patients," (p. 23) outlining tactics for gaining (and regaining) control, even in initial phone contacts, since "treatment is likely to go awry if the therapist is not in control of it" (p. xii). Preserving maneuverability also means that the therapist avoids taking a firm position or making a premature commitment to what clients should do, so that later, if they *do not* do what is

requested, alternate strategies for achieving "less of the same" will still be accessible.

Despite this apparent preoccupation with controlling the course of therapy, this type of stra-tegic therapist rarely exerts control directly in the sense of offering authoritative prescriptions or as-suming the role of an expert. Much more charac-teristic of this approach is what Fisch et al. (1982) call "taking a one-down position." Early in ther-apy, for example, a Columbo-like stance of em-pathic curiosity might be used to track behavioral sequences around the complaint (e.g., "I'm a little slow on the uptake here, so could you help me un-derstand again what it is you *do* when John raises his voice that way?"); later, when intervening to promote "less of the same," a therapist might soft-sell a specific suggestion by saying something like, "I don't know if doing this when he walks through the door will make much difference, but if you could try it once or twice this week, at least we'll have an idea what we're up against." One purpose of these tactics is to promote client cooperation and avoid the common countertherapeutic effects of overly direct or prescriptive interventions.[5]

Empathic restraint, exemplified by the "go slow" messages discussed later in the "Techniques" section, is a related stance characteristic of this approach. Here, too, the therapist aims to avoid apprehension and resistance by conveying that only the client(s) can decide whether and when to change. When the therapist and team are ready to make a specific "less of the same" suggestion, they do so cautiously, without assuming customer-ship (i.e., that clients are ready to change). Once change begins, continued gentle restraint helps the therapist respect the clients' pace and avoid pushing for more change than they can handle. A typical response to clear progress would be for the therapist to compliment clients on what they have done, yet caution them against premature cel-ebration and suggest again that a prudent course might be to "go slow." Similarly, when clients fail to follow a suggestion, a common response is for the therapist to take the blame on him- or her-self (e.g., "I think I suggested that prematurely") and seek alternative routes to the same strategic objective, often within the framework of intensi-fied overt restraint. Nevertheless, even this gen-eral stance of restraint is applied judiciously and guided by ongoing assessment of the clients' cus-tomership, position, and progress.

Although the writings of the Palo Alto group attach little importance to the therapeutic relationship, this does not mean that strategic therapists come across as cold, manipulative, or uncaring. On the contrary, most therapists we have known and seen working this way would likely receive high ratings on client rapport and "therapeutic alliance." A reason may be that practicing this approach requires very close attention to clients' unique language, metaphors, worldviews—and that communicating effectively within the framework of someone else's construct system (if only to frame an intervention) usually entails a good deal of empathy. In fact, if asked what clinical skills or attributes are most essential to successful therapy in this approach, we would put something akin to this conceptual (or constructivist) empathy high on the list. The stance required is not for everyone because, as suggested by Watzlawick (1978), a strategic therapist becomes "more a chameleon than a firm rock in a sea of trouble. And it is at this point that many therapists dig in behind the retort, 'Anything except that,' while for others the necessity of ever new adaptations to the world images of their clients is a fascinating task" (p. 141).

Assessment

The main goals of assessment are to (1) define a resolvable complaint; (2) identify solution patterns (problem–solution loops) that maintain the complaint; and (3) understand clients' unique language and preferred views of the problem, themselves, and each other. The first two goals provide a template for *where* to intervene, whereas the third goal is relevant to *how* to intervene.

The therapist's first task is to get a very specific, behavioral picture of the complaint and assess who sees it as a problem, and why it is a problem now. Because the problem is not assumed to be the tip of a psychological or relational iceberg, the aim of assessment is simply to gain a clear understanding of who is doing what. A useful guideline for this phase is for the therapist to have enough details to answer the question, "If we had a video of this, what would I see?" Later the therapist also tries to get a clear behavioral picture of what the clients will accept as a minimum change goal. For example, "What would he (or she, or the two of you) be doing differently that will let you know this problem is taking a turn for the better?"

The next step requires an equally specific inquiry into the behaviors most closely related to the problem, namely, what the clients (and any other people concerned about it) are doing to handle, prevent, or resolve the complaint, and what happens after these attempted solutions. From this step emerges a formulation of a problem–solution loop, and particularly of the specific solution behaviors that will be the focus of intervention. The therapist (or team) can then develop a picture of what "less of the same" will look like—that is, what behavior, by whom, in what situation, will suffice to reverse the problem-maintaining solution. Ideally this strategic objective constitutes a 180 degree reversal of what the clients have been doing. Although interventions typically involve prescribing some alternative behavior, the key element is stopping the performance of the attempted solution (Weakland & Fisch, 1992). Understanding problem-maintaining solution patterns also helps the therapist be clear about what positions and suggestions to avoid—what Weakland and colleagues called the "mine field." Thus, if a husband has been persistently exhorting a wife to eat or spend less, the therapist would not want to make any direct suggestions that the wife change in these ways, so as not perpetuate "more of the same" problem-maintaining solution. A more helpful "less of the same" stance might entail wondering with the wife about reasons why she *should not* change, at least in the present circumstances, and about how she will know whether, or when, these changes are actually worth making.

The most relevant problem-maintaining solutions are current ones (what one or both partners continue to do about the complaint *now*), but the therapist investigates solutions tried and discarded in the past as well, because these give hints about what has worked before—and may work again. In one of our alcohol treatment cases (Rohrbaugh et al., 1995), a wife, who in the past had taken a hard line with her husband about not drinking at the dinner table, later reversed this stance because she did not want to be controlling. As his drinking problem worsened, he further withdrew from the family, and she dealt with it less and less directly by busying herself in other activities or retreating to her study to meditate. Careful inquiry revealed that the former hard-line approach, though distasteful, had actually worked: When the wife had set limits, the husband had controlled his drinking. By relabeling her former, more assertive stance as caring and reassuring to the husband, the therapist was later able to help the wife reverse her stance in a way that broke the problem cycle.

Along these lines, we have found it useful to distinguish ironic solution patterns that involve action (commission) from those that involve inaction (omission). The solution of pressuring one's partner to change, as in the demand–withdraw cycle described earlier, exemplifies a commission pattern, whereas the indirect stance of the alcoholic's wife in the case just mentioned illustrates problem maintenance based on omission. Although commission patterns are more salient, ironic solutions of omission are surprisingly common, especially among couples coping with health problems, addictions, or both. One such pattern involves "protective buffering," in which one partner's attempts to avoid upsetting a physically ill spouse sometimes inadvertently lead to more distress (Coyne & Smith, 1991).

The distinction between these two types of ironic processes again underscores the principle that no given solution pattern can be uniformly functional or dysfunctional: What works for one couple may be precisely what keeps things going badly for another—and a therapist's strategy for promoting "less of the same" should respect this heterogeneity.

The final assessment goal—grasping clients' unique views, or what Fisch et al. (1982) call the "patient position"—is crucial to the later task of framing suggestions in ways clients will accept. Assessing these views depends mainly on paying careful attention to what people say. For example, how do they see themselves and want to be seen by others? What do they hold near and dear? At some point, the therapist will usually also ask for their best guess as to *why* a particular problem is happening—and why they handle it the way they do. We also find it helpful to understand how partners view themselves as a couple, and typically ask questions, such as "If people who know you well were describing you two as a couple, what would they say?" or "What words or phrases capture the strength of your relationship—its values, flavor and unique style?"

Finally, some of the most important client views concern customership for therapy and readiness for change. Although much can be determined from how clients initially present themselves, direct questions such as "Whose idea was it to come?" (His? Hers? Both equally?), "Why now?," and "Who is most optimistic that therapy will help?" should make this crucial aspect of client position clearer. It is also important to understand how (if at all) the clients sought help in the past, what they found helpful or unhelpful, how the helper(s) viewed their problems, and how the therapy ended.

Goal Setting

Goal setting in this approach serves several key functions. First, having a clear behavioral picture of what clients will accept as a sign of improvement helps to bring the complaint itself into focus. Without a clear complaint it is difficult to have a coherent formulation of problem maintenance (or, for that matter, a coherent therapy). Second, setting a *minimum* goal for outcome supports the therapist's tactical aim of introducing a small but strategic change in the problem–solution patterns, which can then initiate a ripple or domino effect leading to further positive developments. In this sense, the model emphasizes what some clinicians would call "intermediate" or "mediating" goals rather than ultimate outcomes. For some couples, a spin-off benefit of this strategy may be the implicit message that even difficult problems can show some improvement in a relatively short period of time.

Before setting specific goals, it is usually necessary to inquire in detail about the clients' complaint(s) and, if there are multiple complaints, establish which are most pressing. As the complaint focus becomes clear, the therapist at some point asks questions such as the following:

"How will you know the situation is improving?"
"What kinds of change will you settle for? What will need to happen (or not happen) to let you know that, even if you're not out of the woods entirely, you're at least on the right path?"
"What will each of you settle for?"

As clients grapple with these questions, the therapist presses for specific signs of improvement (e.g., having a family meal together without someone getting upset and leaving the table; a spouse showing affection without it seeming like an obligation). It is easy in such a discussion to confuse means with ends, and the therapist aims to keep clients focused on the latter (what they hope to achieve) rather than how to pursue them. Important assessment information does come from queries about what partners think they should do to make things better, but this is much more relevant to formulating problem–solution loops than to goal setting.

Techniques

The Palo Alto group distinguishes "specific" interventions, designed to interdict ironic, case-specific problem–solution loops, from "general" interventions that tend to be applicable across most cases (Fisch et al., 1982). Most of this section is devoted to illustrating specific interventions for common couple complaints. We focus especially on interventions designed to interrupt demand–withdraw interaction, a common couple pattern associated with not only marital distress but also many health complaints and addictions. First, however, we comment briefly on more general aspects of this therapy.

Because interrupting an ironic problem–solution loop usually requires persuading clients either to do less or the opposite of what they have been committed to doing, it is crucial to frame suggestions in terms compatible with clients' own language or worldview—especially with how they prefer to see themselves. Indeed, grasping and using clients' views—what Fisch et al. (1982) call "patient position"—is almost as fundamental to this form of brief therapy as the behavioral prescriptions that interdict problem-maintaining solutions. Some partners, for example, will be attracted to the idea of making a loving sacrifice, but others may want to teach their mates a lesson. Strategic therapists are careful to speak the clients' language, use their metaphors, and avoid argumentation. These therapists not only elicit but also shape and structure clients' beliefs to set the stage for later interventions. For example, a therapist might accept a wife's view that her husband is uncommunicative and unemotional, then extend this view to suggest that his defensiveness indicates vulnerability. The extension paves the way for suggesting a different way of dealing with a husband who is vulnerable, rather than simply withholding (Coyne, 1988). A less direct way to break an ironic pattern is to redefine what one partner is doing in a way that stops short of prescribing change, yet makes it difficult for him or her to continue (e.g., "I've noticed that your reminding him and telling him what you think seems to give him an excuse to keep doing what he's doing without feeling guilty. He can justify it to himself simply by blaming you").

In addition to interventions that target specific problem–solution loops, the model uses several "general interventions" that are applicable to a broad range of problems and to promoting change in all stages of therapy. General interventions include telling clients to go slow, cautioning them about dangers of improvement, making a U-turn, and giving instructions about how to make the problem worse (Fisch et al., 1982).

Most of these tactics are variations of therapeutic restraint, as described in the previous section. The most common is the injunction to "go slow," given with a credible rationale, such as "change occurring slowly and step by step makes for a more solid change than change which occurs too suddenly" (Fisch et al., 1982, p. 159). This tactic is used to prepare clients for change, to convey acceptance of reluctance to change, and to solidify change once it begins to occur. Fisch et al. suggest two reasons why "go slow" messages work: They make clients more likely to cooperate with therapeutic suggestions, and they relax the sense of urgency that often fuels clients' problem-maintaining solution efforts.

Coyne (1988) described several other general interventions that he uses in the first or second session with couples. One intervention involves asking the couple to collaborate in performing the problem pattern (e.g., an argument) deliberately, for the ostensible purpose of helping the therapist better understand how they get involved in such a no-win encounter, and specifically, how each partner is able to get the other to be less reasonable than he or she would be normally. This task is more than diagnostic, however, because it undercuts negative spontaneity, creates an incentive for each partner to resist provocation, and sometimes introduces a shift in the usual problem–solution pattern.

In terms of Bateson's (1958) distinction between complementary and symmetrical interaction patterns[6] (cf. Watzlawick et al., 1967), some of the most common foci for specific interdiction of ironic problem–solution loops involve complementary patterns such as the familiar demand–withdraw sequence described earlier. For example, one partner may press for change in some way, while the other withdraws or refuses to respond; one partner may attempt to initiate discussion of some problem, while the other avoids discussion; one partner may criticize what the other does, while the other defends his or her actions; or one may accuse the other of thinking or doing something that the other denies (Christensen & Heavey, 1993). Each of these variations—demand–refuse, discuss–avoid, criticize–defend, accuse–deny—fits the problem–solution loop formula, because more demand leads to more withdrawal, which leads to more demand, and so on. Although the brief strategic model avoids (normative) a priori assumptions about adaptive or maladaptive family relations, the clinical relevance of demand–withdraw interaction appears well established by research indicating that this pattern is substantially more prevalent in divorcing couples and clinic couples than in nondistressed couples (Christensen & Schenk, 1991), and that couples embroiled in more intense demand–withdraw interaction patterns are less ready for change (Shoham, Rohrbaugh, Stickle, & Jacob, 1998). Interestingly, many authors have described the demand–withdraw pattern and speculated about its underlying dynamics (e.g., Napier, 1978; Wile, 1981), but few have been as concerned as the MRI group with practical ways to change it.

To the extent that the partner on the demand side of the sequence is the main customer for change, intervention focuses on encouraging that person to do less of the same. In the demand–refuse cycle, one spouse may press for change by exhorting, reasoning, arguing, lecturing, and so on—a solution pattern that Fisch et al. (1982, pp. 139–152) call "seeking accord through opposition." If the wife is the main complainant,[7] achieving less of the same usually depends on helping her suspend overt attempts to influence the husband—for example, by declaring helplessness or in some other specific way taking a one-down position, or by performing an observational–diagnostic task to find out "what he'll do on his own" or "what we're really up against." How the therapist frames specific suggestions depends on what rationale the customer will buy. An extremely religious wife, for example, might be amenable to the suggestion that she silently pray for her husband instead of exhorting him. Successful solution interdiction in several cases seen at the Brief Therapy Center (Watzlawick & Coyne, 1976; Fisch et al., 1982) followed from developing the frame that the behavior one partner saw as stubbornness was actually motivated by the other's pride. Because proud people need to discover and do things on their own, without feeling pressed or that they are giving in, it makes sense to encourage such a person's partner by discouraging (restraining) him or her. A demand-side partner who follows suggestions for doing this will effectively reverse his or her former solution to the stubborn behavior.

For some couples, the demand–withdraw cycle involves one partner's attempt to initiate discussion (to get the other to open up, be more expressive, etc.) while the other avoids it. One of us (Varda Shoham) had the experience of being the primary therapist for one such couple during her training at MRI. The wife, herself a therapist and the main complainant, would repeatedly encourage her inexpressive husband to get his feelings out, especially when he came home from work "looking miserable." When the husband responded to this encouragement with distraught silence, the wife would urge him to talk about his feelings toward her and the marriage (thinking that this topic would bring out positive associations on his part and combat his apparent "misery"). In a typical sequence, the husband would then begin to get angry and tell the wife to back off. She, however, encouraged by his expressiveness, would continue to push for meaningful discussion, in response to which—on more than one occasion—the husband stormed out of the house and disappeared overnight. The intervention that eventually broke the cycle in this case came from Fisch, who entered the therapy room with a suggestion: In the next week, at least once, the husband was to come home, sit at the kitchen table, and pretend to look miserable. The wife's task, when she saw this look, was to go to the kitchen, prepare chicken soup, and serve it to him *silently*, with a worried look on her face. The couple came to the next session looking anything but miserable. They reported that their attempt to carry out the assignment had failed because she—and then he—could not keep a straight face, yet they were delighted that the humor so characteristic of the early days of their relationship had "resurfaced." Whereas the intervention served to interdict the wife's attempted solution of pursuing discussion, it also interrupted the heaviness and deadly seriousness in the couple's relationship.[8]

When the demand–withdraw pattern involves criticism and defense, both partners are more likely to be customers for change; in these cases, change can be introduced through either or both partners. One strategy, noted earlier, is to develop a rationale for the criticizing partner to observe the behavior he or she is criticizing without commenting on it. Another is to get the defending partner to do something other than to defend—for example, by simply agreeing with the criticism or helping the criticizer "lighten up" by not taking the criticism seriously ("I guess you're probably right. Therapy is helping me see I'm not much fun and probably too old to change," or "You're right. I don't know if I inherited this problem from my parents or our kids"). In *Change*, Watzlawick et al. (1974) also describe a more indirect interdiction of a wife's attempts to avoid marital fights by defending herself. As homework, the therapist asked the combative husband to pick a fight deliberately with someone outside the marriage. In the next session, the husband recounted in detail how his attempts to do this had failed, because he had not been able to get the other person to lose his temper. In the authors' view, hearing this "made the wife more aware of her contribution to the problem than any insight-oriented explanation or intervention could have done" (p. 120).

Another approach to interdicting accusation–denial cycles is an intervention the MRI group calls "jamming" (Fisch et al., 1982). When one partner accuses the other of something that both agree is wrong (e.g., dishonesty, infidelity, insensitivity), and the other partner's denial seems only to confirm the accuser's suspicions, leading to more accusations and more denials, the jamming intervention aims to promote less of the same by both parties. After disavowing any ability to determine who is right or wrong in the situation, the therapist proposes to help the couple improve their communication (which obviously has broken down), particularly the accuser's perceptiveness about the problem. Achieving this, the therapist continues (in a conjoint session), will require that the defender deliberately randomize the behavior of which he or she is accused (e.g., sometimes acting "as if" she is attracted to other people and sometimes not), while the accuser tests his or her perceptiveness about what the defender is "really" doing. Both partners should keep a record of what they did or observed, they are told in a conjoint session, but they must not discuss the experiment or compare notes until the next session. The effect of such a prescription is to free the defender from (consistently) defending and the accuser from accusing; thus, the circuit is "jammed," because verbal exchanges (accusations and denial) now have less information value.

Sometimes a problem cycle is characterized by indirect demands related to the paradoxical form of communication Fisch et al. (1982) call "seeking compliance through voluntarism." For instance, a wife may complain that her husband not only ignores her needs but that he also should know what to do without her having to tell him, as he would otherwise be doing it only because she asked him and not because he really wanted to. Or a husband may be reluctant to ask his wife to do something because he thinks she may not really want to do it. The brief therapy strategy recommended in these situations is to get the person who is asking for something to do so directly, even if arbitrarily. If clients want to appear benevolent, the therapist can use this position by defining their indirection as unwittingly destructive; for example, "a husband's reticence to ask favors of his wife

can be redefined as an 'unwitting deprivation of the one thing she needs most from you, a sense of your willingness to take leadership'" (Fisch et al., 1982, p. 155). Intervening through the non-requesting partner might also be possible, if that person can be persuaded to take the edge off the paradoxical "Be spontaneous" demand by saying something like, "I'm willing to do it and I will, but let's face it, I don't enjoy cleaning up."

In other complaint-maintaining complementary exchanges, one partner may be domineering or explosive and the other placating or submissive. Here, less of the same usually requires getting the submissive, placating partner to take some assertive action. This was the approach taken in a controversial case reported by Bobele (1987), who describes the interactional analysis and successful interdiction of a cycle of violence involving a woman and her boyfriend. (Woody and Woody [1988] criticized Bobele's approach on legal and ethical grounds, but see the rejoinders by Bobele [1988] and Weakland [1988].)

Symmetrical patterns of problem-maintaining behavior are less common but often offer more possibilities for intervention because customership, too, is balanced. For combative couples embroiled in symmetrically escalating arguments, the strategy could be to get at least one partner to take a one-down position, or to prescribe the argument under conditions likely to undermine it (Coyne, 1988). Another symmetrical solution pattern stems from miscarriage of the (usually sensible) belief that problems are best solved by talking them through. Yet some couples—including some whose members are very psychologically minded—manage to perpetuate relationship difficulties simply by trying to talk about them. In a case treated at MRI, for example, a couple's problem-solving "talks" about issues in their relationship usually escalated into full-blown arguments. Therapy led them to a different, more workable solution: When either partner felt the need to talk about their relationship, they would first go bowling (Fisch, April, 1992, personal communication).

Interestingly, despite their emphasis on interaction, the MRI group acknowledges a "self-referential" aspect of complaints, such as anxiety states, insomnia, obsessional thinking, sexual dysfunction, and other problems with "being spontaneous." These complaints "can arise and be maintained without help from anyone else. This does not mean that others do not aid in maintaining such problems; often they do. We simply mean that these kinds of problems do not need such "help" in order to occur and persist" (Fisch et al., 1982, pp. 136–137).

Treatment of such problems in a couple context may involve simultaneous interdiction of both interactional and self-referential problem–solution loops. For example, with a woman who experienced difficulty reaching orgasm, the Brief Therapy Center's team targeted two problem–solution loops: one self-referential (the harder she tried, the more she failed) and the other interactional (the more the husband inquired about how aroused she was and whether she had had an orgasm, the harder she tried to perform). One strand of the intervention was a prescription that, for the wife to become more aware of her feelings during intercourse, she should "notice her bodily sensations, *regardless of how much or how little* pleasure she may experience" (Fisch et al., 1982, p. 158, emphasis in original). The second (interactional) strand was a version of jamming: In the wife's presence, the therapist asked the husband not to interfere with this process by checking her arousal—but if he did, the wife was simply to say, "I didn't feel a thing." Other strategies aimed at combined interdiction of interactional and self-referential solution patterns have been applied in the treatment of "individual" complaints, such as depression (Coyne, 1986a, 1988) and anxiety (Rohrbaugh & Shean, 1988).

Interventions for marital complaints usually focus on one or both members of the couple, yet there are circumstances in which other people—relatives, friends, or even another helper—figure prominently in this approach to couple therapy, especially when the third party is a key customer for change. For example, a mother, understandably concerned about her daughter's marital difficulties, may counsel or console the daughter in a way that unwittingly amplifies the problem or makes the young husband and wife less likely to deal with their differences directly. In this case, brief therapy might focus first on helping the mother—an important complainant—reverse her own solution efforts, and take up later (if at all) the interaction between the young spouses, which is likely to change when the mother becomes less involved. Brief therapists have also found ways to involve third parties who may *not* be customers for change, particularly for problems related to marital infidelity (Teismann, 1979; Green & Bobele, 1988).

Finally, for a small subset of marital complaints, the goal of brief therapy is to help couples reevaluate their problem as "no problem," or as a problem they can live with; strategies for achieving this goal typically involve some sort of reframing.

Indeed, marriage is fertile ground for what Watzlawick et al. (1974) call the "utopia syndrome":

> Quite obviously, few—if any—marriages live up to the ideals contained in some of the classic marriage manuals or popular mythology. Those who accept these ideas about what a marital relationship should "really" be are likely to see their marriage as problematic and to start working toward its solution until divorce do them part. Their concrete problem is not their marriage, but their attempts at finding the solution to a problem which in the first place is not a problem, and which, even if it were one, could not be solved on the level on which they attempt to change it. (p. 57)

Published case reports notwithstanding, the outcome of brief therapy rarely turns on a single intervention. Much depends on how the therapist nurtures incipient change and manages termination. When a small change occurs, the therapist acknowledges and emphasizes the clients' part in making it happen but avoids encouraging further change directly. The most common stance in responding to change consists of gentle restraint (e.g., "Go slow") and continuation of the interdiction strategy that produced it. Special tactics may be used with clients who are overly optimistic or overly anxious (e.g., predicting or prescribing a relapse), or who minimize change or relapse (e.g., exploring "dangers of improvement"). Termination occurs without celebration or fanfare. If change is solid, the therapist acknowledges progress, inquires about what the clients are doing differently, suggests that they anticipate other problems, and implies they will be able to cope with whatever problems do arise. Otherwise various restraining methods may be used. If clients ask to work on other problems, the therapist suggests taking time out to adapt to change and offers to reassess the other problems later (Fisch et al., 1982; Rosenthal & Bergman, 1986).

Before concluding the section on technique, we should add that this approach has been criticized as "manipulative," because the therapist does not usually make explicit to clients the rationale for particular interventions (Wendorf & Wendorf, 1985) and may say things he or she does not truly believe to achieve an effective framing (Solovey & Duncan, 1992). Proponents of strategic therapy counter that responsible therapy is inherently manipulative (Fisch, 1990), that therapeutic candor can be disrespectful (Haley, 1987), and that good therapy shows profound respect for clients' subjective "truths" (Cade & O'Hanlon, 1993).

CURATIVE FACTORS/MECHANISMS OF CHANGE

The central (and perhaps only) curative factor in this approach is interruption of ironic processes. As we have emphasized, this interruption depends (1) on accurate identification of the particular solution efforts that maintain or exacerbate the problem; (2) on specifying what less of those same solution behaviors might look like; and (3) on designing an intervention that will persuade at least one of the people involved to do less or the opposite of what he or she has been doing. To demonstrate such a process empirically, it is not enough to document changes in the target complaint. One needs to show that changes in attempted-solution behavior precede and actually relate to changes in the complaint. Evidence of such sequential dependencies in couples is at this point limited to case reports, though we are optimistic that quantitative methods can illuminate these processes as well.

A closely related curative factor is avoidance of ironic *therapy* processes—as can occur, for example, when "working through" a couple complaint in supportive individual therapy makes it possible for partners to avoid resolving the problem directly, or when pushing a spouse to change recapitulates a problem-maintaining solution applied by the clients themselves. The latter pattern is illustrated by our recent study comparing two treatments for couples in which the husband abused alcohol (Shoham et al., 1998). The two treatments—cognitive-behavioral therapy (CBT) and family systems therapy (FST)—differed substantially in the level of demand they placed on the drinker for abstinence and change. Although drinking was a primary target for change in both approaches, whereas CBT took a firm stance about expected abstinence from alcohol, using adjunctive Breathalyzer tests to ensure compliance, FST employed less direct strategies to work with clients' resistance. Before treatment began, we obtained observational measures of how much each couple engaged in demand–withdraw interaction, focusing on the pattern of wife's demands and husband's withdrawal during a discussion of the husband's drinking. The retention and abstinence results were striking: When couples high in this particular demand–withdraw pattern received CBT, they attended fewer sessions and tended to have poorer drinking outcomes, whereas for FST, levels of this pattern made little difference. Thus, for high-demand couples, CBT may ironically have provided "more of the same" ineffective solution: The alcoholic husbands appeared to resist a demanding therapist in the same way they resisted their demanding wives.[9]

For better or worse, this brief therapy model attaches little importance to the curative factors, such as alliance, understanding, skills acquisition, and emotional catharsis, that are central to other therapies. The focus is entirely on interrupting ironic processes in the present, with no assumption that insight or understanding is necessary for such interruption to happen. History may be relevant to clients' views, which in turn are relevant to how a therapist encourages less-of-the-same solution behavior; however, "interpretations" (or frames) offered in this context are pragmatic tools for effecting change, rather than attempts to illuminate any psychological "reality."

A common criticism, of course, is that this approach to therapy oversimplifies—either by making unrealistic assumptions about how people change or by ignoring aspects of the clinical situation that may be crucial to appropriate intervention. Some critics find implausible the rolling-snowball idea that a few well-targeted interventions producing small changes in clients' cognitions or behavior can kick off a process that will lead to significant shifts in the problem pattern; others grant that brief interventions sometimes produce dramatic changes, but doubt that those changes last (Wylie, 1990). Not surprisingly, therapists of competing theoretical persuasions object to the fact that these brief therapies pointedly ignore personality and relationship dynamics that, from other perspectives, may be fundamental to the problems couples bring to therapists. For example, Gurman (quoted by Wylie, 1990) suggested that "doing no more than interrupting the sequence of behaviors in marital conflict may solve the problem, but not if one spouse begins fights in order to maintain distance because of a lifelong fear of intimacy" (p. 31). Defenders of this approach to therapy reply that such "iceberg" assumptions about what lies beneath a couple's complaint serve only to complicate the therapist's task and make meaningful change more difficult to achieve. Unfortunately, it is unlikely that research evidence will soon resolve these arguments one way or the other.

APPLICABILITY

In principle, this brief strategic therapy model is applicable to any couple that presents a clear complaint and at least one customer for change. In practice, however, this approach may be particularly relevant for couples and clients who seem *resistant* to change. Published case reports imply that strategic therapy is most indicated when other, more straightforward approaches are unlikely to work (see Fisch & Schlanger's [1999] *Brief Therapy with Intimidating Cases*). Even advocates of other treatment methods have recommended using this model's principles and techniques at points of impasse—either sequentially, when other methods fail (e.g., O'Hanlon & Weiner-Davis, 1989; Stanton, 1981), or as a therapeutic detour to take before resuming an original treatment plan (Spinks & Birchler, 1982). In addition, controlled studies of both individual problems (Shoham, Bootzin, Rohrbaugh, & Urry, 1996; Shoham-Salomon, Avner, & Neeman, 1989; Shoham-Salomon & Jancourt, 1985) and couple problems (Goldman & Greenberg, 1992) suggest that strategic interventions are more effective than straightforward affective or skill-oriented interventions when clients are more rather than less resistant to change.

Of particular note is Goldman and Greenberg's (1992) study of couple therapy that compared a systemic treatment to Greenberg's own emotion-focused couple therapy and a waiting-list control condition. The systemic treatment employed a team format, with a one-way mirror, and "focused almost exclusively on changing current interactions, [positively] reframing patterns of behavior, and prescribing symptoms" (p. 967). Both of the active treatments were superior to the control condition at termination, but at 4-month follow-up, the couples who had received the systemic therapy reported better marital quality and more change in their target complaint than those who had received emotion-focused therapy. This finding, coupled with their clinical observations, led the authors to conclude that the strategic approach may be well suited for change-resistant couples with rigidly entrenched interaction patterns. Goldman and Greenberg's conclusion fits well with the results of our alcohol treatment study, described earlier, in which couples embroiled in demand–withdraw interaction appeared to do better with a therapy focused on interrupting ironic processes than with CBT (Shoham et al., 1998).[10]

Although these studies are encouraging, we should note limitations to the applicability of this approach. This model is probably *least* applicable to couples whose concern is relationship enhancement, prevention of marital distress, or personal growth, because therapy requires a complaint and would rarely continue more than a few sessions without one. Sometimes a discussion of growth-oriented goals such as "improved communication" leads to specification of a workable complaint, but short of this, the therapist would *not* want to suggest or imply that clients could benefit from therapy. In fact, the ironic process idea sensitizes us to therapeutic excess and the possibility of therapy itself becoming a problem-maintaining solution. In this framework, intervention should be proportionate to the complaint—and when in doubt, less is best.

At the same time, because this approach is so complaint-focused, critics have pointed out that therapists may ignore problems, such as spousal abuse and substance abuse, if clients do not present them as overt complaints in the first session (Wylie, 1990). Although couple therapists working in this tradition explore complaint patterns in great detail, and some (like us) routinely meet with partners separately to allow an intimidated spouse to raise a complaint (Rohrbaugh et al., 1995), the focus of intervention remains almost exclusively on what clients say they want to change. The nonnormative, constructivist premise of brief therapy, which rejects the idea of objective standards for what is normal or abnormal, or good or bad behavior, may too easily excuse the therapist from attempting to "discover" conditions such as alcoholism or spousal abuse. According to Fisch (as cited by Wylie, 1990), Brief Therapy Center's therapists would inquire about suspected wife beating only if it were in some way alluded to in the interview. Thus, although brief therapists no doubt respect statutory obligations to report certain kinds of suspected abuse and warn potential victims of violence, they clearly distinguish between therapy and social control, and reserve the former for customers with explicit complaints.

Other ethical dilemmas in couple therapy concern dealing with the (often conflicting) agendas of two adults rather than one. In this particular approach to couple therapy, a further complication arises when a therapist intervenes through only one member of a couple, with the implicit or explicit goal of changing the behavior of not only the motivated client but also that of the nonparticipating spouse (Watzlawick & Coyne, 1976; Hoebel, 1976): What responsibility, if any, does the therapist have to obtain informed consent from other people likely to be affected by an intervention? Such questions have no easy answers.

Application:
A Family Consultation Approach

Most of our own work on interrupting ironic processes has focused on couples coping with health problems or addictions. For example, as mentioned earlier, ironic demand–withdraw interaction was a central focus in our treatment study of alcohol-involved couples (Rohrbaugh & Shoham, 2002; Shoham et al., 1998). Similar ironic couple patterns—some based on direct influence attempts and others on attempted protection—figure prominently in a "family consultation" (FAMCON) model of intervention for couples in which at least one partner continues to smoke cigarettes despite having heart or lung disease (Rohrbaugh et al., 2001; Shoham et al., 2006).

The following vignettes from our work with change-resistant smokers illustrate couple-level ironic patterns more specifically:

• A husband (H) smokes in the presence of his non-smoking wife (W), who comments how bad it smells and frequently waves her hand to fan away the smoke. H, who had two heart attacks, shows no inclination to be influenced by this and says, "The more she pushes me the more I'll smoke!" Although W tries not to nag, she finds it difficult not to urge H to "give quitting a try." (She did this when he had bronchitis, and he promptly resumed smoking.) Previously H recovered from alcoholism, but only after W stopped saying, "If you loved me enough, you'd quit"; when she said instead, "I don't care what you do," he enrolled in a treatment program.

• H, who values greatly his 30-year "conflict-free" relationship with W, avoids expressing directly his wish for W to quit smoking. Although smoke aggravates H's asthma, he fears that showing disapproval would upset W and create stress in their relationship. W *confides* that she sometimes finds H's indirect (nonverbal) messages disturbing, though she too avoids expressing this directly—and when he does this she feels more like smoking. (Rohrbaugh et al., 2001, p. 20)

A central aim of the FAMCON intervention is to identify and interrupt ironic processes such as these. As it turns out, most ironic patterns tend to involve either doing too much, as in the first example, or doing too little, as in the second. They may also bear on smoking either directly (e.g., nagging to quit) or indirectly (e.g., pushing exercise or a particular quit strategy). Accordingly, the FAMCON therapist–consultant attends closely to ironic interpersonal cycles fueled by well-intentioned

attempts to control or protect a smoker, as well as to the role smoking appears to play in the couple's relationship (e.g., promoting cohesion when both partners smoke, preserving distance when only one does). Thus, to interrupt an ironic pattern in which one partner persistently attempts (without success) to control the other partner's smoking directly, the consultant would look for ways to help the spouse back off—for example, by declaring helplessness, demonstrating acceptance, or simply observing the smoker's habits. On the other hand, when an ironic interpersonal pattern involves *avoiding* the issue of smoking, we encourage a more direct course of action (e.g., taking a stand). Compared to the alcohol-involved couples we saw earlier, our sample of health-compromised smokers tended to show ironic patterns centered more on avoidance and protection than on direct influence. Consequently, our interventions aimed more often to *increase* partner influence attempts than to decrease them.

Beyond such case-specific formulations, the FAMCON approach to smoking cessation takes great pains to avoid the kinds of ironic therapy processes that can occur when a counselor's demand for change intensifies client resistance, or when a therapist aligns with failed solutions attempted by others in the smoker's family. Not surprisingly, in the terms of psychological reactance theory (Brehm, 1966; Shoham, Trost, & Rohrbaugh, 2004), many of the smokers we see appear highly motivated to restore "threatened behavioral freedoms"—especially their freedom to smoke. For this reason, an important overarching guideline is to maximize the smoker's *choice* about various facets of the FAMCON process. We also believe that presenting FAMCON as "consultation," a term that connotes collaboration and choice, arouses less reactance than calling it "treatment" (Wynne, McDaniel, & Weber, 1987).

Ideally, FAMCON for change-resistant smokers proceeds through three sequential phases—the preparation phase, the quit phase, and the consolidation phase—that together encompass up to 10 sessions over 3–6 months. The preparation phase includes two assessment sessions, scheduled about a week apart, in which the consultant works to identify ironic couple interaction patterns that may play a role in the persistence of smoking. In the third (intervention) session, the consultant presents a carefully tailored "team opinion," in which he or she provides specific feedback based on information gathered during the first and second sessions. The opinion includes observations about how smoking fits the couple's relationship and why quitting may be difficult, as well as couple-specific reasons to be optimistic about success and issues for the couple to consider in developing a quit plan. The consultant couches the opinion in terms consistent with the clients' preferred views of themselves and their situation, and concludes the session with an invitation for the couple to consider setting a quit date. In addition to helping the partners cope cooperatively with the threat smoking poses to their health and relationship, a key consideration in the quit phase is to encourage quit strategies that interrupt or avoid ironic processes and neutralize any relationship difficulties that could arise in a smoke-free system. When smokers show signs of "cold feet," the consultant may join them with a "go slow" intervention; and when they do quit, the consultant conveys "cautious optimism" and refrains from premature celebration of change. Finally, during the consolidation phase, the consultant adjusts therapeutic suggestions according to the clients' responses to previous interventions.

In addition to basic information from clinical interviews, the preparation/assessment phase draws upon quantitative daily diary data that the two partners provide independently. Specifically, the clients call our voice mail (answering machine) every morning for at least 14 consecutive days to answer a series of questions about the preceding day. The questions concern specific problem and solution patterns relevant to the case, as well as mood and relationship quality (e.g., How many cigarettes did you smoke yesterday? How much did you try to discourage your partner from smoking? How close and connected did you feel?). Because the questions are answered quantitatively, most on a 0- to 10-point scale, it is possible to identify couple-specific trends over time, such as the extent to which what one person does (e.g., frequency of smoking) correlates from day to day with what the other partner does (e.g., intensity of influence attempts). In addition to using this data in research, we find that presenting selected daily diary results in the feedback/opinion session enhances the credibility of the consultant's observations and therapeutic recommendations. Most couples also do a shortened version of the daily call-ins again later, for at least a week before and after their planned quit date, and this provides a basis for regular contact during the critical transition to not smoking.

The smoking cessation outcomes for couples who went through the FAMCON treatment–development project compare very favorably to benchmarks in the literature (Shoham et al., 2006). For example, the 50% rate of stable abstinence achieved by our health-compromised smokers at a 6-month follow-up is approximately twice that found in a meta-analysis of other intensive interventions with mostly shorter follow-ups (Fiore et al., 2000). Moreover, in an area where relapse rates often exceeds 50% (Stevens & Hollis, 1989), it was encouraging to see that only three smokers who quit for at least 2 days relapsed during the next year. It is also encouraging that the FAMCON intervention appeared well-suited to female smokers and to smokers whose partner also smoked—two subgroups at increased risk for relapse (Homish & Leonard, 2005; Wetter et al., 1998). Still, in the absence of a randomized clinical trial, we cannot conclude with certainty that FAMCON is superior to other cessation treatments.

CASE ILLUSTRATION

The following case, seen in a university psychology clinic, illustrates essential elements of the MRI approach to couple problems: (1) specification of a complaint and minimum acceptable change goals; (2) formulation of an ironic problem–solution loop, including what *less* of the same solution would look like behaviorally; (3) focused interruption of the ironic loop in a specific situation; and (4) use of the client's own views and experiences to frame, or sell, the suggestion for less of the same. Because the therapist saw only the female member of the couple, this case also illustrates the Palo Alto group members' willingness to intervene in a relational system unilaterally, without conjoint sessions. [The man in the couple felt he had good reasons for not coming to the clinic, and we respected this; he did, however, give consent for therapy to address his *partner's* difficulties, including her concerns about the relationship, and he was ultimately pleased by the results.] The case may also be of interest because of what the therapist did *not* do in terms of exploring or dealing with bread-and-butter issues of other therapies.[11]

Maria, a 26-year-old graduate student in biology, came to the clinic for "personal counseling." When initially asked about the problem, Maria said, "I just don't feel good about myself, especially the way I am with men." She went on to talk at length about her contributions to the demise of two earlier relationships, including one in which she had been engaged, and worried that she might soon spoil a third, with Harold, whom she lived with and cared for very much. Maria saw herself following a pattern with these men, one she did not like much, because it was reminiscent of how her mother had been with her father: She simply could not succeed in pleasing or sustaining intimacy with a man she loved, no matter what or how hard she tried. At the same time she resented feeling like she *should* please a man and very much wanted to avoid the kind of traditional, subservient relationship her mother had with her Mexican American father. Despite feminist sympathies, Maria felt that "old tapes from childhood" about woman–man relationships had contributed to her difficulties with men. Later in the session, she contrasted her failures in love with successes in other parts of her life: Not only was she beginning to publish in her chosen academic specialty, she felt "less anxious" and "more grounded psychologically" than she had several years earlier, when she entered graduate school. Maria attributed this mainly to her practice of "mindfulness meditation," which she had taken up during her first year in graduate school, shortly after breaking off a brief engagement to Carlos (whom she felt was becoming emotionally abusive), and about 6 months before she became seriously involved with Harold. At the time of the first interview, Maria and Harold had been romantically involved for nearly a year and had lived together (in his house) for 5 months. They did not discuss long-term plans, and Maria's earlier hopes that marriage would be in the offing were beginning to dim.

After listening attentively to Maria's historical account of problems with men, the therapist asked how these difficulties were showing themselves *currently* in her relationship with Harold. To this the client said, "Well, I just seem to bring out the worst in him," then went on to explain how Harold, a 36-year old faculty member in another department, was a very kind, loving, and sensitive man who, unlike the younger, more *machista* Carlos, could appreciate and respect a competent woman. Nevertheless, Harold was sometimes sensitive to the point of insecurity: He had some "jealousy issues," which the couple attributed to "traumatic residue" from his ex-wife's affairs some years earlier. Try as she might, Maria had not been able to provide the reassurance Harold seemed to need. In fact, their attempts to discuss the jealousy issue

sometimes led to "really bad arguments, like the one last week before I called the Clinic"—hence, the fear about "bringing out the worst."

Seeking a more behavioral complaint description, the therapist at this point asked Maria to describe what typically happened when she and Harold tried to discuss the jealousy issue, perhaps using the previous week's incident as an example: "How does the issue come up? Who says or does what? What happens then? If we recorded your interaction on video, what would I see?" From questions along this line emerged the outline of a problem–solution loop: When Harold expresses concern about whether Maria finds him sexually attractive, Maria typically explains (patiently at first) that yes, she does find him attractive, and in fact has never loved a man the way she loves him. Apparently unconvinced, Harold then asks further questions, either about the details of her past sexual experiences (especially with Carlos) or about men she finds sexually attractive now. For her part, Maria responds to this by denying other interests, offering further reassurances that Harold really has nothing to worry about, and expressing her growing frustration with Harold's inability to trust her. Once, in response to persistent questioning, Maria had actually tried to describe her lovemaking with Carlos, calling it "vigorous, at least on his part," but "unsatisfying for me, because I felt used." To Maria's dismay, Harold questioned her about "vigorous orgasms" in a later dispute, and the accuse–deny sequence between them had several times escalated to the point of yelling and name-calling. On one such occasion she stormed out of the house, and on another, Harold threw a book, accidentally breaking a lamp. These "blow-ups" were invariably followed by periods of remorse, in which both partners (but especially Maria) would try to take responsibility for what happened and resolve not to let it happen again. While allowing that Harold's fits of jealousy were often "unreasonable," Maria clearly regarded them as anomalous to his otherwise pleasing personality and felt that the blow-ups mainly reflected her inability to meet his needs. Despite these complications, Maria confided that she and Harold really did have good sex, especially when they had not tried beforehand to talk about it, which was all the more reason to save the relationship.

Toward the end of the first session, the therapist asked what Maria hoped to gain from coming to the Clinic, and what she would take as a tangible sign that the situation with Harold was improving. She said she most wanted to understand *why* she was unsuccessful with men, because this might help her save the relationship with Harold. The therapist did not challenge this, but pressed instead for a minimum change goal: "What, when it happens, will let you know that you and Harold are getting a handle on the jealousy problem? Or that even though he might not have proposed marriage, your relationship is at least heading in the right direction?" Maria said she just did not want him to be jealous, and eventually she agreed that not having arguments about sexual matters, even if Harold brought it up, would be a significant indication that things were improving. After consulting with the team behind the one-way mirror, the therapist closed the session by suggesting that Maria tell Harold at least about her first goal (to understand *her* contribution to problems in important relationships), and to ask whether he might be willing to help with this later, particularly since he knows her so well—assuming that we (the team) could think of something he could do. [The rationale here was to open the door for Harold's possible participation in the therapy, yet to do so in a way that respected Maria's—and perhaps also Harold's view—that the problem was *hers* rather than his or even theirs. [In retrospect, it would probably have been better to ask Maria's permission to call Harold directly, so that we could better assess his customership and control the message. Later, after the next session, the therapist in fact did this.]

Maria opened the second session by announcing that her homework assignment had not gone well. Although Harold had known about the counseling appointment and felt OK about Maria getting help, he had not expected (she said) that so much time would be spent talking about *him*. Furthermore, as for helping with the therapy, there was no way that he, a tenured professor at the university, could be comfortable with the videotaping and observation room setup, or with talking about personal matters to graduate students and faculty from another department. When asked why she thought Harold reacted this way, and how she handled it, Maria said she thought he might have been embarrassed. She had tried to reassure him that she was really coming to work on her own problems, not to complain about him, but this did not work, so rather than risk another argument, she decided to apologize quietly and drop the subject. After a phone-in from the team, the therapist conveyed to Maria the team's apology for putting

her in this awkward position and asked permission for us to call Harold and apologize to him as well. Maria was initially reluctant, but agreed to the call, adding that she would probably warn Harold what was coming.

The rest of the second session was devoted to further investigation of the problem–solution pattern identified in the first session to develop a clearer picture of what less of the same (the strategic objective) might look like on Maria's side. Although characteristic "solutions" such as explaining, reassuring, and denying were already in focus, it was not clear in what situation(s) the escalating interaction sequence most typically occurred. Questions about this yielded few specific answers: In fact, Maria found it disconcerting that she could not predict *when* Harold would ask her a "sexual attraction" question, because if she could, she might better prepare for it: "It can just come out of the blue, like when he's reflecting on things—even good things." Another useful piece of information came from questioning Maria about solutions that did work for her, at least with other problems. Here we were particularly interested in how she used mindfulness meditation, and what this meant to her. Maria did meditation exercises every morning and preferred to do them when Harold was not in the house, so as not to disturb or distract him. She also said that meditations—and more generally, the Eastern idea of "yielding"— had helped her cope with interpersonal stresses, particularly after problems with Harold. When feeling stressed in this way, Maria would try to "yield" by taking a "miniretreat," which amounted to a brief period of private meditation, again away from Harold. These miniretreats were inevitably "healing, at least temporarily," but they were not always possible to arrange. A final line of questions concerned the views and possible solution efforts of people beyond the couple, such as relatives, friends, and colleagues. Here we learned that Maria spoke several times weekly on the phone with her mother, whose opinion was that the relationship with Harold was unlikely to succeed, in part because he was from a different cultural and religious background. Maria did not argue with her mother about this, but at the same time she stiffened her resolve to succeed in love, as well as work. After all, her mother had at first been skeptical about her career plans, too.

The therapist called Harold several days after the second session as agreed, and found him symmetrically apologetic about the misunderstandings surrounding Maria's therapy. Harold said he hoped the counseling could help Maria, who he felt was often "too hard on herself," and maybe if that happened, there would be some indirect benefits for the relationship. He hoped the therapist would understand, however, why he did not want to come in himself. Sensing that this was not a matter for negotiation, the therapist said she did understand and that we, too, wished the best for his and Maria's relationship. Although careful not to comment or ask questions about any particulars of the relationship, the therapist did ask Harold if she might call him again "sometime down the road" to consult, if she and Maria thought that might be helpful. After a brief hesitation, he agreed to this request.

At a staff meeting a few days later, the team reviewed the accumulated information about the case, sharpened its formulation of problem maintenance, and planned the particulars of an intervention for the third session. Focusing on the jealousy sequence, it was clear that the main thrust of Maria's solution effort involved *talking* with Harold about his fears and concerns, notably, explaining and reasoning with him, offering reassurances, and denying that she was sexually attracted to other men. It was equally clear that less of this solution—the strategic objective that, if accomplished, would suffice to break the cycle—should involve *not* trying to talk Harold out of his concerns or, perhaps better, not talking in the face of accusations at all. [The team briefly considered ways Maria might reverse her usual stance (e.g., by agreeing with Harold and amplifying his concerns), but this seemed provocative and much too risky.] Because it is usually easier in such a context for clients to do something than not to do something, the team considered what the therapist could ask Maria to do that would effectively block her usual solution efforts. After some discussion, it was decided that the simple act of meditation, if done at the right time in Harold's presence, could serve this purpose nicely. An advantage was that the behavior of sitting quietly, breathing evenly, and focusing inwardly, with her eyes closed, was familiar to Maria and a proven way of coping with stress. On the other hand, because Maria preferred to meditate alone, so she would not distract or disturb him, it might be difficult to persuade her to do this with Harold not only present but also actively attempting to engage her in conversation. A final consideration was that the target sequence often came "out of the blue," with no predictable

onset. This meant that Maria's strategic meditation would need to occur contingently, and that when to attempt this should be spelled out clearly in the intervention.

As the team pondered how to frame the meditation intervention in a way that Maria would accept, several aspects of her preferred views, or "position," seemed especially relevant: First, saving the relationship and being helpful to Harold were high on Maria's list of concerns. Second, she understood that mindfulness meditation and knowing when to yield can help people cope with stressful situations, so perhaps this idea could be extended to include possible future benefits for Harold and the relationship, as well as for her. Second, because Maria believed that self-understanding was the preferred path to personal growth and change, it might be advisable to frame the meditation task as something likely to provoke unforeseen insights, primarily for her, but perhaps (eventually) for Harold too. Another aspect of client position that the team considered was Maria's resolve not to be constrained by her mother's expectations, but because this did not seem applicable to framing the meditation intervention, it was held in reserve for possible use later in the therapy.

Session 3 began with a report on Harold's reactions to the therapist's phone call, which Maria characterized as more thoughtful and considerate than she had expected. Although the couple had had a good week, with no jealousy or sexual-attraction disputes, Maria was not optimistic that this state of affairs would continue. The therapist agreed with her assessment, adding that the team had given some thought to Maria's situation and had come up with some ideas that might help in her self-analysis. When Maria said she would like to hear about those ideas, the therapist proceeded to frame the intervention: First, she said, it might be helpful if Maria had a way to cope with the jealousy situation on the spot, so it would be less likely to get out of hand. Second, it might be possible to do this in a way that helps us understand more about *why* Maria behaves as she does, at least with Harold, which in turn could give clues about how to change. Finally, though the team was not sure, what they had in mind might also help Harold with the stress he must be experiencing, and perhaps even help him take stock of what he could do to make the relationship better. [Through all of this, both the therapist and team behind the one-way mirror carefully watched Maria's nonverbal expression, particularly her head nods, to see whether she seemed to be accepting the frame. Only the part about Harold taking stock of his own contributions seemed to evoke skepticism, and the therapist quickly downplayed this as "a pretty unlikely possibility."] Taking a position of mild restraint, the therapist then said that although she knew of several small but specific steps Maria could take to accomplish these things, those steps could be difficult, and she (the therapist) was reluctant to add to Maria's burden. After Maria responded by affirming her commitment to "doing whatever is necessary," the therapist, with an air of caution, proceeded to lay out the strategic meditation idea and its rationale.

The key to doing the meditation successfully, the therapist explained, would be for Maria to pay close attention to her own reactions. When she was sure she felt like defending herself or reasoning with Harold about sexual matters, she should do the following: (1) Look toward the ceiling and politely say, "Excuse me, Harold"; (2) ceremoniously assume a comfortable meditation position on the floor; (3) close her eyes; and (4) begin meditating. If Harold attempted to interrupt this or draw her into conversation, she should simply say, without opening her eyes, "The counselor suggested I do this when I feel stressed. I'll be available again in about 15 minutes." If Harold became upset or tried to roust her from meditation, she would simply remain silent and yield, Ghandi style, no matter what the provocation. Afterwards, she might do whatever felt natural, either with Harold or without him. The therapist went on to underscore the potential enlightenment value of this exercise, pointing out that the team was reasonably confident that should Maria have opportunity to do this a few times, some insights would emerge to shed light on either her habitual difficulties with men or what the future might hold for herself and Harold. The team did not know what form these insights might take, what they might mean, or how soon they would emerge after a meditation session, but the therapist expressed confidence that she and Maria would know how to handle them when the time came. The session closed with Maria reassuring the therapist that the meditation experiment would not be too burdensome for her. Maria also noted that, in her experience, important awarenesses usually occurred well after a mindfulness meditation, for example, while taking a hike. The therapist was unsure what Maria meant by this, but she did not explore it further.

When Maria returned for Session 4, two weeks later, she reported there had been no occasions to try the meditation experiment. Although she had considered doing it several times when she was beginning to feel irritated with Harold, these situations were not really related to the jealousy issue, so she held back. Actually, Maria said, knowing what she would do if/when a difficult situation came up had made her feel more confident, and she wondered whether she might have behaved a little differently around Harold because of this. The therapist complimented her on feeling confident, but suggested that she "go slow" with behaving differently around Harold due to uncertainties about how he (and they) might handle it. The therapist also expressed mild chagrin that Harold had not provided Maria with the learning opportunity she had anticipated. After a period of general discussion about parity in man–woman relationships, the therapist returned to the "missed opportunity" problem and suggested the possibility of delaying the next session until Harold had "misbehaved" to the point of allowing Maria to try the meditation experiment. Maria at first seemed puzzled by this, because she thought talking things out would continue to help her, but she agreed to call in a month for another appointment, or possibly sooner, if she had the fortunate (?) opportunity to meditate in front of Harold.

Roughly a month after Session 4, the therapist received a phone message from Maria announcing: "Big news! Harold proposed!!!" And in a session a few days later, she explained what had happened. One evening not long after the last session, Harold had again tried to draw Maria into a discussion of Carlos's sexual prowess, and after only a minute of this, she had invoked the meditation routine. After she began, he had said, "What the hell?" With eyes closed, Maria repeated the brief explanation about feeling stressed. As best she could tell, Harold left the room a minute or so later, then left the house. He came back fairly late, after Maria had gone to bed, but the next morning before she finished her shower he had prepared pancakes (something he had not done since early in the courtship). At breakfast, after a period of silence, Harold proffered an awkward apology for his insensitivity over the past few months, then asked whether Maria might teach him how to meditate. This was something she had urged him to try a number of times in the past, but he had shown little interest, and she had thought better of pursuing it further. In any case, Maria and Harold had good sex that evening; afterwards, she instructed him in mindfulness meditation. Much to her delight, they had meditated together every morning since then, except for a few days when Harold went to a meeting out of town. There had been two potential recurrences of the jealousy sequences, but Maria had nipped each of these in the bud—the first by looking at the ceiling and closing her eyes, and the second by playfully saying "Meditation time." As for "insight and awareness," Maria said that once she and Harold began meditating together, she realized how "enabling" she had been by preventing him from taking a full share of responsibility for the success of their relationship. Again, however, the team was not entirely sure what to make of this realization, so the therapist respectfully validated it without much elaboration.

Finally, when asked why she decided to come back to the clinic, Maria said she had thought about calling to schedule an appointment earlier, around the time of the first potential jealousy recurrence, but she decided not to risk spoiling her success (and upsetting Harold) by doing that. In fact, she would probably not have called when she did except that, this time, Harold had suggested it. Therapy terminated at this point, amid messages that both congratulated Maria (and, through her, Harold) on what they had accomplished and cautioned her against thinking the road ahead would be trouble free. The therapist would be available over the next few months in case she (or they) wanted to visit the clinic again, and Maria could count on a routine follow-up call from the clinic in 6–12 months. A few days later, the therapist received a personal note from Harold, expressing his sincere thanks for "helping Maria come to terms with the stress in her life." Harold felt that this had helped him, too. In the follow-up contact 9 months later, Maria reported no further recurrences of the jealousy complaint. In addition, she was married and pregnant.

ACKNOWLEDGMENTS

This work was partially supported by Grant Nos. R21-DA13121, R01 DA17539, and U10 DA15815 from the National Institute on Drug Abuse. The order of the first two authors is arbitrary.

NOTES

1. The term "ironic process" was first used by social psychologist Daniel Wegner (1994) in connection with his theory of mental control. Shoham and Rohrbaugh (1997) later extended the term to "ironic interpersonal processes," such as those highlighted by the Palo Alto group (cf. Rohrbaugh & Shoham, 2001).

2. Although Haley and Madanes sometimes used interventions similar to those practiced by the MRI group (which should not be surprising given that Haley was an early member of the MRI Brief Therapy Center), their strategic therapy makes assumptions about relational structure and the adaptive (protective) function of symptoms that the Palo Alto group de-emphasized (Weakland, 1992). Useful descriptions of strategic marital therapy drawing on the Haley–Madanes model can be found in Keim (1999) and in Todd's (1986) chapter in the first edition of this *Handbook*.

3. Paul Watzlawick and Jay Haley both passed away in 2007.

4. Beyond these therapeutic contributions, Coyne's (1976) relational model of depression has stimulated much empirical research on the crucial role of interpersonal processes in the maintenance of depression (Segrin & Dillard, 1992).

5. A similar concern with avoiding ironic "therapy" processes has influenced the framing of our manualized couple therapies for alcoholics and change-resistant smokers as "family consultation" (Rohrbaugh et al., 1995, 2001). By connoting collaboration and choice, the term "consultation" arouses less resistance than "treatment" and underscores our assumption that people come to therapy because they are stuck—not sick, dysfunctional, or in need of an emotional overhaul.

6. Bateson (1958) distinguished "complementary" interaction patterns, in which participants exchange opposite behavior (e.g., nagging and withdrawal, dominance and submission), from "symmetrical" patterns, in which they exchange similar behavior (e.g., mutual blame or avoidance).

7. Most studies indicate that women are on the demand side of demand–withdraw interaction more often than men (Christensen & Heavey, 1993), yet who demands and who withdraws in a conflict may depend more on the situational affordances (e.g., who has power and least wants to change) than on essential differences between the sexes (Klinetob & Smith, 1996).

8. The success of this intervention may owe partly to a shared cultural familiarity between Fisch, Shoham, and the wife, with chicken soup as a credible—and potentially nonverbal—remedy for familial distress.

9. These couple-level results parallel findings from attribute × treatment interaction (ATI) studies of individual therapy (e.g., Shoham-Salomon, Avner, & Neeman, 1989). In both clinical contexts—one in which an individual client resists persistent influence from a therapist, and the other in which a male drinker resists influence from his spouse—treatments that exert different levels of direct pressure for change appear to yield different results to the extent that they activate (or avoid) interpersonal ironic processes.

10. In a review of empirically supported couple therapies, Baucom, Shoham, Meuser, Daiuto, and Stickle (1998) concluded that "the findings from this single investigation place systemic couple therapy into the category of possibly efficacious [treatments]" (p. 61).

11. The therapist, also female, was an advanced graduate student in clinical psychology. She was supervised by M. Rohrbaugh in a consultation team format.

SUGGESTIONS FOR FURTHER READING

Fisch, R., Weakland, J. H., & Segal, L. (1982). *The tactics of change*. San Francisco: Jossey-Bass.

Haley, J. (1987). *Problem-solving therapy: New strategies for effective family therapy* (2nd ed.). San Francisco: Jossey-Bass.

Rohrbaugh, M. J., & Shoham, V. (2001). Brief therapy based on interrupting ironic processes: The Palo Alto model. *Clinical Psychology: Science and Practice, 8*, 66–81.

REFERENCES

Bateson, G. (1958). *Naven* (2nd ed.). Stanford, CA: Stanford University Press.

Baucom, D. H., Shoham, V., Meuser, K. T., Daiuto, A. D., & Stickle, T. R. (1998). Empirically supported couple and family interventions for marital distress and adult mental health problems. *Journal of Consulting and Clinical Psychology, 65*, 53–88.

Berg, I. K., & Miller, S. D. (1992). *Working with the problem drinker: A solution-focused approach*. New York: Norton.

Bobele, M. (1987). Therapeutic interventions in life-threatening situations. *Journal of Marital and Family Therapy, 13*, 225–240.

Bobele, M. (1988). Reply to "Public policy in life-threatening situations." *Journal of Marital and Family Therapy, 14*, 139–142.

Brehm, J. W. (1966). *A theory of psychological reactance*. New York: Academic Press.

Cade, B., & O'Hanlon, W. H. (1993). *A brief guide to brief therapy*. New York: Norton.

Christensen, A., & Heavey, C. L. (1993). Gender differences in marital conflict: The demand/withdraw interaction pattern. In S. Oskamp & M. Costanzo (Eds.), *Gender issues in contemporary society* (pp. 113–141). Newbury Park, CA: Sage.

Christensen, A., & Schenk, J. L. (1991). Communication, conflict, and psychological distance in nondistressed, clinic, and divorcing couples. *Journal of Consulting and Clinical Psychology, 59*, 458–463.

Coyne, J. C. (1976). Toward an interactional description of depression. *Psychiatry, 39*, 28–40.

Coyne, J. C. (1986a). Strategic marital therapy for depression. In N. S. Jacobson & A. S. Gurman (Eds.), *Clinical handbook of marital therapy*. New York: Guilford Press.

Coyne, J. C. (1986b). Evoked emotion in marital therapy: Necessary or even useful? *Journal of Marital and Family Therapy, 12*, 11–14.

Coyne, J. C. (1988). Strategic therapy. In J. Clarkin, G. Haas, & I. Glick (Eds.), *Affective disorders: Family assessment and treatment* (pp. 89–113). New York: Guilford Press.

Coyne, J. C., & Smith, D. A. (1991). Couples coping with a myocardial infraction: Contextual perspective on wife's distress. *Journal of Personality and Social Psychology, 61*, 404–412.

de Shazer, S. (1991). *Putting differences to work*. New York: Norton.

de Shazer, S., Berg, I., Lipchik, E., Nunnally, E., Molnar, A., Gingerich, W., et al. (1986). Brief therapy: Focused solution development. *Family Process, 25*, 207–222.

Fiore, M. C., Bailey, W. C., Cohen, S. J., Dorfman, S. F., Goldstein, M. G., Gritz, E. R., et al. (2000). *Treating tobacco use and dependence. Clinical Practice Guideline*. Rockville, MD: U.S. Department of Health and Human Services, Public Health Service.

Fisch, R. (1986). The brief treatment of alcoholism. *Journal of Strategic and Systemic Therapies, 5*, 40–49.

Fisch, R. (1990). "To thine own self be true ... ": Ethical issues in strategic therapy. In J. Zeig (Ed.), *Brief therapy: Myths, methods, and metaphors* (pp. 429–436). New York: Brunner/Mazel.

Fisch, R., & Schlanger, K. (1999). *Brief therapy with intimidating cases: Changing the unchangeable*. San Francisco: Jossey-Bass.

Fisch, R., Weakland, J. H., & Segal, L. (1982). *The tactics of change: Doing therapy briefly*. San Francisco: Jossey-Bass.

Goldman, A., & Greenberg, L. (1992). Comparison of integrated systemic and emotionally focused approaches to couples therapy. *Journal of Consulting and Clinical Psychology, 60*, 962–969.

Green, S., & Bobele, M. (1988). An interactional approach to marital infidelity. *Journal of Strategic and Systemic Therapies, 7*, 35–47.

Gurman, A. S. (2001). Brief therapy and family–couple therapy: An essential redundancy. *Clinical Psychology: Science and Practice, 8*, 51–65.

Gurman, A. S., Kniskern, D. P., & Pinsof, W. (1986). Research on the process and outcome of marital and family therapy. In S. L. Garfield & A. E. Bergin (Eds.), *Handbook of psychotherapy and behavior change* (pp. 565–624). New York: Wiley.

Haley, J. (1967). *Advanced techniques of hypnosis and therapy: Selected papers of Milton H. Erickson, M.D.* New York: Grune & Stratton.

Haley, J. (1980). *Leaving home*. New York: McGraw-Hill.

Haley, J. (1987). *Problem-solving therapy: New strategies for effective family therapy* (2nd ed.). San Francisco: Jossey-Bass.

Hoebel, F. C. (1976). Brief family–interactional therapy in the management of cardiac-related high-risk behaviors. *Journal of Family Practice, 3*, 613–618.

Homish, G. G., & Leonard, K. E. (2005). Spousal influence on smoking behaviors in a U.S. community sample of newly married couples. *Social Science and Medicine, 61*, 2557–2567.

Keim, J. (1999). Brief strategic marital therapy. In J. M. Donovan (Ed.), *Short-term couple therapy* (pp. 265–290). New York: Guilford Press.

Klinetob, N. A., & Smith, D. A. (1996). Demand–withdraw communication in marital interaction: Test of interspousal contingency and gender role hypotheses. *Journal of Marriage and the Family, 58*, 945–957.

Madanes, C. (1981). *Strategic family therapy*. San Francisco: Jossey-Bass.

Madanes, C. (1991). Strategic family therapy. In A. S. Gurman & D. P. Kniskern (Eds.), *Handbook of family therapy* (Vol. 2, pp. 396–416). New York: Brunner/Mazel.

Miller, G., & de Shazer, S. (2000). Emotions in solution-focused therapy: A re-examination. *Family Process, 39*, 5–23.

Napier, A. Y. (1978). The rejection–intrusion pattern: A central family dynamic. *Journal of Marriage and Family Counseling, 4*, 5–12.

Nichols, M. P., & Schwartz, R. C. (2000). *Family therapy: Concepts and methods*. Boston: Allyn & Bacon.

O'Hanlon, W., & Weiner-Davis, M. (1989). *In search of solutions: A new direction in psychotherapy*. New York: Norton.

Rohrbaugh, M. J., & Shean, G. (1988). Anxiety disorders: An interactional view of agoraphobia. In F. Walsh & C. Anderson (Eds.), *Chronic illness and the family* (pp. 65–85). New York: Brunner/Mazel.

Rohrbaugh, M. J., & Shoham, V. (2001). Brief therapy based on interrupting ironic processes: The Palo Alto model. *Clinical Psychology: Science and Practice, 8*, 66–81.

Rohrbaugh, M. J., & Shoham, V. (2002). Family systems therapy for alcohol abuse. In S. Hofmann & M. C. Tompson (Eds.), *Handbook of psychosocial treatments for severe mental disorders* (pp. 277–295). New York: Guilford Press.

Rohrbaugh, M. J., Shoham, V., & Schlanger, K. (1992). *In the brief therapy archives: A progress report*. Unpublished manuscript, University of Arizona, Tucson.

Rohrbaugh, M. J., Shoham, V., Spungen, C., & Steinglass, P. (1995). Family systems therapy in practice: A systemic couples therapy for problem drinking. In B. Bongar & L. E. Beutler (Eds.), *Comprehensive textbook of psychotherapy: Theory and practice* (pp. 228–253). New York: Oxford University Press.

Rohrbaugh, M. J., Shoham, V., Trost, S., Muramoto, M., Cate, R., & Leischow, S. (2001). Couple-dynamics of change resistant smoking: Toward a family-consultation model. *Family Process, 40*, 15–31.

Rosenthal, M. K., & Bergman, Z. (1986). A flow-chart presenting the decision-making process of the MRI Brief Therapy Center. *Journal of Strategic and Systemic Therapies, 5*, 1–6.

Segrin, C., & Dillard, J. P. (1992). The interactional theory of depression: A meta-analysis of the research literature. *Journal of Social and Clinical Psychology, 11*, 4–70.

Shoham, V., Bootzin, R. R., Rohrbaugh, M. J., & Urry, H. (1996). Paradoxical versus relaxation treatment for insomnia: The moderating role of reactance. *Sleep Research, 24a*, 365.

Shoham, V., & Rohrbaugh, M. J. (1997). Interrupting ironic processes. *Psychological Science, 8*, 151–153.

Shoham, V., Rohrbaugh, M. J., & Patterson, J. (1995). Problem- and solution-focused couple therapies: The MRI and Milwaukee models. In N. S. Jacobson & A. S. Gurman (Eds.), *Clinical handbook of marital therapy* (pp. 142–163). New York: Guilford Press.

Shoham, V., Rohrbaugh, M. J., Stickle, T. R., & Jacob, T. (1998). Demand–withdraw couple interaction moderates retention in cognitive-behavioral vs. family-systems treatments for alcoholism. *Journal of Family Psychology, 12*, 557–577.

Shoham, V., Rohrbaugh, M. J., Trost, S., & Muramoto, M. (2006). A family consultation intervention for health-compromised smokers. *Journal of Substance Abuse Treatment, 31*, 395–402.

Shoham, V., Trost, S. E., & Rohrbaugh, M. J. (2004). From state to trait and back again: Reactance theory goes clinical. In R. A. Wright, J. Greenberg, & S. S. Brehm (Eds.), *Motivation and emotion in social contexts* (pp. 167–186). Mahwah, NJ: Erlbaum.

Shoham-Salomon, V., Avner, R., & Neeman, R. (1989). You are changed if you do and changed if you don't: Mechanisms underlying paradoxical interventions. *Journal of Consulting and Clinical Psychology, 57*, 590–598.

Shoham-Salomon, V., & Jancourt, A. (1985). Differential effectiveness of paradoxical interventions for more versus less stress-prone individuals. *Journal of Counseling Psychology, 32*, 443–447.

Solovey, A., & Duncan, B. L. (1992). Ethics and strategic therapy: A proposed ethical direction. *Journal of Marital and Family Therapy, 18*, 53–61.

Spinks, S. H., & Birchler, G. R. (1982). Behavioral–systems marital therapy: Dealing with resistance. *Family Process, 21*, 169–185.

Stanton, M. D. (1981). An integrated structural/strategic approach to family therapy. *Journal of Marital and Family Therapy, 7*, 427–440.

Stevens, V. J., & Hollis, J. F. (1989). Preventing smoking relapse using an individually tailored skills-training technique. *Journal of Consulting and Clinical Psychology, 57*, 420–424.

Teismann, M. (1979). Jealousy: Systematic, problem-solving therapy with couples. *Family Process, 18*, 151–160.

Todd, T. C. (1986). Structural–strategic marital therapy. In N. S. Jacobson & A. S. Gurman (Eds.), *Clinical handbook of marital therapy*. New York: Guilford Press.

Watzlawick, P. (1978). *The language of change*. New York: Basic Books.

Watzlawick, P., Beavin, J., & Jackson, D. D. (1967). *Pragmatics of human communication*. New York: Norton.

Watzlawick, P., & Coyne, J. C. (1976). Depression following stroke: Brief, problem-focused treatment. *Family Process, 19,* 13–18.

Watzlawick, P., & Weakland, J. H. (Eds.). (1978). *The interactional view.* New York: Norton.

Watzlawick, P., Weakland, J. H., & Fisch, R. (1974). *Change: Principles of problem formation and problem resolution.* New York: Norton.

Weakland, J. H. (1988). Weakland on the Woodys–Bobele exchange. *Journal of Marital and Family Therapy, 14,* 205.

Weakland, J. H. (1992). Conversation—But what kind? In S. Gilligan & M. Price (Eds.), *Therapeutic conversations* (pp. 136–145). New York: Norton.

Weakland, J. H., & Fisch, R. (1992). Brief therapy—MRI style. In S. H. Budman, M. F. Hoyt, & S. Friedman (Eds.), *The first session in brief therapy* (pp. 306–323). New York: Guilford Press.

Weakland, J. H., Fisch, R., Watzlawick, P., & Bodin, A. (1974). Brief therapy: Focused problem resolution. *Family Process, 13,* 141–168.

Wegner, D. M. (1994). Ironic processes of mental control. *Psychological Review, 101,* 34–52.

Wendorf, D. J., & Wendorf, R. J. (1985). A systemic view of family therapy ethics. *Family Process, 24,* 443–460.

Wetter, D. W., Fiore, M. C., Gritz, E. R., Lando, H. A., Stitzer, M. L., Hasselblad, V., et al. (1998). The Agency for Health Care Policy and Research Smoking Cessation Clinical Practice Guideline: Findings and implications for psychologists. *American Psychologist, 53,* 657–669.

Wile, D. B. (1981). *Couples therapy: A non-traditional approach.* New York: Wiley.

Woody, J. D., & Woody, R. H. (1988). Public policy in life-threatening situations: A response to Bobele. *Journal of Marital and Family Therapy, 14,* 133–138.

Wylie, M. S. (1990). Brief therapy on the couch. *Family Therapy Networker, 14,* 26–35, 66.

Wynne, L. C., McDaniel, S. H., & Weber, T. T. (1987). *Systems consultation: A new perspective for family therapy.* New York: Guilford Press.

CHAPTER 11

Structural Couple Therapy

George M. Simon

Strictly speaking, structural couple therapy (SCT) does not exist as a distinct approach for the treatment of couples. Structural family therapy, the "parent" model from which SCT derives, was developed, as its name indicates, as a treatment for families, not couples. As I detail here, SCT's application of the conceptual apparatus and interventive technology of structural family therapy to the treatment of couples entails some distinct strengths for the model, but at least one weakness as well.

BACKGROUND

Structural family therapy emerged during the 1960s and 1970s out of the dissatisfaction with psychoanalysis experienced by Salvador Minuchin when he attempted to treat children at the Jewish Board of Guardians, the Wiltwyck School for Boys, and the Philadelphia Child Guidance Clinic (Minuchin & Nichols, 1993). As Minuchin and his colleagues at these institutions began to meet with the families of troubled children, they began to question the core psychoanalytic assumption that human behavior is driven from the inside out, by internal psychodynamics. Following the

lead of early systems theorist Don Jackson (1957), they began to experiment with an "outside-in" understanding of human behavior. For example, rather than viewing a child's impulsive, acting-out behavior as a response to internal dynamics, Minuchin and his colleagues began to experiment with seeing the behavior as a child's response to, say, a parent's overly controlling, intrusive behavior. However, the parent's intrusive behavior could equally be viewed as a response to the child's acting out. Thus, Minuchin and his colleagues found themselves migrating from a psychoanalytic world of "linear causality" (A causes B), in which each person's behavior is caused by his or her internal psychodynamics, to a systemic world of "circular causality" (A causes B, which causes A, which causes B, ...), in which each person's behavior, at one and the same time, is both an effect and a cause of his or her interactional partner's behavior.

As promising as Minuchin's group found the new systemic perspective forged by theorists like Don Jackson and Gregory Bateson to be, they were dissatisfied with the breadth of scope of the conceptual apparatus that these theorists had developed up to that point. Bateson, Jackson, and their colleagues at the Mental Research Institute (MRI) had focused almost exclusively on circular interactional processes involving only two people. Minuchin's group found that the dyadic concepts developed by this team were unequal to the task of comprehensively describing the interactional dynamics in systems comprising more than two people. With no published literature to guide them, Minuchin and his colleagues undertook to develop concepts of their own that would bring a systemic way of thinking to bear on whole families rather than just dyads. They publicized the fruits of their conceptual labor in *Families of the Slums* (Minuchin, Montalvo, Guerney, Rosman, & Schumer, 1967) and *Families and Family Therapy* (Minuchin, 1974).

In these books, the family is depicted as a system that comprises "subsystems," which arise in families as a result of differences. Generational differences, for example, produce parental and sibling subsystems. In some families, perceived differences between the genders can lead to male and female subsystems. Differences in interest and/or skills can also produce subsystems: A given family might have a "practical" subsystem and an "artistic" subsystem. Precisely because they are produced by differences, subsystems were conceived by Minuchin's group as being surrounded by "boundaries," which demarcate subsystems one from another.

The internal differences that give rise to subsystems are potentially a good thing for the family. That this is so becomes clear when we realize that the family is itself only a subsystem—of an extended family, possibly, but certainly a subsystem of the broader society in which it is immersed. A family is functional to the degree that it nurtures in its members the ability to negotiate well the demands of the world outside the family (Minuchin & Fishman, 1981). Performing this task of socialization requires that the family be able to adapt itself to changes in its social environment. However, it also requires that the family, when necessary, be able to exercise some agency in changing its environment, with an eye toward rendering the environment more supportive of the family's functioning.

The family system is better equipped to engage in this kind of complex interaction with the outside world if it has access to as many internal resources as possible. This is why the presence of internal differences that give rise to subsystems is potentially good news for the family. A family with a significant array of complexly cross-linked subsystems should find itself richly endowed with resources to manage its dealings with the outside world. Such will be the case, however, if, and only if, the various subsystems interact with each other in a way that allows the family as a whole to benefit from the resources contained in each subsystem.

To describe and to assess how adaptively family subsystems interact with each other, Minuchin (1974) proposed that we think of the boundaries that demarcate subsystems one from another as varying in permeability, from diffuse to rigid. A "diffuse" boundary between two family subsystems is one that does not adequately differentiate the functioning of the two subsystems, resulting in a deprivation of resources to the family as a whole. The presence of a diffuse boundary can be assessed when two family subsystems have no clear division of labor and/or focus between them. Subsystems separated by a diffuse boundary are said to be "enmeshed."

Equally debilitating to the family is the presence of "rigid" boundaries between subsystems. Here, differentiation has been carried to the point that resources in one subsystem are unavailable to the other. Subsystems separated by a rigid boundary are said to be "disengaged."

The constellation of subsystems in a family, along with the boundaries, whether diffuse, adaptive, or rigid, that separate the various subsystems from each other, are collectively referred to as the *structure* of the family. In *Families and Family Therapy*, Minuchin (1974) provided a scheme to depict family structure graphically. The maps drawn utilizing this scheme allow one to see in a glance all of the subsystems in a given family, and the pattern of interaction among them. Although they serve a useful pedagogical function in helping trainees learn to "see" family structure, most experienced structural therapists do not need physically to draw these structural maps.

It must be kept in mind that in devising the heuristic metaphors of family structure, subsystems, and boundaries, Minuchin and his colleagues were attempting to expand rather than replace the systemic thinking of Bateson's group. Thus, as much as it did for the latter, the notion of circular causality governs the conceptual universe developed by Minuchin's group. Circular causality is seen as governing transactions both within and between subsystems.

FUNCTIONAL–DYSFUNCTIONAL COUPLES

Most readers no doubt realize that this brief overview of structural family therapy's foundational concepts does not include the couple as an explicit unit of analysis. This omission was not an oversight. To reiterate the point I made at the beginning of this chapter, structural therapy is, first of all, a therapy of families, and only derivatively a therapy of couples.

When structural theorists consider couple functioning, they do so after having first articulated a view of family functioning. Inevitably, then, structural theorists' view of couples, functional and dysfunctional, is set against the background of the theory's view of families. The couple is viewed as a family subsystem, no more and no less, and assessment of how well or poorly a couple is functioning is based on the theory's notion of what constitutes adaptive functioning for any and all family subsystems.

This conceptual arrival in the world of couplehood, after a journey through the world of family life, entails a distinct theoretical strength and one practical weakness for SCT. I describe the deficit—and, I hope, begin to remediate it—later in the chapter. Here, I briefly describe the strength.

Because SCT views the couple as a subsystem (perhaps of a family including children, perhaps of an extended kinship network, certainly of numerous societal-level systems), the approach does not base its understanding of the couple on a notion of romantic love. Structural theorizing about the couple recognizes that the ways people couple and their expectations in doing so have varied dramatically from time to time and from place to place over the course of human history (Minuchin, Lee, & Simon, 2006). The notion that optimal couple relating is based on mutually experienced and reciprocally expressed romantic love is of rather recent vintage. Although this notion has almost unquestioned currency among the middle classes of the developed nations of the West, basing an approach to couple therapy on this notion runs the risk of unnecessarily limiting the applicability of the approach.

Precisely because it evaluates couple functioning generically, utilizing the same conceptual repertoire that it employs to evaluate the functioning of any family subsystem, SCT is applicable to couples who have come together and remain together, or perhaps are coming apart, for a whole host of reasons. It can certainly be applied to couples who understand their relationship as based on romantic love. However, it can also be applied to couples who do not expect romantic love to play a significant role in the way the partners relate to each other. It can be applied to couples who seek therapy to facilitate their uncoupling, as well as to couples who desire to remain together.

What, then, in the view of SCT, characterizes a functional couple? Like any functional subsystem, a functional couple is surrounded by a boundary sufficiently defined to demarcate the couple from its environment, yet sufficiently permeable to allow for adaptive exchange with the environment. Functional couples also share with all other functional subsystems the kind of internal differentiation associated with the presence of a significant array of resources. Thus, functional couples not only tolerate but also actively encourage differences between the partners. They are marked by an ethos and a style of interaction that invites each partner to see the other partner's differences as a resource rather than as a threat.

The dysfunctional couple, in distinction, is one whose external boundary is excessively diffuse or rigid. A diffuse boundary deprives the couple subsystem of integrity, resulting in partners' lack of identity as a couple. A rigid boundary, on the other hand, cuts the couple off from its environment. The couple behaves, not as a subsystem, but as a world unto itself, resulting inevitably in functional and emotional overload, and perhaps in debilitating lack of fit between the couple and its social environment as well.

The dysfunctional couple also displays extremes in its approach to internal differentiation. Differences between the partners are either not tolerated or they are rigidified into warring positions, or at least into positions in which partners do not engage in significant dialogue with each other. In both scenarios, the couple subsystem is deprived of resources.

Although these descriptions of functional and dysfunctional couple relating are undeniably abstract, this very abstractness constitutes a major strength of SCT's conceptualization of couple functioning.

To be sure, structural therapists have over the years mined their clinical experience to develop rather more concrete descriptions of some common forms that couple dysfunction takes. Inevitably, these descriptions were shaped by the kinds of client systems with which structural therapists worked at the time the descriptions were formulated. Because structural therapy, for the first 25 years of its existence, was practiced almost exclusively as a family therapy approach in community clinics where children, adolescents, and young adults were almost invariably presented as the identified patient, the forms of couple dysfunction reported in the structural therapy literature of that period were those associated with family structures that tend to elicit and maintain symptomatic behavior in young people.

One such form of couple dysfunction has as its centerpiece a diffuse boundary between the couple subsystem and the sibling subsystem. The boundary between the couple and other subsystems (e.g., extended family, neighborhood, social service agencies) is also likely to be diffuse. In these couples, an integral identity as a couple is virtually nonexistent. Indeed, the only substantial focus shared by the partners is the children. Thus, they place all their relational eggs in the basket of parenting. They parent incessantly and, inevitably, ineffectively. Periodically, the partners become burned out as a result of their overfunctioning in the parental role and abandon the field, disengaging from each other, and leaving the children to be cared for by someone else or to shift for themselves. After a respite from their overparenting, the partners are likely to reengage with each other, but again around their only shared focus—parenting. Although these partners rather easily abandon each other for a time, they do not engage in extended periods of conflict with each other. Their relationship as a couple has too little salience to give rise to the kind of relational dissatisfaction that fuels couple conflict (Minuchin et al., 1967).

Although chronic conflict does not figure prominently in the dysfunctional pattern just described, it is the centerpiece of two other patterns reported in some of the earlier structural therapy literature. In the first, conflict between the partners is overt and chronic, but due to a diffuse boundary surrounding the couple subsystem, it bleeds out of the couple to draw in other members of the family (Minuchin, 1974). One or more children may enter into a stable coalition with one partner against the other. Additionally, one or both partners may find stable allies in one or more members of his or her family of origin. In a particularly virulent form of this pattern, one child shuttles back and forth sequentially between coalitions with both partners.

In the second pattern, chronic couple conflict is once again fueled by a diffuse boundary surrounding the couple subsystem. However, in this pattern, the diffuse boundary is not crossed in a quest for allies. Instead, the conflict between the partners is avoided, and possibly denied altogether, by means of partners' collusive agreement to focus instead on a problem manifested by one or more of the children (Minuchin, 1974; Minuchin, Rosman, & Baker, 1978; Stanton, Todd, & Associates, 1982). This pattern of detoured couple conflict entails the unfortunate need for ongoing dysfunction in one or more children in the family.

In the 1980s and 1990s, structural therapy began to move from the community clinic into the private practice office. Here, structural therapists began to work with couples who presented themselves for treatment precisely as couples rather than as parents of a child identified patient. Frequently, this different mode of presentation for treatment coincided with different patterns of couple dysfunction from those that structural therapists had encountered and described in the preceding decades. By this point, however, Minuchin and other theorists of structural therapy had become less inclined to construct the kind of typological descriptions of dysfunctional family structures produced earlier in the model's development. Such descriptions were now being replaced by lengthy case reports (e.g., see Minuchin & Nichols, 1993, 1998). In these reports, little effort was made to draw detailed connections between one case of couple treatment and another. Instead, each treated couple was described simply as exhibiting some idiosyncratic combination of the generic features that characterize couple dysfunction: an excessively rigid or diffuse boundary surrounding the couple subsystem; inadequate or exaggerated differentiation of role behavior within the couple subsystem; and conflict that either has been avoided or has hardened into a never-ending, ubiquitous power struggle.

So, what is SCT's explanation for the fact that whereas some couples crystallize an adaptive structure, others drift into an organization characterized by the dysfunctional features just listed? Structural theory has something to say about *when* couples are susceptible to developing a dysfunctional structure. Periods in a couple's life when partners experience a press for change, either from a normative life-cycle transition (e.g., the arrival of a first child, the leaving home of a young adult child) or some acute stressor (e.g., the occurrence of a natural disaster, extended unemployment of one of the partners), are seen in structural theory as periods when the couple is at risk of developing a dysfunctional structure. However, as regards *why* some couples respond to such periods adaptively, while others do not, structural theory is relatively mute.

In large measure, SCT's silence on this matter reflects the model's nondeterministic outlook on the development of human systems. Precisely because human systems are *human*, they are complex, multifaceted entities, whose development over time cannot be subjected to the kind of rigorous modeling that is required to make accurate predictions. The structure exhibited by any given couple subsystem at any given point in its development is the product of the complex and largely idiosyncratic interplay of numerous factors, including the family-of-origin histories of the individual partners, the partners' respective biological endowments, the sociocultural environment in which the couple is immersed, chance events that have impacted the couple's life, and not least, the couple's decisions about how to deal with all of these factors.

A corollary of SCT's nondeterministic outlook on couple development is the belief that a given couple's structure at any point in its development could always have turned out to be something different from what it is. A different decision made by the couple, a different response to some exigency of the couple's life, would have resulted in the crystallization of a different structure. This belief entails a crucial implication for the way SCT is conducted. Structural therapy is thoroughly informed by what I have termed an *assumption of competence* (Simon, 1995). No matter how dysfunctional the structure that a couple exhibits at the outset of treatment, it is never assumed that this structure reveals some essential, core quality of the couple. *Because SCT assumes that the couple could have evolved a structure different from the dysfunctional one now being displayed, it also assumes that the couple possesses in its relational repertoire adaptive resources that currently lie dormant.* SCT is not, therefore, an attempt to put something new into a couple viewed as deficient; rather, it is an attempt to activate what is already there, but latent, in a couple viewed as fundamentally competent. I soon demonstrate what a thoroughgoing influence this assumption of competence has on the way SCT is practiced.

THE PRACTICE OF STRUCTURAL COUPLE THERAPY

As is the case with every model of psychotherapy (Held, 1995), the process of therapy prescribed by SCT follows rigorously from the way the model conceptualizes human functioning. The mechanism of therapeutic change in SCT, the structure of the therapy process, the way assessment is con-

ducted and the goals set, the role of the therapist, and the therapeutic techniques employed all flow from the model's systemic conceptualization of couple functioning.

Mechanism of Change

As I noted earlier, structural therapy fully endorses the concept of circular causality developed by Bateson and his colleagues. In the view of SCT, *the most therapeutically relevant cause of a couple member's behavior is not that person's history, biology, thinking, or feeling. Rather, the most proximal cause is that person's here-and-now experience of his or her partner's behavior.* And, of course, the partner's behavior is itself primarily caused by his or her here-and-now experience of the other's behavior.

In the conceptual universe of SCT, here-and-now relational experience elicits and maintains couple members' patterned behavior. Thus, it follows that a therapist who wants to change behavior must change how couple members experience each other. *The mechanism of change in SCT is the production of new relational experiences for clients.* It is the experience of receiving different behavior from his or her partner that induces a couple member to behave differently toward the partner, and vice versa. In SCT, clients change each other by behaving differently toward each other. The job of the therapist is to facilitate this internal change process within the couple subsystem.

It is precisely because SCT is focused entirely on the production of novel, in-session relational experiences for its clients that *enactment* constitutes the centerpiece of the therapeutic process prescribed by the model (Aponte, 1992; Simon, 1995). "Enactment" refers to those moments in therapy when couple members interact directly with each other. It is in this direct interaction with each other during sessions that clients have the new relational experiences that constitute the mechanism of change in SCT.

I have much more to say about enactment later, at various points in this chapter. Here, I want to make clear that enactment is more than simply one technique among many utilized in the practice of structural therapy. Directly linked as it is to structural therapy's understanding of the mechanism of therapeutic change, enactment is better conceived as a leaven that is mixed into every aspect of the therapy process, from assessment to termination. Minuchin, Nichols, and Lee (2007) express this idea by asserting that enactment is more an attitude of the structural therapist than a technique that he or she utilizes. Everywhere, and at all times, the SCT therapist is oriented toward having couple members enact their relational life in the here and now of the therapy session, rather than talk about the relational life they live outside of the session. Thus, enactment organizes the therapy session as a setting in which couple members *have experiences*. Via enactment, couple members experience the futility and dysfunctionality of their current way of relating, and the possibility of relating in new, more functional ways.

Structure of the Therapy Process

SCT's understanding of the mechanism of therapeutic change dictates the manner in which the therapist manages the nuts-and-bolts details of how the therapy process is structured. Matters such as who should attend therapy sessions, how out-of-session contacts with clients should be handled, and whether referrals for medication evaluation and/or individual therapy should be made are all decided in light of SCT's understanding of the nature of couple dysfunction and how such dysfunction is remediated via the therapy process.

As I just described, SCT aims entirely at changing how couple members experience each other. Obviously, one couple member cannot experience the other differently if that person is not in the therapy room with him or her. Thus, in general, both couple members are expected to be present together in every session of SCT.

The only exception to this rule occurs when the therapist suspects that one couple member is behaving violently or abusively toward the other, and that this fact is not being reported openly in session. Under such circumstances, the therapist arranges individual sessions with each partner, thereby providing the abused partner a safe forum to talk about the violence and/or abuse that is occurring. Because violence or abuse that cannot be talked about openly in a conjoint session is likely the kind that is not amenable to change via conjoint treatment, if individual sessions reveal that abuse or violence is occurring, then couple therapy is not continued beyond that point. Rather, the abused partner is referred to services that help to ensure his or her safety. The therapist also provides an appropriate referral to the abusing partner, provided that, in his or her judgment, doing so will not place the abused partner at heightened risk of receiving some kind of retaliatory response from the abuser.

Although holding individual sessions is absolutely necessary in the circumstances just described, it must be noted that, in the view of SCT, any kind of extended contact between the therapist and one couple member outside of the other member's presence entails considerable risk for the therapy process. Recall that a frequently occurring feature of dysfunctional couples is an excessively diffuse boundary surrounding the couple subsystem. Extended contact between the therapist and one couple member outside the presence of the other provides a dangerous opportunity for the therapist to become one of perhaps many people in the couple's ecology who, through overinvolvement with one of the partners, help to maintain a dysfunctional structure in the couple subsystem.

To avoid this risk, the SCT therapist tries wherever possible to avoid extended contact with one couple member outside of the other's presence. Except in the circumstances noted earlier, all sessions are conducted as conjoint sessions, with both partners present in the therapy room. Phone conversations, which are necessarily with one couple member, are kept relatively brief and on-task, usually devoted to the mundane business of scheduling or rescheduling sessions.

It does the therapist little good to avoid becoming party to a couple's dysfunction via extended, exclusive contact with one couple member, if he or she then behaves in a way that sets up another clinician to do the same thing. Referring a couple member for a medication evaluation or for individual therapy would likely have exactly this effect. It is, in my estimation, almost impossible for an individual therapist or a psychiatrist to work with one member of a dysfunctionally structured couple subsystem without being inducted into a position that, unbeknownst to the clinician, winds up buttressing the subsystem's dysfunctionality. Thus, were the SCT therapist to refer one or both members of a client couple to individual therapy or a medication evaluation, he or she would with one hand be reinforcing a dysfunctional structural arrangement, while with the other hand trying to change it.

As it turns out, the SCT therapist is rarely tempted to make referrals for individual therapy. As noted at the beginning of this chapter, SCT rejects the "inside-out" view of human behavior that provides the conceptual justification for individual therapy. Endorsing the "outside-in" view that behavior is elicited and maintained by loops of circular causality, the SCT therapist is organized by this model to see conjoint treatment as the appropriate means to change almost all human behavior.

Similarly, the SCT therapist is slow to see the need to refer a client for a medication evaluation. It is not that that the structural therapist does not recognize the influence of genetics and biology on human behavior. The contribution of genetic endowment to human behavior has by now been too well documented to be ignored. However, structural theory has always assumed that family structure plays a crucial mediating role between genes and their behavioral expression. Adaptive family structure, the model assumes, works to suppress whatever genetic tendency family members might possess to become psychiatrically symptomatic; likewise, maladaptive family structure works to activate such genetic vulnerabilities. This assumption of structural theory has been validated a number of times by research designed to tease out the interaction between genetic endowment and family dynamics (e.g., see Bennett, Wolin, Reiss, & Teitelbaum, 1987; Wynne et al., 2006).

Recognizing the power of relational dynamics both to activate and to suppress psychiatric symptoms, the SCT therapist responds to the presence of such symptoms in one or both members of a client couple by doing what he or she would do with any couple: begin to work to restructure the couple subsystem. The therapist does so, confident that an adaptive restructuring of the couple relationship will result in a significant abatement or even the remission of whatever psychiatric symptomatology was present at the outset of the therapy.

The SCT therapist only sees a need to make a referral for adjunctive treatment in circumstances in which a client's symptoms entail an imminent and substantial threat to harm self or others. Under such circumstances, the therapist cannot wait until an adaptive restructuring of the couple subsystem has ameliorated the client's symptoms. Such circumstances require the more or less "quick fix" that medication might provide. Thus, under these circumstances, the therapist refers the symptomatic client for a medication evaluation.

A story, perhaps apocryphal, told in structural therapy circles exemplifies the model's stance toward the need for referral to adjunctive or alternative treatment. According to the story, Charles Fishman, the coauthor of *Family Therapy Techniques* (Minuchin & Fishman, 1981), was once asked at a conference at which he was presenting, "Under what circumstance is structural therapy not indicated as the treatment of choice for a symptom being exhibited by a client–family

member?" Without missing a beat, Fishman is said to have replied, "When there is not a competent structural therapist within 100 miles of the client family."

Whereas relational dynamics play a crucial role in the activation–suppression of biology-involving psychiatric symptoms, they are not the only contributing factor. Thus, even at the end of a successful course of SCT, some residual expression of such symptoms might remain in one or both couple members. If, at this point, the clients express the desire to see whether psychopharmacological treatment might produce a further reduction in symptoms, the SCT therapist gladly provides a referral for a medication evaluation. The therapist is open to providing such a referral at this juncture, because the adaptive restructuring of the couple subsystem produced by the therapy has significantly reduced the chances that the involvement of one couple member with a psychiatrist, outside of the presence of the other, will negatively impact the functioning of the couple.

Assessment

What the SCT therapist primarily assesses during the initial encounter with a client couple is, of course, the structure of the couple subsystem. Structural assessment of the couple subsystem entails an assessment of the permeability of the boundary surrounding the subsystem and the way differentiation is handled within the subsystem. The SCT therapist expects that most couples presenting for treatment are surrounded by an external boundary that is either excessively diffuse or excessively rigid. The model also predicts that most client couples either avoid differentiation between the partners—"We think alike on almost everything"—or exaggerate differentiation to the point that the only conceivable alternatives for the couple members is either to live in a state of perpetual conflict or avoid significant interaction with each other altogether.

The client couple carries its structure with it into the therapy room. The unarticulated rules and expectations that organize the couple's relational life outside of the therapy room also organize how the partners behave in the therapy room. Thus, all the SCT therapist need do to bring the couple subsystem structure to the fore is to invite the partners to begin interacting with each other in the therapy session. Such direct interaction between couple members is, of course, what SCT refers to as "enactment." Just as enactment, later in the therapy process, will be the SCT therapist's primary medium for changing the couple subsystem structure, so, too, is it the therapist's primary tool early in the therapy process for assessing that structure.

Any enactment the therapist elicits during the first session will probably provide a glimpse into the couple subsystem structure. However, because the SCT therapist is particularly interested in how the couple subsystem handles internal differentiation, and how this differentiation is circularly linked to the permeability of the subsystem's external boundary, certain kinds of enactment are likely to have more assessment value than others. Specifically, enactments in which couple members air and explore differences between them are likely to provide the therapist with the clearest view of the couple subsystem structure. Therefore, relatively early in the first therapy session, the SCT therapist looks for an opportunity to elicit an enactment between the partners on some matter on which they appear to differ.

Some couples cite intractable differences as precisely the problem that led them to seek therapy. Eliciting an enactment focused on differences is usually easy in such cases. After allowing each partner to articulate his or her position on the controversial issues(s) in question, the therapist merely directs the clients to continue their discussion with each other.

The situation is different when a client couple identifies symptoms in one partner as the presenting problem for therapy. In such circumstances, the partners frequently are in substantial agreement about the nature of the symptoms, and even about possible causes of the symptoms. More often than not, they agree in citing the identified patient's biology and/or his or her developmental history as the cause of the symptoms.

Because enactments focused on presenting symptoms are not likely to expose differences between the partners, the therapist needs to broaden the focus of exploration during the first session beyond the symptoms. The therapist can do so by interrupting the client couple's familiar narrative about the presenting symptom. By asking questions about the symptom that are not addressed by the couple's "official" narrative, questions framed in relational terms, the therapist can turn the presenting symptom into a portal into the couple's relationship (Minuchin et al., 2006, 2007), for example, "When she is depressed, are you left feeling high and dry, alone on a desert island?" or "Does his preoccupation with Internet porn sites feel more to you like a camouflaged kick or an abandonment?" As the therapist moves the conversation toward relational themes, differences between the partners that were papered over by their consensus about the presenting symptom are likely to emerge. Once they have emerged, the therapist can elicit enactments focused on these differences.

Wherever they occur in the therapeutic process, enactments are not so much observed by the therapist as they are experienced. There is no one-way mirror between the therapist and the clients as the latter engage in enactments. The therapist is very much present to an enactment, precisely as a third party within easy reach of the clients as they interact with each other. As such, the therapist occupies the same position during enactments that salient third parties occupy in the couple's natural ecology. Thus, how the clients include or exclude the therapist during first-session enactments provides important information about the permeability of the couple subsystem's external boundary, and about how that permeability is circularly linked to the way differentiation is handled within the subsystem.

For example, a couple might respond to the therapist's repeated requests for enactment with exceedingly brief conversations, followed invariably by one couple member's attempt to engage the therapist in an extended dialogue about a matter not pertaining to the couple relationship. Situated at the receiving end of this transaction, the therapist might find him- or herself being pulled into a focal awareness of the couple member who keeps soliciting attention, and into a forgetfulness of the other member. Several repetitions of this pattern suggest to the therapist that the members of this couple are underinvolved with each other, and that this underinvolvement is circularly linked to enmeshment between at least one of the partners and one or more parties outside of the relationship.

In another example, partners might respond to the therapist's request for enactment by escalating fairly quickly into a robust episode of conflict. The therapist notes that one of the partners repeatedly directs knowing, conspiratorial glances at him or her that seem to say, "Do you see what I have to put up with?" Interestingly, the therapist feels drawn to smile back at this partner, as if to say, "You poor thing." The therapist also notices that each conspiratorial glance by that partner is followed within seconds by an increase in expressed anger by the other. That increase in anger provides the first partner with the occasion for the next conspiratorial glance. The therapist uses his or her experience of the enactments to hypothesize that in this chronically conflicted couple, the intractability of conflict is circularly linked to a coalition between one of the partners and one or more parties outside of the relationship.

If some kind of symptom in one or both partners is presented by a client couple as the reason for seeking treatment, first-session enactments also provide the SCT therapist with the means to assess that aspect of the symptom, apart from possible threat to harm self or other, in which he or she is most interested: the manner in which the symptom "fits" into the couple subsystem structure, maintaining and, at the same time, being maintained by the structure.

For example, married partners inform a therapist early in their first session that they have sought therapy because of the wife's depression. The therapist notes near complete agreement between the spouses as they respond to her questions about the particulars of the wife's symptomatology. Differences, however, begin to emerge when the therapist asks whether they have always agreed about how best to handle the depression. The therapist highlights the differences and asks, in an offhanded way, what else the spouses disagree on. "Nothing, really," the wife replies. "Well, I have told you repeatedly that I think you spoil the children," the husband says tentatively. The therapist invites the spouses to talk together about this matter.

As the resulting enactment proceeds, the therapist notes that the husband builds gradually from a halting, tentative presentation of his ideas about parenting to a vigorous, increasingly angry presentation. The wife responds to each increase in her husband's anger by becoming ever more derogatory of his character: "Well, I may spoil the kids, but you're a socially inept jerk." Each jibe from his wife clearly makes the husband even angrier, but he struggles to remain on task, continuing to press his point about how he thinks they should parent, though doing so with barely masked fury toward his wife.

The cycle of escalation continues for several moments until the wife suddenly falls silent and visibly begins to withdraw. Quietly, and, at least as the therapist experiences it, quite pathetically, she begins to cry. The therapist recognizes that the wife is beginning to enact in session that particular combination and sequence of behaviors that the couple described earlier in the session as consti-

tuting her depression. The husband notices the change in his wife. He reaches out to her with a tissue in hand and gently wipes away her tears. He lovingly caresses her cheeks, then pulls her close in an embrace. Still holding her, he turns to the therapist and says, "I think she handles the kids just fine. She's right; I'm really something of a jerk when it comes to dealing with people."

The therapist uses her experience of this enactment to construct the hypothesis that this is a conflict-avoiding couple, hypothesizing that the wife's depression functions effectively to ward off the outbreak of conflict between the spouses, and to quickly short-circuit any episode of conflict that does manage to break the surface of the couple's life. Because the couple subsystem structure, aided and abetted by the wife's depression, does not permit the airing of differences, resources within the subsystem are not being utilized. The wife cannot benefit from her husband's perspective on parenting, and the husband cannot benefit from his wife's insights about his social skills. Meanwhile, the assiduous avoidance of conflict has had the paradoxical effect of causing considerable unresolved conflict to build up within the subsystem. The more conflict builds below the surface of the couple's life, the more necessary the wife's depression to forestall its outbreak. The longer the depression succeeds in forestalling the airing of conflict, the more firmly rooted within the couple subsystem structure the depression becomes.

Goal Setting

Couples enter therapy with the goal of alleviating whatever it is that they have identified as their presenting problem. The SCT therapist thoroughly accepts this goal and considers the therapy successful only if the couple members are satisfied that their presenting problem has been resolved.

Complicating the matter of goal setting in therapy is the fact that, more often than not, couples enter therapy with not only their presenting problem but also a theory about why the problem is occurring. When the presenting problem is a symptom in one or both partners, clients frequently ascribe the problem to the symptom-bearer's biological makeup and/or his or her developmental history. When the presenting problem is defined in relational terms, each partner usually sees the other as the cause of the problem: "We don't have sex because he's preoccupied with work" or "We don't have sex because she's such a nag. Who would want to have sex with a nag?"

The difficulty that clients pose for the SCT therapist is that their causal theories are almost invariably at odds with the therapist's own causal theory. It is a rare occurrence, indeed, when partners enter therapy subscribing to SCT's assumption of circular causality, and seeing their presenting problem as rooted in the dysfunctional structure of their relationship.

This dissonance between clients' causal theories and those of the SCT therapist presents a problem for the therapist, because causal theories necessarily entail therapeutic goals (Held, 1995). If clients believe that a symptom is caused by biology or developmental history, then the "fix" that they look for is a distinctly individualistic one. Similarly, if partners believe that a presenting problem defined in relational terms is caused almost exclusively by the other, then they expect the therapist to proceed by evaluating their competing claims of causality, deciding which of the couple members is "really" at fault, then whipping the offending partner into shape.

Rooted as it is in its own theory of circular causality, SCT bears little resemblance to these expectations about how therapy will proceed. Thus, as soon as the therapist has formulated a working hypothesis about the structure of a given couple subsystem (typically, late in the first session), he or she must address the likely dissonance between the partners' causal theory about the presenting problem and his or her own. The therapist needs to communicate his or her thorough acceptance of the partners' overarching goal of alleviating their presenting problem. However, he or she needs also to communicate an "explanation" for the presenting problem that orients the clients away from whatever expectations about the therapeutic process they might have carried into therapy, toward at least an inchoate grasp of what the process will in fact look like. The provision of such an "explanation" is what SCT refers to as "reframing" (Minuchin & Fishman, 1981).

The "explanation" provided by reframing is in no way conceived of in SCT as an educative intervention. The causal theories endorsed by most clients who enter therapy are not "incorrect" in any absolute sense. To be sure, these linear, individualistic theories do not fit with SCT's circular, systemic worldview. However, there is nothing self-evidently true about that systemic worldview. It is undoubtedly a worldview that the SCT therapist prefers; however, the therapist made a self-defining *choice* when he or she endorsed it (Simon, 2003, 2006a, 2006b). The linear thinking that underlies

clients' causal theories is every bit as intellectually credible as the circular thinking underlying SCT. Indeed, such thinking is more representative of the mainstream of the mental health professions than is systemic thinking.

Thus, the SCT therapist is not trying to educate clients when, late in the first session, he or she offers a reframing of their presenting problem. Rather, the therapist uses reframing as an exercise in informed consent. In the reframe, the therapist shares with the couple his or her preliminary view of the structural features implicated in the genesis and/or maintenance of the presenting problem. Perhaps more importantly, the reframe also provides clients a glimpse into their therapist's systemic worldview.

To decrease the chance that clients experience reframing as a "teaching" intervention, reframes are frequently cast in metaphorical language. Metaphors, by their very nature, produce more an experiential than an intellectual impact. Note the metaphorical language in the following reframe with a couple who presented the wife's auditory hallucinations as the focus for treatment. Minuchin, who was providing a consultation to the couple's therapist, began by talking to the wife Nina about her "voices."

MINUCHIN: Your voices can be tamed. But they need other voices. Voices just as strong, to fight them. Do you hear Juan's voice? . . .

NINA: No. Never.

MINUCHIN: Ah. [His] voice [is] too soft.

JUAN: She doesn't tell me when the voices talk to her. Only afterward. So I don't know when they talk to her.

NINA: He doesn't mean it like that. He means that you should be strong around the house.

MINUCHIN (*to Nina*): If Juan's voice were stronger, he could tame the voices you hear. The ones that tell you to punish yourself. (Minuchin et al., 2006, p. 116)

A very small percentage of client couples respond to the therapist's reframing of their presenting problem in the first session by leaving therapy. These are couples who presumably find the causal theory about their presenting problem conveyed in the reframe, and perhaps furthermore, the systemic worldview informing the reframe, too foreign to be entertained. The therapist who conceives of reframing as an exercise in informed consent is not disheartened by the exit of these couples from therapy. Having found the SCT therapist's view of their situation unacceptable, these couples, in leaving therapy, are doing exactly what they should be doing: rejecting a treatment whose rationale they find spurious, and mounting a search for a treatment whose underlying worldview fits more closely with their own.

Although the client couples who remain in therapy following the reframing—and these comprise the vast majority—presumably do not experience the causal theory expressed in the reframing as being toxic, as do the couples who leave, it would be incorrect to assume that they simply accept the reframe; quite the contrary, in fact. Most couples devote the bulk of their energy during the next few sessions to attempts to refute the reframe. Some do so explicitly, trying to engage the therapist in a debate about the view of the presenting problem contained in the reframe. Most do so behaviorally, continuing to act in ways that are consonant with their original, linear view of their situation.

The SCT therapist not only expects this response from clients, but he or she actually welcomes it. Clients' "resistance," not only to reframing but also to the therapist's ensuing interventions, helps to shape and to particularize treatment that the SCT therapist delivers.

In addition to its assumption of competence, SCT is also characterized by an "assumption of uniqueness," an assumption that "whatever characteristics it may share with other [couples], each [couple] is fundamentally unique" (Simon, 1995, p. 20). The SCT therapist welcomes clients' struggle against reframing and ensuing interventions, because he or she sees this struggle as representing at least in part clients' assertion of their uniqueness. Seeing "resistance" in this way allows the therapist to think of interventions as tentative probes that provide feedback on a given couple's uniqueness, rather than as specifically targeted change attempts that, because of their very specificity, can only be evaluated either as having "succeeded" or "failed" (Minuchin & Fishman, 1981; cf. Giacomo & Weissmark, 1986).

Because, under the influence of the assumption of uniqueness, the SCT therapist conceives of interventions as probes, he or she allows the particular ways a couple struggles with and against interventions to shape the next series of interventions he or she delivers. Without doubt, that next series of interventions will continue to be guided by the therapist's overarching, generic goal of changing the couple subsystem structure. However, by struggling against interventions, client couples progressively "teach" the therapist, as they simultaneously discover for themselves, what idiosyncratic arrangement, drawn from their reservoir of unutilized resources, they will crystallize as an adaptive alternative to the dysfunctional structure being challenged by the therapist's interventions. It is by struggling with and against the SCT therapist's interventions that the client couple collaborates with the therapist in guiding therapy toward an outcome that, in the end, will be as much informed by the couple's idiosyncratic style, outlook, values, and relational resources, as by the therapist's therapeutic ideology. It is by struggling with and against the therapist's interventions that the client couple participates in setting goals for the therapy.

Role of the Therapist

The fundamental task of the SCT therapist is to help the client couple replace its dysfunctional structure, which is maintaining the couple's presenting problem, with a more adaptive structure. SCT's assumptions of competence and uniqueness lead the therapist to expect that this new structure will emerge from the wellsprings of clients' latent, idiosyncratic resources. Thus, the SCT therapist does not function in the change process as a supplier of adaptive alternatives to the couple; rather, he or she is an *activator* of relational resources that are assumed to lie latent in the client couple's repertoire as the couple enters the therapy.

As highlighted earlier, SCT's assumption of circular causality leads to the view that the most therapeutically relevant cause of human behavior is here-and-now relational experience. Thus, the SCT therapist considers the mechanism of change in therapy to be the production, via enactment, of new relational experiences for clients. By providing the opportunity in session for couple members to experience each other in new ways, the therapist acts to dislodge the self-reinforcing, circular interactional loops that maintain the couple's presenting problem and to help the couple to stabilize more functional, problem-free loops.

The desire to make enactment the centerpiece of the change process in therapy places stringent requirements on both the level of activity and the kind of activity in which the SCT therapist should engage. As regards level of activity, the therapist certainly needs to be active enough to induce clients to begin using relational competencies that are currently being suppressed by the couple subsystem's dysfunctional structure. At the same time, however, the therapist must avoid becoming so active as to centralize him- or herself in the therapy process, with the result that clients spend more time talking with the therapist than with each other.

As regards the kind of activity in which he or she should engage, the SCT therapist is once again guided by the assumption of circular causality. Because SCT assumes that here-and-now relational experience is primarily responsible for eliciting and maintaining human behavior, the therapist uses *how clients experience him or her* as the chief means to activate their latent relational resources.

A concrete example helps to illustrate how the SCT therapist functions to elicit change in therapy. Let us imagine a hypothetical couple subsystem, whose lack of internal differentiation manifests itself in a rigid overfunctioning–underfunctioning role structure. This couple's therapist notes how the complementary role structure informs in-session enactments, with the overfunctioning member invariably taking the lead to organize and to keep on-task any conversation that the therapist elicits between the partners. The therapist also notes how the underfunctioning member invites and reinforces this behavior on the part of the partner, by never taking the lead in conversations and never objecting when the partner leaps in to "help" when the underfunctioning member pauses, even briefly, in what he has to say.

The therapist assumes that both partners are fully capable of behaving differently toward each other. He wishes to elicit an enactment characterized by greater symmetry, with both couple members exercising roughly equal initiative in overtly organizing and leading the conversation.

To elicit such a change-producing enactment, the therapist needs to do something in session to induce the underfunctioning member of the couple to surrender the passive posture that he invariably assumes when dealing with his partner. Structural theory informs the therapist that there is little chance of succeeding in this endeavor if the underfunctioning partner experiences the therapist in the same way he experiences his partner. Thus, the therapist must avoid behaving in the highly active, "helpful" way that the partner does. So, the therapist enters into a conversation with the underfunctioning partner. In this conversation, the therapist works hard to maintain a low-key posture, trying always to follow the client's lead rather than leading in a manner that

is isomorphic with the way the partner usually behaves.

The underfunctioning partner does not immediately respond to the therapist's behavior by increasing his activity level. For a couple of awkward minutes, the conversation between therapist and client becomes a stilted contest of competing minimalism. The therapist's experience of the client during these moments exerts a powerful pull to begin behaving in the same way that the overfunctioning partner does. However, the therapist resists the temptation and maintains a low-key posture. In response, the client begins to increase his activity level in the conversation, until, a few minutes later, the underfunction partner is leading and organizing the conversation in a way he almost never does when interacting with his partner.

The therapist does not consider this shift in the client's behavior all that newsworthy. It comes as no surprise that the client is capable of behaving in this way. SCT's assumption of competence predicted as much. All that has been established thus far is that in a relational context different from the one that holds sway between the partners, the underfunctioning client can behave differently and more adaptively. The therapist needs now to produce an interaction between the partners in which the underfunctioning client behaves toward the partner as he has begun behaving toward the therapist. Thus, the therapist allows the conversation with the underfunctioning client to continue only long enough for the client to develop some momentum in the exercise of the new relational behavior displayed toward the therapist. After a couple of minutes, the therapist elicits an enactment, asking the client to continue the conversation with his partner. Once the enactment begins, the therapist falls silent and begins to observe.

The therapist pays very careful attention to the ensuing enactment, of course, and is interested to see whether the couple's interaction in the enactment becomes informed by a new, more adaptive structure, or reverts instead to its old, dysfunctional organization. However, of far greater import to the therapist than the gross "success" or "failure" of the enactment are the details of *how* it "succeeds" or "fails." SCT's assumption of uniqueness leads the therapist to consider the enactment an opportunity to learn about the idiosyncratic features that render this client couple different from all others. If the enactment "succeeds" in eliciting a new structural arrangement for the couple's interaction, the therapist is interested in seeing the particular ways in which the formerly underfunctioning partner and the formerly overfunctioning partner begin to collaborate in implementing a more even distribution of relational responsibility. If the enactment "fails," with the couple reverting to the old structural arrangement, the therapist uses observation of the step-by-step process of this reversion to learn more about this couple's values and belief system, and about the subjective experience of each couple member. Regardless of whether the enactment "succeeds" or "fails," the therapist uses what he gleans from the enactment about this couple's uniqueness to refine his next attempt to activate the couple's latent relational resources.

As illustrated in this hypothetical vignette, the SCT therapist's role as an activator of latent resources causes his or her behavior in therapy to become organized into an oscillating pattern, in which periods of relatively high activity level alternate with periods of relative inactivity (cf. Simon, 1992, 1993). During the former periods, the therapist strategically presents him- or herself to the couple in a manner designed to induce one or both partners to behave differently than they do when they interact with each other. During the latter periods, the therapist functions as observer of enactments in which one or both partners attempt to extend the novel behavior begun during their interaction with the therapist into their relationship with each other.

The SCT therapist's oscillation between engaged activity and relatively disengaged inactivity may aptly be compared to the behavior of a person who is directing a play in which he or she also acts. (Minuchin [1984] has always been a devotee of the theater. It is, therefore, not surprising that the model of therapy that he helped develop has distinctly theatrical characteristics.) The therapist functions much like the director of a play when eliciting enactments between couple members. The therapist functions as an actor during those moments in therapy when he or she strategically assumes a certain relational posture toward one or both couple members, in an effort to elicit novel behavior from them.

Comparing the SCT therapist to the director–actor of a play not only illuminates the role of the therapist but also provides insight into the clinician attributes required to practice this model successfully. The SCT therapist needs to possess components and qualities of both the "director" and "actor" roles.

Though he or she will certainly get a chance to act in the therapeutic play that he or she is di-

recting, the SCT therapist's "onstage" moments are distinctly those of supporting cast. The couple members have the starring roles in the therapeutic play. As a result, the SCT therapist needs to be comfortable spending much of the therapy "offstage," exercising his or her role as director by quietly monitoring enactments between the couple members.

Operating for much of the therapy in this noncentralized position requires that the SCT therapist have a certain temperament. He or she must be comfortable with not always being the center of attention in any group. The therapist whose interactional repertoire does not include the role of interested-but-silent observer will inexorably centralize him- or herself in the therapeutic process, a position that is incompatible with the SCT therapist's role of director.

As an actor in the therapeutic drama—albeit in the role of supporting cast—the therapist needs to be able to manipulate the presentation of him- or herself to clients, varying that self-presentation deliberately and strategically based on the exigencies of the current moment of a given therapy. The therapist needs to be a person who can present him- or herself as either proximal and soft or as distant and critical, as expert or as confused, as jocular or as serious, as vulnerable or as impassable. The SCT therapist needs, therefore, to be in possession of a complex and varied interpersonal repertoire. Moreover, the therapist, just like an actor, needs to be able, or to develop the ability, to activate, more or less on demand, that element in his or her repertoire that fits the "scene" in which he or she is acting (Minuchin et al., 2006).

Even if he or she possesses the requisite personal characteristics I have just outlined, the SCT therapist will not be able to exercise the role as director–actor of the therapeutic drama unless the clients, who are the "stars" of that drama, allow it. Thus, like therapists of all persuasions, the SCT therapist must devote effort to forging an alliance with clients. How the therapist goes about creating this alliance bears the unmistakable imprint of SCT's fundamentally experiential nature. The therapist connects with a couple by modifying his or her manner of self-presentation in such a way that he or she is experienced by the couple as an "insider," someone whose bearing, language, pacing, and all-around "style" fit with that of the couple subsystem.

Achieving this stylistic fit with the client system is what SCT therapists refer to when they talk about "joining" (Minuchin, 1974; Minuchin

& Fishman, 1981), a word that has come to mean many things as it has gained widespread currency beyond the borders of structural therapy in the mental health field. In common clinical parlance, "joining" frequently means being supportive and/ or empathic. However, being supportive and empathic will only join a therapist to a couple subsystem in which supportive and empathic transactions are the coin of the realm. Such behavior will not join a therapist, for example, to couple members who maintain their connection to each other via endless rounds of debate and refutation. To join with such a couple, the therapist needs to join in the debating, understanding that, in this system, disagreement, far from being an indicator of disconnection, is rather a mechanism for connection.

Joining is simultaneously an automatic and a deliberate maneuver on the part of the therapist (Minuchin & Fishman, 1981). Both of these aspects of joining need to be present for it to be effective. When joining is only deliberate and strategic, it is likely to be experienced by clients as lacking in genuineness, and so will fail, perhaps leading the couple to leave therapy prematurely. When, on the other hand, joining occurs in a completely automatic and unconscious way, the therapist likely becomes too much of an "insider" to the couple subsystem and winds up being as constrained as the clients themselves by the subsystem's current structure. The therapist in such a situation loses the freedom to behave strategically in ways that induce couple members to activate the latent relational resources that are currently being suppressed by the couple subsystem structure. The resulting therapy is likely to be comfortable for all the participants, including the therapist, but for that very reason, incapable of producing change.

Technical Aspects of the Therapeutic Process

Because each client couple is unique, every course of SCT is in some ways also unique. Nonetheless, there is sufficient resemblance between courses of SCT that are successful to allow me to make some generalizations about how a "typical" course of SCT evolves over time. To make these generalizations, I return to the theatrical metaphor I employed in the last section to illuminate the role of the therapist in SCT. If a course of SCT is thought of as a play, in which the therapist functions as

director and supporting actor, then it typically is a play in two acts, with a brief prologue.

Prologue: The Director and Actors Meet

The curious thing about the play that is SCT, is that it is already in progress when the director comes on the scene. The script for this play has been provided by the couple subsystem structure, and the couple members have been following this script for an extended period of time prior to the commencement of therapy. The script has given rise to a problem that has motivated the couple to seek treatment.

As the couple members enter the first session, they are substantially focused on their presenting problem, and only minimally, if at all, on the structural script that has elicited and/or is maintaining the problem. The SCT therapist, in distinction, is primarily focused on the couple subsystem structure, because it is by means of a change in that structure that the therapist undertakes to alleviate the clients' presenting problem. Thus, in most cases, the first meeting finds the director and the actors of the therapeutic drama looking in different directions. This state of affairs needs to be rectified quickly, if the therapeutic play is to move toward a satisfying end.

The primary agenda of the first session in SCT is construction of a consensus between director and actors regarding what the therapeutic play is going to be about. Not only is the pending therapeutic drama talked about during the first session, the session itself constitutes the opening scene of that drama, functioning as its prologue.

For the first session to perform its function as prologue to the therapeutic play, the therapist must execute several tasks during the session, many of them simultaneously. The therapist opens the session by asking the couple members to inform him or her about the problem that has brought them into therapy. As the clients begin to tell the story about their presenting problem, the therapist immediately begins the process of joining, allowing him- or herself to feel the "pull" exerted by the couple, by their pacing, their use of language, and their demeanor and carriage; the therapist accommodates, in his or her own idiosyncratic way, to the couple's style, hoping that the couple members quickly begin to experience him or her as someone who "fits" who they are as a couple.

After giving the clients ample time to narrate their view of the presenting problem, but long before a focus on the problem is allowed to dominate the session, the therapist moves the session toward an assessment of the relational structure that, in the view of SCT, is circularly linked to the couple's presenting problem. The therapist looks for and/or creates opportunities to elicit enactments focused on the partners' differences, using his or her experience of these enactments to begin constructing hypotheses about how internal differentiation is handled within the couple subsystem, and how this differentiation is circularly linked to the permeability of the boundary surrounding the couple.

Almost all client couples allow themselves to be nudged by the therapist during this middle part of the first session, away from a focus on their presenting problem toward an exploration of their relational structure. However, most clients expect, and in my view, have the right to expect, that the therapist will make clear sooner rather than later the connection between the relational structure that he or she has been exploring and the presenting problem that the clients entered therapy to resolve. Thus, the necessary finale to the first session is the provision of the therapist's preliminary formulation as to how the client couple's presenting problem is being elicited and/or maintained by the couple subsystem structure. The therapist provides this formulation in the reframe, described earlier.

Act I: Destabilizing the Old Structure

The return of the client couple for the second session marks the opening of Act I of the therapeutic play. The fact that the actors show up for the second session indicates that they have agreed to "play" with the dramatic script proposed by the therapist–director in the reframe. This is certainly not to say, however, that the actors have accepted their director's script lock, stock, and barrel. Many couples enter the second session with revisions to the therapist's script in hand–revisions that render that script less discrepant with the script they have already been following: "You don't understand. It really *is* all her fault that we argue so much" or "You don't understand. In the face of his obsessiveness, I *have* to act the way I do." Even couples who enter the second session expressing complete acceptance of the therapist's reframe have, in all likelihood, spent the entire time since the first session living out their old structural script with little, if any, change.

The SCT therapist is not in the least surprised by or chagrined at the structural inertia that the client couple almost invariably displays at the beginning of the second session. The therapist, after all, did not expect the reframe to impact the structure of the couple subsystem substantially. As noted earlier, the SCT therapist conceives of reframing as an exercise in informed consent rather than as a restructuring intervention.

The therapist begins in the second session, and in the several sessions that follow, to provide couple members with opportunities to enact in session new, more adaptive structural arrangements. Inevitably, however, this experimentation with a new relational script occurs in the context of clients' long experience of having lived out their old script. As problematic as that old script might be, it is familiar and predictable to the client couple. The partners know their lines well, and the long run that their play has had has given them confidence that they can act their assigned parts to perfection.

As a result, clients' predominant experience during the first several sessions of SCT is the unsettling one of being asked by their therapist to leave that which is relationally familiar to them. Almost invariably, clients respond to this unsettling experience with attempts to hold on to their old relational structure. Thus, a polemic of sorts develops between director and actors—a polemic that quickly comes to dominate the first act of the therapeutic play. Whereas the therapist continually asks clients to experiment with new relational arrangements, the clients continually, sometimes subtly and sometimes not so subtly, try to alleviate their discomfort by reverting to their old relational arrangement. As I demonstrate shortly, this polemic usually builds until a crisis point is reached.

Enactment is the primary tool used by the SCT therapist during the first act of the therapeutic play to begin changing the structure of the couple subsystem. Depending on how it is used, enactment can target for change either the external boundary or the internal structure of the couple subsystem.

Recall that an excessively rigid or diffuse external boundary is a common structural characteristic of dysfunctional couple subsystems. During enactments, the permeability of the external boundary of the couple subsystem is manifest in the manner in which the partners include or excludes the therapist from their interaction. Thus, by strategically varying how much he or she enters into enactments, or refuses to enter into enactments, the therapist can begin to influence the permeability of the couple's external boundary.

For example, let us consider a highly reactive, conflict-ridden couple subsystem, whose reactivity is circularly linked to a high disagree of disengagement from the external world. During the first act of the therapeutic play the SCT therapist is likely to elicit numerous enactments between the partners. Left to their own devices during these enactments, the partners tend to escalate quickly into episodes of intense conflict. The partners are so reactive to each other during these episodes of conflict that the therapist as a third party in the room almost disappears from their awareness. The therapist can begin modifying this rigid boundary between the couple and the outside world by frequently inserting him- or herself into the interaction between the partners, and by demanding that the partners accommodate to his or her input. The therapist predictably experiences considerable difficulty making his or her influence felt in the face of the intense emotionality of the couple's interaction. Nonetheless, the therapist must construct interventions that contain sufficient intensity to "puncture" the rigid boundary surrounding the couple subsystem. The content of the therapist's input in these interventions is far less important than the process of inserting him- or herself into the couple's interaction. It is in asking for and gaining the attention of the clients in the midst of their interaction that the therapist begins to modify the rigidity of the boundary surrounding this couple subsystem.

As a second example, let us consider a client couple in which the partners' underinvolvement with each other is circularly linked to their enmeshment with people outside the relationship. Enactments between the partners that are elicited by the therapist during the first act of the therapeutic play are always exceedingly brief, ending with one or both partners exiting the conversation with the other and attempting to talk instead with the therapist. By simply declining to engage with the clients at this juncture, and sending them back into their interaction with each other, the therapist begins to enhance the solidity of the boundary surrounding this couple subsystem.

By simply regulating how much he or she enters into enactments, the SCT therapist can, during the first act of therapy, exert a direct influence on the external boundary surrounding the client couple. Because all structural elements of a system are linked by loops of circular causality, in the process, the therapist also exerts an indirect influence on the internal structure of the couple subsystem. However, the therapist can also use enactments to exert a direct influence on this internal structure.

I have already described, in the section on the therapist's role, the way the SCT therapist uses enactment to exert direct influence on the internal organization of a couple subsystem. Functioning briefly as a supporting actor in the therapeutic drama, the therapist strategically manipulates his or her manner of self-presentation to the clients, with an eye toward inducing one or both of them to begin utilizing relational competencies that are currently suppressed by their maladaptive structure. Once such competencies have been activated in the interaction between therapist and client(s), the therapist, functioning now as director, elicits an enactment so that the competencies can be extended into clients' dealings with each other.

Because each client couple is unique, the way the therapist needs to "act" to activate latent relational competencies varies considerably from case to case. Still, there is sufficient commonality among cases to allow the identification of two "supporting roles" the SCT therapist plays with some regularity during Act I of the therapeutic play.

The therapist frequently encounters couple subsystems in which lack of differentiation between the partners is manifested in extreme conflict avoidance. Faced with such a couple, the SCT therapist would like to elicit enactments that provide the partners with an experience of adaptive, productive conflict. Doing so requires the therapist to instigate a fight that the clients have been avoiding. To "incite" this kind of conflict, the therapist needs to act in a manner designed to "lend" indignation to one of the partners. This manner of self-presentation by the therapist has been termed "unbalancing" in the literature of structural therapy (Minuchin & Fishman, 1981).

Unbalancing is illustrated by the following dialogue between a therapist and a woman whose conflict-avoidant marriage has deteriorated to the point that both spouses have begun to consider divorce. The woman typically assumes a one-down posture vis-à-vis her husband. The therapist begins the dialogue by inserting himself into an enactment in which the one-up–one-down complementarity between the spouses has played itself out, with the husband lecturing his silent wife on how she has brought their marriage to the brink of demise.

THERAPIST: Denise, may I ask you something? I was just listening to the conversation that you and your husband were having. Do you get the impression that he thinks that he's more intelligent than you? It seems to me that he was just lecturing you as if you were his student.

WIFE: (*speaking to husband*) You see, other people see it, too!

THERAPIST: I find it curious that you allow him to speak to you that way. As I see you, you are every bit as intelligent as he, in some ways more so. It seems to me that you have greater awareness of what's going on in your marriage than he does.

WIFE: (*visibly blushing and looking away*) Well, maybe.

THERAPIST: The thing is, the way you deal with your husband allows him to continue in the mistaken impression that he has more on the ball than you. And that is clearly a mistaken notion. Why aren't you more vocal in telling him your point of view?

WIFE: He won't listen.

THERAPIST: I know that you're right, because I have seen him dismiss you. But I think that the survival of your marriage depends on your perspective becoming as visible as his. You need to get him to listen to you. Talk with him now and see whether you can get him to take you seriously.

Having endeavored to "lend" the wife some indignation over her one-down status in the couple subsystem, the therapist elicits an enactment, hoping to see in that enactment the beginning of an airing of the conflict that has been driving the spouses apart but has rarely emerged into the open.

For several reasons, unbalancing is a difficult "role" for the SCT therapist to play well (Minuchin & Fishman, 1981). To begin with, its implementation is at odds with SCT's core assumption of circular causality. In the previous vignette, for example, structural theory assumes that each spouse elicits the behavior of the other. The wife is as responsible for casting her husband in the one-up position he occupies as he is for casting her in the one-down position. Yet to produce an enactment in which the currently avoided conflict is aired, the therapist needs to act as if the husband is the sole culprit. Since the therapist does not believe that such is the case, acting in this way does indeed require quite the job of "acting."

Adding to the difficulty of the "role" of unbalancing is the fact that to "lend" indignation effectively to a client who is reluctant to engage in or prolong conflict, the therapist must behave in fairly provocative ways. Only a therapist who is comfortable engaging in productive relational conflict will have the stomach to engage in such therapeutic provocation.

Finally, unbalancing, if it is effective, inevitably disrupts the therapist's alliance with the "target" partner. To appreciate this fact, just put yourself in the shoes of the husband in the previous vignette and fantasize how you would feel about the therapist at that moment. Thus, effective unbalancing requires of the therapist an exquisite balancing act: to maintain the unbalanced posture long enough to produce the desired effect of eliciting or prolonging in-session conflict, but not so long as to disrupt irreversibly the alliance with the "target" partner. Indeed, to reestablish equilibrium within the therapeutic system, the SCT therapist frequently follows a period of extensive unbalancing on one partner's behalf with a period in which he or she unbalances on behalf of the other.

Avoidance of couple conflict is a common structural characteristic of families with a child identified patient. Because structural therapy was devoted almost entirely to the treatment of such families during the first decades of its development, unbalancing occupied a prominent place in the structural therapy literature of that period. However, when therapists began to apply structural therapy to couples who presented themselves for treatment precisely as couples rather than as parents of a child identified patient, they found themselves facing the need to supplement unbalancing with another kind of intervention.

Many couples that SCT therapists have encountered during the past 20 years are characterized by conflict that is vigorously aired rather than avoided. Indeed, for many of these couples, it is precisely their chronic and intractable conflict that is the presenting problem in the treatment they are seeking. Although unbalancing might be of some use in the treatment of these couples, genuine restructuring of these couple subsystems requires not the amplification of conflict, which is the goal of unbalancing, but the replacement of conflict with more supportive modes of transaction. To elicit this relational competence, the SCT therapist needs to soften the typically harsh transactions between these partners. "Softening," then, constitutes the second "role" that SCT therapists play with some regularity during Act I of the therapeutic drama.

Examples of softening can be cited from the earlier structural therapy literature (e.g., see Minuchin & Fishman, 1981, p. 167). However, due to the limited call for the use of this intervention with the families that were the focus of structural therapy at that time, softening never developed into an explicit category of intervention in this literature. This lack of a detailed understanding of softening as an intervention in structural therapy is the model's practical weakness I mentioned early in this chapter when it is applied to the treatment of couples.

Although softening is not discussed thematically in the literature of structural therapy, it is the centerpiece of another approach to couple therapy. Emotionally focused therapy (EFT), developed by Greenberg and Johnson (1988; Johnson, 2004), utilizes an intervention called "softening" to help clients access and express to their partners soft, vulnerable, attachment-related emotions.

Because EFT has spawned a literature on softening (e.g., see Bradley & Furrow, 2004), it would be foolish for SCT therapists to ignore EFT's conceptualization of softening as they attempt to discern and to describe the role this intervention plays in SCT. However, I have argued that there exist significant differences in underlying worldview between structural therapy and EFT (Simon, 2004, 2006b). These differences in underlying philosophical assumptions render softening in SCT a substantially different intervention than softening in EFT.

Softening in SCT begins with the therapist him- or herself assuming a soft posture to induce—almost hypnotically—one or both couple members to begin acting softly. Just as the SCT therapist "lends" indignation during unbalancing, he or she "lends" vulnerability during softening.

As the SCT therapist engages in a soft exchange with one or both couple members, he or she looks for the first opportunity to move offstage and to cede the therapeutic drama back to its stars. The therapist maintains the dialogue with one or both clients during softening just long enough to produce the kind of soft, affiliative atmosphere that he or she would like to see stabilized within the couple subsystem. Once that atmosphere has been established, the therapist elicits an enactment between the partners, asking them to maintain the softened mood in their interaction with each other. The therapist then retreats offstage to observe the scene.

The following vignette illustrates the use of softening in SCT. A young married couple requested therapy to address the problem of episodes of intense conflict, followed by extended periods of disengagement from each other. During the first-session prologue of this particular therapeutic drama, the therapist noted that during their periods of conflictual engagement, the spouses were rigidly organized into a complementary pattern of attack (wife)–defend (husband). The couple entered the fourth session in the midst of one of these conflictual episodes. The therapist elicited an enactment, so that the episode could play itself out in the therapy room.

During this go-round of the patterned conflict, the wife was attacking her husband for what she saw as his potentially abusive drinking. Had the therapist wanted to modify the way in which conflict was handled within this couple subsystem, he could easily have intervened during this session by unbalancing on the husband's behalf. However, he had not assessed management of conflict to be this couple's most salient structural difficulty. This couple had no problem airing conflict, and the partners contained their conflict within the boundaries of the couple subsystem. The problem here was that conflict was literally almost the only thing these partners did together. When they were not fighting, their disengagement from each other was almost complete. The therapist judged that the structural change most needed to resolve the presenting problem was the establishment of a more affiliative mode of connection between the spouses. He decided to move toward this structural goal by softening the interaction that was taking place before him during the fourth session.

During the enactment, the wife kept talking about how "concerned" she was about her husband's drinking. Her manner as she used this word bespoke fury rather than worry. The therapist interrupted the enactment after it had proceeded for about 5 minutes.

THERAPIST: (*softly, rolling his chair closer to the couple*) Trish, you've been telling Kevin how concerned you are about his drinking. Tell me what scares you about his drinking.

WIFE: (*after a brief pause, looking a bit nonplussed*) It concerns me that he needs to drink to have a good time.

THERAPIST: Do you think he knows how much seeing him drink frightens you? Do you think he knows how scared you get?

WIFE: (*appearing to struggle to hold back some emotion*) No.

THERAPIST: He certainly knows how angry his drinking makes you, but I don't think he has a clue how much it terrifies you. Do you know why it scares you so much?

WIFE: (*wrapping her jacket tightly around her as she begins to cry softly*) My father was an alcoholic.

THERAPIST: Ah, now I see why his drinking scares you so. Can you tell him now about the fear that you feel when you see him drinking?

The wife stares speechless at her husband for about 30 seconds, while she continues to cry softly. Finally she begins to tell him how frightened she feels when she sees him drink, even though she never really has seen him drink to intoxication. As she speaks with him in this vein, he tentatively reaches out and takes her hand in his.

Whether they occur in the context of unbalancing, softening, or some other "role" played by the therapist as supporting actor in the therapeutic drama, enactments during Act I of that drama inevitably have the effect of introducing a wedge between the partners and the familiar structure that informed their transactions when they entered therapy. This is so, despite the fact that the couple subsystem usually reverts to its old structure, sometimes during the enactments themselves, and almost invariably between sessions. However, even when the partners revert in this way, they generally find that they simply cannot play out their old structural script in the same un-self-conscious way they did prior to the onset of therapy, due to the fact that they are now playing it out in the context of having enacted alternatives to the old script. Their experience during the first act of therapy is thus one of living in a kind of limbo. A new structure has not yet stabilized within the couple subsystem, and the old structure has begun to feel a bit alien.

Living in this limbo is a disorienting experience for clients. In most cases, somewhere around the fourth or fifth session, this experience of disorientation exceeds clients' capacity to bear it comfortably. Most couples at this point seek to relieve their discomfort by making a last-ditch attempt to retrieve their old relational structure. This attempt at retrieval is usually enabled by a crisis, marked by the resurgence, perhaps beyond baseline levels, of the presenting problem that served as the occasion for the commencement of treatment. Recall that in the systemic universe of SCT, a loop of circular

causality exists between the presenting problem and the couple subsystem structure, each eliciting and maintaining the other. Precisely because their presenting problem was intimately linked to their old relational structure, a resurgence of the problem provides clients with an opportunity to retrieve the "gusto" in playing out their old structural script of which the therapy has deprived them.

A crisis occurring around the fourth or fifth session of therapy is generally a sign of a course of SCT that is on its way to succeeding. Interestingly, in their research project designed to test the efficacy of structural therapy in the treatment of young adult heroin addicts, Stanton et al. (1982) found that a characteristic shared by most failed cases was the therapy's failure to generate such a crisis.

Although the occurrence of a therapeutic crisis during Act I of the therapeutic drama enhances the prognosis for the therapy, such an occurrence, in and of itself, is not sufficient to ensure a positive outcome. How the therapist responds to the crisis is a crucial factor in determining whether the therapy proceeds to a successful outcome. Should the crisis manage to deter the therapist from continued efforts to dislodge the old structure of the couple subsystem, the therapy will likely fail. If, on the other hand, the therapist continues restructuring efforts in the face of the crisis, then the development of the therapeutic drama toward a successful outcome is likely to continue. Indeed, an appropriate response of the therapist to the crisis usually ushers in the end of Act I of the therapeutic play. Somewhere around the sixth or seventh session, Act II begins.

Act II: Nurturing the New Structure

The therapist–director's maintenance of dramatic vision in the face of the first-act crisis has an important effect on the therapeutic play's actors. Within a couple of sessions of the occurrence of the crisis, the actors finally surrender whatever "nostalgia" they retained for their old structural script. Freed from their lingering loyalty to the old script, clients begin to devote their undivided attention to exercising their competence and uniqueness in the crystallization of a new relational structure that, while different from the one that organized the couple subsystem at the outset of therapy, still expresses those idiosyncratic elements that make this couple different from all others. This disappearance of the actors' divided loyalty between their old script and their director's vision marks the start of Act II of the therapeutic drama.

Several behavioral indicators signal the therapy's transition to Act II. The most telling of these is a palpable shift in initiative between director and actors. During Act I, the client–actors' inertial tendency back toward their old script required that the therapist be prominent in functioning as both director of and as a supporting actor in the therapeutic play. While maintaining an overall posture of moderate activity level, the therapist did engage with some frequency in episodes of relatively high activity, as described in the previous section. When Act II begins, on the other hand, clients' heightened commitment to the therapeutic process reduces the therapist's need to operate as either director or supporting cast. Couple members begin to engage spontaneously in enactments during this act, without the therapist having first to set the mood and to choreograph the scene. During these self-initiated enactments, couple members engage in a kind of self-propelled search for alternative ways of relating that occurs rarely, if ever, during Act I. With the clients having claimed the initiative for the development of the therapeutic drama, the therapist is able to leave aside much of the directorial and acting responsibilities, and to assume instead the position of "audience."

This is not to say, of course, that the therapist is entirely inactive during Act II. However, although the therapist does intervene, that intervening has a very different tonality than it had during the first act. Functioning primarily as audience during Act II, the therapist does what audiences do: applaud. Indeed, applause is the main way that the therapist influences the shape of the play during Act II. Some of the enactments in which clients spontaneously engage during Act II clearly represent adaptive new structural arrangements for the couple subsystem. The therapist occasionally punctuates such enactments with "applause," congratulating the clients for the wonderful job they did during the enactments and noting how adaptive their interaction was in the enactments.

Some of the enactments that occur during Act II are organized by structural arrangements that, though different from the couple's original structure, are, in the estimation of the therapist, not adaptive for the couple in the long run. However, the therapist does not overtly criticize or challenge these enactments. The fluid state of the couple subsystem structure during the second act renders such "gross" interventions unnecessary. All the therapist need do to reduce the chances that the maladaptive structure informing these enactments becomes stabilized within the couple subsystem is to withhold applause at the end of the enactment. Such silence on the part of the therapist is a powerful intervention in the climate of Act II.

The diminished posture of the therapist during Act II makes termination in SCT a relatively brief and uncomplicated process. After the second act has gone on for a few sessions, it becomes obvious to all the members of the therapeutic system that the therapist has grown more or less superfluous to the couple's already incipiently successful efforts to crystallize a new, more adaptive structure. Thus, it feels like an organic development to all involved when, somewhere around the eighth to 10th session, the therapist wonders aloud whether the clients feel that termination of the therapy might be imminent. Generally, clients agree that it is, indeed, time to terminate the treatment. Sometimes, termination occurs during the very session that the issue is raised; other times, clients agree that the next session should be the last.

APPLICABILITY AND EMPIRICAL SUPPORT

SCT, like all psychotherapeutic approaches, is not effective in all cases. It would be convenient if the cases in which the model is not helpful shared some easily discernible demographic or clinical characteristics. Then, referral to some other, more applicable form of treatment could be made before clients and therapist had devoted effort and resources to a failed course of therapy. Unfortunately, at this time, no research identifies readily observable characteristics shared by failed cases of SCT.

It is certain that the nature of a couple's presenting complaint is not correlated with the outcome of SCT. Couples in which one or both partners describe discrete symptoms as their presenting complaint are no less likely to benefit from SCT than couples who define their presenting problem in relational terms. Likewise, demographic variable are not correlated with outcome. Structural therapy developed out of Minuchin and colleagues' work with urban, poor families. However, over the years, the model has proven helpful in work with all social classes, with families and couples representing numerous ethnic groups, with both homosexual and heterosexual couples, and in numerous countries (Greenan & Tunnell, 2003; Minuchin et al., 2006, 2007).

SCT is also not limited in applicability to couples who define themselves as having a shared future. Because the goal of SCT is to produce an adaptive structure for the client system, the model can be applied to divorcing and divorced couples, as well as it can to engaged and married couples, and to unmarried couples whose mutual commitment is not in question. To be sure, an adaptive structure for a divorced couple little resembles that of a married couple, with the result that the therapy of a divorced couple is likely to have a very different feel from that of a married couple. However, one of the strengths of SCT's single-minded focus on systemic structure is that it renders the model applicable to couples at every stage of coming together, staying together, or coming apart.

Despite SCT's broad scope of applicability, a few situations, described earlier in the chapter, require the therapist to refer rather than to begin treatment. If the therapist detects violence or abuse within the couple that is either not openly admitted or not acknowledged as problematic, the therapist needs to refer the abused partner to domestic violence services that will intervene to ensure her or his safety. Such a referral includes no prospect for the commencement of couple therapy any time soon, if at all. Referral is also the SCT therapist's first move if he or she detects psychiatric symptomatology in one or both partners that entails significant threat of harm to self or other. In such circumstances, the therapist makes the commencement of couple therapy contingent upon participation in a medication evaluation by the client(s) in question. Once the therapist is satisfied that the evaluation has occurred, and that the client has complied with recommendations made by the consulting psychiatrist, a normal course of SCT can begin.

The claims that I have made for the broad applicability of SCT find indirect empirical support in the extant outcome research literature about structural therapy. This literature provides only indirect support because, like the model itself, research on structural therapy's efficacy has tended to focus more on the model's application to family treatment, in which a child, adolescent, or young adult is presented as the identified patient, than on its application to couple therapy.

This limitation having been noted, however, the results of outcome research on structural therapy still deserve to be characterized as impressive. Research to date suggests that structural therapy is effective with widely varying populations, in the treatment of a host of widely varying presenting symptoms, including psychosomatic symptoms in children (Minuchin et al., 1975); anorexia in children (Minuchin et al., 1978); heroin addiction in young adults (Stanton et al., 1982); school adjustment, anxiety, depression, and withdrawal in adolescents diagnosed with attention-deficit/hyperactivity disorder (ADHD; Barkley, Guevremont, Anastopoulos, & Fletcher, 1992); conduct-disordered behavior in adolescents (Chamberlain & Rosicky, 1995; Santisteban et al., 2003; Szapocznik et al., 1989); and drug use in adolescents (Santisteban et al., 2003).

The treatment administered in all of these studies was based on the same theoretical assumptions and constructs, utilizing to a large degree the same interventions described in this chapter. Moreover, in the treatment of two-parent families, the therapy almost invariably attempted to restructure the parental subsystem in ways that are very similar to the ways that SCT attempts to restructure the couple subsystem. Thus, it is reasonable to conclude that these studies provide indirect evidence of the efficacy of SCT intervention principles across a broad range of presenting problems and client populations. However, indirect evidence is hardly sufficient in the face of the current quest for empirically supported psychotherapeutic practice. The field of marriage and family therapy stands in need of well-constructed research studies that provide a direct test of structural therapy's efficacy when applied to the treatment of couples.

CASE ILLUSTRATION

Joe, a 35-year-old police officer, contacted me to request couple therapy for himself and Anita, his wife of 10 years. Anita, a teacher, was also 35 years old. The couple had two young children, a 5-year-old boy and an 18-month-old daughter. Joe had been referred to me by a psychologist he had seen for a several-month course of individual therapy. That therapy ended by mutual consent, just about the time that the couple therapy began.

Anita and Joe impressed me early in the first session as a bright and engaging couple. I found the opening moments of ice-breaking chitchat with them genuinely enjoyable. When I came round to asking what had led them into my office, Joe and Anita were of one mind in designating Joe as the identified patient. Both agreed, woefully, that Joe underfunctioned in the familial context. Anita put it quite succinctly: "He doesn't listen, he forgets, he floats through life." Joe's underfunctioning was a problem for Anita, because she had to function for two when it came to executing the day-to-day tasks of running a household—not that Anita did not judge herself to be up to the challenge. She smiled in tacit agreement when Joe characterized her during the first session as "perfect" and "a rock." .

Both spouses linked Joe's underfunctioning to a diagnosis of ADHD that Joe had received from a physician when he was younger. I lightly called the accuracy of that diagnosis into question when a line of inquiry that I instigated with Joe about his work life revealed that he functioned on the job with exquisite attention to detail. I also pointed out how Joe's self-presentation in the session had changed utterly when he began to talk about work, his previous fumbling, self-deprecating posture replaced by calm self-confidence.

My exploration with Joe of his functioning as a police officer introduced an interruption into the couple's seamless, rehearsed narrative about their presenting problem. I recognized an opportunity to begin introducing relational themes into what had been up to that point a relentlessly symptom-focused discussion. I asked, at this point, for the first enactment of the first session: "Why don't the two of you talk together and see if you can solve this mystery of why a calm, cool, collected cop turns into a bumbling, sometimes disobedient child when he walks in the front door of his house?"

In the ensuing enactment, Anita immediately took charge of the conversation. Joe's self-confident posture evaporated in seconds. As Anita restated to Joe her contention that he was beset by cognitive and emotional deficits, he began to act in ways that perfectly fit her description of him. He lost track of the topic of the conversation. He answered several direct questions from Anita with an embarrassed "I don't know." He volunteered reminiscences of famous incidents in the past, when Anita had had to put right some egregious blunder he had made.

This enactment, and others that followed it during the first session, played out before my eyes the radical one-up–one-down, complementary role structure that Anita and Joe had described to me as characterizing their relational life at home. I was very attentive during these enactments to any signs of incipient conflict between the spouses. Indeed, there were moments when the camaraderie that Joe and Anita seemed to share in their scripted portrayal of him as an incompetent fool seemed to be replaced by annoyed frustration on both of their parts. These moments of frustration, however, never segued during first-session enact-

ments into episodes of even low-level conflict. Invariably, the outbreak of possible conflict was forestalled when the couple ended the enactment by turning to engage me in the conversation.

By late in the first session, these enactments, along with what the couple reported to me about their day-to-day life at home, allowed me to construct an assessment of the couple subsystem structure. I judged that Joe and Anita were a conflict-avoiding couple. Differentiation of perspective and skills was not permitted in the ethos of this couple subsystem. Only one perspective and set of skills was allowed to prevail, that belonging to Anita. The apparent differentiation between Anita and Joe, provided by the one-up and one-down roles that each partner so rigidly played, was in fact nothing more than pseudodifferentiation. As organized by this role structure, Joe was not Joe; he was simply the anti-Anita.

Inevitably, the lack of internal differentiation in the couple subsystem had impoverished and overburdened the subsystem. It was Anita who primarily experienced the overburdening, and Joe who primarily experienced the impoverishment. Anita's sense of being overburdened, and Joe's sense of being impoverished, led each partner from time to time to feel frustrated and angry. A good fight or two might have helped to derigidify this couple's relational structure. But the subsystem structure did not permit conflict in which differences would be aired. An extremely diffuse boundary surrounding the couple subsystem enabled Anita and Joe to avoid conflict almost completely. During first-session enactments, they avoided fighting by looking across that boundary to include me in their interactions. At home, the children, a multitude of instrumental tasks, and Joe's erratic work schedule as a police officer performed the same conflict-avoiding function that my presence did during the first session.

As all first sessions in SCT optimally do, my first session with Joe and Anita needed to close with a reframe that communicated my view that their presenting problem was inexorably linked to the relational structure I had discerned. I sensed, as the session was nearing its end, that constructing a reframe that Joe would find acceptable was not going to be much of a challenge. While functioning in the one-down role that he had enacted through most of the first session, Joe was willing to accept practically anything that anyone sent his way. Constructing a reframe that Anita was willing to give the benefit of the doubt was going to be more of a challenge. Inevitably, my reframe would introduce a perspective on the presenting problem that differed from hers. The current structure of the couple subsystem deprived Anita of many opportunities to respond to perspectives that differed from her own. My reframe would ask her to do something that she did not have much opportunity to do. Thus, I felt that I needed to pay careful attention to how I constructed and delivered the reframe.

While I was ruminating about how I would do this, Anita made a chance reference to her parents' troubled marriage. Stalling for time, I invited Anita to tell me more about what it was like for her to be exposed to her parents' marital difficulties. As Anita responded to my invitation, she ceased being the self-assured "rock" that she had been throughout the session to that point. Pain creased her face, and she began to cry. I chose that moment to deliver the following reframe:

"I have seen clearly during this session that you are both complex, three-dimensional people. Yet you consistently turn each other into two-dimensional cartoon characters. Joe, Anita is not a 'rock.' As you can see in this moment, she is, like all of us, a person with sadness, pain, and regrets. Yet the way you behave toward her corners her into being only part of who she is. You corner her into being only a 'rock.' Anita, at work, and when he was talking with me earlier in the session, Joe showed a glimmer of what a 'rock' he can be for you. Yet the way that you relate to him, like a critical mother, almost demands that he behave toward you like a foolish, though sometimes amusing, child. I think that my task with the two of you is to help you relate to each other in ways that will allow both of you to be as complex and three-dimensional with each other as you are with other people."

Both Joe and Anita nodded pensively. And so ended the prologue of this therapeutic drama.

The second session opened with both spouses taking great pleasure in telling me how dramatically things had improved at home since the first session. Anita reported that Joe had exercised greater initiative and displayed greater competence in the execution of household tasks, and Joe reported that Anita had been less critical of him. The spouses were clearly pleased with each other, and with me. All three of us were so pleased with ourselves, in fact, that half the session drifted by before we landed on a topic to focus our attention. Finally, Anita proposed that we focus on her complaint that, because Joe always was the one to initiate sex, she never got to do the initiating.

I did not respond to this content proposed by Anita in the way that I typically would during a second session. Normally, I would have elicited an enactment focused on the content and used the enactment as a platform for interventions designed to elicit new relational experiences for the clients. What I did instead was to use the content raised by Anita simply to amplify and refine the reframe I had delivered during the first session. As the session was ending, I realized that I had not asked Joe and Anita to engage in a single enactment.

I immediately sat myself down and tried to figure out why I had behaved so atypically during the session. Even during the session itself, I had realized that not much was structurally newsworthy in Anita and Joe's report of how things had changed since the first session. Anita was still clearly locked into her one-up position, and Joe into his one-down. The only thing that had changed during the week was that Joe had gone from being a disobedient child to being an obedient one, and Anita had replaced her scolding with congratulation. However, the one-up–one-down organization of their relationship was still firmly in place. Certainly, had I been so inclined, there had been opportunity aplenty to begin the usual Act I task of destabilizing this client system's structure. Instead, however, I had contented myself with doing a reprise of the first-session prologue. Why?

A little more reflection led me to see that my unusual conduct during the second session was the result of my having already become overly joined with this couple. Indeed, I had "caught" their severe allergy to differentiation and conflict. Their emphatically presented pleasure with themselves and with me at the beginning of the session had seduced me into not rocking the boat by intervening in ways that would have provided Anita and Joe with an unsettling experience of relational alternatives to their usual conflict avoidance and lack of differentiation.

I entered the third session, resolved to begin the restructuring that I should have initiated during the second. Given this couple subsystem's extreme conflict avoidance, it seemed to me that the best way to begin this task was to deliver unbalancing interventions. Because Joe's occupation of the one-down position in this subsystem was unvarying, I intended to make him my "ally" in my unbalancing.

Joe proved to be a frustrating ally. Throughout the first half of the third session, he assiduously declined to "borrow" most of the consternation that I was trying to "lend" him in my unbalancing. I did manage a couple of times to get him a little indignant over Anita's unquestioning, almost smug confidence in the rectitude of her perspective on any topic they were discussing. In the ensuing enactments, however, Joe backed down as soon as Anita signaled displeasure because he challenged her point of view. Invariably, he would defuse the tension by dramatically volunteering how wrong-headed his opinion was.

About midway through the third session, I saw that my unbalancing tack was backfiring. Caught between what he sensed I wanted and what his wife wanted of him, Joe was making ever more exaggerated one-down presentations of himself. His groveling at this point would have been comical had it not been so sad. Clearly, maintaining the interventive tack I was on, however correct it might appear in the abstract, would have been a mistake. I cast around for another direction in which to move the session.

At that moment, I recalled how dramatically the mood in my office had shifted late in the first session, when Anita had begun to cry over her recollection of her parents' troubled marriage. The thought occurred to me that eliciting a softened self-presentation on Anita's part, and having Joe respond empathically and supportively to her, would provide this couple with a relational experience that was every bit as novel as the one that I had been trying to produce via my unbalancing. I decided to replace my unbalancing tack with a softening one.

I began the shift by asking Anita whether she ever felt "alone" in her marriage. Gingerly, she admitted that she did. As I gently prompted her to describe to me how it felt to be married and yet alone, Anita began to cry. I asked Joe to take over for me and to help his wife tell him about her loneliness. Joe was clearly aghast at my request, but he complied. The ensuing enactment was clearly difficult for both spouses. Anita was not used to feeling so exposed and vulnerable in Joe's presence, and Joe did not seem to think that he had anything worth giving her in this moment of vulnerability. Numerous times, the spouses tried to exit the uncomfortable enactment by talking with me. I declined to talk and sent them back into conversation with each other. The enactment consumed the rest of the session.

The spouses made a bid to organize the fourth session along lines that were more familiar to them. Anita began the session by criticizing Joe for

having failed to get her a gift for their wedding anniversary, which had occurred during the previous week. Joe responded to Anita with his usual self-deprecation. The stage was set for a session-long reprise of this couple's baseline structure. I decided to use the content Anita had brought into the session to continue the softening tack I had begun during the previous session, which had appeared promising. While inviting Anita to continue talking with her husband about the nonexistent anniversary present, I constantly recast Anita's criticisms of him into relational statements about how unloved and "invisible" his behavior made her feel. Anita accommodated to my reformulations, and before long, she shifted from her usual posture of maternal annoyance into a congruent display of sadness. I was surprised and heartened by Joe's response to this shift in his wife. Abandoning his usual befuddled self-presentation, he made an impassioned speech to Anita about how much he loved her and how much pain it caused him to see her so sad. In an enactment lasting about 10 minutes, I saw, for the first time during the therapy, Joe and Anita arrayed in a symmetrical structure, relating to each other as peers, indeed, as intimates.

Early in the fifth session, I got the distinct sense that Anita had caught on to what I had been doing during the previous two sessions, and that she was counting on me to do it again. Despite the pain of the displays of vulnerability elicited from Anita in the last two sessions, she seemed inclined to allow me to elicit them. Although, typically, she brought an instrumentally focused criticism of Joe into this session, it took only a little prompting from me for her to say to Joe, "I'm beginning not to care about you. I'm beginning not to love you." Joe responded to his wife with the same congruent display of concern he had made at the end of the previous session. Anita looked as touched and consoled by Joe's response as she had during the fourth session.

Because of a combination of holidays and cancellations, a month intervened between the fifth and sixth sessions. The way the sixth session opened convinced me that Act I of this therapeutic play had reached its defining crisis. Joe reported to me, almost before I had closed the door to my office, that things had been "awful" since the last session. Reprising his baseline one-down posture, he narrated to me a series of "screw-ups" that he had perpetrated during the last month. As Joe went on, it became clear to me that what was most agitating him was the way Anita had responded to his foibles. To be sure, she had from time to time reverted to her usual one-up, maternal stance. However, she had spent most of the month in a posture of withdrawn, even depressed, detachment, which Joe found considerably more unnerving than her usual scolding. Detached and depressed was exactly how Anita looked as she entered the session. Unusually for her, she did not say a single word through the first third of the session. When she did speak, it was only to say, "I don't know what to say."

With Anita exercising no leadership in the session, Joe was trying to organize the session by getting me to treat him as the deficit-ridden "patient" he had depicted himself to be back in the first session: "Do you think I need medication? Should I go back into individual therapy?" Recognizing the tug exerted by Act I crises to allow couple subsystems to return to their baseline structure, I responded by resuming my press for Anita and Joe to experiment with a more functional relational organization: "Joe, you're not sick. You are simply a husband with a depressed and lonely wife. Talk with Anita now, and figure out together how you can make her feel loved, and how she can make you feel needed."

Joe's disappointment over the way I responded to their crisis was palpable. Anita, meanwhile, was so withdrawn that she showed no reaction at all. After asking for an enactment, I refused to do anything else, so the couple had no choice but to engage with each other. During the rest of this session, I saw what I usually see when I manage not to be dissuaded from my restructuring agenda by the occurrence of the Act I crisis. Finally convinced that nothing they presented would convince me to aid and abet a return to their original structure, Joe and Anita set themselves to finding a way to resolve their crisis on their own. Joe surrendered his one-down presentation, moved his chair close to Anita's, and with touching gentleness, launched into an attempt to assure her that "together we can get through this, if only we work together." Anita allowed herself to be coaxed out of her depression, and the two talked together for the rest of the session about how they were going to change their marriage.

As I had anticipated might happen, the tone of the seventh session of the therapy was different from that of all the previous sessions. Gone was the ritual of the previous sessions, in which the partners entered the session arrayed in some variant of their baseline structure, and I responded with interventions that elicited new relational experiences for them. This time, they entered the

session already organized into a different structure. Joe sat down and immediately set the agenda for the session, a dramatic departure from his posture when he had entered previous sessions. Without waiting for me to request an enactment, he turned to Anita and entered into conversation with her. Act II of this therapeutic drama had begun.

What Joe wanted to find out from Anita was why, despite successful efforts on his part to be more "there" for her both emotionally and in the execution of household tasks, she had been so stingy during the previous week in acknowledging the changes he had made. Anita sheepishly admitted to Joe that he had changed significantly, and admitted, as well, that she had withheld acknowledging the change. I smiled inwardly as Joe, displaying finally to his wife the self-assuredness he routinely displayed at work, told her that, although he understood her natural reluctance to trust him, the change he had made was so difficult that he felt entitled to demand that she give him the acknowledgment he needed to sustain the change.

Here, finally, was the indignation that I had tried unsuccessfully to "lend" to Joe earlier in the therapy. Were we still in Act I, I likely would have endeavored to amplify his novel stance toward Anita by unbalancing on his behalf. Now that we were in Act II, such an intervention would have been excessively heavy-handed and superfluous. All I did to support the new, adaptively structured transaction that was being enacted in front of me was to say, "This is a very helpful conversation the two of you are having. You're both doing great. Keep at it." By session's end, Anita had acceded to Joe's request that she find ways to acknowledge "the new Joe." For his part, Joe had thoroughly validated the reasonableness of the fear Anita had expressed during the session that if she began to warm up to him, he would feel "off the hook" and revert to his previous ways. He promised her he would do no such thing.

A much more relaxed and available Anita entered the eighth session, which occurred 2 weeks after the seventh. "She's been that way for the last 2 weeks," Joe reported happily. Anita quickly added, "And he has continued to be the 'new Joe' he's been for the past month." It occurred to me that the spouses were as pleased with each other as they had been during the second session. This time, however, their pleasure was rooted in a new, more adaptive relational structure. Throughout the session, I saw them relate to each other with a complexity that was entirely lacking when every one of their transactions was informed by the rigid one-up–one-down role structure with which they had entered therapy. On almost every issue discussed during the eighth session, I heard two distinct perspectives, and Joe and Anita were not afraid to mix it up with each other when those perspectives were widely divergent. Paradoxically, even when they vigorously disagreed with each other, the sense of intimate connection between them was worlds apart from the pseudocamaraderie that they had shared in the depiction of Joe as a childish fool. There was little for me to do in the session, and I told them so. When I raised the possibility of ending the therapy soon, they volunteered that they had concluded before entering the session that this might be the last session. We agreed to end therapy.

In a follow-up phone call 4 months later, I spoke with Joe and Anita separately. Each told me that the new way of relating they had displayed during the last session had not only endured but had also amplified.

SUGGESTIONS FOR FURTHER READING

Heatherington, L., & Friedlander, M. L. (1990). Applying task analysis to structural family therapy. *Journal of Family Psychology, 4,* 36–48.—This article illustrates the use of task analysis, a discovery-oriented research method, to examine the process of structural therapy.

Minuchin, S. (1974). *Families and family therapy.* Cambridge, MA: Harvard University Press.—The classic presentation of the fundamental theoretical concepts of structural therapy.

Minuchin, S., & Fishman, H. C. (1981). *Family therapy techniques.* Cambridge, MA: Harvard University Press.—A comprehensive treatment of the major techniques of structural therapy, except for the technique of softening.

Minuchin, S., Lee, W.-Y., & Simon, G. M. (2006). *Mastering family therapy: Journeys of growth and transformation* (2nd ed.). New York: Wiley.—This book, focused on supervision of structural therapy, includes a chapter detailing Minuchin's supervision of the treatment of a male, same-sex couple.

Minuchin, S., & Nichols, M. P. (1993). *Family healing: Tales of hope and renewal from family therapy.* New York: Free Press.—This book, written for a nonprofessional audience, provides a chapter-long case study of Minuchin's treatment of a couple whose presenting problem included physical abuse.

Nichols, M. P., & Fellenberg, S. (2000). The effective use of enactments in family therapy: A discovery-oriented process study. *Journal of Marital and Family Therapy, 26,* 143–152.—A description of a study designed to identify therapist and client behaviors associated with successful and unsuccessful enactments in structural therapy.

REFERENCES

Aponte, H. J. (1992). Training the person of the therapist in structural family therapy. *Journal of Marital and Family Therapy, 18,* 269–281.

Barkley, R. A., Guevremont, D. C., Anastopoulos, A. D., & Fletcher, K. E. (1992). A comparison of three family therapy programs for treating family conflicts in adolescents with attention-deficit hyperactivity disorder. *Journal of Consulting and Clinical Psychology, 60,* 450–462.

Bennett, L. A., Wolin, S. J., Reiss, D., & Teitelbaum, M. A. (1987). Couples at risk for transmission of alcoholism: Protective influences. *Family Process, 26,* 111–129.

Bradley, B., & Furrow, J. L. (2004). Toward a mini-theory of the blamer softening event: Tracking the moment-by-moment process. *Journal of Marital and Family Therapy, 30,* 233–246.

Chamberlain, P., & Rosicky, J. G. (1995). The effectiveness of family therapy in the treatment of adolescents with conduct disorders and delinquency. *Journal of Marital and Family Therapy, 21,* 441–459.

Giacomo, D., & Weissmark, M. (1986). Systemic practice. *Family Process, 25,* 483–512.

Greenan, D. E., & Tunnell, G. (2003). *Couple therapy with gay men.* New York: Guilford Press.

Greenberg, L. S., & Johnson, S. M. (1988). *Emotionally focused therapy for couples.* New York: Guilford Press.

Held, B. S. (1995). *Back to reality: A critique of postmodern theory in psychotherapy.* New York: Norton.

Jackson, D. D. (1957). The question of family homeostasis. *Psychiatric Quarterly Supplement, 31,* 79–90.

Johnson, S. M. (2004). *The practice of emotionally focused couple therapy* (2nd ed.). New York: Brunner-Routledge.

Minuchin, S. (1974). *Families and family therapy.* Cambridge, MA: Harvard University Press.

Minuchin, S. (1984). *Family kaleidoscope: Images of violence and healing.* Cambridge, MA: Harvard University Press.

Minuchin, S., Baker, L., Rosman, B. L., Liebman, R., Milman, L., & Todd, T. C. (1975). A conceptual model of psychosomatic illness in children: Family organization and family therapy. *Archives of General Psychiatry, 32,* 1031–1038.

Minuchin, S., & Fishman, H. C. (1981). *Family therapy techniques.* Cambridge, MA: Harvard University Press.

Minuchin, S., Lee, W.-Y., & Simon, G. M. (2006). *Mastering family therapy: Journeys of growth and transformation* (2nd ed.). New York: Wiley.

Minuchin, S., Montalvo, B., Guerney, B. J., Jr., Rosman,

B. L., & Schumer, F. (1967). *Families of the slums: An exploration of their structure and treatment.* New York: Basic Books.

Minuchin, S., & Nichols, M. P. (1993). *Family healing: Tales of hope and renewal from family therapy.* New York: Free Press.

Minuchin, S., & Nichols, M. P. (1998). Structural family therapy. In F. M. Dattilio (Ed.), *Case studies in couple and family therapy: Systemic and cognitive perspectives* (pp. 108–131). New York: Guilford Press.

Minuchin, S., Nichols, M. P., & Lee, W.-Y. (2007). *Assessing families and couples: From symptom to system.* Boston: Allyn & Bacon.

Minuchin, S., Rosman, B. L., & Baker, L. (1978). *Psychosomatic families: Anorexia nervosa in context.* Cambridge, MA: Harvard University Press.

Santisteban, D. A., Coatsworth, J. D., Perez-Vidal, A., Kurtines, W. M., Schwartz, S. J., LaPerriere, A., et al. (2003). Efficacy of brief strategic family therapy in modifying Hispanic adolescent behavior problems and substance use. *Journal of Family Psychology, 17,* 121–133.

Simon, G. M. (1992). Having a second-order mind while doing first-order therapy. *Journal of Marital and Family Therapy, 18,* 377–387.

Simon, G. M. (1993). Revisiting the notion of hierarchy. *Family Process, 32,* 147–155.

Simon, G. M. (1995). A revisionist rendering of structural family therapy. *Journal of Marital and Family Therapy, 21,* 17–26.

Simon, G. M. (2003). *Beyond technique in family therapy: Finding your therapeutic voice.* Boston: Allyn & Bacon.

Simon, G. M. (2004). An examination of the integrative nature of emotionally focused therapy. *The Family Journal, 12,* 254–262.

Simon, G. M. (2006a). The heart of the matter: A proposal for placing the self of the therapist at the center of family therapy research and training. *Family Process, 45,* 331–344.

Simon, G. M. (2006b). Why we don't "get" each other: A response to Susan Johnson. *The Family Journal, 14,* 209–212.

Stanton, M. D., Todd, T. C., & Associates. (1982). *The family therapy of drug abuse and addiction.* New York: Guilford Press.

Szapocznik, J., Rio, A., Murray, E., Cohen, R., Scopetta, M., Rivas-Vazquez, A., et al. (1989). Structural family versus psychodynamic child therapy for problematic Hispanic boys. *Journal of Consulting and Clinical Psychology, 57,* 571–578.

Wynne, L. C., Tienari, P., Nieminen, P., Sorri, A., Lahti, I., Moring, J., et al. (2006). Genotype–environment interaction in the schizophrenia spectrum: Genetic liability and global family ratings in the Finnish Adoption Study. *Family Process, 45,* 419–434.

Integrative Approaches

CHAPTER 12

Affective–Reconstructive Couple Therapy

A Pluralistic, Developmental Approach

Douglas K. Snyder
Alexandra E. Mitchell

BACKGROUND

Meta-analyses of couple therapy affirm that various approaches to treating couple distress produce statistically and clinically significant improvement for a substantial proportion of couples, with the average person receiving couple therapy being better off at termination than 80% of individuals not receiving treatment (Shadish & Baldwin, 2003). However, tempering enthusiasm regarding this overall conclusion are additional findings that in only 50% of treated couples do both partners show significant improvement in relationship satisfaction, and that 30–60% of treated couples show significant deterioration 2 years or longer after termination (Snyder, Castellani, & Whisman, 2006). Meta-analyses provide little evidence of differential effectiveness across different theoretical orientations to couple therapy, particularly once other covariates (e.g., reactivity of measures) are controlled (Shadish & Baldwin, 2003). Such findings have fostered two alternative approaches to treating couple distress: (1) distillation and emphasis of common factors hypothesized to contribute to beneficial effects across "singular" treatment approaches (e.g., Sprenkle & Blow, 2004), and (2) pluralistic or integrative models incorpo-

rating multiple components of diverse treatment approaches (e.g., Gurman, 2002, and Chapter 13, this volume; Pinsof, 1995, 2005; Snyder, 1999; Snyder & Schneider, 2002).

Our pluralistic approach to couple therapy incorporating insight-oriented interventions derives from three assertions. First, an important source of couples' current difficulties frequently includes previous relationship injuries resulting in sustained interpersonal vulnerabilities and related defensive strategies interfering with emotional intimacy. Moreover, therapeutic approaches that fail to address developmental experiences giving rise to these vulnerabilities and their associated reactivities deprive individuals of a rich resource for understanding both their own and their partners' behaviors that could help them to depersonalize the hurtful aspects of their interactions and to adopt an empathic stance. However, couples often enter therapy with debilitating crises, deficient relationship skills, or exaggerated defensive postures that preclude their making effective use of an interpretive approach; hence, insight-oriented techniques need to be implemented strategically within a hierarchical, pluralistic model incorporating structural, behavioral, and cognitive interventions earlier in the therapeutic sequence.

In this chapter we emphasize the use of "affective reconstruction"—that is, the interpretation of persistent maladaptive relationship patterns having their source in previous developmental experiences—within a pluralistic approach building on interventions from alternative theoretical modalities. We begin by describing both the rationale and basic strategies for incorporating multiple theoretical approaches into couple therapy. Because structural and cognitive-behavioral components of our pluralistic model have been well articulated by others, we focus instead on diverse interpretive approaches to couple therapy, and place our own techniques of affective reconstruction within this broader theoretical and historical context. Both the pluralistic model and the approach to affective reconstruction advocated here are contrasted with alternative integrative and interpretive approaches to couple therapy. Initial assessment methods and case formulation, structural considerations, and assumptions underlying the therapist's role, as well as the selection and timing of interventions, are considered from the perspectives of both affective reconstruction and our broader pluralistic model. A case example illustrates principles of affective reconstruction and couples for whom this approach may be particularly useful.

The Rationale for Integrative Approaches

What accounts for diverse individual outcomes of couple therapy? Rarely do couples come to therapists with simple, encapsulated complaints amenable to brief interventions that, after a few sessions, restore the couple to individual and relationship health. Too often, couples avoid seeking professional assistance until initial differences or disappointments fester over a protracted period into generalized disillusionment and deeply engrained patterns of negative interaction. By one account, once they start having problems couples wait an average of 6 years before seeking outside assistance (Gottman & Gottman, 1999). Moreover, relationship conflict both contributes to and is exacerbated by emotional, behavioral, or health problems in one or both partners (Snyder & Whisman, 2003). Hence, couple therapists confront a tremendous diversity of presenting issues, marital and family structures, individual dynamics and psychopathology, and psychosocial stressors that characterize couples in distress. Moreover, modest but growing evidence indicates that couple differences in these domains are related to treatment outcome

(Snyder, Castellani, et al., 2006). Because the functional sources of couples' distress vary so dramatically, the critical mediators or mechanisms of change should also be expected to vary—as should the therapeutic strategies intended to facilitate positive change.

The diverse patterns of factors contributing to couples' distress are addressed with varying levels of success by different treatment modalities. Even within the more restricted domain of individual interventions, growing recognition of unique strengths and limitations of competing theoretical approaches has fueled a burgeoning movement toward psychotherapy integration. For example, advocates of various integrative models of psychotherapy have emphasized the strengths of psychodynamic approaches for identifying enduring problematic interpersonal themes, the benefits of experiential techniques for promoting emotional awareness, gains from cognitive interventions targeting dysfunctional beliefs and attributional processes, and advantages of behavioral strategies for promoting new patterns of behavior (Bongar & Beutler, 1995; Norcross & Goldfried, 1992, 2005).

Thus, particularly complex or difficult couples may benefit most from a treatment strategy drawing from both conceptual and technical innovations in diverse theoretical models relevant to different components of a couple's struggles; that is, effective treatment is most likely to be rendered when the couple therapist has a solid grounding across diverse theoretical approaches, has acquired a rich repertoire of intervention techniques linked to theory, engages in comprehensive assessment of the marital and family system, and selectively draws on intervention strategies across the theoretical spectrum in a manner consistent with an explicit case formulation (Lebow, 2003; Snyder, 1999; Snyder, Schneider, & Castellani, 2003).

Eclecticism, Integration, or Pluralism?

In contrast to previous decades, when clinicians often pledged allegiance to a specific theoretical school advocating its own class of therapeutic techniques, a majority of today's clinicians describe themselves as "eclectic" or "integrative," with the latter term now preferred by a margin of nearly 2:1 (Goldfried, Pachankis, & Bell, 2005; Norcross, Prochaska, & Farber, 1993). Although sometimes used interchangeably, there are important differences between "eclecticism" and "integration." Moreover, in distinguishing between the terms, we prefer to add a third construct of "pluralism." Pluralism, eclecticism, and integration are united in their assertion that no single theoretical perspective or therapeutic modality is likely to hold optimal efficacy across all applications. Each draws on information or techniques from multiple domains reflecting alternative theories (e.g., object relations, social learning, cognitive, interpersonal, or systemic), epistemologies (e.g., rational, empirical, or experiential), and therapeutic modalities (e.g., individual, couple, family, or community).

"Eclecticism" refers to therapists' willingness to draw on therapeutic principles and techniques from diverse theoretical systems without an overarching or unifying framework. At its simplest level, such eclecticism may reflect therapists' unsystematic but well-intentioned effort to do what is best for the client at a given moment (Beutler, Consoli, & Williams, 1995). While freeing the clinician from the constraints of theoretical myopia, the expedient borrowing of diverse principles or techniques without regard for their potential inconsistency in directing either the relative importance or timing of interventions renders both treatment and client vulnerable to haphazard, disjointed, and contradictory interventions—a limitation noted throughout the literature (e.g., Goldfried & Norcross, 1995; Lebow, 1997; Mahoney, 1991; Norcross, 1985; Patterson, 1997; Snyder et al., 2003).

By comparison, "integration" entails a commitment to a conceptual synthesis beyond the technical blend of methods. The goal is to create a unified conceptual framework that synthesizes the best elements of two or more approaches of therapy into one (Goldfried & Norcross, 1995; Lebow, 1997). Some integrative approaches are primarily assimilative, in that they explain competing ideas in terms of a preferred theoretical framework. Others are more generative, combining two or more alternative approaches into a novel transtheoretical structure. However, in his review of integrative approaches to couple and family therapy, Lebow (1997) noted that a frequent shortcoming of integrative approaches is their failure to articulate the specific sequence in which various interventions incorporated from diverse theoretical modalities should be implemented. Moreover, he concluded that "no one integrative therapy has emerged as predominant, nor has there even appeared a serious contender for this distinction" (p. 3).

As an alternative to both eclecticism and integration, we advocate an "informed pluralistic" approach. "Pluralism" holds that no single theoretical, epistemological, or methodological approach is preeminent and there is no single, correct integrative system toward which the field of psychotherapy is evolving. Informed pluralism comprises a contextually based approach toward therapy integration (Safran & Messer, 1997). It is distinct from (1) common factors approaches emphasizing active but nonspecific components of therapeutic change processes and (2) transtheoretical approaches attempting to translate diverse theoretical models into a single unifying language. Informed pluralism reflects a systematic conceptual framework that is distinguished from sloppy thinking or simply "doing what feels right." It is similar to constructs of "empirical pragmatism" (Goldfried & Norcross, 1995), "systematic treatment selection" (Beutler & Clarkin, 1990; Beutler, Consoli, & Lane, 2005), and "prescriptive eclecticism" (Norcross & Beutler, 2000), characterized "by drawing on effective methods from across theoretical camps (eclecticism), by matching those methods to particular cases on the basis of psychological science and clinical wisdom (prescriptionism), and by adhering to an explicit and orderly model of treatment selection" (p. 248).

Distinctions among eclecticism, integration, and pluralism exist at both theoretical and technical levels. For example, although integrationists draw on both theories and techniques from diverse approaches, they do so from a smaller universe than eclectics, because contemporary integrative theories typically synthesize only a small number of theoretical perspectives, while leaving many others unaddressed (Lebow, 1997). Whereas eclectics could potentially select from the entire universe of principles and techniques across theoretical modalities, in practice, most clinicians adopting an eclectic approach draw on the few theoretical perspectives encountered in their previous training experiences (Norcross & Beutler, 2000). One could also practice eclectically within an integrative conceptual framework by drawing selectively on techniques congruent with that theory and excluding other interventions; we would predict that a clinician adopting this approach might have greater efficacy with particular kinds of clients benefiting from systematic application of that integrative model, but be less effective with other clients whose needs or symptomatic complexities fall outside the scope of that theoretical framework. Alternatively, one could practice integratively by synthetically incorporating diverse interventions for a given client, but without an overarching theoretical model guiding treatment selection across clients; we suspect that clinicians adopting this approach might be more effective with specific clients presenting with difficulties less well addressed by existing treatment approaches, but be less effective with most clients overall, because of the lack of systematic principles directing their selection and timing of interventions.

We would predict that the relationship of eclecticism to treatment outcome is curvilinear, and that this relationship is further moderated both by degree of integration (i.e., the extent to which techniques or theoretical tenets from diverse treatment approaches are linked by an overarching organizational or conceptual framework) and by level of case complexity (Snyder et al., 2003). At some intermediate range of eclecticism, treatment outcome is optimized by the therapist's ability to draw on diverse interventions targeting unique attributes of clients' individual or relationship functioning that lie outside the domain of any one system or school of psychotherapy. Practicing exclusively from a single theoretical approach potentially restricts the individual complaints or relationship processes on which the therapist is likely to have a significant impact. However, we would also argue that extensive use of techniques from diverse therapeutic approaches, particularly in the absence of any organizing or integrative framework, potentially compromises treatment effectiveness. The negative impact of high levels of eclecticism may derive from either (1) the unsystematic, chaotic, or contradictory use of specific interventions, or (2) the dismantling of interventions within treatment approaches that rely on the synergistic effects of specific components that lose their effectiveness when administered in isolation from one another. Paradoxically, the more difficult the couple, the more likely the therapist may be to draw on increasingly diverse intervention strategies to address multiple individual and relationship problems, and the less likely these interventions are to be integrated within a theoretically coherent system.

Because a pluralistic approach is less constrained than theoretically integrative approaches that are forced to reconcile competing constructs, it benefits from greater opportunity to accommodate diverse theoretical perspectives. By its systematic inclusion of multiple approaches across the theoretical spectrum, a pluralistic approach also promotes greater attention to diverse constructs and interventions than is shown by the typical eclectic clinician. At the same time, theoretical pluralism may avert haphazard, disjointed, or contradictory interventions resulting from expedient borrowing of diverse principles or techniques, without regard for their potential inconsistency or adverse interaction. In the following section we advocate a pluralistic model for selecting, sequencing, and pacing interventions across theoretical approaches when working with difficult couples.

A Sequential Model for Organizing Couple Interventions

The pluralistic approach to couple therapy advocated here and articulated previously (Snyder, 1999; Snyder & Schneider, 2002; Snyder et al., 2003) conceptualizes therapeutic tasks as progressing sequentially along a hierarchy reflecting the couple's overall level of functioning—from the most chaotic relationship rooted in significant behavioral dyscontrol in one or both partners, to the relatively benign but unfulfilled relationship in which conflicts involving issues such as autonomy or trust compromise emotional intimacy. The therapeutic tasks of couple therapy can be conceptualized as comprising six levels of intervention (see Figure 12.1). This model proposes a progression from the most fundamental interventions promoting a collaborative alliance to more challenging interventions addressing developmental sources of relationship distress. Couples enter treatment at varying levels of functioning and require different initial interventions. Because couple therapy often proceeds in nonlinear fashion, the model depicts flexibility of returning to earlier therapeutic tasks as dictated by individual or relationship difficulties.

The most fundamental step in couple therapy involves developing a collaborative alliance between partners, and between each partner and the therapist (Gurman, 1981; Jacobson & Margolin, 1979). The collaborative alliance begins with the therapist establishing an atmosphere of competence by engaging in relevant assessment and modeling appropriate communication behaviors. It also requires establishment of an atmosphere of safety by limiting partners' negative exchanges and clarifying policies governing issues such as confidentiality. Finally, the therapist strengthens the collaborative alliance by offering a clear formulation of the couple's difficulties, outlining treatment objectives and basic strategies, and defining all participants' respective roles.

Couples sometimes present with disabling relationship crises that, until resolved, preclude development of relationship skills and progress to-

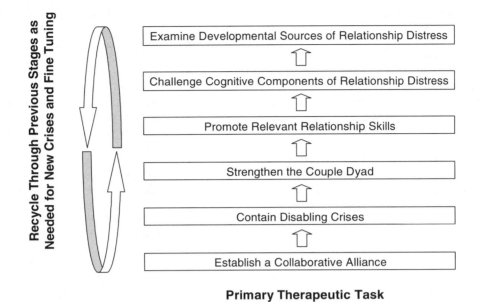

FIGURE 12.1. A sequential, pluralistic approach to couple therapy. The model depicts progression from (1) lower-order interventions aimed at establishing a collaborative alliance and crisis containment, through (2) positive-exchange and skills-building techniques, to (3) higher-order interventions targeting cognitive and developmental sources of relationship distress. Couple therapy may include recycling through earlier stages as required by emergent crises or erosion of individual or relationship skills.

ward emotional intimacy. Occasionally such crises emerge in otherwise healthy couples who experience unexpected job loss or financial hardship, illness or death of a family member, unplanned or terminated pregnancy, and similar events. With such crises, the therapist can assist couples in developing more adaptive attributions regarding their distress by distinguishing between external stressors and relationship characteristics, and by actively promoting intermediate solutions (Hoyt, Chapter 9, and Shoham, Rohrbaugh, & Cleary, Chapter 10, this volume). More often, relationship crises in couples presenting for therapy occur against a backdrop of communication deficits and an impoverished or insecure emotional context. A common crisis involves physical aggression by one or both partners against the other (Holtzworth-Munroe, Marshall, Meehan, & Rehman, 2003; O'Leary, Chapter 16, this volume). Other crises requiring immediate attention involve extramarital affairs (Gordon, Baucom, Snyder, & Dixon, Chapter 14, this volume), substance abuse disorders (Birchler, Fals-Stewart, & O'Farrell, Chapter 18, this volume), and major psychopathology (Snyder & Whisman, 2003). Although such cri-

ses nearly always contribute to and are frequently exacerbated by relationship difficulties, separate treatment for individual partners or other family members is often warranted—including medical/pharmacological, legal, financial, or other psychosocial interventions.

Couples in distress often describe an erosion of positive exchanges that leaves the relationship more vulnerable to subsequent challenges and conflicts. For such couples, reducing conflict is not sufficient for restoring a healthy relationship; increasing positive interactions is also vital. With only a modicum of direction from the therapist, relatively well-functioning couples can sometimes mobilize dormant communication skills in constructing positive change agreements on their own (Jacobson & Christensen, 1996). However, other couples often require direct interventions by the therapist, aimed at strengthening the relationship and securing a foundation of good will, so that the couple can pursue the more difficult task of developing skills of their own. Strengthening the marriage sometimes requires little more than clearly identifying the marital dyad as the primary family unit, promoting a hierarchical organization of responsibility and influence within the family system, and establishing appropriate boundaries with respect to families of origin (Todd, 1986). More often, couples with overwhelming negativity require specific positive exchange agreements that to a large degree are negotiated by the therapist (Epstein & Baucom, 2002; Stuart, 1980); that is, at this earlier developmental stage of the couple therapy, the therapist may need to instigate behavior change directly, before assisting the couple to develop behavior exchange and communication skills of their own.

Sustaining a satisfying marriage requires a broad range of relationship skills. Primary among these are communication skills, including emotional expressiveness, empathic listening, conflict resolution, and decision making (Epstein & Baucom, 2002). However, the essential skills for a satisfying relationship extend beyond communication. In many domains, effective communication presumes a prerequisite knowledge base—something partners often lack and that must be provided by the therapist or through adjunct resources identified by the therapist. Examples include competence related to sexual exchanges (McCarthy & Thestrup, Chapter 21, this volume), parenting (Sanders, Markie-Dadds, & Nicholson, 1997), financial management (Liberman & Lavine, 1998), and negotiation of competing demands on time (Thompson, 1997). As with more basic communication skills, the effective couple therapist provides information, assists the couple in developing relevant new skills, and directs the couple to additional sources of information and support outside of therapy.

A common impediment to behavior change involves misconceptions and other interpretive errors that individuals may have regarding both their own and their partners' behavior (Baucom, Epstein, LaTaillade, & Kirby, Chapter 2, this volume). Such cognitive mediators not only contribute to negative affect but they also result in behavioral strategies that frequently maintain or exacerbate relationship distress. A couple's resistance to interventions aimed directly at strengthening the marital dyad or promoting relevant relationship skills can often be diminished by examining and restructuring cognitive processes that interfere with behavior change efforts. A considerable body of literature has emerged regarding both the nature of cognitive components contributing to relationship distress and strategies for intervention (Epstein & Baucom, 2002).

However, not all psychological processes relevant to couples' interactions lend themselves to traditional cognitive interventions. A primary source of beliefs and expectancies regarding intimate relationships involves partners' developmental experiences within their families of origin and other prior significant relationships (Gurman, 1992, 2002; Snyder, 1999; Snyder & Schneider, 2002). Such expectancies operate at multiple levels of awareness and contribute to both affective and behavioral predispositions that may drive interpersonal exchanges in a distorted or exaggerated manner. Of particular importance are previous relationship injuries that result in sustained interpersonal vulnerabilities and related defensive strategies that interfere with emotional intimacy, many of which operate beyond partners' conscious awareness. Consequently, interpretation of maladaptive relationship patterns evolving from developmental processes comprises an essential component of an informed pluralistic approach to couple therapy.

Affective Reconstruction: Interpreting Maladaptive Relationship Themes

Developmental origins of interpersonal themes and their manifestation in a couple's relationship are explored in a process we refer to as "affective reconstruction" (Snyder, 1999; Snyder & Wills, 1989; Wills, Faitler, & Snyder, 1987), which is roughly akin to traditional interpretive strategies promoting insight but emphasizes interpersonal schemas and relationship dispositions rather than instinctual impulses or drive derivatives. Previous relationships, their affective components, and strategies for emotional gratification and anxiety containment are reconstructed with a focus on identifying each partner's consistencies in interpersonal conflicts and coping styles across relationships. In addition, ways that previous coping strategies, vital to prior relationships, represent distortions or inappropriate solutions for emotional intimacy and satisfaction in the current relationship are articulated.

Theoretical Assumptions

Rather than a single approach to insight-oriented couple therapy, there are many. Theoretical approaches examining affective and developmental components of couples' distress emphasize recurrent maladaptive relationship patterns that derive from early interpersonal experiences either in the family of origin or within other significant emotional relationships (Meissner, 1978; Nadelson & Paolino, 1978). Diverse approaches to examining maladaptive relationship patterns can be placed on a continuum from traditional psychoanalytic techniques, rooted primarily in object relations theory, to schema-based interventions derived from cognitive theory (see Figure 12.2). These approaches vary in the extent to which they emphasize the unconscious nature of individuals' relational patterns, the developmental period during which these maladaptive patterns are acquired, and the extent to which interpersonal anxieties derive from frustration of innate drives. However, these approaches all share the assumption that maladaptive relationship patterns are likely to continue until they are understood in a developmental context. These new understandings and explorations serve to reduce partners' attendant anxiety in current relationships and permit them to develop alternative, healthier relationship patterns.

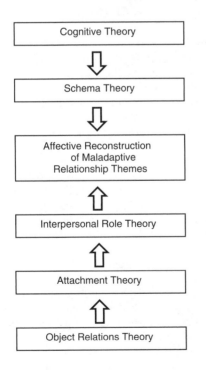

FIGURE 12.2. Theoretical approaches emphasizing affective and developmental components of couples' distress.

Object Relations Theory

Traditional object relations theorists (Fairbairn, 1952; Klein, 1950) argue that the primary drive in infants is to secure attachment to the mother. From interactions primarily with the mother they develop internalized images of the self, images of significant others, and sets of transactions connecting these images or objects. From an object relations perspective, maladaptive relationship patterns of adults reflect enduring pathogenic introjects that give rise to inevitable frustration when these are projected onto relationships with significant others (Scharff, 1995; Scharff & Scharff, Chapter 6, this volume). In a distressed marriage, partners' pathogenic introjects interact in an unconscious, complementary manner, resulting in repeated disappointments that culminate in persistent conflict (Dicks, 1967). Consequently, the goal of psychoanalytically oriented marital therapy is to help partners modify each other's projections, to distinguish these from objective aspects of the self, and to assume ownership of their own projections.

Attachment Theory

Evolving from object relations theory, attachment theory (Bowlby, 1969) emphasizes the importance of emotional closeness to others as an innate survival function from which infants develop information-processing capabilities and emotional responses intended to foster secure emotional bonds. From an attachment perspective, difficulties in intimate adult relationships may be viewed as stemming from underlying insecure or anxious models of attachment (Furman & Flanagan, 1997; Hazan & Shaver, 1987). Partners' dominant emotional experiences drive reciprocal feedback loops that maintain behaviors such as excessive clinging or avoidance (Johnson, 2004). The goal of emotionally focused couple therapy (EFT; Johnson & Greenberg, 1995; Johnson, Chapter 4, this volume), reformulated from an attachment theory perspective, is to help partners gain access to their history of attachment experiences stored in schematic memory and to use this information in moving toward more accurate working models of self and partner. Johnson and Greenberg (1995) described EFT as "one of the few psychodynamic approaches to marital therapy that has been empirically validated" (p. 121).

Interpersonal Role Theory

Interpersonal role theory (Anchin & Kiesler, 1982) regards persistent maladaptive interpersonal patterns to be the result of their reinforcement by the responses of significant others. This emphasis involves an important shift from the initial internal object relations giving rise to these patterns to the current interpersonal exchanges perpetuating them. The concept of role complementarity, derived from interpersonal theory, accounts for some of the same phenomena addressed by early object relations theorists, but in a language more closely linked to current events and at a lower level of abstraction. Thus, rather than stressing constructs of projective and introjective identification, interpersonal theory emphasizes the unconscious assignment of specific roles to oneself and others, "in which feared and anticipated relational events tend to be elicited and enacted by the individual in his or her interactions with others, who, in turn, will tend to respond in ways complementary to the interpersonal actions of that individual" (Messer & Warren, 1995, p. 120).

The brief psychodynamic models of individual psychotherapy developed by Strupp and Binder (1984), Luborsky (1984), and Wachtel (1997) exhibit a strong linkage to interpersonal role theory. These authors use the terms "cyclical maladaptive patterns," "core conflictual relationship themes," and "cyclical psychodynamics" to refer to recurrent strategies used to influence relationships in a way that minimizes expected painful outcomes and maximizes desired outcomes in relationships with significant others. Moreover, these approaches emphasize the interpretation of maladaptive relational patterns within the immediacy of the therapist–client exchange as a vehicle for promoting the client's understanding of how these same maladaptive patterns are enacted outside of therapy.

Schema Theory

Schema theory (Horowitz, 1988; Young, 1999; Young, Klosko, & Weishaar, 2003) emphasizes relationship schemas extending beyond attachment to the mother (object relations theory) or significant others (attachment theory) to consider more generally how early relationship experiences influence adult intimate relationships. For example, Young (1999) conceptualizes early "maladaptive schemas" as enduring themes initially developed in childhood that serve as a set of expectancies or

"template" for processing interactions of oneself with the environment. The greater the conflict between the desired and the anticipated or feared interpersonal state, the more rigid and maladaptive the scripted expression of those expectancies is likely to be. Young conceptualizes his work as an extension of cognitive therapy, but his model overlaps considerably with psychodynamic relational models in its (1) emphasis on interpretation of interpersonal exchanges within the therapy session as a vehicle for change; (2) attention to affect during the processing of schema-related events; and (3) emphasis on the childhood origins of maladaptive schemas and the emotional reformulation or reworking of these early experiences.

Affective Reconstruction of Maladaptive Relationship Themes

Drawing on earlier psychodynamic formulations, Snyder and Wills (1989) articulated an insight-oriented approach to couple therapy emphasizing affective reconstruction of previous relationship injuries that result in sustained interpersonal vulnerabilities and related defensive strategies interfering with emotional intimacy. In affective reconstruction, the therapist explores developmental origins of interpersonal themes and their manifestation in a couple's relationship using techniques roughly akin to traditional interpretive strategies promoting insight, but emphasizing interpersonal schemas and relationship dispositions rather than instinctual impulses or drive derivatives (Snyder, 1999). Previous relationships, their affective components, and strategies for emotional gratification and anxiety containment are reconstructed, with a focus on identifying each partner's consistencies in interpersonal conflicts and coping styles across relationships. In addition, the therapist articulates ways in which previous coping strategies that were vital to prior relationships represent distortions or inappropriate solutions for emotional intimacy and satisfaction in the current relationship.

Affective reconstruction builds on strengths of earlier relational models by capitalizing on features unique to conjoint couple therapy. First, in couple therapy, data reflecting current expression of persistent dysfunctional patterns of interpersonal relating are not confined to the individual's interactions with the therapist but extend more visibly and importantly to *in vivo* observations of the individual and his or her significant other. Thus, core conflictual relationship themes having greatest relevance to each partner are more likely to be apparent than in the context of individual therapy. Second, an individual's understanding of maladaptive relationship themes and reformulation of these in less pejorative terms may extend beyond his or her own dynamics to a more benevolent reinterpretation of the partner's more hurtful behaviors; that is, both individuals can be helped to understand that whereas certain relational coping strategies may have been adaptive or even essential in previous relationships, the same interpersonal strategies interfere with emotional intimacy and satisfaction in the present relationship. Finally, in couple therapy the "corrective emotional experience" (Alexander, 1956) of disrupting previous pathogenic interpersonal strategies and promoting more functional relational patterns has an opportunity to emerge between not only the individual and therapist but also the individual and his or her partner. Thus, interpretation of maladaptive interpersonal themes in the context of couple therapy affords unique opportunities for affective reconstruction of these patterns in individuals' primary emotional relationships.

Comparing Affective Reconstruction with Alternative Approaches

Alternative Psychodynamic and Developmental Approaches

Psychodynamic approaches to couple therapy share a common assumption that current interpersonal difficulties evolve at least in part from maladaptive relationship dispositions acquired during earlier developmental struggles and maintained largely on an unconscious level. However, psychodynamic strategies vary considerably in the extent to which they emphasize the genetic interpretation of instinctual strivings and the projection of intrapsychic conflicts versus the perpetuation of maladaptive interpersonal dispositions as misguided efforts to avoid painful outcomes and to procure relational fulfillment (Barber & Crits-Christoph, 1991; Messer & Warren, 1995).

In its more orthodox application, psychoanalytically oriented couple therapy strives to free the relationship "from the grip of its obligatory projective and introjective identificatory processes" (Scharff, 1995, p. 172). Distressed relationships are viewed as the culmination of frustrated narcissistic needs and an inability to cope with the consequent disillusionment. Thus, interpretive strategies emphasize helping partners to modify each other's projections, to distinguish these from

objective aspects of their self, and to assume ownership of their own projections. By contrast, the relational approach to couple therapy advocated here deemphasizes the intrapsychic components of maladaptive patterns rooted in the first years of development, and instead emphasizes the perpetuating aspects of maladaptive interpersonal strategies in the present relationship. Couples' conflicts are viewed as evolving from a self-fulfilling process in which partners' mutual efforts to minimize or avoid anticipated relationship injuries result in exaggerated or inflexible interpersonal strategies that often elicit and maintain these feared relationship experiences.

In many respects, an emphasis on contemporary relationship dynamics perpetuating each partner's maladaptive relationship dispositions can be discerned in Sager's (1976) formulation of marital "contracts." Working from a psychodynamic perspective, Sager proposed that couples develop an interactional contract incorporating respective conscious and unconscious expectations and needs around themes such as dependence–independence, activity–passivity, closeness–distance, dominance–submission, and autonomy–control. Sager viewed relationship conflicts as resulting from partners' implicit contracts that are internally inconsistent or contradictory. Interventions from this perspective strive to explicate unconscious aspects of partners' implicit relationship expectations and to negotiate interactional contracts that are complementary. Less central to Sager's formulation are the intrapersonal components of maladaptive relationship behaviors that recur across interpersonal relationships, or the need for individuals to gain understanding and emotional resolution of enduring relational anxiety resulting from previous relationship injuries.

Wile (1995, 2002) advocated an ego-analytic approach emphasizing partners' pejorative attitudes toward themselves and their resulting difficulty in communicating "leading-edge" feelings to which they feel unentitled. These unexpressed feelings are viewed as giving rise to more symptomatic relationship behaviors. Wile argued that developmental interpretations focusing on the inappropriateness of partners' affective responses have the effect of invalidating these responses and maintaining their symptomatic expression. Wile's ego-analytic approach emphasizes the universality of partners' feelings and the hidden appropriateness in the person's seemingly inappropriate behavior. Rather than linking current relationship difficulties to partners' developmental struggles and enduring sensitivities, Wile encourages partners to own and disclose their primary emotions, to "appeal to each other as resources in dealing with them, and create a joint platform from which to look at them" (Wile, 1995, p. 118). The approach advocated by Wile offers important strategies for promoting an individual's acceptance of his or her own and the partner's primary affect. However, the ego-analytic approach differs critically from the relational model advocated here in its explicit avoidance of interpretive strategies linking current affect to previous relationship experiences and to partners' inadvertent maintenance of maladaptive relationship patterns.

Indeed, the emphasis of Wile's ego-analytic approach on expression of leading-edge emotions and avoidance of developmental interpretations gives this approach striking similarities to the emotionally focused couple therapy (EFT) described by Johnson (2004; Johnson, Chapter 4, this volume; Johnson & Greenberg, 1995). Based on attachment theory, EFT views distressed relationships as "insecure bonds in which essentially healthy attachment needs are unable to be met due to rigid interaction patterns that block emotional engagement" (Johnson & Greenberg, 1995, p. 121). An important assumption of EFT is that understanding of valid attachment needs promotes more empathic responding and less defensive interactions between partners. Similar to the relational model advocated here that incorporates interpretive techniques, attachment-based couple interventions strive to "access information that couples have selectively excluded from processing, sustain attention to this new information, and facilitate couples' abilities to incorporate and use this information in moving toward more accurate, integrated working models of self and partner" (Kobak, Ruckdeschel, & Hazan, 1994, pp. 60–61).

The distinction of the affective–reconstructive approach we advocate from alternative attachment-based models rests on the extent to which interpretive techniques emphasize previous relationship experiences and the unconscious components of maladaptive relationship patterns. Affective reconstruction emphasizes explication of enduring maladaptive relationship patterns rooted in earlier relationship injuries, with dynamics that result from these developmental experiences operating largely beyond awareness. Nevertheless, even this distinction is often blurred. For example, in discussing couple therapy from an attachment perspective, Furman and Flanagan (1997) noted that when working models from early development appear implicated in current relationship difficulties, the therapist may help partners "address the unfinished business with parents and in effect rework their models of parents" (p. 197). Interestingly, similar to the hierarchical model advocated here, Furman and Flanagan also describe adopting a sequential approach to couple therapy—beginning with behavioral or other structural approaches and using resistance to change diagnostically to explore partners' underlying attachment models that may be contributing to relationship difficulties.

Alternative Integrative Approaches

The pluralistic approach to couple therapy proposed here can also be contrasted with several alternative approaches described by their respective proponents as "integrative." Among the first integrative couple therapies to be articulated was Gurman's (1981, 1992, 2002; Chapter 13, this volume) depth-behavioral integrative approach, drawing on principles of social learning theory, object relations theory, and general systems theory. Gurman emphasizes the critical interrelation of intrapsychic and interpersonal factors in couples' interactions and defines the goal of couple therapy as the loosening and broadening of each spouse's implicit matrix of assumptions, expectations, and requirements of intimate interpersonal contact. This is accomplished through interpretation, cognitive restructuring, and creation of therapeutic tasks to promote each spouse's exposure to those aspects of him- or herself and his or her partner that are blocked from awareness.

Although Gurman's integrative approach to couple therapy has been consistently assimilative, its relative emphasis on psychodynamic versus behavioral theory as the "home theory" in which to assimilate competing constructs has changed significantly over the past 25 years. For example, Gurman (1981) argued that "the most appropriate theoretical foundation for an integrative understanding of marital interaction, dynamics, and change is to be found in psychodynamic thinking, especially in a focused use of certain concepts originating in object relations theory" (p. 453). From this perspective, behavioral techniques such as teaching partners to rely on positive reinforcement for modifying their spouse's behavior may be reconceptualized as "a direct inhibitor of [partners'] proclivities to engage in projective identification" (Gurman, 1980, p. 90). More recently, however, Gurman's depth-behavioral integrative approach emphasizes the centrality of functional behavior analytic theory—overlapping with but distinct from enhanced cognitive-behavioral couple therapy (Epstein & Baucom, 2002) and integrative behavioral couple therapy (Jacobson & Christensen, 1996) (Gurman, personal communication, August 2007).

The pluralistic approach advocated here shares much in common with Gurman's model, including attention to enduring maladaptive relationship patterns that have early developmental origins. However, there are several important distinctions between the two approaches. Unlike Gurman's more assimilative model, the pluralistic approach advocated here regards diverse interventions within their original theoretical contexts rather than reformulating these within a single integrative perspective. Second, although both Gurman's model and our own emphasize the critical role of establishing the therapeutic alliance early in treatment, Gurman appears more likely than we to incorporate a psychodynamic formulation of the couple's difficulties from the outset—suggesting that the couple's presenting problems typically contain the clues to identifying partners' interlocking intrapsychic conflicts, "albeit often in disguised or derivative fashion" (Gurman, 1992, p. 434). By contrast, the pluralistic model described here defers examination of enduring maladaptive relationship themes from a psychodynamic perspective until later in the therapeutic sequence, after limited impact of earlier behavioral and cognitive interventions. Finally, the sequential approach we advocate differs from Gurman's assimilative model, in which interventions from different theoretical perspectives may be combined concurrently more often and earlier in treatment than in our model.

Segraves (1982, 1990) also proposed a combined psychodynamic–behavioral model for addressing both intrapersonal and interpersonal components of chronic relationship discord. Segraves asserts that individuals in distressed relationships are likely to possess internal representational schemas of their partners that are discrepant with objective reality. He attributes distorted schemas both to transference and failure of discriminative learning, resulting in limited conceptual dimensions for perceiving and understanding significant others. Similar to conceptualization from interpersonal role theory (Anchin & Kiesler, 1982), Segraves proposes that individuals reliably elicit behavior from others that confirms their preexisting schemas through a process of stimulus–response chaining. Although conceptualized in part from

a psychodynamic perspective, Segraves' strategies for intervening in relationship difficulties are largely cognitive-behavioral, encouraging each partner to observe behaviors of the other that are discrepant with internal schemas for that partner, with less attention to early developmental experiences giving rise to these schemas or reconstructing these experiences on an affective level.

More recently, Christensen and colleagues (Jacobson & Christensen, 1996; Dimidjian, Martell, & Christensen, Chapter 3, this volume) have proposed an integrative approach combining traditional behavioral techniques for promoting change (specifically, communication and behavior-exchange skills training), with strategies aimed at promoting acceptance. Acceptance techniques are viewed as essential "when direct efforts to change are blocked by incompatibilities, irreconcilable differences, and unsolvable problems" (p. 11). Jacobson and Christensen describe interventions that promote tolerance and encourage partners to appreciate differences and to use these to enhance their marriage. Empathic joining may be facilitated by a "soft disclosure" by the partner or a reformulation by the therapist. Jacobson and Christensen state that acceptance work is sometimes sufficient on its own; at other times, it facilitates behavior-change efforts by promoting a context of collaboration.

In contrast to the interpretive emphasis in affective reconstruction, acceptance interventions in Jacobson and Christensen's (1996) model leave largely unaddressed those developmental experiences giving rise to apparent incompatibilities or exaggerated reactivities. Thus, individuals are potentially deprived of a rich resource for understanding their partners' behaviors that might help them to depersonalize the hurtful aspects of their interactions and to adopt an empathic stance. In addition, Jacobson and Christensen advocate beginning couple therapy with acceptance interventions prior to communication and behavior-exchange skills training. To the extent that acceptance techniques comprise common interventions promoting a collaborative alliance between partners, this recommendation is consistent with the hierarchical model we advocate here, affirming partners' collaborative alliance as a prerequisite to all subsequent interventions. However, to the extent that an individual's acceptance of the partner's behaviors relies on empathic understanding of those behaviors as coping strategies acquired from previous relationship injuries, the sequential approach advanced here proposes strengthening the relationship and challenging cognitive components of distress more accessible to immediate awareness prior to examining developmental sources of enduring relationship dispositions. Premature exploration of developmental issues may heighten defensiveness and exacerbate rather than ameliorate resistance to change.

The sequencing of interventions prescribed by the pluralistic model presented here mirrors the general progression of interventions characterizing Pinsof's (1995, 2005) integrative problem-centered therapy. Pinsof advocates commencing therapy with a focus on the behavioral patterns that prevent a couple from solving their presenting problems. If intervention at that level is not effective, therapy progresses to an exploration of the affective and cognitive components of the maladaptive patterns. Only if interventions at this experiential level fail does Pinsof advocate progressing to a developmental perspective focusing on family-of-origin patterns and specific historical determinants of enduring maladaptive relationship patterns. Although similar in their overall sequencing of interventions, our pluralistic model and Pinsof's integrative approach differ in subtle ways. First, the pluralistic model we articulate here emphasizes the frequent necessity of attending to immediate relationship crises and distinguishes explicitly between strengthening the dyad through structural interventions and specific skills building interventions. Our pluralistic model also draws a sharper distinction between cognitive and affective components of relationship distress and associated interventions, regardless of their temporal origins. Finally, although consistent with techniques of affective reconstruction described here, Pinsof's model does not explicitly address unique benefits of conducting developmental interventions in the context of conjoint couple therapy.

HEALTHY VERSUS DYSFUNCTIONAL RELATIONSHIPS: DIFFERENCES OF DEGREE

From the pluralistic perspective advocated here, no couple is immune to potential relationship difficulties, and no couple is without individual and relational resources. The difference between healthy and dysfunctional relationships is one of degree, not kind. Healthy loving relationships extend beyond the initial emotional idealization characterizing romantic love. Rather, enduring love finds expression in partners' disciplined caring for one another when they least feel generous.

What factors promote healthy relationships and resilience to stress? First are those components of individual functioning that promote self- and other-awareness, emotional regulation, and both the capacity and willingness to defer one's own gratification for the sake of another (Snyder, Simpson, & Hughes, 2006). Although we do not subscribe to the view that relationship dysfunction necessarily implies individual deficits, we do believe that individual deficits necessarily constrain opportunities for relationship health and resilience. In addition to extensive data regarding the comorbidity of relationship distress and individual emotional and behavioral disorders, research indicates that mental health problems can render couple therapy less effective and contribute to premature dropout (Snyder & Whisman, 2004).

Second, healthy relationships prevail when both partners possess specific knowledge and skills essential to couple and family functioning. These include communication skills such as emotional expressiveness, active listening, and conflict resolution, as well as more specific skills in domains such as the couple's sexual relationship, parenting, management of time and financial resources, and routine household maintenance. Despite research indicating that nondistressed couples often engage in low rates of specific communication behaviors promoted in couple therapy (Gottman, 1999), the skills vital to distressed couples' disruption of intense negativity or recovery from relationship trauma likely differ from those processes that protect relatively happy couples from relationship erosion.

Separate from those intrapersonal and interpersonal components that distinguish between healthy and dysfunctional relationships are aspects of the extended family, social network, and community that either support or compromise the couple's relationship. Any individual or couple, despite previous high levels of adaptive functioning, can succumb to changes in situational demands requiring new skills not yet developed or to atypical stressors overwhelming usually adequate adaptive resources. Examples include transitions across family life stages, major mental or physical illness, or unexpected tragedies.

In summary, factors differentiating between healthy and unhealthy relationships have their sources in individual, couple, and broader systemic functioning; may reflect primarily contemporary or historical influences or their interaction; and tend to vary quantitatively rather than qualitatively (i.e., by degree rather than by kind). Distinguishing among these sources of influence, their relative impact on the couple's relationship, and their implications for intervention requires comprehensive assessment strategies reflecting multiple levels and facets from a broad systemic perspective (Snyder, Heyman, & Haynes, 2008).

PURSUING AFFECTIVE RECONSTRUCTION WITHIN A PLURALISTIC APPROACH

Structure of the Therapeutic Process

Participants

From a broad systemic perspective, a pluralistic approach to couple therapy could conceivably target any individual member or combination of members from the broader family or social system. However, when partners define their "relationship" as the focus of treatment when presenting for couple therapy, or when our own assessment confirms the centrality of relational difficulties despite either partner's tendency to focus on shortcomings of the other, our clear preference is to employ conjoint sessions throughout the course of treatment. Although a conjoint format offers unique advantages to promoting partners' shared understanding of each other's developmental contributions to current distress, there may be times when individual therapy provides an important alternative or complement to conjoint sessions.

For example, among couples who have achieved a relatively satisfying relationship, one or both partners may recognize enduring issues of their own that compromise functioning across diverse domains, including their relationship, and elect to address these in individual therapy. In such cases, affective reconstruction of maladaptive relationship patterns may produce substantive relationship gains if the individual in therapy has the capacity to initiate positive changes in his or her own behavior, and the other partner has the capacity to change as the partner in treatment changes. At the other extreme, individual therapy may prove an important alternative or complement to conjoint sessions with highly dysfunctional couples whose persistent antagonism precludes partners' willingness to confront individual issues or initiate unilateral changes that may be essential to restoring a more collaborative foundation to couple therapy. In cases when either partner needs or desires more extended individual treatment, we refer him or her to a colleague for independent collateral work.

Various treatment formats have been described in the literature, each with its own merits and limitations, including mixing of individual and conjoint sessions by the same therapist, referral of partners to separate therapists for individual work, using cotherapists for both conjoint and individual sessions, and so on. The use of alternative formats raises both pragmatic and ethical issues, such as managing confidentiality and negotiating competing individual and couple treatment goals (Gottlieb, 1996; Gottlieb, Lasser, & Simpson, Chapter 26, this volume; Snyder & Doss, 2005). Having cotherapists raises particularly interesting possibilities when implementing interpretive techniques because of the increased potential for transference distortions within the couple therapy, as well as the opportunity for corrective emotional experiences. However, there exists little, if any, empirical basis to date for articulating specific criteria for alternative formats within the hierarchical model prescribed here.

Given research indicating high rates of comorbidity between relationship distress and psychological disorders (especially depression, anxiety, and substance abuse), concurrent psychopharmacological interventions may be indicated for one or both partners. Recommending medication for one partner and not the other can be difficult therapeutically—particularly early in treatment, when partners fear being assigned undue responsibility for relationship problems based on individual deficits. We frame collateral treatments—whether psychosocial or medical/pharmacological—as efforts to maximize each partner's individual resources for change rather than as diagnostic indicators of partners' respective blame for relationship difficulties.

Length, Frequency, and Duration of Sessions

With the exception of manualized treatments under scrutiny in controlled studies, the length of treatment for most disorders—individual, couple, or otherwise—typically reflects both the complexity and severity of presenting difficulties. The insight-oriented couple therapy developed by Snyder and Wills (1989) was designed for implementation within 25 weekly, conjoint sessions lasting 50 minutes each. In fact, couples receiving this treatment averaged 19 sessions, although roughly 10–15% required fewer than 15 sessions and another 10–15% required twice that many.

Not all couples require each of the treatment components outlined in the pluralistic model proposed here. Individual differences in couples' strengths and concerns often dictate that different components of the model be given greater or lesser emphasis. For example, some couples require little more than stabilization and crisis resolution to restore a positive relationship; others require extensive assistance in reworking enduring maladaptive relationship patterns established early in their individual development. With relatively higher-functioning couples we have been able to implement the complete model in as few as 8–10 sessions; with couples exhibiting both significant individual and relational impairment, successful therapy has required a year or more of intensive intervention.

Ground Rules

There are few ground rules that distinguish affective reconstruction or the pluralistic approach advocated here from other couple therapies. Both partners must agree to the format and proposed schedule of sessions. Both must agree that, if physical aggression occurs to any extent in their relationship, strategies for eliminating violence will be the first priority of treatment. Partners must agree in principle to civil behavior in sessions, to allowing the therapist to intervene as necessary to disrupt destructive exchanges, and to a conceptual formulation of the "relationship" as the client.

So long as the treatment is defined as "couple" rather than "individual" therapy, regardless of any individual sessions that might be held within the couple treatment, the therapist enforces an explicit agreement that any communication that occurs unilaterally between either partner and the therapist may be incorporated into conjoint sessions at the discretion of the therapist (Snyder & Doss, 2005). The therapist reinforces this ground rule early in the therapy by refusing to meet with one individual if his or her partner fails to show for a scheduled conjoint session. Any phone calls or notes from either partner to the therapist between sessions are typically shared in the subsequent conjoint meeting. On the infrequent occasion that one partner unilaterally shares information with the therapist outside conjoint sessions but insists on this remaining confidential despite the initial explicit agreement otherwise, the therapist may agree to one or two separate sessions with that individual to assist him or her in bringing the information into conjoint therapy; if the individual persists in demanding confidential treatment of

that information, the therapist asserts his or her inability to continue as a credible and effective couple therapist and assists transfer of the couple's treatment to an alternative therapist not similarly compromised.

Role of the Therapist

In a pluralistic approach, the therapist's roles vary considerably across stages of treatment. Early in therapy, primary roles include the assessment of overall individual and relationship functioning, containment of negativity, disruption of destructive exchanges, and repeated encouragement regarding the couple's collective resources for improving their relationship. The therapist remains highly active, lending his or her own expertise and problem-solving abilities to crisis resolution, and directing structural changes in partners' interactions and within the broader family and social system to strengthen the couple's relationship. An active stance continues during skills building interventions, but emphasis shifts from the therapist's role as problem-solver to dual roles as facilitator and educator in assisting couples to acquire expertise and to implement interventions on their own to resolve conflict and enhance intimacy.

When individual dynamics interfere with the acquisition or implementation of more positive relationship behaviors, the therapist's role shifts to that of "guide" or "auxiliary processor" (Messer & Warren, 1995). Although cognitive components of relationship distress that are reasonably accessible to conscious awareness might be approached from a more psychoeducational stance directed toward both partners, deeper sources of intrapersonal conflict beyond immediate awareness require the therapist to adopt roles more typical of individual psychodynamic therapy. The specific features of these roles become clearer when we examine the specific techniques of affective reconstruction described below.

Assessment and Treatment Planning: Basic Principles

We have previously proposed a comprehensive model for directing and organizing couple assessment strategies that target diverse domains (e.g., cognitive, affective, and behavioral components) across multiple levels of the family system, including individual partners and their relationship, as well as parent–child dyads and the broader, extended family and psychosocial context (Snyder, Cavell, Heffer, & Mangrum, 1995; Snyder, Abbott, & Castellani, 2002). Specific assessment strategies and techniques are necessarily tailored to the couple's unique constellation of presenting difficulties, as well as specific resources of both couple and clinician.

However, regardless of the specific context, several recommendations for assessing couples generally apply (Snyder et al., 2008). For example, assessment foci should progress from broad to narrow—first identifying relationship concerns at the broader construct level, then examining more specific facets of couple distress and its correlates using a finer-grained analysis. Given empirical findings that link couple distress to individual disorders and their respective impact in moderating treatment outcome, partners should be screened for individual emotional or behavioral difficulties potentially contributing to, exacerbating, or resulting in part from couple distress. Certain domains should always be assessed with every couple because of either their robust linkage to relationship difficulties (e.g., communication processes involving emotional expressiveness and decision making) or because the specific behaviors, if present, have a particularly adverse impact on couple functioning (e.g., physical aggression or substance abuse).

Couple assessment should integrate findings across multiple assessment methods. Self- and other-report measures may complement findings from interview or behavioral observation in generating data across diverse domains both centrally or conceptually related to the couple's difficulties, or across those domains that are potentially more challenging to assess because of their sensitive nature or not being amenable to direct observation. Therapists should choose evaluation strategies and modalities that complement each other and follow a sequential approach that uses increasingly narrowband measures to target problem areas that have been identified by other assessment techniques.

Tailoring Couple Therapy to Individual Differences

At the simplest level, tailoring couple therapy to individual differences involves use of assessment findings that match couples to therapeutic approaches or treatment components designed specifically to remediate individual and relationship deficits and build on existing strengths. Matching couples to treatment rests on the premise that individuals or relationships exhibiting particular attributes may respond more favorably to one treatment, or set of interventions, than to an alternative approach. For example, evidence suggests that couples in which one partner exhibits major depression may benefit most from a combination of social learning and cognitive interventions emphasizing increases in positive exchanges, enhanced decision-making and emotional expressiveness skills, and partners' improved understanding of depression and its correlates in facilitating realistic relationship expectations (Beach & Gupta, 2003). By comparison, couples with pervasive and intense negativity, high levels of mistrust, and limited awareness or understanding of emotions may initially be ill-suited for therapeutic approaches encouraging introspection, developmental exploration, and vulnerable self-disclosures (Snyder & Schneider, 2002).

Although the challenge of matching treatments to clients has been examined to a modest degree in individual therapy, less consideration has been devoted to treatment matching in couple therapy. Several factors limit progress in this area. The first involves the relative absence of replicated findings that demonstrate differential effectiveness across different theoretical orientations to couple therapy (Shadish & Baldwin, 2003). A second factor involves the limited findings with regard to aptitude × treatment interaction (ATI) effects, in which individual or couple characteristics influence or moderate therapy outcome. Studies regarding "prescriptive indicators" of differential treatment response to alternative couple-based interventions are infrequent and have generally yielded limited or inconsistent findings (Atkins et al., 2005; Snyder, Castellani, & Whisman, 2006). Finally, available evidence suggests that couple treatments themselves are rarely as distinct as their proponents suggest; that is, although different treatments may be distinguishable by their unique specific interventions, they likely also share a variety of active but nonspecific components (Sprenkle & Blow, 2004; Wills et al., 1987).

Conceptually, tailoring couple therapy to individual differences from a pluralistic perspective involves identifying inclusionary criteria for selecting a specific treatment component for a given couple (i.e., characteristics deemed to be either essential or advantageous for that intervention's efficacy), along with exclusionary criteria (i.e., characteristics determined to result in either diminished efficacy or actual harm in response to that intervention). Different treatment components likely vary in their effectiveness in addressing specific couple concerns, as well as their selection criteria. For example, there is growing evidence that traditional behavioral interventions, although potentially least restrictive in inclusionary and exclusionary characteristics, at times may be less effective than alternative approaches. For example, Johnson and Greenberg (1985) found that EFT produced a better outcome at both termination and at 2-month follow-up compared to a behavioral approach emphasizing communication and problem-solving skills training. In their study comparing behavioral and insight-oriented couple therapy, Snyder, Wills, and Grady-Fletcher (1991a) found that at 4-year follow-up, 38% of couples in the behavioral condition had divorced compared to only 3% in the insight-oriented condition. More recently, in their study comparing traditional and integrative behavioral treatments, Christensen and colleagues (2004) found that couples in the integrative behavioral condition made steady improvements in satisfaction throughout the course of treatment, whereas couples receiving traditional behavior therapy improved more quickly early in treatment but plateaued later in treatment.

However, each of these studies also suggested potential moderator effects that may interact with treatment condition. Johnson and Talitman (1997) found that favorable response to EFT was predicted by a positive therapeutic alliance and women's trust in their partners' caring. Snyder, Mangrum, and Wills (1993) found that couples were more likely to be divorced or maritally distressed 4 years after completing either behavioral or insight-oriented therapy, if partners initially showed high levels of negative marital affect, poor problem-solving skills, low psychological resilience, high levels of depression, or low emotional responsiveness. Atkins and Christensen (2001) found that highly distressed couples improved more rapidly in early stages of traditional behavioral couple therapy compared to integrative behavioral therapy, but subsequently gained less overall in the longer term in the traditional behavioral condition. Overall, these findings suggest that couples characterized by high levels of relationship distress, or partners exhibiting higher levels of defensiveness, greater impulsivity, or diminished capacity for introspection, may initially respond less favorably to more restrictive emotionally focused, insight-oriented, or acceptance-based interventions than to a less restrictive traditional behavioral approach—but

that these more restrictive approaches may ultimately produce more enduring relationship changes once these moderators of treatment response are addressed in treatment and resolved.

Goal Setting

Initial Goals: Addressing Presenting Issues

The initial clinical interview serves as a means to obtain important information, informally observe partners' communication patterns, and establish a collaborative alliance for subsequent interventions. Snyder and Abbott (2002) advocate an extended initial assessment interview lasting about 2 hours, in which the following goals are stated at the outset: (1) getting to know each partner as an individual separate from the marriage; (2) understanding the structure and organization of the marriage; (3) learning about current relationship difficulties, their development, and previous efforts to address them; and (4) reaching an informed decision together about whether to proceed with couple therapy and, if so, discussing respective expectations.

The process of promoting an initial therapeutic alliance takes precedence over any specific content. Partners come to an initial interview primed to talk about their relationship difficulties and, more often than not, to explain why the other partner is primarily at fault. Beginning the interview with an emphasis on getting to know each individual helps to counteract this tendency. While inquiring about the family of origin and previous marriages or similar relationships, inferences can often be drawn regarding patterns of emotional or behavioral enmeshment or disengagement, models of emotional expressiveness and conflict resolution, appropriateness and clarity of boundaries, and standards or expectations about authority, autonomy, fidelity, and similar themes.

Although from a pluralistic model perspective the therapist may speculate either covertly or explicitly about the potential role of intrapersonal conflicts and their inclusion as eventual treatment goals, more typically initial goals are framed in the context of the couple's presenting complaints. What does each partner identify as the primary contributing factors to the current struggles? How do partners agree or disagree on their definition and understanding of their difficulties? What does each individual believe would be required from him- or herself to promote positive change in the marriage? Common themes emerging from the assessment process include (1) repetitive unresolved conflicts that either focus on one issue or generalize across multiple issues; (2) emotional distance or disaffection related to persistent remoteness, excessive demands, relentless criticism, or physical or emotional abuse; (3) stable but devitalized relationships characterized by an absence of intimacy, passion, or joy; (4) difficulties with third parties, including in-laws, affair partners, or children; and (5) acute crises, including alcohol or substance abuse, major psychopathology, sudden financial stressors, death of a family member, or similar concerns (Karpel, 1994).

Self-report measures of relationship functioning can also be useful for delineating and prioritizing initial treatment goals addressing areas of conflict and problematic interactional patterns. Among other advantages, such measures are relatively easy to administer, obtain a wealth of information across a broad range of issues germane to treatment, and allow disclosure about events and subjective experiences partners may initially be reluctant to discuss (Snyder et al., 2008). One such measure is the Marital Satisfaction Inventory—Revised (MSI-R; Snyder, 1997), a 150-item inventory designed to identify both the nature and intensity of relationship distress in distinct areas of interaction. The MSI-R includes two validity scales, one global scale, and 10 specific scales assessing relationship satisfaction in such areas as affective and problem-solving communication, aggression, leisure time together, finances, the sexual relationship, role orientation, family of origin, and interactions regarding children. A computerized interpretive report for the MSI-R draws on actuarial validity data to provide descriptive comparisons across different domains both within and between partners (cf. Snyder et al., 2004).

Emergent Goals: Identifying Core Relationship Themes

An essential prerequisite to affective reconstruction of relational themes is a thorough knowledge of each partner's relational history. Critical information includes not only the pattern of relationships within the family of origin but also family relational themes extending to prior generations. Beyond the family, intimate relationships with significant others of both genders from adolescence to the present offer key information regarding issues such as perceived acceptance and valuation by others, trust and disappointment, stability and resilience of relationships to interpersonal injury,

levels of attachment and respect for autonomy, and similar relational themes. Some of this information may be gleaned from earlier interventions linked to establishing appropriate boundaries with families of origin, discussion of partners' expectancies regarding parenting responsibilities acquired during their own childhood and adolescence, or disclosures of traumatic experiences with significant others prior to the current relationship. Alternatively, in anticipating focused work on developmental issues, the therapy may adopt more structured clinical or self-report techniques.

The family genogram (McGoldrick, Gerson, & Shellenberger, 1999) comprises a graphic means of depicting transgenerational family structures, dynamics, and critical family events potentially influencing family members' interactions with one another. It is constructed from information derived from an extended clinical interview regarding family history, and it both directs the interview content and evolves in response to new information gleaned during the course of therapy. The genogram reflects a family systems perspective, positing that relationship patterns in previous generations may provide implicit models for family functioning in the next generation. As such, it provides a subjective, interpretive tool that helps the therapist to delineate recurrent relationship themes within partners' extended families of origin as a prelude to interpretation of enduring individual relationship patterns.

Developed from Young's schema-based approach to therapy, the Young Schema Questionnaire (Young & Brown, 1999) is a 205-item measure assessing common maladaptive schemas across four general areas of functioning that involve, to varying degrees, perceptions of self, others, and relationships. The four general domains and specific schemas within each include (1) autonomy—with schemas addressing specific issues of dependence, self-subjugation, vulnerability to harm, and fears of losing self-control; (2) connectedness—with schemas regarding issues of emotional deprivation, abandonment, mistrust, and social isolation; (3) worthiness—with schemas concerning specific issues of one's own defectiveness, social undesirability, incompetence, guilt, and shame; and (4) expectations and limits—with schemas that concern unrelenting standards for self or, conversely, exaggerated sense of entitlement. Young (1999) has provided examples of schema maintenance, avoidance, and compensation for each of these early maladaptive schemas and their relevance to couple therapy (Young & Gluhoski, 1997).

Process and Technical Aspects of Affective Reconstruction

Timing Interpretive Interventions

For interpretation of maladaptive relationship themes to be effective with couples, the therapist needs to attend carefully to both partners' preparedness to examine their own enduring relational dispositions. Unlike individual therapy, in which clients often accept at least partial responsibility for their own distress, persons entering couple therapy often focus on their partners' negative behaviors and resist examining their own contributions to relationship difficulties—particularly those linked to more enduring personality characteristics. Distressed couples often have a long history of exchanging pejorative attributions for each other's behaviors that furthers their initial resistance to clinical interventions emphasizing early maladaptive schemas underlying relationship distress. Consequently, examining developmental sources of relationship distress demands a prerequisite foundation of emotional safety, partners' trust in the therapeutic process, partners' ability to respond empathically to the other's exposed feelings of vulnerability, and an introspective stance, initially prompted by examination of dysfunctional relationship expectancies and attributions residing at a more conscious level.

From this perspective, one of the most serious strategic errors the couple therapist can commit is to interpret underlying emotional dynamics in either partner too early in the therapeutic process—before the individual feels sufficiently secure to explore intrapersonal dynamics, or before his or her partner can respond to the interpretation in an empathic rather than attacking manner.

Linking Relationship Themes to Current Conflict

In affective reconstruction, to reduce anxiety and resistance during this exploration phase, previous relationships are initially explored without explicit linkage to current relational difficulties. Often, individuals are readily able to formulate connections between prior relationships and current interpersonal struggles; when this occurs, it is typically useful for the therapist to listen empathically, encouraging the individual to remain "intently curious" about his or her own relational history but to refrain from premature interpretations that may be either incorrect, incomplete, or excessively

self-critical. Just as important is adoption of an accepting, empathic tone by the individual's partner during the developmental exploration, encouraging self-disclosure in a supportive but noninterpretive manner.

Provided with relevant developmental history, the therapist encourages each partner to identify significant relational themes, particularly with respect to previous relationship disappointments and injuries. Gradually, as the partners continue to explore tensions and unsatisfying patterns in their own relationship, both can be encouraged to examine ways that exaggerated emotional responses to current situations have at least partial basis in affective dispositions and related coping styles acquired in the developmental context. Developing a shared formulation of core relationship themes is a critical antecedent to subsequent linkage of these themes to current relationship exchanges. Both individuals can be helped to understand that whereas certain relational coping strategies may have been adaptive or even essential in previous relationships, the same interpersonal strategies interfere with emotional intimacy and satisfaction in the present relationship.

In couple therapy, the therapist's direct access to exchanges between partners affords a unique opportunity to link enduring relationship themes to current relationship events. Rather than interpreting transferential exchanges between either partner and the therapist, the focus is on partners' own exchanges in the immediate moment. Interpretations emphasize linking each partner's exaggerated affect and maladaptive responses to his or her own relationship history, emphasizing the repetition of relationship patterns and their maintaining factors in the present context. Guidelines for examining cyclical maladaptive patterns in the context of individual therapy (Binder & Strupp, 1991; Luborsky, 1984) readily lend themselves to couple work. How does the immediate conflict between partners relate to core relationship themes explored earlier in the therapy? What are each person's feelings toward the other and desired response? What impact do partners wish to have on each other in this moment? How do their perceptions regarding the partner's inner experience relate to their attitudes toward themselves? What fantasies do they have regarding the partner's possible responses? What kinds of responses from the partner would they anticipate being helpful in modifying their core beliefs about the partner, themselves, and this relationship?

Specific therapeutic techniques relevant to examining core relationship themes in individual therapy (cf. Luborsky, 1984) apply to affective reconstruction in couple therapy as well. For example, it is essential that the therapist recognize each partner's core relationship themes, that developmental interpretations link relational themes to a current relationship conflict, and that therapy focus on a few select relationship themes, until some degree of resolution and alternative interpersonal strategies are enabled. It is also important that the extent and complexity of interpretations take into account (1) the affective functioning of the individual and his or her ability to make constructive use of the interpretation, (2) the level of insight and how near the individual is to being aware of the content of the proposed interpretation, and (3) the level of partners' relationship functioning and the extent to which developmental interpretations can be incorporated in a mutually supportive manner.

From a psychodynamic perspective, cognitive linkage of relational themes from early development to the current context is frequently insufficient for reconstructing or modifying these interpersonal patterns. The affective component of interpretation is seen in the reconstruction of these critical emotional experiences in the immediate context; new understanding by both partners often promotes more empathic responses toward both the self and the other, facilitating more satisfactory resolutions to conflict. Often the individuals must be encouraged to work through previous relationship injuries, grieving losses and unmet needs, expressing ambivalence or anger toward previous critical others in the safety of the conjoint therapy, and acquiring increased differentiation between prior relationships and the present one. Similar to individual therapy adopting a relational model, the therapist serves as an auxiliary processor helping to "detoxify, manage, and digest" the partners' relationship themes in a manner that promotes interpersonal growth (Messer & Warren, 1995, p. 141).

Promoting Alternative Relationship Behaviors

Affective reconstruction makes possible but does not inevitably lead to changes in maladaptive relationship patterns. In addition to interpretive strategies, interventions must promote spousal interactions that counteract early maladaptive schemas. Thus, the couple therapist allows part-

ners' maladaptive patterns to be enacted within limits, then assists both partners in examining exaggerated affective components of their present exchange. Partners' exaggerated responses are framed as acquired coping strategies that interfere with higher relationship values. Interpretations of the developmental context underlying the current unsatisfactory exchange help both partners to depersonalize the noxious effects of the other's behavior, to feel less wounded, and consequently to be less reactive in a reciprocally negative manner.

Both individuals are encouraged to be less anxious and less condemning of both their own and their partner's affect, and are helped to explore, then express their own affect in less aggressive or antagonistic fashion. Throughout this process, each individual plays a critical therapeutic role by learning to offer a secure context in facilitating his or her partner's affective self-disclosures in a softened, more vulnerable manner. The couple therapist models empathic understanding for both partners and encourages new patterns of responding that enhance relationship intimacy; that is, by facilitating the nonoccurrence of expected traumatic experiences in the couple's relationship, the therapist enables both individuals to challenge assumptions and expectations comprising underlying maladaptive schemas. Thus, therapeutic change results from experiential learning in which both partners encounter relationship outcomes that are different from those they expected or feared. In response, partners' interactions become more adaptive and flexible in matching the objective reality of current conflicts and realizing opportunities for satisfying more of each other's needs.

Although affective reconstruction seeks to promote new relationship schemas facilitating more empathic and supportive interactions, couples sometimes need additional assistance in restructuring longstanding patterns of relating outside of therapy. In the pluralistic hierarchical model for sequencing interventions advocated here, couples already will have been exposed to communication and behavior-exchange techniques characterizing traditional behavioral approaches. Consequently, alternative relationship behaviors can often be negotiated more readily after schema-related anxieties and resistance to changing persistent interaction patterns have been understood and at least partially resolved.

From a pluralistic model, termination of couple therapy proceeds when the couple has resolved any initial crises potentially precipitating treatment; when partners have acquired information and specific skills essential to maintaining individual as well as relational health; and when each partner understands and resolves individual dynamics previously contributing to exaggerated emotional reactivities, and substantially reduces or eliminates distorted responses to his or her own as well as the other's dynamics. As evidence of these goals being met evolves, the therapist may suggest terminating or "thinning out" the frequency of sessions—with remaining interventions emphasizing an integrative review and consolidation of therapeutic work that has been accomplished, and preparation for anticipated stresses from within or outside the couple relationship that may challenge individual or relationship functioning in the future.

MECHANISMS OF THERAPEUTIC CHANGE

Affective reconstruction strives to bring about critical changes in how individuals view themselves, their partner, and their relationship. In examining recurrent maladaptive relationship themes, partners gain increased understanding of their own emotional reactivity and exaggerated patterns of interacting that contribute to their own unhappiness. Increases in partners' self-understanding can lead to diminished confusion and anxiety about their own subjective relationship experiences. Moreover, insight into developmental influences contributing to current difficulties often facilitates an optimism regarding potential for self-change and restores hope for greater emotional fulfillment in the relationship. Affective reconstruction of maladaptive schemas promotes resolution of persistent dysfunctional relationship patterns through redirected cognitive and behavioral strategies.

In the context of couple therapy, affective reconstruction offers unique advantages over similar therapeutic strategies conducted with individuals. Specifically, as participant–observer in the partner's work on developmental issues, individuals frequently come to understand the partner's behaviors in a more accepting or benign manner—attributing damaging exchanges to the culmination of acquired interpersonal dispositions rather than to explicit motives to be hurtful. This new understanding often facilitates within-session exchanges that challenge existing relationship schemas, reduce defensive behaviors, and promote empathic and mutually supportive interactions.

TREATMENT APPLICABILITY AND EMPIRICAL SUPPORT

Selection of Couples

Affective reconstruction of recurrent maladaptive relationship themes is not appropriate for all couples. Some couples enter therapy with relatively healthy relationship schemas but exhibit difficulties resulting from situational stressors or specific relationship skills deficits. Such couples often achieve significant and enduring gains from traditional behavioral strategies emphasizing communication and behavior-exchange skills training.

Other couples may be inappropriate candidates for interpretive strategies because of persistent hostility, mistrust, inflexibility, and resistance to change. Unless an atmosphere of safety can be established that extends beyond therapy sessions to the couple's interactions outside of therapy, each individual may be reluctant to disclose the intimate and emotionally difficult material from previous relationships that is essential to the process of affective reconstruction of relationship themes. Ultimately, the capacity of each partner to adopt an empathic stance toward the other's feelings may be as critical, or more so, as the therapist's own empathic understanding when implementing interpretive techniques in the context of conjoint couple therapy.

Similar to selection criteria for brief psychodynamic approaches to working with individuals (cf. Luborsky, 1984; Strupp & Binder, 1984; Wachtel, 1997), both partners must be open to examining current relational difficulties from a developmental perspective. Both should exhibit some capacity for introspection, be open to examining feelings, and be able to resurrect affective experiences from previous relationships on a conscious level. Each partner needs to have established a basic level of trust with the therapist, experiencing the exploration of cyclical maladaptive patterns as promoting the individual's own relationship fulfillment. Moreover, both individuals need to exhibit a level of both personal maturity and relationship commitment that enables them to respond to the partner's intimate disclosures with empathy and support rather than seizing details of previous relationships as new and more potent ammunition in a mutual blaming process.

Empirical Support for Efficacy of Affective Reconstruction

Although psychodynamic approaches to couple therapy are among the earliest approaches to treating relationship distress, empirical study of their efficacy has been quite limited. Only one study has examined the effectiveness of affective reconstruction as described here. Snyder and Wills (1989) compared behavioral and insight-oriented approaches to couple therapy in a controlled outcome study involving 79 distressed couples. The behavioral condition emphasized communication skills training and behavior-exchange techniques; the insight-oriented condition emphasized the interpretation and resolution of conflictual emotional processes related to developmental issues, collusive interactions, and maladaptive relationship patterns. At termination, after approximately 20 sessions, couples in both treatment modalities showed statistically and clinically significant gains in relationship satisfaction compared to a waiting-list control group. Treatment effect sizes at termination for behavioral and insight-oriented conditions were 1.01 and 0.96, respectively, indicating that the average person receiving either couple therapy was better off at termination than approximately 83% of individuals not receiving treatment. Moreover, treatment gains for couples in both therapy conditions were substantially maintained at 6-month follow-up.

However, at 4 years following treatment, 38% of the behavioral couples had experienced divorce, in contrast to only 3% of couples treated in the insight-oriented condition (Snyder et al., 1991a). Based on these findings, Snyder and colleagues suggested an important distinction between *acquisition* of relationship skills through instruction or rehearsal versus interference with *implementation* of these skills on a motivational or affective basis. They argued that spouses' views toward their partner's behavior "are modified to a greater degree and in a more persistent manner once individuals come to understand and resolve emotional conflicts they bring to the marriage from their own family and relationship histories" (Snyder, Wills, & Grady-Fletcher, 1991b, p.148).

CASE ILLUSTRATION

Presenting Concerns

Alan and Hannah, ages 51 and 44, respectively, were referred to the first author (D. K. S.) for couple therapy by a pediatrician who had been assisting them with parenting strategies related to their 10-year-old son Jason, who had been diagnosed with attention-deficit/hyperactivity disorder (ADHD). The couple reported significant rela-

tionship problems throughout most of the 23-year marriage. In addition to Jason they had an 18-year-old daughter, April, who would be leaving home to attend college within a few months. Alan and Hannah acknowledged poor communication skills and described intense arguments occurring several times per week—sometimes related to parenting of Jason, but just as frequently related to other household or family management issues, with particularly severe conflicts over finances. Hannah emphasized her repeated frustration and anger over what she described as Alan's irresponsibility, and he countered with complaints about her intrusive and controlling behaviors. Although both partners professed commitment to staying married, each acknowledged substantial and persistent disillusionment with their relationship. The couple had been in couple therapy twice previously, each time for only a few months, terminating both times when the therapy appeared ineffective in alleviating longstanding conflicts.

Developmental Background

The couple met while Alan was completing a master's degree in electrical engineering and Hannah was a college freshman; they married a year later, at which point Hannah withdrew from school. Alan had difficulty finding employment suited to his engineering skills and eventually settled for a job teaching general science to ninth graders at a small private school. The couple had difficulty supporting their household, and Alan pursued various unskilled positions to supplement his teacher's salary—most recently working at a bakery several hours each morning before school, a situation that often left him exhausted by the time he arrived home in the evening. Shortly after April was born, Hannah pursued a part-time position in a tailoring and custom alterations shop, and gradually expanded her work to include alterations from their home. Although averaging only 30 hours per week, absorbing her work schedule into demands of managing their household and contending with Jason frequently left Hannah exhausted as well, and resentful of their financial struggles. She had expected more for them and showed no reluctance in letting Alan know of her disappointment in his apparent lack of career aspirations or drive.

In the initial interview, Hannah reported that she was the seventh of nine children. Her parents divorced when she was 4, and she had seen little of her father since that time. Her father had been physically abusive toward her mother, who never remarried. Hannah described being close to her mother and talking with her weekly by phone, but visiting her out of state only once each summer for a week. She declined to discuss feelings about her father's abuse or her parents' divorce, other than to assert that she had learned early on "to be strong and count only on myself." Alan had grown up in an intact family with three younger sisters. He reported little overt conflict in his family of origin but acknowledged that members of his family had never been close. His father was emotionally distant, and neither parent had set many limits on Alan's behaviors during adolescence—contributing to his experimentation with alcohol and recreational drugs, as well as occasional truancy from school. As an adult, Alan had felt encouraged by his mother, and continued to grieve her death 2 years earlier. Loss of his mother, despair in

his marriage, and lack of efficacy in his career all contributed to clinical depression.

Test Findings

The couple's profiles on the MSI-R confirmed high levels of overall relationship distress experienced by both partners—particularly for Hannah, whose score of 79T on Global Distress placed her at the 99th percentile relative to the community standardization sample for this measure (see Figure 12.3). Neither partner made any effort to conceal marital distress, and Hannah's profile suggested her potential to minimize any positive features of the marriage while attending and reacting primarily to negative characteristics. Alan's responses reflected a moderate level of inconsistency in identifying relationship concerns—suggesting that within vari-

MSI-R Scales			Raw	T	30T	40T	50T	60T	70T
Inconsistency	(INC)	Wife	0	29					
		Husband	9	67					
Conventionalization	(CNV)	Wife	0	34					
		Husband	2	40					
Global Distress	(GDS)	Wife	22	79					
		Husband	15	68					
Affective Communication	(AFC)	Wife	9	62					
		Husband	7	61					
Problem-Solving Communication	(PSC)	Wife	15	64					
		Husband	18	72					
Aggression	(AGG)	Wife	0	40					
		Husband	3	56					
Time Together	(TTO)	Wife	8	64					
		Husband	6	60					
Disagreement about Finances	(FIN)	Wife	10	71					
		Husband	7	64					
Sexual Dissatisfaction	(SEX)	Wife	3	49					
		Husband	9	58					
Role Orientation	(ROR)	Wife	2	37					
		Husband	6	48					
Family History of Distress	(FAM)	Wife	9	70					
		Husband	2	45					
Dissatisfaction with Children	(DSC)	Wife	4	60					
		Husband	5	62					
Conflict over Child Rearing	(CCR)	Wife	8	70					
		Husband	5	64					

Interpretive Key (does not apply to ROR Scale) — Good — Possible Problem — Problem

Client Key ●——● Wife   ▲——▲ Husband

FIGURE 12.3. Initial profiles on the Marital Satisfaction Inventory—Revised (MSI-R) for Alan and Hannah. The MSI-R form is from Snyder (1997). Copyright (c) by Western Psychological Services. Used by permission of the publisher, Western Psychological Services, 12031 Wilshire Boulevard, Los Angeles, California, 90025 USA. Not to be reprinted in whole or in part for any additional purpose without the expressed, written permission of the publisher. All rights reserved.

ous domains of spousal interaction he experienced mixed elements of satisfaction and distress.

Alan's MSI-R profile highlighted his primary complaints about the couple's inability to manage even minor disagreements and his view of Hannah as having become intensely negative and emotionally aggressive. By comparison, Hannah's profile emphasized her immense frustration with the couple's management of finances and conflicts over child rearing—particularly as these related to their struggles in parenting Jason. Upon inquiry, both partners denied any incidents of physical aggression. Both reported significant deficits in emotional intimacy and quality of leisure time together, but only Alan complained of deficits in sexual intimacy—consistent with Hannah's apparent lack of interest in physical closeness. Both partners endorsed somewhat traditional marital and parental roles, with Hannah adopting a pronounced position advocating husbands' responsibility for supporting their family and a leadership role in the home—something she underscored as lacking in Alan. Consistent with her reports in the initial interview, Hannah's profile affirmed her description of extensive disruption in her family of origin, contrasted with Alan's minimization of concerns in his own family.

Initial Interventions

Consistent with the pluralistic model we described earlier, initial interventions with Alan and Hannah emphasized strengthening the therapeutic alliance with both partners and their collaborative stance with each other. Although Alan spoke more often than Hannah, the intensity and negativity of her statements risked dominating the treatment emotionally. Greater balance was achieved by limiting the length of Alan's verbalizations and gently but persistently assisting Hannah in tempering the affective intensity of hers. Although both partners were committed in principle to staying in their marriage, their pessimism about potential for change led each to retreat into familiar patterns rather than risk change in their own behaviors, requiring explicit and modest challenges from their therapist each week to implement at least one meaningful and measurable different behavior before the next session.

Ineffective strategies for managing their son's ADHD contributed to regular crises in their home. Already frustrated with Alan's lack of involvement and feeling overwhelmed herself, Hannah frequently reacted to Jason's noncompliance and temper tantrums with explosive anger of her own—yelling at her son, berating Alan for his lack of support, and alternating between intrusive but ineffective efforts to control Jason and tearful retreats to her bedroom. Hannah benefited considerably from several books provided by her therapist outlining more effective parenting strategies for special-needs youngsters, and she began to use couple sessions as opportunities to explore her emotional responses to Jason and enlist Alan's support in less angry and blaming ways. Their couple therapist consulted with Jason's pediatrician to explore both behavioral and pharmacological strategies for assisting Jason and his parents, and within a month both parents reported significant improvements at home. With their anger at Jason significantly reduced and their empathic awareness of their son's own emotional turmoil enhanced, the parents requested a family session including Jason. During the family meeting, the therapist helped Jason to hear his parents' concerns in a way that felt more supportive, and Jason disclosed his own fears about difficulties in managing his emotions and behaviors in ways that further encouraged his parents' understanding and assistance.

Increased parental collaboration in dealing with Jason generalized to modest but visible collaboration in other domains as well. Hannah developed greater understanding of the physical demands posed by Alan's maintaining two jobs and offered an hour for rest in the evening before requesting his assistance with parenting or other household responsibilities. Feeling somewhat more appreciated, Alan reciprocated by providing Hannah relief and assuming a greater share of responsibilities in the home on the weekend. Both partners took independent steps to address individual challenges: Alan, by acknowledging his enduring depression and pursuing an initial trial of medication; and Hannah, by adopting explicit strategies to monitor and intervene in her own emotion regulation difficulties. The marriage got noticeably better and recurrent feelings of imminent marital crisis abated; however, significant relationship difficulties persisted.

Intermediate Interventions

Alan and Hannah struggled with considerable financial stress—including credit card debt of over $40,000 that had accumulated during the past 5 years, aging vehicles that they were unable to replace but required costly repairs, limited preparations for retirement that loomed larger with each passing year, and a limit on their overall income that constrained efforts to address these various concerns. Their enduring financial strains began to dominate couple therapy sessions and became a medium for pursuing more effective problem-solving and decision-making skills. With considerable effort, they were able to agree on a small number of substantive changes, including refinancing of their mortgage, fewer meals outside the home, and relinquishing a time-share investment property. However, the more Alan and Hannah worked to address enduring financial difficulties, the more intense their respective styles of managing stress became. Hannah pursued harsh, somewhat draconian constraints on their daily lifestyles that had little substantive impact on their overall financial status. She viewed these as essential symbolic representations of their shared commitment to the family. By contrast, Alan experienced her demands for monetary constraint as excessive, largely ineffective, and a daily reminder of his failure to provide adequately for his family.

Efforts to challenge the meanings that each partner attributed to the financial struggles had only modest impact. Hannah acknowledged daily terror surrounding her anticipated demise of the family but remained rigidly unwilling to explore any connection between her current fears and the feelings of abandonment she had experienced as a youngster after her parents divorced and her mother struggled to provide for nine children. Alan at times hinted at his own fears of inadequacy and the guilt and shame he experienced, but Hannah's harsh criticisms more consistently elicited his complaints about her intrusive and excessive control of his and their children's behaviors. Therapeutic injunctions encouraging Hannah to "work less hard at rescuing Alan from his avoidance of difficult financial choices" led to modest but temporary softening in her challenges to Alan and to his equally modest but temporary initiatives in addressing financial difficulties. However, neither partner felt sufficiently secure in the couple therapy to suspend attacks on the other and to examine the developmental sources of his or her own emotional vulnerabilities. Initial therapeutic efforts to highlight the similarity of current emotions to those of earlier experiences yielded only modest gain, as reflected in the following exchange from a typical session:

DKS: Hannah, talk with me about the feelings you're having right now.

HANNAH: It's the same old story all over again.

DKS: The same old story ...

HANNAH: Yeah—the same today, the same last year, the same 20 years ago. He just doesn't get it. He's got his head in the ground.

DKS: Try to describe the feelings ...

HANNAH: It's hopeless. I may as well just give up. There's no point in pursuing this with Alan. He's just not going to step up to the plate.

DKS: That hopelessness—it feels familiar?

HANNAH: Familiar? You bet, daily.

DKS: Since when?

HANNAH: Since practically the beginning of the marriage, when Alan settled for a third-rate job instead of pursuing something he was really trained for.

DKS: You had more hope then ...

HANNAH: Well, it didn't last very long.

DKS: (pausing) What about before then? Do you recall ever feeling hopeless earlier on? I know that your life wasn't an easy one.

HANNAH: I never felt hopeless, because I learned early on to do what had to be done to survive.

DKS: You're a survivor, for sure.

HANNAH: That's right.

DKS: But I'm wondering whether perhaps that also comes with some cost.

HANNAH: Like what?

DKS: Well, I'm thinking that 4- and 5-year-olds aren't supposed to have to survive on their own.

HANNAH: I had my mother.

DKS: You did, and she worked hard to be a good mom. But it must have been a real struggle with nine children—even after moving in with your grandparents ...

HANNAH: We did what we had to.

DKS: Just like now.

HANNAH: That's right—except then at least I had someone else to count on, like my mom or grandparents—not like now.

DKS: (resisting the allusion to Alan) And your dad? What about him?

HANNAH: He wasn't in the picture—like I've told you before—so I don't have any feelings about him at all.

ALAN: (sarcastically) Oh yeah, right—no feelings at all.

HANNAH: (*to Alan*) I never expected anything—never got anything—so I just don't care about him. But I expected more from you. Maybe *that* was my mistake …

DKS: (*to Hannah*) Can you describe the feeling you're having right now?

HANNAH: Yeah, I'm angry at Alan for trying to make out like he's a victim somehow—that I'm blaming him for what happened earlier in my life. That's just a bunch of crap and I'm not buying it. I'm holding you accountable for *you*, Alan, and you keep falling short.

ALAN: (*after a long pause, and looking away*) Right …

DKS: Alan, talk with me.

ALAN: About what?

DKS: Just talk with me about what you're feeling now …

ALAN: There's just no point … (*refusing to re-engage in the session*).

Over the next 2 months, further progress was slow and limited. Alan and Hannah continued to collaborate more effectively in parenting Jason and shared other responsibilities in the home somewhat more effectively. They found ways to support their daughter's college expenses through various loans, college aid, and cost containment strategies. The frequency and intensity of their arguments diminished, but each partner continued to harbor resentments around their enduring financial strains, with Hannah concluding that matters in this respect would never improve, and Alan remaining convinced that nothing he did would ever be sufficient. After several months of maintaining a stable, if not intimate, relationship Hannah announced her decision to discontinue couple therapy—with Alan concurring in a tone of subdued relief. For 2 years, there was no further contact with the couple.

Final Interventions

After a 2-year absence, Hannah called requesting an opportunity to resume couple therapy, stating that they had weathered several crises prompting a renewed commitment to resolve longstanding problems. A year after suspending the earlier therapy, Hannah had been diagnosed with breast cancer that—although successfully treated—contributed to a major depression that eventually required psychiatric hospitalization. Now, 6 months later, the

couple was determined to make the most of their lives together. Hannah's illness had forced her to terminate work outside the home. She recognized all that Alan had done to care for their family while she had been incapacitated and affirmed a newfound respect for his quiet but steadfast manner. Alan showed less intimidation when interacting with Hannah, as well as greater empathy for her emotional vulnerability. Both partners requested assistance in resolving longstanding struggles in dealing with their finances. Both expressed confidence that they could unravel the emotional dynamics that had kept them tied in knots and had rendered previous efforts in this domain ineffective, although both also professed confusion about the nature of their respective dynamics and the effects on their interactions. Insight was acquired slowly over several sessions as both Alan and Hannah explored earlier developmental experiences that had given rise to their respective vulnerabilities. There were no sudden breakthroughs. Rather, there were several series of small discoveries, shared vulnerabilities, supportive affirmations from each other, and modest celebrations as prior antagonisms yielded to a trust in each other's intentions and greater acceptance of their respective emotional struggles. The following excerpt from a typical session reflects the couple's efforts to understand the origins of their feelings more fully.

HANNAH: It's just always been so difficult.
    DKS: Difficult?

HANNAH: Difficult, uncertain—you know—never really feeling confident that things would be OK.

DKS: Help me understand that feeling better, what it's like when you don't feel that basic security.

HANNAH: It's terrifying. I mean, I know other people have it worse—no partner, no job, maybe no home or living on the streets—and I've never had that. But it felt almost as bad …

ALAN: I still have trouble understanding that …

HANNAH: I know, Alan. I know on some level it doesn't make sense, but that's still the way it has felt.

DKS: Terrifying …

HANNAH: Yeah. I remember when we worked together last time you said I should try to remember times when I felt that before, like maybe after my dad left … and I just couldn't. Maybe that was too frightening for me, or maybe I thought Alan wouldn't take my concerns about us seriously if he could blame my parents' divorce.

DKS: And now?

HANNAH: I don't worry about that as much now. I know Alan takes me seriously, even when we see things differently. He's not going to up and leave. We've got some real problems, but when worse came to worst, he stood by and kept things running.

DKS: Ask Alan what that was like for him.

HANNAH: (*looking at Alan*) So, what was that like?

ALAN: Hannah, I'm never going to leave. And I'm not going to let things fall apart, no matter what. I just wish you could trust me to take care of things—to take care of *you*.

HANNAH: That's always been so hard. I wish you could understand how scared I've been …

ALAN: I try, I really do—and sometimes I can see it. It's easier to see you're scared when I don't have to look past your anger. But when you're angry with me, or even when I hear the disappointment in your voice, I just want to run away. You're the one I need to believe in me, Hannah (*tearing up*).

DKS: Alan, where is the hurt coming from?

ALAN: (*after a long pause*) You know, I've always talked about how easy it was growing up—few arguments with my parents, pretty much doing what I wanted. But toward the end of high school I began to see that the freedom I had wasn't because they trusted me. It was more like they just weren't all that concerned about me, that it just didn't really matter.

DKS: *It* didn't matter?

ALAN: That *I* didn't really matter. And then when I dropped out of college after the first year, it was clear that I mattered enough for them to be disappointed in me—especially my dad.

DKS: What happened?

ALAN: It's more like what didn't happen. I mean, I didn't get much encouragement. They didn't really try to figure out what was going on with *me*. My dad's idea of encouragement was to tell me to get a job and not go back to school until I was ready.

DKS: How did you distinguish their indifference from their acceptance?

ALAN: I'm not sure. I mean … my mom essentially told me the same thing, but there was a differ-

ence in how she said it—more caring in her voice—like she knew things would eventually work out for me …

DKS: And your dad?

ALAN: I learned to be more careful with what I told him. I never let him know what my plans were. That way, if they fell through, I didn't have to deal with his disappointment.

HANNAH: But you did the same thing with me, Alan, and so I never knew that things would be OK because you never let me know that you were worried, too, or how you were hoping to fix things.

ALAN: I just couldn't deal with your disappointment (*pause*) or your anger.

HANNAH: I was just scared …

ALAN: I was scared, too—but not about whether we could make it. I was more scared about how you were feeling about me, about no longer looking up to me. I tried to reassure you by not letting anything upset me and not worrying out loud with you.

HANNAH: And I mostly saw that as your not caring—not caring about me, not about us—and that terrified me more than anything else we were facing (*long pause*).

ALAN: I can do a better job of sharing my own concerns so you don't feel as alone with yours.

HANNAH: And I can do a better job of trusting you.

Similar exchanges over several sessions illuminated long histories of recurrent feelings of abandonment for Hannah and inadequacy for Alan, and ways these had contaminated many of their exchanges over the years in not only how they managed their finances but also how they addressed challenges of parenting and approached their sexual relationship. As each reconstructed the developmental experiences that had given rise to these dynamics, the disruptive intensity of their exchanges diminished. Alan and Hannah each recognized his or her own escalating emotions earlier in the midst of problem-solving efforts or stressful events at home, and found more effective ways of labeling and owning their feelings. Each developed greater empathy for the other's struggles in ways that constrained his or her own reactivity. Within a few months, they had reached decisions together that promised to reduce substantially, if not eliminate, financial strains within the next few years. More importantly, they gradually restored trust in each other and began to pursue more effective ways to play together and rediscover joy in being together.

CHALLENGES OF PURSUING AN INFORMED PLURALISTIC APPROACH

To practice effectively from a pluralistic approach, couple therapists must be thoroughly schooled in both the conceptual suppositions and technical interventions linked to diverse theoretical models of relationship distress and treatment. Equally important is the ability of the couple therapist to incorporate these models in a conceptually coherent manner tailored to specific characteristics of individual partners, their relationship, and immediate circumstances of the therapeutic process. In encouraging couple and family therapists to pursue a personal integrative approach, Lebow (1987) noted that technique offers no substitute for therapeutic skill, and that therapists need to adopt a blend of theory, strategies, and specific interventions with which they are both professionally and personally comfortable.

Affective reconstruction comprises a critical component of couple therapy from a pluralistic perspective. Whereas some partners demonstrate a capacity to implement and maintain important relationship changes without undertaking such reconstructive work, others remain significantly, if not permanently, mired in recurrent maladaptive interactions until they understand and resolve the developmental origins of exaggerated or distorted emotional responses to their own concerns or those of their partner. For some couples, affective reconstruction yields rapid and dramatic breakthroughs and resolution of longstanding dysfunctional patterns of interrelating. For others, insights are more gradual and the gains, more circumscribed. Affective reconstruction becomes critical to couple therapy when partners' difficulties arise in part from previous relationship injuries resulting in sustained interpersonal vulnerabilities and related defensive strategies interfering with emotional intimacy. Partners' ability to benefit from insight into these vulnerabilities and defensive strategies is optimized when affective reconstruction is embedded within a broader, comprehensive therapeutic strategy building upon structural, behavioral, and cognitive interventions earlier in the therapeutic sequence.

SUGGESTIONS FOR FURTHER READING

Case Studies

Snyder, D. K. (1999). Pragmatic couple therapy: An informed pluralistic approach. In D. M. Lawson & F. F. Prevatt (Eds.), *Casebook in family therapy* (pp. 81–110). Pacific Grove, CA: Brooks/Cole.

Snyder, D. K. (2002). Integrating insight-oriented techniques into couple therapy. In J. H. Harvey & A. E. Wenzel (Eds.), *A clinician's guide to maintaining and enhancing close relationships* (pp. 259–275). Mahwah, NJ: Erlbaum.

Empirical Studies

Snyder, D. K., & Wills, R. M. (1989). Behavioral versus insight-oriented marital therapy: Effects on individual and interspousal functioning. *Journal of Consulting and Clinical Psychology, 57,* 39–46.

Snyder, D. K., Wills, R. M., & Grady-Fletcher, A. (1991). Long-term effectiveness of behavioral versus insight-oriented marital therapy: A four-year follow-up study. *Journal of Consulting and Clinical Psychology, 59,* 138–141.

Integrative Reviews of Couple Assessment and Intervention Techniques

Snyder, D. K., Castellani, A. M., & Whisman, M. A. (2006). Current status and future directions in couple therapy. *Annual Review of Clinical Psychology, 57,* 317–344.

Snyder, D. K., Heyman, R. E., & Haynes, S. N. (2008). Assessing couple distress. In J. Hunsley & E. Mash (Eds.), *A guide to assessments that work.* New York: Oxford University Press.

REFERENCES

Alexander, F. (1956). *Psychoanalysis and psychotherapy.* New York: Norton.

Anchin, J. C., & Kiesler, D. J. (Eds.). (1982). *Handbook of interpersonal psychotherapy.* New York: Pergamon Press.

Atkins, D. C., Berns, S. B., George, W. H., Doss, B. D., Gattis, K., & Christensen, A. (2005). Prediction of response to treatment in a randomized clinical trial of marital therapy. *Journal of Consulting and Clinical Psychology, 73,* 893–903.

Atkins, D. C., & Christensen, A. (2001, November). Main outcome findings from active treatment: Self-report of marital quality. In K. Sutherland (Chair), *The effects of marital therapy: Posttreatment results of a dual-site clinical trial.* Symposium presented at the meeting of the Association for the Advancement of Behavior Therapy, Philadelphia, PA.

Barber, J. P., & Crits-Christoph, P. (1991). Comparison of the brief dynamic therapies. In P. Crits-Christoph

& J. P. Barber (Eds.), *Handbook of short-term dynamic psychotherapy* (pp. 323–352). New York: Basic Books.

Beach, S. R. H., & Gupta, M. (2003). Depression. In D. K. Snyder & M. A. Whisman (Eds.), *Treating difficult couples: Helping clients with coexisting mental and relationship disorders* (pp. 88–113). New York: Guilford Press.

Beutler, L. E., & Clarkin, J. (1990). *Systematic treatment selection: Toward targeted therapeutic interventions.* New York: Brunner/Mazel.

Beutler, L. E., Consoli, A. J., & Lane, G. (2005). Systematic treatment selection and prescriptive psychotherapy. In J. C. Norcross & M. R. Goldfried (Eds.), *Handbook of psychotherapy integration* (2nd ed., pp. 121–146). New York: Oxford University Press.

Beutler, L. E., Consoli, A. J., & Williams, R. E. (1995). Integrative and eclectic therapies in practice. In B. Bongar & L. E. Beutler (Eds.), *Comprehensive textbook of psychotherapy: Theory and practice* (pp. 274–292). New York: Oxford University Press.

Binder, J. L., & Strupp, H. H. (1991). The Vanderbilt approach to time-limited dynamic psychotherapy. In P. Crits-Christoph & J. P. Barber (Eds.), *Handbook of short-term dynamic psychotherapy* (pp. 137–165). New York: Basic Books.

Bongar, B., & Beutler, L. E. (1995). *Comprehensive textbook of psychotherapy: Theory and practice.* New York: Oxford University Press.

Bowlby, J. (1969). *Attachment and loss: Vol. 1. Attachment.* New York: Basic Books.

Christensen, A., Atkins, D. C., Berns, S., Wheeler, J., Baucom, D. H., & Simpson, L. E. (2004). Traditional versus integrative behavioral couple therapy for significantly and chronically distressed married couples. *Journal of Consulting and Clinical Psychology, 72,* 176–191.

Dicks, H. V. (1967). *Marital tensions: Clinical studies towards a psycho-analytic theory of interaction.* London: Routledge & Kegan Paul.

Epstein, N. B., & Baucom, D. H. (2002). *Enhanced cognitive-behavioral therapy for couples: A contextual approach.* Washington, DC: American Psychological Association.

Fairbairn, W. R. D. (1952). *Psychoanalytic studies of the personality.* London: Routledge & Kegan Paul.

Furman, W., & Flanagan, A. S. (1997). The influence of earlier relationships on marriage: An attachment perspective. In W. K. Halford & H. J. Markman (Eds.), *Clinical handbook of marriage and couples interventions* (pp. 179–202). New York: Wiley.

Goldfried, M. R., & Norcross, J. C. (1995). Integrative and eclectic therapies in historical perspective. In B. Bongar & L. E. Beutler (Eds.), *Comprehensive textbook of psychotherapy: Theory and practice* (pp. 254–273). New York: Oxford University Press.

Goldfried, M. R., Pachankis, J. E., & Bell, A. C. (2005). A history of psychotherapy integration. In J. C. Norcross & M. R. Goldfried (Eds.), *Handbook of psychotherapy integration* (2nd ed., pp. 24–64). New York: Oxford University Press.

Gottlieb, M. C. (1996). Some ethical implications of relational diagnoses. In F. W. Kaslow (Ed.), *Handbook of relational diagnosis and dysfunctional family patterns* (pp. 19–34). New York: Wiley.

Gottman, J. M. (1999). *The marriage clinic: A scientifically based marital therapy.* New York: Norton.

Gottman, J. M., & Gottman, J. S. (1999). The marriage survival kit: A research-based marital therapy. In R. Berger & M. T. Hannah (Eds.), *Preventive approaches in couples therapy* (pp. 304–330). Philadelphia: Brunner/Mazel.

Gurman, A. S. (1980). Behavioral marriage therapy in the 1980s: The challenge of integration. *American Journal of Family Therapy, 8,* 86–96.

Gurman, A. S. (1981). Integrative marital therapy: Toward the development of an interpersonal approach. In S. H. Budman (Ed.), *Forms of brief therapy* (pp. 415–457). New York: Guilford Press.

Gurman, A. S. (1992). Integrative marital therapy: A time-sensitive model for working with couples. In S. H. Budman & M. F. Hoyt (Eds.), *The first session in brief therapy* (pp. 186–203). New York: Guilford Press.

Gurman, A. S. (2002). Brief integrative marital therapy: A depth-behavioral approach. In A. S. Gurman & N. S. Jacobson (Eds.), *Clinical handbook of couple therapy* (3rd ed., pp. 180–220). New York: Guilford Press.

Hazan, C., & Shaver, P. R. (1987). Romantic love conceptualized as an attachment process. *Journal of Personality and Social Psychology, 59,* 511–524.

Holtzworth-Munroe, A., Marshall, A. D., Meehan, J. C., & Rehman, U. (2003). Physical aggression. In D. K. Snyder & M. A. Whisman (Eds.), *Treating difficult couples: Helping clients with coexisting mental and relationship disorders* (pp. 201–230). New York: Guilford Press.

Horowitz, M. (1988). *Introduction to psychodynamics: A new synthesis.* New York: Basic Books.

Jacobson, N. S., & Christensen, A. (1996). *Integrative couple therapy: Promoting acceptance and change.* New York: Norton.

Jacobson, N. S., & Margolin, G. (1979). *Marital therapy: Strategies based on social learning and behavior exchange principles.* New York: Brunner/Mazel.

Johnson, S. M. (2004). *The practice of emotionally focused couple therapy* (2nd ed.). New York: Brunner-Routledge.

Johnson, S. M., & Greenberg, L. S. (1985). Differential effects of experiential and problem-solving interventions in resolving marital conflict. *Journal of Consulting and Clinical Psychology, 53,* 175–184.

Johnson, S. M., & Greenberg, L. S. (1995). The emotionally focused approach to problems in adult attachment. In N. S. Jacobson & A. S. Gurman (Eds.), *Clinical handbook of couple therapy* (2nd ed., pp. 121–141). New York: Guilford Press.

Johnson, S. M., & Talitman, E. (1997). Predictors of success in emotionally focused marital therapy. *Journal of Marital and Family Therapy, 23,* 135–152.

Karpel, M. A. (1994). *Evaluating couples: A handbook for practitioners.* New York: Norton.

Klein, M. (1950). *Contributions to psychoanalysis*. London: Hogarth.

Kobak, R., Ruckdeschel, K., & Hazan, C. (1994). From symptom to signal: An attachment view of emotion in marital therapy. In S. M. Johnson & L. S. Greenberg (Eds.), *The heart of the matter: Perspectives on emotion in marital therapy* (pp. 46–71). New York: Brunner/Mazel.

Lebow, J. L. (1987). Developing a personal integration in family therapy: Principles for model construction and practice. *Journal of Marital and Family Therapy, 13*, 1–14.

Lebow, J. L. (1997). The integrative revolution in couple and family therapy. *Family Process, 36*, 1–17.

Lebow, J. L. (2003). Integrative approaches to couple and family therapy. In T. L. Sexton, G. R. Weeks, & M. S. Robbins (Eds.), *Handbook of family therapy: The science and practice of working with families and couples* (pp. 201–225). New York: Brunner-Routledge.

Liberman, G., & Lavine, A. (1998). *Love, marriage and money*. Chicago: Dearborn Financial Publishing.

Luborsky, L. (1984). *Principles of psychoanalytic psychotherapy: A manual for supportive–expressive treatment*. New York: Basic Books.

Mahoney, M. J. (1991). *Human change processes: The scientific foundations of psychotherapy*. New York: Basic Books.

McGoldrick, M., Gerson, R., & Shellenberger, S. (1999). *Genograms: Assessment and intervention* (2nd ed.). New York: Norton.

Meissner, W. W. (1978). The conceptualization of marriage and family dynamics from a psychoanalytic perspective. In T. J. Paolino & B. S. McCrady (Eds.), *Marriage and marital therapy: Psychoanalytic, behavioral, and systems theory perspectives* (pp. 25–88). New York: Brunner/Mazel.

Messer, S. B., & Warren, C. S. (1995). *Models of brief psychodynamic therapy: A comparative approach*. New York: Guilford Press.

Nadelson, C. C., & Paolino, T. J. (1978). Marital therapy from a psychoanalytic perspective. In T. J. Paolino & B. S. McCrady (Eds.), *Marriage and marital therapy: Psychoanalytic, behavioral, and systems theory perspectives* (pp. 89–164). New York: Brunner/Mazel.

Norcross, J. C. (1985). Eclecticism: Definitions, manifestations and practitioners. *International Journal of Eclectic Psychotherapy, 4*, 19–32.

Norcross, J. C., & Beutler, L. E. (2000). A prescriptive eclectic approach to psychotherapy training. *Journal of Psychotherapy Integration, 10*, 247–261.

Norcross, J. C., & Goldfried, M. R. (Eds.). (1992). *Handbook of psychotherapy integration*. New York: Basic Books.

Norcross, J. C., & Goldfried, M. R. (Eds.). (2005). *Handbook of psychotherapy integration* (2nd ed.). New York: Oxford University Press.

Norcross, J. C., Prochaska, J. O., & Farber, J. A. (1993). Psychologists conducting psychotherapy: New findings and historical comparisons on the psychotherapy division membership. *Psychotherapy, 30*, 692–697.

Patterson, T. (1997). Theoretical unity and technical eclecticism: Pathways to coherence in family therapy. *American Journal of Family Therapy, 25*, 97–109.

Pinsof, W. M. (1995). *Integrative problem-centered therapy: A synthesis of family, individual, and biological therapies*. New York: Basic Books.

Pinsof, W. M. (2005). Integrative problem-centered therapy. In J. C. Norcross & M. R. Goldfried (Eds.), *Handbook of psychotherapy integration* (2nd ed., pp. 382–402). New York: Oxford University Press.

Safran, J. D., & Messer, S. B. (1997). Psychotherapy integration: A postmodern critique. *Clinical Psychology: Science and Practice, 4*, 140–152.

Sager, C. J. (1976). *Marriage contracts and couple therapy: Hidden forces in intimate relationships*. New York: Brunner/Mazel.

Sanders, M. R., Markie-Dadds, C., & Nicholson, J. M. (1997). Concurrent interventions for marital and children's problems. In W. K. Halford & H. J. Markman (Eds.), *Clinical handbook of marriage and couples interventions* (pp. 509–535). New York: Wiley.

Scharff, J. S. (1995). Psychoanalytic marital therapy. In N. S. Jacobson & A. S. Gurman (Eds.), *Clinical handbook of couple therapy* (2nd ed., pp. 164–193). New York: Guilford Press.

Segraves, R. T. (1982). *Marital therapy: A combined psychodynamic–behavioral approach*. New York: Plenum Press.

Segraves, R. T. (1990). Theoretical orientations in the treatment of marital discord. In F. D. Fincham & T. N. Bradbury (Eds.), *The psychology of marriage: Basic issues and applications* (pp. 281–298). New York: Guilford Press.

Shadish, W. R., & Baldwin, S. A. (2003). Meta-analysis of MFT interventions. *Journal of Marital and Family Therapy, 29*, 547–570.

Snyder, D. K. (1997). *Manual for the Marital Satisfaction Inventory—Revised*. Los Angeles: Western Psychological Services.

Snyder, D. K. (1999). Affective reconstruction in the context of a pluralistic approach to couple therapy. *Clinical Psychology: Science and Practice, 6*, 348–365.

Snyder, D. K., & Abbott, B. V. (2002). Couple distress. In M. M. Antony & D. H. Barlow (Eds.), *Handbook of assessment and treatment planning for psychological disorders* (pp. 341–374). New York: Guilford Press.

Snyder, D. K., Abbott, B. V., & Castellani, A. M. (2002). Assessing couples. In J. N. Butcher (Ed.), *Clinical personality assessment: Practical approaches* (2nd ed., pp. 225–242). New York: Oxford University Press.

Snyder, D. K., Castellani, A. M., & Whisman, M. A. (2006). Current status and future directions in couple therapy. *Annual Review of Clinical Psychology, 57*, 317–344.

Snyder, D. K., Cavell, T. A., Heffer, R. W., & Mangrum, L. F. (1995). Marital and family assessment: A multifaceted, multilevel approach. In R. H. Mikesell, D. D. Lusterman, & S. H. McDaniel (Eds.), *Integrating family therapy: Handbook of family psychology and systems theory* (pp. 163–182). Washington, DC: American Psychological Association.

Snyder, D. K., Cepeda-Benito, A., Abbott, B. V., Gleaves, D. H., Negy, C., Hahlweg, K., et al. (2004). Cross-cultural applications of the Marital Satisfaction Inventory—Revised (MSI-R). In M. E. Maruish (Ed.), *Use of psychological testing for treatment planning and outcomes assessment* (3rd ed., pp. 603–623). Mahwah, NJ: Erlbaum.

Snyder, D. K., & Doss, B. D. (2005). Treating infidelity: Clinical and ethical directions. *Journal of Clinical Psychology, 61,* 1453–1465.

Snyder, D. K., Heyman, R. E., & Haynes, S. N. (2008). Assessing couple distress. In J. Hunsley & E. Mash (Eds.), *A guide to assessments that work.* New York: Oxford University Press.

Snyder, D. K., Mangrum, L. F., & Wills, R. M. (1993). Predicting couples' response to marital therapy: A comparison of short- and long-term predictors. *Journal of Consulting and Clinical Psychology, 61,* 61–69.

Snyder, D. K., & Schneider, W. J. (2002). Affective reconstruction: A pluralistic, developmental approach. In A. S. Gurman & N. S. Jacobson (Eds.), *Clinical handbook of couple therapy* (3rd ed., pp. 151–179). New York: Guilford Press.

Snyder, D. K., Schneider, W. J., & Castellani, A. M. (2003). Tailoring couple therapy to individual differences: A conceptual approach. In D. K. Snyder & M. A. Whisman (Eds.), *Treating difficult couples: Helping clients with coexisting mental and relationship disorders* (pp. 27–51). New York: Guilford Press.

Snyder, D. K., Simpson, J. A., & Hughes, J. N. (Eds.). (2006). *Emotion regulation in couples and families: Pathways to dysfunction and health.* Washington, DC: American Psychological Association.

Snyder, D. K., & Whisman, M. A. (Eds.). (2003). *Treating difficult couples: Helping clients with coexisting mental and relationship disorders.* New York: Guilford Press.

Snyder, D. K., & Whisman, M. A. (2004). Treating distressed couples with coexisting mental and physical disorders: Directions for clinical training and practice. *Journal of Marital and Family Therapy, 30,* 1–12.

Snyder, D. K., & Wills, R. M. (1989). Behavioral versus insight-oriented marital therapy: Effects on individual and interspousal functioning. *Journal of Consulting and Clinical Psychology, 57,* 39–46.

Snyder, D. K., Wills, R. M., & Grady-Fletcher, A. (1991a). Long-term effectiveness of behavioral versus insight-oriented marital therapy: A four-year follow-up study. *Journal of Consulting and Clinical Psychology, 59,* 138–141.

Snyder, D. K., Wills, R. M., & Grady-Fletcher, A. (1991b). Risks and challenges of long-term psychotherapy outcome research: Reply to Jacobson. *Journal of Consulting and Clinical Psychology, 59,* 146–149.

Sprenkle, D. H., & Blow, A. J. (2004). Common factors and our sacred models. *Journal of Marital and Family Therapy, 30,* 113–129.

Strupp, H. H., & Binder, J. L. (1984). *Psychotherapy in a new key: A guide to time-limited dynamic psychotherapy.* New York: Basic Books.

Stuart, R. B. (1980). *Helping couples change: A social learning approach to marital therapy.* New York: Guilford Press.

Thompson, B. M. (1997). Couples and the work–family interface. In W. K. Halford & H. J. Markman (Eds.), *Clinical handbook of marriage and couples interventions* (pp. 273–290). New York: Wiley.

Todd, T. C. (1986). Structural–strategic marital therapy. In N. S. Jacobson & A. S. Gurman (Eds.), *Clinical handbook of marital therapy* (pp. 71–105). New York: Guilford Press.

Wachtel, P. L. (1997). *Psychoanalysis, behavior therapy, and the relational world.* Washington, DC: American Psychological Association.

Wile, D. B. (1995). The ego-analytic approach to couple therapy. In N. S. Jacobson & A. S. Gurman (Eds.), *Clinical handbook of couple therapy* (2nd ed., pp. 91–120). New York: Guilford Press.

Wile, D. B. (2002). Collaborative couple therapy. In A. S. Gurman & N. S. Jacobson (Eds.), *Clinical handbook of couple therapy* (3rd ed., pp. 281–307). New York: Guilford Press.

Wills, R. M., Faitler, S. M., & Snyder, D. K. (1987). Distinctiveness of behavioral versus insight-oriented marital therapy: An empirical analysis. *Journal of Consulting and Clinical Psychology, 55,* 685–690.

Young, J. E. (1999). *Cognitive therapy for personality disorders: A schema-focused approach* (3rd ed.). Sarasota, FL: Professional Resource Press.

Young, J. E., & Brown, G. (1999). *Young Schema Questionnaire* (2nd ed.). In J. E. Young (Ed.), *Cognitive therapy for personality disorders: A schema-focused approach* (3rd ed., pp. 59–69). Sarasota, FL: Professional Resource Press.

Young, J. E., & Gluhoski, V. (1997). A schema-focused perspective on satisfaction in close relationships. In R. J. Sternberg & M. Hojjat (Eds.), *Satisfaction in close relationships* (pp. 356–381). New York: Guilford Press.

Young, J. E., Klosko, J. S., & Weishaar, M. E. (2003). *Schema therapy: A practitioner's guide.* New York: Guilford Press.

CHAPTER 13

Integrative Couple Therapy
A Depth-Behavioral Approach

ALAN S. GURMAN

Integrative Couple Therapy (ICT) is a therapeutic approach to the relationship difficulties of couples that attends simultaneously to interpersonal and intrapersonal factors. Although ICT was not originally designed to be time-limited, the model's implicit therapeutic values, intervention focus, and usual techniques tend to render it a relatively brief experience. ICT rests on a foundation of general family systems theory and adult developmental theory, including attachment theory, but it is most pervasively influenced by applied social learning theory (behavior therapy) and object relations theory.

ICT has been developed and refined over the last three decades (Gurman, 1981, 1985, 1992), growing out of a series of works addressing both empirical research in couple and family therapy (Gurman, 1973; Gurman & Kniskern, 1978a, 1978b, 1978c, 1981; Gurman, Kniskern, & Pinsof, 1986) and conceptual considerations (Gurman, 1978, 1980, 1983, 2001; Gurman & Knudson, 1978; Gurman, Knudson, & Kniskern, 1978) in the practice of couple therapy. Although developed independently, ICT is similar in some ways to the integrative models offered by Segraves (1982), Berman, Lief, and Williams (1981), and Gilbert and Shmukler (1996).

BACKGROUND

The Need for Integrative Approaches to Couple Therapy

The most common theoretical orientation among psychotherapists in general (Bergin & Jensen, 1990) and couple therapists in particular (Rait, 1988) is eclecticism. Despite many years of deep conceptual divisions in the field of couple therapy (Gurman & Fraenkel, 2002), Lebow (1997) has appropriately recognized the reality of a profound and pervasive, yet often unacknowledged movement toward integration that he considers a "revolution." And Nichols and Schwartz (2001) observed that "as family therapy enters the twenty-first century, integration is the dominant trend in the field" (p. 413.

The major virtue of integrative approaches to couple therapy is an enhanced understanding of human behavior that enhances treatment flexibility. Specifically, emphasizing either intrapsychic or interpersonal factors in couple relationships, while virtually excluding either domain, can be done only arbitrarily. As Martin (1976) stated over 30 years ago, "Those who prefer to stress either the intrapersonal or the interpersonal aspects alone limit themselves. The separation ... is an artificial separation that does not occur in the nature of the human being" (p. 8). Wachtel (1997), a systems-oriented individual therapist, has argued, "Interpersonal and intrapsychic are not really alternatives but rather two poles of a single ... dialectic process" (p. 338). ICT asserts that therapeutic thinking about couples that is genuinely "systemic" is inherently integrative, in that the relationships of human beings (unlike machines or subhuman species) operate at not only multiple levels of organization but also multiple levels of consciousness. ICT is especially "systemic" in its "attention to organization, to the relationship between parts, to the concentration on patterned rather than linear relationships, [and] to a consideration of events in the context in which they are occurring rather than an isolation of events from their environmental context" (Steinglass, 1978, p. 304).

The evolution of ICT and of some other integrative approaches to couple therapy, especially those that incorporate psychodynamic considerations (e.g., Berman et al., 1981; Feldman, 1979; Segraves, 1982), has occurred to a significant degree in reaction to a historical reification of the notion of "the family as a system" in the field of family therapy (Gurman & Fraenkel, 2002; Schwartz & Johnson, 2000). By their reinclusion of the psychology of the individual, such integrative approaches have provided practical support to Ferreira's (quoted by J. Framo, personal communication, October, 1981) observation that "We had to recognize that the family was a system before we could recognize that it did not always act like a system."

Finally, ICT asserts that treatment approaches attempting to produce change on multiple levels of experience lead to the development and use of interventions that are flexible and responsive to differences between patients, thus leading to more positive and enduring outcomes. Despite its general effectiveness (Lebow & Gurman, 1995), marital therapy has at times been found to yield only moderate rates of improvement and to show some waning in its effects at longer-term follow-up (Bray & Jouriles, 1995; Jacobson & Addis, 1993). Such positive yet somewhat limited effects have been found in studies of "singular" methods of therapy, which typically emphasize change in certain domains of experience over others, often to the exclusion of others. For example, behavioral methods have traditionally emphasized change in overt behavior, whereas more psychodynamic methods emphasize nonobservable intrapsychic change. The method that to date has shown the most enduring benefits from treatment has been couple therapy that attends to both intrapsychic and interpersonal factors, and to both conscious and unconscious factors in marital satisfaction (Snyder, 1999; Snyder & Wills, 1989). Relatedly, the behaviorally oriented couple therapies that have shown the strongest clinical outcomes are those that include treatment elements not contained in more pure form, "traditional" behavioral couple therapy (cf. Dimidjian, Martell, & Christensen, Chapter 3, this volume; Jacobson & Holtzworth-Munroe, 1986), and that balance their attention to both overt behavior change and affective–cognitive change (Baucom, Epstein, LaTaillade, & Kirby, Chapter 2, this volume).

ICT and Integrative Therapy Approaches

Although integrative models are not as common in couple therapy as in individual therapy, they are not uncommon, and they have brought together, for example, structural and strategic approaches (e.g., Stanton, 1980; Todd, 1986), and behavior therapy and systems theory approaches (e.g., Birchler & Spinks, 1980; Weiss, 1980). The most common integrations, however, have involved behavioral and psychodynamic approaches (e.g., Bagarozzi & Giddings, 1983; Berman et al., 1981; Feldman, 1979; Gilbert & Shmukler, 1996).

It is generally agreed that there are four main types of psychotherapy integration (Messer, 2001). "Technical eclecticism" calls upon interventions from theoretically diverse methods, and includes "prescriptive matching"—that is, pairing the use of particular techniques with particular symptoms, syndromes or personality (or, here, relationship) types. "Theoretical integration" attempts to combine different theories, as well as the techniques deriving from those theories, and typically identifies one theory that dominates the other(s). The "common factors approach" to integration emphasizes therapeutic variables and processes that are presumed to be central to the effective conduct of all types of therapy (e.g., Duncan & Miller, 2000).

The great majority of systematic integrations in couple therapy have been of the theoretically integrative type—most often with psychodynamic or object relations theory serving as the conceptual core for understanding marital dynamics, and relying heavily on behavioral techniques, because of the paucity of techniques specific to the practice of psychodynamic marital therapy (Gurman, 1978). This retention of a core or "home" theory and concurrent incorporation of techniques originating outside the home theory constitute "assimilative integration" (Messer, 2001), the fourth type of psychotherapy integration.

ICT explicitly calls upon behavioral and psychodynamic perspectives in both its understanding of functional and dysfunctional couple relationships and its methods of assessment and intervention; as such, it has elements of both theoretical integration and assimilative integration. ICT attempts to integrate the interpersonal with the intrapersonal, and to integrate people, as well as theories and techniques.

ICT and Therapeutic Brevity

Although ICT can be practiced within predetermined time limits, this is not a cardinal feature of the approach. Still, ICT is generally a brief method for two main reasons. First, it adheres very closely to the central values of most brief therapies (Budman & Gurman, 1988), such as clinical parsimony, the use of a developmental perspective, an emphasis on change that occurs outside therapy, and an emphasis on current issues. In addition, ICT's use and view of time, its views of the therapist–patient relationship, the nature of its typical treatment focus, and its most common techniques, which together constitute "the four central technical factors of brief therapy" (Gurman, 2001), generally lead to relatively brief courses of treatment. As emphasized elsewhere (Budman & Gurman, 1988), brief therapy is most usefully defined not by the number of therapy sessions but by the presence of the sorts of active ingredients just enumerated.

THE WELL-FUNCTIONING VERSUS DYSFUNCTIONAL MARRIAGE

ICT accepts as fundamental the assumption that the proclivity of people to form and maintain relational attachments throughout life is probably universal. ICT agrees with attachment-oriented couple therapies (e.g., Johnson, Chapter 4, this volume) that secure connections to accessible and responsive attachment figures allow for interactional flexibility and open communication, while simultaneously fostering autonomy. Conversely, as Karpel (1994) summarizes the matter, "Difficulties in early attachments can lead to an inability to trust, to unmet and therefore excessive needs for attachment, to internal representations that distort perceptions of the partner, and to unconscious

defenses that preclude vulnerability and intimacy" (p. 10). As we shall see, although ICT generally does not focus on early attachment experiences per se, it certainly respects the power of the residue of such experiences to create conditions for the appearance and maintenance of couple conflict.

The Topography of Marital Functioning

Therapists of different theoretical orientations define the core problems of the couples they treat quite differently, ranging from relationship skills deficits to maladaptive ways of thinking and restrictive narratives, to matters of self-esteem, to unsuccessful handling of normal life-cycle transitions, to unconscious displacement onto the partner of conflicts with one's family of origin, to the inhibited expression of normal adult needs, to the fear of abandonment.

Despite such varied views of what constitutes the core of marital difficulties, in recent years, marital therapists of different orientations have sought a clinically meaningful description and understanding of functional versus dysfunctional intimate relationships that rests on a solid research base (Lebow, 1999). Perhaps uniquely in the world of psychotherapy, the major findings from this body of (mostly cognitive, behavioral, and social-psychological) research (especially Gottman, 1994a, 1994b, 1998) have been uniformly praised by and incorporated into the treatment models of an astoundingly wide array of marital therapists, ranging from eclectic (Budman, 1999) to cognitive-behavioral (Baucom et al., Chapter 2, this volume) and behavioral (Dimidjian et al., Chapter 3, this volume), humanistic and experiential (Johnson, Chapter 4, this volume), psychodynamic (Donovan, 2003), and transgenerational (Roberto-Forman, Chapter 7, this volume). These findings, taken as a whole, provide a theoretically and clinically rich, credible description of the typical form and shape of many healthy and unhealthy marital interactions. Therapists of different orientations make sense of and complement such findings in their own ways, with observations about functional versus dysfunctional marriages that are specific to their own perspectives. The overall pattern of these findings is relevant to both treatment planning and the therapeutic process in ICT.

In regard to both marital satisfaction and long-term marital stability, satisfied (functional, happy) couples, compared to dissatisfied (dysfunctional, unhappy) couples, show: higher rates of pleasing behavior and lower rates of displeasing behavior; lower probability of reciprocating nega-tive behavior (e.g., "If you're nasty to me, I'll be nasty to you"); and better communication skills (e.g., expressive skills, such as using positive re-quests for behavior change; receptive skills, such as empathizing) and problem-solving skills (e.g., focusing on solutions via brainstorming, maintain-ing a clear topical focus).

Poor communication and problem solving are characterized by "harsh start-ups" of problem-focused conversations (e.g., "Hey, why are you always so damned late when we're going out to-gether!") and poor ability to repair ruptures, espe-cially early in couple exchanges (e.g., by the use of humor or a show of affection). These interac-tions indicate a focus on affect rather than on problem solving and tend to be accompanied by negative physiological arousal (especially in men), combined with the aroused partner's difficulty in self-soothing. This pattern may culminate in the rapid escalation of two-way aversive experiences, setting up the couple for developing a chronic pat-tern of emotional disengagement and withdrawal via a process of escape/avoidance conditioning fueled by negative reinforcement. In addition, distressed couples tend to become deadlocked over inherently unresolvable differences, known as "perpetual problems" (e.g., core personality or value differences), but mistakenly deal with these differences as though they were resolvable, thereby leading inevitably to feelings of frustra-tion, nonaffirmation, and resentment. Finally, in unhappy couples, partners try to influence each other by using styles characterized by pain control (e.g., "aversive conditioning", providing emotion-ally painful consequences to a partner's undesired behavior via criticism, contempt, stonewalling, and/or defensiveness rather than mutual reciproc-ity). In attempting to control the behavior of one's partner via contempt and criticism (punishment), one simultaneously attempts to reduce one's own pain via stonewalling and defensiveness (avoid-ance, negative reinforcement).

In the cognitive realm, unhappy couples show negative attributional biases in the form of disregarding both the presence of positive partner behavior and even increases in desired partner be-havior (Baucom et al., Chapter 2, this volume). Unhappy couples see negative partner behavior as reflecting permanent characteristics, and positive partner behavior as reflecting temporary states. Negative events have longer-lasting negative ef-fects in unhappy couples than in happy couples. Unhappy partners tend to blame each other for

their couple problems, while taking little responsi-bility for them, and tend to make faulty attributions about their partners' motivations and intentions. They also tend to engage in cognitive distortions, such as all-or-nothing thinking, overgeneraliza-tion, jumping to conclusions, and catastrophizing and magnification. Finally, unhappy individuals are more likely than happy ones to have more un-realistic expectations of both marriage in general and of their actual partners.

The Skills Deficit Hypothesis

As compelling as such findings are, they are mere-ly descriptive and do not address some central clinical questions: Why do dysfunctional couples behave in the particular ways they do? Why do such perceptual/attributional patterns emerge? Why do such patterns persist despite the pain they bring? On this matter, behavioral therapists have generally taken a very clear position. Such patterns exist because the couples who show them have "skills deficits" of various sorts, and, one might say, "cognitive excesses" (e.g., too many cognitive distortions and faulty attributions). The timing of the emergence of significant conflict is understood in light of the ever-changing contin-gencies of adult relationship life that pose new challenges for which couples "lack appropriate skills."

Several studies (Birchler, Weiss, & Wampler, 1972; Birchler, Weiss, & Vincent, 1975; Birchler & Webb, 1975; Vincent, Weiss, & Birchler, 1975) have found that partners in distressed marriages behave more positively in interactions with strang-ers than with their partners in problem-solving situations. Moreover, partners in distressed mar-riages can change their communication styles in a positive direction simply by following an experi-menter's instruction to do so (Vincent, Friedman, Nugent, & Messerly, 1979). Such findings suggest that the "skills deficient" partners from unhappy marriages often can and do exhibit important in-terpersonal skills in other interactional contexts. This observation exemplifies the core distinction within applied social learning theory between problems of "acquisition" (the person has never learned the behavior in question) and problems of "performance" (the person shows the requisite be-havior in some circumstances, but not in others). For example, although Susie complains that Bob "shows no feelings, is cold and distant to me, isn't interested in my point of view, and argues about almost everything," Bob often displays such apparently "missing" people skills with other people (e.g., coworkers and friends).

It is noteworthy that the undisputed pioneer of the behavioral approach, the late Neil Jacobson, acknowledged (but only in passing) that the skills deficit perspective may be a weak one, noting that

> For many of these skill areas, it is likely that the more appropriate label would be 'performance deficit' rather than 'skill deficit' ... it may be that ... the innate abilities are present ... but the enactments are not occurring under the stimulus control of the partner's presence. The term 'skill' may be a metaphor rather than a term to be taken literally. (Holtzworth-Munroe & Jacobson, 1991, pp. 100–101, emphasis added)

And, more recently, Jacobson (Lawrence, Eldridge, Christensen, & Jacobson, 1999) wrote, "Typically, couples know how to communicate effectively, but haven't used these abilities for some time. We elicit the skills they already have" (p. 254).

Moving toward an Alternative Hypothesis

It seems that the skills-focused view of couple difficulties has failed to acknowledge the fundamental nonequivalence and noncomparability of intimate versus superficial relationships, which lack a developmental history, privately shared meaning systems, and implicit transactional "rules." Dicks (1967) noted, "The special feature of such apparent hate-relationships in marriage is that they occur within the framework of a compelling sense of belonging. The spouses are clear in their minds that they would not dream of treating anyone else but each other in this way" (p. 70).

So, *why* do unhappy couples not communicate and problem-solve better, please each other more, repair conversational ruptures, stay calm even in the face of discussing differences, and so on? *Why* do they escalate their conflict, reinforce the very behaviors in each other that they object to so passionately, block out from their awareness the good in their partners and highlight the bad, and attribute the most unkind motivations to each other? *Why* do they go on, as Dicks said, "treating ... each other in this way" (p. 70)? What are they really fighting about? Although research has aided us tremendously in describing the topography of marital conflict, we must turn to other, complementary theoretical perspectives to understand the function of the kinds of observable behavior we see so regularly in marital conflict.

The Unconscious Dimension of Marital Interaction

The Marital Quid Pro Quo

A foundational concept relevant here is Jackson's (1965a, 1965b) notion of family "rules"—that is, inferred patterns of interaction that structure the most defining aspects of a relationship. Among family rules, of greatest importance in marriage is the "marital quid pro quo." In contrast to quid pro quo arrangements in, for example, behavior exchange interventions in behavioral couple therapy, quid pro quo exchanges are "not overt, conscious or the tangible result of real bargaining" (Jackson, 1965a, p. 592), and are not point for point or "time-bound" (Lederer & Jackson, 1968, p. 272). Rather, the essence of the quid pro quo is an "unconscious effort of both partners to assure themselves that they are equals, that they are peers. It is a technique enabling each to preserve his dignity and self-esteem" (Lederer & Jackson, 1968, p. 179). The quid pro quo provides "a *metaphorical* statement of the marital relationship bargain; that is, how the couple has agreed to *define themselves* within this relationship" (Jackson, 1965b, p. 12; emphasis added).

The "unconscious" attribute of quid pro quo exchanges is not the familiar Freudian unconscious or, indeed, the unconscious of any particular theoretical system. It is what we may call the "descriptive unconscious"—that which simply is out of awareness. This descriptive unconscious is an essential notion in ICT, because it allows a bridging of an active and strongly behaviorally influenced therapeutic style with an overriding respect for an awareness of factors that influence marital behavior quite outside the realm of direct observation, including conscious self-observation. This conceptual position is similar to Wachtel's (Wachtel & McKinney, 1992) concept of "cyclical psychodynamics," which emphasizes the repetitive cycles of interaction between people and notes how these cycles reciprocally include both intrapsychic processes and overt behavior, that is, how deep structures and surface structures operate together.

The Important Contribution of Object Relations Concepts

Among the conceptual systems dealing with deeper structures, the one that speaks most directly to couple therapists is object relations theory, which provides for ICT the specific concepts to explain the mechanisms at work in the quid pro quo. ICT does not incorporate the wider belief system associated with object relations theory (e.g., see Dicks, 1967; Meissner, 1978; Scharff & Scharff, Chapter 6, this volume), but draws selectively upon object relations concepts that facilitate the development of an "assimilative" integration.

ICT recognizes "the legacies of early attachment" (Karpel, 1994, p. 10) and assumes that early attachment difficulties from "not good enough" parenting (Bowlby, 1988; Winnicott, 1960) or attachment injuries from later relationships play a significant role in the capacity for healthy relating in intimate adult relationships. But ICT places much more emphasis on the present dyadic reenactment of such unfortunate individual developmental histories—on how, as Bentovim (1979) put it, "interpersonal relationships determine intrapsychic structure and how these structures in the mind come to reactivate such relationships at a later date" (p. 331) and give meaning to interpersonal events.

In this framework, the core source of marital dysfunction is both partners' failure to see themselves and each other as "whole persons" (Dicks, 1967; Gurman, 1981). Conflict-laden aspects of oneself, presumably punished (aversively conditioned) earlier in life, are repudiated and "split off." "Projective identification" evolves when these aspects of self are projected onto (attributed to) the mate, who in turn "accepts" the projection (e.g., by behaving in accordance with it). The problematic aspect of the unconscious quid pro quo is that there is not only a mutually reinforcing process of projective identifications but also, and perhaps even more importantly, an implicit agreement or *collusion* not to talk about or challenge the "agreement." The collusion is a joint, shared avoidance that involves both intrapsychic and interpersonal defenses against various fears (e.g., merger, attack, abandonment). "Collusion" is a bilateral process in which partners seek to maintain a consistent, if maladaptive, sense of self. It represents a pattern of attempted solutions to individual and dyadic problems. Projective identification and collusion are unconscious forms of communication in which important information about oneself is exchanged. Scarf (1986), reminiscent of Jackson's (1965b) quid pro quo, notes that "the exchange of projections is a psychological barter occurring at an unconscious level" (p. 52).

Collusion is especially problematic when partners' relational schemas are very rigid and make it likely that they will see each other, consciously or unconsciously, in terms of past relationships instead of as "real contemporary people" (Raush, Berry, Hertel, & Swain, 1974, p. 25). Such rigidity and associated polarized psychological roles may significantly reduce the capacity of the couple or its individual partners to "adapt to new circumstances" (p. 25; e.g., inevitable changes that occur over the couple's life cycle).

Catherall (1992) emphasizes that the major problem with projective identification is not its existence but "the couple's failure—as a system—to manage the disturbing thoughts and feelings that are the substance of projective identifications" (pp. 355–356). To manage such experiences, couples must be able to engage in effective containing and holding. "Containing" is a self-referential process in which the partner is able to allow painful feelings and thoughts into consciousness, without the need to project them onto the mate. It involves the capacity to self-regulate and self-soothe. "Holding" is a dyadic process in which the listener/recipient can identify with the speaker's feelings (i.e., can empathically hear them as belonging to the speaker), whether they are about the speaker or the listener, without experiencing intolerable anxiety (i.e., he or she is able to contain any discomfort associated with the speaker's behavior). The recipient who is unable to identify with the speaker and contain his or her own feelings is more likely to enact reciprocal, and often rapidly escalating, problematic behavior.

The Functional Value of Marital Conflict and the Functional Value of "Skills Deficits"

Although these unconscious communication processes may seem malevolent, they are in fact both problematic and positive. Repetitive, seemingly nonproductive conflict is goal-oriented: It serves to prevent the awareness of unconscious anxiety stimulated by relationship intimacy. But, in addition to this two-way protective function, collusion is a potentially growthful collaboration—an adaptive effort to resolve individual conflicts through specific, unwittingly accommodating, intimate relationships.

But cooperation via collusion exacts a high toll. Poor communication and problem solving are quite predictable from an observed pattern of paradoxical communication. Moreover, such "unskilled" communication styles are required to maintain unconscious collusion; that is, in the ICT framework, "poor social skills" in intimate relationships more often than not reflect the more basic, unspoken rule of limited intimacy. The unfortunate protective function of "skills deficits" requires that the therapy include explicit attention to the mutually avoidant defensive function of such "deficits" to challenge the joint defenses in the very service of which the "deficits" exist.

The skills deficit hypothesis is also weakened when one recognizes that, as Berman et al. (1981) put it, "marriages are indeed different from other relationships. ... Most people do not project the same internal conflict equally on everyone, but only on the person with whom one allows oneself to be intimate" (p. 11).

There is another important, functional value of marital conflict as conceived in ICT. Although attacking aspects of their mates that in part reflect unwanted self-aspects understandably appears negative and destructive to observers, such perpetual projections at the same time keep the partners in contact with lost or split-off parts of themselves; in this way, they reflect reparative efforts toward growth (Dicks, 1967; Stewart, Peters, Marsh, & Peters, 1975).

The Emergence of Marital Conflict

J. C. Anchin (personal communication, August, 1999) has noted that "a *comprehensive* understanding of a given couple's dysfunctionality must ... capture ... the determinative psychodynamics of the reflective individuals ... and ... the truly fundamental manner in which these problematic individual—intrapsychic and interpersonal— systemic dynamics reciprocally sustain and perpetuate one another" (emphasis in original). Given the centrality in marital satisfaction of self-affirmation and safety, it now becomes clear how marital conflict typically emerges and appears. In large measure, significant conflict—that is, conflict that is both phenomenologically painful and enduring—arises and continues when the "rules" of the relationship that are central to either partner's sense of self or core organizing schema for close relationships are violated, overlapping Gottman's (1999) notion of "perpetual issues." These "rules" can be either explicit and obvious, or implicit and unspoken (cf. Sager, 1976, 1981). When the latter is the case, the conflicted couple is likely to seem quite chaotic and dysregulated, because the partners have no useable cognitive map to allow them to make sense of the pervasive but undeniable tension between them.

People prefer and usually seek to maintain a relatively consistent sense of self, even if the self with which they are familiar is relationally maladaptive. Change, especially change that taps into core aspects of the self, is anxiety-arousing. Such anxiety-arousing violation of central relationship rules can occur in a seemingly endless variety of manifestations, most of which can be subsumed under three headings. The first "violation" of such relationship rules, and perhaps the most common source of difficulty, involves the naturalistic exposure to the reality of the partner beyond the early stage of idealization. Sager (1981) has further differentiated such exposure to the mate's reality by noting that problems may arise when one realizes either that one's partner cannot meet one's needs or that no partner can do so. Sager also emphasizes the commonly found contradictory nature of the needs within partners. The second "violation" of core relationship rules involves changes in one's partner that do not match the real or perceived characteristics of that person that initially contributed to one's romantic attraction (e.g., a partner may seek a good deal more or less closeness than at an earlier point in the relationship). The third common "violation" involves experiences through which one sees unacceptable aspects of oneself that were previously blocked from awareness but are now evoked in the couple interaction. These various "violations" may stimulate and evoke one or more common intimacy fears, such as fears of merger, exposure, attack, abandonment, or expressing one's own aggression (Feldman, 1979). It is important to note that all three of these conflict-generating patterns can be stimulated by externally generated forces, as well as by changing expectations and needs within the couple dyad.

The relevant relationship "rules" include both conscious and unconscious expectations of and anxieties about intimate relating that are brought to the relationship by each partner, including attachment anxieties. The patterned regularities of a marriage do not just evolve randomly or from repeated interactions, but from a subtle interplay of the implicit relationship rules of each individual (Gurman, 1978; Gurman & Knudson, 1978; Gurman et al., 1978). The ICT view is not that problems develop because of interpersonal "skills deficits," but that such apparent deficits very often represent the expression of the fundamental difficulties each partner has in intimate relating and/ or a breakdown of the underlying implicit couple "contracts" (Sager, 1976, 1981) about central aspects of the relationship. "Skills deficits" are viewed as manifestations of more fundamental incompatibilities (Hamburg, 2000), or, more accurately, as the emergence into consciousness of these incompatibilities in one or more of the three relationship rule violation pathways described earlier.

The Maintenance of Marital Conflict: The Synergy of the Interpersonal and the Intrapersonal

When a couple's rule violations occur with such impact (e.g., a single event such as infidelity violates a core symbolic relationship value) or with such frequency and regularity as to negatively affect the overall tenor of the relationship, each partner attempts to shape the other to stay within, or get back within, the limits of behavior "allowed" by that individual's "rules." The circular, problem-maintaining processes that unfold express the inevitable human interconnection among multiple simultaneous levels of experience. These maladaptive circular processes demonstrate that defenses are interactional and maintained only via exchanges with one's partner. These defenses operate so that the person avoids "seeing" behavior inconsistent with his or her internalized image of the ideal mate and/or requirements for maintaining a consistent view of oneself. The utopian and anxiety-based expectations that people bring to marriage sensitize them to slight deviations from these relational "rules" that, when they occur, predictably increase the amplitude and frequency of countercontrol maneuvers.

Bagarozzi and Giddings (1983) clearly articulate the pattern of what they call "mutual shaping toward the ideal," or what I have called "implicit behavior modification" (Gurman, 1992); that is, one partner unwittingly (and wittingly as well) attempts to reinforce and extinguish behavior in his or her mate that is allowed and disallowed, respectively, according to the person's own conscious and unconscious expectations of a marital partner. The other partner does likewise in response to the behavior of his or her mate that is "allowed" and "disallowed," according to the internal "rules" of how the partner needs to "see" him- or herself. This "implicit behavior modification" takes several predictable forms, each of which may provide clues to the therapist about useful points at which, and useful patterns about which, to intervene. Thus, in couple relationships, the mutual processes of reinforcement and punishment occur in such a way that each partner (1) reinforces behavior of the other partner that is consistent with his or her own mate ideal; (2) reinforces behavior of the other partner that is consistent with his or her own self-view; (3) reinforces (covertly) his or her own behavior that is consistent with the required self-view; (4) punishes/extinguishes (e.g., via avoidance, denial) behavior in the other partner

that is inconsistent with his or her own mate ideal; (5) punishes/extinguishes behavior in the other partner that is inconsistent with his or her own required self-view; and (6) punishes/extinguishes (covertly) his or her own behavior that is inconsistent with his or her own required self-view. In addition, partners in chronically conflicted relationships (7) regularly reinforce the very behaviors in their mates about which they complain.

As Goldfried (1995) has pointed out, because this synergistic process is circular, that is, with reinforcing and punishing contingencies provided by both partners, it can be triggered by either partner. This process often involves what Scheinkman and Fishbane (2004) call joint "vulnerability survival strategies," in which one partner's attempt to solve his or her vulnerability problem-of-the-moment activates the other partner's self-protective "survival" strategy in a way that is punishing to the first partner, and the cycle continues on. Moreover, the cycle can be triggered by either publicly observable behavior in either partner, by privately experienced stimuli, or by external "situational" factors. Once begun, the bilateral, interlocking, problematic, implicit behavior modification does not belong to either partner alone; it belongs to, and in therapy must come to be "owned" by, both partners. Ironically, but hopefully, as we shall see, the very complexity of what maintains problematic couple cycles affords the therapist ample possibilities for helpful intervention.

THE PRACTICE OF ICT

The Structure of Therapy

Who Is Included in Therapy

In the ideal practice of ICT all treatment sessions include both couple partners, because the core healing components of ICT are believed to lie within that relationship. Consequently, the ICT therapist is very reluctant to see partners individually and almost never sees one partner alone for the initial interview. When partners are seen alone, the ICT therapist maintains particular awareness of any interactions that may carry significant implications for the alliances already established in the three-way conjoint meetings, and is especially attuned to any interactions that may disturb the husband–wife alliance. Relatedly, except in genuine crises or emergencies, partners are never seen alone when one partner fails to appear for a therapy session—whether this failure is due to a marital argument, acute illness, unexpected work conflicts, or even bad weather or traffic conditions!

Partners are not separated during the initial assessment. The only time the therapist initiates individual sessions is when conjoint sessions regularly have become unmanageable to the point of being counterproductive (rather than merely unproductive, as some sessions inevitably are in any course of therapy). This occasion typically involves couples in which both partners have great difficulty self-regulating their anger or dramatic expressions of emotional turmoil, are not reliably able to be soothed and calmed by the therapist, and/or unyieldingly engage in mutual blaming to the virtual exclusion of seeing their own role in the couple's difficulties. Often, a short-term series of individual sessions with each partner, focused on fostering more cooperative roles in joint therapy, may allow a less inflammatory ambience when conjoint sessions are resumed.

ICT can be conducted by either a single therapist or cotherapists, although current patterns in health care delivery, such as managed care programs, effectively keep the use of cotherapy to a minimum. A cotherapy arrangement is both well suited to the ICT approach, and not without complications. Because ICT emphasizes the importance of the therapist's understanding the couple on multiple levels simultaneously and intervening with an appreciation of the possible effects of an action on multiple levels, the presence of a second therapist may enhance such awareness. At the same time, because ICT therapists regularly intervene at one level of psychological experience with an intent to produce change at another level, cotherapists must be extremely well attuned to each other's thinking; otherwise, a perfectly reasonable intervention by one therapist may lead to confusion or uncertainty in the second therapist, thus disrupting or distracting the flow and focus of the therapy session.

What Is Included in Therapy

SELECTION OF A SESSION FOCUS

Although ICT values thematic consistency and a clear therapeutic focus (or foci), the therapist does not usually impose a topical agenda on therapy sessions. On the contrary, just as couples are seen as the major healing agents, they are also given the responsibility for deciding what is addressed in therapy. Also, because the ICT therapist is sensitive to the factors (Gurman, 2001) that bias most

couple therapy toward brevity, it is not assumed that a couple will wish to address the same secondary, derivative problem from session to session. Indeed, couples regularly are unaware of how seemingly different "problems of the day" are connected thematically. It is the therapist's responsibility to foster such understanding. Thus, partners in ICT are routinely asked at the beginning of the session, "What would you like to focus on today?" This deceptively simple question implies (1) that the partners are in charge of knowing what matters to them; (2) that all therapy sessions must have a focus, purpose, or goal; and (3) that their needs, sensibilities, and struggles are not static, but shift through time. The therapist also distinguishes between the overtly agreed-upon "negotiated focus" that provides continuity across time, and the "operative focus"—the usually unspoken mediating goals the therapist believes need to be achieved for the couple to reach its negotiated ultimate goals (Gurman, 2001). In ICT, as in probably all types of couple therapy, couples regularly bring to the session material from the time since their previous meeting. The ICT therapist is typically quite active in such "troubleshooting" (Jacobson & Holtzworth-Munroe, 1986) conversations, although the form of his or her activity varies (see below).

Not infrequently, some aspects of couple problems become functionally autonomous of their origins. As I pointed out elsewhere (Gurman, 1978),

> Regardless of the extent to which marital conflict may have been initially determined by unconscious forces, current interaction not only reinforces shared collusions, but also offers fertile ground for secondary, but very real and salient difficulties that must be treated independently of the historically underlying dynamic struggle. (pp. 456–457)

These comments referred to what cognitive-behavioral couple therapists (e.g., Baucom et al., Chapter 2, this volume) now refer to as "secondary" (vs. "primary") distress—that is, maladaptive patterns of responding to unfulfilled needs.

INTERPERSONAL VERSUS INTRAPERSONAL FOCUS

ICT, like most couple therapies, strongly emphasizes interpersonal couple process issues. At the same time, it is commonplace in couple therapy for "individual" issues to rise intermittently to the fore. These may be centrally and transparently linked to the major couple problem theme, such as when an emotionally distancing wife talks about the abuse that took place in her family when she was a child. Or such an "individual" issue may at first seem more tangential to the relational focus (e.g., when one partner expresses anxiety about stresses or conflicts in the workplace). When people are in couple therapy, they know they are in couple therapy. Almost nothing that is brought up for the therapist to hear about is brought up randomly or without meaning. Almost always, as unclear as this meaning may be at first to the therapist, it involves the couple's relationship, the process of the couple therapy, or the like. When partners themselves are not able to see such connections, it falls to the therapist to facilitate an understanding of the functional relevance of such topic choices to the central themes of the therapy.

There are two common situations in which such "individual" factors arise. The first occurs when one partner has a diagnosable, and probably diagnosed, psychiatric disorder of a largely symptomatic nature (e.g., depression or anxiety). The second situation occurs when an important aspect of one partner's contribution to the couple problem reflects significant psychopathology that is largely of an interpersonal nature (e.g., a personality disorder), and may not have been formally diagnosed. In both situations, ICT focuses on the functional relationships between an individual's symptoms or personality characteristics and central problematic couple themes. ICT looks upon nomothetic descriptions of psychiatric disorders as a useful source of hypotheses about a given individual, not as a set of "facts." To be of practical use, these hypotheses require verification in the individual case, and once verified must be functionally relevant to the central relational problems (cf. Hayes & Toarmino, 1995). If not, they probably fall outside the purview of ICT, which insists on maintaining a clear treatment focus.

Some sessions in ICT may look to an outside observer like individual therapy being done in the presence of a partner. The guiding principle in ICT is that the implications of such "individual" conversations for the couple's relationship must be made explicit before the end of the session, at the latest. It is especially valuable if this "individual" material can be coherently connected to the central theme(s) of the joint therapy. Not everything that affects the partners' comfort and satisfaction in their relationship is about, or derives from, that relationship. With its simultaneous interpersonal and intrapersonal awareness, ICT respects the relevance of "individual" issues in the couple's life, but insists that since this is couple therapy, virtually everything that is discussed is considered in a relational light. It is not inherently an error to do some "individual" therapy within couple therapy. Doing so can become an error if the treatment emphasis repeatedly centers more on the therapist–partner interaction than on the partner–partner relationship. As already emphasized, there is almost never an emphasis in ICT on one domain of psychological experience "instead of" others. To allow this to happen is not to practice integratively and, therefore, ICT argues, not to practice with optimal clinical effectiveness.

THE THERAPY CONVERSATIONS

The general flow and rhythm of an ICT session often includes a good deal of conversation between each partner and the therapist, with the other partner "just listening." The other partner is never "just listening," of course, but is processing what is heard, as overtly silent as he or she may be. The ICT therapist places no priority on having partners talk primarily to each other, although they may do so selectively. This statement may seem at odds with ICT's emphasis on the centrality of the partner–partner relationship in the couple healing process, but it is not. Because the central mechanism of change in ICT is seen as the creation of new relational learning experiences for the couple, both inside and outside the sessions, the therapy sessions themselves obviously must allow for conditions where such change is possible. Allowing (and sometimes even directing) partners to speak directly to the therapist may help to foster a listening environment that feels safer to the partners than that in everyday life, thus allowing gradual but consistent exposure to the "real" partners.

Because, as noted, ICT assumes that conflicted couples remain locked into painful, recurrent dances for perfectly "good" (i.e., potentially understandable) intrapsychic, as well as interpersonal, reasons, a safe therapeutic environment is essential as the partners encounter each other in new ways. The partners in highly conflicted marriages cannot be expected to trust the safety of the therapeutic situation and, therefore, each other, unless they experience an adequate sense of order. Direct partner–therapist conversation is an important element in the structuring of such order. Of course, as therapy progresses and trust between the partners increases, the therapist can and should encourage more and more partner–partner conversation. Naturally, most couple therapy sessions include a mixture of partner–partner and partner–therapist conversation. It falls to the therapist to be sensitive to the optimal balance at given points in time.

Temporal Aspects of Therapy

LENGTH, SPACING, AND NUMBER OF SESSIONS

ICT sessions are typically 50–60 minutes long, though there is no absolute contraindication to scheduling longer sessions when this is arranged in advance. Likewise, the scheduling of sessions is done flexibly and in response to the partners' needs, their availability, and so on. Some couples, not necessarily those in crisis, are wisely seen weekly at first (e.g., when the therapist experiences difficulty in establishing a working alliance, or senses that one or both partners' commitment to staying in therapy may be tenuous). At the other extreme, couples may be seen only monthly, if circumstances require that, although such a gap between sessions tends to dilute the central focus and lessen the immediacy of the experience. In practice, sessions are most often held on a biweekly basis, because this period between sessions seems optimal for maintaining an adequate therapeutic focus and, at the same time, allowing enough time to elapse for couples to experiment with change, to give adequate consideration to the discussion of the previous session, and so forth. Given ICT's emphasis on the central healing role of the partner–partner relationship, it follows that meaningfully designed change experiences between sessions are important, and the partners must be allowed adequate space and time to carry their new learning into the natural environment.

Although ICT emphasizes therapeutic brevity primarily through its establishment of a thematic focus, it is not formally time-limited. Helpful and effective courses of therapy have occurred in as few as three or four meetings over just a few weeks, or have required as many as 100 sessions or more over periods exceeding several years. On average, ICT, like most marital therapies (Gurman, 1981, 2001), lasts about 12–15 sessions.

It is important to note that couple therapy need not be continuous. In its attempt to be flexibly responsive to developmental changes in a couple's life and to the inevitable waxing and waning of motivation for therapeutic work that is typical of most couples, ICT often includes discontinuous "courses" of treatment, usually for different lengths of time. Indeed, the rationing of time in therapy in this developmentally sensitive, discontinuous way is a hallmark of much effective brief psychotherapy (Budman & Gurman, 1988; Gurman, 2001).

TEMPORAL FOCUS

Although important conversations about the past certainly do occur in virtually all courses of ICT (e.g., when discussing the historical origins of a patient's fear of closeness, or when exploring changes over time in each partner's expectations of marriage and of one's partner), the temporal focus is decidedly biased toward the present. A common occurrence that should cue the therapist to inquire about historical factors is when a seemingly minor event or seemingly inconsequential behavior elicits very intense or uncomfortable feelings, especially when the recipient partner cannot make sense of the first partner's behavior.

As I discuss in the section "Assessment and Goal Setting," ICT's central organizing question is "Why *now*?" Although ICT is sensitive to and interested in partners' developmental trajectories and patterns, it concurs with structural family therapist Aponte's (1992) view that "a therapist targets the residuals of the past in a family's experience of the moment" (p. 326).

CONCURRENT TREATMENTS

As noted, a fair amount of "individual" therapy may occur in ICT; at the same time, ICT therapists are extremely hesitant to schedule actual individual sessions. Carrying on a parallel true individual therapy with a marital partner who is being seen by the therapist in conjoint couple therapy is never an option in ICT. Moreover, concurrent individual psychotherapy done by other therapists during the course of ICT is generally not favored, thought it is often a real-world inevitability. Unless such therapies are clearly focused on discrete symptoms (e.g., phobias or compulsions), there is a great likelihood that during a time of marital crises or at least intense pain, the couple's relationship will become a prime topic for discussion. Therein lies the risk of either duplicated or (more worrisome) contradictory therapeutic aims and interventions. More broadly, such parallel, concurrent individual therapies often dilute a patient's therapeutic energy and focus away from the couple therapy, and may weaken rather than strengthen the needed therapeutic alliance between marital partners to sustain effective work.

On the other hand, concurrent psychopharmacological treatment—for instance, for depression or bipolar disorder—generally poses few such problems. When the couple therapist is also able to prescribe indicated medications, this is preferable to a concurrent treatment arrangement, because it allows immediate, three-way processing of the meaning and implications of such prescribing for the couple's relationship. Moreover, such a practice is a concrete expression of the value within ICT of dealing with couples at multiple levels of experience, including the biological.

The Role of the Therapist

In ICT the therapist serves alternatively, and at times simultaneously, as teacher/consultant, healer, and provocateur. His or her stance toward the couple and toward each partner varies as a result of what seems to be functionally needed at a given time. At times the therapist is supportive and gentle; at other times, confronting and insistent. At times he or she is intense and serious; at other times, playful. At times he or she is empathically centered; at other times, emotionally somewhat distant. Sometimes the therapist closely structures and directs; at other times, he or she hovers above the flow of the session, listening for key words, feelings, or themes. The therapist's stance is flexibly responsive to the current tone and needs of the couple. On the other hand, the variability of the stance is not whimsical or undisciplined. It is always arrived at with caring consideration for what this couple needs and wants at this time, and in a way that is connected to the partners' central and recurring treatment goals. The therapist's varying stance always rests on a consistent primary foundation of what is in the best interests of the couple—not what is in his or her personal best interests, or in the best interests of supporting a particular theory of marital dysfunction or marital therapy.

Although the therapist in ICT is not an expert on how to live life, he or she must be an expert on how to create a therapeutic structure in which the partners can find, create, and implement answers and solutions to their problems. The ICT therapist also assumes responsibility for having and using expert professional knowledge about relationships and relationship change, based on clinical or clinically relevant research and theory development. Because, as we see in the next section, ICT calls upon a wide range of therapeutic techniques, the integrative therapist has an absolute responsibility to be familiar with emerging treatment methods, especially those that are empirically supported.

The Therapist's Three Central Roles

Beyond this overarching stance with couples, the ICT therapist has three particular roles: (1) inculcating systemic thinking and awareness, (2) teaching and coaching relationship skills, and (3) challenging dysfunctional relationship "rules."

The *teaching of systemic awareness* may occur implicitly or explicitly. This style of intervention fundamentally involves enhancing the partners' capacity for doing their own functional analysis (see below in "Assessment and Goal Setting") of their difficulties. It often involves the modeling of context questions (e.g., "What were you doing, Bob, just before Jill told you how anxious she was feeling?" or "Jill, what was the first thing you saw Bob do after you told him how anxious you were?"). By modeling the basic principles of functional analysis (see below) through his or her own questions, reflections, and observations in sessions, the therapist helps the partners become more sensitive to the recurrent circular processes in their relationship that maintain their primary problems, including intrapsychic events and cues. In effect, the ICT therapist conversationally models and encourages the couple to become curious about the "discriminative stimuli" that set the occasion for, or become circularly involved in, problematic interaction patterns. Thus, the partners become more adept at being able to solve problems in ways that are meaningful to them. This kind of systemic or *functional-analytic awareness training* directly fosters the development of a more multicausal, "both–and" couple perspective, which may help to counter the common (and always problematic) single-factor, "either–or" style of thinking in which distressed couples regularly engage in their polarized, mutual projective dance of attributing blame to each other.

The ICT therapist's second major role involves the *enhancement*, via modeling and feedback, *of facilitative relationship skills*, especially those focusing on communication and problem solving. The use of such skills training in ICT is discussed in detail below.

Finally, in ICT the therapist plays the all-important role of *challenging the couple's maladaptive relationship "rules,"* especially those that are centrally linked (i.e., functionally related) to the core thematic problem. The therapist must be particularly attuned to the implicit, out-of-awareness rules that govern pertinent and persistent marital patterns. The therapist's role in ICT in this regard is, in effect, to violate the partners' dysfunctional rules in a safe environment that prevents avoidance of or escape from exposure to new possibilities about one's self and one's partner, therefore increasing the opportunity for new and more satisfying relational learning. Often such a therapeutic "violation" of the couple's rules involves asking the unaskable or saying the unsayable. At times in ICT, this "violation" may require a therapist to express rather forcefully what one or both partners may be thinking or feeling but not directly saying, based on a finely nuanced understanding of each partner. In the process of eliciting and interpreting unexpressed feelings, the ICT therapist must serve as a model of how the partners can provide effective holding for each other.

The Therapeutic Alliances

All methods of psychotherapy appropriately emphasize the central, change-facilitating role of the therapeutic alliance. In marital therapy, there are in effect three alliances that must be attended to (Gurman, 1981, 1982b): (1) the therapist's alliance with each partner, (2) the therapist's alliance with the couple, and (3) the working alliance between the partners. Because couple therapy is usually brief, active change induction needs to be addressed rather early, so that a working alliance with the couple is established to create a safe environment in which change can begin. Thus, early therapist interventions must be aimed at both establishing such an alliance and increasing optimism about problem-relevant change. Thus, all early change-oriented interventions should also facilitate the patient–therapist alliance, or at least not interfere with it.

The three targets of early alliance building usually must be attended to simultaneously, with priority given to the first two areas.

THERAPIST–PARTNER ALLIANCES

Therapist–partner alliances require attention in the very first session. Each partner should feel that something of personal value has been achieved, though how this occurs varies from person to person. Some people feel an alliance emerging when they are offered empathy and warmth, whereas others require insight, beginning directives for behavior change, or reassurance about the viability of their marriage. Consistent with the emphasis on the functional analysis of problems, ICT requires that the therapist quickly discern what is functionally relevant to each partner, in terms of establishing a therapist–partner alliance that is likely to increase the chances that the partner will continue in therapy. One size, or approach, does not fit everybody, and the therapist must also be prepared to offer different bases for an alliance, even within the same couple.

THERAPIST–COUPLE ALLIANCE

In addition to learning how to "speak to" each partner of the couple effectively, the therapist must identify early the paired unspoken "language" that simultaneously bonds the partners together and creates the medium for the emergence of the current and continuing conflict. In ICT, the therapist learns to speak to both partners at once, as it were, even when overtly addressing only one of them. This second alliance area is best established by speaking empathically to the mutually contingent manner in which the partners collude to keep aspects of themselves and of each other out of awareness. In the early phase of therapy, the therapist's aim is to offer a tentative acknowledgment and attribution of the dominant ways the partners' overt struggles reflect the growth-oriented purposiveness of their initial attraction and later commitment.

PARTNER–PARTNER ALLIANCE

Such empathically offered interpretation serves not only to impart insight but also to strengthen the couple alliance. One common and helpful strategy for fostering the partner–partner alliance is for the therapist, while acknowledging the partners' stylistic differences during conflict, to identify and underscore ways the partners show similar relationship strivings. If, however, the therapist forces such a view on the couple, without accurately understanding each partner's relationship fears and aims, such an interpretation will appear not only off-target but also contrived. Psychodynamically and affectively attuned interpretations (e.g., "You show it in very different ways, but you both seem to feel too disconnected from each other") along these lines, in contrast, are regularly met by a sense of relieved acceptance.

Assessment and Goal Setting

Because ICT attends to both individual and relational aspects of couple functioning, it casts a wide net in the opening phase of treatment in an attempt to identify the most salient factors influencing the couple's appearance in the therapist's office, their core conflictual theme(s), and the obstacles to and potentials for change. ICT is generally very problem-focused, pragmatic, and oriented toward brevity, so it may seem inconsistent with this stance of an assessment process that is so wide-ranging. The kind of broad initial assessment in ICT discussed here is conducted, ironically, in the service of heightening the focality of treatment, by creating a rich environment of potential clues for the development of a practical, central focus.

General Considerations and Principles

The assessment process in ICT is almost entirely carried out via traditional clinical interviews. The therapist has the responsibility for creating a clinical formulation that includes "data" not only from patient self-reports and the therapist's direct observations in the interview, but also from the therapist's conceptual understanding of the recursive interplay between the interpersonal and the intrapersonal, and between the conscious and the unconscious forces in couple relationships.

In ICT, no variables or factors are viewed as being inherently more important than others for assessment purposes. ICT does not "privilege" any particular domain of behavior. The core assessment method is the functional-analytic approach of behavior therapists (Kanfer & Phillips, 1970), but with a "twist." As traditionally applied, the functional-analytic method often focuses on rather discrete patient behaviors. In ICT, the functional approach is applied both to highly specific couple behaviors and to broader classes of couple behavior; these are roughly equivalent to what Christensen, Jacobson, and Babcock (1995) call "derivative events" (i.e., specific interactions) versus "controlling themes" (variously referred to in the field as "the dance," "the fight," "the vulnerability cycle," "the mutual activation process," "the core impasse," and, most often, "the underlying issue"). Unlike this distinction within behavioral couple therapy, *the central controlling themes in ICT regularly also include both the implicit unconscious individual and dyadic motivations that play pivotal roles in the maintenance of couple problems. It is this attribute of ICT that renders it a "depth-behavioral approach."*

The functional-analytic approach, which emphasizes case-specific formulation, is seen as the ultimate expression of respect for patients; while certainly incorporating universal principles

of behavior maintenance and behavior change, it fundamentally emphasizes the uniqueness of each couple and of each member of the couple. In this very important way, the functional-analytic foundation of ICT is flexible and inherently responsive to differences between couples based on ethnic, racial, class, religious, and gender differences (Hayes & Toarmino, 1995).

Although the cultural context in which marital problems occur is almost always interesting to consider, it does not necessarily follow that culture-level factors are causally relevant, that is, problem-maintaining, in the given case. Moreover, even when significant cultural determinants of marital problems are at work, and even when they are undeniably so, they are not necessarily able to be influenced via the vehicle of psychotherapy. In the first case, the cultural dimensions of a couple's life might not be addressed at all after the assessment, because they are not seen as part of current problem-maintaining patterns. In the second case, they might likewise receive minimal attention after the initial assessment, because they are seen as being outside the realm of likely therapeutic influence. Cultural factors in couple distress are not seen in ICT as inherently any more or less important than any other set of possibly relevant factors (e.g., individual psychopathology, poor relationship skills, maladaptive cognitive processes, unconscious strivings). *Problematic behavior patterns are targeted not because of their form, but because of their function in the couple's difficulties.* Thus, the therapist's sensitivity to and awareness of cultural differences among couples can serve as a basis for generating useful hypotheses about problem-maintaining factors, as can any body of knowledge that helps to organize complex information about general behavioral tendencies in a particular group of people (e.g., the symptom pattern of a given patient diagnostic group). But the functional emphasis of ICT requires that any potential problem-maintaining variable be considered salient only if it matters in this particular case.

ICT assessment is largely present-oriented, for three reasons. First, a large proportion of couples come to therapists in crisis, and one or both partners in such a couple are often eager to flee the "enforced togetherness" (Brewster & Montie, 1987) of conjoint therapy, so the rapid development of a working therapeutic alliance is essential if the couple is to return to treatment. Conversations in early meetings that focus on the present are usually experienced by patients as more "tuned in" to their perceptions and pain. Second, present-focused conversations generally allow more useful therapist mappings of the problem-maintaining patterns of the couple via the appearance of real-time enactments (whether prompted by the therapist or not) of recurrent interactional difficulties. Third, although some history taking is a standard part of the ICT approach, historically oriented conversations tend to occur in the longer mid-phase of ICT. The core assumptions of the change process in ICT—that *couple therapy can lead to change in both interactional patterns and inner representational models,* and that *such changes often occur via direct behavior change efforts*—reinforce a decidedly present-time emphasis. Even when historical factors are highlighted during the early assessment phase, this occurs, as Yalom (1975) has said, "not to excavate the past, but to elucidate the present" (p. 28).

In ICT, there is no sharp distinction between an "assessment phase" and an "intervention phase." Potentially change-inducing interventions often occur quite early—even in the first session. Naturally, this is more likely to occur when ICT is practiced by a more experienced therapist. Such a therapist may "construct probes, prescribe tasks, offer interpretive reframings of meanings, pose challenges, and so on" (Gurman, 1992, p. 199) as varied means of assessing central problem-maintaining dynamics and of testing a couple's capacity for change.

Universal Areas of Assessment

Although the elements of a comprehensive couple assessment are presented here, all these areas do not require equal emphasis. In most cases, a few areas stand out as especially pertinent to the therapist's understanding of the nature and maintenance of the problem(s) at hand, and some are quickly revealed to be of little or no functional significance. Moreover, whereas in most cases the therapist might need two to four sessions to have a strong sense of understanding the couple in each of these areas, except with the most severely disengaged, enraged, or disorganized couples, a reasonably experienced couple therapist should be able to form at least tentative impressions in most of these areas after one or two sessions. The following "topographical map" of assessment areas is used to help generate practical, relevant foci for the work of therapy. The present categorization of assessment domains overlaps those of Nichols (1988) and Birchler, Doumas, and Fals-Stewart (1999) but was conceived independently.

CONFLICT

Conflict includes the couple's observable *communication* and *problem-solving* skills, emphasizing the distinction, discussed earlier, between problems of acquisition and problems of performance. The conflict domain also necessarily includes the partners' *presenting problem*(s) and their previously unsuccessful *attempted solutions*. Secondary problems, as discussed earlier, must also be considered.

COMMITMENT

Essential for initial treatment planning is the therapist's understanding of both partners' intention to stay in or leave the relationship and discrepancies between them in this regard. Moving ahead with couple therapy versus divorce therapy (see Lebow, Chapter 15, this volume) requires very different emphases. It is also essential to be aware of patterns that may threaten commitment (e.g., affairs, other secrets) or strengthen it (e.g., social support, religious involvement).

CONNECTEDNESS

This is the couple's sense of "we-ness." It involves their basic *compatibility,* their *attachment security,* capacity for mutual *empathy* and *acceptance,* and *sexual expression.*

Although ICT is present-centered, there are at least two strategically important reasons to learn about the couple's connectedness by understanding certain aspects of the *couple's history* together. First, talking to the partners about their shared evolution may help to build a working therapeutic alliance. Such conversations allow them to "tell their stories" to an unbiased, interested third party, as well as to recount positive aspects of the beginnings of their relationship. Second, such conversations often provide the therapist with clues about why and how the couple's central problems have been maintained over (often a very long) time. They may also suggest salient developmental factors that may have negatively influenced either partner's relationship needs and expectations, or diverted the couple from a normal developmental progression.

Because couple difficulties brought to therapists rarely have begun just recently, conversation about the couple's history usually helps to enhance the therapist's understanding of the partners' responses to the central assessment question of all brief therapy: "Why *now* do they seek help?" (Budman & Gurman, 1988). More specifically:

1. How and when did the couple meet? The psychosocial context in which the partners met, and the developmental point in their individual lives at which they met, may provide important hints about the needs each partner hoped to fulfill in establishing this relationship.

2. What attracted the two to each other? Understanding a couple's early connection often sheds light on the partners' current disappointments and dilemmas.

3. How did the couple handle conflict when it first appeared in the relationship? Even a cursory mapping of such interactions after the idealization phase of the couple's relationship often foreshadows present difficulties.

4. Were there any untoward reactions to the couple's dating or marrying from the partners' families of origin, close friends, or other significant persons or institutions (e.g., church)? Are the major presenting problems thematically linked to any such earlier tensions?

5. How has the couple handled nodal events and potential stressors (e.g., deaths, serious illnesses, births of children, shifts in educational/career involvement)?

6. Have there been separations during the relationship (other than those occasioned by outside forces, e.g., military service or work obligations)? How and why did the partners get back together, and did they deal adequately with the issues that lead to the separation?

7. Have there been, and are there now, involvements in extramarital relationships (including nonsexual but emotionally deep involvements)? Are there nonromantic "affairs" (with work, friends, family of origin, etc.) suggesting a primary "attachment" to aspects of life other than the partner? Are these long-term or more recent?

CHARACTER

This area includes all therapeutically relevant aspects of each partner's *personality style* and *individual psychopathology*. In this regard, it is essential that the initial assessment include discussion of whether violence and alcoholism, or other drug abuse, exist. Also included is an assessment of each partner's individual *strengths* and emotional *resilience*, and *capacity for self-regulation*.

CONTEXT

The context domain refers to a wide range of *cultural*, *developmental*, *familial* and *physical* (biological, medical) factors that may both affect and be affected by couple functioning and dynamics. Included here are factors such as various external stressors and *life-cycle challenges* (e.g., job loss, illness in the aging parent of a partner, relocation, childhood developmental delays).

Context importantly also includes answers to the central opening question, "Why now" is this couple seeking help (Budman & Gurman, 1988)? Although many couple therapies are initiated in the context of acute crises, most distressed couples have endured through a longer period of repeated conflict or disengagement, and often there is "something different" in the current context that brings the couple to therapy and is likely to be very relevant to the therapist's initial treatment planning.

A Note on Couple Therapy and the Larger Family. Marriages do not exist in a familial vacuum. The children of distressed marriages are more likely to suffer from anxiety, depression, conduct problems, and impaired physical health (Gottman, 1999). Likewise, the illnesses or other problems of children may create significant stress for couples. While a systemically sensitive couple therapist will keep his or her ears open for child problems, in ICT there is no automatic focus on the couple's children, or on the parent–child relationship. These areas of family life are addressed in ICT when they are functionally relevant to the couple's problems, for example, when the couple regularly fights about parenting differences or a child is evidently caught up in a scapegoated role in the parental conflict. Given the degree to which couple problems and parenting problems covary (Sanders, Markie-Dadda, & Nicholson, 1997), integratively oriented couple therapists are advised to be conversant with methods of behavioral parent training.

Likewise, the ICT clinician pays ongoing attention to other dimensions of family life, such as historically salient family-of-origin issues, and present extended family matters, when either the initial assessment, or later revisions of the assessment, reveal the functional relevance of such aspects of the couple's difficulties. Since a clinically useful functional analysis is not merely descriptive of a problem and what maintains it, but necessarily includes a plan for intervention, the form of ICT intervention in wider family issues may vary widely for pragmatic reasons. Thus, for example, family-oriented discussion of how one partner's childhood experiences help to make sense of his or her present relationship vulnerabilities may be called on to increase his or her spouse's empathy when he or she behaves in ways that are distressing. Alternatively, in the same course of therapy, the therapist might decide to give the husband an out-of-therapy task involving his family of origin, designed to enhance his differentiation from his family. Such intervention decisions flow naturally from functionally relevant case formulation (see below), in which family-level factors are certainly possible candidates for intervention.

CAUSALITY AND CHANGE

It is commonplace for marital partners to enter therapy with very divergent, and often actively conflicting *theories of the origins and maintenance of their problems*. It is important for the therapist to be aware of the degree to which each partner can acknowledge his or her own contributions to the couple's difficulties. It is also essential for the therapist to be aware of similarities and discrepancies in the partners' *treatment goals*. It is quite common for partners to disagree about whether the changes that are needed are more "individual" or "interactional." Failure to do so can carry significant implications for the adequacy of the early therapeutic alliances that are established (see below).

Closely related to partners' treatment goals are the notions of *readiness for change* and *readiness for therapy*. The two may not be the same. In addition to ICT's present focus and interest in the "Why now?" question, it recognizes that marital partners are not necessarily, or perhaps even usually, equally ready to change at the same point in time. The fact that a chronically conflicted couple remains that way through the contributions of both partners does not imply that partners are equally motivated to change (though they may be, or at least see themselves as being, quite receptive to "change"; i.e., to change in each other!). Such motivation may even wax and wane, with the partners motivationally crisscrossing over time.

A partner's low readiness to change may be the result of any of a wide array of factors. Common expressions of this state include a lack of commitment to the marriage, with or without an ongoing affair; a (defensive) belief that marriage should not require "work" to go well; a desire for a "quick fix" (usually of one's mate); a fear of novelty and self-disclosure; a fear that "open communication" may "make things worse" (e.g., by revealing fundamental and unchangeable differences between the partners that are not acceptable); despair regarding the likelihood of meaningful change, whether due to an individual's pervasive pessimism or to a sense that the couple has "waited too long"; a disbelief in the effectiveness or relevance of psychotherapy; and a partner's unspoken anxiety about having to change, which implies a fear that he or she has contributed to the couple's central problems, which in turn may be associated (perhaps not unrealistically) with a fear that all the couple's problems will be blamed (by the mate and/or the therapist) on him or her.

Whatever the phenomenology of a partner's level of readiness to change, what is especially salient is the difference between partners' current relative readiness levels. Note that the therapeutic alliance must be managed and kept in awareness at all times. Early imbalances in the alliance between the therapist and each partner, at times expressed through overt side taking or, more often, unspoken "agreement" that one partner "is" more of the problem than the other, can be deadly for the opening phase of therapy. Psychotherapists are understandably more drawn to patients who are cooperative, easy to engage, and motivated to change. Thus, significant partner–partner discrepancies along these lines threaten essential treatment alliances, and the therapy itself.

Drawing upon Prochaska's (e.g., Prochaska, Norcross, & DiClemente, 1994) stages-of-change model, Budman (1999) exemplifies and illustrates how combinations of different levels of partner readiness for change are typically manifested early in the process of couple therapy, and what action implications these combinations carry for the therapist. Prochaska's stages include "Precontemplation" (in which there is little motivation for change; e.g., a partner is in therapy because of the threat of divorce); "Contemplation" (in which ambivalence dominates—this probably characterizes most couples in therapy); "Preparation" (in which one is committed to change but has not yet begun to make changes); and "Action" (in which one has already initiated change and is eager to try new alternatives). Adequate attention to each partner's readiness to change can help to foster viable therapist–partner treatment alliances (see below).

Interestingly, Miles (1980) and Smith and Grunebaum (1976) have pointed out that marital partners may enter and stay in therapy even though their motivation to work toward a more functional marriage is low. Miles (1980) emphasizes that these partners may have very strong "alternative" motivations for seeing a therapist (e.g., to justify an already decided-upon separation; to ensure that a partner has someone to care for him or her after a separation; or to "take the heat off" the less willing partner). Smith and Grunebaum (1976) also identify the common partner motivation of "looking for an ally" to help stand up to one's mate. Miles stresses that these alternative motivations (to the ones therapists would prefer to encounter) for being in couple therapy are problematic when they are primary motivations, and when the therapist fails to recognize them.

Attention to partners' differential readiness to change is important in and of itself, and acknowledgment of their change readiness levels implicitly points to the importance of intrapersonal factors in ICT.

COUNTERTRANSFERENCE

Couple therapy is a therapy of systems, and the therapist is a part of that system, not outside it. Therefore, the therapist must be aware of his or her own experience as a part of the initial (and ongoing) assessment. For simplicity's sake, the traditional idea of countertransference is used to capture this experience. "Countertransference" is expressed in couple therapy primarily in terms of *ongoing* (vs. occasional) *side-taking* by the therapist (e.g., speaking too much for one partner; having repeated difficulty empathizing with one partner) and, even earlier, by obvious difficulties forming a therapeutic alliance with either partner. Note that what is meant here is not time-limited, intentional, and strategic side taking to unbalance rigid couple patterns. It is the sort of taking sides in which the therapist literally has difficulty seeing the couple's problems from both partners' points of view, or in which the therapist actually believes that one partner is overwhelmingly more responsible/culpable for the couple's difficulties. Especially early in therapy, the therapist must be able to "hold" the couple's anxiety without being drawn into their collusive interplay.

Focal/Functional Assessment

In addition to these universal or molar areas of assessment, a more fine-grained, molecular assessment of the couple's most salient problematic patterns is necessary. To this end, ICT calls upon both an object relations-based understanding of the couple's core conflictual issues and a social learning theory–oriented assessment of these core issues.

THE ROLE OF FUNCTIONAL ANALYSIS

The "molecular" aspect of ICT assessment emphasizes what behavior therapists call "functional analysis" or "behavioral analysis." A functional analysis is concerned not with the topography or form of behavior, but with its effects or functions, roughly equivalent to its contextual purposes. Functional analysis is a method of connecting assessment and treatment planning, including technique selection (Hayes, Follette, & Follette, 1995; Hayes & Toarmino, 1995; Haynes & O'Brien, 1990). The goals of functional analysis are to identify patterns of behavior of clinical concern, to identify the conditions that maintain these patterns, to select appropriate interventions, and to monitor the progress of treatment (Follette, Naugle, & Linnerooth, 2000).

The function of a behavior or behavior pattern is assessed by identifying the factors that control, or maintain, the pattern. This calls for a description of the behavior (or pattern), including its frequency; the conditions, settings, or contexts in which it occurs; and the consequences of its occurrence; that is, the behavior's antecedents (discriminative stimuli, both covert and overt) and consequences (positive or negative reinforcement, punishment, both covert and overt) are tracked. When a functional analyst is asked "why" someone does something, he or she provisionally finds the answer in the particular pattern of antecedents and consequences attendant to the behavior; that is, it is not the "act" that matters, but the "act-in-context," including the meanings attributed to the act. Historical facts or experiences are relevant in a functional analysis to the degree that they establish learned behavior or patterns that continue into the present and are clinically relevant to the problems for which change is sought (as one former colleague put it, "If it doesn't matter now, it doesn't matter").

Typically, couples identify very particular or even singular triggering situations (e.g., a recent argument) as though those situations or events constitute the problem. Whereas this is occasionally appropriate, it is much more likely that the therapist needs to be cognizant of the recurring pattern that is problematic, the latest (or almost any "chosen") instance of which is probably merely an illustration. The patterns or "themes" are referred to as "functional classes" or, more commonly, "response classes"; that is, various behaviors are considered to be members of a larger functional class, in that apparently "different" (i.e., topographically dissimilar) behaviors share the same function (purpose, effect). Response classes are not determined by the degree of similarity of the content or form of particular behaviors or events. The practical implication of thinking in terms of response classes is that because the behaviors that make up the class are functionally equivalent, changing one particularly frequent or salient component of the response class may lead to change in other, topographically "different" behaviors within the class, thus fostering generalization (Berns & Jacobson, 2000) and providing a clearer therapy focus. Moreover, tracking the function of "different" behaviors may help the therapist identify a functional theme that the couple fails to see, instead of seeing each problematic event or interaction as though it were a separate class unto itself. Doing so often helps to establish a coherence to the early phase of therapy, in which the partners feel less overwhelmed by having "so many" problems, which, functionally speaking, often are actually very few.

To facilitate a reasonably coherent experience of therapy, and to have a relatively clear thematic focus, it is essential that the therapist think in terms of such response classes. In most cases, the marital problem will be in a "hot" area—one in which the partners are less likely to respond to change with comfort. Even when a couple's early, chaotic presentation makes it appear that there is but an endless "list" of difficulties with no central, unifying theme, there *is* a theme. It is the therapist's responsibility to make thematic sense out of apparent chaos.

Functional Analysis and Private Events. Although behavior therapy is widely known for its emphasis on overt, external, or environmental factors in controlling behavior, internal or covert events (and their antecedents and consequences) are legitimate subject matter for a functional analysis. Private events include thoughts, feelings, and physiological responses (recall Gottman's [1999] finding of problematic diffuse physiological arousal in men in conflicted marriages).

Kanfer and Saslow (1969) set forth an influential description of "behavioral diagnosis" (i.e., functional analysis). Their analytic model went beyond the standard Antecedents–Behavior–Consequences (A-B-C) assessment model to include variables about the state of the organism, recast as Stimulus–Organism–Response–Consequences (S-O-R-C). Consideration of the "O" factor includes, for example, hunger and arousal. It also includes what Kanfer and Saslow call a "motivational analysis."

For traditional behavior therapists, such a motivational analysis would never include anything that smacks of the unconscious. As Jacobson (1991) noted, "The fundamental enemy of a truly behavioristic system is the hypothetical construct, especially one used to describe an internal process" (p. 441). Jacobson argues that such constructs provide "only the illusion of understanding" (p. 441), because they are attributed causal significance. Thus, a clinically useful "problem story will describe the emotional reactions that we and our partners experience from the problem *without speculating on possible motives* in our partners *that led to their actions*" (Christensen & Jacobson, 2000, p. 150, emphasis added).

Floyd, Haynes, and Kelly (1997) have included among the factors leading to an "invalid functional analysis" (p. 369) the omission of "important causal variables." But note that, very often, as Christensen et al. (1995) wrote, "couples cannot articulate what is bothering them" (p. 36). In the view of object relations theory, or any clinical theory that allows for the relevance of motivation that is out of awareness (i.e., unconscious), such difficulty identifying and describing what is problematic is often quite understandable as involving denial, repression, and similar defense mechanisms. Although "many have abandoned the notion of unconscious motives entirely as a useless construct" (Christensen & Jacobson, 2000, p. 147), the ICT view is that it is just such unconscious motives that may provide useful clues to what is most distressing to a couple. And at the beginning of therapy, it is often only by the use of reasonable therapist inferences and hypotheses about such unspoken, and unspeakable, motives that sense can be made of the underlying pattern of the partners' varied complaints and concerns.

Thus, one may say that to identify the central couple collusions, the ICT therapist must look for the ways in which the S-O-R-C analysis of the marital partners' interactions intersect and mutually affect one another. Marital behavior is as often under the control of (unwitting) self-administered consequences as of partner-administered consequences.

It is the concurrent emphasis on both the "within" and the "between" that renders ICT a "depth-behavioral" or "intrapersonal–interpersonal" therapeutic approach. The kinds of salient intervening cognitive and emotional cues and events, including those that are either implicit or beyond conscious awareness, are of the sorts referred to in Dollard and Miller's (1950) classic concept of "response-produced cues." These are cues associated with thoughts or experiences that, via previous learning, have become signals (discriminative stimuli) for anxiety or other painful affects or negatively valenced cognitions. When such cues are elicited, there is a natural tendency to avoid them (e.g., to remain unaware of them).

A complete statement of the functional analysis, sometimes identified as S-O-R-C-I, necessarily includes the identification of the Intervention(s) that are expected to be helpful, thus producing what is traditionally called a "case formulation." And yet, as Kanfer and Phillips (1970) reminded us decades ago, "In general ... little more than hunches based on observed coincidences of target responses and consequences is available for identification of factors maintaining problem behaviors" (p. 516). The case formulation, is, in effect, the eighth "C" of assessment that unites the thematic coherence of more content-focused areas with a plan for how change may be achieved.

IDENTIFYING MUTUAL PROJECTIVE IDENTIFICATION/COLLUSION

Within the perspective just presented, it becomes essential in ICT to help partners modify not only the overt behaviors about which they complain but also the patterns of reciprocal projective identification around their thematically central concerns. Because the circular process of "mutual projective identification," or collusion, is an inferred one (supported, of course, by overt interaction), "it" cannot be observed directly. Nonetheless, a number of behavioral patterns signify its presence. Mutual projective identification is manifested in many forms, usually with several of the following forms present in the interaction of a particular couple:

- Partners consistently fail to see salient aspects of each other's behavior or personality that are readily perceptible to a third person (e.g., the therapist).
- Partners often fail to see changes in each other that are perceptible to a third party who is familiar with them.
- Partners behave in ways that appear to protect them from behaving in a manner inconsistent with their preferred views of themselves in the relationship.
- Without conscious awareness, partners often reinforce in each other's behavior the very behaviors or characteristics about which they complain.

- Partners largely fail to see, or at least to acknowledge, their own contributions to the problems at hand.
- Partners agree that one or the other of them "is" the problem at times, by virtue of that person's purported personality pathology or psychiatric diagnosis.
- Partners argue over whose personality pathology accounts for their problems.
- Partners exaggerate their differences and minimize their similarities, appearing at first blush to be "totally opposite" from each other.

The ICT therapist tracks, via both partners' reports and his or her own observation, the recurring ways they punish in each other behavior they claim to value, and reinforce in each other behavior they claim to abhor. How the partners consequate "adherence" to and "violation" of the central rules of their relationship is attended to carefully throughout therapy, since these constitute the primary patterns the therapist seeks to disrupt and replace with new patterns. The ICT therapist attempts to have a heightened awareness of what Snyder (1999, p. 358), without implying unconscious intent, refers to as the "inadvertent maintenance of maladaptive relationship patterns." This awareness begins in the very first conjoint encounter.

At the outset of therapy, it is less important for the therapist to have a clear sense of the origins of the couple's collusion, historically speaking, though such understanding may become more important later in therapy. The old family systems theory saw that "a system is its own best explanation" applies equally well to early therapy mappings of couple collusive processes.

Goal Setting

The basic ICT premises about clinical change are that (1) because people shape core relationally relevant aspects of each other's personalities, couple therapy can lead to individual change, both behavioral and intrapsychic; and (2) behavior change can lead to change in relationally relevant inner representational models.

ICT seeks to change both individuals, as well as their interaction; to facilitate more accurate self-perception and more accurate perception of one's partner; and to resolve what the partners define as their presenting problem. The form these changes take varies, of course, as defined by the functional analysis. *Just as ICT does not "privilege" given areas of a couple's relationship to experience for assessment, it also does not privilege given areas for change. ICT respects goals focused on action and reflection, feeling and doing, bonding and bargaining, attachment and differentiation and warmth and assertiveness.*

The functional analysis is inherently responsive to individual differences; thus, it incorporates whatever factors are deemed relevant, whether their origins or present sources are intrapsychic (cognitive or affective, conscious and unconscious), dyadic, larger family systems, sociocultural (e.g., race, ethnicity, class, gender), or biological/physiological. It is not necessary (or usually appropriate) to attempt to address all identifiable areas of couple discord, or all aspects of spouses' individual conflicts that impinge on the couple relationship. As a well-done functional analysis usually reveals, disharmony is usually determined and characterized by a few major issues.

Just as ultimate treatment goals vary, so do early treatment goals. A couple in crisis may require a good deal of containment, structuring, and even practical advice at the outset. Only after the crisis has become muted can the partners fully engage in cooperative exploration of their relationship, and of themselves as individuals within that relationship. Even when the immediate stimulus to the couple's crisis is an external event (e.g., job loss, family-of-origin conflict, recovery from illness), the ICT therapist tries to understand the working relationship models within each partner, without necessarily voicing these inferences and hypotheses. Some couples (with basically flexible styles of interaction, a more robust degree of self-acceptance, etc.) facing "situational" problems can rather rapidly be helped with direct, concrete problem-solving guidance. The couple's view of the "presenting problem" must, of course, be taken seriously. Still, even when externally generated problems constitute the couple's initial problem presentation, it is appropriate for the therapist to include in his or her formulation how the current dilemma or stressor fits within the internal relationship schemas of both partners. The great majority of couples seeking therapy, however, present difficulties that are much more complex both in origin and maintenance, and require a therapist's intervention at multiple levels of experience, using a rather broad array of techniques.

Therapeutic Techniques

The three central ICT therapist roles in teaching systemic awareness, enhancing relationship skills, and challenging dysfunctional relationship rules

are fulfilled in large measure, by following three core principles of intervention: (1) the interruption and modification of collusive processes, (2) the linking of individual experience to relational experience, and (3) the creation of therapeutic tasks for the couple. Because ICT often addresses unconscious experience via rather direct and concrete therapist activity, it is essential that the therapist think with complexity, yet intervene simply. To this end, ICT requires of the therapist an attitude of technical flexibility and a concrete mastery of a rather broad range of intervention skills.

The Three Principles of Intervention and Their Associated Techniques

Each of the three overarching intervention principles just identified has an array of associated techniques.

INTERRUPTION AND MODIFICATION OF COLLUSIVE PROCESSES

The couple therapist must consistently and persistently track, label, and interrupt the marital collusive process as it occurs in therapy sessions. A therapist who intervenes to change this dysfunctional mutual defensive process implicitly challenges the maladaptive rules of the relationship. Typical ways in which collusion may be seen to operate during therapy sessions have been described in the section "Assessment and Goal Setting."

General Guidelines. The limitless ways in which therapists can interrupt and block collusive processes as they occur in the immediacy of the conjoint sessions are probably constrained in their variety only by the therapist's clinical creativity and technical mastery. Some general guidelines can be set forth regarding what the therapist should do (i.e., the therapeutic strategy) as distinct from how to do it (i.e., the therapeutic technique, which is discussed below). In-session interruption and modification of collusive processes are facilitated by taking several sorts of actions:

1. Encouraging each partner to differentiate between the experiential impact of the other's behavior and the intent attributed to it.
2. Interrupting partner behavior that is aimed at reducing anxiety in the other spouse, especially when that partner is behaving in ways that are historically contrary to the couple's collusive interactional contract.

3. Focusing each partner's attention on concrete evidence in the behavior of the other that denies similarly anachronistic perceptions of that partner.
4. Encouraging each partner to acknowledge directly his or her own behavioral changes that are incompatible with the maladaptive ways in which this person has tended to see him- or herself and to be seen by the other partner.

Naturally, as therapy progresses, the therapist ideally fades out his or her initial responsibility for these types of responses, and increasingly encourages the partners to monitor, interrupt, and shift their own formerly collusive process. Indeed, their increasing capacity to do so is probably a reliable, unobtrusive measure of positive therapeutic change.

Specific Techniques: Blocking Problem-Maintaining Interactions. Here, I briefly present some illustrative techniques for interrupting and modifying in-session collusive processes. These methods fall into the first main category of techniques in ICT, "blocking interventions" (Gurman, 1982a), whose aim is to block, interrupt, or divert couple enactments of habitual unconscious contracts in response to observable in-session behavior. Blocking techniques are used reactively and responsively rather than proactively. Their use and its timing cannot be predicted, anticipated, or planned. They are called upon by the therapist in the natural, emerging flow of the therapeutic conversation. In this sense, blocking interventions are explicitly process-oriented.

Two blocking interventions that are central in the practice of other influential couple therapies are used with a different intent in ICT.

Cognitive Restructuring: Unilateral and Bilateral. Techniques derived from cognitive-behavioral therapy, and employed regularly in cognitive-behavioral marital therapy, challenge each person's "automatic thoughts" about and overt reactions to the partner's behavior, and may usefully be incorporated into ICT. Such automatic thoughts are seen in ICT as especially problematic if they center on negative generalizations about the other partner's behavior or character, and particularly if their content implies malevolent purposes or fixed psychological defectiveness. These attributions, along with selective inattention to (or denial of) who the "whole partner" is, are especially likely to reflect underlying projective elements. In con-

trast, functionally maladaptive processes regarding general relationship expectations (i.e., those that would pertain to any partner) are somewhat more likely to reflect consciously held values and the direct effects of relationship modeling—for example, by one's parents. As a result of their usually being less evocative of anxiety, these processes may be clinically addressed by relatively straightforward methods, such as the provision of normative information about relationship functioning or the suggestion of bibliotherapeutic material.

In addition to the use of cognitive techniques that focus on the faulty attributions and selective inattention of individuals, ICT also urges therapists to develop some deftness at "equalizing the dynamic struggle" (Gurman, 1982a). This strategy calls for the therapist to interpret to the couple, rather than to individuals, the salient ways their overt differences reflect similar dynamic themes. Such interpretations, which clearly emphasize conscious cognitive understanding, help to increase empathy and to counter defensive projections.

Shifting Affective Gears. This intervention calls for a refocusing of one partner's negative feelings (e.g., anger) and awareness of the undesirable behavior of the other onto that partner's internal experience (of rejection, sadness, etc.). This shift of affective focus is similar to the refocusing from "hard" to "soft" feelings by emotionally focused couple therapists (Johnson, Chapter 4, this volume) and integrative behavioral couple therapists (Dimidjian et al., Chapter 3, this volume). The latter therapists call upon this approach as a core strategy in acceptance training, and the former see such affective shifting as central to the development of partners' accessibility and responsiveness.

The ICT therapist shifts the focus from "hard" to "soft," and from "outside" to "inside," for two reasons. At a purely pragmatic level, such a shift interrupts (blocks) recurrent negative interactions, thus allowing opportunities for new behavior to replace old, destructive behavior. At the same time, the utility of such a shift is not its only virtue. The ICT therapist also actually believes in the psychological truthfulness of the shift itself; that is, the expression of destructive and pain-inducing feelings really is an indirect cover for, or defense against, the direct expression of feelings involving vulnerability.

Note that the "shifting of affective gears" ("high gears" = "hard" emotions, "low" gears = "soft" emotions) also allows the therapist to attach (i.e., condition) new labels ("high and low gears") to relationally facilitative versus maladaptive expression of feelings in a way that can be seamlessly incorporated into self-control/self-regulation coaching. Such "shorthand" cues can be called upon in self-regulation coaching, discussed below. When the attacking partner shifts focus to softer feelings, the therapist must not only support this frightening movement but also block any behavior by the partner that may switch the attacking partner back into a negative, defensive mode. As noted earlier, out of their own anxiety about change, partners often punish the appearance of "positive" mate behavior, even the very kind behaviors for which they have asked.

Self-Control, Self-Regulation, and Containment Coaching. Recently, a growing intersection of empirical and clinical developments in the areas of neuroscience, attachment theory, and developmental psychobiology (e.g., Atkinson, 2005; Schore, 2002; Tatkin, 2005) have paralleled and occurred during the same period within psychology as the robust interest in self-regulation. Although clinical applications of self-regulation currently are of great interest, they are not really new. "Self-control," a broader behavioral notion that includes both affective and behavioral self-regulation, has been with us for at least three decades (e.g., Mahoney & Thoresen, 1974).

Although Integrative Behavioral Couple Therapy (IBCT; Dimidjian et al., Chapter 3, this volume) places great emphasis on marital partners' enhancement of mutual acceptance in the place of emotional reactivity, in large measure it does not (cf. Halford, 2001) explicitly teach self-regulation skills. As noted earlier, this limited attention within IBCT to self-change (in the sense of both changing conscious affective and behavioral responses, *and* accepting heretofore unconscious urges, fears, drives, and motivations) may have been its major "missing link." To close this breach, Fruzzetti (Fruzzetti & Fantozzi, Chapter 20, this volume; Fruzzetti & Iverson, 2004) has refined the use of many of the methods of dialectical behavior therapy (Linehan, 1993) with affectively dysregulated couples. Interventions such as mindfulness training, building distress tolerance, and teaching emotion regulation skills are comfortably incorporated into ICT. Any of a wide array of arousal down-regulating methods are used. They all serve to block or interrupt problem-maintaining collusive interactions (hence the term "containment coaching").

An interesting strategic matter arises in the use of self-regulatory methods in couple therapy. Calming of the couple by the couple (note that the therapist often serves as both the model of and regulator of affect, especially early in therapy, and often throughout therapy with "difficult" couples) can occur in two ways. In *auto (self)-regulation*, a partner changes his or her own behavior. In *interactive regulation*, a partner serves as the calming vehicle for the affectively overloaded partner (via the use of a soft voice, slowing of speech, providing empathy, etc.). Some (e.g., Schore, 2005) have argued that autoregulation of couple conflict (as it is often done, by the partners separating until they regain composure, then returning to their conversation) is often inferior to interactive regulation, because it isolates the partners and can unwittingly heighten abandonment anxiety in the "left" partner. Although interactive auto-down-regulation also is preferred in ICT because of its relative efficiency, this often must be successively approximated by the following shaping sequence: in phase 1, the dysregulated partner excuses him- or herself to down-regulate, then returns to the conversation; in phase 2, the dysregulated partner engages in down-regulating activities in the presence of his or her partner, without physically separating; in phase 3, the dysregulated partner is calmed by the other partner; and in phase 4, a combination of auto- and other-regulation is used, thus fostering as much a "we" as an "I" experience. Such a progressive down-regulation coaching sequence may require many sessions and a good deal of at-home experimentation and practice. As in all other technical aspects of ICT, there is no inherently superior approach to fostering affect down-regulation: Form always follows function. Here, format also follows function.

A practical note on coaching down-regulation skills: It is sometimes difficult for partners to transfer their down-regulating experience from the therapist's office to home, especially if the therapist has been very active in helping them to contain difficult feelings. At these times, it is helpful for the therapist to offer some kind of verbal "tag" or (conditioned) cue to help initiate their down-regulation process. For example, the author often suggests the use of the familiar children's guide about responding to a fire, "Stop, Drop, and Roll," translated into "*Stop* what you are doing (in the problem interaction). *Drop* your defensiveness (self-justifying comments, attacks on your partner). *Roll* with the punches ('go with the flow' by slowing your breathing, etc.)."

These suggestions illustrate that the countless ways to counter collusion are limited only by the therapist's ability to put form ahead of function. Catherall (1992), for example, offers a perceptive and compelling set of other possibilities that complement those described here.

Anticollusive Questioning: Inquiring about and Commenting on Ambivalent Projections. Integrative couple therapists do a good deal of "anticollusive (or counterprojective) questioning" that (1) points to partners' inferred (hence, unspoken) wishes and fears that help to maintain problematic patterns; (2) directs partners' attention to problem-maintaining behavior that is outside their conscious awareness; (3) hints at the "unwitting" (unconscious) ways the partners "cooperate" in appearing to work toward change, yet maintaining the status quo; and (4) identifies self-contradictions between partners' overt behavior and their stated preference and desires. These sorts of questions, which may be asked in a somewhat rhetorical tone only to plant a seed for later questions, require no direct patient response; or they may be asked with the explicit expectation that the partner(s) consider and address the matter, theme, or issue raised by the therapist's question at the time it is presented. As with all blocking techniques, these anticollusive questions are always asked in immediate response to what a partner (or both partners) does or says in the session. Blocking anticollusive questions forces attention on the problem-maintaining elements of the couple's relational patterns. In so doing, they invite the partner both to disengage from relationally destructive behavior at the moment, and to reflect on the unconscious purposes of the broader pattern of which this present behavior is but a therapeutically convenient example. There is no formal limit on the number or types of blocking, anticollusive questions that can be asked, but there are several recurrent problematic marital themes for which the following illustrative questions seem often to be appropriate. These questions are typically preceded by a therapist's segue, such as "You know, when you say (or do) that, I wonder . . .

- could it be that you fear that you two are really too similar rather than too different?"
- how do you protect each other from even worse pain?"
- can you imagine anything negative that might happen if your couple problems just disappeared? (or if your partner suddenly started to behave exactly the way you say you wish he or she would)?"
- if, despite your complaining about _____ in your partner right now, might there be times when you actually like or admire _____ ?"
- even though you often complain about _____ in your partner's behavior, do you ever find that sometimes you do _____ yourself?"
- are there sometimes moments when your partner is behaving in some way you've really wanted to see more of, and yet you don't 'stroke' him or her for it?"
- what stops you from accepting what your partner is giving you, especially since it seems to be just what you're asking for?"
- where did you first learn to be uncomfortable with [whatever the person is repeatedly complaining about in the partner] in yourself?"
- what do you do to get your partner to behave in ways that, ironically, bother you so much?"
- when you think of some things you could do differently to help solve the problem, how do you stop yourself from doing these things? What do you say to yourself?"
- what would it be like if you were married to a person who was virtually identical to yourself psychologically?"
- how can you help him or her help you to change whatever *you* want to change in yourself?"
- how do you think you would feel if the two of you were to switch [psychological] roles for a while?"
- what can you do to help your partner do less [or more] of what you'd like to be different in your relationship?"

Anticollusive questions such as these cannot be used in a "rote," staged fashion. They must organically and thematically "fit" and be woven into the conversational flow of the session. When appropriately tuned to the affective and substantive context of the session, they appear quite unforced. When the therapist is well-tuned-in to the couple's maladaptive "contract" (Sager, 1976, 1981), evocative questions such as these do, in fact, appear to arise intuitively. When the therapist uses a well-timed anticollusive question that identifies centrally relevant content and is put forth in the couple's usual expressive style, the recipient usually feels both uncomfortably exposed and deeply understood. This dynamic tension facilitates change. As I have noted elsewhere (Gurman, 1992), "One way to lengthen therapy is to not ask painful or anxiety-arousing questions of patients" (p. 190).

A related, more structured gestalt therapy technique known as "leaning into the accusation" (Sunbury, 1980) can be used in a manner that complements anticollusive questioning. Partner A lists a few of partner B's most upsetting qualities that especially focus on what A is complaining about in B in the session. A reads one such description aloud. B acknowledges the partial accuracy of the description and points out ways in which he or she is different from the description as well. A acknowledges how he or she sometimes behaves in a manner very similar to that about which A has complained about or to B. This process is then reversed. This technique is intended to limit projections and splitting.

LINKING INDIVIDUAL EXPERIENCE AND RELATIONAL EXPERIENCE: INSIGHT AND THE PLACE OF INTERPRETATION

The ICT therapist values both cognitive awareness and behavioral change. In ICT the development of insight, and the use of interpretation to foster such insight, are but two of many potentially useful therapist interventions. Specifically (and in contrast to its role in traditional "insight-oriented" psychoanalytic therapies), interpretation is one helpful means of fostering therapeutic exposure and a shifting perception of one's partner, allowing for the development of more adaptive and flexible interactions.

In couple therapy, interpretation is intended to expose partners to hidden feelings (or impulses, etc.) about both themselves and their mates. Whatever their origins, such feelings are hidden in the present, so most therapist interpretations are present-oriented rather than historically or genetically focused. Even when an interpretation is focused on one partner's experience from an individual historical perspective (e.g., regarding one's family of origin), its implications for the current marital relationship must be struggled with or at least identified. This is in keeping with the broader principle described earlier—that all "individual" work within the conjoint session must be translated in terms of its marital meaning, ramifications, or consequences.

It is probably self-evident that the use of exposure-enhancing therapist interpretations requires a solid therapist–partner alliance as a buffer against anxiety. What cannot be overlooked in the process of couple therapy, however, is that therapist interpretations that expose one partner also require an adequate partner–partner alliance and general atmosphere of empathy and safety, lest a therapist's interpretations be used by the second partner as a weapon against the first partner. For this reason, such individually focused interpretations usually are less common early in therapy than later on.

Thus, interpretation has three main purposes in ICT: (1) by naming the previously expressed feeling, to help a person contain the "bad stuff" that would otherwise be projected onto the partner; (2) by helping a person to accept (by exposure) the projected material as being in him- or herself, to decrease blame and increase acceptance of the partner; and (3) by derailing repetitive interactions in the moment, to shift the couple's interaction to allow new relational possibilities that include, prominently, mutual empathy. The value of interpretation also lies in its shifting of couple interactions maintained, in part, by implicit partner "theories" of what constitutes the couple's dysfunctionality.

CREATING THERAPEUTIC TASKS: INSTIGATING CHANGE-PROMOTING INTERACTION

Any number of tasks or therapist directives may facilitate the desired change processes in ICT. There is certainly a place for active and experientially powerful techniques from the gestalt (e.g., Sunbury, 1980), structural (e.g., Minuchin & Fishman, 1981), and strategic (e.g., Stanton, 1980) therapy traditions. Paradoxical techniques such as prescribing symptoms and restraining change (e.g., Papp, 1980), though used sparingly in ICT, may also foster ICT goals (Gurman, 1981) for valid psychodynamic reasons (Skynner, 1981). As Skynner emphasized:

> *All* double-binds and other paradoxical communications are attempts to maintain a fantasy world, different from reality, by expressing *both* fantasy and reality at the same time in a form which conceals the discrepancy between the two, and also by conveying at the same time a "command" to others to collude with the "self-deception" and so preserve the speaker's fantasy world (or the joint fantasy of the marriage or family). Paradoxical *therapeutic* interventions can then be seen not as "tricks" but as expressions of the most essential truth, which subtly break the rule that fantasy and reality must be kept apart, by relating the two in a disguised, seemingly innocent fashion which expresses only the positive aspects. Once the family or couple accept the bait, they cannot avoid seeing more than appeared to be implied in the original paradoxical intervention. (p. 76; emphasis in original)

Thus, an ICT therapist who positively connotes to a couple the function of a symptom or an interaction pattern does so with a belief in the actual veracity of what he or she is saying.

Therapeutic tasks refer to the general category of what in ICT are called "instigative interventions." In contrast to blocking interventions, these interventions typically do not arise out of the immediate natural flow of a therapy session. Rather, in contrast to the more process-oriented blocking interventions, instigative interventions are more goal-oriented and directive; they are "strategic" in Stanton's (1981) sense that "the clinician *initiates* what happens during treatment and *designs* a particular approach for each problem" (p. 361, emphasis added). Thus, these interventions are usually more planned by the therapist, even (and often) to the point of being designed outside the therapy sessions. Although the ICT therapist obviously plans such interventions in a way that is responsive to the treatment needs of partners as the therapist assesses each couple, they typically are not set forth in immediate response to the couple's behavior and are generally experienced as being "brought into" the therapy session. The other major difference is that blocking interventions interrupt, draw attention to, and increase awareness of maladaptive couple patterns, whereas instigative interventions are designed to initiate, prompt or model healthier interactions.

Out-of-session tasks vary from exploring the consequences of new marital behavior to reflecting on particular themes identified during therapy sessions, to pinpointing concrete desires for change in one's partner or in oneself. Tasks may be as loosely constructed as asking each member of a couple to "think about how you yourself contribute to the problems that bother you most in your relationship."

ADDITIONAL INSTIGATIVE INTERVENTIONS

Other instigative interventions have in common the therapist's planful efforts to stimulate positive change along the lines of the couple's central problematic theme(s). Although instigative intervention other than communication and problem-solving experiences can focus on in-session couple behavior (e.g., directing and encouraging a couple to sustain a conversation about an anxiety-arousing topic), most of these interventions emphasize out-of-session experiences. This aspect of instigative intervention highlights two different but related assumptions of ICT that are central to brief therapies, and especially to brief marital and family therapies (Gurman, 2001): (1) The central source of healing is within the partner–partner relationship, not the partner–therapist relationship; and (2) effective brief therapy must include change that is reinforced in the couple's natural environment.

Given these guidelines, many therapist interventions may qualify as instigative. For example, encouraging the use of positive reinforcement for change is a deceptively simple technique. This intervention, which calls for the therapist to coach and encourage partners to reinforce positively (via concrete simple acknowledgment, expression of thanks, etc.) the appearance of behavior each has asked to see more of, by definition, is intended to increase partners' "desired" behavior. In addition, following through on this principle, especially when partners reciprocate, often has the more subtle effect of inhibiting their tendency to engage in projective identification. As discussed earlier, partners in sustained marital conflict often identify behavior that stimulates anxiety about their own impulses, needs, and desires as "unwanted" behavior in their mates. Direct therapist instruction to reinforce positively desired changes in partners' behavior implicitly requires that each partner attend to and acknowledge aspects of the mate that are characteristically minimized or discounted. The couple is put in a "win–win" situation by the therapist's encouragement of reinforcing desired change. If, on the one hand, they follow through as suggested, partners strengthen valued elements of their relationship. On the other hand, a lack of follow-through, even after it is clear in session that the partners understand the rationale for the therapist's idea, may signify the intensity of their "stuck" projective process. The therapist can then redirect attention to the unspoken motivations and attributions that drive each partner, behaviorally speaking, to continue to emphasize negative perceptions of the other. Such a formulation does not universally explain couples' noncompliance with suggested prosocial behavioral reinforcement approaches, but it provides a conceptual framework that is often very useful in helping a therapist make sense of partners' anxieties about change. Once identified, such anxieties, again following a functional-analytic approach, can themselves be addressed.

A Coda on Technique. In ICT, the therapist selects particular interventions, not because of what they "look like," but because of what they may accomplish. As in architecture, form follows function. Like architecture, couple therapy is a blending of art and science.

THE SEQUENCING OF INTERVENTIONS

Just as the sequencing of ultimate and mediating treatment goals varies from couple to couple, so the sequencing of different types of therapeutic interventions varies across couples. Indeed, in ICT, there is a fluid interplay of depth-oriented and behavior change–oriented therapist intervention, and how much of each occurs in any given phase of therapy is more a matter of emphasis than of exclusion. Whereas at times, the ICT therapist may push for highly specific behavioral changes in session or out of session to unblock long-term and rigid interactional obstacles to intimacy, at other times, he or she may "go deep," and work to address the couple's painful, individual vulnerabilities to establish enough of a sense of safety that partners are willing to make visible changes outside the therapy, that is, without the therapist present.

Still, some guidelines can be offered about therapist decision making in the choice, and especially the timing and sequencing, of different types of interventions in ICT. ICT conceives of three levels of therapist intervention into the object relational (OR) realm of couple dynamics and interaction. At Level 1, *Inadvertent OR Intervention*, the therapist uses any therapeutic method with which he or she is familiar, without any intention to produce change in the object representational inner world of the marriage. As I discuss in detail later, many common couple therapy interventions, such as communication and problem-solving training, unwittingly facilitate OR changes. Inadvertent OR interventions are common among what ICT calls "instigative interventions."

At Level 2, *Implicit OR Intervention*, the therapist may use the same kinds of interventions as in Level 1, but with full awareness of the likely inner representational meaning of the interventions, for example, by wondering, "How might use of this particular technique unbalance the couple's particular collusive agreement to avoid exposure and closeness?" Level 2 intervention also includes variations on the use of anticollusive questioning, discussed earlier, in hinting at the functional significance of partners' unconscious strivings, including projective identification, but without explicitly identifying or labeling them.

At Level 3, *Explicit OR Intervention*, the therapist explicitly and directly interprets unconscious experience and its role in the marital dynamics. Accessing the feelings that underlie maladaptive overt behaviors, such as angry criticism, and interpreting its defensive function, is a common example of a Level 3 intervention. Level 3 interventions tend to be both thematic and incident- or event-focused, because they point to recurrent couple patterns, as illustrated by the content of a particular therapeutic moment and interaction.

ICT therapists prefer to begin therapy with a significant use of Level 3 intervention, but clinical reality does not always allow this. Because Level 3 intervention emphasizes functionally relevant themes in the couple's conflict, it includes more of the controlling factors in the couple's tension, or put another way, it emphasizes a larger sampling of the various functionally related ways that different content plays out in the couple's central problems. Moreover, thematic intervention that helps the partners improve their understanding of the unconscious dimensions of their relationship inherently attends to both overt and covert factors in the couple interaction. In these ways, helpful Level 3 intervention is more likely to generalize to the couple's life outside therapy.

What, then, should influence the therapist's decision as to whether Level 3 intervention is appropriate early in therapy? The guide is to be found, once again, in the functional analysis: not the functional assessment of what maintains the couple's core problems, but the "I," or "Intervention," component of the full S-O-R-C-I functional analysis. The therapist's predictions about how the partners may respond to Level 3 intervention, combined with sensitivity to their reactions to such interventions, are key. Essentially, the cues the therapist must stay aware of involve the couple's openness to Level 3 intervention. Openness is influenced by the partners' general psychological mindedness, but especially their level of comfort at dealing with non-surface-level aspects of their relationship. There are no absolute guidelines as to who these "open" couples are. "Difficult" couples—those with marked, intense hostility, individual vulnerability, and chronic marital tension—might at first seem to be too easily dysregulated by Level 3 intervention, but this is not automatically the case. The moderating factor in such cases can be the quality of the therapist–patient alliance or, more specifically, whether strong alliances can be established early in therapy. If not, then more alliance building is needed for the therapist to provide an adequate level of holding for the couple's anxiety. Interestingly, but not surprisingly, although many couples find therapist empathy and support to be key to being adequately held, others find that a therapist's structuring, for example, via behavioral exchanges, or offering of directives, serves the same therapeutic function. Alternatively, partners who appear very open to simple behavior exchanges early in therapy may be so because they are fundamentally well connected, flexible, and open to each other's influence. It is also possible that they are open to focusing only on discrete changes out of a shared avoidance of dealing with deeper issues. Once again, what matters is not the form of the (therapist's or couple's) behavior, but its function.

Transference, Countertransference, and Mechanisms of Change

Unlike the individual therapy setting, in which only one physically real transference pairing (patient–therapist) exists, there are four transference pairs in couple therapy: husband–wife, wife–husband, husband–therapist, and wife–therapist. In addition, triadic transference may emerge (i.e., husband–wife–therapist). Although partner transferences toward the therapist clearly occur in conjoint therapy, their salience is usually quite attenuated for three main reasons. First, the relative brevity of ICT inherently caps the impact of most transferential elements of the patient–therapist relationship by countering the sense of fantasized timelessness that often characterizes long-term intensive individual therapy (Budman & Gurman, 1988). Relatedly, ICT is focused and goal-directed, emphasizing the partners' reality, as well as their unspoken fantasies, and the therapist more often than not participates as a real object. A third common characteristic of transference-inducing therapy is the therapist's relative constancy. As shown earlier, the therapist plays many roles in ICT—from provision and modeling of holding functions to provoking warded-off affect, to "coaching" interpersonal social skills, to providing expert information and knowledge about relationships. Although the ICT therapist certainly provides constant concern, support, and collaborative effort to couples, his or her "job description" includes a describable but widely varying set of action possibilities. Transference reactions in a focused therapy such as ICT include important information on the partners' feelings, perceptions, misperceptions, and attributions of intent, motivation, and loyalties; of course, these must be addressed when they are overt and pose obstacles to the forward movement of the therapy.

At the same time, transference reactions do not typically impede progress in ICT, as they may be more likely to do in longer-term, more uncovering couple therapies based on object relations theory (see Scharff & Scharff, Chapter 6, this volume). In ICT, the most powerful transferences occur between the marital partners, and it is there that therapeutic attention must be focused. As Skynner (1980) crisply put the central issue, "The unconscious conflicts are already fully developed in the mutual projective system between the couple, and could be better dealt with directly rather than by the indirect methods of 'transference'" (pp. 276–277). Working toward the resolution of a limited number of currently relevant, bilateral marital transference patterns serves well as an overriding, orienting aim in ICT.

This emphasis on treating relationship problems in what social learning theorists call the "natural environment" decreases patients' dependency on the therapist and promotes generalization of change from the *in vitro* setting of the therapist's office to the *in vivo* setting of everyday life. Thus, the classical "corrective emotional experience" is to be found within the couple-as-patient. One of the most corrective of such experiences is learning to discriminate the real current partner from the misperceived, past "inner" partner.

ICT asserts that a rather broad range of therapist interventions, including behavioral interventions, can foster such bilaterally corrective experiences. For example, successful communication and problem-solving experiences (usually not requiring "training") often make partners safer, more accessible, and more responsive. At the same time, exposing warded-off (thus, indirectly conveyed) feelings to an increasingly nonattacking, empathic partner requires the taking back of projections and necessarily leads to a decreased punishing of one's partner for one's own strivings, conflicts, and fears. Likewise, the development of relationally relevant insight—for instance, about the childhood or previous adulthood origins of relationship anxieties—facilitates opportunities for bonding.

On the other side of the equation, the potential for the therapist's problematic countertransferential reactions to the couple, or to either partner, is heightened in a brief, active, goal-oriented therapy such as ICT. It is impossible for most couple therapists not to encounter in their own current or past intimate relationships some of the painful issues involved in the relationships of patient couples. Moreover, a therapist's generally high level of activity in ICT—including actively engaging the couple, and engaging with his or her own thought process on multiple levels of experience—does not allow a great deal of time and opportunity for in-session self-reflection.

The most common and most dangerous therapist error in ICT is nonstrategic side taking, that is, side taking, particularly of a recurrent nature, that results from the clinician's failure to appreciate the anxiety and pain behind the "negative" behavior of either partner. Although the therapist can and should use his or her own countertransference reactions as important guides to what is most distressing and fearful for the marital partners, again, the focus must remain on the partner–partner relationship. The therapist's self-awareness should emphasize an understanding of what in the *couple's* relationship draws out the side-taking inclinations of the therapist.

This side-taking error is particularly dangerous very early in therapy, of course. At that time, the partners are likely to be most entrenched in their split, rigidly projected negative views of each other, increasing the possibility that the therapist will be unwittingly taken in by one partner, whose characteristics or (mis)attributions about the mate strike an uncomfortable chord in the therapist. Such unfortunate (though nearly inevitable) problematic countertransference reactions, if they are not recurrent, can be more easily repaired later in therapy.

Behavioral Intervention and Therapeutic Couple Exposure

ICT calls upon the active techniques associated with various marital therapies to facilitate OR ends. This is not a new phenomenon in couple therapy. Indeed, 30 years ago (Gurman, 1978), in a comprehensive comparative analysis of marital therapies, I underscored the fact that "psychoanalytically oriented marriage therapy is largely 'analytic' in the way it organizes the complex material at hand and conceptualizes the nature of marital discord, but is, of necessity, quite pragmatic, if not eclectic, in its selection of actual therapeutic interventions" (p. 466; original emphasis omitted).

In ICT, many common methods associated with traditional behavioral couple therapy, IBCT, and cognitive-behavioral marital therapy are recruited to foster the process of helping partners

reintegrate denied aspects of themselves and their mates—that is, to work toward the fundamental reintegrative goals of the ICT approach. Marital partners in conflict must be exposed to aspects of themselves and their mates that are blocked from awareness. These self-aspects are blocked from awareness because of the anxiety they evoke. As Freud (1909) himself acknowledged almost 100 years ago, people only overcome their anxieties by exposure to that which elicits the anxiety. This exposure can be accomplished in couple therapy in a manner roughly analogous to the antiavoidance behavioral treatment of anxiety and phobic disorders. Therapeutic couple exposure may attend to the kinds of cognitive and physiological anxiety-eliciting cues that constitute the treatment targets of exposure therapy (Barlow, 2002), as well as the overt behavioral avoidance. At the same time, therapists need to keep in mind that not all marital avoidant behavior is "irrational" or unwarranted. The partners in chronically distressed marriages almost always display what behavior therapists would call genuinely "aversive consequences." Marital partners and therapists alike must deal differently with real versus imagined responses to their behavior. Ultimately, for a marital partner to be open to exposing his or her vulnerabilities, there must be good reason for the mate to be seen as "a safe, real person" (Dicks, 1967, p. 43).

Applications of the kinds of principles, strategies, and techniques just described for interrupting and modifying dysfunctional collusive couple behavior in session create opportunities for therapeutic exposure to warded-off aspects of the self and the other. Less obviously, but with equal power, commonplace behavioral couple therapy interventions also create such relational learning opportunities. For example, the traditional methods of communication and problem-solving coaching are common in ICT. Such techniques can facilitate the process of helping partners reintegrate repudiated aspects of themselves and their mates; that is, they can serve as a means of enabling partners to emerge as whole persons in intimate relationships. "Whole persons" are more emotionally available and accessible, and more accepting of differences; active interventions can foster the emergence of more "whole" persons.

I must emphasize that in ICT, rather than quickly attempting to control the dance of projective identification and do away with unpleasant feelings, the therapist often welcomes its real-time enactment in the session. The ICT therapist may even work to intensify split-off feelings in the partner in whom they originated, to gain access to underlying fears and vulnerabilities, as a step that precedes encouraging the couple to "find a different way to get–say–do what you need or want right now." Such intensification (a common structural therapy intervention) often involves the therapist's supportive insistence that the partners sustain their conversation in the face of high levels of discomfort. This is analogous to arranging exposure experiences in the behavioral treatment of phobias, in that the patient is required to feel and to tolerate, rather than to avoid, high levels of anxiety.

Although ICT welcomes the recent shift of emphasis in IBCT toward acceptance, in addition to behavior change, the behavioral approach seems to have incorporated only half of the therapeutic formula for inducing change. That is, IBCT increasingly emphasizes mutual acceptance, that is, acceptance of both "others." In the ICT framework, in contrast, both partners must also come to be more accepting of *themselves* in terms of what they have denied in themselves and projected into their mates. Accepting undesired behavior in one's mate is an important step toward acceptance of oneself, but it is certainly not equivalent to doing so.

The Countercollusive Power of Communication and Problem-Solving Intervention

ICT differs substantially from more traditional applications of object relations theory to couple therapy (e.g., Scharff, 1995) regarding the preferred means of reaching antiprojective ends. Proponents of more traditional approaches assert that these ends are not reached through "the familiar techniques of communications-trained or behavioral couple therapists" (Scharff & Bagnini, 2002, p. 64). By way of contrast, in ICT these very interventions are seen as offering some of the most direct available antidotes to unconscious collusion and splitting. At a "meta" level, the use of these techniques requires that the couple partners (1) speak only for themselves, not for each other; (2) assume responsibility for their own thoughts and feelings; (3) systematically track their own affective and cognitive experience; (4) focus on current intrapersonal and interpersonal events; (5) desist from the idealized, defensive stance that each partner should be able to know what the other wants

without having to be asked; and (6) attend to their own contributions to displeasing couple patterns.

Thus, traditional behavioral couple therapy techniques collectively discourage collusion and promote relationally healthy integration of the self in several important ways:

1. The techniques emphasize self-differentiation—for instance, even through the therapist's intermittent encouragement for partners to state their views and feelings from a time-honored, if a bit overworked, "I" position.

2. The techniques emphasize self-change, and in so doing, counter predictable partner blaming (projective identification). Inner awareness is promoted in place of outer (and other-) attack.

3. The techniques lower partners' needs to escape and avoid aversive arousal, thus increasing intimate, safer engagement.

4. The techniques shift awareness from the unconscious reinforcement of avoidant behavior (in self and partner) to the conscious reinforcement of desired behavior.

5. The empathic emphasis contained in communication skills coaching directly increases partners' mutual acceptance. Moreover, when such empathic relating is focused on a partner exposing the vulnerabilities that motivate his or her undesired behavior, the partner's enhanced acceptance includes acceptance of the "bad" or the unchangeable in the mate, plus acceptance of disavowed parts of the self along similar thematic lines. Catherall (1992), from an object relations perspective, has persuasively argued that empathy neutralizes projective identification. Tellingly, Christensen et al. (1995), from a behavioral perspective, have stressed that often when a couple "empathically joins around a problem" (p. 54), the partners more easily accept differences between them, and often without further skill-oriented guidance; and more cooperatively engage in new patterns of behavior. The object relations and behavioral rationales for the central role of enhancing empathic relating in marital therapy were anticipated almost three decades ago by Gurman (1981), who noted that "the therapist's goal ... is to have spouses learn by experience that unacceptable aspects of themselves and their mates need not be overwhelming. As this aim is being achieved, it often becomes progressively easier for couples to negotiate changes in overt behavior" (p. 446).

6. While improving overt communication, communication "skills training" techniques also

countercollusively decrease each partner's fantasy of who the mate should be and increase the reality of who the mate actually is. As noted in the earlier discussion of communication and problem-solving "skills deficits," poor communication is more often than not both a symptom of collusion and a maintainer of collusion. Poor communication reflects an implicit rule of limited intimacy through shared avoidance of self-disclosure and self-exposure. Improved communication allows real differences to be revealed. Private fantasies about the idealized partner may be a natural part of early romantic attraction, but engagement with the real partner is essential for genuine long-term intimacy.

Resistance

Because time is generally quite limited in the practice of couple therapy, the ICT therapist actively intervenes in situations involving change-resistant behavior between a partner (or both partners) and the therapist only when such events or patterns clearly pose a genuine obstacle to continuing therapeutic progress. Certainly, transferences resembling parent–child relationships can develop in couple therapy, but as already noted, they are not especially common in focused, brief couple work.

Just as ICT views the partner–partner relationship as the source of relational healing, so, too, does it constantly keep an eye open for resistance to change expressed in that relationship. Haley's (1963) well-known "first law of relationships" is relevant here. Haley wrote that "when one person indicates a change in relationship to another, the other will act upon the first so as to diminish and nullify that change" (pp. 223–224). Haley saw such interpartner resistance to change in terms of power and social influence. In ICT, by contrast, the bedrock of resistance to change is the "internal pressure generated by the desire to maintain one's own self-esteem and psychic boundaries" (Gurman & Knudson, 1978, p. 127), which in turn is a function of two factors: first, the level of anxiety aroused in the partners as they become aware of (i.e., exposed to) the split-off and projected aspects of themselves; and second, the frequency and intensity of the partners' unwitting reinforcement of each other's efforts to avoid or escape such reintegration (i.e., to avoid change). When one partner no longer fully plays out his or her half of the implicit collusive marital "script," the other partner will commonly work to shape the former to get "back in character." At such moments, the

therapist's task is to coach, coax, and support the partner to stick to the revised "script" (i.e., to encourage exposure), while identifying and allaying the other partner's discomfort at the wished for/feared changes and urging the other partner to remain open to the change.

Termination

Except for problematic terminations (e.g., those ruptures in the therapeutic alliance caused by errors involving therapist neutrality and side taking), the ending of most ICT work is relatively uneventful and rarely as disequilibrating a termination as that in long-term individual treatment can be. Because the primary attachment and transference in ICT are those between the marital partners, there is little sense of "a wrenching from treatment or a cutting the patient adrift to fend for himself" (Fisch, Weakland, & Segal, 1982, p. 176). Moreover, many couples stop therapy when the central symptoms or problems have been resolved, or at least have abated. As Brewster and Montie (1987) noted, "A family will come in during a crisis and once that is over, its members typically want to back off from the enforced togetherness of the therapeutic session" (p. 34). As much as the therapist may hope to engage with the couple at multiple levels of intervention, there may not be enough time available to do so. As a result, always with the anticipation that termination may not be far away, the ICT therapist seeks to intervene at multiple levels of experience in an active style that evokes, exposes, and modifies problematic, projectively induced, and sustained patterns.

In ICT, contact with the couple often occurs on a brief, intermittent basis, with the partners returning to the therapist about similar or different issues than those for which they were initially seen. One of the hallmarks of effective and practical brief therapy, including couple therapy, is the development of a therapist–patient (couple) relationship not unlike that with a primary care physician to whom the patient returns as life demands and changes require (Budman & Gurman, 1988). Thus, ICT does not usually view termination as "final."

Therapy is generally terminated when the partners either have reached their primary goals or find that although they have not fully achieved their aims, they have lost a significant degree of motivation for continuing at this time. Alternatively, of course, one or both partners may call a halt if they see no progress being made or do not have an adequate alliance with the therapist. The decision to "terminate" is the couple's, although in the interest of directness and efficiency, the ICT therapist occasionally may also suggest "taking a break" from therapy if he or she believes the couple is not adequately committed to the therapeutic task.

In practical terms, the ICT therapist again takes advantage of an opportunity to reinforce the central therapeutic messages about relationship change. First, in the knowledge that one never fully casts off projected aspects of oneself, the therapist may inquire (supportively rather than confrontationally) whether "there is anything problematic about the ways you used to be with your partner that you sometimes feel an urge to return to, even though you mostly don't." This question is not posed "paradoxically," but as an expression of a genuine therapist acceptance of the understandable ambivalence with which people typically engage in meaningful change. Relatedly, in the "termination" session, the ICT therapist not only asks the partners to review what changes have occurred but also (if necessary, pushing) to acknowledge both their own and each other's contributions to the positive changes that have occurred.

APPLICABILITY AND EFFECTIVENESS OF ICT

Scharff (1995) has taken the position that psychoanalytic couple therapy based on object relations theory is "for couples interested in understanding and growth ... not for the couple whose thinking style is concrete" (p. 184). Although this may be true of more traditional psychoanalytically oriented couple therapies, which place great emphasis on interpretation and on transference phenomena, it is not true of the variant of object relations couple therapy that is ICT. ICT always highlights multilevel formulations of couples' problem maintenance and urges therapists to intervene simply, even while holding moderately complex formulations. Thus, a fundamental belief in ICT is that therapists can use their psychodynamic/object relations understanding of problematic couple relationships without necessarily explicitly "speaking the language of psychodynamics," so to speak. One may practice ICT without much interpretive activity (e.g., regarding warded-off feelings), with little or no attention to the past (especially the past of the partners as individuals, outside their relationship) and little or no explicit attention to patient–

therapist transference phenomena. To some, this may then sound as if the "psychodynamics" of the treatment have been entirely purged from the therapy experience. But, as I have emphasized here, many very direct, practical therapist interventions can go a long way to serve object relations therapy aims. Even with partners whose capacity to empathize is severely limited, whose capacity to contain painful feelings is likewise limited, and who cannot therefore participate well in the newer style of behavioral couple therapy that emphasizes acceptance building (Christensen et al., 1995), old or "traditional" behavioral marital therapy interventions emphasizing behavioral exchange, and communication and problem-solving coaching may still be helpful, albeit to a more limited degree. ICT would argue that even in such constraining circumstances, ICT intervention may be able to modify partners' maladaptive inner relationship representations enough to produce a qualitative improvement in the relationship, largely through its feeling safer and more secure to the partners.

Naturally, partners are likely to gain more from therapy if they are able not only to engage with behavioral interventions but also to (1) respond cooperatively to the therapist's interpretive efforts; (2) "go with the flow" in response to the kinds of "anticollusive" questions the therapist may seemingly, at times "out of the blue," throw into the mix of a particular therapy session; and (3) remain in a good working alliance with the therapist, even when the therapist is unmasking the unspoken, hidden couple interaction by interrupting and blocking problem-maintaining couple interactions. Clearly, the capacity to tolerate such affective arousal and relatively deeper interpretation requires a moderate level of cognitive and affective maturity.

Couples who are typically most responsive to the various levels of intervention included in ICT can be identified rather straightforwardly, even early in treatment. They are the couples whose members tend, before any therapy experience, to see life interactively and circularly rather than linearly; are somewhat flexible in their ability to entertain new possibilities for both explaining and changing their conflicted situation; are curious about themselves and about relationships generally; and can and do, with or without therapist prompting, acknowledge their own contributions to the marital tension. A couple with flexibility in the relationship, ego strength in each partner, and a reasonable capacity for "holding" and "containing" may require only extremely brief and practical problem-solving assistance, often for difficulties that originate outside the couple's relationship, even if it is consuming the partners' energy and affect.

Thus, although few particular patient or couple characteristics preclude the applicability of ICT, some do severely limit its role, as with any approach to couple therapy. Such characteristics include most prominently volatile, uncontrollable arguing or otherwise grossly dysregulated behavior in the therapy sessions, or individual psychopathology that simply overwhelms the interaction. Dangerous levels of physical aggression usually render ICT, like other methods, inappropriate.

In addition, in an altogether too common type of couple that appears in therapists' offices, multileveled ICT, or perhaps any method of couple therapy, is difficult. Members of these couples are fundamentally incompatible (Hamburg, 2000) in most major spheres of life and probably should not have married in the first place. Such fundamentally incompatible couples typically got together for one or more universally unwise reasons ("forced marriage" due to a pregnancy, a need to escape a painful family situation, a transitional relationship exit out of another unsatisfying marriage, etc.). As Hamburg argues, such fundamentally incompatible partners may never be able to establish a secure and safe relationship together, because their inherent differences preclude them from feeling mutually validated and valued, and render almost impossible the development of any level of genuine empathy beyond perfunctory and grudging acknowledgment that the two of them have very different feelings and very different views of the world. Some of the behavioral techniques used in ICT, especially behavior exchange and problem-solving coaching, may allow such partners to tolerate and endure each other, but to expect an outright enhancement of their likelihood of genuine acceptance of each other is not realistic.

ICT is ideally suited to couples whose members, despite their pain, either intend to remain together or at least are open to the possibility. Severely estranged or separated couples usually do not have enough relational incentive to anesthetize themselves for a conjoint therapy that not only modifies but may also expose hidden vulnerabilities.

The Efficacy of ICT

The efficacy and effectiveness of ICT have not been tested in controlled clinical trials or in self-report survey research. Still, ICT regularly incorporates many of the central therapeutic interventions that research on cognitive-behavioral marital therapy (Baucom et al., Chapter 2, this volume) and IBCT (Dimidjian et al., Chapter 3, this volume) has shown to make a difference clinically, such as communication and problem-solving coaching, behavioral exchange, and acceptance training. But whereas behavioral methods emphasize acceptance of the *partner*, ICT places an equal emphasis on the acceptance of *self*. Moreover, ICT also regularly includes a number of the core interventions of empirically supported emotionally focused couple therapy (Johnson, Chapter 4, this volume; e.g., the softening of harsh emotions, and the connecting of interpersonal and intrapersonal experience). ICT also includes attention to unconscious psychodynamic forces in marital tensions, as does the affective–reconstructive approach of Snyder (Snyder & Mitchell, Chapter 12, this volume), which has shown very positive treatment effects at long follow-up periods, and ICT pays attention to such factors more consistently during the course of therapy than does Snyder's approach. In summary, ICT is the only marital therapy approach that articulates both the theoretical and technical integration of ideas and strategies from multiple, demonstrably effective methods of working with distressed couples.

CASE ILLUSTRATION

An 11-session course of therapy with Cathy and Steve over a period of 7 months illustrates the ways ICT therapists operate at multiple levels of experience in marital difficulty, addressing current, external situational matters, multigenerational patterns and attachment anxieties, unconscious collaboration in problem maintenance, and individual personality styles. This work with Cathy and Steve also illustrates the flexible yet coherent use of therapist interventions designed to promote change in different domains of the couple's experience.

Steve came to the clinic alone at first, identifying his main problem as being depressed and pessimistic about the viability of his marriage to Cathy, to whom he had been married for 9 years, and with whom he had two children, ages 5 and 2. He was referred to me after an initial evaluation by a staff psychiatrist, who thought that, in light of both his central concerns and his current level of functioning, and a lack of a prior history of mental health treatment, medication did not seem essential, and that couple therapy should be offered first. While Cathy was very supportive of his desire to get help for "his" depression and, indeed, had made most of the initial arrangements (checking insurance, etc.) for Steve to be seen in our clinic, Steve's initial solo appearance exemplified the couple's central marital conflict: Steve was the relationship initiator, the "complainer," and Cathy was the relationship reactor, rarely explicitly expressing her needs or dissatisfactions, but highly reliable in looking out for the welfare of others. Steve referred to her as being "too damned self-sacrificial. She's so focused on other people, that sometimes I feel like I don't even know who she is."

The immediate external stimulus for Steve's initial appearance was career-related. An outgoing and successful midlevel insurance company executive in his mid-30s, Steve was actively being recruited by a larger firm in another city. He saw this job change opportunity as being likely to open exciting and rewarding career possibilities, and he needed to make a decision about it within the next few months. Cathy, a part-time nurse, was less of a risk-taker, describing herself in the first three-way session as more of a "homebody type." Taking care of others in both her professional and private lives was a core part of her identity. She preferred routine, predictability, and order. "It probably has a lot to do with my ADHD [attention-deficit/hyperactivity disorder]. Structure is very important to me. I have to think for myself with patients, but there are rules and protocols to follow all the time. Most nurses hate all that stuff, but to me, it's a relief." The idea of taking care of Steve by moving was more than even she could tolerate, especially given her feelings of responsibility to her patients and to the doctors for whom she worked.

Steve had seen himself in "a kind of competition" with Cathy's work, and long before the new job possibility arose. When he would raise this issue, Cathy would counter that he "should have known better than to think about moving, since I've always been dedicated to my profession." Indeed, Cathy's stance on this matter was hardly news to Steve. Besides representing a perfectly real life-transition decision that the couple had to make, moving also signified Steve's longstanding concern about the emotional distance in the marriage that Cathy seemed to prefer. She also was "devoted" to her young children, regularly placing their needs, interests, and welfare ahead of those of her husband, the marriage, or indeed herself, ra-

tionalizing that "there will be plenty of time for us (later), but the kids need us now."

This pattern of "putting our marriage in second place ... on a 'good' day," as Steve described the problem, was now taking on another form as well. Steve's recent success at work had earned him an all-expense-paid trip for two to Hawaii in January (a most welcome prize in wintry Wisconsin!). He saw this trip as a chance to "recharge" the marriage by "having some 'alone time' without the kids." He also saw it as a sort of yardstick as to whether Cathy "really wants to be involved in this relationship." Cathy was very hesitant about going on the trip for two reasons. First, she had a "flying phobia" (though the couple had taken several flights together during their marriage, before their children were born); second, she was very concerned that "it might be very upsetting for the kids for us to be away from them for 6 days" (though this idea had never been tested, and there were nearby relatives, including similar-age cousins, with whom the children were very familiar and comfortable, with whom they could stay). Although Cathy's travel- and child-related anxieties seemed clearly to be functionally involved in her pattern of avoiding marital closeness, they were also quite real in their own right and needed to be respected as such. On the rare occasions that she had flown, it had always been on domestic flights ("So we could get back to the kids, if we needed to"), and she had required a fast-acting anxiolytic even to board the planes.

Cathy had grown up in a "good Catholic family" of five children, the second oldest child and the oldest daughter. Her parents, preoccupied with their careers, had been largely inaccessible and unresponsive to the needs of their children, often rationalizing their distance from their children as "encouraging them to be able to be self-sufficient." Cathy attended private parochial schools through 12th grade, finding them "repressive and cruel." She learned to take care of herself but in an isolated, conflict-avoiding way. A "self-starter," she had been "a good girl," graduating near the top of her high school class, and earned a scholarship to a local State university, which she attended over the objections of her parents, who "tried to force me to go to Central College," a small evangelical school in the Midwest. It was at the State university that, as a sophomore, she met Steve, a senior, and a garrulous, energetic honor student and business major, a leader in his business-major-dominated fraternity, and the President of his college's "Young Entrepreneurs Club."

As for his part in the marital distance, Steve was, of course, hardly uninvolved. A significant aspect of his outgoing style was a kind of overwhelming neediness, in Cathy's eyes, which she saw as a sort of off-putting dependency ("like a little puppy dog who always needs to sit in your lap and can't be by himself very much"). Steve, though overtly quite different from Cathy, was struggling with very similar conflicts and fears. Raised in a family with a chronically depressed mother and an intermittently alcoholic and abusive father, Steve had "decided" long ago that when he had a family, he would never treat them the way he had been treated. He would foster family relationships, with both his wife and children, at any personal cost ("Family is everything to me"). Cathy had struggled with her attachment fears, protecting herself from further hurt by not exposing her needs, but she was sad and self-contained. Steve handled his fears by seeking contact with people who mattered most to him, but often in a way that felt smothering to Cathy. She found his attentiveness to be "controlling." To that comment, Steve responded, "Yeah, well somebody's gotta pay attention to our relationship."

Of relevance to the possible upcoming family move, Steve's choice of a business career was hardly just because of his being "good with numbers and math from way back." His parents' on-again, off-again marriage had often put them in dire financial straits ("I learned to love peanut butter," Steve said wryly), and when old enough to begin to think about adulthood, he decided he was "going into some kind of work where I could make a lot of money."

It was very easy to form quick "social" alliances with Steve and Cathy. For all their joint difficulty connecting verbally, neither of them lacked "social skills," as was demonstrated regularly in their jobs and with their children. But establishing "therapeutic" alliances was not as easy. With rare exceptions, when our conversation turned to emotions, desires, and needs, Cathy became very laconic and measured in her speech. To her, being "known" was dangerous. It was difficult to draw Cathy out, without her seeing my curiosity and wish to know her better as an attack, as taking Steve's side, or both. Being very explicitly explanatory about why I was doing what I was doing several times each session helped to provide a clear-enough framework for Cathy to be able to stay engaged despite her anxiety. With Steve, the converse was the case, and my challenge was to engage him a way that he did not feel "left alone" by my inviting responses from Cathy, showing interest in her ideas, and so forth. I soon learned that although Steve was "a real talker," he did not always need "talk" to feel connected. Often, as I spoke to and listened to Cathy, a quick glance toward Steve that said, "I know you're still there," was enough.

Steve and Cathy were in a mutually reinforcing cycle of pursuing–distancing. When on the rare occasion that she would express her needs or show affection, which Steve said he wanted her to do, he would often subtly, but perceptibly to her, not support her by turning away and becoming uncharacteristically quiet, which Cathy interpreted as disinterest. At times, he would acknowledge that although he wanted her to be more expressive ("real") with him, because this would mean "she really cares," he felt afraid as she spoke, fearing that his needs would be forgotten, "as if there were two cuddly 'puppy dogs' competing for the same lap," I commented in a "light" tone, while pointing to a central tension over how they could *both* get their emotional needs met in their marriage. Especially in the early part of our therapy together, in effect, I became the "lap" they could learn to share. When Steve reconnected conversationally, Cathy would retreat into a passive listening style that she said was "respectful," but that Steve experienced as "uninvolved." They could take turns expressing their needs and wishes, but doing so usually had the tone of "me," then "you," with little sense of "we." There was little sustained conversation over important issues, and now the possibility of moving was "really in our faces."

The overriding treatment goal, as I proposed it, and as agreed to by the couple, was "to increase your sense of being more of a 'we' in a way that feels safe, so that each of you still knows who *you* are in the process. Then, 'we' can decide about moving or not, or anything else." My interventions to this end took very specific forms that focused on both the couple's in-session process and out-of-session patterns. To decrease their cautious turn-taking style, in which conflict (at the overt level at least) was avoided by passive rather than active listening, I offered the idea that Cathy and Steve needed to learn to get comfortable with having "balanced conversation." Not "balanced" as in "I go, then you go," but as in being more immediately verbally responsive (e.g., allowing interruptions; shortening the speaker's "floor time," paired with invitations [from both the speaker and from me] for responses by the partner; encouraging more direct, eye-to-eye contact; and less speaking to/through me). I began every session by asking, "What shall we focus on today?" Cathy, of course, regularly deferred to Steve about this. The conversational shifts occurred in the context of whatever subject matter the couple brought to the session to focus on. They were not based on structured or planned exercises or formats. My intent was to block, *in vivo*, each partner's recurrent ways of avoiding genuine dyadic exchange, fueled by the fear of neglect (Steve) and reprisal (Cathy). The main antidote to each partner's anxiety about less cautious exchange was my close tracking and acknowledging of the partners' discomfort as they allowed me to guide them in "new ways of speaking, where you can both be heard, without being hurt." My empathic tracking was extended to facilitate Steve's and Cathy's capacity to stay "in tune with yourself, even while you're tuning in to each other." Each partner's being able to acknowledge his or her discomfort aloud also helped to contain anxiety, reducing the internally driven (and externally reinforced) need to escape (e.g., by nonverbally withdrawing) and unwittingly punish the partner for his or her expressiveness. I think now, and thought then of the main process component of my interventions as a kind of systemically sensitive, bilateral, simultaneous "exposure therapy," wherein increasing what to the couple I referred to as the in-session "conversational flow," opened up previously warded-off exposure to both unacceptable aspects of self and feared aspects of the partner. Both partners, though often in fits and starts, became increasingly more adept at providing safety for each other's self-expression, aided at first a good deal by my "managing" parts of their conversation and modeling calm attending and listening, and later in therapy, by providing less defensive "audiences" for each other.

As therapy moved beyond establishing critical working alliances with Cathy and Steve, and beyond the more concrete interventions intended to strengthen their alliance with each other, I felt freer to talk to them about more subtle and implicit aspects of their difficulties. I addressed or at times more tentatively alluded to their ways of "unconsciously collaborating" by "protecting each other from experiencing painful things that each of you sort of intuitively understands but are afraid to let yourselves see, let alone say out loud to each other." Addressing this level of their relationship at times involved offering traditional interpretations of the unconscious strivings and unwitting collusion in their maintaining the paradoxical "change, but stay the same" messages reflected in their overt behavior. At times, addressing this level involved posing reflection-inviting, "anticollusive questions," such as "Steve, even though you complain about Cathy's 'living in her own world' in your marriage, do you yourself ever wish you yourself could be more comfortable when you're all alone by yourself?" and "Cathy, please don't answer automatically, think about this a bit: Can you think of any ways you may actually be ironically 'helping' Steve not feel so comfortable being by himself?"

In addition, I also created out-of-session exposure tasks of the more transitional sort, designed to challenge the couple's rigidities. For example, I addressed Cathy's "flying phobia" with direct coaching in some principles of relaxation training and other relatively easily learned behavioral self-control skills (e.g., rational disputation and "reality checking" via common cognitive-behavioral therapy methods). These were presented to Cathy as "some ways to take care of yourself and the relationship at the same time." On Steve's side, I suggested that he also use common rational (cognitive) restructuring techniques when he became unduly anxious about the (more) apparent (than real) urgency for making his job change decision and that he, as a former successful athlete, renew his involvement in anxiety-reducing (cardiovascular) exercise. For both Cathy and Steve, then, I offered these out-of-session self-soothing and self-care activity ideas not only in an effort merely to reduce each partner's anxiety but also, and more significantly, to remove obstacles to closer and safer couple encounters, and to counter aspects of each partner's externalizing defenses (e.g., "Airplanes make me afraid" and "Employers pressure me"). What at times might to an observer have looked like "individual" therapy with each of them also took place. In addition to Cathy's brief relaxation training and Steve's rational disputation coaching, on several occasions Steve also allowed himself to express a degree of ambivalence about taking a new "high-powered" job that he had not shared with Cathy. While he was clearly a "star" at what he did, he often felt that he was "just faking it," and that he mostly had gotten praise and promotions for his work not because of his expertise in finance, accounting, or actuarial science, but because "I'm a friendly, likable guy." I suspected that he might have been correct about this, but the important aspect of those miniconversations was that this "super self-confident guy," as Cathy referred to him, actually had trouble "finding the right words" to express his self-doubt.

As Cathy experienced this hidden, fearful side of Steve's outgoing, take-charge style, she began to see him in less polarized ways, as a more genuine "man in the middle," as "neither 'puppy dog' or 'alpha dog,'" as I put it. For years, when Steve would directly express self-doubt, Cathy would be unresponsive ("frozen," Steve called it), torn between wanting to be helpful and supportive, of course, on the one hand, yet terrified of the part of herself that could not ask for nurturance, and the part of Steve with which she could not be comfortable in herself; thus, she punished Steve as a way of staying out of touch with similar needs in herself.

Another important early- to midtherapy out-of-session task had a more "structural" emphasis and tone. Its purpose was both to challenge the partners' shared avoidance in a way that complemented the blocking and redirecting of their in-session exchanges, and to do so via a "shared project," in contrast to the "individual projects" of taking on a flying phobia (Cathy) and challenging self-damaging automatic thoughts (Steve). The couple had evolved a bedtime pattern with their children as follows: Cathy and Steve begin the nightly ritual together. Two-year-old daughter Grace is seamlessly soothed by Steve until she falls asleep, while Cathy accommodates 5-year-old Nick, who is "very fussy, and demands more and more stories," (by reading to him in his bed until he falls asleep, followed soon thereafter by her falling asleep there). All the while Steve is becoming impatient (for Cathy to finish) and retreats to his home office to "catch up on some important work stuff" on his computer, finally awakening Cathy as much as 2 hours later. Cathy, who usually begins her nursing shift very early, is "wiped out" and almost immediately goes to bed. Although the intervention in this scenario was "tweaked" several times, it focused on putting Steve in charge of his son Nick and Cathy in charge of Grace. Steve could more readily and consistently set limits than Cathy. On occasion, he even began to use an "I've got to go downstairs now to do some work" "excuse" to facilitate spending some evening time with Cathy, who, over time, was less exhausted and more available to Steve (who also set better limits on his at-home work as a previously all-purpose way to avoid conflict, while simultaneously "reinforcing" his obsessiveness about his competence and adequacy).

A few weeks before therapy came to a close, Steve and Cathy had returned from the Hawaii trip (which she managed with minimal anxiety, bolstered by their children being well taken care of and happy to stay with relatives). They had agreed not to move away, at least not in the near future (with Steve more confident than before that other good, career-enhancing opportunities would come along). Even over the course of a relatively brief treatment, Steve and Cathy had each become more accepting of aspects of the individual experience that each had previously avoided, and more accepting of each other's needs and anxieties. Dealing with similar anxieties about close relationships, expressed and manifest in different compensatory ways, had only added to the couple's ongoing confusion about their difficulties. As they became safer, both to each other and to themselves, they became "more real" and more flexible toward each other, and could more directly address differences as they arose across a variety of different content topics. Although they agreed that other areas of their relationship warranted therapeutic attention, they felt sufficiently closer and sufficiently safe at that point to "try to do some of the work on our own," and so they concluded therapy, with an open door to return at any time.

SUGGESTIONS FOR FURTHER READING
Case Reports

Gurman, A. S. (1985). Tradition and transition: A rural marriage in crisis. In A. S. Gurman (Ed.), *Casebook of marital therapy* (pp. 303–336). New York: Guilford Press.—A Wisconsin farming couple in crisis is worked with in the ICT approach, demonstrating the use of active therapeutic methods to address object-relational impasses.

Gurman, A. S. (1992). Integrative couple therapy: A time-sensitive model for working with couples. In S. Budman, M. Hoyt, & S. Friedman (Eds.), *The first session in brief therapy* (pp. 186–203). New York: Guilford Press.—The therapist's interventions and rationales for those interventions in the first session of ICT are described in detail. Includes couple–therapist dialogue.

Conceptual and Historical Reviews

Gurman, A. S. (1978). Contemporary marital therapies: A critique and comparative analysis of psychoanalytic behavioral and systems theory approaches. In T. J. Paolino & B. S. McCrady (Eds.), *Marriage and marital therapy* (pp. 445–566). New York: Brunner/Mazel.—A detailed comparative analysis of the theoretical and practical aspects of the—then—three dominant perspectives in the field, plus a critique of the strengths and weaknesses of these approaches.

Gurman, A. S., & Fraenkel, P. (2002). The history of couple therapy: A millennial review. *Family Process, 41*, 199–260.—The most comprehensive and in-depth review and analysis to date of the theoretical and clinical history of the field, including an historical account of trends in research since the field's inception.

REFERENCES

Aponte, H. J. (1992). The black sheep of the family: A structural approach to brief therapy. In S. H. Budman, M. Hoyt, & S. Friedman (Eds.), *The first session in brief therapy* (pp. 324–341). New York: Guilford Press.

Atkinson, B. (2005). *Emotional intelligence in couples therapy: Advances from neurobiology and the science of intimate relationships.* New York: Norton.

Bagarozzi, D. A., & Giddings, C. W. (1983). The role of cognitive constructs and attributional processes in family therapy: Integrating intrapersonal, interpersonal, and systems dynamics. In L. Wolberg & M. Aronson (Eds.), *Group and family therapy 1981* (pp. 207–219). New York: Brunner/Mazel.

Barlow, D. (2002). *Anxiety and its disorders: The nature and treatment of anxiety and panic.* New York: Guilford Press.

Bentovim, A. (1979). Theories of family interaction and techniques of intervention. *Journal of Family Therapy, 1*, 321–345.

Bergin, A. E., & Jensen, J. P. (1990). The meaning of eclecticism: New survey and analysis of components. *Professional Psychology, 21*, 124–130.

Berman, E. B., Lief, H., & Williams, A. M. (1981). A model of marital integration. In G. P. Sholevar (Ed.), *The handbook of marriage and marital therapy* (pp. 3–34). New York: Spectrum.

Berns, S., & Jacobson, N. S. (2000). Marital problems. In M. J. Dougher (Ed.), *Clinical behavior analysis* (pp. 181–206). Reno, NV: Context Press.

Birchler, G., Doumas, D., & Fals-Stewart, W. (1999). The seven C's: A behavioral–systems framework for evaluating marital distress. *The Family Journal, 7*, 253–264.

Birchler, G., & Spinks, S. (1980). A behavioral–systems marital and family therapy: Intervention and clinical application. *American Journal of Family Therapy, 8*, 6–28.

Birchler, G., & Webb, L. (1975, April). *A social learning formulation of discriminating interaction behaviors in happy and unhappy marriages.* Paper presented at the annual meeting of the Southwestern Psychological Association, Houston, TX.

Birchler, G., Weiss, R. L., & Vincent, J. P. (1975). A multidimensional analysis of social reinforcement exchange between maritally distressed and nondistressed spouse and stranger dyads. *Journal of Personality and Social Psychology, 31*, 349–360.

Birchler, G., Weiss, R. L., & Wampler, L. D. (1972, April). *Differential patterns of social distress and level of intimacy.* Paper presented at the annual meeting of the Western Psychological Association, Portland, OR.

Bowlby, J. (1988). *A secure base: Parent–child attachment and healthy human development.* New York: Basic Books.

Bray, J. H., & Jouriles, E. N. (1995). Treatment of marital conflict and prevention of divorce. *Journal of Marital and Family Therapy, 21*, 461–473.

Brewster, F., & Montie, K. A. (1987, January–February). Double life: What do family therapists really do in private practice? *Family Therapy Networker*, 33–35.

Budman, S. H. (1999). Time-effective couple therapy. In J. Donovan (Ed.), *Short-term couple therapy* (pp. 173–197). New York: Guilford Press.

Budman, S. H., & Gurman, A. S. (1988). *Theory and practice of brief therapy.* New York: Guilford Press.

Catherall, D. R. (1992). Working with projective identification in couples. *Family Process, 31*, 355–367.

Christensen, A., & Jacobson, N. S. (2000). *Reconcilable differences.* New York: Guilford Press.

Christensen, A., Jacobson, N. S., & Babcock, J. C. (1995). Integrative behavioral couple therapy. In N. S. Jacobson & A. S. Gurman (Eds.), *Clinical handbook of couple therapy* (pp. 31–64). New York: Guilford Press.

Dicks, H. V. (1967). *Marital tensions.* New York: Basic Books.

Dollard, J., & Miller, N. E. (1950). *Personality and psychotherapy.* New York: McGraw-Hill.

Donovan, J. (2003). *Short-term object relations couple therapy.* New York: Brunner-Routledge.

Duncan, B. L., & Miller, S. D. (2000). The client's theory of change: Consulting the client in the integrative process. *Journal of Psychotherapy Integration, 10*, 169–187.

Feldman, L. B. (1979). Marital conflict and marital intimacy: An integrative psychodynamic–behavioral–systemic model. *Family Process, 18*, 69–78.

Fisch, R., Weakland, J., & Segal, L. (1982). *The tactics of change: Doing therapy briefly.* San Francisco: Jossey-Bass.

Floyd, F. J., Haynes, S. N., & Kelly, S. (1997). Marital assessment: A dynamic functional-analytic approach. In W. K. Halford & H. J. Markman (Eds.), *Clinical handbook of marriage and couples intervention* (pp. 367–377). New York: Wiley.

Follette, W. C., Naugle, A. E., & Linnerooth, P. J. N. (2000). Functional alternatives to traditional assessment and diagnosis. In M. J. Dougher (Ed.), *Clinical behavior analysis* (pp. 99–125). Reno, NV: Context Press.

Freud, S. (1909). A phobia in a 5-year-old boy. *Collected Works, 3*, 149–289.

Fruzzetti, A. E., & Iverson, K. M. (2004). Couples dialectical behavior therapy: An approach to both individual and relational distress. *Couples Research and Therapy, 10*(1), 8–13.

Gilbert, M., & Shmukler, D. (1996). *Brief therapy with couples.* Chichester, UK: Wiley.

Goldfried, M. (1995). Towards a common language for case formulation. *Journal of Psychotherapy Integration, 5,* 221–244.

Gottman, J. M. (1994a). *What predicts divorce?* Hillsdale, NJ: Erlbaum.

Gottman, J. M. (1994b). *Why marriages succeed or fail.* New York: Simon & Schuster.

Gottman, J. M. (1998). Psychology and the study of marital processes. *Annual Review of Psychology, 49,* 169–197.

Gottman, J. M. (1999). *The marriage clinic: A scientifically based marital therapy.* New York: Norton.

Gurman, A. S. (1973). The effects and effectiveness of marital therapy: A review of outcome research. *Family Process, 12,* 145–170.

Gurman, A. S. (1978). Contemporary marital therapies: A critique and comparative analysis of psychoanalytic, behavioral and systems theory approaches. In T. Paolino & B. McCrady (Eds.), *Marriage and marital therapy* (pp. 445–566). New York: Brunner/Mazel.

Gurman, A. S. (1980). Behavioral marriage therapy in the 1980's: The challenge of integration. *American Journal of Family Therapy, 8,* 86–96.

Gurman, A. S. (1981). Integrative couple therapy: Toward the development of an interpersonal approach. In S. H. Budman (Ed.), *Forms of brief therapy* (pp. 415–462). New York: Guilford Press.

Gurman, A. S. (1982a). Changing collusive patterns in marital therapy. *American Journal of Family Therapy, 10,* 71–73.

Gurman, A. S. (1982b). Creating a therapeutic alliance in marital therapy. *American Journal of Family Therapy, 9,* 84–87.

Gurman, A. S. (1983). Family therapy research and the "new epistemology." *Journal of Marital and Family Therapy, 9,* 227–234.

Gurman, A. S. (1985). Tradition and transition: A rural marriage in crisis. In A. S. Gurman (Ed.), *Casebook of marital therapy* (pp. 303–336). New York: Guilford Press.

Gurman, A. S. (1992). Integrative couple therapy: A time-sensitive model for working with couples. In S. Budman, M. Hoyt, & S. Friedman (Eds.), *The first session in brief therapy* (pp. 186–203). New York: Guilford Press.

Gurman, A. S. (2001). Brief therapy and family/couple therapy: An essential redundancy. *Clinical Psychology: Science and Practice, 8,* 51–65.

Gurman, A. S., & Fraenkel, P. (2002). The history of couple therapy: A millennial review. *Family Process, 41,* 199–260.

Gurman, A. S., & Kniskern, D. P. (1978a). Deterioration in marital and family therapy: Empirical, clinical and conceptual issues. *Family Process, 17,* 3–20.

Gurman, A. S., & Kniskern, D. P. (1978b). Research on marital and family therapy: Progress, perspective, and prospect. In S. L. Garfield & A. E. Bergin (Eds.), *Handbook of psychotherapy and behavior change* (2nd ed., pp. 817–901). New York: Wiley.

Gurman, A. S., & Kniskern, D. P. (1978c). Behavioral marriage therapy: II. Empirical perspective. *Family Process, 17,* 139–148.

Gurman, A. S., & Kniskern, D. P. (1981). Family therapy outcome research: Knowns and unknowns. In A. S. Gurman & D. P. Kniskern (Eds.), *Handbook of family therapy* (pp. 742–775). New York: Brunner/Mazel.

Gurman, A. S., Kniskern, D. P., & Pinsof, W. M. (1986). Process and outcome research in family and marital therapy. In A. E. Bergin & S. L. Garfield (Eds.), *Handbook of psychotherapy and behavioral change* (3rd ed., pp. 565–624). New York: Wiley.

Gurman, A. S., & Knudson, R. M. (1978). Behavioral marriage therapy: I. A psychodynamic systems analysis and critique. *Family Process, 17,* 121–138.

Gurman, A. S., Knudson, R. M., & Kniskern, D. P. (1978). Behavioral marriage therapy: IV. Take two aspirin and call us in the morning. *Family Process, 17,* 165–180.

Haley, J. (1963). Marriage therapy. *Archives of General Psychiatry, 8,* 213–224.

Halford, W. K. (2001). *Brief therapy for couples.* New York: Guilford Press.

Hamburg, S. R. (2000). *Will our love last?: A couple's road map.* New York: Scribner.

Hayes, S. C., Follette, W. C., & Follette, V. M. (1995). Behavior therapy: A contextual approach. In A. S. Gurman & S. B. Messer (Eds.), *Essential psychotherapies* (pp. 182–225). New York: Guilford Press.

Hayes, S. C., & Toarmino, D. (1995, February). If behavioral principles are generally applicable, why is it necessary to understand cultural diversity? *Behavior Therapist,* pp. 21–23.

Haynes, S. N., & O'Brien, W. H. (1990). Functional analysis in behavior therapy. *Clinical Psychology Review, 10,* 649–668.

Holtzworth-Munroe, A., & Jacobson, N. S. (1991). Behavioral marital therapy. In A. S. Gurman & D. P. Kniskern (Eds.), *Handbook of family therapy* (2nd ed., pp. 96–133). New York: Brunner/Mazel.

Jackson, D. D. (1965a). Family rules: The marital quid pro quo. *Archives of General Psychiatry, 12,* 589–594.

Jackson, D. D. (1965b). The study of the family. *Family Process, 4,* 1–20.

Jacobson, N. S. (1991). To be or not to be behavioral. *Journal of Family Psychology, 4,* 436–445.

Jacobson, N. S., & Addis, M. E. (1993). Research on couples and couples therapy: What do we know? Where are we going? *Journal of Consulting and Clinical Psychology, 61,* 85–93.

Jacobson, N. S., & Holtzworth-Munroe, A. (1986). Marital therapy: A social-learning cognitive perspective. In N. S. Jacobson & A. S. Gurman (Eds.), *Clinical handbook of marital therapy* (pp. 29–70). New York: Guilford Press.

Kanfer, F. H., & Phillips, J. S. (1970). *Learning foundations of behavior therapy.* New York: Wiley.

Kanfer, F. H., & Saslow, G. (1969). Behavioral diagnosis. In C. M. Franks (Ed.), *Behavior therapy: Appraisal and status* (pp. 417–444). New York: McGraw-Hill.

Karpel, M. A. (1994). *Evaluating couples: A handbook for practitioners.* New York: Norton.

Lawrence, E., Eldridge, K., Christensen, A., & Jacobson, N. S. (1999). Integrative couple therapy: The dyadic relationship of acceptance and change. In J. Donovan (Ed.), *Short-term couple therapy* (pp. 226–261). New York: Guilford Press.

Lebow, J. L. (1997). The integrative revolution in couple and family therapy. *Family Process, 36,* 1–17.

Lebow, J. L. (1999). Building a science of couple relationships: Comments on two articles by Gottman and Levenson. *Family Process, 38,* 167–173.

Lebow, J. L., & Gurman, A. S. (1995). Research assessing couple and family therapy. *Annual Review of Psychology, 46,* 27–57.

Lederer, W., & Jackson, D. (1968). *The mirages of marriage.* New York: Norton.

Linehan, M. (1993). *Cognitive-behavioral treatment of borderline personality disorder.* New York: Guilford Press.

Mahoney, M. J., & Thoresen, C. E. (1974). *Self-control: Power to the person.* Monterey, CA: Brooks/Cole.

Martin, P. A. (1976). *A marital therapy manual.* New York: Brunner/Mazel.

Meissner, W. W. (1978). The conceptualization of marriage and family dynamics from a psychoanalytic perspective. In T. Paolino & B. McCrady (Eds.), *Marriage and marital therapy* (pp. 25–88). New York: Brunner/Mazel.

Messer, S. B. (Ed.). (2001). Assimilative integration [Special issue]. *Journal of Psychotherapy Integration, 11,* 1–154.

Miles, J. E. (1980). Motivation in conjoint therapy. *Journal of Sex and Marital Therapy, 6,* 205–213.

Minuchin, S., & Fishman, H. C. (1981). *Family therapy techniques.* Cambridge, MA: Harvard University Press.

Nichols, M. P., & Schwartz, R. (2001). *Family therapy: Concepts and methods* (5th ed.). Boston: Allyn & Bacon.

Nichols, W. C. (1988). *Marital therapy: An integrated approach.* New York: Guilford Press.

Papp, P. (1980). The Greek chorus and other techniques of family therapy. *Family Process, 19,* 45–57.

Prochaska, J. O. (1995). An eclectic and integrative approach: Transtheoretical therapy. In A. S. Gurman & S. B. Messer (Eds.), *Essential psychotherapies* (pp. 403–440). New York: Guilford Press.

Prochaska, J. O., Norcross, J. C., & DiClemente, C. C. (1994). *Changing for good.* New York: Morrow.

Rait, D. (1988, January–February). Survey results. *Family Therapy Networker,* pp. 52–56.

Raush, H. L., Barry, W. A., Hertel, R. K., & Swain, M. A. (1974). *Communication conflict in marriage: Explorations in the theory and study of intimate relationships.* San Francisco: Jossey-Bass.

Sager, C. J. (1976). *Marriage contracts and couple therapy.* New York: Brunner/Mazel.

Sager, C. J. (1981). Couples therapy and marriage contracts. In A. S. Gurman & D. P. Kniskern (Eds.), *Handbook of family therapy* (pp. 85–130). New York: Brunner/Mazel.

Sanders, M. R., Markie-Dadda, C., & Nicholson, J. M. (1997). Concurrent interventions for marital and children's problems. In W. K. Halford & H. J. Markman (Eds.), *Clinical handbook of marriage and couples intervention* (pp. 509–535). New York: Wiley.

Scarf, M. (1986, November). Intimate partners: Patterns in love and marriage. *The Atlantic Monthly,* pp. 45–54, 91–93.

Scharff, J. S. (1995). Psychoanalytic marital therapy. In N. S. Jacobson & A. S. Gurman (Eds.), *Clinical handbook of couple therapy* (2nd, ed., pp. 164–193). New York: Guilford Press.

Scharff, J. S. & Bagnini, C. (2002). Object relations couple therapy. In A. S. Gurman & N. S. Jacobson (Eds.), *Clinical handbook of couple therapy* (3rd ed., pp. 59–85). New York: Guilford Press.

Scheinkman, M., & Fishbane, M. D. (2004). The vulnerability cycle: Working with impasses in couple therapy. *Family Process, 43*(3), 279–299.

Schore, A. (2002). *Affect dysregulation and disorders of the self.* New York: Norton.

Schwartz, R. C., & Johnson, S. M. (2000). Does couple and family therapy have emotional intelligence? *Family Process, 39,* 29–33.

Segraves, R. T. (1982). *Marital therapy: A combined psychodynamic behavioral approach.* New York: Plenum Press.

Skynner, A. C. R. (1980). Recent developments in marital therapy. *Journal of Family Therapy, 2,* 271–296.

Skynner, A. C. R. (1981). An open-systems, group analytic approach to family therapy. In A. S. Gurman & D. P. Kniskern (Eds.), *Handbook of family therapy* (pp. 39–84). New York: Brunner/Mazel.

Smith, J. W., & Grunebaum, H. (1976). The therapeutic alliance in marital therapy. In H. Grunebaum & J. Christ (Eds.), *Contemporary marriage: Structure, dynamics and therapy* (pp. 353–370). Boston: Little, Brown.

Snyder, D. K. (1999). Affective reconstruction in the context of a pluralistic approach to couple therapy. *Clinical Psychology: Science and Practice, 6,* 348–365.

Snyder, D. K., & Wills, R. M. (1989). Behavioral versus insight-oriented marital therapy: Effects on individual and interspousal functioning. *Journal of Consulting and Clinical Psychology, 57,* 39–46.

Stanton, M. D. (1980). Marital therapy from a structural/strategic viewpoint. In G. Sholevar (Ed.), *The handbook of marriage and marital therapy* (pp. 303–334). New York: Spectrum.

Stanton, M. D. (1981). Strategic approaches to family therapy. In A. S. Gurman & D. P. Kniskern (Eds.), *Handbook of family therapy* (pp. 361–402). New York: Brunner/Mazel.

Steinglass, P. (1978). The conceptualization of marriage from a systems theory perspective. In T. Paolino & B. S. McCrady (Eds.), *Marriage and marital therapy* (pp. 298–365). New York: Brunner/Mazel.

Stewart, R. H., Peters, T. C., Marsh, S., & Peters, M. J. (1975). An object-relations approach to psychotherapy with marital couples, families and children. *Family Process, 14,* 161–178.

Sunbury, J. F. (1980). Working with defensive projections in conjoint marriage counseling. *Family Relations, 29,* 107–110.

Tatkin, S. (2005). Psychobiological conflict management of marital couples. *Psychologist–Psychoanalyst: Division 39 of the American Psychological Association, 35*(1), 20–22.

Todd, T. C. (1986). Structural–strategic marital therapy. In N. S. Jacobson & A. S. Gurman (Eds.), *Clinical handbook of marital therapy* (pp. 71–105). New York: Guilford Press.

Vincent, J. P., Friedman, L., Nugent, J., & Messerly, L. (1979). Demand characteristics in observations of marital interaction. *Journal of Consulting and Clinical Psychology, 47,* 557–566.

Vincent, J. P., Weiss, R. L., & Birchler, G. (1975). A behavioral analysis of problem-solving in distressed and nondistressed married and stranger dyads. *Behavior Therapy, 6,* 475–487.

Wachtel, P. L. (1997). *Psychoanalysis, behavior therapy, and the relational world.* Washington, DC: American Psychological Association.

Wachtel, P. L., & McKinney, M. (1992). Cyclical psychodynamics and integrative psychodynamic therapy. In J. C. Norcross & M. R. Goldfried (Eds.), *Handbook of psychotherapy integration* (pp. 335–370). New York: Basic Books.

Weiss, R. L. (1980). Strategic behavioral marital therapy: Toward a model for assessment and intervention. In J. P. Vincent (Ed.), *Advances in family intervention, assessment and theory* (Vol. 1, pp. 229–271). Greenwich, CT: JAI Press.

Winnicott, D. W. (1960). The theory of the parent–infant relationship. *International Journal of Psycho-Analysis, 41,* 585–595.

Yalom, I. D. (1975). *The theory and practice of group therapy* (2nd ed.). New York: Basic Books.

PART II

APPLICATIONS OF COUPLE THERAPY

Special Populations, Problems, and Issues

Rupture and Repair of Relational Bonds

Affairs, Divorce, Violence, and Remarriage

CHAPTER 14

Couple Therapy and the Treatment of Affairs

Kristina Coop Gordon
Donald H. Baucom
Douglas K. Snyder
Lee J. Dixon

Couples who have experienced an extramarital affair in their lifetime are not a rarity; recent studies with large, representative U.S. samples across all age cohorts have found that approximately 25% of men and 15% of women have participated in sex outside of their marriage (Lauman, Gagnon, Michael, & Michaels, 1994). Furthermore, when asked about infidelity in the past year alone, 4.7% of men and 2.3% of women report engaging in extramarital affairs (Davis, Smith, & Marsden, 2005). Infidelity also is the most frequently cited reason for why marriages end, and those couples who experience an affair are twice as likely to divorce (Amato & Rogers, 1997; Atkins, Baucom, & Jacobson, 2001). Given the prevalence of extramarital involvement and its great potential for damage to a marital relationship, it is not surprising that approximately 30% of couples begin marital therapy because of the effects of an affair (Glass & Wright, 1988; Greene, Lee, & Lustig, 1974; Whisman, Dixon, & Johnson, 1997). Given these findings, Reibstein and Richards's (1993) statement that most people fall into one of five categories is no surprise: persons who know someone close who has had an affair; those who have experienced a spouse having an affair; those who have participated in an affair themselves; those who, before being married, were a third party in an affair; and those who either have considered or have come close to having an affair.

Despite a wealth of literature on this topic in the self-help area (e.g., Abrahm Spring, 1996; Glass, 2003; Lusterman, 1998; Snyder, Baucom, & Gordon, 2007), clinicians still report that the aftermath of an affair is notoriously difficult to handle in couple therapy; for example, in a survey, practicing couple therapists ranked extramarital affairs as the third most difficult problem to treat, following lack of loving feelings and alcoholism in the marriage (Whisman et al., 1997). The treatment we outline in this chapter was developed to address the characteristic difficulties that couples affected by an affair experience, by integrating literature from both the fields of interpersonal forgiveness and the response to traumatic events (Gordon & Baucom, 1998).

It is our belief, along with others in the field, that conceptualizing affairs as a form of interpersonal trauma helps therapists to understand the cognitive, behavioral, and emotional disequilibrium that often follows an affair and to better formulate these difficult therapy cases (e.g., Abrahm Spring, 1996; Glass & Wright, 1997; Gordon & Baucom, 1999; Lusterman, 1998). The traumatic response literature suggests that people are most likely to become emotionally traumatized following an event that violates their assumptions regarding how the world and others operate (Janoff-Bulman, 1989; McCann, Sakheim, & Abrahamson, 1988); that is, individuals often hold cherished assumptions about their partners and their relationships, such as "We've promised each other that we would always be faithful" or "I can depend on my partner to be honest with me and look out for my well-being." Similarly, we have found that participating partners also can be traumatized, both by their own actions, which often violate their own values of fidelity and trustworthiness, and by their partners' actions following the affair, which can be uncharacteristically vengeful and sometimes violent. When cherished assumptions are violated by the revelation of an affair, both the injured partner and the partner who participated in the affairs may feel that they cannot predict the future; thus, both partners may experience a loss of control and safety regarding themselves, their relationship partners, and their relationships. Feelings of anxiety, depression, and shame often accompany this loss of control and safety. Therapies based on trauma theory attempt to restructure clients' schemas about how the world operates and to help them regain a sense of control over their lives (e.g., Calhoun & Resick, 1993; Foa & Kozak, 1986).

Forgiveness-based interventions are similar to trauma-based therapies in their approaches to helping people get past the hurt of interpersonal betrayals. These interventions that focus on helping individuals explore the factors surrounding the affair so that they develop a greater understanding about why the betrayal took place, studies evaluating these treatments demonstrate increased levels of empathy and positive feelings, and decreased anger and feelings of hostility (e.g., Freedman & Enright, 1996; Worthington, 2005). Although different theories of forgiveness have unique facets, most are similar with regard to how they define the end result of forgiveness of an interpersonal betrayal. Definitions of forgiveness usually contain three common components: (1) gaining a more balanced view of the offender and the event; (2) decreasing negative affect toward the offender, potentially along with increased compassion; and (3) giving up the right to punish the offender further or to demand restitution.

Both types of treatments mentioned earlier have demonstrated efficacy in guiding individuals through the process of recovering from traumatic experiences; however, neither treatment has focused specifically on how to deal with the intricacies of treating couples in committed relationship who have experienced an affair. To meet couples' specific needs in the treatment of interpersonal trauma from a dyadic perspective, our treatment also is drawn from two empirically supported couple therapy approaches: cognitive-behavioral couple therapy and insight-oriented couple therapy. Cognitive-behavioral couple therapy (CBCT; see Baucom, Epstein, LaTaillade, & Kirby, Chapter 2, this volume) builds on skills-based interventions of behavioral couple therapy by targeting couple communication and behavior exchange, and directing both partners' attention to the explanations they construct for each other's behavior, and to expectations and standards they hold relative to their own relationship and relationships in general (Epstein & Baucom, 2002). Because recent discovery of an affair typically leads to emotional turmoil and destructive exchanges between partners, the structured, directive strategies offered within cognitive-behavioral interventions provide focus and direction to couples at a time when they are needed most. Moreover, in exploring factors that placed their relationship at risk for an affair, couples frequently need to improve their ability to negotiate changes in how they interact and manage daily challenges of their relationship. CBCT is particularly well suited to these therapeutic objectives; however, CBCT's general focus on the present and the future also leaves important gaps in dealing with couples experiencing an affair. Many couples report that they cannot move forward and put the affair behind them; they need some way to process the trauma that has occurred, along with some way to make sense of the past.

It also is useful to draw from insight-oriented couple therapy (IOCT; see Snyder & Mitchell, Chapter 12, this volume), an approach that is designed specifically to help partners have a greater understanding of how the past affects current relationship struggles (Snyder, 1999). This improved understanding of both one's own and one's partner's developmental history and the role that developmental experiences have played in current and past relationships can aid in transforming an injured partner's understanding of how the participating (or betraying) partner could make the decision to engage in an extramarital affair. Furthermore, these revelations of vulnerability may have the added benefit of allowing partners to develop more mutual empathy and compassion. Increased insight and empathy also help partners develop a more coherent narrative regarding the affair, as well as a better perspective on future changes that need to take place to make the relationship more secure. Thus, the couple intervention for addressing infidelity outlined in this chapter draws upon cognitive-behavioral interventions integrated with insight-oriented approaches to provide a treatment strategy that balances the past, present, and future.

FACTORS PREDICTIVE OF RECOVERY FROM AFFAIRS

There are multiple ways that individuals and couples can respond to either the disclosure or the discovery of an affair. With regard to couple functioning, researchers have demonstrated that extramarital affairs often lead to negative marital results, such as marital distress, lowered commitment levels, conflict, violence, and divorce (e.g., Amato & Rogers, 1997; Beach, Jouriles, & O'Leary, 1985; Daly & Wilson, 1988; Janus & Janus, 1993; Lawson & Samson, 1988). However, not all such couples divorce, nor are the long-term effects of affairs on marital relationships always negative. Some research has indicated that, for a few couples, the event can serve as an impetus for tackling issues that have caused difficulties throughout the relationship (e.g., Charny & Parnass, 1995). However, according to a survey of clinicians who conduct couple therapy, whereas an affair might lead some couples to address longstanding relationship difficulties, very few took the view that infidelity is relationship enhancing (Glass, 2002). Furthermore, extramarital affairs have been shown not only to cause difficulties within the dyad but also to be detrimental to individual functioning. Injured partners often experience similar symptoms to those seen in posttraumatic stress disorder (PTSD), and also are likely to experience increased rage, shame, anxiety, and depression, as well as a sense of having been victimized (Beach et al., 1985; Cano & O'Leary, 2000; Charny & Parnass, 1995; Glass & Wright, 1997; Gordon & Baucom, 1999; Gordon, Baucom, & Snyder, 2004).

Although infidelity is often extremely damaging to individuals and their relationships, some people are better able to weather this particular emotional storm than others. We have found in our clinical experiences and our review of the literature on infidelity (Allen, Atkins, Baucom, Snyder, Gordon, & Glass, 2005) that a number of factors regarding the couple's relationship—the injured partner, the participating partner, and other

contextual factors, such as the nature of the affair itself—can affect the couple's ability to recover from the affair. Familiarity with these factors can help the therapist to develop more accurate and effective treatment expectations. Here we review some of the more important factors that we have found to play a role in a couple's recovery.

First, not all committed relationships are the same, and some distinguishing characteristics of committed relationships (most research involves legal marriages) are predictive of how individuals might respond to an affair. For example, unsurprisingly, affairs appear to be most emotionally devastating when they are coupled with the initiation of a divorce or breakup of the relationship (Sweeney & Howitz, 2001). Additionally, individuals who are more satisfied with their marriages are more likely to feel remorseful following an affair (Allen & Baucom, 2005), and greater remorse generally improves the effectiveness of couple therapy. Furthermore, shorter length of marriage, lower commitment to working on the marriage, and lower marital satisfaction all increase the odds of a couple divorcing after an affair (e.g., Blumstein & Schwartz, 1983; Buunk, 1987; Glass, 2003). Thus, the more committed the couple is to the relationship when partners enter treatment, and the more satisfied they are with the relationship, the more likely they are to negotiate successfully the tasks posed during the course of therapy.

Furthermore, many in our field seem to agree that a couple's ability to discuss the affair and its antecedents together openly is a good prognostic indicator for recovery (e.g., Glass, 2002; Gordon, Baucom, & Snyder, 2000, 2004; Vaughn, 2002). Along these lines, one study found that couples who experienced an affair also experienced less intimacy than couples who had not experienced an affair, but only if they did not reveal the affair until after entering couple therapy, as opposed to revealing the affair prior to entering therapy (Atkins, Yi, Baucom, & Christensen, 2005). Although little empirical evidence clarifies what type of disclosure regarding the affair is beneficial, some research suggests that once the affair is disclosed, answering the injured partner's questions about the affair helps the participating partner to bolster the injured partner's sense of predictability and control regarding the relationship (Allen et al., 2005). Thus, partners who can talk openly and freely about the affair in a voluntary, nondefensive, remorseful manner are more likely to recover from the affair than partners who resist discussing the affair or cannot find a way to do so in a constructive manner. Consequently, it is important to assess how well and how openly the couple is able to talk about the affair in the beginning of treatment. If partners are not able to do so, then the therapist will likely need to address this issue relatively quickly in the therapy.

Next, some characteristics of the participating partner have been shown to predict whether a couple will ultimately survive the occurrence of an affair. In particular, the gender of the participating partner seems to play an important role in how an affair affects both partners, as well as the outcome of the relationship. A woman who participates in an affair is more likely than a man to have feelings of guilt regarding the affair (Spanier & Margolis, 1983). Furthermore, depression is more likely to occur in either partner if the wife participated in an affair (Beach et al., 1985). Some researchers and clinicians have suggested that feelings of guilt and depression are more prevalent when the wife has an affair, because most societies are more accepting of men who engage in an affair than of women (Atwood & Seifer, 1997; Lusterman, 1997; Mackey & Immerman, 2001). These societal norms might contribute to the finding that cross-culturally, a wife's affair is more likely to lead both to thoughts of divorce and actual divorce than a husband's affair (e.g., Betzig, 1989; Glass, 2003; Lawson, 1988). However, the higher divorce rates following a wife's affair may be due not only to men's affairs being more socially accepted but may also be affected by the characteristics of the affairs in which women participate (Allen et al., 2005). Indeed, women are more likely than men to characterize their affairs as emotional in nature, and they seem to find it more difficult to separate sexual involvement from emotional attachment (Banfield & McCabe, 2002; Glass & Wright, 1985). Thus, women are more likely to be attached to their affair partners, to experience greater ambivalence and dissatisfaction with their current committed relationship, and to feel more depression, grief, and remorse upon entering therapy. The therapist should be alert to these possibilities and explore them early in the therapy, possibly in individual sessions, as described below.

Certain characteristics of the injured partner also have an effect on a couple's response to the affair. For example, Glass and Wright's clinical experiences (1997) led them to assert that the injured partner's reactions to an affair are more severe if he or she had difficulties with self-esteem and trust prior to the affair. Furthermore, they suggested that the severity of the reaction is exacerbated when the injured partner has strong assumptions regarding the commitment of the other partner to the monogamous aspect of the marriage contract. Thus, the relative strength of the injured partner's assumptions regarding the fidelity of the participating partner might influence the degree of his or her traumatization upon discovery of an affair.

Furthermore, marital assumptions and beliefs are not always limited to the couple's commitment to being sexually monogamous; they can be much broader in scope. For example, many people assume that they will be the only person to whom their spouses are attracted, and that their spouses will refrain from emotional and romantic commitments to anyone else. The disruption of any of these assumptions can lead an individual to feel emotionally devastated. Thus, the injured partner might enter therapy with a strong sense of betrayal, even if the participating partner has engaged in behaviors that the majority of the population would not consider to be infidelity or extramarital sexual behavior. For this reason, many clinicians and researchers have begun to see the utility of expanding how they conceptualize extramarital affairs. Many have adopted something akin to Glass's (2002) definition of infidelity: "a secret sexual, romantic, or emotional involvement that violates the commitment to an exclusive relationship" (p. 489). The notion that *extramarital sexual contact is not necessary for one to feel betrayed* is supported by a study of individuals who had experienced cybersex in their marriages (Schneider, 2002). When asked how the online infidelity had affected their marriages and families, nearly one-fourth of the injured partners in these cases had divorced, and roughly two-thirds had lost interest in sex with their partner as a result of the online behavior. These results help to illustrate the devastation that even nonphysical extramarital involvement can have on a marriage. Understanding the effect of disrupted assumptions can help the clinician to conceptualize these ambiguous situations better and consequently give the partners greater insight into their experiences as well.

The infidelity literature also suggests that not all individuals and couples who have experienced an affair suffer from the "trauma of betrayal" (see Scheinkman, 2005). Scheinkman asserts that affairs are multidimensional, and that *marital therapists risk causing further trauma if they impose their own assumptions and beliefs regarding extramarital affairs onto the couples they see.* For example, a couple recovering from a partner's one-night stand may not experience the same type of disruption as a couple recovering from a recently discovered long-term emotional and sexual affair. This example highlights how important it is that therapists properly assess a couple's specific situation and whether each individual's assumptions regarding his or her partner and relationship have been violated.

Finally, more general contextual factors, such as the nature of the affair and the behavior of the affair partner, also are likely to influence individual and relationship outcomes following an affair. For example, when the threat of the affair continues because the participating partner remains in contact with the former extramarital partner, the injured spouse may experience a more severe and long-lasting traumatic reaction, because it impedes the possibility of regaining a sense of safety (Glass & Wright, 1997). Glass (2003) discovered that there is a higher chance for divorce or separation when the participating partner continues the affair during marital therapy. Similarly, we have found that even if the participating partner ends the affair and stops contact, if the affair partner continues to initiate contact with either partner, then the injured partner can be continually retraumatized. Thus, the therapist should intervene quickly in these cases and help the couple find a way to end this contact if it is traumatizing. Furthermore, the nature of the affair also can influence individual responses; a participating partner who felt close to the extramarital partner and satisfied with that relationship is less likely to feel remorse or guilt for having engaged in the affair (Allen & Baucom, 2005; Spanier & Margolis, 1983). Finally, the type of affair also can determine the course the relationship takes following the event; an affair that involves both sexual and emotional infidelity seems to be the most relationally disruptive. Indeed, a study revealed that husbands rarely left their marriages if they had participated in affairs that were more sexually focused (Glass, 2003).

AN INTEGRATIVE TREATMENT FOR COUPLES RECOVERING FROM THE DISCOVERY OF AN AFFAIR

Given the complexity of affairs and their potentially devastating impact on couple relationships, it is essential that efficacious interventions be developed to assist couples experiencing infidelity. The following sections outline an integrative approach to help couples recover from the discovery of an affair. As previously described, this treatment strategically draws from cognitive-behavioral interventions, insight-oriented approaches, and forgiveness and traumatic response literatures to provide a comprehensive yet flexible approach that allows both therapists and couples to understand their current experiences better, to work through their past hurts, and to make better decisions about the future of their relationship.

The Structure of the Therapy Process

Given that a careful exploration of both partners' contributions to the context of the affair is a central ingredient in this therapy process, this treatment is typically conducted with both partners present. However, obtaining both partners' commitment to treatment can be difficult. Often the participating partner is reluctant to discuss his or her affair and fearful that elaborating upon it in detail might lead to greater damage to the relationship and more unproductive and conflict-laden interactions. Likewise, he or she might be ambivalent about the marriage/committed relationship and reluctant to invest time in attempting to improve it. In these instances, it can be helpful for the therapist to encourage the reluctant partner to come for an initial exploratory visit, clarifying that by doing so, he or she is not committing to an ongoing therapy process. In that initial visit, the therapist can assess and then address the partner's concerns. Ideally, if the therapist is able to demonstrate a neutral, nonjudgmental, supportive, competent, and hopeful atmosphere, and to lay out a compelling rationale for the process of therapy, then the reluctant partner may become more willing to enter into treatment. However, when the participating partner either refuses to attend therapy or cannot participate due to logistical complications (e.g., the couple is now divorced and living in different cities), the principles outlined in this chapter can still be helpful in guiding the injured partner toward a healthy resolution of the betrayal. If one partner decides to drop out of therapy but continue in the marriage, and the other partner wishes to stay in therapy, then the therapist must use his or her clinical judgment as to whether continuing to see the remaining partner is therapeutically appropriate. However, if the therapist decides to continue treatment, then he or she should carefully describe the risks of conducting individual therapy with the remaining partner. For example, the therapist should elaborate on how this new therapeutic relationship might compromise or preclude the therapist's ability to continue the conjoint therapy should the partner that left decide to return to treatment.

Although this treatment is best conducted in a conjoint format, not all sessions are necessarily conjoint. We believe that individual sessions, if handled carefully, can be helpful for a variety of reasons. However, it is critical to clarify the principles regarding confidentiality for the individual sessions to both partners during the conjoint sessions. This requirement is necessary not only to create an atmosphere of safety that allows the partners to air their genuine feelings about the situation and their goals regarding the couple therapy in the individual sessions but also to protect the therapist against the uncomfortable experience of holding secrets. Therapists can handle confidentiality in individual sessions in a number of ways. We typically consider individual sessions to be confidential. However, we also explain that our primary client is the relationship. Therefore, if information arises during individual sessions that is inconsistent with what is discussed during conjoint sessions and has major implications for the progress of therapy (e.g., the affair is ongoing), then the therapist should discuss with the individual disclosing the information how best to address these issues with the other partner. In other words, we make it clear to clients before they disclose potentially explosive material that we will not hold a secret we consider to be detrimental to the couple therapy; thus, these individual sessions are not wholly confidential. However, we also emphasize that if the client needs to reveal information that might compromise his or her physical safety (e.g., reporting severe partner abuse), then we will not disclose information that might harm him or her. If the client chooses to disclose this kind of information but is not willing to discuss it in conjoint therapy, then she or he should be urged to reconsider whether engaging in couple therapy is appropriate at this time. The therapist also should carefully consider whether he or she feels comfortable continuing in therapy with the couple if the partner is unwilling to address this issue. In cases in which it appears best that conjoint therapy be discontinued, either from the client's or the therapist's point of view, the therapist discusses with the client the best way to address this issue. There are clearly many complex issues to address when including individual sessions in this treatment; however, we have found that the benefits of individual sessions overall outweigh the potential difficulties.

As described below, we believe individual sessions can be a critical part of the assessment process. Furthermore, we also schedule individual sessions early in the treatment, if necessary, to work with each partner on his or her individual functioning and emotion regulation strategies, so that both partners are better able to respond constructively in the conjoint sessions. In the context of these sessions, we assess whether the individual might benefit from adjunct individual treatment or a referral for pharmacological treatment. If we do make these referrals, we find it critical to be in touch with the individual therapists to coordinate treatment. It becomes awkward and potentially countertherapeutic if the couple therapist is working to repair the relationship, while the individual therapist is encouraging the person to seek a divorce. The extent to which both therapists can be open about their treatment goals and coordinate efforts can greatly affect the success of both treatments. Finally, occasionally we also schedule individual sessions to restore the therapeutic alliance and provide extra individual exploration and support when the conjoint therapy hits "stuck points" and it becomes clear that the presence of the partner is substantially impeding an individual's ability to process information and/or explore his or her own contributions to the relationship problems. This decision is typically made only when the therapy is clearly "stuck" and one partner becomes so focused upon and dysregulated by the other partner's presence that conjoint therapy is not likely to be effective.

Consistent with most couple therapists' experiences that extramarital affairs are particularly difficult to treat, our interventions for infidelity typically are longer than for many other types of presenting couple complaints. The length of treatment can vary from 6 months to several years, depending on the complexity of the case. However, these longer treatments usually are not solely focused on recovery from the affair. In such instances, couples that typically are able to recover from the affair early in treatment still might have a number of more general issues in their marriages and lives that require additional attention and work. Similar to most other treatments, the length of the therapy has much to do with the overall psychological health of the partners; in couples in which there is a significant degree of psychopathology, particularly Axis II disorders, therapy tends to take longer and be more complex. These couples also may require more balancing of conjoint and individual sessions. Treatment ends when both partners (1) feel that they have come to a thorough understanding of why the affair occurred; (2) are emotionally ready to put the event behind them and can commit to forgiving their partner and themselves; and (3) have a clear sense of what they need to do to make their relationships healthier and less vulnerable to another affair, feel capable of achieving these changes, or decide that the relationship is not likely to be a healthy one and are able to terminate the relationship in a constructive manner.

Furthermore, because addressing infidelity is often quite explosive and crises between the partners can arise on a regular basis, we believe that the therapist should initially meet with the couple at least once a week. If the couple is particularly volatile, and the risk of severe conflict escalation is particularly high, then it is advisable to consider meeting more frequently until the situation stabilizes. As the need for damage control decreases, the therapist and couple can decide together about whether and when to reduce session frequency. Additionally, if the couple comes in several years after the affair occurred, this initial frequency can be negotiable. Even if the partners are calm and crises are not occurring, we believe it is preferable in most cases to see them weekly to maintain treatment momentum and keep the partners engaged in the process. However, once the affair crisis is resolved and the couple is transitioning into more traditional couple therapy, biweekly sessions might also be appropriate, depending upon the therapist's clinical judgment.

Finally, given that these couples often enter into treatment in severe crisis, contacts between sessions also might be needed to minimize damage or destructive interactions at home. However, despite our model's openness to between-session contact for specific purposes, we ask couples to follow some guidelines, so that such contacts are handled appropriately. The purpose of between-session contact is considered to be primarily "coaching" (similar to Linehan's [1991] approach to between session contact in her treatment of borderline personality disorder; see Fruzzetti & Fantozzi, Chapter 20, this volume) to help couples use skills they are learning in sessions or to problem-solve on a specific crisis that has arisen and needs an immediate resolution. These contacts are not a time when one partner can complain, attack, or vent about the other partner or the therapy. We also ask that partners inform the other person if such a contact

has been made. In this way we attempt to avoid the perception of unintended alliances with one partner or to perpetuate secrets from one partner, a pattern that often was a very destructive part of the affair.

The Role of the Therapist

A strong alliance between the therapist and couple can be critical in treating infidelity successfully. We have found that there are several critical ingredients in creating the optimal therapeutic relationship with these couples. The first, most important, task for the alliance is establishing an atmosphere of safety and trust. Both partners need to know that their thoughts and feelings will be heard and respected, and that they will not be attacked or belittled. To achieve this safe atmosphere, the therapist must intervene quickly and directly in the couple's discussions to limit the amount and types of negativity that are expressed during the session. The therapist needs to help partners focus their discussion on productive topics that are most likely to facilitate their recovery. Offering a rationale for interrupting and redirecting partners' destructive exchanges helps to promote tolerance for such interventions. Additionally, both partners need to know that they will not be pushed to disclose or to do things that they are not ready to address, and that the therapist will respect the pace at which partners need to proceed.

The second major task in establishing a productive alliance is to promote the partners' belief and trust in the therapist's competence in helping couples recover from affairs. Couples struggling with the aftermath of infidelity need to feel confident that the therapist's expertise is specific to treating such kinds of relationship trauma. The first way we demonstrate our expertise in treating affairs is by providing a normative context for the couple's struggles. Partners dealing with the aftermath of an affair need a framework understand what is happening to them. Describing common responses to affairs for both injured and participating partners (1) allows them to make better sense of their own and their partner's current behaviors, (2) gives them hope for recovery, and (3) creates more realistic expectations for the course of treatment. Finally, trust in the therapist's expertise allows partners to participate more willingly when they confront difficult situations in the context of treatment.

The third task in developing a strong alliance is affirming fairness to both partners. Even when two partners present simultaneously for couple therapy and agree to identify their relationship as the "client," conflicts of interest may be unavoidable—for example, when partners differ in mental or physical health, or when caring for one partner requires decisions that have negative consequences for the other. For example, when one partner is suicidal, the therapist may have to proceed more slowly and cautiously than he or she normally would; this change in pace can present a challenge when the suicidal client is the participating partner and, consequently, the injured partner might feel that his or her needs are overlooked or not addressed quickly enough. Challenges in ensuring fairness to both partners can sometimes be addressed, at least in part, by clearly articulating the nature of this challenge to both partners.

Finally, a number of ethical issues are particular to the treatment of couples following affairs. For a more extensive treatment of these issues, we refer the reader to Snyder and Doss (2005). However, here we briefly outline a few of the most common issues clinicians face when dealing with this problem. First, the heightened level of negative affect following an affair often means that assessing for physical violence between the partners is of paramount importance. If aggression is present, then the therapist must quickly intervene to terminate aggressive behaviors, both within and between sessions. The therapist should know how to establish a safety plan with any partner who feels that he or she is in danger. If the level of physical force is minor and does not appear to present significant danger to either partner or risk escalation, then the therapist might address this issue through directed problem solving and careful use of time-out procedures (e.g., Epstein & Baucom, 2002). Regardless of the level of aggression, the therapist must set clear expectations that any physical force from the outset of therapy will not be tolerated.

In addition, unique risks posed by sexual exchanges with an outside person also present ethical challenges to the therapist and the couple. Consequently, it is important to evaluate (1) whether the affair involved sexual contact and, if so, whether there was intercourse in which a condom was not used; and (2) whether both partners have been tested for HIV or other sexually transmitted diseases since the affair.

Assessment and Treatment Planning

The first stage of the treatment encompasses assessment and management of the affair's impact.

An array of marital measures (e.g., as described in Epstein & Baucom, 2002) can be used to assess the basic aspects of couple functioning (e.g., satisfaction, communication skills, and commitment level). Typically, we give these measures to the couple at the first session and ask that partners complete them separately and return them at the next session. These measures can help guide the therapist in gathering information about the couple's relationship history. While gathering the history, specific attention should be focused on events and experiences leading up to the affair. In addition, the therapist should gather information about how the couple is currently dealing with the impact of the affair, looking at both partners' strengths and weaknesses. Furthermore, individual assessment sessions, one for each partner, also are beneficial. The focus of the individual session is to obtain an individual history for each partner, if one has not been obtained as part of the conjoint sessions, and to explore this history in more depth, paying particular attention to aspects of development that may have impacted his/her actions surrounding the affair. Examples of these issues may be patterns in past relationships, beliefs about marriage, and parental history and attitudes toward marriages. These elements are explored further in conjoint sessions in the second phase of treatment; however, the information gathered in this session affords the therapist the opportunity to gather initial data in a setting in which the partners might be more revealing and vulnerable.

Assessing the Couple's Relationship

It is important to ascertain what people are central in the partners' lives, as well as how the partners are currently interacting, and how they have interacted in the past. A brief history should include information about (1) the length of the couple's own relationship (if married, both before and since marrying); (2) previous marriages, how they ended, and ongoing contact with former spouse(s); (3) children by this or previous partners, and their current living arrangements; and (4) previous affairs, separations, or experiences in couple counseling—and the circumstances surrounding each of these.

Next, it is important to identify issues or crises requiring immediate attention, such as the extent of disruption in the partners' major patterns of interacting. For example, are the partners still sharing meals or sleeping together? Have their typical patterns of connecting either emotionally or physically been disrupted? If they have children, have both partners been able to maintain essential parenting roles—either separately or collaboratively? What assistance does the couple require immediately for containing the crisis, preventing further damage, and reaching decisions for managing the logistics of household operations? For example, the partners may need help in defining "rules of engagement" with each other to prevent the escalation of their negative interactions (e.g., Epstein & Baucom, 2002).

Additionally, it is important to assess the content and regulation of partners' emotions. To what extent does either partner struggle to manage overwhelming feelings of hurt, anger, fear, loss, guilt, or shame? Does either partner exhibit undercontrol of emotions in ways that contribute to spiraling negative exchanges? For example, the participating partner might be so sensitive to feelings of shame about his or her behavior that he or she stonewalls the injured partner's efforts to discuss the affair, which in turn leads the injured partner to escalate attempts to engage in discussions about the affair. On the other hand, not all couple relationships affected by an affair are emotionally chaotic or out of control. Often, one or both partners may be unable to access their feelings or may avoid uncomfortable interactions in ways that prevent discussion of what happened or how to begin recovery. If so, providing guidelines for expressing feelings and exchanging essential information to reach initial decisions may be warranted (e.g., Epstein & Baucom, 2002).

When inquiring about the couple's abilities to regulate strong feelings, it is critical to assess the level of the partners' verbal and physical aggression and the potential for violence. The clinical literature provides differing guidelines on how to elicit reliable information about physical violence and promoting partners' safety. For example, research indicates that some persons experiencing a partner's physical aggression do not disclose this behavior in early interviews due to embarrassment, minimization, or fear of retribution (Ehrensaft & Vivian, 1996). Conversely, arguments against individual interviews for assessing partner violence emphasize potential difficulties in conjoint therapy if one partner has disclosed information to the therapist about which the other partner remains uninformed. An alternative method is to include measures of conflict tactics in a standard assessment battery for all couples. Some research indicates that couples are most likely to indicate the occurrence of violence using this method (e.g.,

Straus, 1979). However, even if the therapist selects this method, he or she still needs to decide whether to follow-up in a conjoint interview or an individual interview. Whether assessing for partner violence in either individual or conjoint sessions, it is critical to gather information about both the frequency and severity of aggression, to inquire in a tone that conveys concern for both the partners and their relationship, and to be explicit about policies regarding containing physical aggression as a precondition for conjoint therapy. More extended discussions of the complex issues involved in assessing and treating partner violence are available elsewhere (e.g., Holtzworth-Munroe, Marshall, Meehan, & Rehman, 2003; O'Leary & Maiuro, 2001; Rathus & Feindler, 2004).

A major issue that many couples face upon the disclosure or discovery of an affair involves who else to inform regarding the affair. Do they tell their children, extended family, friends, or coworkers? If couples do not handle this issue well, it can cause significant future problems. For example, partners' relationships with their children or with their own or each other's extended family can be irrevocably damaged when family members learn that a partner has had an affair. If the affair happened in a work setting, then punitive actions by the injured partner, such as informing the participating partner's employer, can produce adverse impacts and enduring financial hardships. It is important to assess how the partners are addressing such decisions early in treatment and to provide explicit guidelines as needed to help them navigate these issues (Snyder et al., 2007).

Assessing the Outside-Affair Relationship

Evaluating both previous and current contact with the outside-affair person is critical to understanding factors that potentially influence the nature of the affair trauma, ongoing sources of continued turmoil, and the likelihood of restoring emotional security in the couple's relationship. Obtaining relevant information can be complicated, in some cases, because the participating partner has not yet disclosed the full degree of this contact to the injured partner. It is important to consider the possible impact of eliciting new disclosures in the initial session, because such information could exacerbate the partners' turmoil before they have decided whether to continue with couple therapy.

It is important during the initial assessment to address several questions regarding the outside relationship. The therapist should determine when the affair first began. What was the nature of the affair? Was it primarily emotional, primarily sexual, or both? When did it become sexual, if it was sexual? Next the therapist should explore the current status of the affair. If the affair has ended, is this just for now or permanently? What contact has either partner had with the outside person since the end of the affair? What steps, if any, have been taken to ensure that no further contact takes place, or are there agreements between the partners regarding what types of contact are acceptable at this point? It also is important to gain additional information about the person with whom the participating partner had the affair. What does the outside-affair person want? Is the other person married or in a committed relationship? Does that person's partner know? Finally, the therapist should assess with the couple the potential consequences of the affair. Who else knows about the affair? Are there any complications at work or other legal problems? Could the outside person and/or his or her partner, make the couple's lives more difficult if they decided to do so?

If the affair has not ended, yet its existence is known by the injured partner and both partners wish to continue in therapy, we believe that whether to continue with treatment is up to the therapist's clinical judgment. Our position is that to end therapy at that point might be premature. The partners are likely be in a better position to make decisions about how they want to proceed with their relationship after they complete this treatment. However, in this case, the first stage of therapy should address the kinds of boundaries the couple wishes to place on contact with the affair partner. See Snyder et al. (2007) for an extended discussion of this issue.

Assessing Individual Strengths and Vulnerabilities

Even among individuals with good premorbid individual functioning, emotional and behavioral well-being after the disclosure or discovery of an affair may be substantially disrupted. As described earlier, both research and clinical findings suggest that, following an affair, similar reactions of depression, guilt, and acute anxiety are common effects for both partners, and these reactions may be particularly strong in married couples when the disclosure or discovery of infidelity results in separation or threats of divorce. These intense feelings can lead to other problems, such as misuse of alcohol or other substances, suicidal thoughts or

behaviors, or physical aggression. It is important to assess for these issues in individual sessions and address them or refer the individual for adjunct treatment as necessary. Similarly, negative consequences also may be observed in the couple's children, even if they have not been informed explicitly about the affair. There is ample evidence linking severe or chronic marital conflict to a wide range of deleterious effects on children, including depression, withdrawal, disrupted social functioning, poor academic performance, and a variety of conduct-related difficulties (e.g., Buehler et al., 1998).

Partners' individual functioning, as well as the emotional and behavioral well-being of their children, can be evaluated by asking both partners a series of questions. First, the therapist might ask, "What are you (or your children) struggling with the most right now in terms of thoughts and feelings or just getting through the day?" Similarly, the therapist might ask the partners to explain how they and their children are continuing to manage despite the challenges. What has been the most helpful to them—in terms of their own resources, responses from their partners, or support from others?

Assessing Outside Stressors and Resources

The therapist should have some sense of the specific stressors that impinge on the couple and the partners' individual and joint resources that can be brought to bear on the situation. The primary goal when assessing outside stressors during this initial assessment is to identify immediate stressors that undermine the couple's ability to manage the initial turmoil accompanying disclosure or discovery of the affair. Common stressors that can interfere with initial efforts to contain the impact of the affair include continued contact with the outside person; excessive demands from work or family responsibilities that further drain one or both partners; or concerns related to finances, physical health, or children's well-being that can further add to the partners' difficulties and impinge on their ability to focus on and work through the affair. Common resources that can buffer the adverse impact of an affair on partners or render recovery more promising include a history of strong emotional connection and positive interactions prior to the affair, shared values or commitment to common goals (including caring for the children), support for the couple's relationship from family and friends, and healthy patterns of separate interests or pursuits that facilitate tolerance of current disruption in the couple relationship.

Knowledge of the existing stressors can help the therapist identify when and where to intervene immediately to relieve current stress, and free up resources and emotional energy to engage the difficult task of recovery. Similarly, knowledge of existing strengths gives the therapist and couple ideas about sources of renewal and support to draw upon during the times ahead.

Goal Setting

The first and often the most salient goal when a couple begins treatment is clarifying whether the partners plan to continue the relationship, terminate it, or are uncertain regarding its future. Some degree of ambivalence about the future of the relationship is common, and one or both of the partners may experience ambivalence about entering therapy. For example, the injured partner may fear getting close again to the person who hurt him or her, or may have doubts about continuing a relationship with someone capable of inflicting so much pain. Similarly, the participating partner in the affair may still be grieving the loss of the affair partner and focusing on positive qualities of the affair partner that are not currently present in the marital relationship. We typically address this issue by discussing the process of therapy. The partner should be reassured that the goal of therapy is not to maintain the relationship unless it is a healthy relationship for both of them. The suggestion to partners that it is extremely difficult and perhaps premature to make a decision about the future of their relationship at present can normalize their ambivalence about the marriage. However, we also assert that by going through the process of therapy, the information they gain about themselves and their relationship will allow them to make the best decision about whether to stay together. Essentially, it is important for partners to experience a thoughtful therapeutic process that leads to (1) an increased understanding of why the affair occurred, (2) better insight into themselves and their partners, and (3) we hope, better relationship skills and more positive interactions. After experiencing this process, they can use what they have learned to make good decisions about the future of their relationship.

In addition, each stage of treatment has its own particular set of goals. Table 14.1 gives an overview of each stage of treatment, its goals, and the treatment strategies relevant to these goals.

Given that dealing with an affair first involves addressing the impact of the event, the treatment components for Stage 1 of the therapy are primarily cognitive-behavioral and directly target problems that arise from the immediate impact of the affair (e.g., emotional dysregulation, depression, the need to express feelings of anger and hurt, and "damage control" where necessary). This stage also focuses on problem solving and dealing with immediate issues. The goal of Stage 2 is to understand the meaning or the context of what happened from both a more recent and a historical perspective; therefore, treatment strategies in Stage 2 of the therapy combine cognitive and insight-oriented approaches. Consequently, to the extent possible and where appropriate, partners' empathy for each other's experiences at the time of the affair is promoted between to aid in the reduction of anger and increase understanding of each person's decisions and, if appropriate, to increase feelings of intimacy and closeness between the partners. Finally, in Stage 3, "moving On," the partners are encouraged to (1) address the issue of forgiveness, (2) consolidate what they have learned about each other, (3) reexamine their relationship, and (4) decide how they wish to continue their relationship in the future. The components and challenges of each stage are described in further detail below. Finally, as in all stage models, these stages are not necessarily linear; the therapists and the couple may cycle through elements of the stages at different times throughout treatment.

Stage 1: Dealing with the Impact of the Affair

After evaluating the information gained from the couple's assessment interviews, the therapist should have a good understanding of how the couple is functioning and which of the following treatment components are most likely to be needed for a particular couple. The therapist should then give the partners (1) his or her conceptualization of what led up to the affair, (2) a summary of the problems they are currently facing in their relationship and why they are experiencing them, and (3) a treatment plan. Then the couple should be given an explanation of the stages of the recovery process and the response to trauma conceptualization described in the introduction. This discussion serves several purposes. It orients the partners to treatment and gives them a "map" of where they are likely to go. The formulation, if conducted in a collaborative manner (see Epstein & Baucom,

TABLE 14.1. Overview of Goals and Interventions by Stage of Treatment

Treatment goals	Interventions
Stage 1. Dealing with Impact	
Assessment	One conjoint session; one individual session with each partner
Boundary setting	Conjoint sessions using directed problem solving, instruction in use of time-outs and venting techniques
Self-care and affect regulation	Individual sessions and handouts
Exploring impact of the affair	Conjoint session discussion and supervised letter writing by each partner regarding impact of the affair
Coping with flashbacks	Conjoint session discussion and directed problem solving
Stage 2. Finding Meaning	
Exploration of factors contributing to the affair	Conjoint sessions emphasizing developmental exploration of contributing factors from the couple's relationship, external context (e.g., work, extended family, pursuit by other), aspects of the participating partner, and aspects of the injured partner
Relationship work	Conjoint session discussion, directed problem solving, and targeted homework assignments
Stage 3. Moving On	
Summary and formulation of affair	Conjoint session discussion, letter writing by each partner to the other, therapist formulation, and feedback
Examination of forgiveness and related concepts of "letting go" and "moving on"	Conjoint sessions exploring models of forgiveness, common beliefs about forgiveness, potential benefits and costs of forgiveness, and apprehensions or resistance to moving on
Exploration of factors affecting decision whether to continue the couple's relationship	Conjoint session discussions; directed questioning of ability and commitment to make needed changes
Additional relationship work or preparation for termination	Conjoint sessions involving continued exploration, problem solving, and targeted homework

2002), also can help them feel understood and supported by the therapist, and it can serve the crucial function of helping them begin to see the "big picture" of their relationship and how the affair might fit into it. A discussion of the notion of "trauma" can help partners to understand and reframe the reactions that they are having and can help some partners begin to develop empathy for each other's struggles. This explanatory framework also can normalize their experiences and provides an excellent rationale for the treatment plan and course of therapy.

In addition to assessment, feedback, and formulation, a major goal of Stage 1 of therapy is to contain ongoing damage from the affair and to help the couple regain some equilibrium. Another major goal is helping the couple to explore the impact of the affair; during this exploration, we pay particular attention to ensuring that the injured partner has a chance to communicate the impact of the affair effectively to the participating partner, and the participating partner has the opportunity to respond nondefensively and remorsefully, if he or she is sincere. To accomplish these goals, Stage 1 of treatment incorporates five sets of interventions: (1) problemsolving and damage control, (2) time-out and "venting" techniques, (3) self-care techniques, (4) emotional expressiveness skills and discussion of the impact of the affair, and (5) coping with flashbacks.

Problem Solving and "Damage Control"

The negative emotions following the betrayal may impact many other aspects of the couple's functioning. As described earlier in the section on assessment, a couple's normal functioning and interaction patterns can become severely disrupted. For example, partners who once prided themselves on their ability to parent well together may find themselves arguing bitterly in front of their children. Given that they are likely to experience a high level of conflict that often occurs at a much higher frequency than usual, they are likely to need immediate assistance from the therapist in setting limits, or boundaries, on their negative interactions. During the assessment period, the therapist gathered information on areas of current functioning that are particularly problematic for the couple; these areas should then be the major initial targets of treatment early in therapy. The therapist should help the partners to develop their own solutions for the problems defined in the assessment period by using directed problem solving (Epstein & Baucom, 2002). It is important to emphasize that these solutions are temporary, designed primarily for "damage control." The participating partner may have to agree to some behaviors that would not be healthy in any marriage long term but may be needed in the short term to help the injured partner regain a sense of control or safety, and to demonstrate his or her remorse for the affair. For example, if a common cause of arguments is the husband's insecurity over his wife's whereabouts after learning of her affair, then the wife may agree to be overzealous in checking in with her husband until some trust or security has been reestablished.

Time-Out and Venting Techniques

Due to the often heightened level of negative affect in the period following the discovery of an affair, many partners need a strategy that allows them to disengage when the level of emotion becomes too high. "Time-out" strategies (as described in Epstein & Baucom, 2002; Holtzworth-Munroe et al., 2003) are introduced, and the partners are instructed on how to recognize when they need to call a time-out and how to do so effectively. "Effectively" in this case means agreeing ahead of time on a mutually acceptable way to call the time-out and determining a specified length of time before returning to the discussion at hand.

In addition, instead of using time-outs to fume and plan a counterattack, the partners are instructed in how to a time-out constructively, to "vent" their tension through nonaggressive strategies such as physical exercise, if necessary, then to reduce their emotions to a more manageable level.

Self-Care Guidelines

Research and clinical observations suggest that the emotional sequelae of affairs often involve feelings of anger, anxiety, depression, shame, and lowered self-esteem. Unfortunately, these feelings are occurring at a time when the partners are often least equipped to deal with them. Consequently, partners can become involved in a vicious cycle, wherein these feelings make them less effective in their interactions with each other, which in turn makes them more depressed or anxious. Thus, another major target for this stage of therapy involves helping both partners take better care of themselves to have more emotional resources as they work through the aftermath of the affair.

Our approach offers basic self-care guidelines that encompass three areas: (1) physical care, including aspects such as eating and sleeping well, decreasing caffeine, and exercising; (2) social support, paying careful attention to what is and is not appropriate to disclose; and (3) spiritual support, such as meditation, prayer, and talking with a spiritual counselor, if consistent with the partner's belief system. These guidelines, typically presented in individual sessions with each partner, allow the therapist to assess the degree of each partner's distress and to address this distress appropriately. In addition, these individual sessions allow the therapist to express support for each individual, without worrying about the reactions of the partner; to talk about the upcoming sessions; and to develop a plan for how each partner will attempt to manage his or her emotions during the painful discussions to come and the interactions outside of therapy. We find that in this beginning stage of therapy a partner is sometimes better able to focus on his or her own difficulties and contributions to the relationship problems when the other partner is not in the room. When defensiveness decreases and there is more connection and trust between the partners, these issues then can be better addressed in the conjoint sessions.

It is in these individual sessions that the therapist and the participating partner can discuss feelings of guilt, anger, shame, and ambivalence that the partner may be experiencing, and to develop strategies about how to manage and express these feelings appropriately in the conjoint sessions. In this stage in the therapy, when the injured partner's anger and hurt are likely to be at their highest levels, the participating partner's own anger and ambivalence may cause more polarization between the couple. Thus, we find that these issues may be best addressed and supported in individual sessions in Stage 1 of therapy, then addressed in the conjoint sessions during Stage 2 of therapy as the participating partner begins to examine his or her reasons for the affair. On the other hand, the injured partner is more likely to hear the participating partner's feelings of remorse, shame, and guilt early in the therapy, because these feelings provide evidence that the participating partner is aware of the magnitude of his or her actions and that the affair is having a similarly negative impact on both partners. Therefore, these particular emotions are likely to be explored more successfully in the conjoint sessions.

Discussing the Impact of the Affair

A common need for the injured partner in this situation is to express to the participating partner how she or he has been hurt or angered by the affair. It is likely that this need serves both a punitive and a protective function. This discussion might serve as a way to communicate that what happened was wrong and to ensure that the participating partner also feels as much discomfort as possible as a result of his or her actions. In this sense, the injured partner might feel that expressing hurt and anger helps to ensure that infidelity will not happen again, which in turn protects the injured partner from additional harm in the future. However, despite the injured partner's clear need to express his or her feelings, these interactions between the partners are often rancorous and complicated by feelings of anger and guilt on the part of the participating partner. Consequently, they might not serve the desired purpose, and may leave the injured partner feeling as vulnerable and angry as he or she felt before the interaction occurred. Often, the participating partner has feelings of bitterness about an earlier hurt or betrayal in the relationship that interfere with his or her ability to sympathize with the injured partner's feelings of betrayal. As a result, the injured partner is not likely to feel that his or her feelings have been heard supportively, and may increase his or her demands or comments,

precipitating a negative cycle of interactions between the partners.

The current treatment seeks to interrupt this cycle through three means: First, couples are taught to use appropriate emotional expressiveness skills for both speaker and listener to help the injured person be more effective in communicating his or her feelings and the participating partner to be more effective in demonstrating that she or he is listening (Epstein & Baucom, 2002). Second, couples are given a careful conceptualization of why this step is necessary; The participating partner must understand that his or her own perspective of the affair will most likely not be heard and fully understood by the injured partner unless the injured partner first perceives that the participating partner (a) truly understands the meaning of his or her actions, (b) is remorseful for the effect of his or her actions on the injured person and the relationship, *and* (c) communicates this understanding and remorse clearly to the injured partner. The participating partners are reassured that they will have a chance to address their own issues in Stage 2 of therapy, at which time they are more likely to be heard. We also help them to understand that if the injured partner's feelings of anger, vulnerability, and hurt are not addressed effectively, then the couple will be unlikely to reach a successful resolution of the process. The goal of these rationales is to motivate the participating partner to carefully listen to and acknowledge the injured partner's perspectives in the conjoint session.

Third, the injured partner is encouraged to write a letter, exploring his or her feelings and reactions to the affair, that is first given to the therapist. The therapist pays particular attention to helping the injured partner identify and express any vulnerable and/or positive feelings (e.g., "You matter to me, and it hurts me that I might not matter to you"). After feedback from the therapist, the letter is then revised and read to the participating partner. This process allows the injured partner to explore his or her reactions in a calmer setting, and enables him or her to take time to express these reactions in ways that are not attacking or abusive, and are likely to be understood by the participating partner. It also allows the injured partner some emotional safety away from the participating partner to fully explore their more vulnerable reactions to the affair and possibly link them to earlier developmental experiences, such as a rejection by a parent or another previous relationship partner. Consequently, when the letter is finally read in the conjoint sessions, the participating partner often hears vulnerable, softer emotions and reactions that he or she did not know existed. With support in the session from the therapist, the participating partner can be coached in responding supportively and empathically to these vulnerable emotions, thus providing the couple with a more positive exchange regarding these painful experiences than they are likely to accomplish on their own. For more detail on this intervention see Snyder, Gordon, and Baucom (2004). We have found that couples often dread this session, because they are fearful of each other's reactions, but when they finally read the letters, they almost uniformly find the experience to be powerful and connective.

Coping with "Flashbacks"

A final and important component in Stage 1 is the explanation of "flashback" phenomena and the development of a plan to cope with them. As mentioned earlier, the reaction to an affair strongly parallels the traumatic response; thus, not surprisingly, both partners also are likely to encounter "reexperiencing" phenomena in the course of dealing with an affair. For example, a wife who discovers an unexplained number on a telephone bill may then be reminded about the unexplained telephone calls during the affair, triggering a flood of affect related to her husband's affair. If the husband is not aware of this sequence of events, his wife's emotions may appear inexplicable, which may in turn cause him to question their progress in recovering from the affair. By having their process explained and normalized, the partners may be less likely to misattribute these interactions to lack of progress. Instead, they have a better conceptualization of what is happening, and they are given the opportunity to problem-solve what each person needs to do in coping with these situations effectively. For more information about how to help couples develop plans to cope with these flashbacks, please see Snyder et al. (2007).

Common Problems in Stage 1

DEFENSIVENESS

Defensiveness by either partner is best addressed proactively. In the individual sessions with the participating partner, the therapist attempts to establish a strong therapeutic alliance with him or her, while at the same time clearly laying out ex-

pectations for the sessions to come. Acknowledging that the coming sessions will be extremely hard and that it will be difficult to avoid being defensive helps to support the partner and prepare him or her, while still communicating an expectation that she or he should try to avoid this response. The more the partners understand how these sessions are important to the process, and how crucial managing their defensiveness is to the process, the more motivated they may be to engage in the emotion regulation strategies developed in the individual sessions.

LACK OF AFFECT

Whereas many couples may be quite volatile following the discovery of an affair, others may present as disengaged and minimize their reactions to the affair. This lack of affect from one or both partners regarding the affair (when the affair clearly is a problem in the relationship for either partner) may be addressed in two ways, depending upon its source. First, if lack of affect is due to a fear of exploring the emotions or a misunderstanding of how this could help the couple, then the therapist should address those fears and misunderstandings with a more thorough rationale for and collaborative discussion of this stage of treatment. However, if it is due to an individual's more general difficulty in expressing or experiencing emotion, or engaging with others emotionally, more time should be spent helping this person to feel safe to explore and acknowledge his or her feelings.

CRISES

When a couple arrives and is discouraged by the process or enraged by an argument on the way to the session, the therapist must first assess the extent of the crisis, and whether its resolution is crucial to the progress of the session or more attributable to the couple's general level of functioning. If it is the former, the therapist may spend time addressing that issue; however, if it is the latter, the therapist must avoid being pulled into addressing the crisis. Instead, a more effective approach would be to put the despair or the argument into the larger picture of the couple's functioning and the recovery process itself, thus acknowledging, supporting, and then normalizing the feelings. The primary message should be that the process is not easy for anyone, and nothing will make it easier except to go through it. The couple should then be gently urged to continue with the treatment strategy.

Stage 2: Finding Meaning

After the crisis of the initial response to the affair has quieted down, the couple can address the central question posed by most injured partners: "Why did this happen?" Stage 2 of treatment involves exploring factors that contributed to the affair's occurrence. Toward this end, a comprehensive conceptual model is proposed to the couple that integrates both recent (proximal) and early developmental (distal) factors across multiple domains influencing vulnerability to, engagement in, and recovery from an affair. Domains of potential contributing factors include (1) aspects of the couple's own relationship (e.g., high conflict, low emotional warmth); (2) situational factors outside the relationship (e.g., work-related stressors, pursuit by a potential partner outside the relationship); (3) characteristics of the participating partner (e.g., anger at the injured partner, insecurities about self, unrealistic relationship expectations, developmental history, or enduring personality disorders); and (4) characteristics of the injured partner (e.g., discomfort with emotional closeness, avoidance of conflict, developmental history, and longstanding emotional or behavioral difficulties).

Exploration of the Factors Contributing to the Affair

After the emotional chaos or emotional distance has been addressed in Stage 1, and the partners have had a chance to explore the impact of the affair to the point that the injured partner has become more vulnerable and better able to listen, then the stage is set for Stage 2 of treatment, which focuses on helping the couple to explore and understand the context of the affair. First, the couple must understand the logic behind this exploration and, optimally, be motivated to engage in this process. After this goal is accomplished, then the focus of the therapy turns toward examining the different factors that may have influenced the partner's decision to have the affair. These factors may include (1) aspects of the relationship, such as difficulty communicating or finding time for each other; (2) external issues, such as job stress, financial difficulties, or in-laws; (3) issues specific to the participating partner, such as his or her beliefs about romantic relationships or developmental history; and (4) issues specific to the injured partner, such

as his or her developmental history or relationship skills (Snyder et al., 2007).

This last point is likely to be most problematic for the couple given that it may appear to be blaming the victim. *At this point, the couple needs to understand an important distinction between contributing to the context of the affair and being responsible for engaging in the affair.* In this treatment, the participating partners are held responsible for their choices to have the affair, or to choose that particular solution to their relational or individual dilemmas. However, it is important that the injured partner also be able to look at how he or she may have contributed to the context of the affair or the dilemma that the participating partners attempted to "solve." For example, the injured partner might have "looked the other way" due to his or her fear of conflict, even when it was clear that there was a problem with the participating partner, or the injured partner might have been preoccupied with his or her own issues and ambitions and was unable or unwilling to attend to the participating partner's needs. Furthermore, as mentioned earlier, often the participating partner may feel bitter about hurts the injured partner may have caused. In these instances, it is beneficial to explore these problems as well, and to help the participating partner work toward a resolution of these issues. In this example, the participating partner may have felt hurt and rejected by his or her partner's preoccupation, and as a result may need to come to a better understanding of that preoccupation.

Although the injured partner is not responsible for the participating partner's decision, it is important that *both* partners become aware of the effects of their own actions in the relationship, and how their own behavior can cause their relationship to become more vulnerable to problems. This knowledge, although painful, also may help the injured partner regain a sense of control in the relationship. Identifying weak points in the relationship allows the couple to pinpoint danger signals, which in turn allows partners to feel "safe," thus reducing the need for hypervigilance about the security of the relationship.

In addition, it is important to acknowledge developmental factors that contribute to the injured partner's response to the affair. For example, that person's response to the affair may be stronger if he or she has experienced previous betrayals. The response also may be affected by his or her expectations for relationships. To give an extreme example, his or her response to the affair may be surprisingly calm if the injured partner expects the partner to have an affair, believing "that's what men (women) do."

These sessions typically are conducted in two ways. Depending on the partners' level of skills and their motivation to listen to and understand each other, these sessions may take the form of structured discussions between partners as they attempt to understand the many factors that contributed to the affair. The therapist intervenes as necessary to highlight certain points, to evoke and strengthen positive emotional experiences between the partners, reinterpret distorted cognitions, or to draw the parallels or inferences from their developmental histories that the partners are themselves not able to discern. However, if their communication skills are weak, if either partner is acutely defensive, or if they have difficulty understanding each other's positions, then the therapist may structure sessions that are more similar to individual therapy sessions, focusing primarily on one partner, while the other partner listens and occasionally is asked to summarize his or her understanding of what is being expressed, and contributes his or her own perspective on the issues being discussed.

In both types of sessions, the therapist works to promote empathy between the partners by helping the listening partner draw parallels between what the other is describing and his or her own similar experiences, or by encouraging the partners to use their imagination and put themselves in the other's place as best they can. For example, a husband was able to emotionally resonate with his wife's current feelings of hurt and rejection when the therapist helped him recall times in his adolescence when he had felt painfully outcast by his peers, because his family had recently immigrated to this country. As he drew on his own feelings of rejection, he came to understand his wife's current situation more fully and softened toward her, in spite of her affair. Research indicates that empathy is considered an important mediating factor in people's ability to forgive and move beyond interpersonal betrayals (McCullough, Worthington, & Rachal, 1997). Thus, this treatment pays particular attention to the information the partners have gained about each other and their acknowledgments of vulnerability to promote an atmosphere of mutual support and empathy, without approving of the affair.

In addition, the therapist also looks for patterns and similarities between what the partners have reported in their individual histories and the problems they report in their relationships. It is in these aspects of the therapy, promotion

of empathy and developmental exploration, that the treatment borrows most heavily from insight-oriented approaches (Snyder, 1999; Snyder & Schneider, 2002). Understanding how historically based needs and wishes influence an individual's choices in the present can be a critical element in understanding why a participating partner chose to have an affair, or how an injured partner has responded to this event. Often, choosing to have an affair as a possible solution to present problems is influenced by strategies that have worked in previous relationships, or by developmental needs that were not met in the past. For example, a man who was repeatedly rejected sexually in early adolescence and young adulthood, and consequently sees himself as unlovable and undesirable, may be particularly vulnerable to choosing a sexual affair to solve his feelings of rejection and abandonment in his marriage. Helping the man and his partner to see that pattern and to understand the reasons behind it may serve to increase both empathy between the partners, by changing his partner's attributions about why the affair occurred, and his ability to choose new behaviors to meet his needs. Directing both members of the couple to explore these influences helps them to gain a deeper understanding of each other's vulnerabilities and may promote a greater level of empathy and compassion between them.

Problem Solving or Cognitive Restructuring of Problematic Issues in the Relationship

Throughout the sessions, the need to make changes in numerous aspects of the relationship and themselves as individuals may become evident to partners, and they may naturally begin to engage in problem solving. However, it also is beneficial to build in separate problem-solving sessions for two reasons. First, over time, partners may become frustrated with daily ongoing difficulties that are separate from the affair, or that may have contributed to the affair; therefore, they often need structured time in the sessions to address these current relationship difficulties and arrive at a good resolution. As a result, the therapist needs to balance the work of therapy between focusing on the affair and focusing on ongoing relationship issues. Second, giving partners opportunities to work on these issues and to have small successes together may make them feel more hopeful about the relationship, and the resultant positive feelings might fuel the additional insight-oriented exploration sessions. For example, during this phase of treatment, members of one couple began to realize that their relationship became vulnerable to an affair because they were not making it a priority in their lives. Consequently, they developed some new solutions to safeguard their time together on a daily basis to maintain a stronger connection. Success in following through with the strategies they created made them more hopeful about the future of the relationship and gave them renewed energy for continuing treatment.

Additionally, the couple might require cognitive restructuring, as well as behavioral changes. If the therapist observes that one or both partners hold problematic beliefs about their relationship or relationships in general, he or she should bring these thoughts or interpretations to their attention and help them explore the effects of these beliefs on their relationships (Epstein & Baucom, 2002). For example, whereas one partner might believe that romantic partners should spend all of their free time with each other, the other partner might expect to have both joint activities and "alone time." Although neither belief by itself is problematic, these differing expectancies are likely to cause conflicts for the couple. Consequently, the therapist needs to address these beliefs in therapy and help the partners both to evaluate the impact of these beliefs and to decide how or whether they can modify them to be more adaptive for the relationship. For more information about this technique, please see Baucom et al., Chapter 2, this volume.

Problems Encountered in Stage 2

RESISTANCE TO EXPLORING THE CONTEXT OF THE AFFAIR

Initially the couple, or more likely one partner, might exhibit reluctance to explore factors contributing to the development of the affair. Often partners feel that these discussions may reopen old wounds, or they may have difficulty separating "understanding" the context of affair and "excusing" the affair. Consequently, it is helpful to set the stage for this phase of treatment by explaining the difference between understanding and excusing, and by first exploring thoroughly partners' fears and concerns about this process. After the therapist has addressed the concerns, the focus of treatment turns to an examination of the benefits of partners' increased understanding of each other and their relationship that they gain through this

process. Some examples of possible benefits are (1) a change in the injured partner's initial inaccurate explanations of why this event occurred (e.g., realizing that the affair did not happen because he or she was a bad partner, or unattractive, or boring); (2) an injured partner's understanding of why this event happened, which makes the future seem less frightening and unpredictable; (3) a decrease in the injured partner's sense of anxiety about the relationship that helps to set the stage for rebuilding trust; and (4) the participating partner might come to a clearer understanding of his or her own behavior, as well as his or her partner's behavior, and thus have increased ability to make needed changes.

LACK OF EMPATHY

Another potential difficulty in Stage 2 of treatment is the inability of either partner to experience empathy for the other. As mentioned earlier, empathy plays an important role in the process of forgiveness (McCullough et al., 1997); therefore, the therapist should take care to promote greater empathy between partners during this process, as is appropriate. Again, there may be resistance to this concept, particularly if the partners associate empathy with excusing the behavior. In addition, before the partners begin to explore the context of the affair, it is useful to ask questions designed to prime them to experience empathy in reaction to the other partner's experiences. For example, some questions may be designed to prompt both partners to think about times in their own lives when they hurt others and to reflect on their own reasons for doing so, or to think about times when they were under a great deal of stress or difficulty and consequently made bad decisions. Engaging in these exercises can help partners to gain a different perspective on the other's dilemmas and to become more open to exploring reasons for his or her decisions.

RELUCTANCE TO ACKNOWLEDGE PROGRESS

In addition, an injured partner might show reluctance to acknowledge any progress in the therapy or any efforts at change on the part of the participating partners. A large part of this reluctance to acknowledge change might be due to the injured partner's need to stay angry at, or be protected from his or her partner. One motivation for this reluctance may be punishment; the injured partner may feel that acknowledging the other's efforts is the same as letting the participating partner "off the hook." If this is the reason behind the injured partner's reluctance, then the therapist should explore these concerns and help the injured partner to see how acknowledging the good qualities or effort of the participating partner might not mean having to "erase" the effects of his or her inappropriate behaviors. The therapist should help the injured partner to understand that it is acceptable and normal to feel good about progress or change, yet still feel angry or hurt about what happened and perceive that what happened was wrong.

Similarly, the injured partner also might be afraid to acknowledge positive changes, because he or she feels that recognition would imply choosing to stay in the relationship. The therapist also should gently challenge this belief. Instead, the injured partner should be encouraged to note the changes occurring in the present, with the understanding that this is important information about what his or her partner has been able to do. However, the injured partners also should be told that despite the changes that occur, he or she has the freedom to decide not to live with what happened in the past and may choose to end the relationship. This permission is given in the hope of freeing the injured partner from a need to protect him- or herself, allowing him or her to become a more impartial observer of the changes occurring in the relationship.

Stage 3: Moving On

In the third stage of treatment, the therapist begins by integrating information obtained in previous sessions as a method to prepare the couple to reach an informed decision about how to "move on." Verbal and written summaries by the therapist, along with letters written by each partner to the other, are used to converge on a shared formulation regarding factors that contributed to the affair's occurrence. During the construction of this formulation, particular attention is paid to how the couple now understands previously violated assumptions. Similar to the cognitive processing therapy for PTSD described by Resick and Calhoun (2001), any remaining questions or fears about the relationship are then addressed, and reconstructed beliefs about the relationship are evaluated. Once this goal is achieved, handouts and written exercises are used to promote partners' evaluation and discussion of their relationship's viability, its

potential for change, and partners' commitment to work toward change based on what they have learned about themselves and each other. Partners explore the process of moving on by examining the meaning of this construct as it relates to both their personal and relationship values and belief systems. Specific issues pertaining to this phase of the treatment process are described below.

Summary and Formulation of the Affair

After the couple has carefully and systematically explored the factors contributing to the affair, the couple's and the therapist's job is to summarize this exploration and weave these different factors into a coherent "story" explaining how the affair came about for the couple (Snyder et al., 2007). In addition, the therapist and the partners discuss what aspects of their relationship may need additional attention and how this can be accomplished to help them avoid future betrayals. In this respect, the therapy begins to move from a focus on the past to a focus on the present and future of the relationship.

Discussion of Forgiveness

Although the entire process outlined in this treatment is based on our model of forgiveness and can be conceptualized as the process of coming to forgiveness, this concept is not introduced to the couple until near the end of the treatment. This delay in addressing forgiveness explicitly is necessitated by the injured partner's likely reluctance to engage in a process of forgiveness when he or she has recently discovered an affair. Mentioning forgiveness to someone who recently has been hurt and is extremely angry at his or her partner is unlikely to elicit a positive response. However, introduction of this concept at a later point in the treatment, when the anger has died down and the person's understanding of the betrayal has increased, is more likely to have a successful outcome, and the injured partner is likely to be more willing to consider this possibility. In addition, we have found that when partners are introduced to Gordon and Baucom's (1998) three-stage model of forgiveness, they are able to recognize that they have largely completed the work of the first two stages, which can motivate them to continue the process and consider forgiveness as an appropriate and possible choice.

During the discussion of forgiveness, four

basic points are covered: (1) a description of the forgiveness model; (2) common beliefs about forgiveness; (3) consequences of forgiving and not forgiving; and (4) blocks to forgiving and "moving on." The description of the forgiveness model is presented in terms of its similarity to the process of exploration that the partners have just completed, and they are informed that by acknowledging and exploring the impact of the betrayal, and the reasons and context behind the betrayal, they may already have taken significant steps towards being able to forgive each other (Enright & the Human Development Study Group, 1991; Gordon & Baucom, 1998; Hargrave & Sells, 1997). Partners are then encouraged to examine and to reevaluate their beliefs about forgiveness in comparison to the definition of forgiveness presented to them in the treatment. For example, often couples report difficulty with forgiveness out of beliefs that forgiving their partners is "weak" or is equivalent to saying that what happened is acceptable or excusable. Challenging this belief by presenting couples with the definition of forgiveness described earlier and by allowing that people may forgive, yet appropriately hold partners responsible for their behaviors, may result in a new conceptualization of forgiveness that feels more possible for couples to achieve.

However, if these discussions do not help the couple feel more open to forgiveness, then the therapist may wish to help the couple evaluate the consequences of not forgiving. Recent research has indicated that continuous anger and bitterness can have a detrimental effect on individuals' physical and emotional health (e.g., Seybold, Hill, Neumann, & Chi, 2001; Toussaint, Williams, Musick, & Everson, 2001) and on relationships with their children and future relationships (e.g., Ashleman, 1997; Gordon, Hughes, Tomcik, & Litzinger, 2006; Holeman, 1998). It is important that these issues be discussed with the couple in a balanced manner. The therapist should avoid communicating to partners that they should or must always forgive. Indeed, some research indicates that immediate forgiveness in abusive relationships might lead individuals to stay in or return to unhealthy situations (Gordon, Burton, & Porter, 2004; Katz, Street, & Arias, 1997). In these cases, forgiveness before the injury is rectified or stopped may be premature or inappropriate. It is possible that these individuals might need encouragement to admit fully to themselves that this abuse is destructive and that they have a right to be angry. This anger may serve as a motivating force to help them make important changes in their relationships. Thus, moving these individuals too quickly to the end of the forgiveness process might be inappropriate. Furthermore, in some cases, people may not be ready to forgive. In this case, the therapist must examine what purpose the anger and negative affect, behaviors, and cognitions still serves for the couple, then, based on what is uncovered, appropriately address these blocks to "moving on."

Exploration of Factors Affecting the Partners' Decision to Continue Their Relationship

In addition, the partners also should be encouraged to decide whether they wish to recommit themselves to this relationship on the basis of what they have learned about themselves, their partners, and their relationship. In other words, forgiveness does not require reconciliation. Partners may make appropriate decisions that they cannot stay with each other, yet still be able to separate and not harbor intense anger and resentment toward each other. To this end, they are encouraged to discuss together within the sessions a series of questions designed to help them evaluate their relationship. A number of these questions relate to whether either member of the couple has shown the desire or the ability to make the needed changes in their relationship to ensure that the betrayal does not happen again, and whether the partners are able to regain a measure of trust and safety within the relationship. A list of possible questions for the couple to consider appears in Table 14.2.

Problem Solving or Cognitive Restructuring on Problematic Issues in the Relationship or Issues Relating to a Decision to Separate

If the partners decide to recommit to each other, then the remainder of treatment is focused on addressing problematic issues in the relationship that may directly arise from the affair, such as rebuilding trust or physical and emotional intimacy issues, and/or on addressing more general ongoing issues in the relationship that may or may not be indirectly related to the affair, such as power and control issues, communication problems, or difficulty finding time together. Common cognitive-behavioral techniques, such as skills training, homework assignments, and cognitive restructuring, are used to accomplish these goals (Epstein & Baucom, 2002; for a discussion of rebuilding intimacy in marriage, see Johnson, 2004; Prager, 1999) for a more complete description of these techniques.

TABLE 14.2. Viewing Your Relationship from the Larger Perspective

What were our reasons for becoming a couple?

- What initially attracted us to each other?
- Why did we marry or make a long-term commitment to this relationship?

How have we grown individually and as a couple?

- How have my partner and I helped each other to grow as individuals?
- How have we brought out the best or the worst in each other?
- How has our relationship grown to accommodate new or difficult challenges?

What have we done the best?

- What are our best achievements as a couple?
- What would I miss most if we end our relationship now?

What challenges have we overcome together?

- What have been the most difficult times we've faced together in the past?
- How did we manage to get through those times?
- In what ways did previous challenges make us stronger as a couple? In what ways did they leave us feeling hurt, disappointed, or more vulnerable?
- How have we reconnected in the past after feeling particularly hurt?

How does the current crisis fit into the big picture?

- Has your partner been truthful in the past prior to this affair?
- Did this affair occur at a time when your marriage was particularly vulnerable?
- Looking back prior to the affair, was there more good in this marriage than bad?

If the partners decide to separate, then the focus of therapy moves to helping them to do so in a way that involves the least amount of acrimony. Partners are encouraged to consider how they can use what they have learned during the treatment to maintain respect and, we hope, empathy, for each other during the difficult process of separation. Again, they are encouraged to evaluate the consequences of maintaining bitterness versus the benefits of letting go of the anger and recrimination. Furthermore, in addition to helping them plan how to maintain a sense of forgiveness, the therapist also helps partners problem-solve the myriad issues that can arise during separation, such as child custody arrangements, finances, and other decisions.

Problems Encountered in Stage 3

RESISTANCE TO THE IDEA OF FORGIVENESS

Many of the problems encountered in Stage 3 already have been described in the previous section. First, the couple may be resistant to the idea of forgiveness. This resistance may arise out of mistaken beliefs about forgiveness or hidden agendas that are served by a continuation of anger and bitterness. In these cases, the therapist must carefully assess for these hidden goals, a process that is best accomplished in individual sessions. Once uncovered, these goals should be addressed as the therapist deems appropriate; however, the individual also should be encouraged to consider other means to meet these goals and previously unacknowledged or unknown consequences of continuing to hold onto the bitterness. One common example of such a hidden agenda is when individuals believe that forgiveness places them at risk for the injury to happen again; thus, in these cases anger serves as a protective mechanism against future hurt. Helping clients to articulate this belief, then to examine both its accuracy in their current relationship and its consequences can be a useful strategy in this case. In addition, the therapist can help clients to think through other means of creating a sense of safety in the relationship.

DIFFICULTIES WITH REBUILDING TRUST

A second problem that may occur in Stage 3 is that if the partners have recommitted themselves to the relationship, they may still have difficulties with trust. Although the injured partner may have agreed to forgive and to work on the relationship, he or she may still have difficulty to trusting the partner again. This difficulty is understandable in light of the betrayal and is a common occurrence in couples who have experienced an affair. The couple should be given a conceptualization that makes this hesitation understandable to both partners, yet also clearly indicates that if the injured partner plans to remain in the relationship, he or she must begin to take small, manageable, increasingly risky stops with the partner to rebuild the trust. To elaborate further, in keeping with the view of this intervention as a trauma-based program of recovery, trust building is viewed as following an exposure-based paradigm. The injured partner is encouraged to identify a series of small hierarchical steps that involve increasing levels of emotional risk taking in the relationship. This hierarchical exercise might enable the injured partner to "test the waters" without taking a risk that feels too overwhelming and might invite failure.

The therapist must then explain to the partner who had the affair that he or she has to follow through on these steps or else risk major damage to the relationship. For example, if the injured partner has been checking frequently on his or her whereabouts, then the first step may be to decrease the amount of checking from 100 to 50%, yet still do some random checks to reassure him- or herself that the partner is acting in a trustworthy manner. After the partner has proven that he or she is where he or she reported being, then the injured partner may be encouraged to take a risk and decrease the checking even more.

RESISTANCE TO FORGIVENESS IN SEPARATION AND DIVORCE

A third problem that may occur in Stage 3 often arises when the couple decides to separate. This decision may not always be mutual, and even if it is, it may still engender anger and bitterness between the partners. At this point, it is crucial that the therapist continue to provide the partners with the "big picture" (i.e., the balanced view of each other and the relationship that emerged during their exploration of the context of the affair). In addition, the therapist should also continue to point out the benefits of forgiveness and the consequences to the partners and to others if they continue to harbor bitterness regarding the end of the relationship.

CURATIVE FACTORS AND MECHANISMS OF CHANGE

There are several aspects of this treatment that we believe are necessary factors for the couple's recovery and change. Most importantly, given that much of this treatment is based on a theoretical understanding that disrupted assumptions about self, partner, and relationship are what make an affair traumatic, we believe that the crucial ingredient in recovering from an affair is partners' ability to reconstruct their views about themselves, each other, and their relationships in a way that promotes a feeling of security and ability to interact effectively with one another in the present. Even if the partners decide not to stay together, we believe that this reconstruction process is critical in ensuring that the partners not allow the affair to poison their parenting relationships, if they have children

together, and not experience lasting effects from this affair in future relationships. What they learn about themselves and their relationships in this treatment should help them to avoid making the same mistakes in future relationships.

Furthermore, the insights they gain into each other's developmental histories also can have the effect of promoting greater empathy for each other in their current struggles to feel close, and to feel safe in their current relationships. We believe that this combination of insight into each other's struggles and developmental needs, and experience of empathy for one another is a critical ingredient for treatment success if the partners plan to stay together, because it will promote a stronger connection and greater sense of emotional safety within the couple.

Even as the partners come to understand each other more deeply, many couples also need help in translating these insights into new ways of interacting with one another. Communication skills training can be a starting point for helping partners to examine the strengths and weaknesses in their current interactions and encouraging them to try new ways of interacting with each other. As partners become more trusting and understanding of each other, they are more likely to use their new skills. In turn, as they use their skills, their interactions improve, and trust and hope in their relationship may be further enhanced. Thus, the degree to which couples are able to access old or to learn new communication skills is a critical curative factor.

The therapist's ability to remain neutral and to frame a couple's issues systemically is a factor in the majority of couple treatments. However, it also is an ability that takes on particular salience when dealing with infidelity. Infidelity can elicit a number of negative thoughts and emotions in the general population, and therapists are not necessarily exempt from these reactions. These negative and, at times, judgmental reactions can be heightened in therapists who themselves have been the "victim" in an affair. We have received feedback from couples who have engaged in therapy with therapists who, unable to work through these personal reactions, failed to maintain a more neutral stance. Although these therapists might have perceived these interventions as being supportive of the injured partner, injured partners have told us that the ultimate result of these efforts was that participating partners refused to continue treatment. Many of our participating partners expressed their belief that the impartiality shown by the therapists in our treatment project was a crucial factor in their decision to fully engage in the treatment and in their experience of safety in the sessions. Therefore, we believe that another critical ingredient of this therapy is a neutral, empathic, nonjudgmental therapist.

There are several couple factors that might moderate the success or failure of this treatment. Thus, they are not essential curative ingredients of this therapy, but they are factors that can affect the success of the treatment. The first major factor is the personalities of the partners. One of the most striking individual differences that affects the recovery process is the presence of psychopathology in either member of the couple, particularly the presence of antisocial and narcissistic personality traits. As with most treatments, these characteristics are a poor prognostic indicator for successful recovery. Furthermore, when either partner has preexisting difficulties with emotional fragility or affect regulation, or had a fragile sense of self-worth prior to the affair due to other abandonment or negative relationship experiences, the treatment may be less effective and may progress more slowly. Additional time must be taken to help that partner contain his or her negative affect enough to participate in treatment; the strategies described in Stage 1 of treatment can be useful for these situations. Discomfort with and avoidance of affect is another individual difference that is likely to have implications for treatment. We discussed strategies to address this discomfort with affect earlier in the Stage 1 interventions. However, it may also be important to address the developmental source of this problem in Stage 2, particularly if it is a major contributor to the affair. Often, these individuals have had either direct or vicarious experiences with intense emotions that had frightening or devastating outcomes.

Issues related to commitment levels in the relationship also may be pertinent in two ways. In a more immediate sense, as discussed previously, partners' levels of commitment to their relationship when they enter treatment clearly are important factors in their ability to recover. However, in a more distal sense, the issue of commitment in the treatment of infidelity also may be related to a developmentally based fear of intimacy or feelings of being "trapped" in a stable relationship. Attachment theorists describe a pattern of attachment that is characterized by approach–avoidance (e.g., Hazan & Shaver, 1994). Individuals with this pattern may need intimate relationships and seek them out, yet fear them to such an extent that they find it difficult to feel safe in long-term intimate relationships. Affairs may then serve as a means to create a safe level of distance from their partners (Allen & Baucom, 2005). In this case, the participating partner may need adjunctive individual treatment that targets this issue before the marital relationship is able to recover.

TREATMENT APPLICABILITY AND EMPIRICAL SUPPORT

Treatment Applicability

This treatment approach has been created explicitly to address the difficulties that couples experience following an affair. However, the affair need not be limited to a sexual relationship; as we mentioned earlier, extramarital *sexual* contact is not always necessary for one partner to feel that the other's relationship with someone outside the marriage breaks the agreed-upon commitment to monogamy in the marital contract. Additionally, because this model is based on both the traumatic response literature and the interpersonal forgiveness literature, it can be tailored to treat couples recovering from other, severe interpersonal betrayals that are not classified as extramarital affairs. Any event that severely disrupts either partner's assumptions regarding the relationship has the potential to cause great emotional distress and destroy the experience of safety within their relationship (e.g., perceived abandonment, financial deception). These disruptive events often require the same therapeutic process described in this chapter.

Although this approach can be used to address myriad types of relationship betrayals, it is not well-suited for couples in which the involved partner denies having participated in an affair; nor is it useful when neither partner feels that he or she has been betrayed. This approach has been designed specifically to address recovery from betrayal, and it is doubtful that a couple would benefit from this therapy if neither partner felt that a such a betrayal had taken place. Furthermore, if a couple presents with more general relational problems, but neither partner particularly feels that a betrayal has occurred, the couple may be served best by a more traditional type of therapy that is not affair-specific. This approach also is not well-suited to couples who abuse alcohol or drugs, or experience severe physical violence; in particular, if the threat of significant violence looms over the relationship, then no conjoint therapy is recommended (Holtzworth-Munroe et al., 2003).

Empirical Support

Initial findings provide some empirical support for this treatment approach. A replicated case-study was conducted with six couples in which one of the partners had participated in an affair (Gordon, Baucom, et al., 2004). Initially, the majority of injured partners were found to have significantly elevated symptoms of depression and PTSD. Furthermore, the couples reported low levels of commitment, trust, and empathy, and clinically elevated levels of marital distress, and all injured partners reported difficulties forgiving the affair. After participating in the intervention outlined in this chapter, gains were greatest for injured partners in the domains specifically targeted by this treatment. Responses on the Forgiveness Inventory (Gordon & Baucom, 2003) demonstrated that feelings of anger, revenge, and avoidance were reduced greatly following treatment, whereas feelings of understanding, release, and peace increased. There also were substantial decreases in symptoms associated with PTSD and depression. General marital distress of injured partners also decreased, but less so for the participating partners; however, participating partners initially reported less marital distress than did the injured partners. Furthermore, although this study found that the treatment was most advantageous for the injured partners, it also was beneficial for the partners. Upon completing the treatment, such partners expressed that the treatment was critical to their improvement in several domains, including a better understanding of why they participated in the affair and increased ability to tolerate their partners' initial negativity and subsequent flashback reactions.

Effect sizes in this study were found to be moderate-to-large and were comparable to effect sizes of empirically validated marital therapies not created specifically to target the difficulties couples experience following an affair (see Baucom, Shoham, Mueser, Daiuto, & Stickle, 1998). Additionally, a recent article by Baucom, Gordon, Snyder, Atkins, and Christensen (2006) found that the infidelity-specific intervention outlined in this chapter had larger effect sizes for decreasing global individual symptoms and depression in both the participating partners and injured partners than integrative behavioral couple therapy (IBCT). However, this approach was equal to IBCT with regard to changes in global marital distress. Final-ly, additional empirical support for this treatment stems from the fact that the two treatments that serve as the basis for this current treatment, CBCT and IOCT, have been empirically validated (Baucom et al., 1998; Snyder, 1999), as discussed in Baucom et al., Chapter 2, and Snyder and Mitchell, Chapter 12, this volume.

CASE ILLUSTRATION

To demonstrate how our principles of treatment are applied to a specific couple, we present the following case example. Brian, a 31-year-old white man, and Liz, a 28-year-old white woman, entered treatment 8 months after the discovery of Liz's affair with a mutual friend. Liz had moved out of the home, but she returned and decided to try to repair her relationship with Brian a week before they presented for treatment. During their initial assessment, the couple reported a 2-year marital history that included stressors such as a major move and a period of unemployment for Liz. Liz had difficulty finding a new job and, as she met with more rejection, her efforts toward finding a job dwindled. In response, Brian attempted to support her by clipping out help-wanted ads from the newspaper and asking her daily about the success of her search. Unfortunately, these efforts served only to increase Liz's distress and to create resentment toward Brian. Meanwhile, Brian was very successful, but his job required long hours and a great deal of travel. When Brian was home, he often went out for drinks with his colleagues after work and came home late. Liz made few friends, and most of her social circle was made up of Brian's friends.

Brian and Liz began to get close to one couple in particular and spent a great deal of time with them. The husband of the couple worked at home as a freelance writer, so he and Liz began to meet for lunch. At first, the purpose of these lunches was to provide moral "support" for her job search, but their relationship deepened, and soon they became involved in an emotional and sexual affair, which began after they had had a couple drinks at lunch and gave into their mutual attraction. Liz soon felt too guilty to continue the affair, so she broke it off and confessed to Brian. They initially decided to separate, and Liz chose to move back to her parents' home. However, they stayed in touch with each other, and discovered that they were even more miserable apart than together. Consequently, they decided to try to rebuild their marriage and enter couple therapy to deal with the aftermath of the affair. At intake, both partners reported a clinically elevated level of marital distress, particularly Liz. Furthermore, Brian reported a clinically elevated level of PTSD symptoms and very little forgiveness toward Liz.

When Brian and Liz presented for treatment, they required very little "damage control." Because they had already worked out much of their day-to-day life and were not engaging in much overt fighting, treatment focused more on uncovering Brian's reactions to the affair and helping him to express emotions other than anger toward Liz. Prior to entering treatment, Brian engaged in a number of sarcastic, cutting remarks about Liz's loyalty and moral character that hurt her deeply and increased her defensiveness and guilt. Liz felt unable to respond to these comments, because she thought she deserved them and did not want to provoke Brian further. The therapist gathered information about the partners' history and introduced them to the treatment in the first two conjoint sessions, after which she met with each partner separately to assess how they were functioning individually and to give each an opportunity to express his or her experiences in the relationship without fear of the partner's responses. Brian reported that he was more irritable with everyone around him and disliked who he was becoming. After some discussion of his hurt and disillusionment following the affair, he and his therapist developed some strategies to manage some of his irritation when it boiled over (e.g., using time-outs, talking with supportive and safe friends). In turn, Liz was having trouble managing her own reactions to Brian's irritability; thus, her individual session focused on support and on helping her to understand Brian's reactions. She also problem-solved how to (1) care for herself to reduce her own emotional vulnerability, (2) respond to Brian's comments nondefensively, and (3) not react in ways that would inflame the situation. Both partners found these individual sessions to be helpful and felt supported by the therapist.

In the next few sessions, the therapist taught the couple emotional expressiveness skills (Epstein & Baucom, 2002) and used these skills to explore the impact of the affair on each partner and the relationship. Brian was very resistant and bitter during these sessions, and Liz was often tearful and hurt by his hostility. He reported in his narratives that the experience of the affair was "surreal" and nothing he had ever expected in his marriage, which was the source of much of his bitterness. However, after a great deal of coaching by the therapist, Brian wrote and read a letter to Liz in which he was able to identify and express some of his more vulnerable experiences, such as his fear of losing her, and how her behavior had caused him to question himself and to feel worthless. Also after coaching by the therapist, Liz was able to reflect nondefensively a deep understanding of these feelings to Brian; he found this very gratifying, and the couple experienced an increase in intimacy after this experience. Liz particularly found that this session eased much of her tension; she noted that in previous discussions, all she had heard from Brian had been his anger and scorn. Hearing his more vulnerable side and seeing how much she mattered to him helped Liz to listen to Brian less defensively and to feel closer to him. In turn, when Brian saw that Liz could express understanding and acceptance of his feelings, and that this expression of his vulnerability drew her to him, he began to soften toward her and to experience more hope for the relationship.

Finally, the therapist introduced the partners to the idea of PTSD-like flashbacks and helped them problem-solve how to handle these instances. Liz found this to be very helpful, because it reframed for her Brian's moodiness as part of the process and something to be expected. They still had some difficulty recognizing when flashbacks occurred, because the reality was not as clear as the examples used in the session, but after some repeated discussion of this issue in later sessions, they became more effective in identifying these situations, and less reactive and hopeless when they occurred.

Despite their progress in Stage 1, Brian displayed a great deal of defensiveness and frustration in the early part of Stage 2, and was often unable to listen to Liz's descriptions of her thought processes at the time of her affair, because they made him feel inadequate and guilty for not "solving her problems." He was under a period of intense stress at work, and this stress spilled over in his feelings toward Liz; he coped with this issue by staying out late with coworkers and avoiding Liz as much as possible at home. Both members of the couple felt worn out and frustrated that their relationship was not "fixed" by this point. In fact, as they began to explore the context of the affair, this work brought issues to light that they had tried to ignore over the course of their marriage, such as differences in career goals and expectations regarding intimacy and conflict. Furthermore, although Brian vehemently wanted to understand why the affair occurred and to explore its context, he evidenced at the same time a great deal of resistance to the process, often subtly denigrating the therapist and the treatment, and "forgetting" his homework.

Consequently, the therapist again conducted separate sessions with each person individually to strengthen her therapeutic alliance with each partner and boost their motivation to continue treatment. In addition, these sessions provided each partner a place to express hopelessness and frustrations safely and to receive support, encouragement, and advice from the therapist. These sessions relieved a great deal of the tension, and Brian became much more engaged in the process. In addition, the therapist introduced problem-solving skills in the conjoint sessions during Stage 2 to help them begin to address some of the issues they were uncovering in the sessions. Both partners were grateful for these tools and put them to use, and they were particularly successful in addressing Brian's tendency to stay out late and Liz's resulting feelings of abandonment.

As the treatment proceeded, Brian's defensiveness further decreased when the therapist helped both partners draw links between their behaviors in their marriage and their developmental histories. In one session, Liz read a letter describing her role in her family of origin, and how that influenced her behavior in her own marriage. She explored how her need to play the "peacekeeper" in her family kept her constantly smoothing over problems; if she did not do so, then she often saw her family erupt into chaos and rage. Therefore, when she encountered emotionally charged issues that needed to be addressed in her own marriage, she was fearful of confrontation and avoided the issues as her dissatisfaction grew. Brian developed considerable empathy regarding Liz's vulnerability, and became sad and regretful about her experience. They discussed how disclosing their vulnerabilities made them feel more "real" to each other; yet both were fearful of this vulnerability and the risk it posed for being emotionally hurt by each other. However, each expressed a desire to make the relationship "safe" to express these feelings to each other. This shift in affect appeared to be a turning point for Brian, allowing him to move beyond the affair and helping him better understand why Liz had not turned to him when she was upset about their marriage. He also had a clearer insight into how alone and unsupported Liz had felt right before she became attracted to the male with whom she had the affair.

Finally, the third key issue for Liz and Brian in Stage 2 was their continued ambivalence about their relationship, with lack of clarity being highly anxiety-provoking and draining for them. They spent a great deal of energy between sessions ruminating on whether to stay together. Eventually, the therapist relieved this pressure by giving them "permission" to work on the relationship one day at a time, promising that they would revisit the issue of their future relationship in Stage 3. The permission to focus only on the present was comforting, and the couple experienced immediate emotional relief and noted, consequently, more positive interaction at home.

When Brian and Liz finally addressed their future together during Stage 3, they had made enough improvements in their marriage that they eventually committed to stay together and to forgive. As the therapist and the couple constructed their narrative about the affair, it became clear that Brian and Liz's understanding of the affair had shifted a great deal over the course of treatment. In particular, Brian's final description of its development moved from blaming Liz completely and stating that she would never change, to a more nuanced understanding that took into account their avoidant communication styles, their differing expectations for marriage, Liz's peacemaking tendencies and fear of conflict, and his own difficulty in responding supportively to his partner's emotional state and needs. After they discussed these issues, both partners felt hopeful that they could make progress on changing these patterns of interaction, and could point to instances throughout the treatment where they had managed to interact differently and had success in engaging more intimately. This opportunity to reflect on where they had been and where they were currently gave them more hope that they could make the necessary changes in their relationship. It also gave Brian a feeling of greater security about moving forward with Liz.

When the therapist discussed the idea of forgiveness, both partners were receptive to the idea but felt that any specific ritual would be "corny" and unlike them. Brian expressed a desire to forgive Liz and felt that he was "mostly there"; however, Brian felt that he needed more time and evidence that Liz was really committed to him and the marriage to resolve his remaining hesitation. At the same time, he felt willing to forgive and was able to express this willingness to Liz and commit to working actively on letting go of his anger and bitterness about the affair. Specifically, he would concentrate on not bringing up the affair continually during disagreements and try to decrease his ongoing tendency to withdraw. In turn, Liz said she understood that this was a process, and she committed to dealing constructively with any frustration or resentment she might feel if Brian slipped and inappropriately brought the affair up again. Both agreed that there might be times when flashbacks would occur, or other unresolved issues regarding the affair might resurface, and they decided they could deal with these issues without jeopardizing the forgiveness process itself, as long as they could discuss these instances openly and nondefensively. In a sense, the therapist helped them develop their own relapse prevention plan by framing these issues as normal incidences in the recovery process and helping them proactively to develop a plan to cope with these potential setbacks.

The couple then spent several sessions developing ways to express negative emotions safely to each other, and discuss their goals and interests as a couple. At the end of treatment, they still reported some relationship distress and did not feel that all of their relationship issues were completely addressed, but they felt committed to the process of recovery and capable of addressing these remaining issues on their own. By the end of treatment, Brian's PTSD symptoms had decreased, and his forgiveness measures had all greatly improved to within one standard deviation of the normal community population. In addition, both partners' global marital distress levels had decreased, although they were still reporting some distress. All treatment gains were maintained or improved at follow-up 6 months later. At treatment end and at follow-up, both members of the couple reported that the treatment had a positive impact on their relationship. It is important to note that treatment ended here because Brian and Liz were part of a research study attempting to standardize treatment across couples; whereas there was some flexibility in number of sessions across treatment, they had come to the end of the specified treatment; thus, therapy was terminated. If they had been in a more typical therapeutic context, the therapist would have continued working on their current relationship issues until they reported less distress. However, this couple was offered a referral for additional treatment at our clinic but declined, because they felt the skills they had gained from treatment would allow them to address their remaining problems successfully, and their narrative data indicated that they had made some progress in these areas 6 months later.

Both Brian and Liz said that the treatment led to greater understanding between them and provided tools to improve their relationship. However, both also agreed that the treatment at times was extremely painful; Brian in particular said that the treatment often "caused more stress than it [relieved]." This effect was particularly evident in the early stages of treatment, when both members remarked in their posttreatment narratives that they got along better when they just ignored their problems. At the same time, the treatment helped both of them to see how ignoring or smoothing over real difficulties ultimately caused them to experience more distance and disconnection from each other. Liz expressed much relief and gratitude for opportunities within treatment to problem-solve on difficult, longstanding issues in a safe and supportive environment. By the end of treatment, she was expressing hope that they could use what they had learned to continue improving their relationship. Whereas Brian also felt that the intervention was helpful, and was more positive in general about his relationship with Liz, his final words at the 6-month follow-up were more bittersweet as he expressed awareness of his vulnerability to pain in his relationship, and his difficulty in ever fully trusting that Liz would always be there unconditionally for him. He stated:

"[The] treatment definitely aided with getting through that period and better coming to understand myself, [my wife], and us. Life and marriage are not easy. ... I love my wife and want to be with her but through this experience, the affair and counseling, the concept of death do us part is questioned. ... I wish [that weren't true.]"

These words indicate both the potential for healing through treatment, and how difficult and traumatic recovering from an affair can be for a couple. Some lasting cracks and flaws may remain, but therapy ultimately can help couples piece their shattered worlds back together and move on in a healthier and forgiving manner.

SUGGESTIONS FOR FURTHER READING

Allen, E. S., Atkins, D. C., Baucom, D. H., Snyder, D. K., Gordon, K. C., & Glass, S. (2005). Intrapersonal, interpersonal, and contextual factors in engaging in and responding to infidelity. *Clinical Psychology: Science and Practice*, *12*, 101–130.—An exhaustive list of empirical and some theoretical research on infidelity in committed couples.

Baucom, D. H., Snyder, D. K., & Gordon, K. C. (in press). *Treating couples recovering from affairs*. New York: Guilford Press.—This treatment manual provides an extensive description of our treatment, along with sample therapy transcripts and extended case studies. It will also include handouts to give to couples and may be used in conjunction with the trade book below.

Gordon, K. C., & Baucom, D. H. (1998). Understanding betrayals in marriage: A synthesized model of forgiveness. *Family Process, 37*, 425–450.—A detailed description of the forgiveness model that underlies this intervention.

Gordon, K. C., Baucom, D. H., & Snyder, D. K. (2004). An integrative intervention for promoting recovery from extramarital affairs. *Journal of Marital and Family Therapy, 30*, 213–232.—This article provides detailed case studies and empirical findings on the replicated case study that tested the efficacy of this treatment model.

Snyder, D. K., Baucom, D. H., & Gordon, K. C. (2007). *Getting past the affair: How to cope, heal, and move on— together or apart.* New York,: Guilford Press.—This trade book is for individuals to use either individually or in conjunction with their partner to work through the issues involved in recovering from an affair. It is based on our treatment model and provides worksheets for couples to complete alone and/or together. It is intended also to be a resource for clinicians who help couples recover from infidelity.

REFERENCES

Abrahm Spring, J. (1996). *After the affair: Healing the pain and rebuilding trust when a partner has been unfaithful.* New York: HarperCollins.

Allen, E. S., & Baucom, D. H. (2005). Dating, marital, and hypothetical extradyadic involvements: How do they compare? *Journal of Sex Research, 43*, 307–317.

Amato, P. R., & Rogers, S. J. (1997). A longitudinal study of marital problems and subsequent divorce. *Journal of Marriage and the Family, 59*, 612–624.

Ashleman, K. (1997, April). *Forgiveness as a resiliency factor in divorced families.* Paper presented at the Biennial Meeting of the Society for Research in Child Development, Washington, DC.

Atkins, D. C., Baucom, D. H., & Jacobson, N. S. (2001). Understanding infidelity: Correlates in a national random sample. *Journal of Family Psychology, 15*, 735–749.

Atkins, D. C., Yi, J., Baucom, D. H., & Christensen, A. (2005). Infidelity in couples seeking marital therapy. *Journal of Family Psychology, 19*, 470–473.

Atwood, J. D., & Seifer, M. (1997). Extramarital affairs and constructed meanings: A social constructionist therapeutic approach. In J. D. Atwood (Ed.), *Challenging family therapy situations: Perspectives in social construction* (pp. 41–70). New York: Springer.

Banfield, S., & McCabe, M. P. (2001). Extra relationship involvement among women: Are they different from men? *Archives of Sexual Behavior, 30*, 119–142.

Baucom, D. H., Gordon, K. C., Snyder, D. K., Atkins, D.

C., & Christensen, A. (2006). Treating affair couples: Clinical considerations and initial findings. *Journal of Cognitive Psychotherapy, 20*, 375–392.

Baucom, D. H., Shoham, V., Mueser, K. T., Daiuto, A. D., & Stickle, T. R. (1998). Empirically supported couple and family interventions for marital distress and adult mental health problems. *Journal of Consulting and Clinical Psychology, 66*, 53–88.

Beach, S. R., Jouriles, E. N., & O'Leary, K. D. (1985). Extramarital sex: Impact on depression and commitment in couples seeking marital therapy. *Journal of Sex and Marital Psychology, 11*, 99–108.

Betzig, L. (1989). Causes of conjugal dissolution: A cross-cultural study. *Current Anthropology, 30*, 654–676.

Blumstein, P., & Schwatz, P. (1983). *American couples.* New York: William & Morrow.

Brown, E. M. (2001). *Patterns of infidelity and their treatment* (2nd ed.). Ann Arbor, MI: Brunner-Routledge.

Buehler, C., Krishnakumar, A., Stone, G., Anthony, C., Pemberton, S., Gerard, J., et al. (1998). Inter-parental conflict and youth problem behaviors: A two-sample replication study. *Journal of Marriage and the Family, 60*, 119–132.

Buunk, B. (1987). Conditions that promote breakups as a consequence of extradyadic involvements. *Journal of Social and Clinical Psychology, 5*, 271–284.

Calhoun, K. S., & Resick, P. A. (1993). Post-traumatic stress disorder. In D. H. Barlow (Ed.), *Clinical handbook of psychological disorders: A step by step treatment manual* (2nd ed., pp. 48–98). New York: Guilford Press.

Cano, A., & O'Leary, K. D. (2000). Infidelity and separations precipitate major depressive episodes and symptoms of nonspecific depression and anxiety. *Journal of Consulting and Clinical Psychology, 68*, 774–781.

Charny, I. W., & Parnass, S. (1995). The impact of extramarital relationships on the continuation of marriages. *Journal of Sex and Marital Therapy, 21*, 100–115.

Daly, M., & Wilson, M. (1988). Evolutionary social psychology and family homicide. *Science, 242*, 519–524.

Davis, J. A., Smith, T. W., & Marsden, P. V. (2005). *General social surveys, 1972–2004: Cumulative codebook.* Chicago: National Opinion Research Center.

Ehrensaft, M. K., & Vivian, D. (1996). Spouses' reasons for not reporting existing marital aggression as a marital problem. *Journal of Family Psychology, 10*, 443–453.

Enright, R. D., & the Human Development Study Group. (1991). The moral development of forgiveness. In W. Kurtines & J. Gewirtz (Eds.), *Handbook of moral behavior and development* (pp. 123–152). Hillsdale, NJ: Erlbaum.

Epstein, N. B., & Baucom, D. H. (2002). *Enhanced cognitive behavioral therapy for couples: A contextual approach* (pp. 507–515). Washington, DC: American Psychological Association.

Foa, E. B., & Kozak, M. J. (1986). Emotional processing of fear: Exposure to corrective information. *Psychological Bulletin, 99*, 20–35.

Freedman, S. R., & Enright, R. D. (1996). Forgiveness as an intervention goal with incest survivors. *Journal of Consulting and Clinical Psychology, 64,* 983–992.

Glass, S. P. (2002). Couple therapy after the trauma of infidelity. In A. S. Gurman & N. S. Jacobson (Eds.), *Clinical handbook of couple therapy* (3rd ed., pp. 488–507). New York: Guilford Press.

Glass, S. P. (2003). *Not "just friends": Protect your relationship from infidelity and heal the trauma of betrayal.* New York: Free Press.

Glass, S. P., & Wright, T. L. (1985). Sex differences in type of extramarital involvement and marital dissatisfaction. *Sex Roles, 12,* 1101–1120.

Glass, S. P., & Wright, T. L. (1988). Clinical implications of research on extramarital involvement. In R. A. Brown & J. R. Field (Eds.), *Treatment of sexual problems in individual and couples therapy* (pp. 301–346). Costa Mesa, CA: PMA Publishing Corp.

Glass, S. P., & Wright, T. L. (1997). Reconstructing marriages after the trauma of infidelity. In W. K. Halford & H. J. Markman (Eds.), *Clinical handbook of marriage and couples interventions* (pp. 471–507). Hoboken, NJ: Wiley.

Gordon, K. C., & Baucom, D. H. (1998). Understanding betrayals in marriage: A synthesized model of forgiveness. *Family Process, 37,* 425–449.

Gordon, K. C., & Baucom, D. H. (1999). A multitheoretical intervention for promoting recovery from extramarital affairs. *Clinical Psychology: Science and Practice, 6,* 382–399.

Gordon, K. C., & Baucom, D. H. (2003). Forgiveness and marriage: Preliminary support for a measure based on a model of recovery from a marital betrayal. *American Journal of Family Therapy, 31,* 179–199.

Gordon, K. C., Baucom, D. H., & Snyder, D. K. (2000). The use of forgiveness in marital therapy. In M. E. McCullough, K. I. Pargament, & C. E. Thoresen (Eds.), *Forgiveness: Theory, research, and practice* (pp. 203–227). New York: Guilford Press.

Gordon, K. C., Baucom, D. H., & Snyder, D. K. (2004). An integrative intervention for promoting recovery from extramarital affairs. *Journal of Marital and Family Therapy, 30,* 213–231.

Gordon, K. C., Burton, S., & Porter, L. (2004). Predicting the intentions of women in domestic violence shelters to return to partners: Does forgiveness play a role? *Journal of Family Psychology, 18,* 331–338.

Gordon, K. C., Hughes, F. M., Tomcik, N. D., & Litzinger, S. (2006, November). *Widening circles of impact: The role of forgiveness in individual, marital, and family functioning.* Paper presented at the annual meeting of the Association for Behavioral and Cognitive Therapies, Chicago, IL.

Greene, B. L., Lee, R. R., & Lustig, N. (1974). Conscious and unconscious factors in marital infidelity. *Medical Aspects of Human Sexuality, 8,* 97–105.

Hargrave, T. D., & Sells, J. N. (1997). The development of a forgiveness scale. *Journal of Marital and Family Therapy, 23,* 41–62.

Hazan, C., & Shaver, P. R. (1994). Attachment as an organizational framework for research on close relationships. *Psychological Inquiry, 5,* 1–22.

Holeman, V. T. (1998). Effects of forgiveness of perpetrators on marital adjustment of survivors of sexual abuse. *The Family Journal, 6,* 182–188.

Holtzworth-Munroe, A., Marshall, M. A., Meehan, J. C., & Rehman, U. (2003). Physical aggression. In D. K. Snyder & M. A. Whisman (Eds.), *Treating difficult couples: Helping clients with coexisting mental and relationship disorders* (pp. 201–230). New York: Guilford Press.

Janoff-Bulman, R. (1989). Assumptive worlds and the stress of traumatic events: Applications of the schema construct. *Social Cognition, 3,* 113–136.

Janus, S. S., & Janus, C. L. (1993). *The Janus report on sexual behavior.* Oxford, UK: Wiley.

Johnson, S. M. (2004). *The practice of emotionally focused couple therapy* (2nd ed.). New York: Brunner-Routledge.

Katz, J., Street, A., & Arias, I. (1997). Individual differences in self-appraisals and responses to dating violence scenarios. *Violence and Victims, 12,* 265–276.

Laumann, E. O., Gagnon, J. H., Michael, R. T., & Michaels, S. (1994). *The social organization of sexuality: Sexual Practices in the United States.* Chicago: University of Chicago Press.

Lawson, A. (1988). *Adultery: An analysis of love and betrayal.* New York: Basic Books.

Lawson, A., & Samson, C. (1988). Age, gender and adultery. *British Journal of Sociology, 39,* 409–440.

Linehan, M. (1991). *Cognitive-behavioral treatment of borderline personality disorder.* New York: Guilford Press.

Lusterman, D. D. (1997). Repetitive infidelity, womanizing, and Don Juanism. In R. F. Levant & G. R. Brooks (Eds.), *Men and sex: New psychological perspectives* (pp. 84–99). Hoboken, NJ: Wiley.

Lusterman, D. D. (1998). *Infidelity: A survival guide.* Oakland, CA: New Harbinger.

Mackey, W. C., & Immerman, R. S. (2001). Restriction of sexual activity as a partial function of disease avoidance: A cultural response to sexually transmitted diseases. *Cross-Cultural Research, 35,* 400–423.

Makinen, J. A., & Johnson, S. M. (2006). Resolving attachment injuries in couples using emotionally focused therapy: Steps toward forgiveness and reconciliation. *Journal of Consulting and Clinical Psychology, 74,* 1055–1064.

McCann, I. L., Sakheim, D. K., & Abrahamson, D. J. (1988). Trauma and victimization: A model of psychological adaptation. *Counseling Psychologist, 16,* 531–594.

McCullough, M. E., Worthington, E. L., Jr., & Rachal, K. C. (1997). Interpersonal forgiving in close relationships. *Journal of Personality and Social Psychology, 73,* 321–336.

O'Leary, K. D., & Maiuro, R. D. (2001). *Psychological abuse in violent domestic relations.* New York: Springer.

Prager, K. (1997). The intimacy dilemma: A guide for couples therapists. In J. Carlson & L. Sperry (Eds.),

The intimate couple (pp. 109–157). Philadelphia: Brunner/Mazel.

Rathus, J. H., & Feindler, E. L. (2004). *Assessment of partner violence: A handbook for researchers and practitioners.* Washington, DC: American Psychological Association.

Reibstein, J., & Richards, M. P. M. (1993). *Sexual arrangements: Marriage and the temptation of infidelity.* New York: Macmillan.

Resick, P. A., & Calhoun, K. S. (2001). Posttraumatic stress disorder. In D. H. Barlow (Ed.), *Clinical handbook of psychological disorders* (3rd ed., pp. 60–113). New York: Guilford Press.

Scheinkman, M. (2005). Beyond the trauma of betrayal: Reconsidering affairs in couples therapy. *Family Process, 44,* 227–244.

Schneider, J. P. (2002). The new "elephant in the living room": Effects of compulsive cybersex behaviors on the spouse. In A. Cooper (Ed.), *Sex and the Internet: A guidebook for clinicians* (pp. 169–186). New York: Brunner-Routledge.

Seybold, K. S., Hill, P. C., Neumann, J. K., & Chi, D. S. (2001). Physiological and psychological correlates of forgiveness. *Journal of Psychology and Christianity, 20,* 250–259.

Snyder, D. K. (1999). Affective reconstruction in the context of a pluralistic approach to couple therapy. *Clinical Psychology: Science and Practice, 6,* 348–365.

Snyder, D. K., Baucom, D. H., & Gordon, K. C. (2007). *Getting past the affair: How to cope, heal, and move on—together or apart.* New York: Guilford Press.

Snyder, D. K., & Doss, B. D. (2005). Treating infidel-ity: Clinical and ethical directions. *Journal of Clinical Psychology, 61,* 1453–1465.

Snyder, D. K., Gordon, K. C., & Baucom, D. H. (2004). Treating affair couples: Extending the written disclosure paradigm to relationship trauma. *Clinical Psychology: Science and Practice, 11,* 155–159.

Snyder, D. K., & Schneider, W. J. (2002). Affective reconstruction: A pluralistic, developmental approach. In A. S. Gurman & N. S. Jacobson (Eds.), *Clinical handbook of couple therapy* (3rd ed., pp. 151–179). New York: Guilford Press.

Spanier, G. B., & Margolis, R. L. (1983). Marital separation and extramarital sexual behavior. *Journal of Sex Research, 19,* 23–48.

Straus, M. A. (1979). Measuring intrafamily conflict and violence: The Conflict Tactics (CT) Scales. *Journal of Marriage and the Family, 41,* 75–88.

Sweeney, M. M., & Horwitz, A. V. (2001). Infidelity, initiation, and the emotional climate of divorce. *Journal of Health and Social Behavior, 42,* 295–309.

Toussaint, L. L., Williams, D. R., Musick, M. A., & Everson, S. A. (2001). Forgiveness and health: Age differences in a U.S. probability sample. *Journal of Adult Development, 8,* 249–257.

Vaughn, P. (2002). *Help for therapists (and their clients) in dealing with affairs.* La Jolla, CA: Dialogue Press.

Whisman, M. A., Dixon, A. E., & Johnson, B. (1997). Therapists' perspectives of couple problems and treatment issues in couple therapy. *Journal of Family Psychology, 11,* 361–366.

Worthington, E. L. (2005). *Handbook of forgiveness.* New York: Brunner-Routledge.

CHAPTER 15

Separation and Divorce Issues in Couple Therapy

JAY LEBOW

BACKGROUND

A paradoxical aspect of the practice of couple/marital therapy[1] is the frequent presence of divorce as a possible outcome. Many clients enter marital therapy with the explicit purpose of utilizing this venue as a step in the process of leaving their partners, whereas others reach the conclusion that divorce is the best option based at least in part on their lack of success in achieving personal goals for their marriage during treatment. How then does the marital therapist deal with the slippery and controversial slope of this possible outcome, and what can a therapist do to help those who want to divorce do so successfully? This chapter has two purposes related directly to these issues: (1) to examine the ways marital therapists best deal with discussion of divorce during the course of treatment focused on the marriage, and the place of divorce as a possible outcome of marital therapy; and (2) to look at the ways marital therapists can best help those who have decided to divorce to divorce.

DIVORCE IN OUR SOCIETY: FUNCTIONAL VERSUS DYSFUNCTIONAL PATTERNS

Divorce and the wisdom of divorcing remains a highly controversial topic in North America and Western society, one of the markers of the difference between what in American politics are referred to the red states (with socially conservative notions) and blue states (with socially liberal values). Before discussing how this interface about values does, can, or should impact treatment, I begin with a brief review of research about divorce, which mostly is unambiguous. What does the now large body of excellent research about divorce tell us?

For almost everyone experiencing divorce, there are short-term negative consequences. Both children and adults show more role strain, a greater number of behavioral problems, and, in Mavis Hetherington's provocative words, a feeling of this not "being me" (Hetherington & Elmore, 2003; Hetherington & Kelly, 2002, 2003).

After an initial period of 1–2 years, most family members in divorcing families do well and cannot be distinguished from families who did not go through divorce on measures of functioning, symptoms, or happiness (Hetherington & Kelly, 2002).

Over time, rates of problems in those who have experienced divorce in their families remain higher than those who have not, but only marginally higher (Hetherington & Kelly, 2002; Hetherington & Stanley-Hagan, 2000). The majority of children of divorce fall within the normal range on all measures of functioning and symptoms. When writers cite these data, their conclusions often make a stronger statement about their position about divorce than about the impact of divorce. It is true that there are somewhat more frequent problems in children of divorce than in those from intact families, and that the vast majority of these children are well within the normal range (Amato & Booth, 2002; Emery, 2004).

It is crucial to bear in mind that when research involves comparisons of families that experience divorce and those who do not, the comparison group comprises families with happy marriages and those with unhappy marriages. Thus, even the small differences between the rates of difficulty in families experiencing divorce and in those who do not may be inflated, because the comparison is not fully to those who experience marriage difficulty. Said another way, it is hard to sort out how much of what effect stems from divorce and how much stems from simply having marital difficulties. There is no specific evidence that family members who go through divorce do any worse than those who remain in families in which the marriage is unhappy but the parents remain together (Greene, Anderson, Hetherington, Forgatch, & DeGarmo, 2003).

High conflict in marriage is a major risk factor for children in families with marriages that last over time and in divorced families (Grych & Fincham, 1990, 1992; Grych, Fincham, Jouriles, & McDonald, 2000). It is not clear whether high conflict is more deleterious in nuclear or in divorced families. However, it is clear that in both contexts, high conflict is quite deleterious for everyone.

Other factors, beyond whether parents divorce, also have an enormous impact on whether children do well or do poorly in divorce. For example, it appears clear from Hetherington's research that adding too many other life changes (e.g., moving several times, change in financial status, and parental remarriage within a short span) to changes associated with divorce vastly increases children's risk from divorce (Hetherington, 1979;

Hetherington & Clingempeel, 1992; Hetherington & Elmore, 2003). Financial strain, parental depression, and low levels of child monitoring, in addition to going through divorce, increase children's level of vulnerability.

Even though children in divorced families on average do not do worse in life than those who do not experience divorce, such children almost universally describe challenging affective experiences about which they have continuing feelings. When Emery surveyed college students at the University of Virginia about their experiences with divorce in their families (Emery, 2004, 2006), he found that even among these academically successful young people who had gained admission to a prominent university, stories of family life were filled with pain. For example, nearly 50% believed they had a harder childhood than others (compared to 14% among adults whose parents' marriage remained intact), and 28% wondered whether their fathers loved them (compared to 10% among adults whose parents' marriage remained intact). Such statements of painful feeling have also dominated the widely circulated but flawed research of Wallerstein[2] and Marquardt (Emery, 2006; Marquardt, 2005; Wallerstein, Lewis, & Blakeslee, 2002; Wallerstein & Blakeslee, 1989; Wallerstein, Corbin, & Lewis, 1988; Wallerstein & Kelly, 1975, 1980).

Some researchers have identified a group of children that they believe clearly do worse when their parents divorce rather than remain together: children in families where parental unhappiness is not transparent to their children. Researchers such as Amato and Afifi (2006) suggest that because these children lived in low-conflict, benign environments, they would be expected to be like children from happy families were it not for the divorce, that is, overwhelmingly to do well. They also suggest that the sense of loss for these children is great, causing them to be especially vulnerable. However, others (Ahrons & Tanner, 2003) argue against this supposition, because one does not in fact know how their lives would have progressed if their parents had not divorced, especially given that being in an unhappy marriage presents a risk factor for parents' mental health over time.

Protracted conflict over child custody and visitation is especially deleterious for all involved (Emery, 2006; Hetherington & Stanley-Hagan, 2002; Johnston, Walters, & Olesen, 2005; Kelly, 2003b). High levels of parental conflict almost always accompany disputes over child custody and visitation (Johnston & Campbell, 1988b). The child-centered conflicts engendered are particularly upsetting for children (Buchanan, Maccoby, & Dornbusch, 1996; Grych & Fincham, 1999; Johnston, 1993, 1994).

In summary, divorce is painful, but it represents a life challenge rather than necessarily a pathway to difficulty. Most people recover full functioning after a period of time, even though most retain painful memories of that time. The data are ambiguous as to whether divorce is better or worse for adults and children than continuing to live in a family in which unhappily married parents stay together, though indications are that the answer to this question has much to do with the nature of those family lives, that is, whether life is overtly smooth or filled with conflict, anxiety, violence, or depression.

The research also suggests that divorce represents not so much a single event but a developmental process. Families undergo a number of challenges and transitions in the process of adaptation to divorce. The first phase, typically lasting 1 to 2 years postdivorce, is a period of high stress and turmoil. Because most families are more distressed after 1 year than immediately after the divorce, many families feel overwhelmed and discouraged at that time. However, longitudinal research (Hetherington, Cox, & Cox, 1982) indicates a remarkable recovery for most families by the end of the second year. Most families stabilize in 2 years, and most parents and children are functioning well when followed up 6 years later. Still, many families undergo multiple transitions as residences and custody arrangements change over time. When remarriage of one or both partners occurs, other complexities are introduced, some that promote better coping and others that involve further challenges. Nearly two-thirds of women and three-fourths of men remarry after divorce (Weitzman et al., 1992). In most families, divorce and remarriage merge into a continuous process.

Added to these complexities is the ambiguity of norms regarding the degree of involvement between former spouses, between parents and children, and with new partners/stepparents during and after divorce (Ahrons & Rodgers, 1987). Divorce, like other major life transitions, disrupts a family's paradigm, the worldview and basic premises that underlie the family identity and guide its actions. When individuals share unrealistic expectations that the postdivorce family should function like a nondivorced two-parent family, there is a sense of disappointment and deficiency when those fantasies cannot be met (Ahrons & Rodgers, 1987).

Research and clinical experience also suggest that there are better and worse ways of divorcing. The divorce process goes best when there are opportunities for divorcing partners to communicate; when there is a sense of having a chance to work through the problems; when extramarital involvements or marital violence are not part of the picture; when children are not triangulated into the parental conflicts; and when there is an orderly process of making decisions relevant to the divorce. I should add that the interface with the judicial system makes a good deal of difference as well. Situations in which lawyers act in aggressive ways and partners are pushed to reside together for unusually long amounts of time after a decision to divorce often lead to the degeneration of the process.

THE DECISION TO DIVORCE AS AN ASPECT OF COUPLE THERAPY

Probably no issue in couple therapy is as contentious as how to handle the decision to divorce. In couples that enter marital therapy, often at least one person is seriously considering the costs and benefits of divorce as a possible course. Moreover, divorce represents a very special outcome. Although divorce can be taken as obvious evidence of the failure of couple treatment to improve marital satisfaction, it also can be the occasion for one or both partners to feel better and improve individual functioning. Client self-reports of the wisdom and value of this outcome are in most cases divided, with one partner regarding this transition as necessary and helpful, and the other seeing it as a negative outcome.

The prescribed strategies for intervention in the wake of one or both partners stating a desire to divorce vary enormously across couple therapists. However, I first accentuate the commonalities that most couple therapists share in the wake of these issues. All couple therapists strongly support marriage; therefore, they listen carefully to the basis for the decision to divorce and first explore whether there remains any possibility for reconciliation. All good couple therapists also take the wish to divorce seriously and work to establish an empathic connection with both parties in the process of working with this issue.

However, there remains a major divide between couple therapists about the message delivered in the wake of the presentation of a desire to divorce. On one extreme are the self-designated marriage savers and "divorce busters" (Weiner-Davis, 1987, 1992), who suggest that the therapist should strongly side against a decision to divorce or separate. Doherty (1999, 2001) offers a somewhat more tempered version of this position, suggesting that therapists begin with a strong family-centered declaration on the side of marital stability, followed by a focus on reviving the marriage, supporting divorce only if all possible efforts to produce a viable marriage are exhausted. At the other extreme are the writers of popular books such as *Creative Divorce* and *The New Creative Divorce* (Krantzler, 1973; Krantzler & Krantzler, 1999), which support divorce as an acceptable and even growth-enhancing outcome. Ahrons (1994, 2004; Ahrons & Rodgers, 1987) suggests a moderate version of this position, pointing to the differences between those who divorce well and those who do so poorly, and the reality that some individuals' marriages either never worked or lost their viability long ago. Many writers also distinguish between marriages in which divorce occurs early in a childless marriage and those in which divorce occurs later.

Those strongly identified with marriage preservation see therapists and, for that matter, our society as too easily condoning decisions to divorce, whereas those at the opposite pole shudder at the vision of therapists who bring their own moral agenda to clients. Between these poles lie the majority of couple therapists that range along a continuum, but most of whom strongly support marriage yet also see divorce as an option.

There are a few situations for which the specifics of individual circumstances transcend ideology. For example, it is widely regarded that severe marital violence is a circumstance under which divorce is strongly preferable to remaining married.[3] However, in the majority of situations in which one or both partners consider divorce, the shadow of personal values of the therapist is very powerful.

It would be inappropriate to suggest that there are correct or incorrect positions relative to such personal values. However, there is consensus regarding to a both–and position among most marital therapists at this point in supporting marriage but also remaining open to consideration of the life stories and feelings of the partners in treatment. Some marriages clearly appear to be highly likely to remain mired in problems regardless of intervention (Gottman, 1993). When the sorts of marital patterns that have been identified indicate the complete erosion of marital connection, such

as the presence of contempt or stonewalling (Gottman & Notarius, 2000), serious questions must be raised about the viability of the marriage. Furthermore, when one partner unequivocally states that he or she is leaving the marriage, there is little to be gained from anything other than exploring how absolute this feeling is, observing whether it remains over time, and, if this remains the reality, helping the couple and family cope best with divorcing.

ASSESSING READINESS TO DIVORCE

Although discussions about divorce push heavily on therapist values in terms of how to intervene, assessment of the degree to which one or both partners are ready to divorce potentially remains more objective. Typically, the strength of stated beliefs that divorce is the best option provides a clear indication of how close parties are to divorcing. Yet it is important to bear in mind that statements about the possibility of ending the relationship also can represent efforts to exert influence or experience catharsis in people who are, in fact, far from taking this action. Actions that signal the process of disengagement, such as separating, engaging new partners, having serious discussions with divorce attorneys or filing, or separating finances, provide what may be more telling, unobtrusive measures of divorce readiness. So, too, may the frequent presence of those behaviors that, as Gottman (1999) suggests, predict divorce, such as contempt, belligerence, and stonewalling. For those wishing to utilize a self-report instrument to assess readiness to divorce, Weiss and Cerreto (1980) have developed the Marital Status Inventory, which assesses the presence of thoughts and behaviors related to divorcing.

The assessment of readiness to divorce is, of course, only part of the assessment of a couple. This information can be paired with whatever system the therapist has for assessing couple relationships (e.g., those presented in numerous chapters in this volume), allowing each couple to be placed in an informative 2 × 2 matrix of divorce readiness by relationship quality.

WORKING WITH COUPLES WHO HAVE DECIDED TO DIVORCE

Many couples seek therapy to deal explicitly with the process of divorcing; many others remain in a marital therapy that morphs into divorce therapy when one person has decided to leave the relationship. It is a good thing that couples participate in divorce therapy; the differences between couples who divorce well and those who do not are pronounced. In particular, high-conflict divorce is toxic for the mental health of divorcing partners, their children, and the extended family. There are numerous other, high-risk circumstances, such as when children are triangulated into parent conflict, or when a marriage ends with little communication and much unfinished business. This is a time for which few people are prepared, when intervention can make a significant difference.

There are three major methods for intervention with divorcing couples: prevention programs, mediation, and divorce therapy. "Prevention programs" teach about the process of divorce, providing guidelines about what to expect and how best to deal with problems that typically arise, and sometimes also involve the sharing of personal experiences in a group format. A number of evidence-based programs for adults, children, and families experiencing divorce clearly have been demonstrated to have a positive impact on the divorce process and to mitigate potential problems (Braver, Hipke, Ellman, & Sandler, 2004; McKinnon & Wallerstein, 1988; Pedro-Carroll, Nakhnikian, & Montes, 2001; Pedro-Carroll, 2005; Pedro-Carroll, Sutton, & Wyman, 1999; Silliman, Stanley, Coffin, Markman, & Jordan, 2001). Such programs conducted by educators or mental health professionals focus on coparenting and child resilience, and are brief in duration.

"Mediation" involves a formal process of negotiating differences about issues, such as the division of money, child support, child custody, and the postdivorce time with each parent. The typical process involves meetings with each partner and the partners together to define the issues, followed by negotiation sessions that typically are 2 hours in length. Mediators do not have the power to make decisions, only to promote a positive exchange in the process of resolving differences. Mediators do at times, however, provide feedback to third parties about typical arrangements and/or face the likelihood of having their position supported by the Court, if the dispute reached that stage. The success of mediation in promoting positive outcomes in divorce for both parents and children has been well established (Emery, 1999; Emery, Sbarra, & Grover, 2005; Folberg, 1991; Folberg, Milne, & Salem, 2004; Milne & Folberg, 1988). For example, Emery has shown that 75% of couples were able to resolve conflicts over child custody in mediation. As an offshoot of mediation, in many U.S. jurisdictions and in some other countries, a new profession called "parent coordinators" has also recently emerged. Parent coordinators have the ability to arbitrate when mediation fails, thus avoiding the legal process (Kelly, 2003a). As yet, there is no evidence on the impact of these methods, though clinical experience has been favorable.

Divorce therapy differs from prevention and mediation in that therapists are able to engage in the full range of typical intervention strategies in psychotherapies. Whereas prevention programs focus almost exclusively on psychoeducation and mediation focuses on negotiation, divorce therapy adds to these processes the ability to explore the couple relationship and the individual process of the partners. This chapter examines divorce as it is dealt with in psychotherapy. The reader is referred to Pedro-Carroll (2005; Pedro-Carroll & Alpert-Gillis, 1997; Pedro-Carroll, Sandler, & Wolchik, 2005) for a consideration of psychoeducational programs and to Emery (1994) and Folberg and Milne (1988; Folberg et al., 2004; Milne & Folberg, 1988) for a discussion of mediation.

GOAL SETTING

In the territory of possible or probable divorce, goal setting becomes perhaps the crucial aspect of treatment. It is common to have partners with disparate goals occupy different life spaces (e.g., working with the children about the divorce vs. working on the marriage); thus, the negotiation of these goals becomes crucial. Furthermore, the both–and attitude so helpful in much of conjoint therapy often does not work here. Working on the issues of separating lives and on being together are often incompatible.

The negotiation of disparate goals is one of the key skills in divorce therapy. Even if both parties agree about the decision to divorce, it is rare for them to have the same notion of the process and content of the therapy.

When one partner wants a divorce and the other does not, the first phase of treatment focuses on finding a collective focus. The first operation almost invariably involves seeing whether the partner who is ready to divorce will agree to work on the marriage for a time. As an offshoot of this exchange, a compromise may be reached to see whether feelings change over that time, and if they do not change, to proceed with divorce. However, in numerous cases one partner enters treatment fixed in a plan to divorce. When signs of that sort of fixed plan are present, the focus must shift to working with the second party to accept the reality that divorce will occur, given that only one party is required to obtain a divorce.

Negotiation of the content of sessions is much like any other in couple therapy. Each party lists his or her concerns, and an agreed-upon agenda is generated.

STRATEGIES IN DIVORCE THERAPY

My method of practice is an integrative therapy, drawing from a wide range of theories and strategies of intervention adapted to the particular treatment context. I envision creating a treatment contract, building a therapeutic alliance, and forming an assessment as therapy begins as setting the stage for the choice of a set of treatment strategies that is likely to impact the particular problem and life situation of the clients. Within this viewpoint, there is no single, "right" way of approaching particular clients; rather there are ways that are more and less likely to be effective given this set of clients, this problem, and this therapist. Functioning as what Stricker calls the "local clinical scientist" (Stricker & Trierweiler, 1995), strategies are adapted and changed as needed in relation to the acceptability of treatment interventions for the clients and their responses to treatment (Lebow, 1984, 1987, 1997, 2006a). Therapy is seen as drawing from the best evidence available (albeit, today, mostly imperfect evidence) to determine what are likely the most effective paths for intervention (Lebow, 2006b).

In the context of divorce, I have developed an integrative treatment for high-conflict divorce based in the special life situations of these families (Lebow, 2003, 2005). Below I review both the high- and low-conflict core intervention strategies most relevant to the treatment of divorcing families, which I combine in my integrative therapy.

Just as there is no single way to divorce, there is no single way to do divorce therapy. The strategies for intervention must have an ecological fit with the system at hand. Some couples want merely to use treatment to make for a fragile peace, so that divorce can occur with the least conflict possible; others enter with specific goals, such as working with particular high-risk children, and still others look to this couple therapy as a format to take a deeper look at their life and relationship, hoping to use it to achieve the best possible end-

ing and learning that will be useful in the future. Although most therapists (including myself) view the work involved in exploring the deeper feelings as a better way to leave what was thought to be a lifelong relationship, partners' wishes to keep treatment simple and direct are common and must be taken seriously.

The family context of the divorce also makes a considerable difference in terms of the goals of therapy. Partners without children typically disconnect and have almost no further contact after divorce, whereas those with children typically have some sort of partnership about the children over many years. This makes the tasks of therapies with these two types of couples quite different.

Treatment must vary with the ecology of the couple's relationship. As Carl Whitaker highlighted long ago (Whitaker & Miller, 1969), feelings of emotional connection do not cease just because a relationship ends. Most people can call up feelings toward former partners long after divorcing, even toward partners they have not seen for many years. In low-conflict situations in which the desire to divorce is mutual, and cooperation remains high and may even involve a positive postdivorce connection (Ahrons, 1994), the possibilities are quite different from those in a high-conflict divorce in which minimizing conflict and achieving parallel lives may be the only achievable goal (Johnston, 2005).

What follows is a generic list of useful strategies from which therapists can draw from and adapt to the case a hand in working with divorcing couples. For most of these operations, variations for high- and low-conflict divorce are explicated.

Establishing the Therapeutic Contract

The establishment of a clear therapeutic contract is essential in any psychotherapy (Orlinsky & Howard, 1987), but clarity about that contract is even more crucial in this clinical context. As already noted, partners may have very different goals, with one thinking of "marriage therapy" to resuscitate a relationship, and the other of "divorce therapy" to end it. Furthermore, a client may often bring inappropriate frames for this work, believing the therapist will act as a moral judge who will cajole and/or shame the partner into moving to the client's position, or even act as custody evaluator or parent coordinator. And in high-conflict cases, the involvement of lawyers and the Court in almost all aspects of clients' lives adds even greater importance to a clear, agreed-upon contract.

Confidentiality is an expectation in this therapy, as in other mental health treatment. However, special constraints on confidentiality should clearly be recognized. Given the life crisis, partners often tend to discuss therapy sessions with friends and family, and frequently no rule or agreement can constrain this. In high-conflict divorce in which a dispute over child custody or time to be spent with children is at issue, the couple may also have no real option but to address issues in the context of the therapy, knowing that the therapist will possibly share this information with a custody evaluator and/or the Court (Gould, 1998). Although each individual has the right to insist on confidentiality, there are powerful pressures in the name of the best interest of children in these contexts to share information (Greenberg & Gould, 2001). There also are times when the leverage of informing the Court is essential to maintaining both parties' participation and cooperation in the treatment (Lebow, 2005).

Establishing a Therapeutic Alliance

Establishing a working alliance is an essential aspect of any couple therapy. In the context of divorce therapy, especially when partners' goals differ, establishing such an alliance is difficult. Partners lack what Pinsof calls a "within system" alliance with each other (Knobloch-Fedders, Pinsof, & Mann, 2004), making the formation of a working alliance connecting the partners and the therapist much more difficult. Success in building a good working alliance is an art given the virtual certainty that partners see the issues quite differently. The principal ingredients in most cases lie in conveying a nonjudgmental connection with each partner and creating a holding environment that allows a sense of safety in which to share feelings (also, intervention by the therapist to protect therapy sessions from becoming pathogenic). Given the stories of victim and victimizer, and the frequent presence of questionable behavior on the part of at least one party (e.g., extramarital involvements or triangulation of children into marital disputes) that often are active in divorcing couples, ruptures of alliances are frequent. Thus, the repair of such ruptures is an essential part of most divorce therapy.

Psychoeducation

Psychoeducation about divorce, and about better and worse ways of divorcing, a cornerstone of most

intervention in divorce, constitutes the essence of most prevention programs and is central in divorce therapy and divorce mediation as well. Although everyone knows someone who has divorced, inaccurate information proliferates. Furthermore, the emotional pulls of being in the process of divorce are powerful and can block out adequate consideration of balanced information. For example, the parent who sees his or her child being upset about a transition between households in the early stages of divorce, a very normal reaction among children, frequently interprets the child's reaction as being about the behavior of the other parent (thus, he or she may look to minimize the time the child spends with the other parent) instead of recognizing this as normal development.

One focus of psychoeducation is on the range of feelings and behaviors that typify families going through divorce. Hetherington (1999) succinctly described a core aspect of divorce for divorcing partners as being what she termed the "not me" experience, the feeling that "I am not feeling or acting in the usual way I experience myself." Divorce and separation is a time of numerous overlapping changes not only in the ending of what is the core anchoring relationship in our culture, but also in changes in living arrangements, finances, daily routines, relationships with extended family (some of whom technically are no longer family), and innumerable other factors. Understanding that such feelings of disequilibrium are typical and do, for most people, pass over a period of six months to two years helps promote a sense of balance.

A second important focus of psychoeducation with couples who have children centers on the typical reactions of children. Perhaps most crucial here is to deal with the common mythology about the inevitable damage inflicted on children by divorce. Such research (Hetherington & Elmore, 2003) shows that most children who experience the divorce of their parents cope and do not develop psychopathology or social–emotional difficulties. This same research also shows, however, that there is a higher risk (typically about double) for the development of problems in children in divorcing families compared to those in families where the parents do not divorce (Amato, 2003; Hetherington & Elmore, 2003), and that children almost invariably have strong feelings and considerable pain about their parents' divorce. Therefore, the most useful psychoeducational message orients parents to children's feelings and how to communicate about those feelings, helping them understand the likely short-term impact on their children and monitor for the emergence of problems, yet ultimately remaining hopeful about children's resilience in the wake of this life stress.

Couples in divorce therapy typically look for professional input about how to deal with their children relative to the divorce. Although suggested guidelines for parents vary with the situation (e.g., high- and low-conflict families differ in the advisability of having family meetings to discuss the divorce), some clearly transcendent principles are broadly applicable.

Perhaps foremost is avoiding persistent, acrimonious conflict in the presence of or over the children and/or setting up triangles in which they are involved. Another guideline is to maintain as much stability in the children's lives as possible. Considerable research has shown that multiple changes increase risk for children (Hetherington & Kelly, 2003). A plan for a stepwise process of absorbing change is preferable to having a child suddenly find him- or herself in a remarriage family in a new house and school.

Finding good ways to communicate about the divorce to children and to discuss feelings also makes a difference. It is crucial for parents to grasp that children process the concept of divorce through the lens of their developing understandings, and that explanations must take into account the developmental stage of the children. Because children often tend to blame themselves for the divorce of parents and fear a rupture in their connection with one or both parents, it is helpful for parents to reassure children that the parents are not divorcing because of them, and that the future involves the parents not being together, not a separation between parents and children. It should be added that children ultimately tend to become as upset about parents' denial that life is changing as they are about their overreactions. Messages that minimize anything major happening fly in the face of the obvious understanding that close relationships are in the process of changing. The best communication both empathizes and reassures.

Another focus of psychoeducation is about typical feelings that partners have toward soon-to-be former partners. The task involved in divorce is unique among human challenges: to disconnect from the person to whom one formed (at least at one time) a primary bond. Feelings such as anger and contempt are helpful in this radical act of excising such a core attachment, yet such feelings, especially when accompanied by hostile action, readily lead to a symmetrical sequence of escalating conflict that is bad for everyone. This translates into messages in therapy that promote the exploration of feelings and disengagement, while also monitoring and intervening to prevent what look to be the establishment of fixed symmetrical conflicts.

Negotiation

Negotiation, which represents another set of core competencies for successful divorce, not only is the central ingredient in mediation but it is also an aspect of divorce therapies. The challenges in negotiation are clear. Partners who typically have not negotiated well in marriage are now called upon to settle many issues, such as time with children after divorce.

Mediators offer highly structured processes for negotiation. In a typical mediation, each partner first meets alone with the mediator, stating his or her view of the issues to be negotiated and hopes for the outcome. Mediation then involves moving through the list of differences, typically beginning with the ones most readily amenable to solution. Custody and residence arrangements for children, and division of money and property (including child support and/or maintenance) are most often the focus of mediation. Mediation is done with complete confidentiality that, if successful, leads to a document that spells out the results of the mediation and is then passed on to attorneys to re-draft as a legal document. Mediators are neutral on matters of divorce, though they do offer information about common guidelines that are accepted by the Court in a geographic area and feedback to clients whose positions are not in keeping with typical guidelines. The results of studies of mediation show that three out of four couples heading toward legal conflicts reach working arrangements in mediation (Emery, 1994, 1995; Emery et al., 2005; Folberg, 1991; Folberg et al., 2004).

The application of negotiation principles in the therapy room mirrors much of what I have described about mediation. However, therapists typically look to do more than just reach a working agreement. Therapists teach partners negotiation skills that they hope clients can employ in future negotiations (an irony of the process of negotiating a divorce decree is that, for most parties, negotiation about matters must continue over time lest one be left with an arrangement appropriate for young children, with no adaptation to the current age of the children).

Establishing Reliable, Rule-Driven Methods of Communication and Good-Enough Coordination

As partners begin to divorce, ground rules for their life as a couple change. It is essential that one of the first matters to be negotiated be these ground rules: What are the expectations over the short run about such matters in terms of other partners, financial responsibilities, time together, and communication? If anything, establishing such ground rules through negotiation is even more important when partners differ in their attitudes toward the impending divorce.

When couples have children, communication has to transcend the time of the divorce or the divorce therapy. In low-conflict situations, this may merely involve reviewing possible formats and deciding on a structure for communicating. However, in high-conflict situations or when there is a high level of disengagement, a crucial aspect of the treatment is being able to build reliable and agreed-upon methods of communication and coordination.

The working expectation in high-conflict cases is for the households to function independently, with only a minimum of communication and coordination, except in those special circumstances that necessitate coordination. In this context, it is useful to teach and practice a speaker–listener technique involving only a few crisply delivered, rule-governed exchanges (Renick, Blumberg, & Markman, 1992). Too much communication often is as risky in these families as too little, easily degenerating into off-subject fights that frequently involve children. When differences between households present special difficulties (e.g., about radical differences in family rules), or when children present with issues that render coordination imperative (as in diabetes or attention deficit disorder), the therapist aims to create just enough coordination for children to go on with their lives successfully.

Disengagement Skills and Anger Management

In high-conflict situations, the ability to disengage is as important as the ability to engage. Intrusive behavior is often justified as only an attempt to communicate about important matters. Anger management skills training is crucial in high-conflict divorce. In such high-conflict situations, clients are taught skills to respectfully disengage from conflict, such as ways of responding to challenging behaviors and statements. Anger management may involve learning to control indirect forms of provocation, such as passive–aggressive action, as well as angry outbursts. The therapist models and role-plays conflict situations and helps clients practice these skills. Often, achieving these ends requires not only behavioral practice but also a focus on attributions, emotions, and individual dynamics (see below).

Reattribution and Narrative Change

Negative attribution plays an essential role in most couples' divorces, and is best regarded as simply a part of creating the distance needed to leave a partner. However, there are often times when such attributions extend well beyond a simple distancing and come to be an essential part of intractable conflict. In such cases, each parent comes to view the actions of the other through a negative filter, in which problematic actions by one parent are invariably viewed as evidence of character flaws and/or hostile action, whereas constructive behavior is seen as disingenuous or transitory. In one example, a mother, faced with evidence that her separated spouse had become abstinent in the use of alcohol and a faithful attendee of Alcoholics Anonymous, attributed these changes to his desire to win his court case, and remained convinced that the alcoholic behavior would return as soon as the court proceeding was completed. Children, extended family, and friends in high-conflict cases often easily become caught up in similar patterns of selective attribution (Johnston & Campbell, 1988).

Integrative therapy with these high-conflict cases draws on techniques from cognitive (Beck & Freeman, 1990) and narrative therapies (Combs & Freedman, 1990) to create new ways of thinking about the problems that are occurring. For example, when parents see their children's upset as a direct function of the other parent's behavior, but this interpretation does not appear to be based in actual events, the therapist frames a new narrative that emphasizes other sources for the distress, such as children's powerful feelings about separation, the natural difficulties in learning to live in two households, or memories of old events. The therapist actively questions "irrational" beliefs and works to build new narratives that are neither blaming nor destructive. Such a reattribution is not therapeutic if the parent in question continues to present dangers for the children; in that case, the focus must be on helping that parent to become less dangerous and the other parent and children to differentiate between behaviors the present threats and those that do not.

Catharsis

Divorcing couples typically feel traumatized and injured. Therapy can be a safe place to share such strong feeling. Such sharing can have great benefit. For example, when one's partner is leaving for another relationship, the "left" partner often is benefited by sharing feelings that are witnessed by the therapist. When a partner has not been able to express his or her feeling about divorce, that expression may be a key event in his or her working through feelings about the divorce. Other couples work through their grief by expressing their sadness, showing that they can still connect around that, if around little else.

However, I must also highlight that such a collective catharsis may or may not be helpful, depending on the couple. In high-conflict couples, such shared feelings often devolve into conflict and despair. In such couples, catharsis is better reserved for separate, individual sessions (with a goal of expressing feeling there, so that less such expression is directed toward the partner) or in individual therapy with another therapist whose agenda at least in part is to express and master feelings of hurt and anger.

Resolving Past Conflicts

This is a time of ending the story of a couple's life together. In the best of circumstances, couples can fully experience their history together, and the decision to part in the wake of that history. Of course, this expectation is beyond the capability of most partners at a time of such powerful feeling, but for those who can revisit the whole of their relationship, there is the possibility of deconstructing the problems and using this forum at least to heal as individuals.

Exploring Individual Issues

Addressing past histories of the partners and their internal conflicts and processes represents a complicated territory in divorce couple therapy. Few clients enter such a therapy looking to do this kind of exploration; other issues predominate.[4] Furthermore, in high-conflict situations and many other

variations on the demise of a marriage, the context of couple therapy is not likely to be a safe place for such exploration.

Having said this, the transition of divorce is a time in which reflection about self is central; and the ability to explore what this divorce means often is a crucial aspect of therapy at this time. In many divorces, it may be that only work at this level actually impacts on the strong feelings invoked. At its most cooperative and profound, therapy can focus on how the couple reached this point and what each partner contributed to the demise of the marriage. Such insights can then be the focus of later exploration, in and out of therapy, of the ramifications and resolution of these feelings.

In most cases, such exploration of "deeper" individual feelings about self and the meanings of life events best occurs in a concurrent individual therapy. In some cases, the couple therapist can utilize a limited number of individual client sessions to focus on the most powerful of such issues that clearly constrain the progress of the therapy.

Working with Children

Divorce is an event that affects not only the couple but also the family. It is common, but unwise, to separate couple divorce therapy from divorce therapy involving children. There are a number of ways that the needs of children can be reflected in couple divorce therapy: They may be brought directly into sessions; their parents may work with them, with coaching from the therapist; or a collaborative relationship may be established with another therapist who sees the whole family. However, it is essential to emphasize that children are very much part of most divorcing systems, whatever the format, and whether present or not, they are inevitably affected by and a part of divorce therapy.

The need to involve children directly is greater in high-conflict situations or when the children themselves manifest strong signs of problems in relation to the divorce. In these instances, expanding the sessions to include the children in family therapy and/or individual child therapy is clearly indicated.

Building Parent–Child Understandings

High parental conflict that focuses on children is sometimes an associated result or product of problematic relationships between parents and children. In these instances, family sessions with the therapist or a colleague involving parents and children can best promote good parenting and the parent–child connection, thereby reducing levels of interparental conflict. In cases of high levels of parent–child conflict, meetings between parent and child focus on rebuilding their bond and reducing the level of conflict. Such meetings also may focus on helping to structure crisp boundaries that limit conversations about cross-household conflict and reduce alienating behaviors (Kelly & Johnston, 2001).

Working with Extended Family

The families and new partners of parents often are strongly affected by and influence the level of conflict in divorce (Johnston & Campbell, 1988). In general, it is important to keep in mind the systemic understanding that divorce affects and is affected by extended family, not just the partners. In high-conflict situations these effects may be so pronounced that involvement of extended family in treatment may be necessary. Such involvement is most beneficial when partners who are subject to conscious or unconscious pressure from families to remain in conflict are unable to deal with such pressures, and when family members are able to have a calming effect on the conflict.

Combining Strategies in Treatment

Combining the strategies I have described with divorcing couples is the art of working with these cases. Divorcing couples are alike only in that they are getting divorced; they come to treatment as very different people and with a wide array of issues, difficulties at various systemic levels, and vast differences in the acceptability of various kinds of intervention. Thus, treatment plans vary enormously with reference to the strategies and when they are utilized in treatment.

However, a few generalizations are possible. Almost all couples benefit from some psychoeducation and from the generation of behavioral agreements. In high-conflict only situations, strategies at the behavioral and structural end of the spectrum may be possible. Anger management, based in a combination of emotion-focused and cognitive strategies, is an essential ingredient in treatment of these high-conflict cases. In more psychologically minded couples who want to mourn the loss of their relationship and learn from it, strategies that access feeling, emotion, and insight are both possible and preferable.

SPECIAL CHALLENGES AND ARRANGEMENTS

Separation as a Treatment Option

Some therapists, such as Lee Raffel (1999) in a recent trade book, proactively advocate a controlled separation as an option. These therapists argue that distance allows more thoughtful consideration of the advantages and disadvantages of divorce. However, this solution must also be considered in the light of the fact that the vast majority of couples who separate get a divorce. Because this possibility is extremely high, this solution as a therapist-suggested intervention is best reserved for couples who are in the midst of a cascade of negative feeling and are initiating divorce, and for whom a bit more contemplation time might help.

Of course, whatever the wishes of the therapist, many couples do separate. When they do, clearly established rules and expectations for the separation becomes a crucial task early in treatment. At this time, it is easy for one party to see him- or herself as mostly divorced, while the other sees him- or herself as mostly married. Ground rules for seeing one another, dating others, communication, the handling of money, time with children, and participation in treatment are crucial to easing this painful time and allowing some chance for reconciliation.

Difficulties over Child Custody and Visitation

Conflicts over child custody and visitation are among the most pathogenic situations for families. There is a great deal of discord. The family structure is unclear. Children are triangulated between parents, and others (including family, friends, and lawyers) readily become involved in these complex disputes. This subset of divorcing parents (estimated at 5–10%) remains mired in intractable conflict. For these high-conflict families an intensive strategy is necessary. Typical methods of therapy, and the mental health treatment and judicial systems, such as unmitigated support and uncoordinated efforts at helping, become iatrogenic in these cases.

A number of adaptations in treatment that need to be made in these cases are discussed in greater detail elsewhere (Lebow, 2003, 2005). Most important are those concerned with the coordination with other mental health and the judicial system, and with setting goals for a good-enough parent system, with little contact between the parents.

Leverage with the court is essential in these cases. Often clients are in treatment primarily because of a desire to make a good impression in court or to respond to the court's orders. The court can and typically does make it very difficult not to engage in or cooperate with treatment. This, in turn, leads to adaptations in the therapy contract with these cases. Clarity about the kinds of information that are shared is essential, as is the signing of appropriate releases for sharing information. The contract calls for confidentiality to be maintained in relation to others, outside the legal system, as it would in other cases, with the understanding that a special relationship will be established with the court. The contract also specifies that the general level of client cooperation will be reported to the court and attorneys, and that there will be more specific sharing with the attorney for the children (if there is one) about the status of the therapy and court case, and with each adult client and his or her own attorney (there is no sharing about one parent with the other parent's attorney).

A second crucial aspect of these cases is coordination with attorneys and mental health treatment providers. Such coordination is preferable in all cases, but here negative effects abound whenever there is a lack of coordination. It is not atypical for an individual therapist involved in treating one partner to become convinced of the aggressive nature of the behavior of his or her client's partner and to support behavior that to the couple therapist looks provocative and destructive.

The other crucial difference is the need to set realistic, attainable goals. In these systems, it is rare that conflicts are ever actually resolved. Goals of distance between parents, minimal communication, and maintenance of quiet mutual dislike are most achievable. Achieving even these ends requires much change at many levels and the use of a variety of the treatment strategies described earlier (also see the case illustration at the end of this chapter).

The Interface between Divorce Therapy and the Judicial System

Divorce occurs in various venues, one of which is the legal system. Therefore, the interface with the legal system is significant, particularly when legal matters over child custody or money become intense or stalled. The adversarial context of much of the judicial system provides endless opportunities for confrontations in pleadings, subpoenas, depositions, and court appearances, frequently engendering conflict. Furthermore, what transpires on these occasions becomes evidence for negative attribution. In the context of interviews with judges and attorneys, children also can become highly polarized about their best interests. Although attorneys and judges often do intervene to mitigate conflict, such measures are frequently met with resistance, sometimes even leading to parents' engagement of new attorneys or petitioning for a change in judges.

In my integrative therapy for high-conflict divorce, therapists work closely with lawyers and judges to understand what is transpiring within the judicial process and help the court understand the therapy process. By working in concert with the judicial system, the therapist can anticipate court appearances and develop ways of dealing with these events to minimize trauma that may occur around court appearances. Attorneys for the children, in particular, typically welcome such coordination and are prepared to intervene actively to support the therapy process. Attorneys for the parents and the court frequently are also prepared to provide such support.

Of course, utilizing the leverage of the court has risks. Biases from countertransference with clients (particularly those who are frustrating in treatment) may readily affect and color reporting to the court. Furthermore, such reports, even with the best of communication, entail risk for inaccurate transmission in the therapist–attorneys and court–clients pathway; this readily can produce alliance ruptures in which the accuracy of information or meanings conveyed are questioned. And there also are other risks to the therapeutic alliance. The presence of such feedback can engender overt cooperation on the part of one or both partners, coupled with covert hostility, or at times a run-away, symmetrical escalation of conflict between the therapist and one partner.

Yet such leverage is almost always needed in high-conflict cases. Greenberg and Gould (2001) have nicely commented on the important role of what they term the "treating expert," who interfaces with the judicial system in these cases, serving both the judicial system and the treatment. The value of transmitting such information in writing, with clear, concise terminology, cannot be underestimated. It also is essential for clients to know the information being transmitted about them and to understand as fully as possible to whom the information is being transmitted. Some lawyers clearly use such information better than others. As a rule of thumb, such sharing is far easier when dealing with attorneys for children or with the court, and riskier with attorneys for the partners.

Residing in the Same House

One of the most problematic situations encountered in divorce therapy occurs when a couple shares a single household over a lengthy period of time, while in the active process of divorcing. As Gottman (1999) suggests, so much of the success of couples in relationship depends on positive sentiment override. These life situations lack positive sentiment override, and there are lots of problems to process. Yet the legal system often makes it next to impossible to alter such a situation, and lawyers frequently advise not leaving the marital home until matters of money and child custody are resolved. In such instances, even the most motivated couples typically wear down and conflict ensues.

Such situations call for clear negotiation of rules and roles. When conflict is high, it is best that ground rules divide time as if the partners do not live together, with time with children and other responsibilities clearly specified and contact between the partners kept to a minimum.

Violence

When one or both partners present with histories of violence, special measures must be taken to minimize contact between the parents, in and out of sessions. In such cases, conjoint meetings may be contraindicated. It is important to bear in mind that divorce is often a time when even persons with no history of violence engage in violent confrontations, and that rates of marital violence are typically underreported (Feldbau-Kohn, Schumacher, & O'Leary, 2000). In high-conflict treatment that involves child custody disputes, the therapist also works with the court to ensure the safety of children in at-risk situations.

The Possible Transition from Couple Therapy to Individual Treatment in Cases Ending in Divorce

When couple therapy ends in divorce, what is the responsibility of the couple therapist to the respective partners? This question represents one of the most complex ethical issues confronting the couple therapist.

From the Olympian heights of most theories of couple therapy, the couple therapist is the therapist to the couple system, with coequal re-

sponsibilities to both partners. Based in this well-considered viewpoint, the couple therapist should remain the therapist to the couple, regardless of how the couple relationship develops or whether both partners are willing to remain in couple therapy, therefore referring partners to someone else for individual therapy as needed. In this way, triangulation is kept to a minimum, and the alliances remain balanced if the couple chooses to return to treatment.

Yet when divorce ensues, a vicissitude of situations and feelings may be launched that at times renders such a decision clinically questionable. For example, when one partner abandons the other and the therapy, by being unwilling to continue to see the abandoned partner, the couple therapist leaves that partner subject to a second abandonment by the therapist—a decision that cannot feel "therapeutic" and usually is not. Indeed, some partners even enter couple therapy with a covert agenda, so that their at-risk partner is engaged with a therapist when the bad news comes. Such situations call for something more than simple, absolute boundaries around the transition from couple to individual therapy. The subsequent work in individual therapy often turns out to be quite special, because the therapist has been witness to a major life trauma and has seen the real-life relationship.

Having said this, it is essential to add that not all couple therapists would agree with the wisdom of making such a transition. Many do not see clients in individual therapy after couple therapy in any situation. Additionally, I cannot state too strongly that even for those open to making such a decision to continue with a partner in individual therapy, this transition should only occur with a full consideration of the ethics of the situation. An abandoning partner also has feelings and an alliance with the therapist. It is always wise to obtain the partner's consent to this transition before making it. It also is essential for the therapist to convey a sense of choice as to who the client will see in individual therapy, by helping the client consider alternative care providers: The therapist must carefully consider whether he or she is considering this transition because of the client's needs or his or her own needs, financial or emotional. This transition is ripe with opportunities for transference and countertransference (particularly insofar as the demise of the marriage may be seen as the therapist's failure), and such potential transferences and countertransferences need to be examined carefully. And a final consideration is that couple and individual therapies differ in their formats and assumptions, and the transition always requires some reorientation.

CURATIVE FACTORS/MECHANISMS OF CHANGE

Curative factors in all of these cases depend on the therapist establishing an alliance to be able to process heightened emotion and addressing the numerous tasks of this time of life. The simpler strategies of intervention, skills development, psychoeducation, and promoting positive exchange are useful in every case. The other strategies I have described are invoked as suggested in the assessment and in the feedback that occurs when attempting various intervention strategies. The success of these intervention strategies often depends on the willingness of the parties to engage fully in therapy rather than merely stay with the more superficial aspects of divorce negotiation. In high-conflict situations, success almost invariably involves some shift (often in the client's narrative about his or her partner, and clearly with some emotional change) that allows the anger and hurt to be processed enough to allow other considerations, such as coparenting, to move to the foreground.

TREATMENT APPLICABILITY/EMPIRICAL SUPPORT

Perhaps due to a climate that renders government funding of research on divorce virtually nonexistent, to date there have been no studies of the impact of divorce therapy. Research on psychoeducation in prevention programs (Pedro-Carroll, 2005) and mediation (Beck, Sales, & Emery, 2004) indicate that when there is research on at least some of the strategies described here, that research does show an impact. For the present, all we can do is note that clients, judges, and lawyers often come to regard divorce therapy as essential, and marital therapy often is the key ingredient in avoiding divorce.

CASE ILLUSTRATION: HIGH-CONFLICT DIVORCE WITH CONFLICTS OVER CHILD CUSTODY

Margaret and Tony had a great deal of conflict throughout their 15-year marriage. Margaret saw Tony as selfish, leaving her with most of the house-hold tasks, in addition to her job. Tony felt that Margaret was too angry and critical, and he frequently complained about the low level of sexuality in their marriage. After many fierce confrontations, each partner became convinced that divorce was the only acceptable option. Margaret had filed for divorce, but 9 months passed in which there had been very little progress toward a divorce, with each partner remaining in the martial home. Litigation was moving slowly through the court, and no determination had been made as to custody or residence for their children: Ron, age 12, and Sandra, age 10. Each parent had filed to be custodial parent and to have his or her home be the primary residence for the children.

Therapy was initiated at the suggestion of the attorney for their children in the divorce. Because the couple had continued to reside in the marital home together, there had been frequent arguments that verged on getting out of control. Although there was no marital violence, these arguments included a great deal of name-calling and yelling, and often ended with one partner withdrawing and the other pursuing that partner through the house to continue the argument. Many of these arguments centered on Margaret's concern about Tony's permissive and passive way of parenting the children.

With my input, a structured court order mandated the participation of the parents, as well as some involvement of the children, in therapy. Because participation in therapy was a central concern of the court, as in many of these cases, all parties were fully cooperative with scheduling sessions once the order was entered, even though they had not engaged in any previous therapy.

I began the therapy with individual meetings with Tony and with Margaret. During these meetings, I listened to each partner's narrative about the events and outlined the therapeutic contract. All the parties would be involved in treatment. A schedule for the first few meetings was agreed to, and I let them know about how the plan was likely to evolve over time. I described the ways information would be shared with the attorney for the children, their attorneys, and the court, and had the parents sign appropriate releases for this sharing of information. I also clearly explained the focused task for our sessions. This was not to be a child custody evaluation in the form of a report, in which I made recommendations to the court for how custody and residence were to be shared.

Instead, our goals would focus on finding ways to reduce the conflict and make the present situation more viable for everyone, whether or not we (or they) could resolve the larger issues about child custody.

My primary goals in these initial meetings were to build an alliance with each of the parties and to assess problems. It was strikingly easy to build a therapeutic alliance with both Margaret and Tony (always a positive sign in cases like this). Both were very frustrated with their present circumstance and saw therapy as a place to vent their feelings and to gain support for their view of the conflict. Both Margaret and Tony were in the precontemplative stage in assessing their roles in creating and maintaining the problem, but each partner was open to participating in therapy sessions. The children were also cooperative in a session I had with them by themselves. Both Ron and Sandra indicated that they simply did not like the conflict and wanted it to end.

My initial assessment was that this couple was clearly on the way to divorce. Neither partner had any desire to consider staying married and had held to these positions over several months. Clearly, the task was to help the couple divorce, reduce the level of conflict, and arrive at a postdivorce working arrangement. Both Tony and Margaret were experiencing a profound sense of loss, anger, and betrayal about the end of their relationship and about the escalating conflict.

After these initial sessions, I felt I had enough information to form an initial assessment that became the basis for the creation of a set of proximate and ultimate goals, and a specific treatment plan for this family. At the systems level, there was a need to calm the frequent crises and break the circular chains of accusation and counteraccusation that were being unleashed. In turn, this depended on being able to create mutual understanding about the handling of this phase of life and to begin preparing for the next phase, during which time with and responsibility for the children would need to be divided. Both parents would need to learn to control their anger, and we would need to negotiate arrangements involving them and their children. To make this goal feasible, Tony's parenting skill would need to develop further, and both parents would need to establish good-enough communication about these issues. Given the agenda, I decided that the work would principally involve Tony and Margaret. A few sessions would be scheduled to help the children cope

with being in the presence of these conflicts, but the major thrust of the work would be to reduce the conflict.

Although the first meeting between the parents evolved as one might expect, with both partners arguing their positions and not much real communication, there did seem to be some signs for hope. Each partner could see that the arguments in the home had a negative impact on everyone, especially the children. Both partners seemed very interested in the welfare of their children, notwithstanding their argument about how best to parent.

Therefore, I suggested a first goal of reducing the conflict in the home, a problem that everyone seemed to identify (even though Tony and Margaret each blamed the other for the conflicts). I explained how easy it was to have such conflicts in their cohabiting arrangement and the problem of symmetrical escalation, in which each party blames the other for conflict. I suggested some simple behavioral deescalation steps, so that either partner would be able to suggest a time-out at any point in a discussion. Over two sessions, we also created a plan for where and how they would discuss issues that emerged, so that, ideally, they would have a structure for discussion and help available when they needed it.

Remarkably, this alone had an immediate effect on the frequency and destructiveness of their arguments. It seemed that the behavioral steps I suggested, coupled with the frame that blamed neither partner for the problem but allowed each of them to feel understood for their position, freed them up immeasurably. We followed up with my having a meeting with each partner alone to discuss anger management techniques. Although we could have been discussed these techniques in conjoint sessions, the separate meetings allowed each partner to speak freely, without the specter of raising the level of conflict, and to explore the cognitions and narratives each had about the other. In this work, I did not seek to change how they experienced each other, but instead just focused on how easy it was to adopt the worst view of each other. With each, I combined working on self-talk about the other, and focusing on self-regulation and self-soothing. This led to a further reduction in the frequency of arguments.

With the situation calmer, the sessions moved toward negotiate about parenting and parenting styles. We were able to develop a set of principles for how the each parent would be involved with the children during the other parent's designated parenting time in the home, which had already been set by the court. Although setting such boundaries in a divorcing couple living together presents challenges (e.g., when one child has math homework and the parent who is not the math expert is the designated parent), establishing such ground rules mostly worked and helped a good deal. I also moved the focus to Margaret and Tony both learning to live with their differences in parenting styles. This led to discussion of the parts of parenting that each partner saw as essential. In these discussions, Margaret and Tony were able to identify a number of aspects of parenting they agreed about, such as the importance of doing homework, and they negotiated other aspects that they considered essential, such as when the children came home at night.

A couple of additional individual sessions with each partner focused on building acceptance of the reality that Tony and Margaret differed (and would always differ) in some significant ways. I also was able to engage Tony in a discussion of his parenting. With the conflict reduced and with my setting the frame that he was a good, well-intentioned parent who needed to learn a bit more about parenting, he was able to engage about ways he could improve as a parent, such as learning to set better limits. The changes that evolved led Margaret to feel more comfortable with Tony's parenting.

With a new spirit of cooperation, the couple began to talk in sessions about how they might divide parenting time after the divorce. Preliminary discussions seemed positive, and the partners had meetings with their attorneys in which they negotiated a joint parenting agreement with joint custody and the children spending 5 out of 7 days with their mother. In our sessions, we developed a plan for them to support each other in parenting and communicate about the children when necessary.

This led to Tony moving out of the marital home. At the end of therapy, Tony and Margaret still had a good deal of negative feeling toward one another. We had not touched the reservoir of bad feeling that developed over years of marriage. However, we had developed a good-enough way of resolving differences, achieved a successful separation of their homes, and a good-enough method of communicating. This allowed Tony and Margaret and their children to go on with their lives, without the specter of ongoing conflict.

NOTES

1. The words "couple" and "marital" in this chapter are presented interchangeably, referring to participation in committed relationships, regardless of legal status. Thus, gay, lesbian, and other longstanding relationships not recognized by law are also included under these terms. However, the legal aspects of divorce and their impact are unique to marriages recognized by the state.

2. This research has been widely criticized for its lack of a control group, unrepresentative sample, and likely affects attributed to the effect of the experimenter in shaping subject's life stories.

3. Here the research strongly supports the dissolution of marriage, because the rate of success in changing these forms of marital violence is very poor (Jacobson, Gottman, & Shortt, 1995). Nonetheless, it also must be recognized that women mostly return to such situations; therefore, even feminist-based therapies have been developed are based in this reality (Goldner, 1998).

4. This work is typically easier to initiate when a marital therapy has morphed into divorce therapy, and the precedent and alliance for this kind of work is already established.

SUGGESTIONS FOR FURTHER READING

Ahrons, C. R. (1994). *The good divorce: Keeping your family together when your marriage comes apart.* New York: HarperCollins.

Emery, R. E. (1999). *Marriage, divorce, and children's adjustment* (2nd ed.). Thousand Oaks, CA: Sage.

Hetherington, E., & Clingempeel, W. (1992). Coping with marital transitions: A family systems perspective. *Monographs of the Society for Research in Child Development, 57*(2–3), 1–242.

Hetherington, E. M., & Kelly, J. (2002). *For better or for worse: Divorce reconsidered.* New York: Norton.

Kelly, J. B. (2003). Parents with enduring child disputes: Focused interventions with parents in enduring disputes. *Journal of Family Studies, 9*(1), 51–62.

Lebow, J. (2003). Integrative family therapy for disputes involving child custody and visitation. *Journal of Family Psychology, 17*(2), 181–192.

REFERENCES

Ahrons, C. R. (1994). *The good divorce: Keeping your family together when your marriage comes apart.* New York: HarperCollins.

Ahrons, C. R. (2004). *We're still family: What grown children have to say about their parents' divorce.* New York: HarperCollins.

Ahrons, C. R., & Rodgers, R. H. (1987). *Divorced fami-*

lies: A multidisciplinary developmental view. New York: Norton.

Ahrons, C. R., & Tanner, J. L. (2003). Adult children and their fathers: Relationship changes 20 years after parental divorce. *Family Relations: Interdisciplinary Journal of Applied Family Studies, 52*(4), 340–351.

Amato, P. R. (2003). Reconciling Divergent perspectives: Judith Wallerstein, quantitative family research, and children of divorce. *Family Relations, 52*(4), 332–339.

Amato, P. R., & Afifi, T. D. (2006). Feeling caught between parents: Adult children's relations with parents and subjective well-being. *Journal of Marriage and Family, 68*(1), 222–235.

Amato, P. R., & Booth, A. (2002). A generation at risk: Growing up in an era of family upheaval. *Journal of the American Academy of Child and Adolescent Psychiatry, 41*(4), 486–487.

Beck, A. T., & Freeman, A. M. (1990). *Cognitive therapy of personality disorders.* New York: Guilford Press.

Beck, C. J., Sales, B. D., & Emery, R. E. (2004). Research on the impact of family mediation. In J. Folberg, A. Milne, & P. Salem (Eds.), *Divorce and family mediation: Models, techniques, and applications* (pp. 447–482). New York: Guilford Press.

Braver, S. L., Hipke, K. N., Ellman, I. M., & Sandler, I. N. (2004). Strengths-building public policy for children of divorce. In K. I. Maton, C. J. Schellenbach, B. J. Leadbeater, & A. L. Solarz (Eds.), *Investing in children, youth, families, and communities: Strengths-based research and policy* (pp. 53–72). Washington, DC: American Psychological Association.

Buchanan, C. M., Maccoby, E. E., & Dornbusch, S. M. (1996). *Adolescents after divorce.* Cambridge, MA: Harvard University Press.

Combs, G., & Freedman, J. (1990). *Symbol, story, and ceremony: Using metaphor in individual and family therapy.* New York: Norton.

Doherty, W. J. (1999). Morality and spirituality in therapy. In F. Walsh (Ed.), *Spiritual resources in family therapy* (pp. 179–192). New York: Guilford Press.

Doherty, W. J. (2001). *Take back your marriage: Sticking together in a world that pulls us apart.* New York: Guilford Press.

Emery, R. (2006). Book review of Elizabeth Marquardt's *Between Two Worlds*: The inner lives of children of divorce. *Family Court Review, 44*(3), 498–500.

Emery, R. E. (1994). *Renegotiating family relationships: Divorce, child custody, and mediation.* New York: Guilford Press.

Emery, R. E. (1995). Divorce mediation: Negotiating agreements and renegotiating relationships. *Family Relations, 44*(4), 377–383.

Emery, R. E. (1999). *Marriage, divorce, and children's adjustment* (2nd ed.). Thousand Oaks, CA: Sage.

Emery, R. E. (2004). *The truth about children and divorce: Dealing with the emotions so you and your children can thrive.* New York: Viking.

Emery, R. E. (2006). *Custody disputes in high-conflict*

families: PsycCRITIQUES 2006. Washington, DC: American Psychological Association.

Emery, R. E., Sbarra, D., & Grover, T. (2005). Divorce mediation: Research and reflections. *Family Court Review, 43*(1), 22–37.

Feldbau-Kohn, S., Schumacher, J. A., & O'Leary, K. (2000). Partner abuse. In V. B. Van Hassett & M. Hers (Eds.), *Aggression and violence: An introductory text* (pp. 116–134). Needham Heights, MA: Allyn & Bacon.

Folberg, J. (1991). *Joint custody and shared parenting* (2nd ed.). New York: Guilford Press.

Folberg, J., & Milne, A. (1988). *Divorce mediation: Theory and practice.* New York: Guilford Press.

Folberg, J., Milne, A. L., & Salem, P. (2004). *Divorce and family mediation: Models, techniques, and applications.* New York: Guilford Press.

Goldner, V. (1998). The treatment of violence and victimization in intimate relationships. *Family Process, 37*(3), 263–286.

Gottman, J. M. (1993). A theory of marital dissolution and stability. *Journal of Family Psychology, 7*(1), 57–75.

Gottman, J. M. (1999). *The marriage clinic: A scientifically based marital therapy.* New York: Norton.

Gottman, J. M., & Notarius, C. I. (2000). Decade review: Observing marital interaction. *Journal of Marriage and the Family, 62*(4), 927–947.

Gould, J. W. (1998). *Conducting scientifically crafted child custody evaluations.* Thousand Oaks, CA: Sage.

Greenberg, L. R., & Gould, J. W. (2001). The treating expert: A hybrid role with firm boundaries. *Professional Psychology: Research and Practice, 32*(5), 469–478.

Greene, S. M., Anderson, E. R., Hetherington, E., Forgatch, M. S., & DeGarmo, D. S. (2003). Risk and resilience after divorce. In F. Walsh (Ed.), *Normal family processes: Growing diversity and complexity* (3rd ed., pp. 96–120). New York: Guilford Press.

Grych, J. H., & Fincham, F. D. (1990). Marital conflict and children's adjustment: A cognitive-contextual framework. *Psychological Bulletin, 108*(2), 267–290.

Grych, J. H., & Fincham, F. D. (1992). Interventions for children of divorce: Toward greater integration of research and action. *Psychological Bulletin, 111*(3), 434–454.

Grych, J. H., Fincham, F. D., Jouriles, E. N., & McDonald, R. (2000). Interparental conflict and child adjustment: Testing the mediational role of appraisals in the cognitive-contextual framework. *Child Development, 71*(6), 1648–1661.

Hetherington, E. (1979). Divorce: A child's perspective. *American Psychologist, 34*(10), 851–858.

Hetherington, E., & Clingempeel, W. (1992). Coping with marital transitions: A family systems perspective. *Monographs of the Society for Research in Child Development, 57*(2–3), 1–242.

Hetherington, E., & Elmore, A. M. (2003). Risk and resilience in children coping with their parents' divorce and remarriage. In S. Luthar (Ed.), *Resilience and vulnerability: Adaptation in the context of childhood adversities* (pp. 182–212). New York: Cambridge University Press.

Hetherington, E., & Kelly, J. (2003). For better or for worse: Divorce reconsidered. *American Journal of Psychiatry, 160*(3), 601–602.

Hetherington, E., & Stanley-Hagan, M. (2002). Parenting in divorced and remarried families. In M. Bornstein (Ed.), *Handbook of parenting: Vol. 3. Being and becoming a parent* (2nd ed., pp. 287–315). Mahwah, NJ: Erlbaum.

Hetherington, E. M. (1999). *Coping with divorce, single parenting, and remarriage: A risk and resiliency perspective.* Mahwah, NJ: Erlbaum.

Hetherington, E. M., & Kelly, J. (2002). *For better or for worse: Divorce reconsidered.* New York: Norton.

Jacobson, N. S., Gottman, J. M., & Shortt, J. W. (1995). The distinction between Type 1 and Type 2 batterers—Further considerations: Reply to Ornduff et al. (1995), Margolin et al. (1995), and Walker (1995). *Journal of Family Psychology, 9*(3), 272–279.

Johnston, J. R. (2005). Clinical work with parents in entrenched custody disputes. In L. Gunsberg & P. Hymowitz (Eds.), *A handbook of divorce and custody: Forensic, developmental, and clinical perspectives* (pp. 343–363). Hillsdale, NJ: Analytic Press.

Johnston, J. R., & Campbell, L. E. (1988). Tribal warfare: The involvement of extended kin and significant others in custody and access disputes. *Conciliation Courts Review, 24*, 1–16.

Johnston, J. R., Walters, M. G., & Olesen, N. W. (2005). The psychological functioning of alienated children in custody disputing families: An exploratory study. *American Journal of Forensic Psychology, 23*(3), 39–64.

Kelly, J. B. (2003a). Parents with enduring child disputes: Focused interventions with parents in enduring disputes. *Journal of Family Studies, 9*(1), 51–62.

Kelly, J. B. (2003b). Parents with enduring child disputes: Multiple pathways to enduring disputes. *Journal of Family Studies, 9*(1), 37–50.

Kelly, J. B., & Johnston, J. R. (2001). The alienated child: A reformulation of parental alienation syndrome. *Family Court Review, 39*(3), 249–266.

Knobloch-Fedders, L. M., Pinsof, W. M., & Mann, B. J. (2004). The formation of the therapeutic alliance in couple therapy. *Family Process, 43*(4), 425–442.

Krantzler, M. (1973). *Creative divorce: A new opportunity for personal growth.* New York: Evans.

Krantzler, M., & Krantzler, P. B. (1999). *The new creative divorce: How to create a happier, more rewarding life during—and after—your divorce.* Holbrook, MA: Adams Media.

Lebow, J. L. (1984). On the value of integrating approaches to family therapy. *Journal of Marital and Family Therapy, 10*(2), 127–138.

Lebow, J. L. (1987). Integrative family therapy: An overview of major issues. *Psychotherapy: Theory, Research, Practice and Training, 24*(3S), 584–594.

Lebow, J. L. (1997). The integrative revolution in couple and family therapy. *Family Process, 36*(1), 1–17.

Lebow, J. L. (2003). Integrative family therapy for disputes involving child custody and visitation. *Journal of Family Psychology, 17*(2), 181–192.

Lebow, J. L. (2005). Integrative family therapy for families experiencing high-conflict divorce. In *Handbook of clinical family therapy* (pp. 516–542). Hoboken, NJ: Wiley.

Lebow, J. L. (2006a). Integrative couple therapy. In G. Stricker & J. Gold (Eds.), *A casebook of psychotherapy integration* (pp. 211–223). Washington, DC: American Psychological Association.

Lebow, J. L. (2006b). *Research for the psychotherapist: From science to practice.* New York: Routledge/Taylor & Francis.

Marquardt, E. (2005). *Between two worlds: The inner lives of children of divorce.* New York: Crown.

McKinnon, R., & Wallerstein, J. S. (1988). A preventive intervention program for parents and young children in joint custody arrangements. *American Journal of Orthopsychiatry, 58*(2), 168–178.

Milne, A., & Folberg, J. (1988). The theory and practice of divorce mediation: An overview. In J. Folberg & A. Milne (Eds.), *Divorce mediation: Theory and practice* (pp. 3–25). New York: Guilford Press.

Orlinsky, D. E., & Howard, K. I. (1987). A generic model of psychotherapy. *Journal of Integrative and Eclectic Psychotherapy, 6*(1), 6–27.

Pedro-Carroll, J., Nakhnikian, E., & Montes, G. (2001). Assisting children through transition: Helping parents protect their children from the toxic effects of ongoing conflict in the aftermath of divorce. *Family Court Review, 39*(4), 377–392.

Pedro-Carroll, J. L. (2005). Fostering resilience in the aftermath of divorce: The role of evidence-based programs for children. *Family Court Review, 43*(1), 52–64.

Pedro-Carroll, J. L., & Alpert-Gillis, L. J. (1997). Preventive interventions for children of divorce: A developmental model for 5 and 6 year old children. *Journal of Primary Prevention, 18*(1), 5–23.

Pedro-Carroll, J. L., Sandler, I. N., & Wolchik, S. A. (2005). Special issue on prevention: Research, policy, and evidence-based practice. *Family Court Review, 43*(1), 18–21.

Pedro-Carroll, J. L., Sutton, S. E., & Wyman, P. A. (1999). A two-year follow-up evaluation of a preventive intervention for young children of divorce. *School Psychology Review, 28*(3), 467–476.

Raffel, L. (1999). *Should I stay or go?: How controlled separation (CS) can save your marriage.* Lincolnwood, IL: Contemporary Books.

Renick, M. J., Blumberg, S. L., & Markman, H. J. (1992). The prevention and relationship enhancement (PREP): An empirically based preventive intervention program for couples. *Family Relations, 41*(2), 141–147.

Silliman, B., Stanley, S. M., Coffin, W., Markman, H. J., & Jordan, P. L. (2001). Preventive interventions for couple. In H. A. Liddle, D. A. Santisteban, R. F. Levan, & J. H. Bray (Eds.), *Family psychology: Science-*

based interventions (pp. 123–146). Washington, DC: American Psychological Association.

Stricker, G., & Trierweiler, S. J. (1995). The local clinical scientist: A bridge between science and practice. *American Psychologist, 50*(12), 995–1002.

Wallerstein, J., Lewis, J., & Blakeslee, S. (2002). The unexpected legacy of divorce: A 25 year landmark study [Book review]. *Journal of the American Academy of Child and Adolescent Psychiatry, 41*(3), 359–360.

Wallerstein, J. S., & Blakeslee, S. (1989). *Second chances: Men, women, and children a decade after divorce.* New York: Ticknor & Fields.

Wallerstein, J. S., Corbin, S. B., & Lewis, J. M. (1988). Children of divorce: A 10-year study. In E. M. Hetherington & J. D. Aratch (Eds.), *Impact of divorce, single parenting, and stepparenting on children* (pp. 197–214). Hillsdale, NJ: Erlbaum.

Wallerstein, J. S., & Kelly, J. B. (1975). The effects of parental divorce: Experiences of the preschool child. *Journal of the American Academy of Child Psychiatry, 14*(4), 600–616.

Wallerstein, J. S., & Kelly, J. B. (1980). *Surviving the breakup: How children and parents cope with divorce.* New York: Basic Books.

Weiner-Davis, M. (1987). Confessions of an unabashed marriage saver. *Family Therapy Networker, 11*(1), 53–56.

Weiner-Davis, M. (1992). *Divorce busting: A revolutionary and rapid program for staying together.* New York: Summit Books.

Weiss, R. L., & Cerreto, M. C. (1980). The Marital Status Inventory: Development of a measure of dissolution potential. *American Journal of Family Therapy, 8*(2), 80–85.

Weitzman, L. J., Dixon, R. B., Arendell, T., Krantz, S. E., Riessman, C. K., Ahrons, C. R., et al. (1992). Divorce and remarriage. In A. Skolnick & J. Skolnick (Eds.), *Family in transition: Rethinking marriage, sexuality, child rearing, and family organization* (7th ed., pp. 217–289). New York: HarperCollins.

Whitaker, C. A., & Miller, M. H. (1969). A reevaluation of "psychiatric help" when divorce impends. *American Journal of Psychiatry, 126*(5), 611–618.

CHAPTER 16

Couple Therapy and Physical Aggression

K. Daniel O'Leary

BACKGROUND

Mental Health Professionals' Acknowledgment of the Problem of Physical Aggression

Marital couple and therapy approaches to address problems of psychological and physical aggression in relationships are accepted by many professionals (e.g., Geller, 2007; Hamel & Nichols, 2006; Stith & McCollum, in press). And, by 2020, it is likely that all licensed mental health professionals will be ethically mandated to assess for the presence of physical aggression in relationships. Many hospitals already conduct such assessments. By 2020, almost all mental health professionals will be required to take courses in their clinical training programs or continuing education courses to show that they have received some training in intimate partner violence (IPV). California and Florida already require such training. By 2020, marital therapists will be much more conversant with the IPV literature because of its relevance to them.

Currently, many marital and family therapists do not see IPV as a relevant issue because they do not believe that they have cases that involve partner aggression. Indeed, until the 1980s, partner aggression was almost completely ignored

by mental health professionals. Fortunately, in 1979, there were two important books published that gradually had some impact on mental health professionals. Murray Straus, Richard Gelles, and Susan Steinmetz published *Behind Closed Doors: Violence in the American Family*, which presented the first U.S. representative sample survey of physical aggression directed toward family members. The study showed that approximately 12% of men *and* women in the past year had engaged in physical aggression against their partners. Lenore Walker, in her now classic book *The Battered Woman* (1979), showed how women become entangled in a "cycle of violence" in which there is initial closeness, followed by psychological and sometimes physical aggression. After the physical aggression, there is an apology by the male, though often with denial of responsibility. Walker argued that without intervention, the abuse or battering cycle in which men use power and control tactics will not stop.

Mental health professionals were influenced by these books and by subsequent articles published in peer reviewed journals only gradually. In the 1980s and 1990s, very few graduate curricula contained readings on IPV or other, similar titles such as wife abuse, battering, or family violence.

However, because of the greater concern about protection of children, many states required that all professionals who deal with children (e.g., teachers, mental health professionals, and physicians) take courses related to the identification and mandated reporting of abuse of children. The issue of mandated reporting of physical abuse of partners is still debated because of concern about whether reporting such abuse may actually place women at even greater risk than not reporting it. In addition, there is concern that a woman, often called the "victim," should have the power to make her own decisions about whether to report such aggression. Sometimes issues such as mandated reporting of physical abuse and the need for women's shelters as a result of partner aggression seem largely irrelevant to the day-to-day lives of mental health practitioners, who say that these issues are so infrequently relevant to them. My goal by the end of this chapter is to show all mental health professionals, especially marital and family therapists, that physical aggression in intimate relationships is quite common in couples in the community and even more common in couples seeking marital therapy. Furthermore, marital and family therapists need to know the kinds of interventions that are helpful to such clients. I discuss these interventions in this chapter.

It is important to give feminists and grassroots organizers their due respect for helping to awaken the public to the issue of domestic violence (Schecter, 1982) when mental health professionals ignored it. Even the mental health professionals who addressed the issue of partner violence, or what was called "physical abuse" or "battering," often angered women's groups, because they were attempting to ascertain why "battered women stay." Some characterized abused women as masochistic (Hilberman, 1980). Only a few mental health professionals, such as Ganley (1981), provided input that was accepted by women and organizers of shelters and facilities for abused women. In short, the women's movement took on the issue of battered women, while most mental health professionals ignored it.

Although mental health professionals ignored the problem of partner abuse, they were later were forced to accept (or at least to address) prevailing views of IPV that largely had one view about the cause of such aggression or violence. For years, physical aggression in relationships was seen as being caused by one major factor, a patriarchical society that taught men to use and abuse power and control tactics with women (e.g., Pence

& Paymar, 1993; Yllo, 1993). Men were seen as the abusers and women, as the victims. In turn, these views lead to the rejection of marital therapy as an accepted intervention for men and women in relationships characterized by physical aggression. Consequently, the field thus far has relatively few research-based treatment outcome studies in which men and women are assigned to couple and/or other interventions. Thus, this chapter initially provides a historical context for the current status of couple treatment of relationships in which there is some physical aggression.

Why Mental Health Professionals Have Ignored the Problem

With a few notable exceptions, mental health professionals did little to address the problem of IPV in the 1970s. They ignored the problem, because they did not think that physical aggression occurred in the couples and families they assessed and treated. I felt similarly in 1978, when I began to conduct research on physical aggression in relationships. A graduate student, Alan Rosenbaum, asked if I would supervise a dissertation on the treatment of "wife abusers." I told Rosenbaum that I did not know anything about "wife abusers," but I would be glad to learn with him, and I suggested that we start by trying to ascertain how men who engaged in physical aggression against their spouses differed from men who were maritally discordant but not physically aggressive. Rosenbaum came to me because I had been conducting research on marital treatment with Hillary Turkewitz (Turkewitz & O'Leary, 1981), though we did not even assess for the presence of physical aggression in our marital cases at that time. Rosenbaum encountered the problem of physical aggression at his internship in a county mental health facility on Long Island, where he was providing therapy to a woman who was considered leaving her husband because of marital discord and physical aggression. One day when Rosenbaum was not at the clinic, the husband of the woman Rosenbaum was seeing came after him brandishing a knife, though Rosenbaum had never seen the man before. That eventful day prompted Rosenbaum to enter the IPV field, and he has been in it ever since, as have I (Rosenbaum & Kunkel, in press). And his dissertation was perhaps the first to use a contrast approach comparing three groups: (1) physically aggressive and maritally discordant men; (2) maritally discordant but were not physically aggressive men; and (3) happily married men who were not physically aggressive

(Rosenbaum & O'Leary, 1981). He found that the physically aggressive men, compared to the happily married men and the maritally discordant but not physically aggressive men, were less assertive, abusive to children, and more likely to have witnessed parental spouse abuse. They were also more likely to be conservative and alcoholic. The physically aggressive men in that study were recruited at a facility that provided court-mandated interventions and interventions for men who volunteered for help. These were men who have traditionally been called wife abusers, and even then, research with them did not seem particularly relevant to the day-to-day lives of therapists who provided services for couples and families.

The problem of physical aggression in relationships was not seen as an issue by marital therapists in the 1970s and early 1980s. Marital therapists did not assess for the presence of physical aggression in relationships, and frankly, when I started the University Marital Clinic at Stony Brook in the 1980s, we did not ask specifically about whether physical aggression was a problem. Susan Geiss and I asked a sample of marital therapists to name the most frequent problems in the marital relationships of couples they were seeing. Physical aggression or abuse was mentioned as occurring in only 12% of couples, and it ranked 26th in terms of occurrence (Geiss & O'Leary, 1981). In fact, the most frequent problems were communication difficulties (84%), unrealistic expectations of spouse (56%), and lack of loving feelings (55%) and demonstrations of affection (55%). In 1997, Whisman, Dixon, and Johnson conducted a systematic replication of the Geiss and O'Leary (1981) study sampling members of the Family Therapy Division of the American Psychological Association and members of the American Association of Marriage and Family Therapists (AAMFT). They used the same list of 29 problems used by Geiss and O'Leary to assess the stability of presenting problems in couple therapy. The mean number of years in marital therapy practice was 18, so the sample clearly represented experienced marital therapists. The correlation between the rank order of the presenting problems in the two studies was .95, indicating remarkable stability of presenting problems over a 15-year period. Communication (87%), power struggles (62%), unrealistic expectations of spouse (50%), and sex (47%) were most frequent problems. Physical abuse, however, was reported as occurring in only 12% of the cases seen by the marital therapists—the identical percentage found by Geiss and O'Leary. However,

in terms of treatment difficulty, therapists in both studies ranked physical abuse as very difficult to treat. It was ranked seventh in terms of difficulty in the 1981 study, and sixth in the 1997 study. By comparison, alcoholism was ranked first in terms of difficulty in 1997, and second in 1981. In summary, based on marital therapists' reports about their clients, one could conclude that aggression is infrequently reported as a major issue about which the clients are seeking help.

What If Clients Are Asked Specifically about Aggression?

Based on the previously discussed studies by Geiss and O'Leary (1981) and Whisman et al. (1997), one might expect that physical abuse is an infrequent problem in relationships. At a minimum, one can state the men and women seeking marital therapy do not see physical abuse as a problem. However, there is a very big difference between "abuse" and "aggression." In fact, *physical aggression may be present in couples seeking marital therapy, but physical abuse may not be reported, because men and women seeking therapy may not perceive the physical aggression as abuse.* In 1992, when we had become more interested in the problems of physical aggression and abuse in close relationships, we asked men and women who came to our clinic for help with their marital problems to list the five major problems in their marriage and to write several sentences about each problem (O'Leary, Vivian, & Malone, 1992). The major problems were as follows: (1) lack of communication; (2) lack of love and caring; and (3) differences over child rearing and discipline. Only 6% of the women reported any problem regarding physical aggression. However, following completion of the initial assessments noted earlier, we also gave the men and women, the Conflict Tactics Scale (CTS; Straus, 1979), which, among other things, contains a list of physically aggressive behaviors, such as pushing, grabbing, shoving, slapping, kicking, and beating. To our surprise, when we examined the percentage of men and women who reported at least one act of physical aggression by themselves or their partner, we found that 53% of the women and 53% of the men reported that spouse had engaged in some act of physical aggression against them. When we analyzed composite data, 67% of couples reported male-to-female aggression. Furthermore, 25% of couples in this sample (21% of women, 17% of men) reported the occurrence of severe male-perpetrated aggression (e.g., kicking, beating, biting, hitting). The bottom line is that on an objective checklist approximately two-thirds of the couples indicated some physical aggression in their relationship, but very few even mentioned physical aggression as a problem in their relationship.

In an attempt to recruit nonviolent or non-physically-aggressive subjects as controls in studies of intimate partner violence, Holtzworth-Munroe et al. (1992) were surprised to find that many more control subjects than they anticipated had reported physical aggression. Across five different studies in which subjects were recruited via newspaper advertisements, up to one-third of the maritally nondistressed subjects and one-half of the maritally distressed subjects reported that violence had occurred in their relationship. Amy Holtzworth-Munroe (2000) provided some historical context to this research in her memorial statement for Neil Jacobson. She stated that in response to early publications, such as those of Straus et al. (1979) and Rosenbaum and O'Leary (1981), she and Neil Jacobson had conducted an informal survey on the prevalence of violence in his marital clinic, and "we were shocked to find that over half of the couples reported the occurrence of husband physical aggression in their relationship" (p. 1). She went on to say that Jacobson was a leading authority on marital therapy "who had never considered the problem of husband violence" (Holtzworth-Munroe, 2000). Fortunately, Jacobson entered the field of partner violence and contributed significantly to it, as exemplified in his 1998 book with Gottman, *When Men Batter Women: New Insights Into Ending Abusive Relationships.*

Cascardi, Langhinrichsen, and Vivian (1992) assessed 93 consecutive couples who sought psychological treatment and the University Marital Clinic at Stony Brook. They evaluated the prevalence, impact, and health correlates of marital aggression in a clinic sample of maritally discordant couples seeking psychological treatment. Overall, 71% of clinic couples reported at least one act of marital aggression during the past year. Although 86% of the aggression reported was reciprocal between husbands and wives, impact and injuries sustained as a function of this aggression differed between husbands and wives. Specifically, wives were more likely than husbands to be negatively affected and to sustain severe injuries. Additionally, wives who experienced marital aggression reported clinical levels of depressive symptomatology.

In 2004, when Doss, Simpson, and Christensen assessed 147 men and women seeking marital therapy in Los Angeles and Seattle, they asked them for the reasons they were seeking such help. As in the previous study, participants were asked to write down the reasons they were seeking help in response to the simple, straightforward question, "Please list the main factors that led you personally to seek marital therapy." On average, spouses wrote three reasons. Wives listed communication, affection, and separation/divorce concerns. Men listed affection, separation/divorce concerns, and desire to improve the relationship. Physical aggression/abuse was reported by less than 5% of the couples. However, they asked respondents to complete the CTS to assess for the presence of physically aggressive acts in the relationship, and such aggression was reported in 52% of the couples. Moreover, severe aggression had occurred in 24% of the couples in the past year. Thus, Doss, Simpson, and Christensen (2004) concluded, "Treatment plans should not be based solely on couples' reasons for seeking therapy; instead psychologists should inquire directly about important areas such as physical abuse." I fully agree with the general point except that it is best to ask about the presence of specific acts of physical aggression, not whether there are problems of physical abuse in the relationship.

Research by Murphy and O'Farrell (1994) on a sample of 107 couples found a rate of physical aggression identical to that in the O'Leary et al. (1992) study, namely, 66% of the couples reported husband-to-wife aggression. Couples in this study were entering marital therapy for recovering alcoholic males at the Veterans Hospital in Brockton, Massachusetts, and researchers used the CTS (Straus, 1979) to report the occurrence of physical aggression in the previous year. Fifty-four percent of the women in the study reported being victimized by their partners in the past year. Additionally, 48% of men in this study reported perpetration, and composite rates indicated that, when combined, 66% of couples reported husband-to-wife aggression.

At the University of Maryland Marital and Family Program, LaTalliade and Epstein (personal communication, June 20, 2007) also assessed men and women who were seeking marital therapy because of the physical aggression in their relationships. Using the CTS, they found that 46% of the males and 43% of the female reported that they engaged in some act of physical aggression against their partners in the past year, and that 48% of the males and 51% of the females reported that their partners engaged in physical aggression against them. Of special interest to those concerned about the protection of women, 13% of the women reported that their partners engaged in some severe acts of physical aggression against them, and 8% of the men reported that they engaged in such aggression. In short, again, we see that physical aggression reportedly occurred in approximately half of all couples seeking marital therapy.

In summary, based on these studies, it appears that between 40 and 70% of couples who seek marital therapy at clinics report that there is some physical aggression in their relationship if they are asked about the presence of specific physical behaviors, such as pushing, slapping, shoving, kicking, hitting, and beating. Based on these survey studies of practicing marital therapists, it is possible that the clients who seek marital therapy from private practitioners are somewhat less aggressive than those clients who seek marital therapy at clinics. However, it is not known whether therapists who serve private clients have the same therapist biases as those who serve clients at clinics; that is, therapists serving private clients likely do not ask specifically about the presence of physical aggression, though it may well be there.

Are Most Community Couples between Ages 20 and 35 Physically Aggressive?

In 1980, this question would have seemed ridiculous to most marital and family therapists. First, such aggression was rarely reported to therapists, and, as noted earlier, few therapists asked about such aggression. However, in 1979, Straus et al. reported that in a representative sample of U.S. citizens, the National Family Violence Survey (NFVS), 12% of males and 12% of females reported that they engaged in some act of physical aggression in the past year. Though developmental phenomena certainly were not a major focus of this book, a table in the appendix documented that aggression differed across three age groups: 20–35; 36–55; and 56–70. Specifically, based on Straus et al.'s table (p. 141), one could estimate the rates of aggression for couples across three broad age groups: under 30, 15%; 31–50, 6%; and 51–65, 2%. As Straus et al. concluded, partner aggression was highest in couples under age 30, and, as age increased, violence decreased.

For purposes of presenting data by age groupings for men alone (rather than as couples as was done by Straus et al., [1979]), O'Leary (1999) analyzed reports of husband-to-wife physical aggression from the NFVS, and showed that prevalence of physical aggression against a female partner declined markedly with age. There were 10 age groupings: 20–24, 25–29, 30–34, 35–39, 40–44, 45–49, 50–54, 55–59, 60–64, and 65–69 years. Pearson's correlation between the average age in each age group and the proportion of men who used any physical aggression within each age group was $r = -.87$. Overall, the prevalence of husband-to-wife physical aggression declined from 37% in 20- to 24-year-olds to 2% in the 65- to 69- year-olds. In addition, O'Leary and Woodin (2005) were able to use a very large, representative married U.S. Army sample. There we again found a steady downward projection of aggression across age groups. In fact, using the above described aggregate approach with 5-year age groupings, I found a negative correlation of $-.82$ for age and partner aggression, the exact association found in the civilian population noted earlier (O'Leary, 1999). In short, in representative samples of both civilians and military personnel male physical aggression against female partners declines with age.

Anyone with some knowledge of partner violence might ask how these conclusions square with the notion that some men appear to start being physically aggressive at a very early stage in the relationship and that their aggression often escalates across time. Indeed, Lenore Walker (1979) warned women that partners who engage in physical aggression against them early in the marriage would almost certainly continue to do so. Walker recruited a sample of women who had some problems with psychological and physical aggression in their relationship. Although it is unclear exactly who they represent, the women reported that physical aggression escalated in their relationships. The issue of how and whether individual physical aggression escalates or desists in intimate relationships is very complicated, and to address it in any detail is beyond the scope of this chapter. However, it appears that whereas the majority of individuals who are physically aggressive early in relationships desist in their use of aggression, some individuals' aggression escalates. Fortunately, based on the population-based studies I referred to earlier, it also appears that the percentage of individuals who maintain or escalate their use of physical aggression is relatively small, because only 4–10% of the overall population appears consistently to be physically aggressive and abusive (Straus et al., 1979; Straus & Gelles, 1990; O'Leary & Jacobson, 1997; Heyman & Slep, 2006).

However, let us now return to the question about the prevalence of physical aggression in couples between 20 and 35 years of age. We now know that at approximately 50% of young couples in a representative sample are physically aggressive. For example, consider our representative sample of parents of 3- to 7-year-old children in Suffolk County, New York. These couples (N = 453) recruited through a phone sampling procedure called "random digit dialing," appeared to be reasonably representative of the population of young parents in the area who had phones (Slep, Heyman, Williams, Van Dyke, & O'Leary, 2005). All had to have been coparenting for at least a year, the vast majority of the sample (94%) was married, and the average age of the husbands and wives was 37 and 35 years, respectively. The couples were assessed quite extensively over a 6-hour period with self-report assessments, physiological measures, and observations of marital interactions. The self-report questionnaire that is relevant to this discussion, the CTS, assessed the presence and frequency of physical aggression toward a partner. Approximately 28% of the males and 37% of the females reported that they had engaged in some act of physical aggression against their partner in the past year. Furthermore, use of a method called either–or reporting, in which physical aggression is counted as present if either the male or the female report it, determined that 37% of males and 44% of females had been physically aggressive in the past year (O'Leary & Williams, 2006). Now let us turn to the question, "In what percentage of couples does physical aggression occur?" In this particular sample, physical aggression in which the individual was *either* perpetrator *or* recipient of the aggression, was reported in 48% of the couples (Slep & O'Leary, 2005). Thus, when we return to question, "Are the majority of couples between 20 and 35 years of age physically aggressive?" the answer is almost, but not quite a "yes."

Policies and Positions against Couple Treatment

A number of states have agencies that provide services to women in physically aggressive relationships but forbid these agencies and affiliates to provide any services for couples. Specifically, marital counseling and marital treatment are forbidden as interventions for couples and families in which there has been any report of physical aggression by a male toward a female partner (e.g., Healy, Smith, & O'Sullivan, 1998). In at least 12 states, including Massachusetts, Colorado, Florida, Washington, and Texas, state guidelines effectively preclude any treatment other than feminist therapy for domestic batterers. They do not permit couple counseling unless the man has participated in a profeminist-based men's intervention first.

Basically, feminist approaches to treatment, especially as exemplified in one of the most prominent batterer programs in the Duluth model (Pence & Paymar, 1993) emphasize concepts such as gender, power/control, and patriarchy (Gondolf, 2002; Yllo, 1993). As Satel (1997) noted, another 12 states, among them Maine and Illinois, drafted similar guidelines. Satel went on to describe the position of profeminists who reject joint counseling, the traditional approach to marital conflict. As she stated, joint counseling and other couple-based treatments violate the feminist certainty that it is men who are always and solely responsible for domestic violence. According to individuals with such positions, any attempt to involve the batterer's mate in treatment amounts to "blaming the victim."

In another review of U.S. programs and services for men in relationships characterized by aggression, Austin and Dankwort (1998) noted that the majority of states have guidelines on the certification of programs into which the Court may direct domestic violence offenders. They stated that in at least 20 states and many smaller jurisdictions, certification requirements explicitly and specifically include compliance with the feminist model. They also mentioned that their review of 31 sets of standards currently in use in the United States, patriarchy was cited as causing and/or maintaining men's violence against women in 70% of the standards. And, not surprisingly, joint counseling for couples in violent relationships was identified as inappropriate in 73% of the standards.

It may now seem anachronistic to have such a policy that bans couple counseling/treatment for all individuals, but an analysis of two reasons that, in my opinion, have merit help to provide some appreciation for the policy. First, if couple treatment is offered, it is asserted that when the man and woman receive counseling, topics are discussed that lead to arguments, and those arguments in the counseling session in turn lead to arguments and physical fights after the counseling sessions. This argument, in fact, makes reasonable sense and is an issue to be considered by any mental health provider who offers couple counseling or treatment. Anyone who has provided couple treatment for at least a few years also wonders whether arguments that start in the therapy session may escalate when the couple goes home.

Another reason that is advanced for the ban on couple counseling/treatment is that discussion of factors that lead to arguments and ultimately physical aggression may lead the wife to believe that she is partly the cause of the marital problems and, ultimately, the physical aggression. This position also deserves serious attention, because, in a dyadic model of partner aggression, physical aggression in a relationship often is caused or influenced by relationship discord (O'Leary & Slep, 2003; Riggs & O'Leary, 1996); that is, instead of trying to decry this argument, marital therapists who see many couples, even some couples who engage in physical aggression, may believe that the marital problems, and the couples' inability to communicate about the marital problems, are the root of their problem. I return to these concerns about marital or couple counseling in the discussion of the outcomes of such interventions.

There appears to be a major difference between the philosophies of agencies serving "battered" women and men who are batterers, and marital and family agencies. If they were to take the recommendations seriously, marital and family therapists would only be able to serve about half their clientele. Yet if one referred the clients who report some aggression in the form of pushing, slapping, and shoving, it is extremely unlikely that these individuals would go to such agencies, or if they went, they would drop out quickly. The vast majority of these women in relationships with some physical aggression do not even see themselves as abused women, and they do not fear their partners. With very few exceptions, the men in these relationships are not what Jacobson and Gottman (1998) called "batterers," because they do not act in a fashion that makes their wives fearful of them and, in the vast majority of cases, they do not cause any injury to their partners (Cascardi et al., 1992).

It seems that the majority of individuals in public and private agencies that serve women in relationships that involve some aggression are not well informed about existing epidemiological studies on the presence of partner aggression (which I discuss later). Many are not able to put the prevalence studies in perspective, and they do openly address the fact that women often are unilaterally aggressive and often act aggressively in a fashion that is not in self-defense. Furthermore, they do not address the relatively high prevalence of physical aggression in the marital therapy studies I reported earlier.

Why Don't Clients See Physical Aggression as a Major Problem?

Clients do not consider the problem of physical aggression to be as important as other problems in their relationship. Might they be correct? Consider a couple in which one or both partners have engaged in one or two acts of physical aggression against the other in the past year. The acts of psychological aggression would be much more important than the physical aggression, because the acts of psychological aggression occur much more frequently. And there is now evidence that the psychological aggression is perceived to be more important than the physical aggression in a majority of cases (Arias & Pape, 2001; Dutton, Goodman, & Bennett, 2001; Follingstad, Rutledge, Berg, Hause, & Polek, 1990).

In 1996, Ehrensaft and Vivian gathered self-report questionnaires and conducted clinical interviews, revealing that over 60% of the 136 couples (272 spouses) seeking marital therapy experienced physical violence in their relationship (a finding that overlaps some with the results noted earlier in this chapter (Cascardi et al., 1992). However, of special interest, less than 10% of these couples spontaneously reported or identified the violence as a presenting problem. An almost identical finding reported by O'Leary et al. (1992) indicated that although partner aggression was reported in the relationships of about 60% of couples, only 6% of the women at intake reported that physical aggression was a problem in their relationship. Ehrensaft and Vivian (1996) took the issue of lack of reporting of physical aggression a step further. Specifically, they examined the reasons couples gave for not reporting physical aggression as a problem in the relationship. The top three reasons were as follows: (1) It is not a problem; (2) it is inconsistent or infrequent; and (3) it is secondary to or caused by other problems. There were no gender differences in this regard. However, as might be expected, spouses who said that aggression was a marital problem were in relationships characterized by severe aggression. As Ehrensaft and colleagues noted, mild aggression, especially when it occurs only a few times per year, may be discounted because it is less salient than other, less intermittent problems. This interpretation is consistent with the finding that a large proportion of spouses reported that aggression was secondary to or caused by other marital problems. Indeed, they simply stated that the physical aggression was "not a problem." Furthermore, spouses who said that physical aggression was not a problem were less likely to have been injured and were the targets of fewer acts of aggression than spouses who did not give this reason.

Many other issues may also be of greater concern to clients than physical and/or psychological aggression. Issues of infidelity, sexual problems, or threats of separation or divorce are likely to be much more important than the presence of physical aggression. Recalling the surveys by Geiss and O'Leary (1981) and Doss et al. (1997), remember that the problems seen most frequently were communication problems, lack of caring/affection/sex, and unrealistic expectations of the partner. The label "communication problems" may represent many different things to clients, but among them is the likely culprit "psychological aggression" and the negativity associated with it. A study with results relevant to the issue of couple differences is a meta-analysis of 66 observational studies of couple interactions by Woodin (2007). One of the three most common differentiators of overall marital distressed and maritally satisfied couples was negativity. This meta-analysis of 66 studies (4,613 couples) examined behaviors observed during marital conflict. Wives were slightly more negative than husbands, and husbands were slightly more withdrawn than wives. However, negativity and withdrawal were equally detrimental for marital satisfaction, regardless of gender. Surprisingly, positivity was related to satisfaction at a similar but opposite magnitude as negativity, whereas withdrawal was less closely linked to satisfaction.

ASSESSING FOR PHYSICAL AGGRESSION

Based on the evidence from both community and clinical samples, it seems crucial that all marital and family therapists assess for the presence of physical aggression in relationships. It may even be unethical not to do so, although there is no ethical mandate in the American Psychological Association or AAMFT ethics codes to do so. However, some states, such as Florida, now require that practitioners take a course documenting that they have some exposure to partner violence issues, and California has recently increased the training needed in the assessment of partner violence to 15 hours to be able to sit for the Psychology Licensure Exam. Regardless of the specific requirements of states and licensure boards, it seems prudent and ethically sound to assess for partner aggression. Not doing so would allow one to begin marital treatment without having any sense that aggression has occurred or might occur in the future.

One need not engage in a detailed assessment of all cases for partner aggression, because most individuals are not physically aggressive. However, in all cases, it is useful at least to ask about the presence of aggression against partners. Whether the initial assessment is via written self-report or individual interviews does not seem crucial. However, it is important to assess for such aggression individually, not in a conjoint interview, because women may be fearful of reporting such aggression in the presence of their male partners.

One could simply ask the following general question in a written or verbal form in an interview, "In the past year, when you had a disagreement or argument with your partner, have you engaged in any acts of physical aggression against your partner such as pushing, slapping, shoving, hitting, beating, or some other acts of aggression?" If the individual responds in the affirmative, then it is also useful to follow-up the question in an interview in which one obtains the context of the aggressive incident(s). In addressing the context, the partner should be asked whether there has been any injury and what functions the aggression served. A brief assessment of overall marital satisfaction and physical aggression that could be given to each partner (Table 16.1).

TABLE 16.1. Relationship and Marital Assessment

I. Marital satisfaction

All things considered, overall how do you rate the level of your marital satisfaction?

> Extremely unhappy; very unhappy; unhappy; neutral; happy; very happy; extremely happy

II. Partner aggression

In the past year, when you had a disagreement or argument with your partner, have you engaged in any acts of physical aggression against your partner such as pushing, slapping, shoving, hitting, beating, or some other acts of aggression?

III. Ability to express your opinion without fear of reprisal from your partner

All things considered, overall how do you rate your ability to express your opinion without fear of reprisal from your partner?

> Extremely unable; very unable; unable; neutral; able; very able; extremely able

III. Commitment to partner

Overall, from 1 to 100 (with 100 being the most), how committed are you to remain in your marriage?

IV. Commitment to make changes in marriage

Overall, from 1 to 100 (with 100 being the most), how committed are you to make changes yourself to make your marriage better?

There seems to be a slow but growing acceptance of marital therapy for men and women in relationships characterized by physical aggression, but under certain conditions. There are seven such conditions specified by Aldarondo and Mederos (2002) in their book *Programs for Men Who Batter*, and the authors suggest couple counseling only if all of these conditions have been met:

1. The abused partner has chosen to enter couple counseling after being informed of all other intervention options, including support groups for abuse victims and individual psychotherapy.
2. The abusive man's violence is limited to only a few (no more than one or two) incidents of minor violence, such as slaps, shoves, grabbing, and restraining, without bruising or injury.
3. The man's use of psychological abuse has been infrequent, mild, and has not created a climate of constant anger or intimidation. This guards against attempting therapy when the effect of powerful intimidation and psychological abuse is still present.
4. No risk factors for lethality are present, even in the absence of severe physical and psychological abuse.
5. The man admits and takes responsibility for his abusive behavior.
6. The abusive man has made an unshakable commitment to refrain from further violence and intimidation. He understands that at times he may feel "provoked" or "justified" to abuse his partner again in response to participation in couple counseling; despite this, he must demonstrate an ongoing commitment to contain his explosive feelings, without blaming others or acting them out, so they do not provide a justification that propels him into a relapse of violent behavior during the course of treatment.
7. The abuse victim reports in a confidential interview (when the abuser is not present) that she is not afraid of speaking honestly in therapy and does not fear retaliation by the abusive partner.

Almost all of the items noted are conditions with which I agree. Conditions 2–7 are in fact variants of conditions we have outlined for marital therapy with couples involved in physical aggression (O'Leary & Cohen, 2006). However, these conditions reflect a view of intimate partner violence that is perpetrated by men only—a view, as

documented in this chapter with a number of studies, that is not defensible. As amply documented in scores of studies, women engage in physical aggression as often as men (Archer, 2000). It is also important to note that mutual physical aggression by men and women at the nonsevere level (e.g., pushing, slapping, and shoving), is not associated with injury or fear. The vast majority of women in community samples who report that their partners engaged in physical aggression against them do not report injuries (Stets & Straus, 1990). More specifically, in a large representative community sample, Stets and Straus found that 3.0% of females and 0.4% of males who were recipients of physical aggression by their partners reported that they needed to see a doctor about injury resulting from a violent incident. Nonetheless, men's aggression is seen as having a greater impact than women's, especially at the severe level, and I now address that issue.

GREATER IMPACT OF MEN'S AGGRESSION

Fear

Abused women display and report significantly more fear of their spouses than maritally discordant, nonabused women (O'Leary & Curley, 1986; Cascardi, O'Leary, Lawrence, & Schlee, 1995). On the other hand, as might be expected from data already presented in this chapter, similar rates of partner fear were reported among men and women in a community-based sample of young couples who were dating, cohabiting, or married (Capaldi & Owen, 2001). However, from a clinical standpoint, it is important to know that women's own ratings of fear were more effective at predicting future violence than a set of 25 risk factors drawn from the literature (Weisz, Tolan, & Saunders, 2000); thus, women's fears must be taken seriously.

Presently, no standardized assessment instrument measures levels of partner fear. However, we have developed a Fear of Partner Scale that displays three internally consistent factors (Cohen & O'Leary, 2007). The scale appears to measure reliably fear of various forms of aggression, including physical, sexual, and emotional abuse, as well as fear of expression in front of one's partner. We recommend that a clinician screen out couples in which one partner is fearful of the other in one or more of these realms (physical aggression, emotional abuse, and expression of opinions in therapy and consequences thereof), because treatment in a dyadic context relies on the ability of partners to be able to communicate with one another. Our assessment, a 25-item, self-report scale, has high internal consistency (total scale: Cronbach's a = .90; subscales: physical/sexual abuse, a = .72; emotional abuse, a = .90; expression, α = .92) and good construct validity (Cohen & O'Leary, 2007).

Injury

Compared to injuries of men, injuries of women are more likely to occur in dating (Foshee, 1996), community (Stets & Straus, 1990), marital therapy (Cascardi et al., 1992), and military settings (Cantos, Neidig, & O'Leary, 1994). For example, in one study of young couples from a representative sample with no overall difference in percentages of men and women who engaged in physical aggression (Ehrensaft et al., 2004), women who reported being in a physically abusive relationship were significantly more likely than men to have needed medical care (24% of women vs. 3% of men, $p < .05$).

Sexual Coercion

Males engage in more sexual coercion than do females (Straus, Hamby, Boney-McCoy, & Sugarman, 1996; Hines & Saudino, 2003; O'Leary & Williams, 2006). For example, in a representative sample of parents of children between ages 3 and 7, we found that men's sexually aggressive behaviors were about twice as likely to occur as women's sexually aggressive behaviors (O'Leary & Williams, 2006). Furthermore, rape of women is much more common than rape of men (Tjaden & Thoennes, 2000).

Partner Homicide

More women than men are killed by their intimate partners. In fact, in 1998, whereas approximately 1,317 females were killed by their partners in the United States, only 512 men were killed by their partners (Rennison & Welchans, 2000). Fortunately, the absolute number of men and women killed per year by intimate partners has declined since 1976. However, the number of women killed was 1,600 in 1976, and the number of men killed was 1,357. Thus, the decline in deaths from in intimate partner homicide have been must greater for men than for women, and, in fact, the decline for women did not occur until the period from 1993 to 1997. Risk factors for being an IPV victim in both men and women include being African American, being separated or divorced, and living in rental housing.

OUTCOMES OF COUPLE TREATMENT WHEN PHYSICAL AGGRESSION HAS OCCURRED

Substance of Couple Treatments

All of the interventions I describe in this section on couple treatments involve monitoring one's thoughts, using "cool" thoughts to lessen one's anger, recognizing one's anger cues, cognitive restructuring, and time-outs. In addition, most of the programs had a goal of improving communication by teaching interpersonal skills, such as paraphrasing and reflection. In addition, most programs placed some focus on issues of gender roles and issues of misuse of power and control, especially by males. Although most of the outcome research has been on couples groups, there is no need to have the couple in a group; in fact, individual attention to a couple seems preferable.

Therapy Goals and Means of Achieving Them

Although specific treatment goals vary somewhat depending upon individual and couple needs, most typically fit into one of the following: (1) decreasing psychological aggression; (2) decreasing/eliminating physical aggression; (3) increasing hope for and commitment to the relationship; (4) increasing overall satisfaction with the relationship; and (5) increasing positive/loving feelings (O'Leary & Cohen, 2006). Couple therapy for individuals who have been in relationships characterized by physical aggression is not generic marital therapy. It is not a simple variant of a communication or problem-solving approach to couple problems. As characterized herein, it is a therapy process designed to reduce psychological and physical aggression in the relationship, and those targets are paramount.

The need to decrease psychological aggression outside and inside the sessions is crucial. In fact, it so crucial that it is not fruitful to see the couple until both individuals can control their emotional outbursts and highly vocal criticism. The emphasis on decreasing psychological aggression is based on the evidence that physical aggression is almost always preceded by high levels of psychological aggression. In a very real sense, clients may be told that couple therapy is a process that can help, but only if they are ready and able to address issues in a civil manner; that is, sometimes individuals must work for the privilege to be in couple therapy. Anger is usually reflective of one individual feeling slighted or hurt by the actions of the other, and it is important to verbalize such hurt rather than to have anger outbursts. Finally, individuals who feel that an argument with the partner is getting out of hand, should state that they will take up the issue again within 24 hours, or at the next therapy session. If an action of one partner, such as an affair or secretive use of family money, has led to mistrust, the individual who engaged in those behaviors must demonstrate through day-to-day behaviors that the undesired actions will not occur again and that he or she is truly sorry for engaging in the behaviors and for causing hurt. In some cases, it is also crucial that a genuine apology be made, and that the person who engaged in the undesired action take full responsibility for the behavior.

It is often useful for a therapist to indicate why he or she feels that there is hope for the relationship (if, in fact, the assessment phase indicates that such hope is reasonable). Like other therapy endeavors, there is value in the belief that things can get better, and if one finds in the initial assessment that each individual is committed to working on the relationship, then this very positive sign can be emphasized by the therapist. If both partners verbalize caring for one another, then that should be emphasized as well. And, based on evidence I present later, one can utilize the generally positive evidence of the effectiveness of couple therapy with many clients who very likely had some physical aggression in their relationship.

There is a need to work on increasing general levels of satisfaction in a relationship, because the degree of relationship discord is one the largest predictors of marital aggression (or the lack thereof). The general level of satisfaction is likely enhanced by helping individuals in the couple session verbalize the traits and behaviors they like/respect in the other. Furthermore, it is important to help individuals show respect for their partners' efforts in the day-to-day life of the relationship and family. Women who care for children and do not work outside the home often do not feel that they get respect from their husbands for their daily efforts with child care, cooking, and housekeeping. Husbands often need special encouragement to show respect for their wives' behavior.

Throughout the therapy process, it is important to focus on establishing a therapeutic bond with both partners. Treatment dropout has been

one of the most crucial problems associated with traditional treatments for men in physically aggressive relationships. Many men simply do not like the emphasis on the male's misuse of power and control. The formation of a positive alliance has proven to be of value in predicting decreases in husband-to-wife psychological aggression, as well as mild and severe physical aggression (Brown & O'Leary, 2000).

Who Is the Target of the Intervention?

It might seem to some that there is a natural tendency to identify with the plight of the female in a relationship characterized by some physical aggression, and that the primary target of the therapy is the male. However, in the vast majority of the cases, the physical aggression in couples is mutual (i.e., both individuals engage in the aggression) and not in self-defense. Nonetheless, because male aggression is more likely to engender fear and injury (even though it is not highly probably in couples seeking couple therapy), there should be a clear emphasis that partners' physical aggression should cease, and that male aggression usually has a more negative impact. As in generic marital therapy, the therapist needs to build an alliance with both partners. Often this means that the therapist needs to pay special attention to forming a bond with the opposite-sex partner, because clients often assume that the therapist will identify with the same-sex client. Overall, however, there should be an emphasis on the couple as the client, with added attention to the possible need to address certain individual issues per se, such as alcohol abuse (see Chapter 18, this volume, by Birchler, Fals-Stewart, & O'Farrell) and depression, over and above the couple issues.

Initial Case Study

One program is mentioned here because of its historical significance. The evaluation by Lindquist, Telch, and Taylor (1983) was the first published study of a couple intervention designed to reduce psychological and physical aggression in men. Their pilot study evaluated a couple-based group intervention, with eight completers. Their results (based on a very small number of participants and a 40% dropout rate) suggested that the completers were less angry and less jealous. And, at the end of treatment, none of the women reported any reoccurrence of abuse. Given that there were only eight completers and a 50% recontact rate at the

6-month follow-up, the study is largely of historic precedence in providing couple-based treatment for aggression.

Initial Comparative Evaluation

Shupe, Stacey, and Hazlewood (1987) conducted one of the largest studies comparing individual couples, couple groups, and gender-specific couples (total N = 241). However, because only a subsample (148) of the participants (241) could be contacted after treatment, conclusions about the effectiveness of the interventions are equivocal. More specifically, of the 148 participants who were contacted, 102 were completers and 42 were dropouts. Of special interest from a substantive and treatment policy standpoint, however, this program for men (one-third were mandated to treatment) in Austin, Texas, is significant because of its specially tailored interventions following couple-based programs. The interventions based on the couple programs were for drug and/or alcohol problems and continuing marital discord. Individuals in all three programs showed reductions in physical aggression, but there were no differences across the couple-versus the gender-based interventions.

Individual Couples versus Groups for Couples

In one of the early studies evaluating a couple treatment designed to reduce physical and psychological aggression of a husband, Harris, Savage, Jones, and Brooke (1988) compared group counseling and individual counseling (one couple) with the overall purpose to reduce psychological and physical aggression. The group counseling program was better able to retain and/or track clients, locating 89% of couples in the couples group compared to 41% of the couples (or at least one partner from the dyad) in the individual counseling. Most couples remained together, but of those who separated, 63% said they left because of the continued abuse. Physical aggression ceased in 54% of the cases, and decreased in 14% of the cases. There were no differences across the treatment groups among persons who remained with their partner.

Gender-Based and Couple-Based Groups

Deschner and McNeil (1986) compared gender-specific and couples groups. They included individuals who had aggressed against their partners, with individual counseling for approximately half

the individuals in both groups throughout the intervention. In both interventions, anger control was a focus of treatment. They had 82 treatment completers and a dropout rate of 39%. Six to 8 months later, 85% of those contacted (54% of the group members) were violence free. There were no differences across the treatments, but this study is instructive, because the clinicians obviously decided that individual counseling might be a needed adjunct to the couples or gender-based group treatments.

Treatment Outcome Studies with Systematic Replication

There are two relatively large, controlled studies of a couple intervention designed specifically to reduce physical aggression, with a specific intervention for couples compared to a specific, gender-based intervention; that is, in two different studies with comparable treatments, couples were assigned to couple-based group treatment, and men and women in the gender-based treatments were assigned to men's and women's groups, respectively (Brannen & Rubin, 1996; O'Leary, Heyman, & Neidig, 1999). Thus, the treatment comparisons involve evaluating the effects of two different group approaches to helping cease/reduce physical aggression in both men and women. Because the treatments were developed with the collaboration of Drs. Peter Neidig and Daniel O'Leary with Dr. Steve Brannen, and because the interventions had a great deal of substantive overlap, the comparison of the treatments can be considered a systematic replication.

Brannen and Rubin (1996), who had the first published study, provided services to men mandated to treatment by a judge in Texas, but the wives were asked to join the husbands in the treatment. The couple-based treatment was based on a program initially developed by the late Peter Neidig for use with the Marine Corps (Neidig & Friedman, 1984) at Paris Island, South Carolina. The gender-based treatment involved having the men attend men's groups, while their female partners attended women's groups. The gender -specific program was based on a variation of the Duluth model (Pence & Paymar, 1993). The couples were randomly assigned to the two treatments provided in a group format, and the judge facilitated monitoring of the men's participation in the treatment. The treatments in both studies lasted approximately 15 sessions of 1.5 hours (sometimes more, depending upon client needs).

The men mandated to treatment in the Brannen and Rubin (1996) study were also mandated to a 10-week stress management course following the couple or gender-specific treatment, a requirement of the criminal justice system in Austin, Texas. To allow comparability across treatments, Brannen conducted the stress management module. Thus, in interpreting the long-term follow-up of the Brannen and Rubin results, one must bear in mind that there were in effect two interventions.

There were no differences in the sizes of the reductions in psychological and physical aggression across the gender-specific and couple treatments. Both groups showed significant reductions in mild and severe physical aggression. However, those assigned to the couples groups showed a greater reduction in mild physical aggression than those in the gender-specific treatment. In addition, for individuals with alcohol problems, the couples groups fared better. For those without a history of alcohol abuse, both groups fared equally well. There were no significant differences postintervention for communication and marital satisfaction. This latter result seems surprising, because the couples groups focused on communication and improving couple interaction.

In the second controlled study, O'Leary et al. (1999) evaluated a couple intervention for 75 couples to reduce partner aggression. Like the Brannen and Rubin (1996) study, this study compared a gender-specific intervention for men and women to a couple intervention designed to reduce partner aggression. Unlike the Brannen study, however, this study involved all volunteer couples, and included selection criteria to exclude couples in which husband-to-wife aggression had led to injury requiring medical attention. Additionally, wives were assessed (in individual interviews) for fear of their partners; in cases when a partner was fearful of participating, both partners were referred to local domestic violence centers for intervention. Both interventions resulted in significant reductions in psychological and physical aggression, both at posttreatment and at a 1-year follow-up.

The key components of the couple-based intervention included partners taking responsibility for their own psychological and physical aggression, using time-outs from discussions and arguments that were getting out of hand, doing things for one another that showed caring (e.g., assuming household tasks usually completed by the other partner), making supportive comments to the partner, listening to the other without interruption, praising the other, and recognizing that psychological aggres-

sion is often a precipitant of the physical aggression, and consequently has to be reduced.

Based on both wives' and husbands' reports, the gender-specific and the couples groups had significant reductions in psychological and physical aggression at posttreatment and at 1-year follow-up. In addition, there were no differences in the dropout rates across the two treatments. Based on reports of wives, there was a 56% cessation rate of mild and severe physical aggression during treatment. At pretreatment, severe physical aggression was reported in 81% of the cases, whereas at posttreatment, only 31% reported any severe aggression. Wives showed decreases in accepting responsibility for their partners' aggression, and husbands showed decreases in blaming wives for their own aggressive behavior. Finally, there were increases in the marital satisfaction of both groups.

In addition to measuring reductions in psychological and physical aggression, we also measured changes in attributions about responsibility for the aggression by men and women, those who argued against couple treatment were concerned that wives in couple treatment would increase their self-blame for aggression. Instead, wives showed decreases in accepting blame or responsibility for their partners' aggression, and husbands showed decreases in blaming wives for their own aggressive behavior. In addition, we measured aggression between sessions, because another concern was that talking about marital problems could lead to arguments within the couple sessions and that fights would ensue following the sessions. There were no differences across the groups in instances of aggression between sessions.

Because of these concerns, we took several important steps to address these issues. First, regarding responsibility for aggression, all individuals, whether in a couple-based or gender-specific treatment, got the message that they were responsible for any aggression that they perpetrated against a partner. There were no acceptable excuses for aggression, not even being sworn at, slapped, or ridiculed—nothing. Men and women alike were responsible for their own aggression. Second, we also took specific precautions to minimize the likelihood that aggression would occur between sessions. The therapist was responsible for keeping an individual after a session if he or she thought that the individual's anger level was high and there was any concern about the individual venting the anger against a family member. In addition, the therapist was asked to call the client's home later in the evening to make certain that everything was peaceful. Although there were very few times this precaution had to be taken, there were a few instances in which a therapist kept a client after the session and called the client's home later that evening.

When we looked at predictors of change at posttreatment and follow-up, we found that pretreatment levels of physical aggression predicted levels of physical aggression at posttreatment and at 1-year follow-up. The pretreatment levels of physical aggression for *both* men and women predicted continued use of aggression and the severity of such aggression. Moreover, women's psychological state at pretreatment predicted such outcomes (Woodin & O'Leary, 2006).

It should not come as a surprise that levels of a pretreatment variable would predict status levels at postintervention and at follow-up. Such results are found in evaluation of treatments for many different clinical disorders. The severity of pretreatment symptomatology has been shown to predict reduced responsiveness, higher dropout rates, and greater relapse for many psychosocial and psychopharmacological interventions, social phobia (e.g., Otto et al., 2000), depression (e.g., Shea, Elkin, & Sotsky, 1999), and eating disorders (e.g., Fairburn et al., 1995). A common finding is that few, if any, pretreatment indices improve prediction of treatment outcome over initial symptom severity alone (e.g., Otto et al., 2000; Peterson et al., 2000). The conclusion often reached from these diverse fields is that although higher pretreatment symptomatology does not necessarily contraindicate proven treatments, it may be that more intensive or focused interventions should be used with severely symptomatic individuals (e.g., Hamilton & Dobson, 2002). If level of pretreatment aggression plays a similar role in predicting treatment outcome, a comparable conclusion may be warranted for very aggressive individuals entering treatment for aggression against their partners.

These results support the position that one should exclude couples from conjoint treatment when the levels of physical aggression are in the severe range and levels of psychological aggression are very high. In fact, the level of psychological aggression may be as important as the level of physical aggression, in part because it occurs much more often than the physical aggression.

Treatment versus No-Treatment Controls

There are no controlled outcome studies with random assignment to waiting-list control groups or no-treatment groups for physically aggressive behavior, but Stith and her colleagues (Stith, Rosen, & McCollum, 2003; Stith & McCullough, in press) compared treatment in a couple context with a non-randomly-assigned control group of nine couples who were eligible but did not attend the treatment. Couple treatment took place in a multicouple group therapy and in an individual-couple format. At 6-month follow-up, relative to recidivism, the multicouple treatment fared better (25%) than the comparison group (66%). However, the recidivism (43%) in individual couple treatment ($N = 14$) did not differ from that in the comparison ($N = 9$) group (66%). And the individual and multicouple groups did not differ at 6-month follow-up. In the 2-year follow-up, recidivism was much higher in the control group compared to the treatment groups. N's in the different groups were small, but data suggest that the couple therapy in either format has positive effects on reducing men's aggression against their partners. In addition, the data suggest that a nontreated group does not improve spontaneously.

Since their original evaluation, Stith and McCollum (in press) have modified their intervention, so that it now involves an individual component before the couple-based intervention. More specifically, men and women are seen individually for a number of sessions in which anger issues are addressed, and if the therapist judges that they are ready for a couple- based treatment, they move ahead to that intervention. If not, they receive additional therapeutic assistance in addressing anger and other individual issues. This sequencing of individual to marital treatment is in accord with our recommendation about when marital treatment is suitable (O'Leary & Cohen, 2006). Basically, we now assess individuals for couple and individual problems for at least two sessions, then begin marital therapy if we think the individuals in the dyad are ready and can profit from such treatment.

This intervention by Stith and McCollum (in press) may facilitate a rapprochement between the feminist groups who provide services to women in various agencies and those who decry the use of marital therapy with couples who have been physically aggressive; that is, Stith and colleagues try to get anger issues under control before addressing couple issues. Although some feminists argue that rather than anger management and anger control issues, power and control issues are the central problem, there is sufficient evidence that anger issue often do need to be addressed (Murphy & Eckhardt, 2005). This approach can also be related to the Deschner and McNeil (1986) study in which individual counseling was provided simultaneously with couple counseling. The approach in which individuals are carefully screened and provided some individual therapy before couple therapy also is in accord with the therapy approach recommended by O'Leary and Cohen (2006).

In addition, Christensen and his colleagues (Doss, Thum, Sevier, Atkins, & Christensen, 2005) have compared marital therapy of an acceptance-oriented variety (called integrative behavior couple therapy) and a standard cognitive-behavioral marital therapy. Couples were accepted into treatment if they were maritally discordant, and screened out if they had moderate to severe violence as reported by the wife (more than six episodes of mild levels of physical aggression in the past year [pushing, shoving, grabbing]; more than two episodes of moderate physical aggression in the past year [slapping] or any episode of severe physical aggression [beating, use of a knife or gun] ever in the relationship). The study was a large outcome intervention. In an analysis presented at a conference (Simpson & Christensen, 2004), physical aggression was used as a predictor of treatment outcome. Both the acceptance therapy and the standard behavior marital therapy led to significant improvements in marital satisfaction. A dichotomous measure of physical aggression did not predict outcome when outcome was measured as either marital satisfaction or divorce. Psychological aggression decreased in the intervention, although physical aggression did not (probably because it was at such a low level initially). Thus, therapy can take place in couple contexts in which some levels of physical aggression exist, without its having adverse consequences, and it may in fact have positive outcomes.

The research by Doss et al. (2005) raises the issue of whether the marital therapy outcome literature in general can be applied to many couples in which some physical aggression has been present. For example, in a review of 17 behavioral couple therapy (BCT) studies published between 1977 and 1990, Baucom, Hahlweg, and Kuschel (2003) presented evidence that marital therapy has been successful with nonselected marital cases. The Baucom et al. review indicated that five studies published in the 1970s, 10 in the 1980s, and one in the 1990s; as noted earlier, marital therapists were not systematically assessing for the prevalence of partner aggression at those times. However, at those times, marital therapy was quite successful (mean effect size = 0.82) and the control groups did not improve at all (mean effect size

= −0.06); that is, given data on couples seeking marital therapy presented earlier on the 40–60% likelihood of physical aggression in a relationship within the past year, presumably there was some physical aggression in the relationships of couples we had been treating, but such aggression was not specifically assessed. Thus, it appears that couple therapy of a generic behavioral variety has been successful with many couples in which some physical aggression has been present. Indeed, if 66% of couples improve in marital therapy, it is certainly likely that physical aggression would have been present in a significant percentage of those cases.

Alcohol Abuse and Wife Abuse

According to Schecter (1982), prior to the battered women's movement, a few shelters were established to house victims of alcohol-related violence. She stated that the first women's shelter in California was established in 1964 by women from Al-Anon. The fact that one impetus for shelters came from the need to protect family members from alcoholic husbands and fathers should not be a surprise, except that for approximately the last two decades, the role of alcohol in wife abuse has been minimized by the mainstream of the battered women's movement. This minimization comes largely from the concern that batterers would be able to excuse their physical abuse as a result of their drinking. Alcohol has been conceptualized as secondary to a more central issue, namely, misuse of power and control tactics. If power and control tactics are held to be central to the physical abuse, then the cessation of drinking would have little, if any, influence on the likelihood of physical abuse. Nonetheless, regardless of one's view of the ultimate causes of physical abuse of women by their husbands, at least some temporary refuge had to be provided for the wife and family.

However, even today there is a bias among many mental health professionals working with battered women to minimize the role of alcohol as an etiological factor or as a precipitant of physical aggression and abuse. Indeed a search of the Web confirms this bias. For example, an argument addressing this issue is presented by Zubretsky and Digirolamo, in their manuscript on the Web called, "The False Connection between Adult Domestic Violence and Alcohol" (*thesafety zone. org/alcohol/article/html*). They address "Harmful, False Assumptions," such as "Alcohol use and/or alcoholism causes men to batterer." They state the following:

The belief that alcoholism causes domestic violence is a notion widely held both in and outside of the substance abuse field, despite a lack of information to support it. Although research indicates that among men who drink heavily, there is a higher rate of perpetrating assaults resulting in serious injury than exists among other men, the majority of men are not high-level drinkers and the majority of men classified as high-level drinkers do not abuse their partners. (Straus & Gelles, 1990)

Basically, these authors also argue that alcohol can be used as an excuse for being unaccountable or less accountable for their behavior, and that alcohol provides a socially acceptable excuse for their behavior. Use of the Straus and Gelles representative sample study must be kept in context. It was a sample of average citizens in the United States, and it was true that the majority of those drinkers were not drinking at the time of their use of physical aggression. However, we have used the same data from Straus and Gelles (a publicly available dataset) to show that there is a small but linear relationship between alcohol use and men's physical aggression (O'Leary & Schumacher, 2003; O'Leary & Woodin, 2005). Moreover, as the use of alcohol increases to a problematic level, physical aggression against a partner increases dramatically. Specifically, heavy drinkers and binge drinkers were the individuals with elevated risk for being physically aggressive to their wives.

Combined Marital Treatment and Alcohol Treatment

At the Brockton, Massachusetts, Veterans Administration Hospital, O'Farrell, Fals-Stewart, Murphy, and Murphy (2003) demonstrated that if one can reduce alcohol use and increase marital satisfaction, then the likelihood of physical aggression is significantly reduced. The treatment, developed with male veterans and their spouses, to stop alcohol abuse was the medication Antabuse, a drug that induces vomiting almost immediately after ingestion of alcohol. The medication must be taken daily, because it does not have any major cumulative effects. Of course, there is some self-selection for this treatment given that one must truly want to cease drinking, because taking a drink while using the medication has immediate, punishing effects. The couple treatment teaches skills that promote partner support for abstinence and also emphasizes amelioration of common relationship problems in these couples. Regarding partner violence, the non-substance-abusing partner is taught certain coping skills and measures to increase safety if the partner uses alcohol and the likelihood of violence increases (e.g., to leave, if possible, if the partner is drinking, and definitely to avoid arguments with an intoxicated partner). The effects of the combined intervention showed clearly that reduction in drinking and increases in marital satisfaction lead to a reduction in physical aggression in the relationship. Moreover, they showed that relapse into use of aggression was predicted by alcohol use. This result is not in accord with the view of many in the domestic violence field that alcohol use is not central to the issue of partner aggression. In fact, the relapse data made clear that, at least in couple relationships in which alcohol use was problematic, reductions in alcohol use are associated with reductions in physical abuse.

Alcohol and Drug Treatment: A Means to Reduce Partner Aggression

This type of research has been replicated by others who used alcohol and drug treatments, along with marital therapy, to reduce partner aggression. This research, summarized by Fals-Stewart, Klostermann, and Clinton-Sherrod (in press) basically shows quite clearly that for couples who experience alcohol/drug abuse and partner abuse, a reduction in alcohol or drug use leads to a reduction in physical aggression. Furthermore, couple treatment, as exemplified by Fals-Stewart and colleagues, is designed to reduce partner violence even if a relapse occurs. Specifically, the non-substance-abusing partner develops a safety plan and methods of avoiding the partner who is drinking, to minimize the likelihood of relapse. In a comparison of several treatments and an attention control, when the male partner was drinking, the likelihood of male-to-female physical aggression was significantly reduced (i.e., approximately 50% lower on average) for couples who received BCT compared to the couples in the two other conditions.

One should not necessarily conclude that the reduction in alcohol use is clinically sufficient to address all the problems in the relationship. When alcohol use has escalated to some significant problematic point, there are usually marital and family problems as well. For example, often a man with significant alcohol problems will be deficient in paying bills, assuming varied household responsibilities, and interacting with the children and other family members. Thus, a clinician should help clients face the varied individual and relationship issues.

DIFFERENT KINDS OF INTERVENTIONS FOR PARTNER AGGRESSION

Given that treatment of men who are physically aggressive in relationships has not proven very effective compared to court monitoring alone (Babcock, Green, & Robie, 2004), there is a clear need to be open to new conceptualizations of the problem of partner aggression. The dominant theme of male power and control that has permeated so many treatment programs simply has not facilitated the development of successful treatments. And, even individuals such as Ellen Pence, a leader in the batterer's treatment area, now admits that power and coercive control simply do not capture the essence of all relationships in which there is physical aggression. Battering may include physical and sexual abuses but is definitely not limited only to such brutalities. However, over time, the term "battering" has come to be used more or less synonymously with "physical violence by an individual against an intimate partner." This restriction of the term has to a certain degree obscured the complexity of its original meaning and its connection to the real experiences of survivors of ongoing IPV. Of special interest, Pence and Dasgupta (2006) have described four different categories of violence perpetrated against intimate partners: (1) battering; (2) resistive–reactive; (3) situational; and (4) pathological.

Pence and Dasgupta (2006, p. 2) said that situational violence often occurs when partners use violence against each other to express anger or disapproval. They also noted that battering is frequently misdiagnosed as a form of situational violence, because practitioners often tend not to investigate whether there is any pattern of abuse in the relationship. They stated a reluctance to suggest couple counseling for such problems, but noted that it might not be dangerous. Rather, they recommended several other interventions, as follows: (1) Create new behavioral options; (2) resolve circumstances leading to the use of violence; and (3) provide counseling programs, such as anger management.

Need for More Individualized Assessment and Treatment

As Hamberger and Holtzworth-Munroe (in press) argued, "The consistent finding that men who batter their partners are a heterogeneous group, with varying levels of psychopathology, calls for a move away from 'one size fits all' treatment approaches to models that emphasize pretreatment evaluation

of therapy needs and development of individualized treatment plans." If one accepts this view, a problem ensues regarding what interventions should be offered: Should there be an array of interventions for a practitioner to offer that might address various individual psychopathologies? If so, what are those interventions? Until such time that those options exist, Murphy and Eckhardt (2005) suggest using a case-based approach that addresses problems of a given individual or couple. They describe a cognitive-behavioral model for conducting in-depth, individual assessments and developing individual case conceptualizations.

Need for Treatment Outcome Research

As I have argued elsewhere (O'Leary & Vega, 2005), there is a strong need for more outcome research evaluating marital and couple approaches to address the problem of psychological and physical aggression in relationships. Not a single couple-based study for aggression meets the widely accepted standards of the American Psychological Association for an "empirically supported intervention" (Chambless & Ollendick, 2001). There needs to be random assignment of couples to treatments and comparison to a waiting-list control or an accepted, empirically documented alternative treatment. The use of waiting-list controls has been avoided because of ethical concerns, but there is no reason why such controls cannot be used with some careful planning and selection of mild levels of physical aggression in which the partner (usually the female) is without fear and injury. Marital discord is remarkably stable, and careful use of control groups might show convincingly that marital and couple interventions are efficacious.

CONCLUSIONS

1. Mental health professionals in general, and marital therapists in particular, largely ignored the problem of partner aggression and abuse until the mid-1980s and early 1990s.

2. In clinical intake assessments, only 5–10% of marital clients reported that physical aggression is a problem in their relationships.

3. Marital researchers and therapists did not assess regularly for the presence of physical aggression in relationships until research in the 1990s showed that between 40 and 70% of marital therapy couples reported physical aggression in their relationships.

4. Physical aggression occurs in almost half of community couples between ages 20 and 35 when they are sampled representatively.

5. Agencies that serve battered women have taken stances against the use of marital therapy by any intervenors when there is physical aggression in relationships.

6. There is a need to differentiate between cases of battering associated with intimidation, control, and fear of a partner and cases of physical aggression in relationships in which the aggression is mutual and not severe (e.g., pushing, slapping, and shoving).

7. It is important to screen individuals who seek marital therapy carefully for the presence of physical aggression and injury, and to determine whether one partner (usually the woman) fears the other. If injury, fear, and a pattern of intimidation are present, marital therapy is not appropriate.

8. Marital therapy approaches have proven useful in reducing physical aggression in relationships, but gender-specific approaches have also proven to be equally effective in head-to-head comparisons. The gender-specific approaches that have been compared to standard Court monitoring have shown little effectiveness over the court monitoring, but both have also been associated with reductions in physical aggression. These head-to-head comparisons of interventions strongly illustrate the need for control groups that receive some lesser intervention in terms of time and effort, or are assigned to a waiting-list control group (when ethically justified).

9. The presence of infrequent mild to moderate physical aggression in relationships has not impeded therapy progress in behavioral marital couple therapy, and one may infer that many past marital therapy outcome studies that demonstrated the effectiveness of marital therapy probably reduced aggression indirectly even without directly targeting it.

10. Alcohol and drug treatment programs combined with behavioral marital therapy have proven effective in reducing male physical aggression against a wife and in lessening its likelihood if a relapse occurs.

11. Given the relatively small and often nonsignificant gains in traditional interventions emphasizing power and control for batterers, it is time for openness in conceptualizing the problem of physical aggression in intimate relationships. Fortunately, there is definitely a growing acceptance of the view that physical aggression occurs in different types of relationships, and that there is a need for different types of interventions to address this problem.

12. There is a strong need for treatment outcome research comparing marital therapy approaches with waiting-list controls and/or alternative empirically supported treatments.

SUGGESTIONS FOR FURTHER READING

Holtzworth-Munroe, A. (2000). Domestic violence: Combining scientific inquiry and advocacy. *Prevention and Treatment, 3*.

Jacobson, N. S., & Gottman, J. (1998). *When men batter women: New insights into ending abusive relationships*. New York: Simon & Schuster.

O'Leary, K. D., & Cohen, S. (2006). Treatment of psychological and physical aggression in a couple context. In J. Hamel & T. L. Nichols (Eds.), *Family interventions in domestic violence* (pp. 363–380). New York: Springer.

REFERENCES

Aldarondo, E., & Mederos, F. (2002). Common practitioner's concerns about abusive men. In *Programs for men who batterer: Interventions and prevention strategies in a diverse society* (pp. 2-2–2-20). New York: Civic Research Institute.

Archer, J. (2000). Sex differences in aggression between heterosexual partners. A meta-analytic view. *Psychological Bulletin, 126*, 651–680.

Arias, I., & Pape, K. T. (2001). Psychological abuse: Implications for adjustment and commitment to violent leave partners. In K. D. O'Leary & R. D. Maiuro (Eds.), *Psychological abuse in violent domestic relations* (pp. 137–151). New York: Springer.

Austin, J., & Dankwort, J. (1999). Standards for Batterer Intervention Programs: A review and analysis. *Journal of Interpersonal Violence, 14*, 152–168.

Babcock, J., Green, C. E., & Robie, C. (2004). Does batterers' treatment work?: A meta-analytic review of domestic violence treatment. *Clinical Psychology Review, 23*, 1023–1053.

Baucom, D., Hahlweg, K., & Kuschel, A. (2003). Are waiting-list control groups needed in future marital therapy outcome research? *Behavior Therapy, 34*, 179–188.

Brannen, S. J., & Rubin, A. (1996). Comparing the effectiveness of gender-specific and couples groups in a court-mandated-spouse-abuse treatment program. *Research on Social Work Practice, 6*, 405–424.

Brown, P. D., & O'Leary, K. D. (2000). Therapeutic alliance: Predicting continuance and success in group treatment for spouse abuse. *Journal of Consulting and Clinical Psychology, 68*, 340–345.

Cantos, A. L., Neidig, P. H., & O'Leary, K. D. (1994).

Injuries of women and men in a treatment program for domestic violence. *Journal of Family Violence, 9,* 113–124.

Capaldi, D. M., & Owen, L. D. (2001). Physical aggression in a community sample of at-risk young couples: Gender comparisons for high frequency, injury, and fear. *Journal of Family Psychology, 15,* 425–440.

Cascardi, M., Langhinrichsen, J., & Vivian, D. (1992). Marital aggression: Impact, injury, and health correlates for husbands and wives. *Archives of Internal Medicine, 152,* 1178–1184.

Cascardi, M., O'Leary, K. D., Lawrence, E. E., & Schlee, K. A. (1995). Characteristics of women physically abused by their spouses and who seek treatment regarding marital conflict. *Journal of Consulting and Clinical Psychology, 63,* 616–623.

Chambless, D., & Ollendick, T. L. (2001). Empirically supported psychological interventions: Controversies and evidence. *Annual Review of Psychology, 52,* 685–716.

Cohen, S., & O'Leary, K. D. (2007). *Fear of partner measure.* Unpublished manuscript, State University of New York, Stony Brook.

Daly, J. E., & Pelowski, S. (2000). Predictors of dropout among men who batter: A review of studies with implications for research and practice. *Violence and Victims, 15,* 137–160.

Deschner, J. P., & McNeil, J. (1986). Results of anger control training for battering couples. *Journal of Family Violence, 1,* 111–120.

Doss, B. D., Simpson, L. E., & Christensen, A. (2004). Why do couples seek marital therapy? *Professional Psychology: Research and Practice, 35,* 608–614.

Doss, B. D., Thum, Y. M., Sevier, M., Atkins, D. C., & Christensen, A. (2005). Improving relationships: Mechanisms of change in couple therapy. *Journal of Consulting and Clinical Psychology, 73,* 624–633.

Dutton, M. A., Goodman, L. A., & Bennett, L. (2001). Court-involved battered women's responses to violence: The role of psychological, physical, and sexual abuse. In K. D. O'Leary & R. D. Maiuro (Eds.), *Psychological abuse in violent domestic relations* (pp. 177–195). Springer: New York.

Ehrensaft, M., & Vivian, D. (1996). Spouses' reasons for not reporting existing marital aggression as a marital problem. *Journal of Family Psychology, 10,* 443–453.

Ehrensaft, M. K., Moffitt, T. E., & Caspi, A. (2004). Clinically abusive relationships in an unselected birth cohort: Men's and women's participation and developmental antecedents. *Journal of Abnormal Psychology, 113,* 258–271.

Fairburn, C. G., Norman, P. A., Welch, S. L., O'Connor, M. E., Doll, H. A., & Peveler, R. C. (1995). A prospective study of outcome in bulimia nervosa and the long-term effects of three psychological treatments. *Archives of General Psychiatry, 52,* 304–312.

Fals-Stewart, W., Klostermann, K., & Clinton-Sherrod, M. (in press). Substance abuse and intimate partner violence. In K. D. O'Leary & E. M. Woodin (Eds.), *Understanding psychological and physical aggression in*

couples. Washington, DC: American Psychological Association.

Follingstad, D. R., Rutledge, L. I., Berg, B. J., Hause, E. S., & Polek, D. S. (1990). The role of emotional abuse in physically abusive relationships. *Journal of Family Violence, 5,* 107–119.

Foshee, V. (1996). Gender differences in adolescent dating abuse prevalence, types, and injuries. *Health Education Research, 11,* 275–286.

Ganley, A. (1981). *Court-mandated counseling for men who batter: A three day workshop for mental health professionals. Participants manual.* Washington, DC: Center for Women's Policy Studies.

Geiss, S. K., & O'Leary, K. D. (1981). Therapist ratings of frequency and severity of marital problems: Implications for research. *Journal of Marital and Family Therapy, 7,* 515–520.

Geller, J. (2007). Conjoint therapy for the treatment of partner abuse: Indications and contraindications. In A. R. Roberts (Ed.), *Battered women and their families: Intervention strategies and treatment programs* (3rd ed., pp. 76–97). New York: Springer.

Gondolf, E. W. (2002). *Batterer intervention systems: Issues, outcomes, and recommendations.* New York: Sage.

Hamberger, L. K., & Holtzworth-Munroe, A. (in press). Psychopathological correlates of male aggression. In K. D. O'Leary & E. M. Woodin (Eds.), *Understanding psychological and physical aggression in couples.* Washington, DC: American Psychological Association.

Hamel, J., & Nichols, T. (2006). *Family approaches to domestic violence: A guide to gender-inclusive research and treatment.* New York: Springer.

Hamilton, K. E., & Dobson, K. S. (2002). Cognitive therapy of depression: Pretreatment patient predictors of outcome. *Clinical Psychology Review, 22,* 875–893.

Harris, R., Savage, S., Jones, T., & Brooke, W. (1988). A comparison of treatments for abusive men and their partners within a family-service agency. *Canadian Journal of Community Mental Health, 7,* 147–155.

Heyman, R. E., & Slep, A. M. S. (2006). Relational diagnoses: From reliable rationally derived criteria to testable taxonic hypotheses. In S. R. H. Beach, M. Wamboldt, N. Kaslow, R. E. Heyman, M. First, L. G. Underwood, et al. (Eds.), *Relational processes and DSM-V: Neuroscience, assessment, prevention, and treatment* (pp. 139–156). Washington, DC: American Psychiatric Press.

Hilberman, E. (1980). Overview: The wife beater's wife reconsidered. *American Journal of Psychiatry, 137,* 1336–1347.

Hines, D. A., & Saudino, K. J. (2003). Gender differences in psychological, physical, and sexual aggression using the Revised Conflict Tactics Scales. *Violence and Victims, 18,* 197–217.

Holtzworth, A., Waltz, J., Jacobson, N. S., Monaco, V., Fehrenbach, P. A., & Gottman, J. M. (1992). Recruiting nonviolent men as control subjects for research on marital violence: How easily can it be done? *Violence and Victims, 7,* 79–88.

Holtzworth-Munroe, A. (2000). Domestic violence: Combining scientific inquiry and advocacy. *Prevention and Treatment, 3,* Article 22.

Jacobson, N. S., & Gottman, J. (1998). *When men batter women: New insights into ending abusive relationships.* New York: Simon & Schuster.

Lindquist, C. U., Telch, C. F., & Taylor, J. (1983). Evaluation of a conjugal violence treatment program. *Behavioral Counseling and Community Intervention, 3,* 76–90.

Murphy, C. M., & Eckhardt, C. I. (2005). *Treating the abusive partner: An individualized cognitive-behavioral approach.* New York: Guilford Press.

Murphy, C. M., & O'Farrell, T. J. (1994). Factors associated with marital aggression in male alcoholics. *Journal of Family Psychology, 8,* 321–335.

Neidig, P. H., & Friedman, D. (1984). *Spouse abuse: A treatment program for couples.* Champaign, IL: Research Press.

O'Farrell, T. J., Fals-Stewart, W., Murphy, M., & Murphy, C. M. (2003). Partner violence before and after individually based alcoholism treatment for male alcoholic patients. *Journal of Consulting and Clinical Psychology, 71,* 92–102.

O'Leary, K. D., & Cohen, S. (2006). Treatment of psychological and physical aggression in a couple context. In J. Hamel & T. L. Nicholls (Eds.), *Family interventions in domestic violence* (pp. 363–380). New York: Springer.

O'Leary, K. D., & Curley, A. D. (1986). Assertion and family violence: Correlates of spouse abuse. *Journal of Marital and Family Therapy, 12,* 281–290.

O'Leary, K. D., Heyman, R. E., & Neidig, P. H. (1999). Treatment of wife abuse: A comparison of gender-specific and conjoint approaches. *Behavior Therapy, 30,* 475–505.

O'Leary, K. D., & Jacobson, N. S. (1997). *Partner relational problems with physical abuse. In DSM IV Sourcebook* (pp. 673–692). Washington, DC: American Psychiatric Association.

O'Leary, K. D., & Slep, A. S. (2003). A dyadic longitudinal model of adolescent dating aggression. *Journal of Child and Adolescent Psychology, 32,* 314–327.

O'Leary, K. D., & Vega, E. M. (2005). Can partner aggression be stopped with psychosocial interventions? In W. M. Pinsof & J. L. Lebow (Eds.), *Family psychology: The art of the science* (pp. 243–263). New York: Oxford University Press.

O'Leary, K. D., Vivian, D., & Malone, J. (1992). Assessment of physical aggression against women in marriage: The need for multimodal assessment. *Behavioral Assessment, 14,* 5–14.

O'Leary, K. D., & Williams, M. C. (2006). Agreement about acts of physical aggression in marriage. *Journal of Family Psychology, 20,* 656–662.

O'Leary, K. D., & Woodin, E. M. (2005). Partner aggression and problem drinking across the lifespan: How much do they decline? *Clinical Psychology Review, 25,* 877–894.

Otto, M. W., Pollack, M. H., Gould, R. A., Worthington, J. J., III, McArdle, E. T., & Rosenbaum, J. F. (2000). A comparison of the efficacy of clonazepam and cognitive-behavioral group therapy for the treatment of social phobia. *Journal of Anxiety Disorders, 14,* 345–358.

Pence, E., & Dasgupta, S. (2006, June). *Re-examining "battering": Are all acts of violence against intimate partners the same?* Unpublished manuscript, Praxis International, Inc.

Pence, E., & Paymar, M. (1993). *The Duluth Domestic Abuse Intervention Project.* New York: Springer.

Peterson, C. B., Crow, S. J., Nugent, S., Mitchell, J. E., Engbloom, S., & Mussell, M. P. (2000). Predictors of treatment outcome for binge eating disorder. *International Journal of Eating Disorders, 28,* 131–138.

Rennison, C. M., & Welchans, S. (2000, May). Intimate partner violence. [Bureau of Justice Statistics, Special Report No. NCJ178247]. Washington, DC: U.S. Bureau of Justice.

Riggs, D. S., & O'Leary, K. D. (1996). Aggression between heterosexual dating partners: An examination of a causal model of courtship aggression. *Journal of Interpersonal Violence, 11,* 519–540.

Rosenbaum, A., & Kunkel, T. (in press). Group Interventions for Intimate Partner Violence (With Contributions by Alyce LaViolette, Steven Stosny, and Ellen Pence). In K. D. O'Leary & E. M. Woodin (Eds.), *Understanding psychological and physical aggression in couples.* Washington, DC: American Psychological Association.

Rosenbaum, A., & O'Leary, K. D. (1981). Marital violence: Characteristics of abusive couples. *Journal of Consulting and Clinical Psychology, 49,* 63–71.

Satel, S. (1997, Summer). It's always his fault: Feminist ideology dominates perpetrator programs. *The Women's Quarterly.*

Schechter, S. (1982). *Women and male violence: The visions and struggles of the battered women's movement.* Boston, MA: South End Press.

Shea, M. T., Elkin, I., & Sotsky, S. M. (1999). Patient characteristics associated with successful treatment: Outcome findings from the NIMH Treatment of Depression Collaborative Research Program. In D. Janowsky (Ed.), *Psychotherapy indications and outcomes* (pp. 71–90). Washington, DC: American Psychiatric Press.

Shupe, A., Stacey, W., & Hazlewood, L. (1987). *Violent men, violent couples: The dynamics of domestic violence.* Lexington, MA: Lexington Books.

Simpson, L. E., & Christensen, A. (2004, November). *Low-level violence among distressed couples: What is the impact on treatment outcomes?* Symposium presented at the 38th annual meeting of the Association for the Advancement of Cognitive and Behavior Therapy, New Orleans, LA.

Slep, A. M. S., Heyman, R. E., Williams, M. C., Van Dyke, C. E., & O'Leary, S. G. (2006). Using random telephone sampling to recruit generalizable samples for family violence research. *Journal of Family Psychology, 20,* 680–689.

Slep, A. M. S., & O'Leary, S. G. (2005). Parent and partner violence in families with young children: Rates, patterns, and connections. *Journal of Consulting and Clinical Psychology, 73*, 435–444.

Stets, J. E., & Straus, M. A. (1990). Gender differences in reporting marital violence and its medical and psychological consequences. In M. A. Straus & R. J. Gelles (Eds.), *Physical violence in American families: Risk factors and adaptations to violence in 8,145 families* (pp. 151–165). New Brunswick, NJ: Transaction.

Stith, S. M., & McCollum, E. E. (in press). Couples treatment for psychological and physical aggression. In K. D. O'Leary & E. M. Woodin (Eds.), *Understanding psychological and physical aggression in couples.* Washington, DC: American Psychological Association.

Stith, S. M., Rosen, K. H., & McCollum, E. E. (2003). Effectiveness of couple treatment for spouse abuse. *Journal of Marital and Family Therapy, 29*, 407–426.

Straus, M. A. (1979). Measuring intrafamilial conflict and violence: The Conflict Tactics (CT) scales. *Journal of Marriage and the Family, 41*, 75–86.

Straus, M. A., & Gelles, R. J. (Eds.). (1990). *Physical violence in American families: Risk factors and adaptations to violence in 8,145 families* (pp. 151–165). New Brunswick, NJ: Transaction.

Straus, M. A., Gelles, R. J., & Steinmetz, S. K. (1979). *Behind closed doors: Violence in the American family.* New York: Anchor/Doubleday.

Straus, M. A., Hamby, S. L., Boney-McCoy, S., & Sugarman, D. B. (1996). The revised Conflict Tactics Scales (CTS2): Development and preliminary psychometric data. *Journal of Family Issues, 17*, 283–316.

Tjaden, P., & Thoennes, N. (2000). Prevalence and consequences of male-to-female and female-to-male intimate partner violence as measured by the National Violence Against Women Survey. *Violence against Women, 6*, 142–161.

Turkewitz, H., & O'Leary, K. D. (1981). A comparative outcome study of behavioral marital therapy and community therapy. *Journal of Marital and Family Therapy, 7*, 159–169.

Walker, L. E. (1979). *The battered woman.* New York: Harper & Row.

Weisz, A. N., Tolman, R. M., & Saunders, D. G. (2000). Assessing the risk of severe domestic violence: The importance of survivors' predictions. *Journal of Interpersonal Violence, 15*, 75–90.

Whisman, M. A., Dixon, A. E., & Johnson, B. (1997). Therapists' perspectives of couple problems and treatment issues in couple therapy. *Journal of Family Therapy, 11*, 361–366.

Woodin, E. (2007). *Positivity, negativity, and withdrawal during marital conflict: A meta-analytic review.* Unpublished manuscript, Vancouver University, Vancouver, Canada.

Woodin, E. M., & O'Leary, K. D. (2006). Partner aggression severity as a risk-marker for male and female violence recidivism. *Journal of Marital and Family Therapy, 32*, 283–296.

Yllo, K. (1993). Through a feminist lens: Gender, power, and violence. In R. Gelles & D. Loseke (Eds.), *Current controversies on family violence* (pp. 47–63). Newbury Park, CA: Sage.

CHAPTER 17

Couple Therapy with Remarried Partners

JAMES H. BRAY

BACKGROUND

Remarriage is not a new phenomenon, but the number of remarried couples has dramatically increased during the past 30 years. This increase is due to the large divorce and remarriage rates, and to increases in the number of children born outside marriage (Bray, 1999; Bray & Easling, 2005). Working with remarried couples has all of the difficulties and demands of couple therapy for first-marriage couples but in a more complex and challenging context. Remarriages and stepfamilies are inherently different from first marriages, and it is imperative that clinicians be aware of these differences. Because remarriages often involve children from previous relationships, ex-spouses, and former in-laws, many more sources of influence and possible conflicts can impact the remarriage relationship. This chapter reviews these unique aspects and suggests appropriate models and interventions for couple therapy with remarried partners.

Research and clinical interest in stepfamilies grew out of general interest in family therapy and the large increase in numbers of stepfamilies following the divorce revolution of the 1960s and 1970s. The early pioneers in this area of practice were Emily and John Visher, psychologist and psychiatrist, respectively, who became interested in the area after they remarried (Visher & Visher, 1979). In addition, Brady and Ambler (1982) developed a psychoeducational group for remarried couples that was a forerunner of other support groups for remarried couples and families. Sager, Brown, Crohn, Engel, Rodenstein, and Walker (1983) developed additional clinical ideas and techniques for working with remarried families and couples. Their work further advanced the field by clearly delineating the unique aspects of remarriages and stepfamilies, and the need for unique treatment models.

In 1979 the Vishers established the Stepfamily Association of America (SAA) to help people in remarried families understand and cope with life after remarriage. SAA was the only nonprofit organization that focused on the dissemination of research-based resources for stepfamilies and professionals who work with them. In 2006, because of financial limitations, SAA merged with the National Stepfamily Resource Center (NSRC) at Auburn University and ceased operations as an independent organization. The primary objective of the NSRC (2007) is to serve as a clearinghouse of information, linking family social science research on stepfamilies and best practices in work with couples and children in stepfamilies.

Despite these early clinical contributions, no systematic research demonstrated how remarried couples differed from other types of couples. The research literature still focused primarily on the divorce process (cf. Hetherington, Cox, & Cox, 1982; Wallerstein & Kelley, 1980). It was completely assumed that "couples are couples," and that remarriages are just like first marriages. This idea, now referred to as the "nuclear family myth," is one of the common unrealistic expectations of therapists and couples that interfere with effective functioning (Bray, 1995; Visher & Visher, 1988). There continues to be a lack of research on remarriage couples, because most of the work on marriage and divorce focuses on first-marriage couples (cf. Gottman, 1994, 1999; Markman, Floyd, Stanley, Storaasli, 1988; Markman, Renick, Floyd, Stanley, & Clements, 1993). Although there is groundbreaking and increasingly sophisticated research on couple relationships and interventions, most of these findings have not been replicated with remarriages and stepfamilies.

This chapter draws on the literature on stepfamilies and remarriages, and some of the findings from the Developmental Issues in Stepfamilies (DIS) research project, which investigated the longitudinal impact of divorce and remarriage on children's social, emotional, and cognitive development (Bray, 1988, 1999; Bray & Berger, 1993; Bray & Kelly, 1998). The DIS project was a multimethod, multiperspective study of parents, children, and extended family members that included extensive interviews, psychological assessments, family assessments, and videotapes of family interactions. The data provide an excellent source of information about divorce and remarriage, and their impact on remarried adults.

HEALTHY AND DYSFUNCTIONAL REMARRIAGES

There are an estimated 15–20 million remarried, repartnered, and stepfamily couples in the United States, and the number continues to increase each year (Bramlett & Mosher, 2001, 2002; Robertson, Adler-Baeder, Collins, DeMarco, & Fein, 2006). There is no reliable estimate of the number of these couples, because the 2000 U.S. Census failed to include information about marital status, and many states no longer report information about marriage and divorce. The rise in the number of stepfamilies is linked to major demographic changes: increases

in cohabitation with more childbearing outside marriage, high divorce rates, and high remarriage rates (Bramlett & Mosher, 2001, 2002; Bray, 1999; Kreider, 2005). The divorce rate for second and subsequent marriages is higher (5–10%) than for first marriages and has been attributed partially to the presence of children from previous relationships (Bramlett & Mosher, 2001). It is estimated that between 65 and 75% of women and between 75 and 85% of men eventually remarry. The percentages vary; whereas younger people are more likely to remarry, older adults are less likely to do so. White and Hispanic women are more likely than Black women to remarry (Smock, 1990). The first year is the most stressful, and if the remarriage makes it through that year, then the probability of divorce drops to that of first marriages.

There are three distinct but related groups of remarried partners. Figure 17.1 presents a matrix of possible types of remarried couples. First are couples in which one or both partners were married previously and had no children in their marriage(s) or relationships. The prior marriage(s) ended because of divorce or death of a spouse. These couples are referred to as "remarried couples." Second are couples in which one or both partners have been previously married, and one or both had children in their previous marriage(s). The prior marriage(s) may have ended because of divorce or death of a spouse. One or both partners may also have been involved in a nonmarital relationship that produced one or more children. These couples are referred to as "stepfamily couples." The third group comprises couples who have had prior relationships or marriages with children, and live together in a stable committed relationship but are not legally married. These couples are referred to as "repartnered couples." They are similar to stepfamily couples, except they are not legally married (Forgatch & Rains, 1997). This chapter focuses on stepfamily couples but also points out differences and similarities in remarried and repartnered couples. Discussion is limited to therapy with heterosexual couples, because there is very little research about same-sex repartnered couples.

The most common type of remarriage couple is the divorce-engendered stepfather family, in which a man, who may or may not have been previously married, marries a woman who has children from a previous marriage or relationship (Bray & Easling, 2005). However, women in remarriages are more likely to seek out psychotherapy. Most stepfamilies are created after a remarriage, but

Partner	Relationship status			
	Not previously married—no children	Not previously married with children	Previously married—no children	Previously married with children
Female or wife				
Male or husband				

FIGURE 17.1. Matrix of remarriage relationship types.

with increases in cohabitation, many repartnered families form without the legal sanction of matrimony. Most existing research and clinical writing about stepfamilies focuses on those with minor children, but stepfamily couples are also created later in people's lives (Hetherington, Henderson, & Reiss, 1999).

Ethnicity

Most research and clinical writings are based on remarried and stepfamily couples from samples of White, middle-class people (Bray & Easling, 2005). Differences due to ethnic diversity of couples have not been adequately studied, although there is some new attention to low-income, predominantly minority stepfamilies and couples in programs funded by the federal government (Robertson et al., 2006). Further research is needed to examine ethnic and economic diversity in response to marital and nonmarital transitions because of the differences in marriage, divorce, and remarriage rates among ethnic groups. For example, for many lower-income African American families, children may come from nonmarital unions, and the role of the nonresidential parent and his or her family may vary in relationship quality and access. We also know that in these families, grandparents and nonbiological kin (often called Aunties) play an important role in child rearing. It is unclear how these multigenerational and nonkin relationships impact stepcouples and what role they play in successful couple relationships. Differential treatment of children from previous marriages compared to children in the current marriage may also impact the remarried couple. We need to understand better how different cultures accept or reject biological and nonbiological relationships, and their impact on the couple. Given the increasing diversity of the U.S. population, these potential differences warrant further exploration, as well as the devel-

opment of culturally specific marital interventions (Robertson et al., 2006).

In the DIS project we identified common development issues that stepfamilies face. We use this information to educate stepfamilies about what to expect, and to begin the change process. The following is a brief overview of common developmental issues that we encounter in clinical work with stepfamilies. For a more complete discussion of these issues, see Bray (1995, 1999, 2001) and Bray and Kelly (1998).

Planning for Remarriage

There are several critical issues for couples to consider as they plan for remarriage. It should be noted, however, that because most couples do not discuss these issues prior to remarriage, the following are common concerns often bring couples into therapy. These include preparing for the financial and living arrangements for the family, resolving feelings and concerns about the previous marriage, and planning for changes and necessary continuities in parenting children. Whereas many couples who plan to remarry address these issues before marriage, unfortunately, many do not. Some couples discuss their remarriage with their children, including them in their plans, whereas children in some families are not even aware of the wedding until after it has occurred!

The adults have to decide where they will live and how they will share money. In general, adults report that it is advantageous to move to a new residence, so that it becomes "their home." Living in the home of one of the adults, particularly if it was the home of the previous marriage, makes it more difficult to establish a new family identity. However, many families cannot afford to move to a new home. In this case, it is important that the partners make this "their" home, so that they both feel comfortable with the living arrangement.

Families generally decide either to share all of their funds and be a "one-pot family" or to keep separate funds and be a "two-pot family." Both methods can work, although couples using a "one-pot" method generally report higher family satisfaction than those using a "two-pot" method (Bray & Kelly, 1998). The most important aspect of sharing money is that the partners agree on how to do it, thus avoiding fights about money issues. Over time, more stepfamilies become "one-pot" families.

Postremarriage Issues

In the first few years of remarriage, couples commonly face several important issues. First, the couple needs to form a strong marital bond (Bray, 1995; Browning, 1994; Visher & Visher, 1994). This is particularly challenging for stepfamily couples with residential stepchildren. The couple with children faces challenges in finding the time and energy to nurture and attend to their marital and adult needs. However, it is critical that couples form a good, strong marriage, as it is difficult to handle the other issues if the marriage is rocky. Helping couples develop a common ground and understanding in their marriage, taking time to meet their adult needs, and having fun and enjoyment in the marriage are essential. Homework assignments include scheduling regular dates and time alone without the children (at least once a week is recommended). Household chores and responsibilities need to be more equally shared, so that the woman feels she has the time and energy to attend to the marriage (Bray, Berger, & Boethel, 1994; Gottman, 1999). It is often important that couples actually schedule their time together, so that other issues and demands do not get in the way. Therapeutically, it is important to help parents deal with their common concern that taking time away for the sake of their marriage is good for the stepfamily and not destructive to the children.

In addition to forming a new marriage, remarriages have the added stress of bringing unresolved and old patterns from previous marriages into the current one. We refer to these as the "ghosts at the table," because they often operate in unseen ways and pop up to create problems in the relationship. Helping couples identify these "old ghosts" and how they operate in the current relationship is an important step in ridding themselves of "ghosts" or at least changing them to "friendly ghosts."

Developing a parenting plan is another critical issue. The biological parent and the stepparent have to come to an agreement about how to discipline and parent the children. As with first-marriage families, the essential part is that they *agree* with and support each other in the parenting. In the early months after remarriage, it is important for the biological parent to play the primary parental role and for the stepparent to focus on developing a relationship with the stepchildren. Helping the biological parent monitor their stepchildren's lives is useful, but more active parenting and discipline by the stepparent usually needs to wait until there is a solid relationship between the stepparent and stepchildren. Helping parents in stepfamilies develop a consistent set of rules, and consequences for violating rules, is a key step in developing a parenting coalition. Bray (1995) and Visher and Visher (1988) describe exercises to help develop parenting plans.

A third issue is integrating the nonresidential parent and his or her kinship into the stepfamily. Unlike first-marriage families, children in stepfamilies live in two families and can have up to four sets of grandparents. There is wide variety in visitation and access plans between nonresidential parents and children. However, even when children do not see the nonresidential parent often, they have loyalty feelings toward that parent. In addition, children are sensitive to criticism of the nonresidential parent, and it is important not to denigrate that parent, because the children may internalize such negative perceptions or feel that they need to defend that parent.

Making transitions between households smooth and conflict free is very important for children's adjustments. This is often a source of problems in stepfamily couples and a focus of therapy. A common problem in the transition between households involves interparental conflict at the pick-up and drop-off points. Arguing about past or current issues in front of the children is especially problematic for the children and often results in marital conflict for the stepcouple. It is best to avoid these situations or to communicate at times when the children are not present. Using written communications (letters or email) can sometimes reduce this type of conflict. This will be discussed more in later sections.

In addition, children often behave differently after a visit with their nonresidential parent for multiple reasons, such as being in a different environment or missing the parent. Sometimes children are more challenging when they return from a visit. In this case, the couple may attribute the child's change in behavior to the nonresidential parent's negativity toward them (i.e., bad-mouthing them, and trying to influence the child against the stepparent). Such attributions set up conflict for the couple. If the stepparent comments on this, the biological parent is likely to defend the child against the stepparent (a type of triangulation). If the biological parent defends the stepparent, then the child may feel hurt and alienated. It is sometimes best to see these changes as normal transition issues for the children, and to allow them time and space to readjust to their home environment.

All stepfamily couples have some unrealistic expectations, but many lead to destructive processes if they are not recognized. Because of prevailing social myths and stories, such as the "wicked stepparent," family members often enter a remarriage with negative emotions and expectations that are unconsciously reinforced by societal descriptions and names for stepfamilies (Bray & Berger, 1992). Adults and children often hold unrealistic expectations about life in a stepfamily (Visher & Visher, 1988). Common problem-generating expectations include the myth of instant love between children and stepparents, the nuclear family myth of trying to mold a stepfamily into a first-marriage family, the view that trying harder will eliminate the potential of a "wicked" stepparent, and the belief that stepparents should love and care for stepchildren just as they would their biological children. Assessment of both adult and child expectations for relationships in stepfamilies is useful in uncovering unrealistic expectations. Helping family members replace unrealistic expectations with more realistic perspectives is a useful process in resolving many stepfamily problems. Overall, nonclinical stepfamilies have better parent–child relations, better marital adjustment, and more marital individuation than clinical stepfamilies (Bray, 1992).

A Developmental–Systems Framework for Working with Stepfamilies

Stepfamilies continue to evolve over time and have their own developmental life cycles that are different from those of first-marriage families (Bray, 1999; Bray & Berger, 1992; Bray & Kelly, 1998; McGoldrick & Carter, 1988; Papernow, 1993). Previous individual and family experiences (i.e., the divorce experience), developmental is-

sues within the stepfamily, and developmental issues for individual family members all impact relationships in stepfamilies. Couple therapy with remarried partners needs to consider the multiple, intersecting developmental paths of family members and the stepfamily life cycle.

Stepfamily life has three major transition points, and two of the three transition points throw a family into temporary crisis (Bray & Kelly, 1998). Cycle 1 includes the first year or year-and-a-half mark and appears to be the most challenging time period. In cycle 2, 3- to 5-year mark, families' identities and patterns are solidified and stress tends to decrease. Cycle 3 occurs after the first 5 years and, for many couples, coincides with the children's adolescent years. This cycle is also challenging, because adolescents' identity needs create new conflicts and challenges in the stepfamily couple (Bray, 1999; Bray & Berger, 1993).

A stepfamily is at greatest risk for divorce during the first 2 years (Bray & Kelly, 1998). Nearly one-third of stepfamilies fail in this period. This finding also has a corollary that is noteworthy because it illustrates the danger of applying a nuclear family map to stepfamily life. Typically, in a first marriage, the level of marital satisfaction begins high, then declines. In a stepfamily marriage, the opposite flow occurs: The marital satisfaction level starts low, then climbs (Bray & Berger, 1993; Hetherington & Clingempeel, 1992).

We use a developmental–systems model to understand a couple's current context and to work with stepfamilies (Bray, 1995; Bray & Harvey, 1995). We define "context" as family members' interactional patterns and styles, the expectations of family relationships, and their attributions or understanding about family relationships and patterns. Strategic–intergenerational interventions are also used to facilitate change in family patterns, interactions, expectations, and meanings (Bray, 1995; Bray & Harvey, 1995; Williamson & Bray, 1988). These interventions are designed to consider the interactions between the life-cycle tasks of the stepfamily and those of the individual family members.

THE PRACTICE OF REMARRIED COUPLE THERAPY

The Structure of the Therapy Process

Our work with remarried couples is primarily provided for individual couples in an outpatient setting. We have provided groups for couples, but these are usually for support and psychoeducation, rather than for therapy. There are many educational and support groups that seem to be helpful (Adler-Baeder & Higginbotham, 2004; Ganong & Coleman, 2004). Our therapy approach with couples is a brief therapy orientation in which we try to help the couple as quickly as possible. Most couples attend between 6 and 10 sessions, but some come for longer periods, and many couples return at different developmental stages for additional help.

We request that both members of the couple come to the first session so that we may observe their interactions and understand the partners' perspectives on their problems. We may also invite the children to get a broader perspective of the family functioning and how parent–child relations impact the marriage. Our preference is to work with both partners throughout the therapy process, although in some cases we are willing to work with only one partner. We are willing to work with one partner if the other partner refuses and our assessment indicates that we can help the couple while only seeing one member of the couple. In these cases we usually invite the other member in for at least one session as a consultant, so that we can get his or her perspective on the problems and issues. We let this person know that we consider both partners to be in therapy and that we will work to improve their relationship, but it usually works better if both members attend the sessions.

Because we take a systems perspective and view the couple as the client, we have found that individual therapy may interfere with our couple work. We also tell clients that research indicates that the chance of divorce is greater if clients engage in individual therapy rather than couple therapy (Bray & Jouriles, 1995). Therefore, we request that partners stop individual therapy during our couple treatment. There is a greater chance of dysfunctional triangling when another therapist is involved. Furthermore, we find that if the other therapist does not have a good understanding of remarriage and stepfamilies, he or she may be recommending things to the client that contradict what we are recommending.

We usually see couples on a weekly basis in the beginning of therapy, then space sessions further apart. We discourage telephone calls between sessions and usually request that people schedule an extra appointment if they feel it is necessary. We frequently see couples at different points in the stepfamily life cycle for new issues that may develop.

Our stance for working with both partners is that we do not want to be more intimate with either member of the couple than his or her partner is; that is, we view sharing individual information (past relationship issues, family of origin information, etc.) between the partners as a way of fostering understanding, healing, and intimacy. This stance also likely avoids marital secrets and minimizes triangling the therapist into the relationship.

Because of our setting in a medical clinic, we often receive individual referrals of people with individual psychological diagnoses. If we determine during the initial session that clearly facing a couple problem, we ask that the partner be involved in the therapy. If we see one partner alone, we usually offer to see the other partner alone also, to provide a balance in the couple therapy. We carefully clarify confidentiality issues prior to working with the individual partners to avoid marital secrets or triangling. We tell clients the limits of confidentially according to state laws and explain that we do not want to become more intimate with them than they are with their spouse by sharing secrets that cannot be discussed with their spouse. If the client insists on discussing a secret, then we may ask the client to discuss it with his or her spouse, if it interferes with therapy. In this way we usually avoid being limited or triangled by information from one member of the couple.

With this understanding stated clearly, we are willing to work with only one member of the couple when one partner refuses to come into therapy or stops coming but the other partner wants to continue to work on the relationship. We always tell the person that therapy is more likely to succeed if both partners participate. However, we are clear with the person about whether we are helping him or her with the marriage or with individual issues. If the focus is on the marriage, then the client is the marriage, even though only one partner attends therapy. This systemic perspective helps the therapist to avoid taking sides and to continue to focus on the couple and the relationship.

Because we work in a medical setting, many of our referrals are from physicians. These clients may have been diagnosed with a mental disorder (the most common diagnoses are depression and anxiety) and placed on a psychotropic medication. We work collaboratively with the physician to monitor the progress of the medical treatment and may make recommendations for changing or stopping medications (Frank, McDaniel, Bray, & Heldring, 2004). This evidenced-based perspective drawn from recent research on depression and marital relations indicates that depression in the presence of marital problems is most effectively treated with marital therapy rather than individual therapy (Beach & Gupta, 2005).

Role of the Therapist

The therapist is an active agent for change and stands for the couple's relationship. This role may include being an educator, when there is discussion about common issues in remarriage. The therapist may also serve as a consultant or coach in helping the couple make important decisions or practice new skills.

It is critical to establish an effective therapeutic relationship with each member of the couple but maintain a neutral stance regarding the relationship. A systems perspective in which problems are seen in an interactional context facilitates this stance. The relevant contexts are the interactional patterns of the couple, their interpretations of those interactions, and the broader stepfamily system. The other central role of the therapist, particularly in the beginning stages of therapy, is to help create new possibilities for the couple and positive expectations for change. The therapist routinely ends the first session by complimenting the partners for seeking therapy at this time and giving feedback to reassure them that their relationship is not hopeless, and that possibilities for positive change are good. Statements such as "I think you are very wise to seek help at this time" or "I have not seen anything today that makes me think you cannot resolve your problems and have a great marriage" or "The problems you present with today are very common and normal for couples at your stage in remarriage. We can help you with those problems" are offered to the partners.

The most common detrimental problems throughout therapy are for the therapist to be perceived as taking sides in the relationship and/or applying a nuclear family model to a remarried couple. If one party feels that the therapist is against him or her or favors one partner over the other, therapy is frequently doomed. Whereas it is sometimes important to support one partner more than the other during a particularly session, it is critical that, overall, there is balance and neutral-ity in the therapist's stance. In addition, trying to help a remarried couple act and feel like a first-marriage couple is usually counterproductive.

The therapist is an active director of the sessions. Based on the work of Alexander (1973), Gottman (1994, 1999), and others on conflict and interactional patterns in couples, therapists no longer encourage or allow couples to fight and argue during sessions. We assess the couple on the Gottman "divorce cascade" of criticism, contempt, defensiveness and stonewalling, and whether they have recast the relationship as totally negative. The exceptions are during the first few sessions, when it is vital to assess how couples argue, what their interpersonal skill level is, how they recover from arguments, and where they are on the "divorce cascade" (Gottman, 1994; Gottman & Gottman, Chapter 5, this volume). After this the therapist usually says, "Thank you for showing me how you argue. I have a clear picture of how you do this and don't need to see it anymore in therapy." This usually engenders a laugh, and the therapist explains that the focus is on positive interactions and improving the relationship rather than allowing therapy to be a place to argue.

Clients are sometimes encouraged to talk to each other and other times, to the therapist. They are encouraged to talk to each other to try out new skills and to facilitate positive nonverbal connection. Partners talk to the therapist to decrease conflict, and so that the therapist can reinterpret and reframe statements.

The therapist sometimes uses self-disclosure to make a point about the challenges facing the couple or to normalize current issues. However, rather than using self-disclosure, we usually frame the comments as "I had a recent client who ... ," then use the information from our own experience as if it happened to another client couple. We find that this type of self-disclosure enables us to communicate the information without crossing therapeutic boundaries. In addition, if the partners do not like the story or see it as irrelevant to their situation, then they can more easily disagree without concern about hurting the therapist's feelings.

It is essential that the therapist have solid couple therapy skills from a variety of approaches covered in this volume. No single approach to working with remarriage couples is seen as the best, *except the therapist must be knowledgeable and skilled in understanding the unique aspects of remarriage and stepfamilies, and apply interventions within this context.*

Assessment and Treatment Planning

A first step in working with remarried and step-couples is to assess which family members have an impact on the presenting problem(s). Stepfamily couples are inherently more complicated than first-marriage couples because of the multiple family systems and contexts that impact their functioning. The stepfamily system comprises the current residential stepfamily, the nonresidential parent's family system, and the stepparent's family system. Issues from previous marital and divorce experiences, and particularly unresolved emotional problems and attachments, and issues from the family of origin, are central areas of focus in this work. We use genograms to conduct our family assessment (Bray, 1994; Bray & Berger, 1992). McGoldrick, Gerson, and Shellenberger (1999) provide an excellent overview of the use of genograms in family assessment, and Bray (1994) and Visher and Visher (1988) provide examples of how to use genograms specifically with stepfamilies. We do not normally use more formal assessments, such as marital satisfaction instruments, but we do have the couple engage in semistructured conversations, so that we can assess their communication and problem skills. We use the codes developed in the DIS project research and in that of other marital researchers to evaluate these interactions (Bray, 1999; Gottman, 1994; Hetherington & Clingempeel, 1992).

In addition to knowing who is in the family, it is important to assess the kind of stepfamily with which we are dealing. In our research, we have found that stepfamilies usually fall into one of three categories: Neotraditional, Matriarchal, or Romantic (Bray, 2005; Bray & Kelly, 1998).

"Neotraditional" stepfamilies are most representative of the popular image of the happy stepfamily. The adults remarry to have a new family *and* a new marriage. The neotraditional stepfamily is usually a close-knit, loving family and works well for a couple with compatible values. Overall, the partners cope well with the stress and changes experienced in forming a stepfamily. This is not to say that they have less stress, but they just seem to "flow with issues" more successfully. They also form relatively quickly a strong marital bond that supports the development of a parenting coalition. On average, Neotraditional couples score very high on important markers of success, such as marital satisfaction and conflict resolution.

"Matriarchal" stepfamilies are rarely mentioned in the popular literature. The adults remarry because they love each other, but not because they want to have a "family life" together. The chief characteristic of the Matriarchal stepfamily is the dominant role of the woman. Matriarchal women usually have powerful personalities, a high degree of domestic competence, and a strong desire to be the family leader. This stepfamily is also frequently successful if the matriarchal woman is married to a man with compatible values. These stepfamilies resemble single-parent families in the beginning, because the woman maintains her primary role as parent and keeper of the household, while the stepfather tends to be in the background and to remain disengaged from the children.

"Romantic" stepfamilies are sometimes seen in the popular literature. The adults remarry because they want a second marriage and family life. Romantic stepfamilies often look like Neotraditional stepfamilies in the early months after remarriage. Romantics expect everything from stepfamily life that Neotraditionalists do, except Romantics expect it immediately and have many unrealistic expectations. They particularly suffer from the "nuclear family myth"—that a stepfamily should be just like a nuclear family. They expect feelings of love, harmony and closeness between not only the parents but also the stepparents and stepchildren to begin flowing as soon as the couple and the children become a stepfamily. This results in many unrealistic expectations. We found that the early conflict-prone period of the stepfamily cycle is particularly difficult for Romantic stepfamilies. Indeed, Romantic stepfamilies had the highest family breakup rate in the DIS project.

A third area to assess is the relevant developmental cycles of the family and family members. As discussed previously, life-cycle issues for the stepfamily as a whole interact with the individual life cycles of family members. It appears to be easier to form a stepfamily with younger children than with adolescents (Bray, 1999), but all stepfamilies face a common set of developmental issues.

We also assess the couple's strengths and positive characteristics. Based on Gottman's (1994) research, we believe that therapy goes best when positive interactions and qualities are enhanced, while problem behaviors and interactions are changed. We assess the degree to which the partners have moved toward divorce, and the degree to which they negatively construe their relationship. We inquire about the "Big Three" areas of couple relations: sex, money, and communication. If they have children, we ask about parenting issues and how the children influence the marriage. We also determine how much time the partners

Stepfamilies have different histories and experiences. List your expectations and ways of handling issues in the following areas. Discuss them with your spouse and children.

1. Mealtimes
2. Discipline
3. Sharing things between family members
4. School/career
5. Areas of interest for each family member
6. Plans for the future

What are your children's and stepchildren's expectations and interests in these areas? Discuss ways that you can share and interact in these areas.

FIGURE 17.2. Worksheet for developing common ground in stepfamilies.

devote to their relationship and whether they create sufficient time to meet their adult needs.

Individual problems and psychopathology, health issues, and special needs are also assessed during this phase. We work collaboratively with our clients and their physicians regarding health and medications needs (Frank et al., 2004). We also assess historical issues (i.e., "ghosts at the table") to see how they are impacting the current marriage. We ask that couples complete worksheets we have developed to help them identify these areas (see Figure 17.2 for an example). We find that these worksheets speed up the process of therapy as the partners continue therapy work at home between sessions.

Goal Setting

The therapist's goals during the first session are to start the couple/family assessment and genogram, understand the presenting problems, decide with the couple which problems to focus on, and begin at least one intervention and assign some homework. The overall goals of therapy are negotiated between the therapist and clients. We use our developmental model to help set the types and pace of goals for therapy.

The therapist focuses on helping newer couples build a common ground in their marriage by developing a common understanding of their marital expectations and ideas for the marriage. Because most partners have been in other intimate relationships, it is important for them to make explicit their expectations about what a good marriage looks like and how they would like

to build a successful and happy relationship. For stepfamily and repartnered couples, this discussion always includes issues related to their children and parenting. In addition, we frequently find that this view of marriage has to be altered to fit a stepfamily, rather than a first-marriage couple.

We help to identify "ghosts at the table" that might interfere with the current relationship. The amount and degree of focus on this issue varies depending on unresolved issues from prior relationships. This is a central focus of therapy for many couples, but other couples have to deal with relatively few ghosts.

We ask people what their relationship would look like if they had a "great" marriage. We tell them that research indicates that about 25% of couples report really being happy and satisfied in their marriages (Gottman, 2004). We want to help them be in that upper 25%. We ask them to write down between sessions what their "great" marriage would look like. This information is used in subsequent sessions to identify goals and issues to be resolved. We talk about what it takes to do this and how it means devoting time and energy to the relationship.

If the couple is in a crisis due to violence, threat of separation, or infidelity, we focus on these issues first to help decrease the emotionality in the relationship, to stop the destructive conflict, and to help partners decide whether to work on the relationship or end it. We assume that if the couple is asking for therapy, the partners want to work on their relationship, unless one or both partners explicitly state otherwise. Even in these cases we take a stand for their relationship, especially if they have children together.

For example, if one or both partners continually call into question the relationship (i.e., threaten to end it), we work on helping them decide or commit to be in or out, even if it is for a specific period of time. We provide psychoeducation about the destructiveness of threatening to end the relationship and explain to them how ambivalence tends to drive a couple apart. We also talk with them about how it is impossible to develop trust and intimacy if there is a covert or overt threat to end the relationship. We ask that they make a commitment, even if only for a limited time period of a few weeks, to see whether we can improve the relationship, so that the partners want to remain in it. This is where we use "possibility thinking" with the couple. We ask about possibilities the partners would like to consider in the relationship, then how we might achieve those possibilities.

Individuals sometimes ask whether they should get divorced or stay together. We tell them we cannot answer that question for them. However, we have found that 70% of individuals regret getting divorced after the first year (Bray & Jouriles, 1995), and that those who did not regret getting the divorce had tried everything reasonable to save their marriage. We add that only they can decide if they have tried everything reasonable to save their marriage. If they have not tried everything reasonable, then we focus on those possibilities in therapy.

We reassess the goals and progress toward goals about every three to four sessions. At that time, we check on the partners' views as to progress and whether we are accomplishing what they want to accomplish, or if we need to change some of our goals. We find that this process assessment helps us to keep on track and enhances the therapeutic alliance.

Process and Technical Aspects of Remarried Couple Therapy

Therapeutic Orientation

We use a variety of interventions developed within the broad field of family therapy and psychology, including communication skills training, problem-solving training, reframing, behavioral tracking, parenting skills, family-of-origin work, and others. It is important to emphasize that all of these interventions are applied within the context of life in a stepfamily. Thus, it is always important to remember the influence of the previous marriage when helping remarried couples to work on their marriages, because the unresolved issues, or "ghosts," are often operating in the present relationship. In addition to psychoeducation and other interventions, we ask family members to do homework assignments outside of sessions to facilitate and hasten the change process. We emphasize couples' positive qualities and strengths and focus on enhancing these throughout the therapy process.

Therapeutic Modalities

Psychoeducation

Stepfamily couples can benefit greatly from education about the stresses and issues they face in the normal stepfamily developmental cycle (Bray, 1995; Visher & Visher, 1990). "Psychoeducation" is the provision of information in a counseling or therapeutic context to promote the change process (Levant, 1986). In addition, information about the unique aspects of marital relations, parenting, and extended family relationships is often included. There are several structured programs available: Burt (1989), Currier (1995), Visher and Visher (1990).

Bibliotherapy

"Bibliotherapy" involves using books, pamphlets, and other written materials as an integral part of the therapy process (Bray, 1993). Some adults and children in stepfamilies read recommended books and other materials or attend lectures to obtain relevant information. See Coleman, Ganong, and Fine (2000), and Ganong and Coleman (2004) for further resources. We recommend our book *Stepfamilies: Love, Marriage, and Parenting in the First Decade* (Bray & Kelly, 1998) and Visher and Visher's, *How to Win as a Stepfamily* (1991), for most couples.

Support Groups

These excellent peer resources for stepfamilies usually meet once or twice a month and provide a forum for discussion of problems and development of solutions. Some groups invite outside speakers (Visher & Visher, 1990).

Couple Therapy

Because most problems experienced by individuals in a stepfamily are related to the interactions within the stepfamily or extended family, family and couple therapy approaches are frequently used with stepfamilies (Bray, 1995; Martin & Martin, 1992). There is relatively little outcome research on such stepfamily-specific therapy, although many therapy outcome studies have included stepfamilies in their samples.

Skills Training

Techniques used and taught in other forms of family therapy are also useful for stepfamilies, with appropriate adaptation to their needs. Parenting skills include discipline methods and resolution of differences in parenting styles (Forgatch & Rains, 1997). Communication skills training is useful for both marital partners, and parent–child, and stepparent–child communications. Bray (1988) found that newly remarried couples had less effective communication skills than first-marriage couples. Training such as the Prevention and Relationship Enhancement Program (PREP) (Renick, Blumberg, & Markman, 1992) and relationship enhancement training (Guerney, 1977), modified for stepfamilies, are useful resources.

The process of therapy varies, depending on whether problems are generated between the partners or are a result of individual factors, such as "ghosts" or family-of-origin issues. As previously stated, we prefer to have both partners attend all sessions, even if we are focusing primarily on individual issues of one partner. The key issue is to maintain a balance with both partners, so that one partner does not get labeled as "the problem." Because we use a family systems orientation, we do not focus on or foster transference. We view transference as an opportunity to do family-of-origin work and let the partners know this needs attention (Williamson & Bray, 1988). We help the partners understand how family-of-origin issues impact the current relationship, and how resolving or changing these relationships may positively impact the current marriage.

We regularly assign homework, which may include completing genograms and worksheets we have developed on aspects of the relationship, such as "ghosts at the table" or parenting, or tracking behaviors that are a focus for change. In addition, we ask partners to practice the skills covered in the sessions at home and to create couple time for fun and positive activities. We may also ask them to read books about stepfamilies or couple relationships. We find that all of these tasks speed up the process of therapy.

We do not usually have a formal termination process for therapy, because we frequently work with couples at different points in the stepfamily life cycle. A couple's decision to stop therapy is based on partners' reaching their goals, and feeling happy and satisfied with their relationship.

Common Pitfalls in Treating Remarried Couples

The most common pitfall in working with a remarried couple is applying a first-marriage model to their relationship. This may occur when a therapist reinforces the couple's ideas about marriage that are not based on an appropriate stepfamily model. For example, new stepparents commonly become too involved in disciplining the children, before they are a relationship with the children and work out a parenting plan. Couples argue about these issues, without recognizing the presence of loyalty issues between the biological versus steprelationships.

A second common problem in working with stepcouples is to ignore the influence of prior relationships. Unresolved hurt and grief or sensitivities developed in the prior marriage often give rise to conflict in the stepfamily couple.

A third common problem occurs when remarried couples do not recognize other sources of influence on the marriage, such as the impact of children, ex-spouses, and other family members. For example, it is common for a remarried couple to plan a weekend or evening alone, without the children, only to have the nonresidential parent refuse to take the children.

In first-marriage families it takes two people—the partners—to make the marriage happy. In stepfamily couples, it takes three—the two partners and the children. Children in a stepfamily exert more influence and control on marital happiness than do children in first-marriage families (Bray & Berger, 1993; Hetherington & Clingempeel, 1992). In addition, parenting is the most stressful aspect of life in a stepfamily and a potential source of conflict—much more so than in first-marriage families. The stress of parenting continues throughout the stepfamily life cycle and increases when the children reach adolescence (Bray & Harvey, 1995).

The added parenting stress is the result of inherent differences in loyalty between biological children, and parents and stepparents. The old adage that blood is thicker than water is true. Biological parents usually defend their children against their spouse and are willing to sacrifice their marriage for them. The reverse is sometimes true as well, as children in stepfamilies are more likely to be ejected or "kicked out" of their families in a stepfamily than in a first-marriage family.

CURATIVE FACTORS/MECHANISMS OF CHANGE

Our work is based on a developmental–systems approach to therapy, as described in previous sections. As such, this approach shares the views of systems approaches in terms of mechanisms of change, which include changing perceptions of individual partners who contribute to conflict and unhappiness, changing the dominant interaction problematic patterns in the couple's relationship, changing the behavior of one or both partners, and helping to heal unresolved grief and loss from prior relationships. These common factors are the same as those in other forms of couple therapy—again, the unique aspect is the stepfamily or remarried context.

The focus on healing past relationships is often a central issue that may not be found in work with first marriage couples. The therapeutic techniques of Enright and colleagues (Enright, 2001; Reed & Enright, 2006) on forgiveness and healing are very useful in our work. This often involves focus on prior marriages/relationships and family of origin issues. Helping the couple see how these unresolved hurts are impacting the current relationship is a key first step to the healing process.

We use psychoeducation about the unique aspects of remarried couples and how they are different than first marriage couples to help couples develop more realistic expectations about remarriage. Pointing out unrealistic expectations and helping the partners develop more realistic ones is a central focus in working with remarried couples during the first few years after remarriage. Normalizing some of their concerns is also a way to decrease stress and conflict. Although this process may resemble cognitive-behavioral therapy (CBT), rather than use CBT or rational–emotive worksheets, we have developed out own that consider the unique stepfamily context.

We start with the assumption that clients have good or adequate communication skills rather than skills deficits, but that emotional factors are blocking clients' use of them in the relationship. If this is not the case, then we help clients develop the necessary skills needed to have a successful relationship. We teach these skills during the therapy process rather than having specific didactic skills training sessions. In a few cases, we refer couples to specific workshops in which these skills are taught. Although such skills training is important, it does not replace a good therapeutic relationship. Therapists with extensive knowledge and understanding of the unique aspects of remarriage cannot be helpful unless they are able to form a solid working relationship with both members of the couple, even when the partners' own differences may at times be extreme.

TREATMENT APPLICABILITY AND EMPIRICAL SUPPORT

There is relatively little outcome research on specific therapeutic approaches for remarried or stepfamily couple therapy. Although traditional family therapy methods may be useful in working with stepfamilies, these methods need modifications that take into consideration unique aspects of remarried couple dynamics and issues (Kelley, 1995). However, there is a shortage of treatment programs for stepfamilies, and few have been empirically evaluated (Michaels, 2000).

Guidelines for clinicians providing therapy to stepfamilies have been based on clinical experience and research findings (Bray, 1995; Browning, 1994; Browning & Bray, in press; Martin & Martin, 1992; Pasley, Dollahite, & Ihinger-Tallman, 1993; Visher & Visher, 1979). Despite the widespread agreement that the first 2 years are usually the most difficult for stepfamilies, intervention programs for this period also have been neglected (Kelley, 1992, 1995).

Initially, a focus on the marriage and spousal relationship, rather than on the whole family, may be more beneficial (Bray, 1995; Browning, 1994; Browning & Bray, in press; Visher & Visher, 1994). Once the marriage becomes stable, group therapy with other stepfamily couples can provide support and help to resolve issues (Brady & Ambler, 1982; Mandell & Birenzweig, 1990; Papernow, 1993; Sager et al., 1983). Family therapy may also be helpful at this stage.

Another recommended therapeutic approach is to link the chosen modality to the developmental stage of the stepfamily (Pasley, Rhoden, Visher, & Visher, 1996). Papernow (1993) identified seven stages of stepfamily adjustment: fantasy; immersion; awareness; mobilization; action; contact; and resolution. For the first three stages, she suggested interventions focused on putting fantasies in perspective, replacing them with more realistic expectations.

The Stepfamily Parent Education Program (Nelson & Levant, 1991) is an example of a skills training program for adults in stepfamilies. Generic communication and parenting skills were taught and then applied to stepfamily-specific situations. One parent (biological or stepparent) from each participating family took part in the program. Improved communication skills were illustrated in the trained stepfamily parents' reflection and expression of feelings. However, some undesirable parenting responses, such as lecturing and giving orders, were still evident. The children of trained stepfamily parents perceived positive changes in their relationship with their parents, as shown in family drawings. On the other hand, children did not notice increased acceptance and decreased rejection from the trained parents. Nelson and Levant found the results generally encouraging, although the program had several limitations, including small sample size, and they recommend that more stepfamily members participate in future training programs.

The objective of the Stepfamily Enrichment Program was to assist stepfamilies during the family formation stage (Michaels, 2000). Pretested in a large metropolitan area and in a smaller college town, the program had the following objectives: to normalize the stepfamily experience; to understand how such families develop; to strengthen the marital relationship; to define and nurture the stepparent– and biological parent–child relationship and to maintain the noncustodial parent–child relationship; and to assess the progress of families and their future plans. Each group was led by two therapists/facilitators, and five weekly 2-hour sessions comprised didactic presentations, group discussions, and experiential exercises; homework was also given. Weekly process evaluations were conducted, and a focus group session was held during the last session.

Program objectives were generally met with regard to normalizing the stepfamily experience. Limitations of the pilot study included its small sample size, lack of a control group, and lack of diversity among the participants, all of whom were white, middle-class, and had no serious relationship problems.

Evaluation of Therapy for Stepfamilies

To gain insights into stepfamilies' therapy experiences, members of the SAA were surveyed (Pasley et al., 1996). The survey responses of 267 currently married individuals who had been in stepfamily therapy were examined. Most of the respondents (54.7%) had stopped therapy more than 12 months previously, and the others were almost evenly divided between those who had terminated therapy less than 6 months earlier and those who had terminated between 6 and 12 months previously. Most study participants had begun therapy within the first 4 years after remarriage.

Stepfamily functioning ("depression or anxiety about how things are working in the stepfamily") and parenting/stepparenting were the two principal areas of concern for the participants in the beginning of therapy. Within the latter category, the discipline of children and stepchildren and stepparent–stepchild interaction were the priorities. Academic and/or behavior problems of stepchildren and behavior of the former spouse were also important.

The majority of participants (82.4%) reported that the therapy was helpful or very helpful, whereas 12.7% found it unhelpful or very unhelpful; 4.9% of participants thought that it had no impact on them. The therapy components considered most helpful were affective support (21.9%), clarification of issues (19.6%), and the process and structure of the therapy (18.1%). The therapist's perceived lack of training and skills in treating stepfamily issues was the most frequently reported unhelpful aspect of therapy.

It is clear from this brief review that more research is needed both to develop programs that address the unique needs of stepfamilies and to evaluate the effectiveness of those programs. Because children in stepfamilies are at greater risk for behavioral and emotional problems, prevention efforts targeted at reducing this risk are needed for. Furthermore, adaptation of existing programs and development of new ones to support and enhance marriages in stepfamilies are also needed.

CASE ILLUSTRATION: STARTING OFF ROUGH

The following case illustrates many of the common problems and issues that arise in the early phase of remarriage. Due to such varied types and structures of remarried and stepcouples (see Figure 17.1), it is not possible to illustrate therapy with all of the different types of couples.

Ms. Y contacted the clinic after being referred by her primary care physician. Ms. Y stated that she had recently seen her doctor, who told her that she had eight out of nine of the symptoms of major depression, and recommended that she take an antidepressant and enter counseling. Ms. Y did not want to take medication, because she thought that rather than being depressed, she was stressed out due to the many problems following her recent remarriage 6 months ago. She stated, "This is just too hard—and not what I expected! I am so upset, I can't sleep or concentrate." Sobbing, she said, "I just don't know what to do—I just got married and I can't tolerate the idea of quitting this early." Ms. Y was asked to bring her husband to the first appointment, because it appeared that her difficulties were related primarily to her recent remarriage. After some discussion and explanation about this request, she reluctantly agreed to ask him to come in with her.

During the first session I learned the following about the couple: Married about 6 months, although they had known each other through their work for over 6 years, they had only dated for about 6 months prior to marriage. Mr. G stated that perhaps they married too soon and did not know each other well enough. Ms. Y responded, "Its too late now—we are already married—you just want out!" He responded with tears in his eyes, "I just don't know. This is not what I expected and it is just so hard. My life has been totally disrupted." Although both partners were clearly upset, Ms. Y was much more emotionally expressive.

Ms. Y had been married and divorced once before. She had one son, age 12, who had a learning disability, from that marriage. She had been divorced for about 5 years. She had joint custody with her son's father, and they appeared to have a good working relationship. The divorce had involved a high-conflict and intense custody battle, and it had taken Ms. Y several years to overcome this conflictual history with her former husband. Her former husband had been remarried for several years and there were no issues reported after his remarriage. Ms. Y was a successful professional, with a demanding career. She owned her own home and was very proud that she was able to finally come out of her first marriage and establish herself independently and successfully. She stated that her husband had had a very difficult time living with her son because of his learning disability and behavior related to this. She stated and her husband concurred, that the relationship had taken a turn for the worse after the marriage.

Mr. G had also been married and divorced once before. His first marriage had ended about 10 years earlier. He had two children, a boy and girl, from that marriage. The children lived with their mother in another state and only visited during the summer and holidays. He reported that he had a good relationship with his former wife and his children. Ms. Y concurred with his assessment. The couple also agreed that Ms. Y had a good relationship with his children, and she stated that they were "wonderful kids and I wish we could spend more time with them." Prior to his marriage to Ms. Y, Mr. G had cohabitated with a woman for several years in his home.

Mr. G was also a successful professional in a field related to his wife's profession. He also worked long hours and traveled frequently as part of his job. Although both partners were successful, Mr. G made considerably more money than Ms. Y. Because he lived in a bigger home, the couple decided to move into his house after the marriage. During the courtship, they had primarily stayed at Ms. Y's home because of her son. Ms. Y did not feel that she was welcome at her husband's house, and that he had not made it "their" home. He countered that he had tried, but she was unwilling to move her things into his house and sell her home. Ms. Y stated that she could not sell her home now, because of all of the conflict in the marriage.

The couple was a "two-pot family"; that is, they did not share their financial resources and they split their bills. This was a source of conflict for both of them. Ms. Y felt she was paying for a lot more than she should, and her standard of living had actually declined after her remarriage. She also paid for things for his children (clothes and presents) that she felt they needed. Mr. G had lived a frugal lifestyle prior to remarriage and had placed a high priority on saving money for retirement. In summary, money was a source of conflict, and the partners had not worked out how to share their resources.

The couple appeared to be a matriarchal stepfamily. They decided to marry because of their relationship. Each member of the couple had strong views on the "right way" to handle situations. Because both partners were independent professionals, used to debating and being right, this was a sensitive arena for their marriage. The "right way" ranged from minor things, such as how to handle the trash, to major issues, such as how to parent their children. I used this as an opportunity to educate them about the diversity of stepfamilies and how there was not just one right way to be happy and successful. They each continued to push this issue so we had the following conversation.

I said, "You know, when you are arguing about some of these issues, you are both right."

Mr. G responded, "What do you mean we are both right—how can that be?"

"Well, as I told you before, our research indicates that there are many ways—not just one way—to have a happy successful stepfamily and marriage. Some of what you are talking about is values differences and both sets of your values can lead to good outcomes."

Ms. Y chimed in. "But my son and I were doing just fine before this marriage, and now that he wants to change everything, we are having all of these problems."

I said, "I know. This is not about being right or wrong, this is about *getting along*. You two are going to have to decide whether it is more important to be right or more important to get along. You probably can't do both. In your professions it is important to be right, but in marriage, it is all about getting along. We need to work on you developing a set of shared values and goals for your family, so you can work on getting along."

The couple had a number of strengths. Despite the conflict and stress, each partner held the other in high esteem and expressed strong feelings of love and affection. Mr. G stated that his wife was a "very special person," whom he "admired greatly." They stated that they had a great sex life and that sex often helped them overcome their arguments and hurt feelings. In addition, each partner was willing to look at his or her role and contribution to the conflict. Furthermore, they had good communication and problem-solving skills but were not using them in their marriage. These strengths would be very helpful in the therapy process.

High Stress—Will It Last Forever?

Both partners repeatedly talked about how stressful their relationship and life had become after remarriage. Mr. G was especially upset about his work routines being disrupted and the added demands to be with his wife and to help with her son. His routine was to be in the office around 9 A.M. and work until 7–8 P.M. He was used to staying up later than his wife. Ms. Y had to rise earlier to get her son ready for school and finish her work earlier to be available to take care of her son after work. Mr. G stated that because of the changing sleep patterns, he did not sleep well. Such increased stress is common in new stepfamily couples, especially during the first year after remarriage (Bray & Berger, 1993). This was an opportunity to educate the couple about our research. After I told them that the stress would likely decrease in a few months, they were visibly relieved.

I ended the session by asking them to do the following homework: first, to complete some of our worksheets that help to identify unresolved relationship issues and bring them in for discussion next session; second, to start preparing a budget, so that we could discuss how they would share their money and resources; and finally, to make time for at least one date in which they focused on enjoying each other. The date was an important way to enhance positive interactions.

I started the second session with the standard question, "How were things this past week—how were they different?" They indicated that they had gotten along much better the first few days, then had a big argument over her son and some financial issues. I first asked what was different, and Ms. Y stated that she felt relieved knowing that the stress in the relationship might decrease significantly in the next few months. Mr. G said he also felt more hopeful and was able to overlook several things that had been bothersome to him. They had not done the worksheets. He had started working on a budget, but Ms. Y said that she had had too many work demands that week to get it done. They did have a successful date, but the positive feelings from the date were undone by the conflict that started the next day.

We then moved on to the conflict. I wanted to see how the couple argued and engaged in conflict. What I heard and saw was that when they had conflict, their arguing escalated quickly. Mr. G said that he really "hated conflict" and tried to avoid it. Ms. Y said that she felt he was ignoring her, and she would continue to pursue him to get some resolution. Whereas she tended to be critical and sarcastic, he would become defensive. His way of ending arguments was to question whether they should be together (i.e., call into question the relationship). This hurt Ms. Y: "It's like having a knife stuck in me each time he does this." This couple was already headed down Gottman's "divorce cascade."

I took this opportunity to discuss two important issues with them. First, I discussed the problem with calling into question the relationship. I explained how and why this is so destructive, especially in partners who have already experienced divorce, and recommended that they only do it if they were serious about ending the relationship. Mr. G seemed to understand the issue, which led to a discussion about how he could share his concerns and feelings about being overwhelmed, without implying that he wanted out of the marriage. Mr. G stated that he did not want out of the relationship. Ms. Y started crying and said, "I hope this is true—it just kills me when you say you want out."

I then discussed the second issue about the supportive–defensive cycle. I explained that when one person feels criticized, the normal human way of responding is to defend oneself. Usually when one defends oneself, the partner experiences this as a criticism. The criticism is defended, and the cycle escalates. I use a set of "Newton's balls" to demonstrate the reverberation of the conflict, and that if one person does not respond in the usual way, the conflict will stop or at least be different. I suggested that each partner try to do two things when the other made a critical statement. First, I urged them to listen to understand (i.e., be empathic) rather than listening to respond. Second,

I emphasized the idea that a partner's comment is more a statement about him- or herself than about them. It is the partner's opinion and concern, and not necessarily true. Because you care about your partner, it is important to listen to his or her concern.

I explained that this is not always easy, as the natural tendency of humans is to fight, flee or shut down. I role-played several situations and ways to respond in this manner. The couple was again asked to do the homework from the first session and to practice this method of responding during the next week. Because of their travel schedule we were not able to meet for a couple of weeks.

They returned for the third session, again feeling very upset. The lack of change in the relationship was very concerning to me, and I wondered what I was missing. Both partners stated that they had gotten along much better for about a week, then had a fight that continued until this session. The fight started when Mr. G got upset with Ms. Y's son and "got after him" for not turning off some lights and for leaving a door unlocked. Ms. Y said that this was a common occurrence, and that his way of handling the situations was impacting her son negatively. She also stated that Mr. G did not understand that her son forgot to do some things because of his learning disability, and that she did not see it as "a big deal." The couple continued to argue over these issues. Once again, the arguments escalated into talk of separation by Mr. G, which really upset Ms. Y.

This problem illustrates a unique issue for stepfamily couples, namely, that the marriage is highly influenced by issues related to the children, more so than in first-marriage families (Bray & Berger, 1993). In this case there were several issues operating. First, there was the loyalty issue of Ms. Y protecting her son against Mr. G. Second, Mr. G was trying to parent and discipline too early, and without the support of Ms. G. Third, the son's talk of living with his biological father more was potentially activating issues with the ex-spouse. As previously discussed, parenting is the most stressful aspect of life in a stepfamily, and the partners have to develop a joint parenting plan. In addition, the stepparent needs to establish a good relationship with the children prior to trying to be a disciplinarian (Bray, 1995; Bray & Berger, 1993). This is difficult to do when there is not a strong marital relationship. I spent the bulk of the session helping them to develop a parenting plan. I touched briefly on the money and budget issue. The partners indicated that they had started talking about these issues, but that it had broken down when they started fighting again. Their homework assignment was to complete the worksheets I had previously assigned. I also gave them some new worksheets on developing a parenting plan, and reminded them about the importance of listening to the partner differently to stop the escalating conflict. I restated the importance of increasing the positive interactions.

They agreed to do these tasks, but I sensed their ambivalence about doing so. I used this as an opportunity to educate them about the importance of giving and keeping their word and commitments.

I said, "It seems to me that you are not committed to doing the homework, and I just want to clarify your intentions."

"Well, I will try, but I have a busy week ahead," replied Mr. G. Ms. Y nodded in agreement.

"To me, 'trying' means that you will not do it, so I would like you to commit to either doing or not doing the tasks. It is OK with me if you don't do them—just say which way it will be. This is a like a light switch. It's on or off—that is, you will either do the tasks or not do them. Either way is OK with me, but if you tell me you are going to do them, then I will hold you accountable for your commitment."

Ms. Y replied, "Well, he often says one thing and then does not follow through. It really upsets me when he does this."

Mr. G started to react and I stopped him. I could tell that he was angered by this statement.

"I asked each of you to do homework and you said you would do it. Then, the next session, you said you were unable to do it. I understand you each have very busy lives and demanding careers, but if you want to have a great marriage, I am suggesting that you need to make your marriage a priority, and if you say you are going to do something, then you will keep your commitments. It is OK with me for you to say no, or not to agree to do something, but one of the problems that you are having in your marriage is that your partner asks you to do something and then you don't do it. This is causing a lot of conflict in the marriage."

They seemed to understand what I was saying and nodded in agreement.

I asked, "What homework will you agree to do between now and the next session?"

Mr. G said he would complete the budget and do both worksheets. Ms. Y said she would complete her budget but that she had time to do only one of the worksheets.

I asked, "Which one?"

She smiled, "Boy, you are tough—I guess I will do the parenting one, since I am most concerned about my son."

I reiterated our agreement, and we ended the session.

At the beginning of the next session, they seemed calmer. Each indicated that things were better overall and that when an argument had started, they had intentionally tried different ways to deescalate and stop the conflict.

Ms. Y said they started saying to each other, "Remember the balls—let's don't reverberate." They seemed to have had a breakthrough in stopping the conflict. The next three sessions focused on money issues and how they were going to share resources, and on developing a parenting plan.

These were not easy discussions, because they involved "ghosts" for both partners around money issues from their prior marriages and families of origin. Although they had signed a prenuptial agreement prior to their marriage, they had not worked out a plan for sharing money during the marriage. Mr. G had grown up in a modest family, and his parents had struggled financially, especially in old age, because they had not prepared sufficient retirement savings. He was very sensitive about saving money, so that he would not end up like his parents. In addition, because he had had to give up half of his retirement savings to his former wife, he felt that he was not adequately prepared for retirement.

Ms. Y felt that her previous husband had overcontrolled their money. She had trusted him with their accounts, but when they divorced, she felt that he had "stolen" a lot of their money and run up large debts with which she was stuck. Thus, she was concerned about placing all of their money in one pot. She also believed that they should not sacrifice so much for their retirement. Ms. Y had a more "live in the moment" attitude about money. Although these are common issues in many marriages, their unique flavor in stepfamilies is often related to unresolved matters from earlier marriage and divorce experiences.

We also focused on developing a parenting plan for their children. Mr. G was a very part-time parent; he only saw his children on holidays and during the summer for 30 days, whereas Ms. Y's son was with her about 60% of the time. Mr. G was more structured and authoritarian than Ms. Y about parenting. In addition, neither of his children had any special needs or behavioral problems.

Ms. Y's son had learning and memory problems, so he was more likely to forget small things, such as turning off the lights or TV. This greatly upset Mr. G, who felt that the boy was just misbehaving or using his learning problem as an excuse. I suggested that Mr. G talk with the boy's tutor and doctor, so that he could better understand his limitations. After Mr. G spoke with these professionals and better understood the issues, he was able to be more understanding and less demanding.

I suggested that they bring in Ms. Y's son for one of the sessions, but they declined. Ms. Y said that she did not want her son or her ex-husband to know about their therapy. She said they were getting along, and that this might create more problems with her ex-husband. Because of the increased conflict, her son had been talking about living with his father, and she felt that the son's involvement might fuel this idea. She was very afraid that her son might leave and live full-time with his father. I told her that I understood, and that developing a parenting plan should decrease the conflict and make their home more welcoming to her son.

I developed a parenting plan with just the couple, using methods I outlined (Bray, 2001, 2005). Creating the parenting plan significantly decreased the couple's conflict and enhanced the interactions between Mr. G and Ms. Y's son. The work also helped them to feel closer, to reestablish good communication, and to develop effective problem solving for future issues. I suggested that they read some books about stepfamilies to help them understand how they were unique (Bray & Kelly, 1998; Visher & Visher, 1991).

Because of scheduling conflicts, we were not able to meet for several weeks. At the next session, the partners indicated that they were still doing much better overall, with fewer conflicts that were short-lived. However, Ms. Y was still very concerned about a few issues. First, she did not feel at home in "his house." She said that although he had invited her to move more of her things in to make her feel comfortable, when she asked for his help or opinion, either he was not supportive or he criticized her choices. This had been a significant area of conflict during the first session, so I was eager to help them address it now.

Mr. G said, "You know, I don't think I handled this situation very well. She's right, I butted out when I was suppose to help her move some things, and when she asked me for my opinion, I gave it to her, not realizing that it would sound critical to her."

Ms. Y looked a little stunned by his statements. In a sarcastic tone, she said, "I can't believe you are saying this." I could see him bristle.

I jumped in, thinking there was about to be an argument. "It seems he is trying to acknowledge his role in this problem."

Ms. Y started to tear up. "I know. It is the first time I have ever heard this from him—thank you for saying that." She reached over and gave him a hug.

The second issue that concerned Ms. Y was the amount of time they spent together. She felt that he put his work ahead of everything else, and he wanted her to adapt her schedule to his and be "at his beck and call." As Mr. G started to defend himself, I stopped him and said, "I think your wife misses you and would like to spend more time with you—it's a compliment."

Mr. G was upset that Ms. Y would cancel time with him to do things with her son. For example, Mr. G had planned a nice dinner with his wife. It was clear that he had put a lot of thought into the plans. He had secured a reservation at a restaurant where it was difficult to get a reservation. A few hours before the dinner, Ms. Y's son called and said he needed his mother's help with a project that was due the next day. Without consulting Mr. G, she told her son to come over and she would help him. The project ended up taking most of the evening and the dinner was cancelled.

When Mr. G approached Ms. Y about his concern, she said, "Well we don't have plans tomorrow night—we can just go then." He felt furious and snapped back, "We can't go tomorrow, and it took weeks to get this reservation." She responded, "Well, what to you want me to do, ignore my son and let him fail?" Mr. G responded, "Maybe he needs to learn to plan ahead and not wait until the last moment—and why can't his dad help him?" They continued back and forth for a few minutes until her son arrived. Mr. G left the house and went to his office.

This problem is also a unique stepfamily issue. First, it is very difficult for biological parents to turn down time with their children or requests for help. This goes back to the loyalty issue previously discussed. Second, there is more unexpected change in stepfamilies, often out of the remarried couple's control. Our research indicated that the happiest stepfamily couples make contingency plans to handle these types of situations (Bray & Kelly, 1998).

These issues led to discussions that were the focus of the next several sessions about how they could make their marriage a priority and still get their professional responsibilities accomplished and attend to their children. These were very big issues for Mr. G, because he felt that his life had been totally disrupted after the remarriage. Still, he had wanted to get married so that he could have more intimacy and social life outside of work. He also felt that Ms. Y was unwilling to compromise her schedule and meet his requests to spend time with him. Because Ms. G more often than Mr. Y had to juggle both work and her child, she was able to talk about the choices she had to make to do both things. The ensuing discussions were beneficial, because they learned more about their partner's work styles and ways of handling these situations. I told them that it was important to make time for their marriage and to schedule other things around their marital time (i.e., the marriage should not be put on the back burner).

After these discussions, they compromised on several issues and developed a plan to ensure that they had adequate couple time in their lives. This involved scheduling some regular time together, learning to make clear requests for time with each other, and developing ways to decline requests in a way that was loving and supportive.

There were again several weeks before we met. In the ensuing time, they had read the books I recommended. We discussed their questions about stepfamilies. It was still a challenge for them to schedule time for their marriage, but they were able to keep most of their couple time. Ms. Y had discussions with her son about this. She was surprised when her son said he understood and was pleased that she had remarried.

They were working on a budget but still finalizing all the details. I offered to help, but they thought they could handle it on their own. They still had some arguments, but these were short-lived and did not have the strong emotionality of previous arguments. Ms. Y said that she had put her house up for sale and already had some interested buyers. She was still scared about selling her house but looked forward to having this issue resolved. They also mentioned that they were looking into selling his house and building one of their own. They said they would like to call me if they needed more help.

I would liked to have had more sessions with Ms. Y and Mr. G to ensure that they had completed the financial discussions and integrated their families, but they felt they could handle this on their own. I suggested that we schedule a time (the way they scheduled time for their marriage) for a follow-up session in a couple of months. I talked to them about relapses and how follow-up sessions helps make the changes more durable. They cancelled their follow-up visit, and it took a month to reschedule them. At this visit, Ms. Y was all smiles because she had sold her house, and they had decided on a builder for their new home. Mr. G was close to selling his home. They said they had had a few rough periods in the previous months but had used the ideas and skills we had addressed to resolve their conflicts.

Mr. G continued to have some difficulty cutting down on his work, so that they could make all their dates. They had worked out small ways to stay connected and to do things together, as recommended by Gottman (2000). Ms. Y said she would like to have more time with her husband, and that she was willing to continue to work on this. We ended with the agreement that they could call if they needed more help or just wanted to come in for a "checkup."

Our developmental–systems model fit well with several aspects of this couple's problems. First, it addressed the developmental issues of stepfamily partners and the various intersections with their individual life cycles. Second, the model helped inform both the couple and me about potential stress points or areas of conflict, so that they could understand and, I hope, plan for them.

ACKNOWLEDGMENTS

The research reported in this chapter was supported by Grant Nos. R01 HD22642 and RO1 HD18025 from the National Institute of Child Health and Human Development.

SUGGESTIONS FOR FURTHER READING

Bray, J. H. (1999). From marriage to remarriage and beyond: Findings from the Developmental Issues in StepFamilies Research Project. In E. M. Hetherington (Ed.), *Coping with divorce, single-parenting, and remarriage: A risk and resiliency perspective* (pp. 253–271). Hillsdale, NJ: Erlbaum.—This is an overview of our research on stepfamilies and its relationship to other research in the area.

Bray, J. H. (2001). Therapy with stepfamilies: A developmental systems approach. In D. D. Lusterman, S. H. McDaniel, & C. Philpot (Ed.) *Integrating family therapy: A casebook* (pp. 127–140). Washington, DC: American Psychological Association.—Provides an overview of our work with stepfamilies and a case example of our therapy approach.

Bray, J. H. (2005). Family therapy with stepfamilies. In J. Lebow (Ed.), *Handbook of clinical family therapy* (pp. 497–515). New York: Wiley.—Provides an update of clinically related research on stepfamilies and a case example of therapy for stepfamilies.

Bray, J. H., & Easling, I. (2005). Remarriage and stepfamilies. In W. Pinsof & J. Lebow (Eds.), *Family psychology: State of the art* (pp. 267–294). New York: Oxford University Press.—Reviews research on stepfamilies and areas for further inquiry.

Bray, J. H., & Kelly, J. (1998). *StepFamilies: Love, marriage, and parenting in the first decade.* New York: Broadway Books.—Provides an overview of our research. It is written for professional and lay audiences.

REFERENCES

Adler-Baeder, F., & Higginbotham, B. (2004). Implications of remarriage and stepfamily formation for marriage education. *Family Relations, 53*, 448–458.

Alexander, J. F. (1973). Defensive and supportive communications in normal and deviant families. *Journal of Consulting and Clinical Psychology, 40*, 223–231.

Beach, S. R. H., & Gupta, M. E. (2005). Marital discord in the context of a depressive episode: Research on efficacy and effectiveness. In W. Pinsof & J. Lebow (Eds.), *Family psychology: The art of the science* (pp. 451–470). New York: Oxford University Press.

Brady, C. A., & Ambler, J. (1982). Use of group educational techniques with remarried couples. *Family Therapy Collections, 2*, 145–157.

Bramlett, M. D., & Mosher, W. D. (2001). *First marriage dissolution, divorce, and remarriage: United States* (Advance Data from Vital and Health Statistics No. 323). Hyattsville, MD: National Center for Health Statistics.

Bramlett, M. D., & Mosher, W. D. (2002). *Cohabitation, marriage, divorce, and remarriage in the United States* (Vital and Health Statistics, Series 23, No. 22). Hyattsville, MD: National Center for Health Statistics.

Bray, J. H. (1988). *Developmental Issues in StepFamilies Research Project: Final Report* (Grant No. RO1 HD18025). Bethesda, MD: National Institute of Child Health and Human Development.

Bray, J. H. (1992). Family relationships and children's adjustment in clinical and nonclinical stepfather families. *Journal of Family Psychology, 6*, 60–68.

Bray, J. H. (1993). Bibliotherapy for divorced and remarried families. *The Family Journal, 1*, 170–172.

Bray, J. H. (1994). Children in stepfamilies: Assessment and treatment issues. In D. Huntley (Ed.), *Understanding stepfamilies: Implications for assessment and treatment* (pp. 59–71). Washington, DC: American Counseling Association.

Bray, J. H. (1995). Family oriented treatment of stepfamilies. In R. Mikesell, D. D. Lusterman, & S. McDaniel (Eds.), *Integrating family therapy: Handbook of family psychology and systems therapy* (pp. 125–140). Washington, DC: American Psychological Association.

Bray, J. H. (1999). From marriage to remarriage and beyond: Findings from the Developmental Issues in StepFamilies Research Project. In E. M. Hetherington (Ed.), *Coping with divorce, single-parenting, and remarriage: A risk and resiliency perspective* (pp. 253–271). Hillsdale, NJ: Erlbaum.

Bray, J. H. (2001). Therapy with stepfamilies: A developmental systems approach. In D. D. Lusterman, S. H. McDaniel, & C. Philpot (Eds.), *Integrating family therapy: A casebook* (pp. 127–140). Washington, DC: American Psychological Association.

Bray, J. H. (2005). Family therapy with stepfamilies. In J. Lebow (Ed.), *Handbook of clinical family therapy* (pp. 497–515). New York: Wiley.

Bray, J. H., & Berger, S. H. (1992). Stepfamilies. In M. E. Procidano & C. B. Fisher (Eds.), *Contemporary families: A handbook for school professionals* (pp. 57–79). New York: Teachers College Press.

Bray, J. H., & Berger, S. H. (1993). Developmental issues in stepfamilies research project: Family relationships and parent–child interactions. *Journal of Family Psychology, 7,* 76–90.

Bray, J. H., Berger, S. H., & Boethel, C. L. (1994). Role integration and marital adjustment in stepfather families. In K. Pasley & M. Ihinger-Tallman (Eds.), *Stepfamilies: Issues in research, theory, and practice* (pp. 69–86). New York: Greenwood Press.

Bray, J. H., & Easling, I. (2005). Remarriage and stepfamilies. In W. Pinsof & J. Lebow (Eds.), *Family psychology: The art of the science* (pp. 267–294). New York: Oxford University Press.

Bray, J. H., & Harvey, D. M. (1995). Adolescents in stepfamilies: Developmental and family interventions. *Psychotherapy, 32,* 122–130.

Bray, J. H., & Hetherington, E. M. (1993). Families in transition: Introduction and overview. *Journal of Family Psychology, 7,* 3–8.

Bray, J. H., & Jouriles, E. (1995). Treatment of marital conflict and prevention of divorce. *Journal of Marital and Family Therapy, 21,* 461–473.

Bray, J. H., & Kelly, J. (1998). *StepFamilies: Love, marriage, and parenting in the first decade.* New York: Broadway Books.

Browning, S. (1994). Treating stepfamilies: Alternatives to traditional family therapy. In K. Pasley & M. Ihinger-Tallman (Eds.), *Remarriage and stepparenting: Current research and therapy* (pp. 175–198). New York: Guilford Press.

Browning, S., & Bray, J. H. (in press). Treating stepfamilies: A subsystems-based approach. In J. H. Bray & M. Stanton (Eds.), *Handbook of family psychology.* London: Blackwell

Burt, M. (1989). *Stepfamilies stepping ahead: An eight-step program for successful family living.* Lincoln, NE: Stepfamily Association of America.

Coleman, M., Ganong, L., & Fine, M. A. (2000). Reinvestigating remarriage: Another decade of progress. *Journal of Marriage and the Family, 62,* 1288–1307.

Currier, C. (1995). *Learning to step together: A course for stepfamily adults.* Lincoln, NE: Stepfamily Association of America.

Enright, R. D. (2001). *Forgiveness is a choice: A step-by-step process for resolving anger and restoring hope.* Washington, DC: American Psychological Association.

Forgatch, M. S., & Rains, L. (1997). *MAPS: Marriage and Parenting in Stepfamilies* [parent training manual]. Eugene: Oregon Social Learning Center.

Frank, R., McDaniel, S. H., Bray, J. H., & Heldring, M. (Eds.). (2004). *Primary care psychology.* Washington, DC: American Psychological Association.

Ganong, L. H., & Coleman, M. (2004). *Stepfamily relationships: Development, dynamics, and interventions.* New York: Kluwer.

Gottman, J. M. (1994). *Why marriages succeed or fail.* New York: Simon and Schuster.

Gottman, J. M. (1999). *The marriage clinic: A scientifically based marital therapy.* New York: Norton.

Gottman, J. M. (2000). *Seven principles for making marriage work.* New York: Random House.

Guerney, B. G. (1977). *Relationship enhancement.* San Francisco: Jossey-Bass.

Hetherington, E. M., & Clingempeel, W. G. (1992). Coping with marital transitions: A family systems perspective. *Monographs of the Society for Research in Child Development, 57*(2–3, Serial No. 227).

Hetherington, E. M., Cox, M., & Cox, R. (1982). The effects of divorce on parents and children. In M. Lamb (Ed.), *Nontraditional families* (pp. 233–288). Hillsdale, NJ: Erlbaum.

Hetherington, E. M., Henderson, S., & Reiss, D. (1999). *Adolescent siblings in stepfamilies: Family functioning and adolescent adjustment.* Malden, MA: Blackwell.

Kelley, P. (1992). Healthy stepfamily functioning. *Families in Society, 73,* 579–587.

Kelley, P. (1995). *Developing healthy stepfamilies.* Binghamton, NY: Haworth.

Kreider, R. M. (2005). *Number, timing, and duration of marriages and divorces: 2001* [Current Population Reports, P70-97]. Washington, DC: U.S. Bureau of the Census.

Levant, R. F. (1986). An overview of psychoeducational family programs. In R. F. Levant (Ed.), *Psychoeducational approaches to family therapy and counseling* (pp. 1–51). New York: Springer.

Mandell, D., & Birenzweig, E. (1990). Stepfamilies: A model for group work with remarried couples and their children. *Journal of Divorce and Remarriage, 14,* 29–41.

Markman, H. J., Floyd, F. J., Stanley, S. M., & Storaasli, R. D. (1988). The prevention of marital distress: A longitudinal investigation. *Journal of Consulting and Clinical Psychology, 56,* 210–217.

Markman, H. J., Renick, M. J., Floyd, F. J., Stanley, S. M., & Clements, M. (1993). Preventing marital distress through communication and conflict management training: A four and five year follow-up. *Journal of Consulting and Clinical Psychology, 62,* 70–77.

Martin, T. C., & Martin, M. (1992). *Stepfamilies in ther-*

apy: Understanding systems, assessment, and intervention. San Francisco: Jossey-Bass.

McGoldrick, M., & Carter, E. A. (1988). Forming a remarried family. In E. A. Carter & M. McGoldrick (Eds.), The changing family life cycle (pp. 399–429). New York: Gardner.

McGoldrick, M., Gerson, R., & Shellenberger, S. (1999). Genograms: Assessment and intervention. New York: Norton.

Michaels, M. L. (2000). The Stepfamily Enrichment Program: A preliminary evaluation, using focus groups. American Journal of Family Therapy, 28, 61–73.

National Stepfamily Resource Center. (2007). A division of Auburn University's Center for Children, Youth, and Families. Retrieved May 21, 2007, from www.stepfamilies.info.

Nelson, W. P., & Levant, R. F. (1991). An evaluation of a skills training program for parents in stepfamilies. Family Relations, 40, 291–296.

Papernow, P. (1993). Becoming a stepfamily: Patterns of development in remarried families. San Francisco: Jossey-Bass.

Pasley, K., Dollahite, D., & Ihinger-Tallman, M. (1993). Bridging the gap: Clinical applications of research findings on the spousal and stepparent role in remarriage. Family Relations, 42, 315–322.

Pasley, K., Rhoden, L., Visher, E. B., & Visher, J. S. (1996). Successful stepfamily therapy: Clients' perspectives. Journal of Marital and Family Therapy, 22, 343–357.

Reed, F. G., & Enright, R. D. (2006). The effects of forgiveness therapy on depression, anxiety, and post-traumatic stress for women after spousal emotional-abuse. Journal of Consulting and Clinical Psychology, 74, 920–929.

Robertson, A., Adler-Baeder, F., Collins, A., DeMarco, D., & Fein, D. (2006). Marriage education services for economically disadvantaged stepfamilies [Report for Office of Planning, Research and Evaluation] Washington, DC: Administration for Children and Families.

Sager, C. J., Brown, S. K., Crohn, H., Engel, T., Rodenstein, E., & Walker, L. (1983). Treating the remarried family. New York: Brunner/Mazel.

Smock, P. J. (1990). Remarriage patterns of black and white women: Reassessing the role of educational attainment. Demography, 27, 467–473.

Visher, E., & Visher, J. (1979). Stepfamilies. New York: Brunner/Mazel.

Visher, E. B., & Visher, J. S. (1988). Old loyalties, new ties: Therapeutic strategies with stepfamilies. New York: Brunner/Mazel.

Visher, E. B., & Visher, J. S. (1990). SAA Workshop manual. Lincoln, NE: Stepfamily Association of America.

Visher, E. B., & Visher, J. S. (1991). How to win as a stepfamily (2nd ed.). New York: Brunner/Routledge.

Visher, E. B., & Visher, J. S. (1994). Avoiding the mind fields of stepfamily therapy. In K. D. Huntley (Ed.), Understanding stepfamilies: Implications for assessment and treatment (pp. 25–34). Alexandria, VA: American Counseling Association.

Wallerstein, J. S., & Kelly, J. B. (1980). Surviving the breakup: How children cope with divorce. New York: Basic Books.

Williamson, D. S., & Bray, J. H. (1988). Family development and change across the generations: An intergenerational perspective. In C. J. Falicov (Ed.), Family transitions: Continuity and change over the life cycle (pp. 357–384). New York: Guilford Press.

Couple Therapy and the Treatment of Psychiatric and Medical Disorders

CHAPTER 18

Couple Therapy for Alcoholism and Drug Abuse

GARY R. BIRCHLER
WILLIAM FALS-STEWART
TIMOTHY J. O'FARRELL

BACKGROUND

Historically, alcoholism and drug abuse have been viewed by the treatment community, as well as by the public at large, as individual problems most effectively treated on an individual basis. However, during the last three decades, awareness of family members' potentially crucial roles in the etiology and maintenance of addictive behavior has grown. In particular, as understanding of how partner interaction influences substance use and abuse has evolved, treatment providers and researchers alike have placed increased emphasis on conceptualizing drinking and drug use from a systemic perspective and, in turn, on treating the couple to address partners' substance abuse. We and others participated in the early call for and provided descriptions of work with couples to address alcoholism (O'Farrell & Cutter, 1984; Paolino & McCrady, 1977) and drug abuse problems (e.g., Fals-Stewart, Birchler, & O'Farrell, 1996).

Since the mid-1970s, three theoretical perspectives have come to dominate family-based conceptualizations of substance use and are the foundation for the treatment strategies most often used with substance users (for a review, see Fals-Stewart, O'Farrell, & Birchler, 2003). The best

known of these, the "family disease approach," conceptualizes alcoholism and other drug abuse as a family "illness" of not only the substance user but also his or her family members (who are viewed as being codependent). Treatment drawn from this perspective involves the substance-abusing patient and his or her family members, addressing their respective disease processes individually; formal couple or family treatment is largely deemphasized. The "family systems approach" applies the principles of general systems theory to families, paying particular attention to ways that families maintain a dynamic balance between substance use and family functioning, and whose interactional behavior is organized around alcohol or drug use (cf. Edwards & Steinglass, 1995; Steinglass, Bennett, Wolin, & Reiss, 1987). Accordingly, family therapy has the goal of modifying family dynamics and interactions to eliminate the family's need for the substance-abusing patient to drink or use drugs. "Behavioral approaches" assume that family interactions serve to reinforce alcohol- and drug-using behavior. The goal of couple or family therapy from this perspective is to eliminate reinforcement for substance use and to promote behavior that serves to reinforce abstinence.

The forerunner of the behavioral couple therapy (BCT) approach to the treatment of alcoholism and drug abuse, which is described in this chapter, was a social learning theory approach to the treatment of marital distress, originally called behavioral marital therapy (BMT). BMT originated in the late 1960s and early 1970s, and has continued to the present as one of very few empirically validated approaches for the treatment of couple distress. Early scientist–practitioners who developed and investigated BMT over the past four decades have included Richard Stuart (Stuart, 1969, 1980); Robert Weiss, associates, and students (Birchler, Weiss, & Vincent, 1975; Christensen, 1987; Jacobson & Margolin, 1979; Weiss, Hops, & Patterson, 1973); and John Gottman and his students (Gottman, Markman, & Notarius, 1977). Since its origination, BMT has featured a functional analysis of distressed and nondistressed couples' antecedents and consequences of partners' social exchanges (i.e., relationship rewarding and nonrewarding behaviors), and their positive and negative communication and problem-solving behaviors. These elements constitute the very foundation of BCT for substance abuse.

In this chapter, we provide a brief discussion of (1) the definition of alcohol and drug use disorders, (2) the theoretical rationale for the use of BCT with substance-abusing patients and their partners, (3) typical treatment methods used as part of the BCT intervention with substance-abusing couples, (4) research findings that support the effectiveness of BCT, and (5) a case illustration of the BCT approach.

THE HEALTHY/WELL-FUNCTIONING VERSUS PATHOLOGICAL/DYSFUNCTIONAL COUPLE/MARRIAGE

Defining Alcohol and Drug Use Disorders

Before examining the interrelationship of substance abuse and relationship functioning, it is important to provide contemporary diagnostic definitions of alcoholism and drug addiction. There are actually several different definitional frameworks for these disorders that have been described in the literature. The most widely used is the "psychiatric diagnostic approach," exemplified in the fourth edition of the *Diagnostic and Statistical Manual of Mental Disorders* (DSM-IV; American Psychiatric Association, 1994) and the tenth edition of the *International Classification of Diseases* (ICD-10; World Health Organization, 1992). Using the

DSM-IV system as an example, the diagnosis of alcohol or psychoactive substance use disorders includes two general subcategories: abuse and dependence. "Substance dependence" is marked by a cluster of cognitive, behavioral, and physiological symptoms indicating that the individual continues to use a given psychoactive substance despite significant substance-related problems. To meet diagnostic criteria for dependence, an individual must display at least three of the following seven symptoms: (1) physical tolerance; (2) withdrawal; (3) unsuccessful attempts to stop or control substance use; (4) use of larger amounts of the substance than intended; (5) loss or reduction in important recreational, social, or occupational activities; (6) continued use of the substance despite knowledge of physical or psychological problems that are likely to have been caused or exacerbated by the substance; and (7) excessive time spent using the substance or recovering from its effects. The essential feature of "substance abuse" is a maladaptive pattern of problem use leading to one or more of the following adverse consequences: (1) failure to fulfill major social obligations in the context of work, school, or home; (2) recurrent substance use in situations that creates the potential for harm (e.g., drinking and driving); (3) recurrent substance-related legal problems; and (4) continued substance use despite having persistent social or interpersonal problems caused or exacerbated by the effects of the substance.

In contrast to the disease-oriented model, behavioral scientists have proposed an alternative approach (e.g., Adesso, 1995; Nathan, 1981). In this framework, symptoms are viewed as acquired habits that emerge from a combination of social, pharmacological, and behavioral factors. Emphasis is placed on environmental, affective, and cognitive antecedents, and reinforcing consequences of substance use. The outgrowth of this functional conceptualization is that drinking and drug use are seen as ruled by motivation and learning principles, as are other behaviors (Wulfert, Greenway, & Dougher, 1996).

Without question, the disease model of addiction is the dominant view held by the vast majority of treatment providers in the substance abuse treatment community. Thus, from a practical standpoint, any widely used intervention for alcoholism and substance abuse (couple-based or otherwise) in most treatment settings must be acceptable to clinicians and clients who define and treat these disorders from a disease perspective. However, it should be noted that the behaviorally oriented treatment approach broadly assumes a "problems perspective," in which problem behaviors presented by couples seeking help are modified to promote sobriety. In fact, the intervention methods we espouse herein actually fit rather easily into a disease model framework if clients and treatment providers accept the premise that behavioral change is the fundamental ingredient to modifying the manifest behaviors that characterize the disease of alcoholism and drug abuse.

Theoretical Rationale for Use of Couple Therapy to Treat Substance Use Disorders

The relationship between substance use and couple dysfunction is complex and appears to constitute a type of "reciprocal causality." For example, compared to well-functioning dyads, couples in which one partner abuses drugs or alcohol usually have extensive relationship problems, often characterized by comparatively high levels of relationship dissatisfaction, instability (i.e., partners taking significant steps toward separation or divorce), high prevalence and frequency of verbal and physical aggression (e.g., Fals-Stewart, Birchler, & O'Farrell, 1999), significant sexual problems (O'Farrell, Choquette, Cutter, & Birchler, 1997), and often significant levels of psychological distress in both partners and other family members, such as children (Fals-Stewart, Kelley, Cooke, & Golden, 2003; Kelley & Fals-Stewart, 2002; Moos & Billings, 1982).

Although chronic substance use is correlated with reduced marital satisfaction for both spouses, relationship dysfunction also is associated with increased problematic substance use and is related to relapse among alcoholics and drug abusers after treatment (e.g., Maisto, O'Farrell, McKay, Connors, & Pelcovitz, 1988). Thus, as shown in Figure 18.1, the relationship between substance use and marital problems is not unidirectional, with one consistently causing the other; rather, each can serve as a precursor to the other, creating a "vicious cycle" from which couples that include a partner who abuses drugs or alcohol often have difficulty escaping.

There are several relationship-based antecedent conditions and reinforcing consequences of substance use. Marital and family problems (e.g., poor communication and problem solving, arguing, financial stressors) often serve as precursors to excessive drinking or drug use, and unfortunately, resulting family interactions can inadvertently facilitate continued drinking or drug use once these

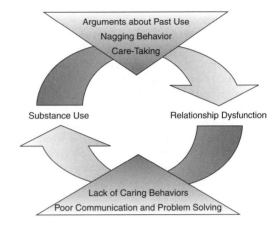

FIGURE 18.1. Vicious cycle between relationship dysfunction and substance abuse.

behaviors have developed. For example, substance abuse often provides more subtle adaptive consequences for the couple, such as facilitating the expression of emotion and affection (e.g., caretaking when a partner has a hangover). Finally, even when recovery from the alcohol or drug problem has begun, marital and family conflicts can, and very often do, precipitate relapses.

Factors That May Influence Substance Abuse Recovery, Couple Functioning, and/or Relationship Longevity

Alcohol and drug abuse are maintained by their consequences at the physiological, individual, and interpersonal levels. From a clinical perspective, a number of risk factors seem to influence the prognosis for successful substance abuse treatment and relationship satisfaction outcomes. The probability of success for a given couple can be diminished if (1) the partner's alcohol or substance abuse is very severe and debilitating, (2) both partners are involved with substance abuse, (3) there is severe partner violence or chronic and highly conflicted couple interactions, or (4) there is in one or both partners the presence of psychiatric comorbidity, such as clinical levels of anxiety, depression, antisocial personality disorder, or psychosis. Additional threats to maintaining sobriety include high-risk occupational or social contact situations (e.g., persistent alcohol or drug use by coworkers within the friendship circle and the community at large, or within extended families of either the user or the nonusing partner). Unfortunately, many couples are challenged by one or more of these risk factors. Whenever possible, the therapist must be active in addressing these problems and in helping to minimize their influence on substance abuse and relationship recovery. Indeed, typically, stand-alone couple therapy is not successful in these cases. Along with couple therapy, referrals to other appropriate treatment providers are indicated.

Finally, there is evidence that client gender plays a role in the development of and treatment strategies used for substance abuse. Given traditional male–female, husband–wife social values, female substance abusers may be more secretive about their substance use. Women and their male partners may be motivated to minimize the problem or to delay treatment to avoid disrupting the family. Interviews of alcoholic wives suggested that they very often drink to function within their marriages, to be able to be more assertive, and to manage the sexual demands of their husbands (Lammers, Schippers, & van der Staak, 1995). Additionally, women are much more likely to have substance-abusing husbands than vice versa, and husbands of drinking wives are relatively uninvolved and uninterested in their wives' sobriety (McCrady & Epstein, 1999). Therefore, when the female is the identified substance abuser, it is important to address such gender-related factors. Fortunately, there is emerging evidence that BCT works about as well with both alcoholic and drug abusing women and their nonsubstance-abusing male partners as it does with alcoholic and drug-abusing men, in terms of maintaining sobriety and improving the couple relationship (Fals-Stewart, Birchler, & Kelley, 2006; Winters, Fals-Stewart, O'Farrell, Birchler, & Kelley, 2002).

THE PRACTICE OF COUPLE THERAPY

The Structure of the Therapy Process

BCT is not a suitable intervention for all substance-abusing individuals involved in intimate relationships. Because BCT attempts to harness the influence of the dyadic system to promote abstinence, it is important that potential participants indicate some evidence of relationship commitment to be successful. Thus, one general criterion is that the partners be married or cohabiting in a stable relationship for at least 1 year or separated but attempting to reconcile. A second criterion, given that BCT is skills-based, is that neither partner can have conditions, such as gross cognitive impairment or psychosis, that would significantly in-

terfere with learning new information, practicing skills, or completing assigned tasks.

Implicit in the BCT model is the assumption that both partners have abstinence from drugs or alcohol as a primary goal; thus, BCT is most effective with couples in which only one partner has a problem with drugs or alcohol. The relationships of dyads in which both partners abuse drugs, sometimes referred to as "dually addicted couples," are often not supportive of abstinence; in fact, if substance use is a shared recreational activity of the partners, the relationship may serve to promote continued drinking or drug use, and may be antagonistic to its cessation (e.g., Fals-Stewart, Birchler, & O'Farrell, 1999). Treating only one of the partners in these relationships creates conflict that is typically resolved either through relationship dissolution or continued use by both partners, resulting in treatment failure.

Couples are excluded from participation in BCT if there is an extensive history of severe partner physical aggression. For example, couples who report recent episodes (i.e., in the last year) of partner violence that resulted in the need for medical attention or hospitalization, or in which a partner describes being physically afraid of his or her significant other, would not be appropriate candidates. In such circumstances, partners would be referred to treatment for domestic violence in conjunction with the substance-abusing partner receiving individualized counseling for his or her substance abuse (Fals-Stewart & Kennedy, 2005).

Among substance-abusing patients entering outpatient treatment, approximately 30% are currently cohabitating in primary couple relationships and may be good candidates for BCT. Typically, if offered the intervention, roughly 80% of such couples choose to participate. Children are not included in conjoint sessions; however, BCT has been offered in formats that include parent training elements of intervention. Currently under investigation are adaptations of BCT formats that provide counseling to only one member of the couple and to users seen with other members of cohabiting units (i.e., the user is treated with his or her mother, father, or other adult not in a romantic relationship with the user; O'Farrell & Fals-Stewart, 2006).

BCT most often has been delivered as an adjunct to standard, individual substance abuse counseling in outpatient and inpatient substance abuse treatment programs. However, BCT can and has been delivered as a stand-alone intervention. It has been offered in 6- and 12-session manualized treatment formats, in individual-couple and small-group formats, and also in outpatient mental health clinics or private practice settings with solo practitioners. Individual conjoint sessions usually last 50–60 minutes; group sessions range from 60 to 90 minutes in length. Generally, within the organized substance abuse treatment programs in which most of the relevant research on BCT models, formats, and treatment outcomes has been conducted, the number of sessions is manualized and therefore time-limited. Couples typically are seen weekly for 12–20 weeks over 5–6 months.

The Role of the Therapist

BCT is a highly structured, behaviorally oriented, skills-based, often manualized, and largely psychoeducational approach. Therefore, the role of the therapist follows strongly in the tradition of cognitive-behavioral therapies; that is, typically there is a psychoeducational and skills-based agenda set for the conjoint treatment sessions. Accordingly, the therapist takes on the integrated roles of teacher, consultant, and subject matter expert regarding behavior modification, substance abuse recovery, relationship improvement, and relapse prevention.

Early on, the therapist also takes certain opportunities to establish a working alliance with the couple at hand, in a collaborative atmosphere fostered by (1) offering frequent validation for what the substance abuser and his or her partner have gone through to get to the point of treatment, (2) constantly offering step-wise guidance and encouragement for the challenging journey ahead, (3) providing clear and defined expectations for the partners' program-related attitudes and behaviors, and (4) maintaining effective control of emotional expression, especially volatile escalation and the expression of destructive negative affect. The latter intervention may require the therapist to interrupt escalating interaction, institute a time-out, validate partners' feelings one at a time, and perhaps even to terminate the conjoint meeting in favor of separate, individual meetings to calm the participants' emotions and make a plan for reconciliation.

Essential Clinical Skills

The BCT therapist must have education, supervision, training, and ultimately independent expertise in several important areas. First, he or she needs knowledge about the principles and patterns

of multiple substance abuse. Different drugs have different effects on the user, different cultural contexts in which the abuser operates to maintain his or her habit, and different social and legal consequences for use. For example, consider the experiences of a user and his or her nonusing partner depending on whether the user abuses alcohol, prescription drugs, or illegal drugs; or whether the user gets high on stimulants versus opiates, or both. The therapist, as resident subject matter expert, should be knowledgeable about all these drugs, their interactions, and related cognitive-behavioral psychotherapeutic interventions to help the user achieve and maintain sobriety.

Second, the therapist must be trained to be an effective couple therapist; in the case of BCT, this means having the ability to assess and to provide treatment planning to initiate positive behavioral exchanges, reducing or eliminating partner behaviors and dyadic interactions that negatively affect the relationship, teaching effective communication and problem-solving skills, and, throughout the course of therapy, monitoring and shaping partners' motivations and attitudes to achieve and maintain sobriety.

Third, it should be noted that these are multiproblem couples; in addition to solid diagnostic and intervention skills for the areas noted earlier, the therapist must know the limits of the BCT approach. More than likely, one or both partners (or the couple) will possess one or more of the risk factors described earlier. This finding has not been subjected to empirical study, but is a well-known clinical fact in the alcoholism and drug abuse treatment field. Indeed, dealing with severe partner violence, compromised physical and mental health issues, and often occupational and legal problems requires the therapist to have in his or her network many healthcare providers to address the needs of the couple (e.g., doctors for medical care and psychiatric medications, individual and group therapists for individualized psychological care, and access to occupational and legal agents to address any major problems outside of the couple dynamics).

Common and Important Therapist Errors

In addition to a failure to assert the recommended therapist role, and to acquire and utilize the clinical skills noted earlier, there are a few more caveats. At the least, couples present to the therapist with a substance abuse problem and a more or less distressed relationship. First, it is important to address the substance abuse issue. Even though it is often tempting in many cases to treat the relationship first, this sequencing rarely is effective. Continued substance abuse seems to destroy any hopes for relationship improvement. Second, the therapist should be careful not to impose his or her own values on the couple. A collaborative approach to goal setting and therapeutic activities leaves room for the couple's values and beliefs. Just because "90 meetings in 90 days" worked for the therapist does not mean that the present client must do the same thing. Third, given that many couples typically have struggled for years with substance use and dysfunctional relationships, there seems to be plenty of blame to go around. Although the therapist needs to be directive and firm, he or she also needs to help the partners to avoid blaming. A long-term perspective suggests a need for repeated efforts to gain and maintain sobriety, and perhaps a realistic necessity for learning to cope with failed attempts along the way. Therapists should not underestimate the degree of anger and resentment that has built up in many couples; usually they need remedial interpersonal skills to process and/ or forgive this history.

Finally, to reach the goals of treatment, partners need an effective balance of individual motivation and competence, and mutual cooperation. Accordingly, the therapist can avoid problems by not overestimating the initial competence and coping skills of these couples (who often look more interpersonally competent than they are). In BCT, couples are encouraged strongly to complete agreed upon homework (i.e., skills acquisition) and to learn how to talk effectively about their substance abuse issues and patterns (i.e., without minimization, denial, or conflict). The therapist should also be careful not to underestimate the tremendous ambivalence on the part of the substance abuser and the partner to change. Typically, the user is reluctant to stop using and the partner is reluctant to trust sufficiently in change to give up familiar patterns of coping and control (even if they are maladaptive).

Assessment and Treatment Planning

BCT for alcohol and drug abuse typically has featured a multimethod assessment process for case conceptualization and treatment planning. The ideal package is described briefly; a similar version of this package has been employed most frequently when research investigations were ongoing and in large, well-subsidized substance abuse treatment

settings. Unfortunately, many community and solo practitioner settings do not provide the time and manpower resources to employ the multimethod system. The best practice assessment methods include (1) clinical interviewing with partners, together and separately; (2) paper-and-pencil assessment measures pertaining to substance abuse and relationship quality; and (3) behavioral observation of the couple's communication and problem-solving skills.

Clinical Interviewing

Clinical interviewing is the most important and sometimes the only assessment method employed. Our semistructured interviews are designed to engage and to form a working alliance with the couple, to provide a subjective understanding of the couple's past and current substance abuse and relationship functioning, and to learn about partners' readiness, expectations, and goals for treatment.

INTERVIEW ASSESSMENT OF SUBSTANCE USE

The assessment of substance use involves inquiries about recent types, quantities, and frequencies of substances used, whether the extent of physical dependence on alcohol or other drugs requires detoxification, what led the couple to seek therapy at this time, outcomes of prior efforts to seek help, and goals of the substance abuser and the family member (e.g., reduction of substance use, temporary or permanent abstinence). Along with alcohol and drug use severity, it is strongly recommended that assessment include an evaluation of problem areas likely influenced by substance use, including (1) medical problems, (2) legal entanglements, (3) financial difficulties, (4) psychological distress, and (5) social/family problems (McLellan et al., 1985). If helping couples with any of these issues falls within the professional skills and scope of the therapist and also fits within any time-limited aspects of the particular BCT program, these problems are addressed in BCT. Certain issues that affect the couple (e.g., legal difficulties, significant medical problems) also may require referral to the appropriate professionals for assistance.

INTERVIEW ASSESSMENT OF RELATIONSHIP PROBLEMS

Often, a behaviorally oriented framework called "the 7 C's" is used to help assess current couple functioning (Birchler, Doumas, & Fals-Stewart,

1999). In any couple therapy setting, the 7 C's framework has proven to be a popular and fairly comprehensive system for relationship evaluation and treatment planning. As the evaluation meetings progress, the 7 C's may be informed by any or all of the assessment methods mentioned in this section. Briefly, couples are evaluated according to their functioning in seven areas of interaction that are prerequisites for long-term intimacy:

1. *Character features.* This dimension refers to the basic type of person and the personality that one brings to the relationship. A person who has a sense of humor, personal integrity, honesty, loyalty, a positive upbringing and outlook on life, and is free of significant mental or physical health problems is rated more favorably for character features. More challenging character features related to maintaining an intimate relationship may include a negative attitude about life, substance abuse, significant mental or physical health problems, dishonesty, untrustworthiness, and so on.

2. *Cultural and ethnic factors.* This domain refers to the developmental and contextual environments in which each partner was raised and the traditions and his or her preferences for living life. Couples can either benefit from or be in conflict about one or many of the following factors: cultural, ethnic, racial, and religious differences; male and female gender roles and responsibilities; appreciation and responsibility for working; the importance of money and its management; handling and expressing anger; disciplining children; and frequency of time spent with extended family; and so forth.

3. *Contract.* This dimension refers to the difference between what each partner wants and gets in the relationship. How close do one's experiences match his or her expectations? Contract features may be explicit and openly understood, for example, "We are going to have a baby, and you will stay at home while I go to work." Or, as is more likely the case in intimate relationships, contract features may be implicit and more vulnerable to misunderstandings: "I expect that you will help me care for the baby, and we will accomplish the housework as equals." Couple contracts evolve inevitably over the relationship life cycle; most couples need to be able to revise or renegotiate their relationship contracts to maintain growth and satisfaction.

4. *Commitment.* There are two important aspects of commitment to consider. One important aspect is "stability." Relationships last longer when partners are loyal and committed to one another for the long run—for better or for worse—and entertain little or no desire to separate despite inevitable problems. The second important aspect is commitment to "quality"; that is, partners are willing to invest effort, to do the work that is required to make the relationship healthy and personally satisfying for both partners. Couples who have a commitment to stability but not to quality can experience long, unhappy marriages. Couples who are committed to quality and personal happiness, but who disengage at the first signs of difficulty, put forth little effort to work through the inevitable problems. Couples who are committed to stability and to quality have the best chance for developing a satisfactory, long-term intimate relationship.

5. *Caring.* "Caring" is a broad term that incorporates several important aspects of an intimate relationship. Partners rated high in caring actively demonstrate support, understanding, and validation of their mates; they have and show appreciation for their mates as people. In addition, the partners demonstrate sufficient activity and compatibility in their affection with one another. Greeting, touching, intimate talking, and companionship activities are all desired and expressed in compatible ways. Their individual and mutually rewarding activities are balanced, in contrast to the activities of partners who may feel abandoned, trapped, or possessed by their respective mates' preferences. Finally, the couple's sex life is satisfactory, healthy, trustworthy, and active at a level satisfactory to both partners. Couples rated lower in caring have identified problems and need improvement in one or more of these areas of function.

6. *Communication.* This is the basic skill that allows a relationship to function and to evolve. Couples who develop and maintain effective communication skills are much more likely to be able to address all the other concerns identified by the 7 C's framework. Effective communication occurs when both partners possess the competence and the motivation to share with one another important information about their thoughts, feelings, and actions. When the messages truly intended and sent by the speaker are fully understood by the listener, effective communication results.

7. *Conflict resolution.* In addition to basic conversation and communication skills, couples also have to be able to work effectively together to make decisions, to solve daily problems in living, and to manage the inevitable relationship

conflicts that arise. Elements of accommodation, assertiveness, negotiation and compromise, emotional expression and regulation, and anger management all come into play. Some couples get into trouble by being too conflict-avoidant; therefore, they do not address important issues; other couples tend to escalate conflicts into patterns of verbal and sometimes physical abuse. Both styles in the extreme can result in damage to the relationship. Couples need to be able to resolve disagreements, or agree to disagree, without becoming disconnected or abusive.

From clinical experience, we have found that, compared to distressed couples in general, couples coping with substance abuse have a significantly higher probability of having difficulties with the 7 C's and a greater degree of dysfunction. Accordingly, couple therapy is not only indicated in most of these cases but its provision may also be critical to the partners' longevity as a couple and the maintenance of sobriety.

INDIVIDUAL INTERVIEWS

Along with the ongoing analysis of the 7 C's, we advocate getting a comprehensive psychosocial history from each partner. Typically, we conduct one early interview session separately with each partner to obtain his and her personal developmental history. In these individual sessions, we usually advocate a policy of "limited confidentiality," whereby the therapist indicates that he or she will not keep secrets that may affect the integrity and ethical allegiance of the couple. At the therapist's discretion, personal history items may indeed be held in confidence, but not if the information compromises the basic goals of the couple contract for relationship therapy. The most likely (and explicitly discussed) exception to this "no secrets" policy relates to partner safety, as in the case of domestic violence. For the record, we also tend not to disclose to the other spouse any "history" of affairs, so long as the affair is neither ongoing nor in any way actively compromises the present therapeutic effort.

The situation may arise in which the therapist is told that one partner is engaged in a current affair and refuses to terminate it or to tell the partner. In practice, it seems equally likely that the substance abuser or the partner may be extramaritally involved. We would find ourselves in an ethical bind of being unable to divulge the affair legally to the partner without the perpetrator's permission, yet not wanting to initiate or conduct BCT while keeping such a potentially damaging and therapeutically success-limiting secret. When faced with this dilemma, we almost always suggest strongly that we will not conduct BCT while a secret affair is ongoing, and we are usually able to persuade the perpetrator either to terminate the affair or deal with the matter openly within BCT. If the perpetrator declines both options and this situation becomes known during the assessment process, we will not start BCT treatment. If it becomes known after treatment starts, then we terminate BCT at a predesignated evaluation point (e.g., after 4 to 6 therapy sessions). Note that the therapist advises every couple at the outset of contact that in the many sources of information acquired, he or she may discover something that would prevent beginning BCT. If so, he or she tells the couple that a referral will be made to a different program for reassessment. When the therapist stops a case in this manner, the perpetrator is informed and must take responsibility for the premature termination; his or her partner may or may not suspect the real reason for stopping and being referred on. Some therapists may have other confidentiality standards.

Paper-and-Pencil Measures

The second assessment method is paper-and-pencil measures. Briefly, instruments are available to assess partners' substance abuse (e.g., Michigan Alcoholism Screening Test), individual psychological function (Beck Depression Inventory), and relationship function (Dyadic Adjustment Scale). Information provided by these instruments supplements and confirms information learned in other assessment methods, and helps to inform treatment planning and quantitative baseline measures of function to compare with post-treatment and follow-up repeated measurements. Although a discussion of such measures is beyond the scope of this chapter, Fals-Stewart, Birchler, and Ellis (1999) provide a detailed description of assessment inventories and procedures often recommended for couples in which partners abuse alcohol or drugs.

Communication Sample

Communication and conflict resolution behaviors can most readily be observed by having the partners provide a live sample of communication as they attempt to resolve a conflict they have identified, with assistance from the therapist. In the now classic BMT/BCT procedure, partners are asked to discuss a moderate-intensity conflict issue for 10–15 minutes while the therapist observes. In this manner, the couple typically offers the therapist an opportunity to analyze real-time behaviors related to effective or ineffective communication and problem solving. There is no good substitute for obtaining such important, skills-related information. It has been demonstrated that certain behaviors observed during this type of interaction can predict the likelihood of separation and divorce several years later (Gottman, 1994).

In summary, an analysis of the 7 Cs, combined with other assessment information from the interviews and optional inventory measures, provides ample information for the therapist to understand the (dys)function of the couple and to formulate a master treatment plan. After all assessment information has been gathered, the clients and therapist meet for a feedback session, which we refer to as a "roundtable discussion," in which the therapist provides an overview of the evaluation's findings. Partners are asked to be active participants in this discussion, sharing their impressions and providing any critical information that they deem to be missing, inaccurate, or incomplete. The goals of this feedback session are (1) to provide the partners with objective, nonjudgmental information about their dyadic functioning and the negative consequences of the substance misuse and (2) to increase motivation for upcoming treatment, if appropriate.

Typically, couple therapy is indicated and the goals of such treatment are delineated. Couple therapy is not recommended if there is potential for moderate-to-severe partner violence; an ongoing affair; or severe substance abuse, physical, and/or mental problems. Additionally, the couple may have too little commitment to sobriety and/or the relationship for the therapist to recommend going forward. In such cases, appropriate referrals are made to people and programs able to address extant problems.

Goal Setting

Inherent in the BCT approach for all substance-abusing couples is the dual focus of eliminating substance abuse and strengthening couples' relationship skills. The former includes providing partners with coping skills to avoid psychological and situational risks to sobriety, and developing resources to enjoy substance free activities. The couple's goals include maintaining sobriety and preventing relapse, learning effective communication, problem solving and conflict management skills, initiating caring behaviors and developing shared rewarding activities, and perhaps learning parenting skills, if appropriate. Although the dual goals of sobriety and improving relationship function are inherent in this approach, stipulation of these goals needs to come from collaboration between the partners and the therapist to be effective. However, it should be noted that third parties may also have a say regarding the urgency for the required goal of abstinence (the courts, employers, etc.).

Generally, abstinence is the goal of treatment. Even when the client will not commit to permanent abstinence, and some form of harm reduction is the ultimate goal (i.e., using legal substances responsibly), abstinence is still the initial goal of treatment. The reason for encouraging at least temporary abstinence in the course of the program is so that the user, and the couple, can experience a period of abstinence and better relationship functioning as a basis for considering future substance use. Accordingly, early in treatment, for most couples, emphasis is first placed on achieving and maintaining sobriety, then therapeutic efforts shift to strengthening the relationship, and finally a dedicated program for relapse prevention is developed. All components (see Figure 18.2) receive several sessions of work. However, in some cases, the relative emphasis placed on these three areas or the sequence may be altered to meet special needs of a given couple.

Process and Technical Aspects of Couple Therapy

In virtually all extant applications and formats of BCT for alcoholism and drug abuse, and in most couples, the goals are enhancing sobriety, dealing with relative levels of comorbid individual psychological issues, and rehabilitating distressed couple relationships. There is some flexibility within the approach to emphasize certain areas over others, as needed by a given individual, couple, or group. As is typical in all couple therapy, the prognosis for a given couple is improved to the extent that the couple is better functioning at the outset of treatment.

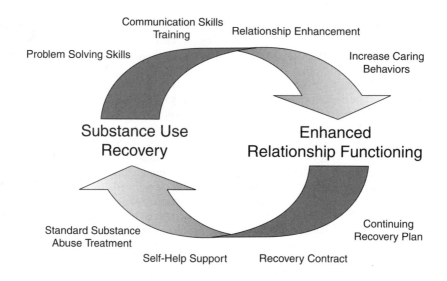

FIGURE 18.2. "Virtuous cycle" illustrating concurrent treatment for substance use and relationship functioning.

Interventions Focused on Substance Abuse

LIMITING EXPOSURE AND RISKY SITUATIONS

The first purpose of couple treatment is to establish a clear and specific agreement between the substance abuser and partner about the goal to deal with the substance use and each partner's role in achieving that goal. It is important to discuss possible exposure to alcoholic beverages, drugs, and substance-use-related situations. With regard to alcohol use, for example, the spouse should decide whether he or she will drink alcoholic beverages in the abuser's presence, whether alcoholic beverages will be kept and served at home, whether the couple will attend social gatherings involving alcohol, and how to deal with these situations. Partners should identify particular persons, gatherings, or circumstances that are likely to be stressful. Also addressed are couple and family interactions related to substance use, because arguments, tensions, and negative feelings can precipitate more abusive behavior. The therapist discusses these patterns and suggests specific counter-measures for partners to use in difficult situations.

BEHAVIORAL CONTRACTING

Written behavioral contracts to promote abstinence have a number of useful common elements. The substance use behavior goal is made explicit. Specific behaviors of each spouse to help achieve this goal are detailed. The contract provides alternative behaviors to negative interactions about substance use. Finally, and quite importantly, the agreement decreases the nonalcoholic spouse's anxiety and need to control the substance abuser and his or her use behavior. The contract we recommend is called the "sobriety trust discussion." In it, the patient reports the status of his or her sobriety during the past 24 hours and states his or her intent not to drink or use drugs that day (in the tradition of "one day at a time"). The spouse expresses appreciation for the patient's efforts to remain abstinent the previous day and offers any needed support for the next 24 hours. The spouse records the performance of the daily contract on a calendar provided. Both partners agree not to discuss past drinking or fears about future drinking at home to prevent substance-related conflicts that can trigger relapse. These discussions are reserved for the therapy sessions. At the start of each BCT session, the Sobriety Contract calendar is reviewed to see how well each spouse has done his or her part. If the Sobriety Contract includes 12-step meetings, urine drug screens, or the taking of medication designed to inhibit substance use, these actions also are marked on the calendar and reviewed. The calendar provides an ongoing record of progress that the therapist rewards verbally at each session. The partners practice the behaviors of their sobriety trust discussion in each session to highlight its importance and to allow the therapist to observe how they carry it out.

ATTENDANCE AT SELF-HELP MEETINGS

Although there is little empirical evidence available regarding the effectiveness of Alcoholics Anonymous (AA)-type support groups (e.g., AA, Narcotics Anonymous [NA], Al-Anon), there also is little doubt in the substance abuse treatment community that such activity is probably very helpful in maintaining sobriety. Accordingly, whenever possible, regular attendance at such meetings is recommended. We encourage that at least the substance abuser participate regularly, and that the partner attend appropriate meetings, if he or she so desires. As noted earlier, the attendance plan and performance records are usually a part of the Sobriety Contract established between partners engaged in BCT.

MEDICATION DESIGNED
TO HELP MAINTAIN SOBRIETY

Antabuse (disulfiram) is a drug that produces extreme nausea and sickness when the person taking it consumes alcohol. As such, it is an option for drinkers with a goal of abstinence. Naltrexone is a medication prescribed to opioid abusers because the drug inhibits the subjective high associated with opioids. Methadone is used to ease the symptoms of heroin or opiate withdrawal. It is taken daily, and its use is supervised by a hospital or outpatient clinic that is a federally licensed methadone clinic. When taking these medications is incorporated into the Sobriety Contract as a component of BCT, research has demonstrated that patient compliance improves significantly, which results in better abstinence rates. The routine medication-taking procedure also decreases alcohol- and drug-related arguments between the drinker and his or her spouse. In respective Sobriety Contracts, the substance abuser agrees to take the appropriate drug each day while the spouse observes. The spouse, in turn, agrees to reinforce the patient positively and to record the observation on the calendar provided. Each spouse should view the agreement as a cooperative method for rebuilding lost trust, not as a coercive, checking-up operation. In the event that the patient objects to his or her partner having to observe medication-taking, we usually try to renegotiate this trust-building exercise for the sake of cooperation, but we do not insist so long as the patient agrees to take the medication.

In summary, helping couples to anticipate risky social situations, to establish new behav-ioral patterns and certain coping skills to avoid such situations, to construct behavioral contracts that serve to reward and support sobriety and encourage attendance at relevant AA-type support groups, and perhaps to use medications that help to deter substance use—all constitute the primary substance abuse-related interventions associated with BCT. Reviewing and maintaining these procedures constitute the basics of initial and continuing recovery plans.

Relationship-Focused Interventions

ADJUSTMENTS TO RECOVERY

Once the substance abuser has decided to change his or her abuse, the focus can shift to improving marital and family relationships. Family members often experience resentment about past abusive behavior, and fear and distrust about the possible return of abusive behavior in the future. The substance abuser often experiences guilt and a desire for recognition of current improved behavior. These feelings experienced by the substance abuser and the family often lead to an atmosphere of tension and unhappiness in marital and family relationships. There are usually secondary problems caused by substance abuse (e.g., bills, legal charges, and embarrassing incidents) that still need to be resolved. Moreover, there is often a backlog of other, unresolved marital and family problems that the substance abuse obscured. Interestingly, these longstanding problems may seem to increase as abuse declines, when actually the problems are simply being recognized for the first time, now that substance abuse cannot be used to obscure and excuse them. Unfortunately, the partners frequently lack the communication skills and mutual positive feelings needed to resolve these problems. As a result, many marriages and families are dissolved during the first 1 or 2 years of the substance abuser's recovery. In other cases, marital and family conflicts trigger relapse and a return to drinking or drug use. Even in cases in which the substance abuser has a basically sound marriage when he or she is not drinking or drugging abusively, the initiation of sobriety can both produce temporary tension and role readjustments and provide the opportunity for stabilizing and enriching the marriage and family. For these reasons, many substance abusers can benefit from assistance to improve their marital and family relationships once changes in substance abuse have begun.

RELATIONSHIP PROMISES DURING TREATMENT

Over the course of the development of BCT, we have found it advantageous to ask couples to make four types of promises regarding their participation in the individualized or group programs. Couples are first asked to "Attend Therapy Sessions and Do Homework as Assigned." Partners promise to renew their relationship through education and skills training. For change to occur, both partners must be active in working toward change. Renewing the relationship takes time, and personal dedication to the process is an important initial promise.

"No Threats of Divorce or Separation" is the second couple promise that partners are encouraged to make. Threatening separation or divorce can interfere greatly with both relationship improvement efforts and feelings of commitment to the relationship. Making this promise discourages the use of threats as ammunition during arguments or as a result of overall frustration. This promise does not require a lifetime commitment or mean that consideration of separation is not valid; rather, during BCT, the topic is reserved for discussion when the therapist is present to facilitate.

The third important couple promise is "Focus on the Present, Not the Past or the Future." The objective of this promise is that partners refrain from bringing up past problems or grievances in anger or in a manner that discourages couple cooperation and maintenance of sobriety. Although the tendency is great, there is little to gain from rehashing past problems: The non-substance-abuser most likely becomes resentful and angry; the substance abuser becomes guilty, shameful, and resentful. This promise helps partners to focus on positive changes for the present and hope for the future.

Finally, the fourth promise is "No Angry Touching." Each partner promises not to threaten or to use any violence with his or her partner. The use of force of any kind to deal with conflict is not only ineffective but also very destructive to the relationship. This means no pushing, shoving, hitting, and so forth. Making this promise encourages the practice of positive communication and conflict resolution skills.

Two major goals of interventions focused on the substance abuser's couple relationship are (1) to increase positive feelings, goodwill, and commitment to the relationship; and (2) to resolve conflicts and problems, and promote a desire for change. Even though these goals often overlap in the course of actual therapy sessions, we describe useful procedures in achieving these two goals separately. The general sequence in teaching couple skills to increase positive interactions and resolve conflicts and problems is (1) therapist instruction and modeling, (2) couple practice with therapist supervision, (3) assignments for homework, and (4) review of homework, with further practice.

INCREASING POSITIVE EXCHANGES

A series of procedures can increase spouses' awareness of benefits from the relationship and the frequency with which they notice, acknowledge, and initiate pleasing or caring behaviors on a daily basis. The couple is told that caring behaviors are "behaviors that show you care for the other person," and is assigned homework called "Catch Your Partner Doing Something Nice" to help partners notice the daily caring behaviors in the relationship. This requires each spouse to record one caring behavior performed by the partner each day on forms provided. The partners read the caring behaviors recorded during the previous week at the subsequent session. Then the therapist models acknowledging caring behaviors ("I liked it when you _____. It made me feel _____."), emphasizing the importance of eye contact; a smile; a sincere, pleasant tone of voice; and expression of only positive feelings. Each spouse then practices acknowledging caring behaviors from his or her daily list for the previous week. After the partners practice the new behavior in the therapy session, homework is assigned for a 5-minute daily communication session at home, in which each partner acknowledges one pleasing behavior he or she noticed that day. As partners begin to notice and acknowledge daily caring behaviors, each begins initiating more caring behaviors. In addition, many couples report that the 5-minute communication sessions result in more extensive conversations. A final assignment is that each partner gives the other a "caring day" during the coming week, by performing special acts to show caring for the spouse. Partners are encouraged to take risks and to act lovingly rather than wait for the spouse to make the first move.

SHARED REWARDING ACTIVITIES

Many couples have discontinued or decreased shared leisure activities, because the substance abuser has in the past frequently sought enjoyment only in situations involving alcohol or drugs and has embarrassed the partner by using. Reversing this trend is important, because participation by the couple and family in social and recreational activities improves outcomes. The therapist has the couple plan and engage in shared rewarding activities (SRAs), with spouses making separate lists of possible activities. Each activity must involve both spouses, either by themselves, or with their children or other adults, and it can occur at or away from home. The couple is instructed to refrain from discussing problems or conflicts during the planned SRAs.

COMMUNICATION SKILLS TRAINING

Inadequate communication is a major problem for substance abusers and their spouses (O'Farrell & Birchler, 1987). Inability to resolve conflicts and problems can cause abusive drinking or drugging and severe marital/family tension to recur (Maisto, McKay, & O'Farrell, 1995). We have regularly employed a now-classic BMT approach to couple communication training (Gottman, Notarius, Gonso, & Markman, 1976; Jacobson & Margolin, 1979). Accordingly, we define "effective communication" as message intended (by speaker) = message received (by listener), or intent = impact, and we emphasize the need to learn both "listening" and "speaking" skills. Two types of miscommunication "filters" are introduced, which can interfere with intent = impact: (1) situational variables (a headache, rough day, happy hour, stressful freeway driving, grouchy children, late night, etc.) and (2) relatively enduring vulnerabilities (e.g., one's negative beliefs, expectations, prejudices, biases, and persistent assumptions) that serve to distort the intended or received communication. Therapists use instructions, modeling, prompting, behavioral rehearsal, and feedback to teach couples how to communicate more effectively. Learning basic communication skills of listening and speaking, and how to use planned communication sessions are essential prerequisites for problem solving and negotiating desired behavior changes. This training begins with nonproblem areas that are positive or neutral and moves to problem areas and emotionally charged issues only after the couple has mastered basic skills.

Communication sessions are planned, structured discussions in which spouses talk privately, face-to-face, without distractions, and take turns expressing their points of view, without interrupting one another. Communication sessions can be introduced for 5 minutes daily when couples first practice acknowledgment of caring behaviors and in 10- to 15-minute sessions three to four times a week in later sessions, when the partners discuss current relationship concerns. The partners set the time and place they plan to have their assigned communication practice sessions, once the therapist assesses the success of this plan at the next session and suggests any needed changes. Establishing a regular communication session as a method for discussing feelings, events, and problems can be very helpful for many couples. Partners are encouraged to ask each other for a communication session when they want to discuss a problem, keeping in mind the behavioral ground rules that characterize such sessions.

Listening skills help each spouse to feel understood and supported, and slow down couple interactions to prevent the quick escalation of aversive exchanges. Spouses are instructed to repeat both the words and the feelings of the speaker's message and to check to see whether the message received was the message intended by the partner ("What I heard you say was. Is that right?"). When the listener has understood the speaker's message, they change roles, and the first listener then speaks.

Speaking skills (i.e., expressing both positive and negative feelings directly) are alternatives to the blaming, hostile, and indirect responsibility-avoiding communication behaviors that characterize many substance abusers' relationships. Speakers express and take responsibility for their own feelings and do not blame the other person for how he or she feels. This reduces listener defensiveness and makes it easier for the listener to receive the intended message. The use of statements beginning with "I" rather than "you" is emphasized. After presenting the rationale and instructions, the therapist models correct and incorrect ways of expressing feelings and elicits the partners' reactions. They then role-play a communication session in which they take turns being speaker and listener, with the speaker expressing feelings directly and the listener using the listening response. Similar homework communication sessions that last 10 to 15 minutes each are assigned three to four times weekly. Subsequent therapy sessions involve more practice with role playing, both during the sessions and for homework. Partners are helped to gain the ability to appreciate each other's experience and point of view, and to express understanding and empathy with their positions.

NEGOTIATION FOR REQUESTS

A fairly straightforward and very effective communication skill that we teach couples is how to make a request of one's partner. Typically, partners, especially in distressed couples, tend to make complaints, criticisms, and so-called "you" statements when they want something from each other. Reliably, these behaviors tend to put the message receiver on the defensive, and an argument may well ensue. Teaching partners a "soft start-up" strategy, along with how to ask for what they want or would prefer in a positive "I" statement, is much more likely to bring success and satisfaction with the process.

PROBLEM-SOLVING SKILLS TRAINING

After they first learn these basic communication skills, partners next learn specific skills to solve problems stemming from both external stressors (e.g., job, extended family) and relationship conflicts. In solving a problem, the couple should first define the problem and list a number of possible solutions. Then, while withholding judgment regarding the preferred solution, the couple considers both positive and negative, and short- and long-term consequences of each solution. Finally, the spouses rank the solutions from most- to least-preferred and agree to implement one or more of the solutions. Using problem-solving procedures can help spouses avoid polarizing on one solution or another. It also avoids the "Yes, but … " trap, with one partner pointing out problems with the other's solution.

In summary, at this point, we have discussed the primary elements of the basic interventions in BCT for substance abuse rehabilitation and relationship improvement. Now, we consider certain interventions to maintain therapeutic gains and to prevent relapse.

Relapse Prevention: Posttreatment Activities to Maintain Therapy Gains

Three methods are employed in BCT to ensure long-term maintenance of the changes in alcohol or drug abuse problems. First, plans for maintenance occur before the termination of the active treatment phase. This involves helping the couple complete a Continuing Recovery Plan that specifies which of the behaviors from the previous BCT sessions they wish to continue in a planned activity program (daily sobriety trust discussion, a Sobriety Contract, medications, AA/NA meetings, SRAs, planned couple communication sessions, etc.). Second, the therapist helps the couple anticipate high-risk situations for relapse to abusive drinking or drugging that may occur after treatment. Possible coping strategies are discussed and rehearsed that the substance abuser, partner, and other family members can employ to prevent relapse when confronted with such situations. Third, discussion includes how to cope with a lapse or potential relapse, if and when it occurs. A specific relapse episode plan, written and rehearsed prior to ending active treatment, can be particularly useful. Early intervention at the beginning of a lapse or relapse episode is essential, and the couple must be impressed with this point. Often, spouses wait until the substance abuse again reaches dangerous levels before acting. By then, much additional damage has been done to the couple relationship and to other aspects of the substance abuser's life.

We suggest that the therapist take responsibility for initiating continued contact with the couple via planned in-person and telephone follow-up sessions at regular and then gradually increasing intervals up to 5 years after a stable pattern of recovery has been achieved. Couples are told that contact is continued because substance abuse is a chronic health problem that requires active, aggressive, ongoing monitoring to prevent or to treat relapses quickly for up to 5 years after an initial stable pattern of recovery has been established.

Termination

As mentioned previously, in many settings and applications, a set number of sessions is offered. Accordingly, termination is applied on a time- and session-limited basis. In other settings, the number of sessions allowed to reach the goals of treatment is more flexible. When confidence, skills sets, and stability have been reached regarding substance misuse and supportive relationship quality, termination is completed. Of course, not all terminations end positively. "Bad" terminations occur when couples drop out of therapy early and/or when neither sobriety nor relationship success and satisfaction is achieved, and treatment is terminated prematurely for any reason.

CURATIVE FACTORS/MECHANISMS OF CHANGE

Although the results of multiple randomized clinical trials indicate that BCT is effective, no studies to date have empirically established *how* it works. More precisely, the mechanisms of change that produce the observed outcomes have not been empirically tested. As described earlier, the general theoretical rationale for the effects of BCT on substance abuse has been that certain dyadic interactions serve as inadvertent reinforcement for continued substance use or relapse, and that relationship distress in general is a trigger for substance use. In turn, the BCT intervention package that has evolved from this rationale involves (1) teaching and promoting methods to reinforce sobriety from within the dyad (e.g., engaging in the Recovery Contract), (2) improving communication skills to address problems and conflict appropriately when it arises, and (3) encouraging participation in relationship enhancement exercises (e.g., shared rewarding activities) to increase dyadic adjustment. Additionally, from an experiential and clinical perspective, it is believed that implementing certain therapist clinical skills and avoiding the central therapist errors we enumerated earlier contribute significantly to the success of BCT.

However, it is not clear whether participation in any or all of these aspects of the BCT intervention results in the improvements observed. For example, although most BCT studies have found that participation in BCT results in improvements in relationship adjustment and reductions in substance use, none has conducted a formal test of mediation to determine whether changes in relationship adjustment (i.e., either during treatment or after treatment completion) partially or fully mediate the relationship between type of treatment received (e.g., BCT, individual counseling, and attention control) and substance use outcomes. Indeed, it is important to highlight that most studies have generally failed to find strong relationships between theoretical mechanisms of change in different interventions and subsequent outcomes, both in general psychotherapy (e.g., Orlinsky, Grawe, & Parks, 1994; Stiles & Shapiro, 1994), and in substance abuse treatment (e.g., Longabaugh & Wirtz, 2001). Thus, it is important for future studies to test the theoretical mechanisms thought to underlie the observed BCT effects.

TREATMENT APPLICABILITY AND EMPIRICAL SUPPORT

BCT for alcohol and drug problems is particularly relevant for committed couples who have been married or cohabitating for at least 1 year, and one of the members has a defined substance abuse problem that both partners are motivated to reduce or eliminate to support that member's sobriety and to improve their primary intimate relationship. In this context, BCT has been demonstrated to enhance the ability of partners to achieve and maintain sobriety by improving their primary relationship.

Research on BCT with Alcoholism

A series of studies has compared drinking and relationship outcomes for alcoholic clients treated with either BCT or individual alcoholism counseling. Outcomes have been measured at 6-month follow-up in earlier studies and 18–24 months after treatment in more recent studies. The studies show a fairly consistent pattern of more abstinence and fewer alcohol-related problems, happier relationships, and lower risk of marital separation for alcoholic clients who receive BCT compared to clients who receive only individual treatment (Azrin, Sisson, Meyers, & Godley, 1982; Bowers & Al-Rehda, 1990; Hedberg & Campbell, 1974; McCrady, Stout, Noel, Abrams, & Nelson, 1991; O'Farrell, Cutler, Choquette, Floyd, & Bayog, 1992). Domestic violence, with more than 60% prevalence among alcoholic couples before entering BCT, decreased significantly in the 2 years after BCT and was nearly eliminated with abstinence (e.g., O'Farrell & Murphy, 1995). Cost outcomes in small-scale studies show that reduced hospital and jail days after BCT save more than five times the cost of delivering BCT for alcoholic clients and their partners (O'Farrell et al., 1996). Finally, for male alcoholic clients, BCT improves the psychosocial adjustment of couples' children more than does individual-based treatment (Kelley & Fals-Stewart, 2002), even though children are not directly treated in either intervention. Thus, there may be a "trickle down" effect of the communication skills training used as part of BCT, with improved methods of interacting permeating the entire family system.

Research on BCT with Drug Abuse

The first randomized study of BCT with drug-abusing clients compared BCT plus individual treatment to an equally intensive individual-based treatment (Fals-Stewart et al., 1996). Clinical outcomes in the year after treatment favored the group that received BCT relative to both drug use and relationship outcomes. Compared to those who participated in individual-based treatment, BCT participants had significantly fewer relapses, fewer days of drug use, fewer drug-related arrests and hospitalizations, and longer time to relapse. Couples in BCT also had more positive relationship adjustment on multiple measures and fewer days separated due to relationship discord than couples whose partners received individual-based treatment only.

Cost–benefit outcome analyses of participants in this study also favor BCT over individual treatment (Fals-Stewart, O'Farrell, & Birchler, 1997). Social costs in the year before treatment for drug-abuse-related health care, criminal justice system use for drug-related crimes, and income from illegal sources and public assistance were reduced by 60% for the BCT group in the year after treatment. Moreover, results of cost-effectiveness analyses also favored the BCT group. BCT produced greater clinical improvements (e.g., fewer days of substance use) per dollar spent to deliver BCT than did individual treatment. Finally, domestic violence outcomes in this same study also favored BCT (Fals-Stewart, Kashdan, O'Farrell, & Birchler, 2002). Although nearly half of the couples reported male-to-female violence in the year before treatment, the number reporting violence in the year after treatment was significantly lower for BCT (17%) than for individual treatment (42%).

In a second randomized study of BCT with drug-abusing clients (Fals-Stewart, O'Farrell, & Birchler, 2001), 30 married or cohabiting male clients in a methadone maintenance program were randomly assigned to individual treatment only or to BCT plus individual treatment. The individual treatment was standard outpatient drug abuse counseling for the drug-abusing partner. Results during the 6 months of treatment favored the group that received BCT on both drug use and relationship outcomes. A third study (Fals-Stewart & O'Farrell, 2003) randomly assigned 80 married or cohabiting men with opioid addiction to equally intensive naltrexone-involved treatments: (1) BCT plus individual treatment (i.e., the client had both individual and couple sessions, and took naltrexone daily in presence of his spouse) or (2) individual treatment only (i.e., the counselor asked the client about naltrexone compliance, but there was no spouse involvement or compliance contract). In the year after treatment, subjects who had BCT plus individual treatment had significantly more days abstinent from opioids and other drugs, longer time to relapse, and fewer drug-related legal and family problems than did subjects who received individual treatment alone.

Barriers to Dissemination of BCT into Community-Based Programs

Although BCT has very strong research support for its efficacy, it is not yet widely used in community-based alcoholism and drug abuse treatment settings. Fals-Stewart and Birchler (2001) conducted a national survey of 398 randomly selected U.S. substance abuse treatment programs. In general, BCT was viewed as too costly to deliver, requiring too many sessions in its standard form. In addition, whereas most BCT studies use master's-level therapists as treatment providers, most community-based alcohol and other drug abuse programs employ counselors with less formal education or clinical training. A series of more recently completed studies addressed each of these concerns. First, Fals-Stewart, Yates, Klostermann, O'Farrell, and Birchler (2005) evaluated the effectiveness of a briefer version of BCT and found that 6 versus 12 BCT sessions combined with 6 versus 12 Individual-based treatment (IBT) sessions were equally effective, and more effective than 12 IBT sessions alone in terms of male partners' percentage of days abstinent and other outcome indicators during the year after treatment. Second, Fals-Stewart, Birchler, and O'Farrell (2002) demonstrated that combined with 12 sessions of group drug counseling for the substance abuser, BCT delivered in a 12-session small-group format versus the standard 12-session individual couple format was equally effective and, again, more effective than 24 sessions of group drug counseling for the substance abuser alone in reducing substance use and improving relationship outcomes during a 12-month posttreatment follow-up period. Third, Fals-Stewart and Birchler (2002) examined the differential effect of BCT based on counselors' educational background, comparing outcomes of couples that received BCT who were randomly assigned to either a bachelor's- or master's-level counselor. Results for 48 alcoholic men and their female partners showed that, in comparison to master's-level counselors, bachelor's-level counselors were equivalent in terms of adherence ratings to a BCT treatment manual, but were rated slightly lower in terms of quality of treatment delivery (although treatment quality was rated in the excellent range for both groups of counselors). Taken together, the results of these studies suggest that treatment providers in community-based substance abuse treatment programs can deliver BCT effectively and more efficiently using groups and/ or 50% fewer sessions.

CASE ILLUSTRATION

To illustrate some of the procedures we have described thus far, our case example is based on a couple treated by a therapist under the supervision of Fals-Stewart. Although selected background data have been altered to protect the confidentiality and mask the identities of the participating partners, the methods used and the results obtained have not been changed.

John, a 38-year-old African American male, was referred to outpatient substance abuse treatment by his physician after repeated problems due to excessive alcohol and other drug use (e.g., job losses, concerns about health, minor altercations leading to a recent arrest for fighting in a bar). During a psychosocial assessment, he described an extensive history of problematic alcohol and other drug use. John reported that he drank nearly every day in his early 20s, usually consuming three to five beers on each occasion. By his mid-20s, he began drinking greater quantities of alcohol on weekends (i.e., 8–10 drinks on Fridays and Saturdays, and on days when he went to local sporting events or watched them on television) and experienced occasional blackouts. He began experimenting with cocaine in his mid-20s but was not a regular user; however, during the last year, he had begun snorting it three to four times per week, or "whenever I could get my hands on it!"

John had previously been treated in two separate outpatient treatment programs, both within the last 3 years. However, he left both programs against medical advice. He said he had prolonged sobriety (1–2 months) on three different occasions in the last 3 years in an effort to "prove" to himself and his wife he could control his use. He noted that each of these periods of abstinence ended after verbal fights with his wife, whom he described as "critical, demanding ... and she doesn't forgive or forget anything."

John reported that his drinking and cocaine use had gotten progressively worse in the last 6 months, with daily use of one or both substances. He reported he was on the verge of losing his job,

which was causing conflict with his wife, not to mention clear financial strain. John also reported he had driven his car while intoxicated a few times a week during the months prior to the assessment. John met DSM-IV criteria for both alcohol and cocaine dependence.

John was asked if he would be willing to participate in marital assessment with his wife Cynthia. He was very reluctant, emphasizing that his wife was often his "biggest critic" and would only use the assessment as an avenue to highlight his shortcomings as a husband. It was explained that the purpose of seeing the couple together was not to allow the assessment to become a forum for criticism, but rather to assess how his marriage might be contributing to his use, and how it might help in his recovery. It was also emphasized that early sessions were only for assessment; he, his wife, and the therapist were not committing to formal treatment. With this explanation, John agreed to participate in the assessment. He signed a release of confidentiality form to allow his therapist to discuss the possibility of participation with Cynthia.

John attended Cynthia's initial session; the assessment procedures were described to the partners. The therapist again emphasized to both partners that this was only an assessment, and that participation in this evaluation did not commit either the couple or the therapist to a course of treatment. Both partners agreed to complete the assessment.

The therapist collected background data from Cynthia and information about the partners' marriage. Cynthia, a 35-year-old white female, was employed part-time as an accountant assistant in an attorney's office. She reported that she had never abused alcohol or used other drugs. John and Cynthia married after a 1-year courtship, when she became pregnant with their one and only child Davy, and have been married for 10 years. Cynthia said she knew John drank "heavily," but she was not aware of the extent of his drinking or that he used cocaine until his recent admissions to her. She said she was "in shock" about these revelations and did not "want to hang around and see the end of this story."

Both partners described their relationship as unstable and reported that they had recently discussed divorce for the first time in their relationship. John said the only reason he stayed in the relationship was for his son. John's primary complaint was that Cynthia was "always nagging, as if that is going to fix things or make it better" and "is never satisfied—everything is either neutral or bad." Cynthia described John as "irresponsible," and as someone who "needs a mother." She argued that if he would stop drinking and using drugs, the problems in their marriage would lift. She added that John spent money "they did not have" and was untrustworthy.

Along with financial problems, Cynthia said she felt "neglected," because John spent so much time drinking with his friends. She added that they rarely spoke "more than 10 minutes," unless John was drunk, when he would be more affectionate, want to have sex, and so on. She also reported that they had not spent any time engaging in recreational activities they enjoyed (e.g., going to the movies, eating out) in the last few years. Neither partner reported any episodes of physical intimate partner violence; however, there was a good deal of arguing that deteriorated into shouting matches two or three times a month.

As part of the assessment, the partners completed a communication sample. The topic they chose was "financial problems." As part of this conflict resolution task, they were asked to describe the problem and to work toward a solution. The following partial transcript of their discussion occurred about 1 minute after the task was initiated:

WIFE: You have stayed straight for 2 months in a row in the last year? Where was I? Ray Charles can see through those lies.

HUSBAND: We get nowhere. If I use, you are pissed. If I don't use, you are pissed I didn't stop earlier. When is it enough? It is ...

WIFE: I'll let you know when it is enough.

HUSBAND: You have me one down and will forever. What does Davy think? What does he think? Can't we just try for him?

WIFE: Don't lay it on him. He has seen enough, don't you think?

HUSBAND: Yes, I do. That is why I am here.

WIFE: Let's not get crazy; you are here because you are scared of losing everything. Once you think you have everyone fooled, you will be back to your old s--t!

HUSBAND: I know. For all I know, I thought you would be happy doing this.

WIFE: I am ... you think I like all of this. I hate it! I just want to stop all of this. Everyone talks about change being so exciting. I want there

to be no excitement or change for a good long time. Please, please ... try to stop. Commit to me and Davy.

HUSBAND: (Whispers.) Leave him out of this (long pause).

WIFE: We have not saved dime one for him; we can't. You are damning him with this s--t and it makes me sick. You know, he is a great student. He can go to college, but we need to get money. You are blowing it away, up your nose. ... You are using his future to be with your friends.

HUSBAND: You don't get this thing.

WIFE: No, I get it ... the bills, the school, the worries, the fear. You are going to lose your job and then we are really f--ked. What is the plan?

HUSBAND: What plan?

WIFE: You know, the one where you get us out of the mess?

HUSBAND: You won't let me off the canvas. ... If I stop, you spend all of your time accusing me of being drunk anyway. It is a mess, but don't think you are not a star in it. You are not just a victim, although you like playing one. Now you can play victim for these people and show them what a dog I am.

WIFE: I am the victim here. But so is your son. I thought you would be such a good dad, but it didn't change you at all. You still go out, hang out with the boys.

HUSBAND: Who said it would change? When you change the game, please let me know the new rules, all right?

WIFE: All right. (Yells.) The game changed when Davy came along. You are supposed to help out; I didn't know you needed a f--king memo!

This exchange, along with other assessment data from the paper-and-pencil interviews and the clinical interviews, revealed multiple deficits across many of the 7 C's described earlier. This discussion revealed not only significant deficits in the partners' *communication* patterns but also a lack of mutual *caring* and a general level of interpersonal antagonism. The approach the couple used for *conflict resolution* can best be described as "kitchen sinking"; although the agreed topic was "financial problems," they introduced several other conflict areas without addressing the problem at hand. The partners described clear deficits in *commitment*, noting on a few occasions that they were only staying together for the sake of their only child. Last, the communication sample revealed a *contract* problem. Cynthia thought John would be involved as a parent once Davy was born; John believed it should not have changed his lifestyle very much.

The partners ultimately agreed to participate in treatment. John realized that conflict and stress in his marriage was making it difficult for him to maintain sobriety. Cynthia agreed to participate, hoping that she would get a better understanding of why John drank and used drugs. Early sessions involved introducing and following through with a negotiated Sobriety Contract, which included five primary components: (1) John agreed to take Antabuse (for which he was medically evaluated) while being observed by Cynthia; (2) the couple agreed to a positive verbal exchange (i.e., a sobriety trust discussion) when John took the Antabuse (i.e., John reporting that he had stayed abstinent from alcohol and drugs during the previous day and promising to remain abstinent for the ensuing day, and Cynthia thanking him for remaining sober); (3) Cynthia agreed not to bring up negative past events concerning John's drinking and drug use; (4) John agreed to attend AA meetings daily; (5) the partners would not threaten to divorce or separate while at home and would, for the time being, bring these thoughts into the sessions; and (6) John would provide urine samples each week to determine whether he had used any cocaine or other drugs.

Cynthia reported that John's consumption of Antabuse gave her great comfort, because she knew that he was not drinking when he was taking it. The positive verbal exchange between the partners made the daily sobriety contract a caring behavior rather than a "checking up" procedure. John said there was less stress in the home, because Cynthia did not bring up his past drinking (although there were occasions when Cynthia lapsed into bringing up the past). John's AA involvement provided him with a support network that did not include friends with whom he drank or used drugs. Urine screens were negative for all drugs tested, which was consistent with John's reports that he was clean and sober.

Communication skills training focused on slowing down the partners' verbal exchanges, with an emphasis on staying on a single topic. Session time was also spent training the partners to make positive specific requests and using "I" statements as a way to own their feelings rather than attributing how they felt to one another.

Later sessions addressed identified relationship problems. Assignments such as "Catch Your Partner Doing Something Nice" and SRAs served to increase positive verbal exchanges and mutual caring, along with reestablishing a long-term commitment to the relationship. Toward the end of therapy, the partners reported that BCT helped them learn to "enjoy each other again." They noted that their sex life had improved dramatically and, with the help of the therapist, they had sought the services of a credit counselor to assist them with some of their financial problems.

During the latter phase of treatment, the focus shifted toward John's parenting and work with Cynthia to allow John to play a more active role in their son's life. Since Cynthia had been doing most of the parenting for the last few years, it was difficult for her to relinquish any control to John, even after extended sobriety. John and Cynthia agreed to allow John to do separate recreational activities with Davy that did not include her. This gave John time to reestablish his relationship with Davy, without involvement and interference from Cynthia. This issue remained a longstanding, ongoing struggle for the partners during and after treatment.

During the 2-year posttreatment follow-up interviews, John reported that he had remained sober except for a 1-week relapse with alcohol. However, he contacted his sponsor, returned to AA, and reestablished abstinence. Both partners reported that they made a point of doing something fun together at least once a week. John was attending AA meetings three to four times weekly. Although the partners continued to have money problems, Cynthia received a work promotion, which helped to alleviate some of the stress.

SUGGESTIONS FOR FURTHER READING

Addiction and Family Research Group (*www.addictionandfamily.org*).—This website provides training materials, multiple therapy manuals, articles, and videotape examples, all related to the use of couple therapy with substance-abusing patients and their partners.

Birchler, G. R., Doumas, D., & Fals-Stewart, W. (1999). The Seven C's: A behavioral systems framework for evaluating marital distress. *The Family Journal: Counseling and Therapy for Couples and Families, 7,* 253–264.—This article provides an excellent and easily understandable road map for organizing the assessment of couples (substance-abusing and distressed couples more broadly) along the dimensions of the 7 C's.

Fals-Stewart, W., Birchler, G. R., & Ellis, L. (1999). Procedures for evaluating the marital adjustment of drug-abusing patients and their intimate partners: A multi-method assessment procedure. *Journal of Substance Abuse Treatment, 16,* 5–16.—This article describes multiple types of assessment procedures used in conjunction with partner-involved treatments for substance abuse.

Fals-Stewart, W., O'Farrell, T. G., Birchler, G. R., Cordova, J., & Kelley, M. L. (2005). Behavioral couples therapy for alcoholism and drug abuse: Where we've been, where we are, and where we're going. *Journal of Cognitive Psychotherapy, 19,* 231–249.—This article provides a comprehensive review of the empirical literature supporting the use of behavioral couple therapy with alcoholic and drug-abusing patients, across primary outcomes (e.g., substance use, relationship adjustment) and secondary outcomes (e.g., children's adjustment, intimate partner violence, cost–benefit and cost-effectiveness).

O'Farrell, T. J., & Fals-Stewart, W. (2006). *Behavioral couples therapy for alcoholism and drug abuse.* New York: Guilford Press.—This comprehensive textbook provides not only a comprehensive overview of the theory and empirical literature supporting behavioral couples therapy with substance-abusing patients and their partners but also a step-by-step guide (including handouts and other materials) for implementing the approach in practice.

REFERENCES

Adesso, U. J. (1995). Cognitive factors in alcohol and drug use. In M. Galizio & S. A. Maisto (Eds.), *Determinants of substance abuse: Biological, psychological, and environmental factors* (pp. 179–208). New York: Plenum Press.

American Psychiatric Association. (1994). *Diagnostic and statistical manual of mental disorders* (4th ed.). Washington, DC: Author.

Azrin, N. H., Sisson, R. W., Meyers, R., & Godley, M. (1982). Alcoholism treatment by disulfiram and community reinforcement therapy. *Journal of Behavior Therapy and Experimental Psychiatry, 13,* 105–112.

Birchler, G. R., Doumas, D., & Fals-Stewart, W. (1999). The Seven C's: A behavioral-systems framework for evaluating marital distress. *The Family Journal, 7,* 253–264.

Birchler, G. R., Weiss, R. L., & Vincent, J. P. (1975). Multi-method analysis of reinforcement exchange between maritally distressed and nondistressed spouse and stranger dyads. *Journal of Personality and Social Psychology, 31,* 349–360.

Bowers, T. G., & Al-Rehda, M. R. (1990). A comparison of outcome with group/marital and standard/individual therapies with alcoholics. *Journal of Studies on Alcohol, 51,* 301–309.

Christensen, A. (1987). Detection of conflict patterns in couples. In K. Hahlweg & M. J. Goldstein (Eds.), *Understanding major mental disorders: The contribution of family interaction research* (pp. 250–265). New York: Family Process Press.

Edwards, M. E., & Steinglass, P. (1995). Family therapy treatment outcomes for alcoholism. *Journal of Marital and Family Therapy, 21,* 475–490.

Fals-Stewart, W., & Birchler, G. R. (2001). A national survey of the use of couples therapy in substance abuse treatment. *Journal of Substance Abuse Treatment, 20,* 277–283.

Fals-Stewart, W., & Birchler, G. R. (2002). Behavioral couples therapy for alcoholic men and their intimate partners: The comparative effectiveness of master's- and bachelor's-level counselors. *Behavior Therapy, 33,* 123–147.

Fals-Stewart, W., Birchler, G. R., & Ellis, L. (1999). Procedures for evaluating the marital adjustment of drug-abusing patients and their intimate partners: A multi-method assessment procedure. *Journal of Substance Abuse Treatment, 16,* 5–16.

Fals-Stewart, W., Birchler, G. R., & Kelley, M. L. (2006). Learning sobriety together: A randomized clinical trial examining behavioral couples therapy with alcoholic female patients. *Journal of Consulting and Clinical Psychology, 74*(3), 579–591.

Fals-Stewart, W., Birchler, G. R., & O'Farrell, T. J. (1996). Behavioral couples therapy for male substance-abusing patients: Effects on relationship adjustment and drug-using behavior. *Journal of Consulting and Clinical Psychology, 64,* 959–972.

Fals-Stewart, W., Birchler, G. R., & O'Farrell, T. J. (1999). Drug-abusing patients and their partners: Dyadic adjustment, relationship stability and substance use. *Journal of Abnormal Psychology, 108,* 11–23.

Fals-Stewart, W., Kashdan, T. B., O'Farrell, T. J., & Birchler, G. R. (2002). Behavioral couples therapy for drug-abusing patients: Effects on partner violence. *Journal of Substance Abuse Treatment, 22,* 87–96.

Fals-Stewart, W., Kelley, M. L., Cooke, C. G., & Golden, J. (2003). Predictors of the psychosocial adjustment of children living in households in which fathers abuse drugs: The effects of postnatal social exposure. *Addictive Behaviors, 28,* 1013–1031.

Fals-Stewart, W., & Kennedy, C. (2005). Addressing intimate partner violence in substance abuse treatment. *Journal of Substance Abuse Treatment, 5,* 5–17.

Fals-Stewart, W., & O'Farrell, T. J. (2003). Behavioral family counseling and naltrexone for male opioid-dependent patients. *Journal of Consulting and Clinical Psychology, 71,* 432–442.

Fals-Stewart, W., O'Farrell, T. J., & Birchler, G. R. (1997). Behavioral couples therapy for male substance abusing patients: A cost outcomes analysis. *Journal of Consulting and Clinical Psychology, 65,* 789–802.

Fals-Stewart, W., O'Farrell, T. J., & Birchler, G. R. (2001). Behavioral couples therapy for male methadone maintenance patients: Effects on drug-using behavior and relationship adjustment. *Behavior Therapy, 32,* 391–411.

Fals-Stewart, W., O'Farrell, T. J., & Birchler, G. R. (2003). Family therapy techniques. In F. Rotgers, J. Morgenstern, & S. T. Walters (Eds.), *Treating substance abuse* (pp. 140–165). New York: Guilford Press.

Fals-Stewart, W., Yates, B., Klostermann, K., O'Farrell, T. J., & Birchler, G. R. (2005). Brief relationship therapy for alcoholism: Clinical and cost outcomes. *Psychology of Addictive Behaviors, 19*, 363–371.

Gottman, J. M. (1994). *What predicts divorce?* Hillsdale, NJ: Erlbaum.

Gottman, J. M., Markman, H., & Notarius, C. (1977). The topography of marital conflict: A sequential analysis of verbal and nonverbal behavior. *Journal of Marriage and the Family, 39*, 461–477.

Gottman, J. M., Notarius, C., Gonso, J., & Markman, H. (1976). *A couples guide to communication.* Champaign, IL: Research Press.

Hedberg, A. G., & Campbell, L. (1974). A comparison of four behavioral treatments of alcoholism. *Journal of Behavior Therapy and Experimental Psychiatry, 5*, 251–256.

Jacobson, N. S., & Margolin, G. (1979). *Marital therapy: Strategies based on social learning and behavioral exchange principles.* New York: Brunner/Mazel.

Kelley, M. L., & Fals-Stewart, W. (2002). Couples- versus individual-based therapy for alcoholism and drug abuse: Effects on children's psychosocial functioning. *Journal of Consulting and Clinical Psychology, 70*, 417–427.

Lammers, S. M. M., Schippers, G. M., & van der Staak, C. P. F. (1995). Submission and rebellion: Excessive drinking of women in problematic heterosexual partner relationships. *International Journal of Additions, 30*, 901–917.

Longabaugh, R., & Wirtz, P. W. (2001). *Project MATCH hypotheses: Results and causal chain analyses* [Project MATCH Monograph Series, Vol. 8]. Bethesda, MD: National Institute on Alcohol Abuse and Alcoholism.

Maisto, S. A., McKay, J. R., & O'Farrell, T. J. (1995). Relapse precipitants and behavioral marital therapy. *Addictive Behaviors, 20*, 383–393.

Maisto, S. A., O'Farrell, T. J., McKay, J., Connors, G. J., & Pelcovitz, M. A. (1988). Alcoholics' attributions of factors affecting their relapse to drinking and reasons for terminating relapse events. *Addictive Behaviors, 13*, 79–82.

McClellan, A. T., Luborsky, L., Cacciola, J., Griffith, J., Evans, F., Barr, H. L., et al. (1985). New data from the addiction severity index: Reliability and validity in three centers. *Journal of Nervous and Mental Disease, 173*, 412–423.

McCrady, B., Stout, R., Noel, N., Abrams, D., & Nelson, H. (1991). Comparative effectiveness of three types of spouse involved alcohol treatment: Outcomes 18 months after treatment. *British Journal of Addiction, 86*, 1415–1424.

McCrady, B. S., & Epstein, E. E. (1999, November). *Alcohol-dependent women in treatment: The women,* *their partners, their relationships.* Paper presented at the annual meeting of the Association for Advancement of Behavior Therapy, Toronto, Canada.

Moos, R. H., & Billings, A. G. (1982). Children of alcoholics during the recovery phase: Alcoholic and matched control families. *Addictive Behavior, 7*, 155–163.

Nathan, P. E. (1981). Prospects for a behavioral approach to the diagnosis of alcoholism. In R. E. Meyer, T. F. Babor, B. C. Glueck, J. H. Jaffe, J. E. O'Brian, & J. R. Stabenau (Eds.), *Evaluation of the alcoholic: Implications for theory, research, and treatment* (DHHS Publication No. ADM 81-1003, pp. 85–102). Washington, DC: National Institute on Alcohol Abuse and Alcoholism.

O'Farrell, T. J., & Birchler, G. R. (1987). Marital relationships of alcoholic, conflicted, and nonconflicted couples. *Journal of Marital and Family Therapy, 13*, 259–274.

O'Farrell, T. J., Choquette, K. A., Cutter, H. S. G., & Birchler, G. R. (1997). Sexual satisfaction and dysfunction in marriages of male alcoholics: Comparison with nonalcoholic maritally conflicted and nonconflicted couples. *Journal of Studies on Alcohol, 58*, 91–99.

O'Farrell, T. J., Choquette, K. A., Cutter, H. S. G., Floyd, F. J., Bayog, R. D., Brown, E. D., et al. (1996). Cost–benefit and cost-effectiveness analyses of behavioral marital therapy as an addition to outpatient alcoholism treatment. *Journal of Substance Abuse, 8*, 145–166.

O'Farrell, T. J., & Cutter, H. S. G. (1984). Behavioral marital therapy for alcoholics: Clinical procedures from a treatment outcome study in progress. *American Journal of Family Therapy, 12*, 33–46.

O'Farrell, T. J., Cutter, H. S. G., Choquette, K. A., Floyd, F. J., & Bayog, R. D. (1992). Behavioral marital therapy for male alcoholics: Marital and drinking adjustment during the two years after treatment. *Behavior Therapy, 23*, 529–549.

O'Farrell, T. J., & Fals-Stewart, W. (2006). *Behavioral couples therapy for alcoholism and drug abuse.* New York: Guilford Press.

O'Farrell, T. J., & Murphy, C. M. (1995). Marital violence before and after alcoholism treatment. *Journal of Consulting and Clinical Psychology, 63*, 256–262.

Orlinsky, D., Grawe, K., & Parks, B. (1994). Process and outcome in psychotherapy. In A. E. Bergin & S. R. Garfield (Eds.), *Handbook of psychotherapy and behavior change* (4th ed., pp. 270–376). New York: Wiley.

Paolino, T. J., Jr., & McCrady, B. S. (1977). *The alcoholic marriage: Alternative perspectives.* New York: Grune & Stratton.

Steinglass, P., Bennett, L. A., Wolin, S. J., & Reiss, D. (1987). *The alcoholic family.* New York: Basic Books.

Stiles, W. B., & Shapiro, D. A. (1994). Disabuse of the drug metaphor: Psychotherapy process–outcome correlation. *Journal of Consulting and Clinical Psychology, 62*, 942–948.

Stuart, R. B. (1969). Operant–interpersonal treatment

for marital discord. *Journal of Consulting and Clinical Psychology, 33,* 675–682.

Stuart, R. B. (1980). *Helping couples change: A social learning approach to marital therapy.* New York: Guilford Press.

Weiss, R. L., Hops, H., & Patterson, G. R. (1973). A framework for conceptualizing marital conflict, a technology for altering it, some data for evaluating it. In L. A. Hamerlynck, L. C. Handy, & E. J. Mash (Eds.), *Behavior change: Methodology, concepts, and practice* (pp. 309–342). Champaign, IL: Research Press.

Winters, J., Fals-Stewart, W., O'Farrell, T. J., Birchler, G. R., & Kelley, M. L. (2002). Behavioral couples therapy for female substance-abusing patients: Effects on substance use and relationship adjustment. *Journal of Consulting and Clinical Psychology, 70,* 344–355.

World Health Organization. (1992). *International classification of diseases and related health problems* (10th rev.). Geneva: Author.

Wulfert, E., Greenway, D. E., & Dougher, M. J. (1996). A logical functional analysis of reinforcement-based disorders: Alcoholism and pedophilia. *Journal of Consulting and Clinical Psychology, 64,* 1140–1115.

CHAPTER 19

Couple Therapy
and the Treatment of Depression

STEVEN R. H. BEACH
JESSICA A. DREIFUSS
KAMERON J. FRANKLIN
CHARLES KAMEN
BARBARA GABRIEL

BACKGROUND

Marital therapy for depression began as an adjunctive treatment for depressed patients, and as such it has steadily gained adherents over the past 20 years. Its popularity is driven by the need for, and the potential benefits of, enhanced social functioning for depressed patients, particularly in the context of their closest relationships. Initially, the conceptual foundation for marital therapy for depression was provided by the empirical literature on stress and social support in depression, which suggested that addressing social difficulties in depression would be palliative for most depressed individuals and might in some cases be curative (cf. Beach, Sandeen, & O'Leary, 1990). Marital therapy for depression was also offered as a treatment for depressed persons with marital role disputes, highlighting its similarity to interpersonal psychotherapy (IPT; Klerman, Weissman, Rounsaville, & Chevron, 1984) which also has gained adherents over the past 20 years. For this reason, marital therapy for depression is typically presented as having a more focused target population and more modest claims for its range of applicability than do individual treatments for depression. Early on, we adopted the position that marital therapy

for depression is probably best limited to persons with significant marital disputes, particularly those related to the onset or exacerbation of the depressive episode (cf. Klerman & Weissman, 1991), and subsequent data, which we review below, appears to support this view. However, it also appears that limited positive interactions with close others is a general problem in depression, so there may be a need for some supportive marital interventions even with depressed persons who do not report distressed relationships.

Brief History of the Approach

A variety of theorists from a range of theoretical positions have suggested that marital therapy may be useful as a treatment for depression (Beach, 1996). Likewise, some empirically oriented therapists made relatively early forays into the area of marital therapy for depression. Friedman's (1975) early work on the use of marital therapy in the treatment of depression is the most commonly cited example, with results that suggest some potential additive benefits of medication and marital therapy. A somewhat less familiar example is Lewinsohn's description of a conjoint marital treatment for depression (Lewinsohn & Shaffer, 1971).

Early insights and suggestions regarding the use of marital therapy with depressed patients were hampered, however, by the lack of empirical research. Before marital therapy for depression could be embraced, the field needed data that indicated the prominence of marital disputes and marital relationship problems among many persons presenting for treatment of depression, and the role of social events and social context as causal variables in the etiology of depression. First, Weissman's (1979) summary of the literature and her call for clinical trials helped launch the modern era of marital therapy for depression and directly influenced our own decision to attempt to work with a depressed population using marital therapy. Second, Brown and Harris (1978) similarly provided the earliest comprehensive, conceptual starting point for our work. Brown's work highlighted the marital relationship as a context that could occasion severely threatening events or severe difficulties, with the potential to provoke an episode of depression. However, his work also highlighted the marital relationship as a context that could potentially be protective against depression. A third major influence on the development of marital therapy for depression was ongoing clinical observation at the Marital Therapy Clinic at the State University of New York at Stony Brook. In the context of hundreds of couples presenting for treatment, many couples that were depressed became less depressed as their relationships improved. This suggested a robust clinical effect of marital therapy on depression and gave researchers hope that the effect of marital therapy on depression could be studied systematically.

The work that led to marital therapy for depression, is a variant of behavioral marital therapy formulated by O'Leary and Beach, designed to be useful in the treatment of depression, which was later published in manual form (Beach et al., 1990). These authors hypothesized that spouses selected for the presence of marital discord and depression, particularly if the marital problems appeared to precede and precipitate the depression, would be most likely to respond well to marital therapy for depression. They used behavioral marital therapy, because it seemed to be a particularly good source of techniques from which build a focused marital intervention for depression. At the time, behavioral marital therapy, the best tested form of marital therapy, had already been demonstrated to relieve marital discord and to maintain effects over a follow-up period (Hahlweg, Bau-

com, & Markman, 1988); furthermore, and it had been shown that higher levels of depressive symptoms predicted better response to intervention (Jacobson, Follette, & Pagel, 1986). In addition, behavioral marital therapy was the only form of marital therapy to have documented cross-cultural efficacy (Hahlweg & Markman, 1988), suggesting its potential to work in a wide range of populations.

The variant of behavioral marital therapy that was eventually developed for the treatment of depression (Beach et al., 1990) focused on the elimination of stressful and distressing transactions in the marriage and the enhancement of social support provision within the marriage, particularly attempting to enhance the view of the partner as a reliable person who could be counted upon to listen to and work with the depressed patient. It was hypothesized that a decrease in level of depression would occur primarily as a function of improvement in the quality of the relationship, a prediction that has been supported in controlled research.

The marital discord model has continued to evolve since its initial presentation in 1990. In particular, there has been increasing attention to the broader interpersonal context of depression and the development of more sophisticated causal models linking social processes and depression (e.g., Hammen, 2005), and increasing interest in the family and relationship context of mental health in general (Beach et al., 2006).

Recent Empirical Influences on the Development of the Model

In our most recent presentations of the marital discord model of depression, we have adopted a variant of Hammen's (1991) stress generation framework. "Stress generation" describes a particular a bidirectional pattern of causation between family relationships and depression. The model posits that depressed individuals can generate stress in their interpersonal environments in a variety of ways, and that the interpersonal stress that is generated can also "feed back" to exacerbate or maintain their depressive symptoms.

In one empirical illustration of the vicious cycle that characterizes marital discord and depression, Davila, Bradbury, Cohan, and Tochluk (1997) found that depression predicted greater negativity in support behavior toward the spouse, which in turn predicted greater marital stress. Finally, closing the vicious cycle, level of marital stress predicted subsequent depressive symptoms (controlling for earlier symptoms). This work highlights the vicious cycle that can operate to erode positives in relationships over time. Likewise, in his review of self-propagating processes in depression, Joiner (2000; see also Joiner, Brown, & Kistner, 2006), highlighted the propensity for depressed persons to seek negative feedback, to engage in excessive reassurance seeking, to avoid conflict and to withdraw, and to elicit changes in their partners' view of them, illustrating as well the potential for vicious cycles that lead to more stressful marital events. In each case, the behavior resulting from the individual's depression carries the potential to generate increased interpersonal stress or to shift the response of others in a negative direction. As a consequence of these converging lines of research, we currently view depression and marital discord as components of a larger vicious cycle that creates a self-sustaining loop.

Recent research also provides illustrations of the way in which particular stressful marital or family events can precipitate or exacerbate depressive symptoms among the vulnerable, initiating the stress generation process. For example, Cano and O'Leary (2000) found that humiliating events, such as partner infidelity and threats of marital dissolution, resulted in a sixfold increase in diagnosis of depression, and that this increased risk remained after they controlled for family and personal history of depression. Furthermore, Whisman and Bruce (1999) found that marital dissatisfaction increased risk of subsequent diagnosis of depression 2.7-fold in a large, representative community sample and, again, the increased risk remained significant after they controlled for demographic variables and personal history of depression. Likewise, marital conflict with physical abuse predicted increased depressive symptoms over time, after controlling for earlier symptoms (Beach et al., 2004). As these studies suggest, marital distress and specific types of marital events may be sufficiently potent to precipitate a depressive episode. In keeping with this growing literature, the targets of marital therapy for depression have been broadened, and the goal of marital therapy for depression has been conceptualized as the interruption of vicious cycles perpetuating both marital discord and depressive symptoms.

Given our longstanding interest in direct empirical support for our treatment approach, another major influence on our thinking about marital therapy for depression has been the evolving outcome literature on marital approaches for depression.

Outcome of Marital Interventions for Depression

Early Investigations of Dyadic Treatment with Heterogeneous Populations

A number of case studies and group comparisons over the years have addressed the issue of spousal involvement in therapy and its potential utility in alleviating depressive symptomatology (see Beach, 1996, for a more complete review). These early studies, although encouraging, had various limitations. In general, of course, case studies provide examples of successful treatment but cannot be taken as evidence that a treatment will generalize across an entire population. In the early group studies, the limitations typically took the form of employing a nonstandard or very loosely specified marital intervention and/or including as subjects persons who were quite heterogeneous diagnostically. So, whereas these studies and case reports provided encouragement of further study, they did not, by themselves, provide a satisfactory answer to the question of the potential effectiveness of marital therapy in the treatment of depressed persons.

Brief Review of the Outcome Research

Several studies have examined well-specified approaches and their efficacy in reducing symptoms of depression and in enhancing marital satisfaction. Three trials compared a standard couple therapy, behavioral marital therapy (BMT), to individual therapy (Beach & O'Leary, 1992; Emanuels-Zuurveen & Emmelkamp, 1996; Jacobson, Dobson, Fruzzeti, Schmaling, & Salusky, 1991). Two clinical trials involved adaptation of individual therapies for depression to a couple format (Emanuals-Zuurveen & Emmelkamp, 1997; Foley, Rounsaville, Weissman, Sholomaskas, & Chevron, 1989). There has been one trial of cognitive couple therapy (Teichman, Bar-El, Shor, Sirota, & Elizur, 1995) and one trial comparing marital therapy to antidepressant medication (Leff et al., 2000), but these did not examine change in marital satisfaction. In addition, a published pilot test of emotionally focused therapy (EFT) for depression (Dessaulles, Jonson, & Denton, 2003) indicated the likelihood of positive effects using this approach, but its very small sample size precluded reliable statistical analyses. Finally, there is also an interesting, unpublished study of marital therapy for depression that offers some new ideas for the marital treatment of depression focused on support provision (Bodenman, 2007).

The three studies comparing BMT to individual therapy all produced similar results. Consistently across the three studies, behavioral marital therapy and individual therapy yielded equivalent outcomes when the dependent variable was depressive symptoms, and a better outcome in marital therapy than in individual therapy when the dependent variable was marital functioning. In addition, in one of the studies, marital therapy was found to be significantly better than waiting-list control (Beach & O'Leary, 1992).

However, it does not appear that the potentially positive effects of marital therapy for depression are confined to behavioral approaches. Foley and colleagues (1989) tested a conjoint marital format for interpersonal psychotherapy (IPT-CM). In their study, 18 depressed outpatients were randomly assigned either to individual IPT or a newly developed, couple-format version of IPT. Consistent with the findings of the studies comparing BMT and an individual approach, Foley et al. found that participants in both treatments exhibited a significant reduction in depressive symptoms, but they found no significant differences between treatment groups in amount of reduction in depressive symptoms. Consistent with observations in BMT, participants receiving couple IPT-CM reported marginally higher marital satisfaction scores on the Locke–Wallace Short Marital Adjustment Test and scored significantly higher on one subscale of the Dyadic Adjustment Scale (DAS) at session 16 than participants receiving IPT with no marital component. Similarly, the investigation of EFT in the treatment of depression provided suggestive evidence that EFT provides a useful framework for intervention with depressed couples as well (Dessaulles et al., 2003).

Because we suspect that enhancement of relationship quality and interruption of vicious cycles maintaining depression are key to any successful approach to marital therapy for depression, it follows that any efficacious marital therapy approach has the potential to be efficacious in the treatment of depression as well. Accordingly, our approach to marital therapy for depression is open to the potential for alternative formats and innovative developments that may be useful depending on particular couple characteristics.

THE NATURE AND ROLE OF ROMANTIC LOVE IN DEPRESSION

Romantic love is an important component of most marital relationships, and discussions of romantic love have become more prominent in the marital area over the past several years, as the field has shifted toward greater attention to positive aspects of marital relationships (Fincham, Stanley, & Beach, 2007). One of the difficulties faced by depressed marital partners is that they often feel they have fallen "out of love" with their partners, or at least they no longer experience the positive feelings they once experienced toward their partners. Clinicians conducting marital therapy for depression may discover this in early, split sessions (if they conduct these), or they may infer it based on the depressed partner's response to suggested homework or feedback during therapy sessions. When marital therapists become aware of this concern in their depressed patients, they typically should reassure couples that loss of feelings of love is a normal aspect of depression and is often accompanied by loss of other positive motivations and feelings. It should be emphasized that the goal of marital therapy for depression is to help couples develop "functional" marriages that meet basic needs for support, companionship, security, coparenting, cooperation, and sexuality. Positive feelings are expected to return, along with the capacity to enjoy positive events, to anticipate positive future interactions, and to recall past positive experiences more easily.

Because romantic love is dominated by feeling tone, it is assumed it will be impaired in the context of marital discord, and even more impaired in the context of depression. In the context of marital therapy for depression, romantic love may be talked about in a manner consistent with attachment theory (i.e., suggesting that feelings of love are influenced by attachment, caregiving, and sexual motives; Shaver, Hazan, & Bradshaw, 1988), all of which may temporarily be impaired by the depressive episode. Alternatively, it may be talked about as a set of feelings that may be deactivated as a protective response to relationship stress (Johnson & Greenman, 2006). Finally, feelings of love may be talked about in the context of emphasizing acceptance, tolerance, and compromise as important responses that may help couples exit from the vicious cycles that trap them in relationships, with little opportunity to experience love for each other (Dimidjian, Martell, & Christensen, 2002). Common to all presentations would be an effort to convey the strong expectation that, for many couples dealing with depression, feelings of romantic love will reemerge as the couple deals with the conflict, the loss of positive relationship interactions, and the relationship stressors that are suppressing it.

Although we expect loss of feelings of romantic love, a history of having felt romantic love for the partner is viewed as a positive prognostic sign, as is romantic love reflected in the couple's courtship accounts. The presence of romantic love in courtship accounts provides a good starting point for the early phases of marital therapy for depression and can provide an initial basis for instilling hope for the future (Beach et al., 1990).

The Healthy versus the Depressed Couple

There is a strong empirical basis for understanding the biological, psychological, and social variables involved in both depression and the development and maintenance of marital discord. Four identifiable patterns distinguish the depressed, dissatisfied couple from the nondepressed, satisfied couple: high levels of distressed behavior, less marital cohesion and intimacy, cognitive and behavioral asymmetry, and deficits in problem solving and communication. However, with the exception of distressed (i.e., depressive) behavior, these patterns are shared with other martially discordant couples.

High Levels of Depressive Behavior

In addition to prototypical behavioral and cognitive symptoms of marital discord, such as endorsing more negative relationship events and greater reactivity to spousal negative behaviors, the couple experiencing marital discord in the context of depression may display unique, additional levels of behavioral negativity. A depressed partner may express negative affectivity about not only him- or herself but also his or her partner. This self-derogation may include negative self-statements, endorsement of negative well-being, negative statements about the future, and general complaints. Self-derogation is not more common in the partners of depressed individuals, nor has

this pattern been shown in discordant dyads with a nondepressed partner, implying that these statements may be unique to depression (Hautzinger, Linden, & Haufmann, 1982).

Depressive behaviors, including negative self-statements, have been hypothesized to be critical to the maintenance of certain types of marital discord. In particular, it has been hypothesized that depressive behavior may have a "suppressive" effect on interpersonal aggression during conflict discussions (Coyne, 1976), but the degree of suppression may decrease as the duration and intensity of marital discord increases (Nelson & Beach, 1990). Accordingly, displays of depressed affect, which include sighing, lack of eye contact, and long latencies between speech utterances (Biglan et al., 1985), may change the tenor of marital discussions and decrease the efficiency of problem-solving discussions. Because of their potential to interrupt the flow of discussion, these behaviors are typically attended to during the course of couple therapy for depression. In particular, both members of the couple are helped to increase eye contact and nonverbal signs of attention and agreement, and to decrease latency of responses to the partner—all of which may predict positive response to treatment (Greden & Carroll, 1980).

Less Marital Cohesion and Intimacy

Other marital interaction patterns are also targeted for treatment, because they are often disturbed in the marriages of maritally discordant and depressed couples. However, these patterns may not distinguish between distressed dyads with a depressed member and other distressed dyads. Long-standing patterns of negative interaction over time can have profound implications for many distressed couples' sense of closeness and intimacy. Negative patterns may lead both members of a discordant couple struggling with depression to feel isolated and distant, to sense that their relationship has lower cohesion than it once did, and, in some cases, to suspect that their relationship never had closeness and intimacy.

Depressed/distressed couples are significantly less satisfied with their level of marital intimacy than are nondepressed/distressed couples (Cordova & Gee, 2001). In addition, because depression may restrict expression of affect, including expressions of intimacy and cohesion, partners in depressed/distressed couples exhibit less interest in enhancing intimacy than do nondepressed/

distressed couples. Consistent with the broad, vicious cycle of stress generation, lack of cohesion and intimacy appears both to result from and to exacerbate depression. Women reporting low marital intimacy are at higher risk for depression (Schweitzer, Logan, & Strassberg, 1992), and couples experiencing conflict over levels of expressed intimacy are more likely to experience depression. Marital therapy for depression usually interrupts this pattern early in therapy by increasing shared pleasant activities, and increasing communication around positive interactions.

Cognitive and Behavioral Asymmetry

Depressed spouses tend to blame themselves, and although nondepressed partners often disagree with depressed spouses' self-blaming statements, their response to their spouses may be interpreted as either criticism or reinforcement of negative self-perceptions. The depressed spouse may in turn generalize partner criticisms and take them as reinforcement of global, stable, and negative attributions (Sher, Baucom, & Larus, 1990). Depression can also result in less self-confidence during marital discussions, such that a depressed spouse may withdraw after a hostile exchange (Mitchell, Cronkite, & Moos, 1983) and avoid further contact with the partner. Marital therapy for depression counteracts the tendency toward withdrawal by helping spouses identify and verbalize positive aspects of the partner and ways that they show their caring for each other, thereby encouraging greater positive contact. At the same time, marital therapy for depression may interrupt patterns in which the nondepressed partner inadvertently confirms the negative self-image of the depressed partner (Katz & Beach, 1997).

Deficits in Problem Solving and Communication

Depressed/distressed couples' difficulty in resolving marital problems is greater than the difficulties associated with problem solving in marital distress uncomplicated by depression (for a more comprehensive review, see Beach, 1996). Depressed couples may also show deficits in their ability to define their problems prior to initiating a resolution strategy, particularly depressed wives who have difficulty identifying and describing relationship problems. Depressed couples' problem-solving discussions are likely to be characterized by high levels of conflict, overt hostility, avoid-

ance, and withdrawal. Depressed individuals may have difficulty being decisive and assertive, but both partners in a depressed couple are likely to use aggressive behaviors in the course of a marital discussion. This can lead to relationship discussions that end either without resolution or with an unresolved escalation. In addition, the depressed spouse is likely to evince high levels of anger and avoidance, and to offer fewer suggestions for problem solving, leading the nondepressed spouse to respond with negativity and rejection. As a consequence, marital therapists working with couples with a depressed partner often need to help couples enhance problem-solving skills while learning to express disagreement productively.

How Does Marital Discord Come to Be Linked to Depression?

As we suggested earlier, the marital discord model has evolved over the past few years to focus on the role of vicious cycles in maintaining the link between marital discord and depression. As a consequence, along with many of our systemically oriented colleagues, we have come to view the disruption of vicious cycles as the key to successful treatment. Many of the interventions utilized in our approach (Beach et al., 1990) focus on changing either the key interactional patterns described earlier, or enhancing social support and reducing marital stress. These latter two foci of intervention have been highlighted as exemplars of the positive (social support) and negative (marital stressors) poles of patterns targeted in treatment, because they are believed to be etiologically important in the link between marital discord and depression.

Loss of Social Support

Several theoretical perspectives have highlighted the potential for loss of critical elements of interpersonal support, resulting in greater risk for the development of depressive symptomatology (Beach, 1996). Some of the supportive processes that are lost when couples experience depression in the context of marital discord include (1) couple cohesion and shared pleasant activities; (2) acceptance of emotional expression and disclosure of personal feelings; (3) actual and perceived coping assistance in dealing with environmental and relationship stressors; (4) self-esteem support and positive, noncritical feedback; (5) perceived spousal dependability, availability, and commitment; and (6) intimacy and confiding in the spouse. Assessment of these areas may identify useful targets of intervention for martially discordant and depressed couples. In addition, depressed individuals who act in ways that elicit rejection and negative support behaviors from others, including spouses, may further contribute to the cycle of depression and maritally discordant behavior.

Extreme Stress

As noted earlier, stress is a well-known etiological factor in the genesis of depression. Stress-generating patterns include (1) verbal and physical aggression; (2) threats of separation and divorce; (3) severe spousal denigration, criticism, and blame; and (4) severe disruption of marital routines, including failure to share household chores and avoidance of physical contact. Depressed individuals may generate further stress for themselves by selectively seeking out and attending to self-verifying negative feedback (Swann, Wenzlaff, Krull, & Pelham, 1992), so that even the support offered by the spouse is viewed through the lens of depression.

THE PRACTICE OF COUPLE THERAPY

Getting the Process of Therapy Underway

Marital therapy for depression may not be appropriate for every couple in which one partner is depressed. As a consequence, therapists must decide whether marital therapy makes sense for a couple, given the particular circumstances, the particular symptom picture for the depressed person, and the state of the marriage at this particular point in time. Marital therapy for depression is often appropriate, either as a stand-alone intervention or in conjunction with other interventions, when (1) the risk of suicide or suicidal behavior is relatively low; (2) the depressed patient is not experiencing bipolar disorder or any delusional disorder; (3) marital discord is present and appears to have played an etiological role or a potentially maintaining role in the current episode of depression; (4) neither spouse has indicated an immediate desire to divorce, has refused to work on improving the relationship, or has indicated the intention to start or maintain an extramarital sexual relationship; and (5) there is no evidence of spousal battering.

To conduct the initial assessment, it is customary for the therapist to meet with each spouse individually and to have both partners complete self-report inventories. This provides multiple perspectives on the couple's current difficulties and allows the therapist to enter the therapeutic process with some indication of treatment alternatives that likely make sense for the couple.

There is no prohibition against including other family members in the initial assessment, and there is increasing evidence that a focus on parenting may be useful in many cases, suggesting the value of broad coverage of family issues in the initial assessment. However, the treatment itself, as long as the focus is on the marital relationship, is primarily dyadic. Individual partner sessions are used only to explore and potentially resolve problems related to therapy process, such as no progress in therapy, concerns of the therapist about hidden agendas, or repeated failure by one partner to participate effectively in therapy sessions.

When the depressive episode appears to have preceded and caused the current episode of marital discord, it is considered appropriate either to refer the couple for individual therapy or antidepressant medication, or to provide both forms of intervention concurrently. Routine, interim assessment should be conducted by the sixth session to examine whether progress is being made on any of the couple's presenting problems related to marital discord and to the depression. Consideration of other treatment options should also be initiated if the couple has shown no positive response in the first 4–6 weeks of treatment.

There is little evidence that cotherapists produce better results than those achieved by a single therapist. We commonly use cotherapy, but the rationale relates training rather than treatment. We also typically recommend that therapy last a specific amount of time (12–16 weeks), with weekly sessions on average, and that our progress be assessed periodically to determine whether we are on track or need to shift course.

When there is concurrent individual therapy, it is essential that the therapists maintain contact with each other. The potential for individual therapy to interfere with marital therapy—even if the former is focused on medication maintenance—is substantial. For example, individual therapists quite commonly agree with spousal blame and encourage an assertive/aggressive reaction to the partner, potentially throwing off the timing of interventions with the dyad. Ideally, a concurrent therapy is conducted by a therapist well known to the marital therapist and with whom collaborative treatment and consultation are possible.

Of course, the potential for additive effects of individual and marital approaches seems high given their differing foci of attention. However, the only empirical examination of this combination of approaches (Jacobson et al., 1991) was disappointing. The finding that marital therapy and cognitive therapy for depression both appear to work, but that they reduce depression through somewhat different mechanisms, again suggests the possibility that combined marital and cognitive therapy should be possible. There are, however, a number of reasons to expect complex issues to arise in formulating a strategy that combines individual and marital therapy sessions, and it would certainly be premature to rule out the eventual success of this approach on the basis of only one attempt. An example of the complexity of the issues involved in combining marital and individual approaches may be found in the Jacobson et al. study, in which "a typical pattern was to begin with individual treatment and then to involve both spouses in the treatment plan" (p. 550). It may be that the weakness of this approach was due to husbands feeling less involved and less motivated to participate actively in marital therapy, or being defensive in the face of their expectation that the therapist had already aligned with the wife. As these observations suggest, at present there is not a good model for concurrent treatment, but the approach cannot be ruled out given several indications that suggest its promise.

Between-session phone calls are encouraged early in therapy to support the initial process of change. Therapists are encouraged to set a time for couples to check in with regard to progress on homework assignment. However, such contacts are typically designed to be brief (no more than 15 minutes). If a longer time is required due to new events or couple crisis, a session is scheduled.

The Role of the Therapist

Stuart (1980) suggested five primary dimensions for the role of the therapist in marital therapy, and his analysis has guided our development of marital therapy for depression. These five dimensions are administration, mediation, reeducation, modeling, and celebrating. We also suggest that there is another important dimension to marital therapy, namely, maintaining a dual alliance. These dimensions suggest that, as with other forms of therapy, key therapist attributes are likely to include warmth, humor, and an ability to structure sessions.

Administration

The marital therapist, as therapy administrator, is responsible for collaborating with the couple to plan treatment, to structure therapy sessions, and to set therapeutic goals. The therapist should create a tentative agenda for each treatment session, begin each session by reviewing the proposed agenda with the couple, and request feedback from the clients about the agenda. The therapist should also be sure to use therapeutic time wisely by pacing therapy content within each treatment session, as well as across the entire course of therapy.

The marital therapist must strike a balance between structuring treatment and providing adequate flexibility. Structure can be particularly important for depressed clients, because it can help to alleviate feelings of hopelessness and to instill confidence in the therapist's abilities. However, it is also essential to be flexible enough to accommodate individual desires and goals to treat each couple most effectively. Furthermore, depressed clients may be reluctant to mention problems that need to be addressed in therapy if the therapist does not provide them an opportunity to add items to the therapy agenda.

As administrator, the therapist must also skillfully adapt the therapeutic model to make it relevant for each couple. For example, the therapist is responsible for choosing homework assignments that both fulfill the goals of the model and are meaningful for each individual couple. Thus, specific details of homework assignments cannot be decided in advance and must emerge from the specific problems and strengths of the couple.

Mediation

In the role of mediator, the therapist is responsible for creating a therapeutic alliance with the clients as a couple. The therapist must be neutral in relation to both partners, and must never align him- or herself with either individual. Alliances between the therapist and one partner can be particularly harmful to therapy, even in cases in which one spouse appears to be "the bad one." Instead, the therapist should adopt the role of mediator, assisting the couple in communication and problem solving. The therapist ensures that spouses express themselves clearly to one another and come to mutually agreeable solutions. The therapist must be alert to any perception of favoritism toward one partner. To that end, the therapist should attempt to make all therapeutic activities and feedback symmetrical with regard to both individuals. For example, if one partner is given critical feedback or is asked to change his or her behavior, the other partner should also receive feedback or an equivalent task.

Reeducation

As a reeducator of depressed clients, the therapist is responsible for both normalizing and validating clients' beliefs about marriage and depression. The therapist should communicate the reasonableness of individuals' beliefs and simultaneously provide psychoeducation on the symptomatology associated with depression. For example, the therapist should tell clients that many factors contribute to depression; that "anhedonia," or loss of pleasure in activities one used to enjoy, is common in depressed individuals; and that initiating behavioral change can be difficult. The therapist may also indicate that decreased sexual libido is often associated with depression and may also be a side effect of some antidepressant medications, and that resumption of sexual desire may take some time. In providing reeducation, the therapist attempts to substitute more adaptive and/or accurate information for clients' beliefs that are problematic or inaccurate.

Modeling

A primary role of the marital therapist is that of a model. The therapist models as teaching devices both specific skills, such as problem solving and effective communication, and generally calm, problem-focused behavior. Because the therapist is "on display" to the clients during therapy sessions, he or she must be sure to remain calm and composed, even in the face of difficult or upsetting client behavior. By doing this, the therapist models how to discuss complicated issues and to problem-solve calmly and effectively.

Celebrating

Another important role of the therapist in marital therapy for depression is celebrating the partners' progress with them. By celebrating progress, the therapist acts to reinforce positive changes in the couple. Distressed spouses are not often adept at acknowledging and celebrating positive behaviors or changes in themselves or their partners. Thus, the therapist is responsible for taking on this role and gradually leading individuals to initiate the celebration of changes in themselves and their spouses. Depressed clients, in particular, often need extra assistance in feeling good about positive changes they have made. The therapist notices, discusses, and compliments clients who display new positive behaviors, reinitiate previously rewarding positive patterns, or approximate desired outcomes. In this way, the therapist models the role of celebrant, so that clients can begin to celebrate changes in each other. To this end, the therapist should also structure homework assignments to maximize the likelihood of success and the opportunity to celebrate with the couple. In particular, assignments should be worded in such a way that clients' attempts to do them result in success. The therapist should gradate assignments, so that each is a successive approximation of larger changes that are desired.

Maintaining the Dual Alliance

In marital therapy for depression it is important that each spouse feels that he or she has a therapeutic alliance with the marital therapist. A situation in which only one spouse feels such an alliance, while the other feels left out, can lead to serious problems in the ongoing process of therapy. Therapy likely breaks down and yields relatively few positive results when there is not a dual alliance. In the context of depression, however, it may be extremely tempting for the therapist, even one who is experienced with marital therapy in other contexts, to establish a differential alliance with the two participants. On the one hand, it may be tempting for the therapist to side with the nondepressed spouse, seeing this partner as the long-suffering and aggrieved partner in the relationship. On the other hand, it may be tempting to side with the depressed partner, seeing him or her as a victim of spousal insensitivity. When these temptations arise, the therapist should remember that the depressed, discordant couple is not very different from other discordant couples when it comes to the importance of the dual alliance. There is always more than enough blame to share in dysfunctional relationships, differing possible perspectives on the "correct" way to partition blame, and little to be gained by encouraging partner blame. Maintaining the dual alliance is as important, if not more so, in the context of depression as in other marital therapy cases.

Assessment and Treatment Planning

Before beginning a course of treatment with any couple or individual, it is important to define the parameters of the presenting problem and establish goals for treatment. When treating comorbid problems, such as depression and marital discord, thorough assessment with a multimethod approach is particularly critical. With such couples, a four-stage assessment process can be undertaken that involves ruling out other severe psychopathologies, assessing suicide risk, establishing the presence of marital discord, and linking depression and marital discord chronologically and etiologically.

Rule Out Other Severe Psychopathologies

A careful initial assessment of each partner's history of psychopathology is necessary before applying a model of marital discord to depressed and discordant couples. Although psychotic features sometimes co-occur with mood symptoms, actively psychotic clients are generally not capable of the dyadic focus required in marital therapy (Clarkin, Haas, & Glick, 1988). Similarly, clients with bipolar disorder may need to seek psychopharmacological intervention to manage their mood dysregulation before they can fully benefit from the marital model. Depression arising from an organic cause or a stable, trait-like personality disorder may also present difficulties for a marital therapist (cf. Beach et al., 1990). Whereas complications associated with mildly dysfunctional personality features may resolve themselves over the course of treatment, severe organic or trait-like pathology can block effective implementation of the marital model and limit the gains made by the depressed individual in remission of depression symptoms. A full medical history or use of a standardized scale, such as the Millon Clinical Multiaxial Inventory–II (MCMI-II; Millon & Green, 1989) or the DSM diagnostic system (e.g., Structured Clinical Interview for DSM-III-R [SCID-II]; First, Spitzer, Gibbon, & Williams, 1995), may at times be appropriate.

Assess Suicide Risk

Given the lack of support and extreme stress inherent in relationship discord, depression in the context of such discord is particularly likely to result in suicidal ideation and behavior. Assessment of suicide risk must be ongoing throughout the course of marital therapy. Self-report measures, such as the Beck Scale for Suicidal Ideation (Beck, Kovacs, & Weissman, 1979), can be used regularly to assess the various facets of suicidal behavior. In the presence of severe suicidal ideation or intent, it can be particularly difficult to maintain therapeutic focus on marital issues (O'Leary, Sandeen, & Beach, 1987). In cases in which suicidal behaviors are prominent, then, it may be clinically advisable to begin individual work with the depressed, suicidal spouse and to incorporate marital work only when suicide risk has been reduced.

Establish the Presence of Marital Discord

Thorough assessment of a couple's marital environment is also critical in the initial stages of treatment. Establishing the chronology of a couple's commitment and initial attraction can be useful in cementing motivation for therapy, though clinicians must be prepared in the event that a depressed spouse reports largely negative perspectives on him- or herself, the partner, and the relationship as a whole. The presence of current marital distress should be established through a clinical interview and, if warranted, general and focused self-report inventories. It is important to meet with each spouse individually to assess for hidden agendas, such as plans for separation or divorce that may derail the treatment (Beach & Broderick, 1983), any ongoing extramarital affairs (Beach, Jouriles, & O'Leary, 1985), the presence of domestic violence or emotional and psychological abuse (O'Leary & Cano, 2001), as well as to establish commitment to the therapy process. Ongoing extramarital affairs can severely curtail the gains made in short-term marital therapy. Similarly, treatment in a dyadic format (Vivian & Malone, 1997) is not appropriate for couples engaging in domestic violence.

Self-report measures can also be an efficient means of gathering data. The DAS (Spanier, 1976) can be a useful tool for measuring overall level of discord when beginning a course of therapy. More focused questionnaires, such as the Areas of Change Questionnaire (ACQ; Margolin, Talovic, & Weinstein, 1983), the Marital Status Inventory (MSI; Weiss & Cerreto, 1980), the Broderick Commitment Scale (Beach & Broderick, 1983), and the Spouse Observation Checklist (Broderick & O'Leary, 1986), may provide a more precise depiction of specific areas of a couple's functioning.

Link Depression and Discord Chronologically and Etiologically

Depression and marital discord, when comorbid, can interact in ways that make it difficult to establish a complete picture of the sequence of the pathologies. Use of a semistructured interview, such as the SCID-II (First et al., 1995) can help establish this temporal relationship. The Beck Depression Inventory–II (BDI-II, Beck, Steer, & Garbin, 1988) may be used to assess level of current depressive symptoms, along with current marital conflict. The clinical interview can address the issue of temporality by examining the ways depressive symptoms and marital conflict have interacted for a specific couple, and establishing precedence in interpersonal stressors and loss of supportive relationship behaviors. Evidence of sequential etiology may influence a clinician's treatment plan in deciding between individual therapy for depression and marital therapy. For example, depressed wives with healthier marital environments are likely to report reduced symptomatology following individual cognitive therapy (Beach & O'Leary, 1992). However, for clients who see relationship problems as strongly impacting their depression, or clients who view relationship problems as preceding their depression, individual cognitive therapy may not be as effective as marital therapy in addressing depressive symptoms (O'Leary, Riso, & Beach, 1990; Addis & Jacobson, 1996).

Goal Setting

The overarching goals of marital therapy for depression are to enhance marital quality and reduce depressive symptoms. To accomplish these goals in a time-limited manner, couple concerns are carefully assessed and prioritized. A collaborative approach is used to set the goals for each session, with a strong emphasis on those interventions most likely to result in couples reaching the primary objectives of enhanced marital quality and reduced depressive symptoms. Because of similarity across couples presenting with marital discord and depression, it is possible to predict the most likely areas of difficulty, which makes this form of marital therapy relatively easy to manualize.

As we discuss in the next section, the early sessions of therapy emphasize creating a foundation of trust and positive change; accordingly, goals in the first several sessions focus on ways to increase displays of caring, companionship, and self-esteem support, while simultaneously attending to any stressful negative interactional patterns that may preclude symptomatic recovery.

The goals of the middle section of therapy emphasize restructuring the relationship to include more responsive, empathic listening; enhanced problem resolution; and an enhanced ability to function as a team.

The goals of the final sessions of therapy emphasize maintenance of gains and disengagement of the therapist in the context of couples assuming greater responsibility for their own continued progress.

Process and Technical Aspects of Couple Therapy

In the following material we focus primarily on the initial phase of marital therapy for depression. Our clinical experience suggests that the initial phase of therapy is critical, because the couple with a depressed partner is prone to become demoralized and to give up if the partners do not see concrete evidence of progress in the first several sessions. Likewise, such a couple may respond more positively than other distressed couples to high levels of session structure and clear homework assignments that instigate change. Once positive momentum has been established, it is possible to shift the focus to other aspects of the relationship. Most typically in our work this involves attention to various aspects of listening, support provision, and joint problem solving. However, if a focus on problems in the relationship comes too early in therapy, there is greater potential for the couple to feel overwhelmed and hopeless. Possibly, this observation may hold more generally for the distressed couple in which one partner has a diagnosable disorder, particularly if it is chronic or recurrent. For this reason we view therapy as having three distinct phases. The initial phase of therapy, which focuses on instigating positive behavior change, is the one we view as critical. The middle phase of therapy, which focuses on addressing longstanding concerns and issues in the dyad, may utilize any efficacious approach to marital therapy, even though in our case it typically involves behavioral marital interventions. Finally, the end phase of marital therapy may be viewed as relapse prevention and anticipation of future challenges. Both marital discord and depression are known to have relatively high rates of relapse. So preparation to respond effectively to any future recurrence is essential for long-term well-being.

When initiating work with discordant or depressed couples, it is important that the therapist structure sessions in such a way that allows both members of the couple to feel safe as they discuss their distress while working toward specific goals. Both spouses should know that the therapy session is not a time in which they can attack or be attacked. Creating this safe environment may include ground rules or guidelines that help couples to communicate in adaptive ways in session, and planning for the prevention of destructive interactions outside of session. The level of structure that is provided is influenced by level of discord within the couple, the couple's desired level of direction, and the level of structure that will facilitate progress toward the couple's goals.

The structure of the therapy session should also be a model for the therapy process overall. Each session includes a plan for action to be carried out before the next session, which includes problem-solving techniques, such as identifying problems, discussing alternatives, choosing an alternative to implement, and evaluating its degree of success. Although problem-solving skills are not an explicit focus until later in therapy, the initial phase of therapy presents an opportunity to model action-oriented intervention.

Couples learn about the importance of homework during the beginning stages of therapy. Selecting appropriate assignments, explaining them to clients, and evaluating the degree of success with the previous week's assignment is an integral component to the structure of each session. When introducing the concept of homework assignments, the therapist emphasizes the individual responsibility of each spouse in completing his or her part of the assignment. The therapist emphasizes completion of homework assignments, because much of the work of therapy takes place between sessions.

Depending on each spouse's commitment level to the relationship and to the therapy process, getting the couple to work toward common goals can be a difficult task. The therapist usually addresses this by increasing the couple's expectations for positive change in the relationship. Helping clients to define their problems and goals in a specific manner is one method to induce an expectation for change. Therapists also give couples information on the research background of the cognitive-behavioral marital therapy approach, emphasizing that many couples' marital satisfaction is increased within a relatively brief time frame. Another way that the therapist can influence the perception of

positive change is by helping couples to monitor how far they have progressed since the beginning of therapy, and pointing out the positive changes that have taken place.

The initial three to five sessions of therapy focus on increasing marital cohesion, increasing self-esteem and marital support, and reducing severe, recurrent marital stressors. Unlike the later phases of therapy that require a greater level of tailoring to the needs of a particular couple, approaches in the initial phase of therapy are useful with almost all discordant and depressed couples, and resonate well with the goals they bring to therapy. These approaches have been found to be helpful in elevating the mood of the depressed patient, instilling a sense that change is possible for both partners, and preparing for the more difficult tasks involved in restructuring the relationship.

Increasing Marital Cohesion

CARING GESTURES

One way to initiate increased marital cohesion is by encouraging couples to engage in gestures that are performed with the goal of communicating through behavior one's love and caring. The activities are typically structured so that no new learning is required. Instead, couples are encouraged to increase a range of small caring gestures that are already available to them but that have been underused for various reasons. The therapist's rationale for increased caring gestures typically emphasizes the benefits of both engaging in pleasant interactions and caring gestures as a foundation for future gains in communication with each other. When couples show caring for each other, a positive context facilitates problem solving and learning new skills. In addition, partners practice showing their feelings for each other, creating a foundation for cumulative change over time.

An important foundational component of increasing caring behavior is to have both partners correctly identify concrete gestures that they perceive as pleasing. Having each mate identify his or her preferences gives the couple the opportunity to participate in behaviors have the intended positive impact upon the relationship. If each partner's preferences are not well-established and understood, then there is the possibility that caring gestures can be perceived as less than positive. To avoid this, partners individually generate a small list of gestures that they would like to have the partner to perform, as well as things they themselves can do to show caring. The lists are then combined to create an easy method of tracking change. It is important for the couple to understand that the lists are a menu of options from which each partner can choose when attempting to do something pleasing, not a list of required activities.

It is also important that the gestures involve small, specific acts that require no new learning on the part of the partner. In keeping with the standard logic of all behavioral assignments, the focus of the assignment involves increasing positive gestures rather than decreasing negative behaviors. Items that are too vague or are framed in a negative manner, or that are not currently in the partner's repertoire or involve a tremendous amount of effort or resources are rejected from the caring gestures list, even though they might be kept as items for future discussion. Items likely to be rejected include asking for expensive gifts or asking a mate to change longstanding, ingrained behavior patterns. Conversely, gestures that can be performed frequently, require little monetary expenditure, and are under the giver's total control are encouraged.

Examples of appropriate list items might include giving backrubs, sending love notes, giving compliments, and doing a chore for the other person. These types of gestures not only are more feasible as an initial step to increasing marital cohesion but they are also more likely to create reinforcing experiences of success as each partner attempts to please the other. Because it can be difficult for couples to generate lists of pleasing behavior, the therapist should act as a guide in the list-making process by offering suggestions if the partners have trouble coming up with ideas.

Three aspects of the caring assignment have been found to be essential for depressed and discordant couples. The first is emphasizing that the caring gestures should be performed daily. The rationale behind this is that daily caring gestures create enough experiences to be observed and recalled despite the depressive episode. Depressed persons often tend to underestimate the frequency of positive events and have difficulty recalling positive things that have happened to them. By encouraging frequent events, this tendency is partially addressed. Second, each spouse is responsible for performing caring gestures independently of the partner's success in performing gestures for him or her. The independence of the caring gestures assignment is established to preclude disruption of the assignment due to either the perception or the reality of one partner getting off to a slow start.

This approach also has the advantage of making it clear that "caring" is not a quid pro quo activity. Third, the therapist emphasizes the importance of giving recognition to the partner that performs caring gestures. To monitor the impact of the intervention, it is important for the clients to keep a record of what gestures are being done, when, and by whom. It is also important for the partners to recognize caring gestures when they occur and to take time to feel good that their spouse has done something positive for them. To stimulate these activities, each spouse is asked to record the caring gestures he or she performs. Each spouse records the gestures he or she performs to facilitate a sense of responsibility for increasing interactions, but both record their gestures in the same place to help each spouse recognize that positive things are happening and to feel the positive change in the marriage.

COMPANIONSHIP ACTIVITIES

Increasing pleasant shared activities can also impact dyadic cohesion. Thus, therapeutic interventions should emphasize increasing companionship by encouraging conjoint activities such as dating, recreational activities, and activities with other couples. Because the purpose of the assignment is to give the couple a sense of hope and mastery, the therapist should support the couple in selecting activities that are likely to create a positive emotional climate and are not likely to fail. One way to do this is to collaborate with the couple in determining each partner's role in planning the activity, and to assign very detailed homework that addresses the specifics of how the activity will be carried out.

Although sexual interactions can be shared positive events, it is essential that the therapist carefully assess the status of sex in the couple's relationship before accepting sexual and sensual items as part of the caring gesture and companionship activity lists. Because many depressed couples experience sexual problems and loss of libido, it is possible that attempts at sexual interactions may not be a positive experience for one or both spouses. If sexual interactions are a significant problem for the couple, sex therapy and other techniques may be implemented at a later stage in therapy.

INCREASED INDIVIDUAL ACTIVITIES

When one spouse expects all of his or her satisfaction to derive from activities involving the partner, it can be particularly stressful to the relationship. This can serve as a barrier to couple cohesion, because the nondepressed spouse may withdraw due to the pressure of being solely responsible for the depressed partner's satisfaction. It also prevents the depressed partner from using individual resources in combating depression. Thus, the depressed spouse is encouraged to pursue individual interests more actively, while concurrently engaging in increased joint activities.

Although the goal is to increase positive events early in therapy, this strategy may not work for all couples. This may especially be the case if the couple is dealing with a large, overwhelming concern that makes it difficult to focus on increasing positive events. The therapist initially encourages the couple to work on increasing positive interactions before addressing larger issues that usually are addressed later in therapy. If this attempt fails, the therapist proceeds with helping the partners address their major concern with the goal of temporary resolution. The therapist does not attempt to teach any skills-building interventions, such as problem solving or communication skills, in a formalized manner. Instead, the therapist makes the couple aware that the issue will probably need to be revisited later in therapy, when skills are taught and applied to the problem situation. The more immediate goal is to address major, idiosyncratic stressors that hinder the progress of therapy.

Increasing Self-Esteem Support

A second aspect of the marriage that is targeted early in therapy is self-esteem support. Positive communication in which one spouse appreciates the positive qualities or behaviors of the other is one major component of self-esteem support. As with caring gestures, positive communication is encouraged as a unilateral behavior, independent of partners' perceived reciprocity or behavior change. This independence makes positive communication less susceptible to failure compared to more complex interactions, such as problem solving or empathic listening.

The concept of positive communication is usually presented as "expressing what you normally take for granted." Hence, the goal is for spouses to verbalize thanks for the many things their partners do for them; to acknowledge desired change in their partners; to give compliments; and to express positive beliefs and feelings about their partners. If couples are reluctant to participate in positive communication, the therapist can explain

that being able to express positives, compliments, and appreciation in a sincere and honest manner is important in keeping the relationship on the best course and providing a more accurate view of the partners and their relationship. The therapist can model positive communication through role plays and allow the partners to practice with each other in session. As they do with caring gestures, couples monitor their use of positive communication to give the therapist a good idea of how they implement these skills at home.

Reducing or Eliminating Major Stressors: An Initial Focus on Negative Patterns

Because marital distress is often an active source of stress, salient, ongoing negative behavior is a pinpointed target of immediate change. This is a necessary first step in the process of healing the relationship, because the damage inflicted by some negative patterns can serve as a barrier to positive change in the relationship. In general, negative behavior has a stronger association with satisfaction levels than does positive behavior (e.g., Broderick & O'Leary, 1986). Thus, a relatively low number of very negative interactions may eliminate the effects of a greater number of positive interactions. For some very severely discordant couples, it may be necessary to alter the course of therapy by using structured individual interventions to increase each spouse's self-control of disruptive behavior before a dyadic focus can be useful. We do not recommend this in the typical case, but if severe negative interactions persist after the first two to three sessions, it should be considered.

DENIGRATING, CRITICIZING, AND BLAMING SPOUSAL REFERENCES

Blaming and devaluing a partner through excessive criticism is seen as a major and chronic stressor in the marriage. To avoid the detrimental effects of name-calling and spousal putdowns, it is often helpful for the therapist to give the couple explicit feedback regarding the dangers of this type of negative communication. He or she may also help the critical partner reattribute negative behaviors and recognize that there are ways other than his or her own perspective to look at the situation. Helping the partner reattribute the cause of problems from internal, stable, blameworthy attributes of the spouse to situationally determined, changeable, nonblameworthy factors it may promote more positive affect and a willingness to let go of the blame and spousal denigration. Alternatively, the therapist can encourage the couple to explore the meanings attributed to certain behaviors. Once partners recognize that every negative interaction is not necessarily the result of negative intent, negative motivation, or selfishness, the feelings of anger and rejection that accompanied the original misunderstanding are likely to be diminished. Another method of reducing spousal blame and criticism that is especially appropriate for couples with a depressed member is to discuss the nature of the syndrome of depression. It is likely that some couples' primary martial complaints may be related to symptoms of depression, such as lethargy, lack of concentration, sleep disturbance, self-focus, irritability, and loss of sexual appetite. These symptoms easily become the focus of marital discord if the couple is not informed that behaviors plausibly attributed to the depression rather than to the depressed person will probably improve as the depression lifts. When a spouse better understands the partner's behavior, it often becomes possible for him or her to change the maladaptive pattern of criticism, blame, and denigration.

VERBAL AND PHYSICAL ABUSE

When verbal and physical abuse is a problem in the relationship, it is helpful for partners to learn specific techniques to limit their anger and to stop abusive escalation before it starts. Although the stimuli for abusive reactions are addressed later in therapy, it is essential to deal with abusive exchanges immediately due to the physical and motivational destructiveness of abusive events. If a couple reports frequent verbal abuse, then time-out procedures are introduced in the first session. This consists of having the each spouse monitor his or her own anger level and calmly asking for a physical separation when anger is escalating. Once calm, the partners can attempt to resume the discussion. It is important for them to know that the goal is to prevent an angry escalation. This means that they should err on the side of calling a time-out too early rather than too late. Partners should also be reminded to respect the other's request for a time-out, even if one spouse is not angry. Because the goal of taking a time-out is not to avoid discussion, partners must attempt to discuss the issue after they have calmed down or make an appointment with the therapist to do so in the future. The therapist should model how to call a time-out appropriately and have the couples practice by performing role plays in session.

THREATS TO LEAVE THE RELATIONSHIP

For depressed and discordant couples, occasional thoughts of divorce are natural. However, therapists remind couples of the evidence that they care about each other and are deeply invested in each other's lives, and ask them to consider that their threats of divorce reflect only temporary feelings. Therefore, couples are encouraged not to verbalize thoughts of leaving, because these thoughts occur in an inconsistent, vacillating pattern and do not represent a final decision.

After the first phase of therapy is complete, it is likely that the couple will show observable signs of change. There may be some initial lifting of the depressed partner's symptoms, and the therapist may notice some softening in each partner's attitudes and communication with the other. At the same time, it should be possible to discern that the partners have some hope that their marriage might be different in the future than in the past, and that it might be more satisfying for both of them.

If the initial stage of marital therapy for depression has gone well, then partners show enhanced cohesion and self-esteem support. Concern that one or both partners might precipitously terminate the relationship, engage in denigrating behavior or physical aggression, or disrupt each other's routines should have subsided as well. This is important, because whatever techniques are used, the second phase of therapy is likely to focus more explicitly and directly on couple problems and issues. Our clinical experience suggests that as partners are encouraged to refocus on more problematic aspects of their relationship, they will experience a temporary increase in felt marital dissatisfaction. We believe this should be predicted and interpreted for the couple as a normal aspect of the progression in marital therapy for depression. Approaching the shift to a problem focus in this manner helps couples to view any fluctuations in marital satisfaction in context and helps to preempt catastrophizing.

An alternative but conceptually consistent approach for restructuring the relationship is suggested by Bodenmann (2007). This approach focuses on training spouses to work together to process stressful events more effectively. Training partners to provide effective social support can potentially supplement the focus on conflict reduction and problem solving that characterizes the middle phase of marital therapy for depression. In addition, given the loss of positive interactions that is common in depression, it may be that marital approaches focusing on the enhancement of social support would be universally applicable to depressed patients, and not be restricted only to those in discordant relationships.

The final phase of therapy focuses primarily on longer-term maintenance of change. We also often recommend booster sessions at longer-term follow-up (e.g., 1 and 2 years after formal therapy has concluded) to assess changes that have occurred and to continue the process of relapse prevention. The key goals in the final phase of therapy include fading out the role of therapist and gradually narrowing the scope of therapy, so that new material is not presented for consideration. Conjoint couple problem solving is viewed as one primary method of relapse prevention, and couples are encouraged to tackle new issues on their own, using the problem-solving strategies they have refined in therapy.

Curative Factors/Mechanisms of Change

Process and Prediction of Response

Given that marital therapy offers some potential to help in the treatment of depression, questions regarding the mechanisms of change in marital therapy for depression immediately arise. In particular, one may question whether change in marital satisfaction is a sufficient explanation for the change in depression brought about by marital therapy. This issue is particularly interesting, because if marital therapy changes depression by changing marital functioning, then it apparently works through a somewhat different process than either individual cognitive therapy or pharmacotherapy, which both appear to have little or no effect, on average, on marital functioning.

Change in Marriage as a Mediator of Change in Depression

Does change in marital satisfaction mediate the effect of marital therapy on depression? The answer appears to be "yes." In both of the studies that have examined this issue, results are consistent with the hypothesis that the effect of marital therapy on depression is mediated by changes in marital adjustment. Beach and O'Leary (1992) found that posttherapy marital satisfaction met all the conditions of mediation (Baron & Kenny, 1986), and accounted fully for the effect of marital therapy on depression. Likewise, Jacobson et al. (1991) found that differences in marital adjustment and

depression severity scores covaried for depressed individuals who received marital therapy, but not for those who received cognitive therapy. So it appears that marital therapy may reduce the level of depressive symptomatology primarily by enhancing the marital environment, and not for some other reason. This implies that if one enhances marital therapy outcome, one might also enhance the effectiveness of marital therapy in the treatment of depression. In a somewhat more speculative vein, one might infer that as couples reconnect and experience their relationship as collaborative and supportive, there is a reversal of the processes that previously maintained depressive symptoms.

Prediction of Response to Treatment

Variables that predict a relatively better response to one sort of treatment than to another are of great interest clinically. To the extent that predictors of differentially good or poor response to a given intervention can be found, therapists can assign patients more readily to treatments that are likely to be most effective. We have attempted to predict differential response to treatment in various ways. Perhaps the most interesting attempt is the one that most closely reflects IPT clinical guidelines.

O'Leary, Riso, and Beach (1990) addressed the question of a clinically immediate and intuitively appealing predictor of outcome by examining the depressed patient's own account of the time precedence and causal relationship between his or her marital problems and depression. Specifically, they asked depressed wives to say which problem came first, the marital discord or the depression, and to indicate the primary cause of their depression. The two judgments were correlated ($r = .8$). When the ratings of temporal ordering were correlated with residualized gains in marital satisfaction, the correlation in the cognitive therapy condition was a highly significant ($-.65, p < .001$). However, for marital therapy subjects the correlations were nonsignificant. Depressed patients whose marital problems arose prior to the onset of their depression had poor marital outcomes when assigned to cognitive therapy but positive marital outcomes when assigned to marital therapy. Ratings of temporal ordering were not predictive of change in depressive symptomatology for either condition.

The O'Leary et al. (1990) analysis, then, suggests an intuitively obvious approach to matching depressed patients to treatment (i.e., on the basis of their perceptions of which came first). Given the strong correlation between reports of temporal ordering and perceptions of whether marital factors were the primary cause of the depression ($r = .8$), and in keeping with the tradition of IPT, these results also suggest that it is reasonable to assess patients' views of the factors contributing to their depression and assign them to a treatment approach that reflects their primary concerns. Conversely, for a depressed wife who believes that her marital problems preceded her depression, and is able and willing to work on marital concerns, a treatment plan that relies entirely on individual cognitive therapy may produce unnecessary deterioration in marital functioning.

Effects of Initial Severity of Depression on Response to Treatment

The results of the National Institute of Mental Health Treatment of Depression Collaborative Research Program (Elkin et al., 1989) raised the possibility that cognitive therapy might be less effective in the treatment of more severely depressed outpatients. We also had hypothesized that more severely depressed patients might respond more poorly to marital interventions (Beach et al., 1990). Using a score of 30 on the pretherapy BDI as the cut point between more and less severe depressions, we examined the recovery rate for both cognitive and marital therapy. However, we found that rate of recovery did not differ as a function of severity for either cognitive therapy or BMT in the Beach and O'Leary (1992) sample. Again, the marital therapy condition produced better results in terms of marital outcomes but had no advantage over cognitive therapy in terms of recovery from depression at either level of severity.

CASE ILLUSTRATION

The following case material is taken from session transcripts but does not identify a single couple. The excerpted material is only slightly edited for coherence and illustrates setting the stage for marital therapy for depression and laying the groundwork for a later focus on communication. In the case of the couple we call Jim and Teresa, the wife met criteria for major depression and the husband did not. Both reported significant marital distress and scored below 98 on the DAS. Teresa had a history of depression, but her most recent episode had begun shortly after the couple relocated and it

became clear that Jim was planning an academic career. Teresa believed her current depressive episode began after the relationship problems began. Their relationship, which was quite positive, had been deteriorating for the past year, and this was a concern to both of them. At the start of therapy, both were feeling frustrated and at an impasse. Despite Jim's reluctance to seek marital therapy, they had recently decided that something had to be done.

As the case of Jim and Teresa illustrates, even when a couple no longer displays feelings of overt caring and there is significant relationship conflict, often a deep reservoir of positive connection in the couple can be tapped by the alert therapist early in treatment. Doing so is critically important to the success of marital therapy for depression, because it is an antidote for the global pessimism about the relationship that may otherwise cause therapeutic efforts, particularly those focused on resolving problems and disagreements, to bog down.

Getting Marital Therapy for Depression Started

THERAPIST: I would like to start off by summarizing what I know about the two of you from your questionnaires and giving you a chance to correct or add to the things I have summarized from them. Then I would like to get a better sense of how the two of you met and how your relationship developed. Finally, I would like to talk about some possible initial constructive steps the two of you may be able to take in getting started. How does that sound?

JIM: That sounds fine. (*Teresa nods*)

THERAPIST: OK. The two major issues highlighted in the questionnaires were conflict around finances and conflict around career decisions. You, Jim, are pretty happy with what you are doing careerwise. You recognize that staying with you current career choice, an academic career, involves moving around the country and in the long run might involve making less money than some other options, but these are both consequences that seem OK to you. But you, Teresa, would much prefer settling down in one place, and the possibility of greater long-term income also is important. Moving around has negative implications for your personal career options and you feel isolated. The two of you also raise problems related to differences in personality, and different backgrounds. You,

Jim, describe yourself as more gregarious and outgoing, whereas you, Teresa, describe yourself as more at ease with a few stable friends and more comfortable with a stable, constant lifestyle. Teresa, you also said that you have been moody and brooding about your upset with the way things are going, and may have started to withdraw. On the other hand, Jim, you may have come to dominate the discussion of these issues. So, neither of you feels that your discussions have gone very well. So those are some of the issues that struck me. How am I doing so far?

TERESA: Very good.

JIM: Right.

THERAPIST: OK. Well, instead of me continuing further, what I would like to do now is invite the two of you to tell more about the problems that are bringing you in, maybe even things you haven't told each other before. And I will leave it up to you as to who starts—but I do want to make sure you both have a chance to add things.

TERESA: You can start.

JIM: Well, everything you said is true except for one thing about my current income. It is actually higher now than if I went into business for myself. Of course, in the long run I agree that I would make more money in business for myself. But it's not so much the money as the style of life that …

THERAPIST: The hours?

JIM: No, the hours are infinitely better the way I do it now, except this month is bad. Really there are many, many advantages to the job I have now, except that we have to live here.

THERAPIST: Where are you from originally?

JIM: I am from Pittsburgh, and we met in St. Louis. We talked about living in California or Texas, or maybe Washington, D.C.

THERAPIST: And is it fair to say that you (*looking at Teresa*) would like to go back to Texas?

TERESA: Very much.

JIM: Well, we could go live in Texas, but I would have to give up my career entirely, and I find that completely unpalatable.

THERAPIST: Teresa, could you tell me a little more about your views on this? You have heard what Jim has been saying and I assume this is not new ground for you, or is it?

TERESA: No, we have these conversations all the time. This particular issue didn't come to a head until this past year. I had always assumed that Jim would go into business for himself and that we would move, maybe back to Pittsburgh, and that's where we would establish roots and become part of a community, and our boys would go to school. This business of his wanting an academic career, to me, sort of came out of left field.

JIM: Though that's not exactly true, because you knew I was thinking about a fellowship. You just didn't believe I was really going to do it.

TERESA: Right.

JIM: (*to therapist*) We talked about this and I mentioned getting a fellowship where I could make more money and stay in Pittsburgh, and she said, "No. If you are going to do a fellowship you should do the best one you can. We will move anywhere and I'll take a job and we'll do anything we need to do to get you the fellowship."

TERESA: That's true. But I guess I didn't think the idea of going into academics would really win in the end. And then we had a very traumatic move here. Looking at a lifetime of moves was something else that was entirely unpalatable to me. So this is now looking at "the rest of our lives," and I am not happy with what I am seeing. Let's say that I do get back into the job market. It's not unlikely that we would then move to another part of the country, and that is all very unpleasant for me.

THERAPIST: So would it be fair to say that the issue of careers and moving is the main issue right now for the two of you?

TERESA: Yes, and what we are doing right now is just sweeping it under the carpet. We aren't doing anything about it. We are just living day to day.

JIM: That's right.

TERESA: (*to Jim*) We don't talk about it, because you don't like unpleasantness, so we try not to confront unpleasant issues.

JIM: (*to therapist*) We talked about it for 6 hours on the way to Pittsburgh, but it gets Teresa upset. So I don't like to pursue it too much. [*Note.* Jim goes on to describe a number of nuances about their situation and gives both his own view of the problem and Teresa's view of the problem. During this time Teresa is silent and a little withdrawn.]

THERAPIST: (*turning to Teresa*) Well, Teresa, let me ask you a couple of tough questions. Sorry they are tough, but first, how do you feel about Jim saying so much about all this and actually speaking for you at times? And second, do you think he is accurately understanding your view, or is he missing some things?

TERESA: Well, Jim speaks for me all the time. Jim is always speaking for me, so I am used to that.

THERAPIST: How do you feel about that?

At this point in the session, the therapist shifts the discussion to process and affect. By moving away from the impasse itself, and toward the issue of process and associated feelings, the therapist has both laid the groundwork for communication training later in therapy and demonstrated to the couple that there are new possibilities to be explored. At the same time, this can be seen as an early direct attempt to change habitual patterns, and so it requires some persistence by the therapist. When successful, as in this case, a shift to process and affect has the beneficial effect of opening the couple to a shift toward a positive focus as well; that is, it suggests the possibility that things can change, and that the therapist can help the partners effect this change.

Later in the session, the therapist moved to initiate a positive focus. In most cases, this is done by reviewing courtship history and using that focus to draw out things about the partners that were attractive and led to the relationship deepening. Because a number of positive elements, and positive beliefs about the partner, seemed buried just below the surface, and because it appeared these positive views were being missed by both partners, in this case the therapist moved in a more direct manner to elicit a positive focus.

THERAPIST: Let me stop you there and switch gears. What I would like you to do now is to describe the best aspects of each other. Just for a few minutes, and I would like to start with you, Jim. What are Teresa's best aspects? What are her best qualities, the one's that you have admired most or that you still admire the most? Just focus on those things with no "buts" like "yes, but." Just say what you admire most.

JIM: Well, I have always been physically attracted to Teresa. I know she doesn't believe it anymore, but it's true. And she's interesting and different. We also share some joint interests like cooking and traveling, which is fun.

THERAPIST: What makes her interesting and different?

JIM: She has something I never had before. … She has helped me be a better person, a better father, helped me be more mature about my studies. She also loves our boys, and I love them too. I really love her family. I enjoy visiting with them. And she does take good care of me, and I guess I like that. Maybe I was looking for someone to take care of me. And she is intelligent, and we can have intelligent discussions.

THERAPIST: (*to Teresa*) What are your views about Jim, about his best attributes, things that you like about him?

TERESA: One of the things that attracted me to Jim is that he is genuinely a good person. I see that every day. It is not just a facade. He is genuinely a good person, and he is charismatic and he attracts people. He is also very good verbally. I like to listen to him talk. As much as I complain about it, I do enjoy listening to him. I think he is very intelligent, and I enjoy listening to his discussions of various things. He also makes a good gin and tonic … and he takes care of me too. He's a romantic, and that was the other thing that I liked about him. He swept me off my feet when we met.

THERAPIST: What were the circumstances? How did you first meet?

At this point the therapist returned to the more usual pattern of exploring the courtship and relationship history with the couple. However, the tone of the session was noticeably changed. The therapist had found a broad vein of positive affect that could be used to shift the momentum in therapy toward building cohesion, approach, and support. At the end of the session, the therapist gave the couple an assignment for the intervening week before their next session.

THERAPIST: OK. Now I would like to tell you a little more about what you can expect from this experience, and what you can do this week. Perhaps each of you could write down things you could do that you think would have a positive impact on the other. These would be little things that would show the caring the two of you clearly have for each other. You might also try one or two of the things out; also see if you notice the things your partner does. If you bring lists next time, I will ask about them first thing at the beginning of the session. [For a more complete discussion of the "caring items" intervention see Beach et al., 1990].

Jim and Teresa went on to rebuild a positive focus in the relationship. In the fourth session they began to focus on their communication and developed ways to help Teresa feel that her concerns were being heard and dealt with. As they worked through a process of problem solving, the partners reported growing closer and continuing to engage in caring activities. By the end of therapy, Teresa was no long depressed; her BDI score had fallen from 35 to 2. Both reported that their relationship was strong, and they were optimistic about the future. At 1-year follow-up, Teresa continued to be nondepressed, and both partners continued to report high levels of relationship satisfaction.

SUGGESTIONS FOR FURTHER READING

Beach, S. R. H., Sandeen, E. E., & O'Leary, K. D. (1990). *Depression in marriage: A model for etiology and treatment*. New York: Guilford Press.
Whisman, M. A. (2005). *Couple therapy for depression* [VC APA Series WM 171 C832.83, 105 minutes]. Retrieved May 14, 2007, from *www.mimh.edu/library/videobytitle.htm*.—Dr. Mark A. Whisman discusses couple therapy for depression. Includes an actual therapy session with real clients and Dr. Whisman.

REFERENCES

Addis, M., & Jacobson, N. (1996). Reasons for depression and the process and outcome of cognitive-behavioral psychotherapies. *Journal of Consulting and Clinical Psychology, 64*(6), 1417–1424.
Baron, R. M., & Kenny, D. A. (1986). The moderator–mediator variable distinction in social and psychological research: Conceptual, strategic, and statistical considerations. *Journal of Personality and Social Psychology, 51*, 1173–1182.
Beach, S. R. H. (1996). Marital therapy in the treatment of depression. In C. Mundt, M. J. Goldstein, K. Hahlweg, & P. Fiedler, (Eds.), *Interpersonal factors in the origin and course of affective disorders* (pp. 341–361). London: Gaskell Academic, Royal College of Psychiatrists.
Beach, S. R. H., & Broderick, J. (1983). Commitment: A variable in women's response to marital therapy. *American Journal of Family Therapy, 11*(4), 16–24.
Beach, S. R. H., Jouriles, E. N., & O'Leary, K. D. (1985). Extramarital sex: Impact on depression and commitment in couples seeking marital therapy. *Journal of Sex and Marital Therapy, 11*, 99–108.
Beach, S. R. H., Kim, S., Cercone-Keeney, J., Gupta, M., Arias, I., & Brody, G. (2004). Physical aggression and depressive symptoms: Gender Asymmetry in Effects? *Journal of Social and Personal Relationships, 21*, 341–360.
Beach, S. R. H., & O'Leary, K. D. (1992). Treating depression in the context of marital discord: Outcome and predictors of response for marital therapy vs. cognitive therapy. *Behavior Therapy, 17*, 43–49.
Beach, S. R. H., Sandeen, E. E., & O'Leary, K. D. (1990). *Depression in marriage: A model for etiology and treatment*. New York: Guilford Press.
Beach, S. R. H., Wamboldt, M., Kaslow, N. J., Heyman, R. E., & Reiss, D. (2006). Describing relationship problems in DSM-V: Toward better guidance for research and clinical practice. *Journal of Family Psychology, 20*, 357–368.
Beck, A., Kovacs, M., & Weissman, A. (1979). Assessment of suicidal intention: The Scale for Suicide Ideation. *Journal of Consulting and Clinical Psychology, 47*(2), 343–352.
Beck, A., Steer, R., & Garbin, M. (1988). Psychometric properties of the Beck Depression Inventory: Twenty-five years of evaluation. *Clinical Psychology Review, 8*(1), 77–100.
Biglan, A., Hops, H., Sherman, L., Friedman, L. S., Arthur, J., & Osteen, V. (1985). Problem solving interactions of depressed women and their spouses. *Behavior Therapy, 16*, 431–451.
Bodenmann, G. (2007). Dyadic coping and the 3-phase-method in working with couples. In L. VandeCreek (Ed.), *Innovations in clinical practice: Focus on group and family therapy* (pp. 235–252). Sarasota, FL: Professional Resources Press.
Broderick, J., & O'Leary, K. (1986). Contributions of affect, attitudes, and behavior to marital satisfaction. *Journal of Consulting and Clinical Psychology, 54*(4), 514–517.
Brown, G. W., & Harris, T. (1978). *Social origins of depression: A study of psychiatric disorders in women*. New York: Free Press.
Cano, A., & O'Leary, K.D. (2000). Infidelity and separations precipitate major depressive episodes and symptoms of non-specific depression and anxiety. *Journal of Consulting and Clinical Psychology, 68*, 774–781.
Clarkin, J. F., Haas, G. L., & Glick, I. D. (1988). Inpatient family intervention. In J. F. Clarkin, G. L. Haas, & I. D. Glick (Eds.), *Affective disorders and the family* (pp. 134–152). New York: Guilford Press.
Cordova, J., & Gee, C. (2001). Couples therapy for depression: Using healthy relationships to treat depression. In S. R. H. Beach (Ed.), *Marital and family processes in depression: A scientific foundation for clinical practice* (pp. 185–203). Washington, DC: American Psychological Association.
Coyne, J. C. (1976). Depression and the response of others. *Journal of Abnormal Psychology, 85*, 186–193.
Davila, J., Bradbury, T. N., Cohan, C. L., & Tochluk, S. (1997). Marital functioning and depressive symptoms: Evidence for a stress generation model. *Journal of Personality and Social Psychology, 73*, 849–861.

Dessaulles, A., Jonson, S. M., & Denton, W. H. (2003). Emotion focused therapy for couples in treatment of depression: A pilot study. *American Journal of Family Therapy, 31*, 345–353.

Dimidjian, S., Martell, C. R., & Christensen, A. (2002). Integrative behavioral couple therapy. In A. S. Gurman & N. S. Jacobson (Eds.), *Clinical handbook of couple therapy* (3rd ed., pp. 251–277). New York: Guilford Press.

Elkin, I., Shea, M. T., Watkins, J. T., Imber, S. D., Sotsky, S. M., Collins, J. F., et al. (1989). NIMH Treatment of Depression Collaborative Research Program: General effectiveness of treatments. *Archives of General Psychiatry, 46*, 971–982.

Emanuels-Zuurveen, L., & Emmelkamp, P. M. (1996). Individual behavioral-cognitive therapy vs. marital therapy for depression in maritally distressed couples. *British Journal of Psychiatry, 169*, 181–188.

Emanuels-Zuurveen, L., & Emmelkamp, P. M. (1997). Spouse-aided therapy with depressed patients. *Behavior Modification, 21*, 62–77.

Fincham, F. D., Stanley, S. M., & Beach, S. R. H. (2007). The emergence of transformative processes in marriage: An analysis of emerging trends. *Journal of Marriage and the Family, 69*, 275–292.

First, M., Spitzer, R., Gibbon, M., & Williams, J. (1995). The Structured Clinical Interview for DSM-III-R Personality Disorders (SCID-II): I. Description. *Journal of Personality Disorders, 9*(2), 83–91.

Foley, S. H., Rounsaville, B. J., Weissman, M. M., Sholomaskas, D., & Chevron, E. (1989). Individual versus conjoint interpersonal therapy for depressed patients with marital disputes. *International Journal of Family Psychiatry, 10*, 29–42.

Friedman, A. (1975). Interaction of drug therapy with marital therapy in depressive patients. *Archives of General Psychiatry, 32*, 619–637.

Greden, J., & Carroll, B. (1980). Decrease in speech pause times with treatment of endogenous depression. *Biological Psychiatry, 15*(4), 575–587.

Hahlweg, K., Baucom, D. H., & Markman, H. J. (1988). Recent advances in therapy and prevention. In I. R. H. Falloon (Ed.), *Handbook of behavioral family therapy* (pp. 413–448). New York: Guilford Press.

Hahlweg, K., & Markman, H. J. (1988). Effectiveness of behavioral marital therapy: Empirical status of behavioral techniques in preventing and alleviating marital distress. *Journal of Consulting and Clinical Psychology, 56*, 440–447.

Hammen, C. (1991). *Depression runs in families: The social context of risk and resilience in children of depressed mothers.* New York: Springer-Verlag.

Hammen, C. (2005). Stress and depression. *Annual Review of Clinical Psychology, 1*, 293–319.

Hautzinger, M., Linden, M., & Hoffman, N. (1982). Distressed couples with and without a depressed partner: An analysis of their verbal interaction. *Journal of Behavior Therapy and Experimental Psychology, 13*, 307–314.

Jacobson, N. S., Dobson, K., Fruzzeti, A. E., Schmal-ing, D. B., & Salusky, S. (1991). Marital therapy as a treatment for depression. *Journal of Consulting and Clinical Psychology, 59*, 547–557.

Jacobson, N. S., Follette, W. C., & Pagel, M. (1986). Predicting who will benefit from behavioral marital therapy. *Journal of Consulting and Clinical Psychology, 54*, 518–522.

Johnson, S. M., & Greenman, P. S. (2006). The path to a secure bond: Emotionally focused couple therapy. *Journal of Clinical Psychology, 62*, 597–609.

Joiner, T. E. (2000). Depression's vicious scree: Self-propagating and erosive processes in depression chronicity. *Clinical Psychology: Science and Practice, 7*, 203–218.

Joiner, T. E., Brown, J. S., & Kistner, J. (2006). *The interpersonal, cognitive, and social nature of depression.* Mahwah, NJ: Erlbaum.

Katz, J., & Beach, S. R. H. (1997). Self-verification and depression in romantic relationships. *Journal of Marriage and the Family, 59*, 903–914.

Klerman, G. L., & Weissman, M. M. (1991). Interpersonal psychotherapy: Research program and future prospects. In L. E. Beutler & M. Crago (Eds.), *Psychotherapy research: An international review of programmatic studies* (pp. 33–40). Washington, DC: American Psychological Association.

Klerman, G. L., Weissman, M. M., Rounsaville, B. J., & Chevron, E. S. (1984). *Interpersonal psychotherapy of depression.* New York: Basic Books.

Leff, J., Vearnals, S., Brewin, C. R., Wolff, G., Alexander, B., Asen, E., et al. (2000). The London Depression Intervention Trial. *British Journal of Psychiatry, 177*, 95–100.

Lewinsohn, P. M., & Shaffer, M. (1971). Use of home observations as an integral part of the treatment of depression: Preliminary report and case studies. *Journal of Consulting and Clinical Psychology, 37*, 87–94.

Margolin, G., Talovic, S., & Weinstein, C. D. (1983). Areas of Change Questionnaire: A practical approach to marital assessment. *Journal of Consulting and Clinical Psychology, 51*, 944–955.

Millon, T., & Green, C. (1989). Interpretive guide to the Millon Clinical Multiaxial Inventory (MCMI-II). In C. S. Newmark (Ed.), *Major psychological assessment instruments* (Vol. 2, pp. 5–43). Needham Heights, MA: Allyn & Bacon.

Mitchell, R., Cronkite, R., & Moos, R. (1983). Stress, coping, and depression among married couples. *Journal of Abnormal Psychology, 92*(4), 433–448.

Nelson, G. M., & Beach, S. R. H. (1990). Sequential interaction in depression: Effects of depressive behavior on spousal aggression. *Behavior Therapy, 12*, 167–182.

O'Leary, K., & Cano, A. (2001). Marital discord and partner abuse: Correlates and causes of depression. In S. R. H. Beach (Ed.), *Marital and family processes in depression: A scientific foundation for clinical practice* (pp. 163–182). Washington, DC: American Psychological Association.

O'Leary, K. D., Riso, L. P., & Beach, S. R. H. (1990).

Attributions about the marital discord/depression link and therapy outcome. *Behavior Therapy, 21,* 413–422.

O'Leary, K. D., Sandeen, E., & Beach, S. R. H. (1987, November). *Treatment of suicidal, maritally discordant clients by marital therapy or cognitive therapy.* Paper presented at the 21st Annual Meeting of the Association for Advancement of Behavior Therapy, Boston, MA.

Schweitzer, R., Logan, G., & Strassberg, D. (1992). The relationship between marital intimacy and postnatal depression. *Australian Journal of Marriage and Family, 13*(1), 19–23.

Shaver, P. R., Hazan, C., & Bradshaw, D. (1988). Love as attachment: The integration of three behavioral systems. In R. J. Sternberg & M. L. Barnes (Eds.), *The psychology of love* (pp. 68–99). New Haven, CT: Yale University Press.

Sher, T., Baucom, D., & Larus, J. (1990). Communication patterns and response to treatment among depressed and nondepressed maritally distressed couples. *Journal of Family Psychology, 4*(1), 63–79.

Spanier, G. B. (1976). Measuring dyadic adjustment: New scales for assessing the quality of marriage and similar dyads. *Journal of Marriage and the Family, 38,* 15–28.

Stuart, R. B. (1980). *Helping couples change: A social learning approach to marital therapy.* New York: Guilford Press.

Swann, W., Wenzlaff, R., Krull, D., & Pelham, B. (1992). Allure of negative feedback: Self-verification strivings among depressed persons. *Journal of Abnormal Psychology, 101*(2), 293–306.

Teichman, Y., Bar-El, Z., Shor, H., Sirota, P., & Elizur, A. (1995). A comparison of two modalities of cognitive therapy (individual and marital) in treating depression. *Psychiatry, 58,* 136–148.

Vivian, D., & Malone, J. (1997). Relationship factors and depressive symptomatology associated with mild and severe husband-to-wife physical aggression. *Violence and Victims, 12*(1), 3–18.

Weiss, R. L., & Cerreto, M. C. (1980). The marital Status Inventory: Development of a measure of dissolution potential. *American Journal of Family Therapy, 8,* 80–85.

Weissman, M. M. (1979). The psychological treatment of depression: Evidence for the efficacy of psychotherapy alone, in comparison with, and in combination with pharmacotherapy. *Archives of General Psychiatry, 36,* 1261–1269.

Whisman, M. A., & Bruce, M. L. (1999). Marital distress and incidence of major depressive episode in a community sample. *Journal of Abnormal Psychology, 108,* 674–678.

CHAPTER 20

Couple Therapy and the Treatment of Borderline Personality and Related Disorders

Alan E. Fruzzetti
Barrett Fantozzi

BACKGROUND

The often severe problems of borderline personality disorder (BPD) are long-lasting and result in suffering for not only the individual with BPD but also his or her loved ones. Partners and other relatives of people with BPD often have very limited knowledge about the disorder and often exhibit significant distress about their loved one's problems and suffering (Hoffman, Buteau, Hooley, Fruzzetti, & Bruce, 2003). About 75% of people with BPD engage in suicidal and nonsuicidal self-injury, and people with BPD typically have multiple co-occurring problems, such as depression and anxiety disorders, substance abuse problems, eating disorders, posttraumatic stress disorder (PTSD), and an assortment of health and other problems (Zanarini, Frankenburg, Hennen, & Silk, 2004). This set of severe and chronic problems often is associated with emergency room visits, psychiatric hospitalization, problems at work (or disability), and chaos and conflict in relationships. It is easy to see the strain these problems can put on a partner and on a couple, in addition to the obvious suffering of the person with BPD.

There is some good news, however, despite the rather serious problems associated with BPD: Effective treatment for BPD is increasingly available. Dialectical behavior therapy (DBT), developed by Linehan (1993a, 1993b), has been shown consistently to improve significantly the safety and stability, and decrease the distress, of patients with severe difficulties across multiple randomized controlled trials in the United States and abroad (Robins & Chapman, 2006). In addition, two other treatments under development (mentalization therapy and schema-focused therapy) have shown promise in the treatment of people with BPD, each with one published, randomized controlled trial suggesting successful outcomes (Bateman & Fonagy, 2001; Giesen-Bloo et al., 2006).

Unfortunately, the couple and family relationships of people with BPD have mostly been neglected. However, recent advancements involving adaptations and extensions of the principles and practices of DBT to couples and families have shown promise. In two studies, parents and partners of people with BPD who participated in a time-limited group program called Family Connections showed significant reductions in grief, depression, burden, and increases in mastery and empowerment, all of which were maintained at follow-up (Hoffman et al., 2005; Hoffman, Fruzzetti, & Buteau, 2007). Adding a DBT couple intervention to ongoing individual DBT resulted in reduced suicidality, substance use, and self-reported negative affect. A mixed group of couples (with and without a partner with BPD or significant BPD features) who participated in a pilot DBT couple therapy study showed significant improvements in relationship satisfaction and communication (decreased invalidating and increased validating responses), whereas individual partners reported lower individual distress and depression, all of which were maintained at follow-up (Fruzzetti & Mosco, 2007).

This chapter explores many of the issues and challenges that confront therapists treating couples in which one partner (or both) has the characteristics of BPD, in particular, high levels of emotional reactivity or dysregulation, which can lead to conflict and emotional distance. Interestingly, partners in relationships that do not include a BPD member may also develop (usually temporarily) the core characteristics of BPD when in severely distressed relationships, albeit typically only in interactions within that relationship. Over time partners can become acutely sensitive and highly reactive to each other, and chaos and negative emotion flow in abundance. Thus, the treatment approach described in this chapter may be quite useful for many such "borderline couples" in which neither partner has BPD or any characteristics of BPD historically, but in which partners have developed patterns of high conflict or other destructive patterns of interaction (e.g., mutually destructive patterns, mutual avoidance patterns, or engage–distance/demand–withdraw patterns; Fruzzetti & Jacobson, 1990).

Details of the essential structure of treatment, targeting processes, skills, and treatment processes of DBT with couples will be described. DBT is an integrative treatment and is compatible with (and indeed includes) both behavioral and systems interventions (Fruzzetti, 2002), yet also includes some aspects of treatment that are quite uncommon, such as a focus on emotion regulation. The DBT approach will provide the core of the chapter, but many of the concepts, techniques and strategies may be incorporated into other approaches (e.g., Baucom, Epstein, LaTaillade, & Kirby, Chapter 2; Gottman & Gottman, Chapter 5; and Gurman, Chapter 13, this volume).

UNDERSTANDING BORDERLINE PERSONALITY DISORDER AND COUPLE INTERACTIONS

It is important to understand the "transactional" model for the development and maintenance of BPD, and how BPD and related problems manifest in couple interactions. This is useful in understanding both couples who have a partner with diagnosed or diagnosable BPD and the larger population of distressed couples whose partners react strongly and quickly with high negative emotion (often referred to as "borderline couples").

BPD Basics

BPD is characterized by high levels of emotional distress, sensitivity, reactivity, and impulsivity, including suicidality and self-harming behaviors, interpersonal difficulties, fears of abandonment, along with occasional transient paranoia and difficulties with experiencing "emptiness" or maintaining a consistent and independent sense of self. About 1% of the population technically meets full diagnostic criteria for BPD, but a much greater proportion of persons has significant features that include high negative affectivity in a significantly distressed relationship.

The best evidence suggests that these kinds of difficulties develop in a complicated transaction between an individual with high emotional vulnerability (e.g., sensitivities, reactivity, and a slow return to emotional equilibrium) and invalidating responses from his or her social and family environment (Fruzzetti, Shenk, & Hoffman, 2005). The essence of this model is that "emotion dysregulation," the core problem of BPD, may also be the core problem of many entrenched distressed and negatively reactive couples.

As show in Figure 20.1, high negative emotional arousal results from a combination of the ongoing events in life plus vulnerability to negative emotion. These events are usually quite "small" and occur throughout every day (e.g., getting a slightly less than desired reaction after saying "hello" to a neighbor, coworker, or family member; finding that one's partner is not as interested in taking a walk or watching a film as one hoped), but they may also be more significant, less regular, and carry more impact (e.g., having a major argument with a partner, receiving a poor job review, or getting a parking or traffic ticket). When emotional arousal is sufficiently elevated, partners commonly focus increasingly on *escape* from this painful experience

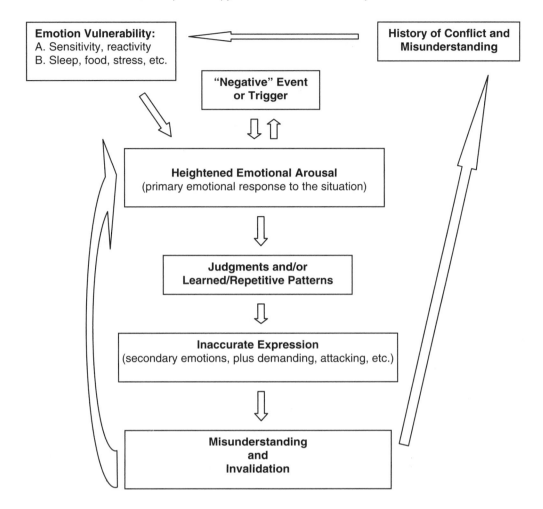

FIGURE 20.1. Relationship between individual emotion dysregulation and couple distress with points of intervention.

and focus less and less on effective problem solving or tolerating the experience, and are instead more focused on simply getting rid of (escaping from) this high level of aversive, negative emotional arousal (Fruzzetti & Jacobson, 1990). Dysfunctional behaviors, such as self-harm, substance abuse, and even aggression, develop as effective means of escaping aversive emotional arousal.

When partners are focused on escape, their ability to express or describe their private experiences accurately (emotions, wants, thoughts) is limited. They are more likely to get stuck in a pattern of being judgmental, further fueling their arousal, and expressing a great deal of negativity rather than simply describing these initial or primary responses to the situation. Most often, they become judgmental, finding extreme fault ("wrong" or "bad") with the other person or with themselves. When they are judgmental of themselves, shame ensues, typically followed by withdrawal. When they are judgmental of others, such as a partner or spouse, anger grows and typically leads to an attack (in tone, emotions, facial expression, and words) on the other person. Both of these scenarios [judgment → emotional arousal (shame or anger) → inaccurate expression (including demanding, criticizing, blaming, nagging, withdrawing, etc.)] are common in distressed couples in general, and in "borderline" couples in particular (Fruzzetti, 2006).

Of course, the person under attack sees, hears, and feels the attack, and it is extremely difficult for him or her to notice that the attacker's expression is not an accurate reflection of what started this progression of emotion dysregulation, which likely was a softer emotion (disappointment, longing, loneliness, worry or concern) or relationally reasonable desire (wanting to spend more time together, to receive or to provide more closeness or support, etc.).

It is extremely important not to pathologize either partner, including the partner with BPD; rather, it is essential for the therapist and the partner (and others) without BPD to understand this disorder as a logical outcome of rather extreme but understandable factors over time, including ordinary temperament and pervasive invalidation. Many people may become increasingly negatively reactive following consistent invalidating responses from others, and they may have had such experiences with boyfriends or girlfriends, family members, supervisors, or others.

Part of the problem in these transactions is that partners' primary emotions are missed, and instead they express secondary emotions (Fruzzetti, 2006; Greenberg & Johnson, 1988, 1990). "Primary" emotions are typically universal, healthy responses to situations or stimuli. In contrast, "secondary" emotions may be learned escape reactions from primary emotions or indirect reactions that are mediated by judgments. For example, if Maria is looking forward to Roberto coming home for dinner, but he calls to say he has to work late and will not be home until after dinner, Maria's primary emotion is almost certainly disappointment (she is not getting what she wants). However, if Maria becomes judgmental of Roberto ("He's inconsiderate" or "What a jerk to abandon me like this"), then the energy of her disappointment quickly transforms into anger. Here, anger is a secondary emotion. Similarly, if Roberto has often been late and the partners have had many negative interactions around this, Maria may simply feel angry (no judgment is required; it is just a learned pattern from repeated similar experiences) when she learns he will be late again tonight. Again, the anger is a secondary emotion. In DBT with couples we emphasize the accurate expression of primary emotions (which is similar in this way to emotionally focused couples therapy; Johnson, Chapter 4, this volume). Expressing a secondary emotion, which is considered an inaccurate expression, is an important part of the dysregulated expression of emotion.

Conflict Patterns

Couples develop fairly consistent patterns of interacting in conflict situations. Although partner behaviors may vary somewhat in different situations, they often form predictable patterns. Here, "conflict" simply means situations of disagreement, such as when partners are unhappy with one another or do not like something the other has or has not done.

Constructive Engagement Pattern

This pattern is, of course, the goal. Here, partners bring up issues that bother them and express themselves in a nonattacking way that reflects an accurate description of what they feel, think, or want, including accurate expression of primary emotions. The other partner listens, tries to understand, and communicates that understanding, even if he or she disagrees. With this beginning, many problems are solved, but even if they are not solved immediately, each person understands the other better and may be able to be more emotionally responsive (provide soothing, be more validating, etc.). Sometimes simply exploring the conflict can bring couples closer by increasing mutual understanding. But, to do this constructively, both partners must be aware of their emotions and wants, and be able to regulate their emotions effectively (Fruzzetti & Iverson, 2006).

Mutual Avoidance and Withdrawal Pattern

When one partner has a negative reaction to the other and starts to become more highly negatively emotionally aroused, the other partner reacts to this and starts to "spike" emotionally as well (typically into secondary emotions, often anger and sometimes fear). Each partner may be aware of the other's accelerating negative arousal and potential to become dysregulated quickly, and may consequently avoid bringing up important issues altogether and/or avoid any interaction for a period. Of course, problems that cannot be discussed cannot be solved, so over time this pattern exacerbates the couple's problems. Closeness and intimacy decrease even though arguments may be infrequent.

Mutual Destructive Engagement Pattern

In this pattern, partners express a great deal of anger (secondary emotion) and engage in mutual attacks. They become so emotionally aroused that they briefly fail to remember (or care) that the person they are attacking is the person they are in partnership with and love. Furthermore, arousal interferes with each partner's ability to listen to and understand the other's point of view, which is already obfuscated by inaccurate expression, mostly in the form of anger and judgmental attacks. Both partners behave in a maladaptive manner (often hurtfully toward each other) and typically regret doing so later. Importantly, this kind of interaction heightens partner vulnerability to negative emotional reactivity the next time a conflict situation arises.

Engage–Distance Pattern

In what is sometimes called the "demand–withdraw" pattern, as one partner moves toward the other, the other resists this increased engagement and may even seek more distance. One partner wants to discuss a topic, be together, and so forth, but the other does not want to do this, at least not at that moment. Often, the conflict is over something related to closeness in the relationship (being heard, spending more time together, etc.). Either the "engager" or the "distancer" can start out doing his or her part in either an effective, constructive way or in a more destructive way (aversive and avoidant, respectively), but eventually the pattern becomes aversive, resulting in more distance between partners.

THE TREATMENT MODEL

The role of negative emotional arousal and dysregulation is clear in each of the problematic patterns we noted earlier, and helping partners regulate their emotions vis-à-vis each other is an ongoing treatment target. In DBT for couples, the larger treatment goals, of course, include reducing these negative patterns and creating more constructive interaction patterns. Regulating one's own emotion is one key part of these changes. To do this, the problems the couple has are arranged in a treatment target hierarchy, with more severe and destructive (and dangerous) behaviors treated before less severe ones. "Small" interactions leading to the chosen treatment targets are examined to find the "links" in the chains of actions and reactions that send the interaction in the dysfunctional direction. At these junctures, the therapist helps partners both to understand

(accept) and to problem-solve (change) these interactions, and to learn specific skills (e.g., emotion self-management, accurate expression, validation) to alter destructive patterns. The therapist models this "dialectic" of synthesizing acceptance and change, providing *both* consistent acceptance and validation (e.g., acknowledging how problem behaviors and destructive reactions make sense, providing "cheerleading," and supporting and validating attempts to engage more constructively), *and* a consistent push to change negative reactions and incorporate more skillful alternative responses into partners' interactions (e.g., blocking dysfunctional responses, insisting on trying new and more skillful responses, pushing each partner to take responsibility for his or her part of the ongoing transaction).

Balancing acceptance and change interventions is also a cornerstone of integrative behavioral couple therapy (Jacobson & Christensen, 1996; Dimidjian, Martell, & Christensen, Chapter 3, this volume). However, the dialectical process is more central and explicit in DBT for both clients and therapists. For example, in DBT the client is explicitly taught both acceptance skills (e.g., mindfulness) and change skills (e.g., emotion regulation, problem solving), while the therapist utilizes a broad repertoire of both acceptance and change interventions, as noted earlier. In addition, DBT with couples emphasizes the role of dysregulated emotions in the breakdown of communication and the escalation of conflict, and includes many interventions to help partners regulate emotion as a means (or mediator) to either acceptance or change.

This dialectic of acceptance and change is the primary dialectic in DBT (cf. Linehan, 1993a), and acting within a dialectical framework is essential for the DBT couple therapist. However, other dialectical tensions when working with couples, in addition to the tension between acceptance and change, are important in DBT. For example, two distressed partners always have quite different experiences, attributions, and perspectives. Each has validity, and the ability of the therapist to synthesize the perspectives of two partners and reduce their polarization is essential (Fruzzetti & Fruzzetti, 2003a).

This form of therapy is very flexible. Some couples prefer a more structured approach, and for them the therapy can be presented as a semistructured "skills training" class, heavy on psychoeducation and learning and practicing new skills. This kind of couple therapy can be offered in groups or individually, and therapists can teach the skills using handouts or a therapy guide (Fruzzetti, 2006), and couples learn the skills in a progressive fashion. In a group, there are typically two therapists, to allow modeling of the management of multiple perspectives. In addition, while one therapist focuses on skill content, the other can attend to more idiosyncratic application of the skills with specific couples.

Other couples either prefer a more traditional and less-structured approach, or cannot stay regulated sufficiently to appreciate a structured approach or learn new skills that way. For them, treatment is offered traditionally (one couple, one therapist), taking the current "hot topic" and examining it, and teaching the needed skill in that moment. Over time, all the skills required are covered, and the partners receive considerable practice in changing the steps in their "dance" to be more constructive, including managing their own emotions more successfully.

Regardless of format, learning both individual emotion self-management skills (e.g., mindfulness, emotion regulation, accurate expression) and more relationship-oriented skills (e.g., relationship mindfulness, validation) are at the core of this approach. However, although different couples may demonstrate quite similar skills deficits and interaction patterns, they may present with different overt (content) problems. For example, some partners are safe and stable even after a nasty argument, whereas for others a particularly unpleasant fight might include violence, or one partner might get drunk afterwards, or might attempt suicide. For partners with BPD and the associated negative emotional reactivity they often experience, it is important to establish a treatment structure that matches the severity of the disorder present, thereby reducing the risk of dangerous behaviors and negative outcomes. We now turn our attention to creating an effective treatment structure, then discuss the practical details of conducting the treatment: assessment, identifying change targets and arranging them in a hierarchy, teaching skills, and other treatment strategies.

TREATMENT CONTEXT

It is important to consider the severity of BPD (or any other individual disorder) in structuring couple therapy. If one or both partners have severe individual problems, concurrent individual treatment may be required. There may be times when

individual treatment should begin, and progress should be demonstrated clearly, before initiating conjoint sessions. Let us consider some guidelines for making these decisions.

Concurrent Individual Treatment

The circumstances that would require concurrent individual treatment can best be described as occurring when one or both partners have "out-of-control" behaviors that may be life-threatening. This includes being suicidal or having recently made a suicide attempt, recent nonsuicidal self-harm (e.g., cutting or burning), severe substance abuse, recent child abuse or neglect, or other severe and destructive impulsive behaviors. In all of these cases, if there were no individual therapist to address these problems, the severity of the individual partner's difficulties would require the immediate and ongoing attention of the couple therapist, therefore precluding, or at least severely limiting, him or her from addressing couple issues.

Of course, one might argue from a systemic perspective that these individual, out-of-control behaviors might be directly related to couple problems and couple interactions. This may often also be true from a DBT perspective. However, couple therapy requires raising difficult issues that often include a good deal of emotional pain. If the partner does not have the requisite skills to manage his or her own behavior without engaging in severe and dangerous or extremely destructive acts, doing the couple work could be iatrogenic. In addition, from a dialectical perspective, although a partner's behavior is always related to his or her social and environmental context and may have an important function vis-à-vis his or her partner, this must be assessed to be determined. Even when relationship problems or one partner's behavior is functionally related (e.g., a relevant antecedent or consequence) to the other partner's out-of-control behavior, DBT emphasizes each individual's responsibility for his or her own behavioral self-control.

The problems of partner abuse and violence provide a good example of this dialectic. On the one hand, there is the valid argument that to treat the abuse or violence conjointly (and to conceptualize it systemically) implies that the abuse victim has at least partial responsibility for the abuse and bears partial responsibility for changing to help the perpetrator cease the abuse. To avoid blaming the victim, this perspective typically requires that the perpetrator (typically a male in heterosexual couples) be treated first individually, and only then would the couple enter therapy together to work on couple problems. On the other hand, many have noted that it is common for both partners to conceptualize partner abuse systemically, at least implicitly, and they often want to work on reducing the conflict that they conceptualize as precursor to the aggression and violence. Especially when the violence is "moderate" or less severe, some therapists argue that conjoint sessions are not only acceptable but also useful (see O'Leary, Chapter 16, this volume).

From a dialectical perspective, we frame the issue as safety. Because DBT maintains that individuals must be responsible for their own behavioral self-control, the targets at this stage of treatment are individual, and the treatment is typically delivered one on one. However, this is conceptualized simply as the first stage of the overall couple therapy. Thus, the DBT couple therapist may refer the perpetrating partner for individual therapy and require significant progress in self-control prior to initiating conjoint sessions, or he or she may choose to treat the couple comprehensively, including the domestic abuse, but engage the abusing partner alone for however long it takes to establish safety and self-control. How the partner abuse is treated in DBT is beyond the scope of this chapter, but is discussed elsewhere (cf. Fruzzetti & Levensky, 2000).

Coordinating Care with Other Treatment Providers

In many cases, one or both partners may be involved in individual psychotherapy of some kind, and both partners seem to be safe and stable enough for couple work. In these cases, it is important to make sure that the individual therapist is not working at cross-purposes to the couple therapy, and to hold a meeting (in person or by telephone) that includes both therapists and both partners, in which treatment goals and targets are clarified for each therapy component.

Many treatment modalities may virtually always be compatible with DBT for couples. Obviously, individual DBT would be completely compatible with couple DBT. In addition, psychoeducation programs designed for family members of someone with BPD, such as Family Connections (Hoffman et al., 2005, 2007), might augment DBT with couples, because so much information about BPD is provided and skills for managing emotionally intense and reactive situations are taught.

However, some individual treatments could be incompatible with couple DBT, particularly in the way that emotions and emotion regulation are conceptualized and treated. Of course, such conflicting treatments should be avoided to provide clients with coherent help.

DBT with Couples May Be Comprehensive Treatment

Finally, if the individual problems of a partner are not out of control (neither partner engages in suicidal behavior, self-harm, partner violence, etc.), then DBT with couples may be provided as a comprehensive treatment; that is, distressed couples are likely to include partners with a variety of problems, including depression, substance abuse, eating disorders, and so on, and the relationship between individual distress and psychopathology, and relationship distress has been well documented (cf. Fruzzetti, 1996). The couple DBT treatment model suggests that both individual and relationship targets should show improvement, and some early data support this, demonstrating reduced individual distress and depression, along with improved communication and relationship satisfaction and reduced conflict following DBT couple therapy (Fruzzetti & Mosco, 2007).

ASSESSMENT, ORIENTING, AND COMMITTING TO THERAPY

There are two primary goals of an initial assessment with couples: (1) identifying treatment targets, and (2) quantifying a baseline to measure progress. Of course, posttreatment assessment allows us to quantify the same domains at a later time, thereby allowing a more objective measure of outcome. In addition, daily or weekly (ongoing) assessment may be an important additional tool to help monitor progress, adjust treatment targets, and keep partners and the therapist focused and collaborating on the same treatment goals or targets. Let us briefly consider both types of assessment.

Assessment during the Pre- and Posttreatment Phases

As noted previously and described in more detail below, DBT with couples follows a treatment target hierarchy paralleling that of individual DBT (Fruzzetti & Fruzzetti, 2003a; Linehan, 1993a). Consequently, it is essential to assess for relevant problems at each point in the hierarchy. This may be accomplished by a combination of self-report questionnaires, both individual and conjoint interviews, and direct observation of partner behaviors (Fruzzetti & Jacobson, 1992).

Questionnaires

Any number of psychometrically sound questionnaires is available for use with couples. It is particularly important to assess important overall dimensions of both individual and relationship functioning. Utilizing a gross measure of couple satisfaction is important. Similarly, including standard measures of individual distress can be quite useful. Measures of conflict, including partner abuse, are quite important to include. Perhaps the most common and sound among these measures is Straus, Hamby, Boney-McCoy, and Sugarman's (1996) Revised Conflict Tactics Scale (CTS2). The specific questionnaires used perhaps matter less than whether they are psychometrically sound, have established norms, and are clear about the domain being evaluated.

Recorded Behavior Samples

Many couple therapists still believe that videotaping couples is something that only researchers can do. On the contrary, clinicians should attempt to include videotaping routinely in their practice for a variety of reasons: (1) It provides more objective opportunities to quantify couple communication and, therefore, valid indices of outcome; (2) videotaped material also may be used therapeutically later on; (3) this may be the only practical way to receive consultation from colleagues about the couple; and (4) videotaped interactions may have more external/ecological validity, because what couples actually do when left alone for a while may be quite different than what they do in front of the therapist, and what they report. For example, people with BPD typically have quite discrepant views from those of their family members about their own and their family members' behavior (Hoffman, Buteau, & Fruzzetti, 2007). Thus, it may be important to observe whether these differing views reflect distortions or misunderstandings on the part of the partner with BPD, the other partner, or both, or whether they simply reflect normative but different experiences.

It may be useful to ask couples to have several different conversations for videotaping. Top-

ics might include satisfaction with emotional closeness and intimacy, time together, or recurring problems. Each partner should be allowed to bring up a relationship-relevant problem for discussion, with the couple left alone in the room with minimal distractions. If taping is not possible, the couple can be observed as inconspicuously as possible by the therapist, who gives the couple minimal instructions, arranges the chairs so that partners are facing each other, and then sits quietly and unobtrusively to the side, out of direct visual sight lines, where he or she can observe the interactions and take notes.

These conversations can be "coded" formally with an established rating or coding system. However, it may be even more practical or useful for the therapist to be able to observe the conversations in "real time," perhaps with consultation from a colleague, to understand each partner's experience in the couple transactions and to help identify treatment targets. Rating or coding the conversations has the added benefit of providing an objective measure of treatment outcome if similar conversations are recorded at the end of therapy.

Interviews

There are many standard parts to any couple interview, including DBT with couples. Although there is not sufficient space to detail all aspects of a standard couple interview here (see Fruzzetti & Jacobson, 1992), it is important that we note several targets of the interview process.

First, it is important to include separate interviews with the partners, along with interviews of partners together. The advantages of including individual interviews (e.g., more accurate or complete information, establishing rapport with each person as an individual, as well as with them as a couple) seem clearly to outweigh the potential disadvantages (e.g., unbalancing the therapy by allying, or appearing to ally, with one partner more than the other; risking the disclosure of a "secret"). During the separate interviews, partners should have the opportunity to discuss both life and relationship successes and failures, and some of their individual history, particularly as it may affect treatment targets. This should include history of problems and treatment (including suicide attempts and other self-harm, substance abuse, etc.); previous or current infidelities; physical and sexual abuse histories; experience of conflict in the relationship, including aggression and violence; commitment to therapy; and commitment to the relationship. Incongruities between partners' verbal descriptions and their questionnaires, of course, must be clarified.

There also should be one or more conjoint interviews that include information about the couple's relationship history, strengths and problems, and any matters pertaining to safety. However, the most important strategy here is to begin to conduct a "chain analysis" of specific targets (Fruzzetti, 2006; Fruzzetti et al., 2007). This is described in more detail below.

Orienting and Committing to Therapy

Given the chaos that often runs through the lives of high-conflict, highly distressed, couples, there are many things in their lives that may interfere with successful engagement in couple therapy. Clearly specifying what the couple may expect from the therapist, and what the therapist expects from the couple, allows partners to make a well-informed choice about participation. Because couple DBT requires more active partner participation (e.g., daily self-monitoring, between-session practice of new skills, and commitment to what for many is a new conceptualization of their problems and interactions), a clear orientation to therapy is essential to receive meaningful commitment.

In addition to orienting partners to the steps involved in the treatment, the therapist may also assess problems that are likely to interfere with or even preclude collaborative engagement in therapy. Have they dropped out of therapy before? If so, why? What would make this different (or the same)? Can the therapist and couple collaboratively anticipate problems in the therapy and problem-solve them before they occur? Common problems include one (or both) partners conceptualizing the therapy as a means of "fixing" the spouse to improve the relationship, rather than taking a more reciprocal or transactional view of their difficulties; wanting the therapist also to function de facto as an individual therapist for one or both partners; perceiving therapy simply as a place to vent, rather than as a program for changing important problematic interactions (with bilateral responsibility for improvements); and preferring a "free-flowing" type of therapy, in which they can talk about whatever is on their minds as opposed to the flexible but still semistructured DBT approach, in which a specific treatment target hierarchy informs each session's agenda, and in which specific skills are learned and applied.

In particular, because DBT with couples is organized according to a hierarchy of targets, it may be useful at times to make an initial contract for just a few sessions to see whether the partners can engage meaningfully in the treatment. One or both partners may be quite reluctant to make an open-ended or long-term commitment to couple therapy, but they may be willing to commit for 6–10 sessions. We can take that commitment and work within the hierarchy to make as much progress as possible within the available time. If this initial commitment is successful, the couple may be willing to recommit later for additional sessions to work on additional targets.

Thus, the couple's initial commitment to therapy may be relatively brief (e.g., 6–10 sessions), or much longer (e.g., 15–20 sessions or more). If partners make improvements, then they may be satisfied and stop therapy at the end of their agreement, or decide to renew their commitment to work on additional problems. Because of the nature of the treatment target hierarchy, the most important problems always are addressed first, so the therapist need not be too concerned with the length of the initial commitment. The DBT therapist is typically willing to renew an agreement (or "contract"), for additional sessions, if the therapy is demonstrably working and partners are showing meaningful improvement.

Data from one study demonstrate that significant improvements can occur after relatively few sessions. For example, Fruzzetti and Mosco (2007) found overall significant improvements in relationship quality and decreased individual distress after six sessions of a couples group program (2-hour sessions), with a mixed sample that included partners with relatively less severe BPD. With more severe BPD and greater couple distress, couple therapy may be expected to go on much longer, perhaps as long as the BPD partner is in individual therapy (a year or more). However, sessions typically are held less frequently after the initial phase of couple therapy. After a period of weekly sessions, especially after some of the more severe and destructive behaviors have been curtailed, it may be possible for a couple to attend therapy on alternating weeks, giving the partners more time to practice between sessions.

Part of the orientation to treatment also includes an orientation to what BPD is and how it develops and is maintained. Psychoeducation is important in part because the transactional model employed in DBT is nonblaming (it also may be considered developmental or systemic; cf. Fruzzetti et al., 2005) and "sets the stage" for the consistently nonblaming framework of the treatment. Utilizing a transactional model is also important because it promotes the understanding that both partners play important roles in the relationship and take an active role in therapy. Some partners of people with BPD see BPD as "the problem" and therapy as a way for the partner with BPD to get "fixed," rather than as a bilateral or joint approach to relationship enhancement that is good for both individuals. This view is problematic from a DBT perspective and must be challenged early on in treatment to orient clients to the model and to obtain a meaningful commitment to therapy.

Psychoeducation may be provided early in treatment in one or two sessions or be spread out over many sessions as topics naturally come up over the course of therapy. Essential psychoeducation topics include (1) understanding the components ("symptoms") of BPD, and how problems regulating emotion are central features of the disorder; (2) understanding how BPD and emotion dysregulation overlap with other diagnoses, such as depression, anxiety, eating disorders, and even other personality disorders; (3) understanding BPD as chronic emotion dysregulation that results from complex transactions of individual vulnerabilities (temperament, emotional sensitivity, and reactivity) and invalidating social and family responses (see Figure 20.1; Fruzzetti et al., 2005; Linehan, 1993a); and (4) knowledge about the natural course of BPD, including the fact that BPD is treatable (Hoffman & Fruzzetti, 2005). Because knowledge about BPD is often limited and frequently is not accurate (Hoffman et al., 2003), it is also important to answer questions that partners might have and to disabuse them of their misconceptions about BPD (see also Gunderson & Hoffman, 2005).

In DBT, the therapist approaches commitment (both to treatment targets and to treatment itself) in a manner similar to how he or she approaches other targets; that is, the therapist must simultaneously assess strength of commitment and validate partner experiences (e.g., worries about commitment, disappointments about prior failures, hopes for improvement), and what is needed to strengthen commitment, targeting these behaviors for change. Therefore, the therapist demonstrates the dialectical balance of acceptance and change that clients will face throughout the ther-

apy, which further helps them assess their comfort with the approach and make a well-considered decision about their commitment.

Ongoing, Daily Assessment and Monitoring: Diary Cards

To continue to work within a treatment target hierarchy, it is essential to know what the couple is doing day to day. Having each partner monitor his or her own behaviors (actions, emotions, judgments, skills, etc.) increases the accuracy of weekly assessment, minimizes guesswork about the most important target on which to focus, and provides a more accurate "snapshot" of the couple's daily life than retrospective reporting, which is affected by memory decay or recency effects bias. Therefore, self-monitoring has the added benefit of bringing the work of therapy into partners' daily lives, reminding them of the importance of their work as well as some of the specific skills they are learning, and possibly enhancing practice.

Ideally, partners monitor their key targets every day. This can be accomplished simply on a piece of paper, or the couple may utilize more advanced technology (e.g., personal data assistants, Web-based daily questions, or an e-mail to the therapist). A typical diary card for a nonviolent couple is shown in Figure 20.2. Targets vary over time.

Note that each partner monitors only his or her own thoughts, actions, emotions, and so on, and may record entries with words, numerical ratings, or even plus and minus signs. Some partners may enjoy keeping track of many different things (a kind of semistructured journal or diary), whereas others may prefer only to record the most important, current targets. The therapist may think of the diary card in the same way that a dentist utilizes an X-ray: It provides important information about what to treat right now, and what needs immediate attention in the context of a larger, overall treatment plan.

CHAIN ANALYSIS AND SOLUTION GENERATION

Conducting chain analyses is one of the core activities of a DBT couple therapist, and at least one chain analysis (or part of one) is conducted in nearly every session. This method of assessment is also an intervention in a variety of ways. The therapist not only identifies key points to change along the

DIARY CARD   Name: _____   Date started: _____

Date	Accurate expression (+ or −)	Level 2 Validation (how many times)	Quality of time together (+10 to −10)	Practiced relationship mindfulness (Y/N)	Satisfaction (+10 to −10)	Note primary emotions and rate intensity (1 to 10)	Describe important situations
Mon							
Tues							
Wed							
Thurs							
Fri							
Sat							
Sun							

FIGURE 20.2. Sample daily diary card.

"chain" of behaviors (emotional reactions, overt actions, judgments, appraisals, verbalizations, etc.) that resulted in dysfunctional or problem behavior (screaming at or invalidating the other partner, suicidal urges, drinking, emotion dysregulation, etc.), but he or she also provides a method for both partners to understand, accept, and validate the other partner and his or her experience. Thus, a chain analysis provides the opportunity for both acceptance and change.

The steps in conducting a chain analysis are actually rather straightforward:

1. The therapist (in collaboration with the couple) selects a clear target in the treatment target hierarchy that has occurred since the last session (the most severe in the hierarchy that has occurred).
2. They identify one specific instance of this problem, or episode (a specific day, time, and place).
3. They identify the beginning, or trigger, for the episode.
4. They "walk through" the chain, with each partner identifying what he or she was feeling, thinking, and doing at each step along the way.
5. They attempt to identify (if needed) what happened so quickly in that moment that one or both partners missed it (e.g., a partner reacted so quickly that he or she missed a primary emotion and went right to a secondary emotion).
6. The therapist validates the valid thoughts, wants, and emotional responses along the way, modeling skillful alternatives for the clients (Linehan, 1997).
7. The therapist helps each partner to understand and validate the other's experience (emotion, wants or desires, etc.).
8. The therapist urges each partner to identify at least one skillful alternative that he or she could do the next time the couple is in a similar situation, instead of whatever he or she did this time.
9. Each partner commits to practice whatever solutions are generated in preparation for the next opportunity to respond differently.

Thus, the analysis flows easily into solutions and results in identifying skills to learn and then practice between sessions, and possible reenactment the following session, using the new skills to change the sequence of the old chain. Of course, the "change" required along the chain may be as

varied as "acceptance" of one's own emotion or the partner's emotion, acceptance of other behaviors, changes in ones' own behavior (e.g., regulating an emotion, engaging the partner more constructively), or other skillful alternatives. When enough "chains" are altered, the recurrent interaction pattern has been rechoreographed. Thus, a chain analysis is both a key intervention tool and an assessment tool, utilizing all of the other interventions common to this treatment.

TREATMENT TARGET HIERARCHY

Treatment targets are organized hierarchically according to the severity of the behavior in question. This hierarchy is a cornerstone of both individual and couple DBT (Fruzzetti & Fruzzetti, 2003a; Linehan, 1993a). The treatment target hierarchy posits that more severe and problematic behaviors must be resolved and brought under control before less severe behaviors can be addressed. Because the overall goal is to help clients establish a satisfying life together, including couple and/or family relationships that are supportive, validating, and satisfying, the treatment target hierarchy identifies targets depending upon how much they interfere with (1) safety, (2) active and collaborative participation in treatment, (3) basic individual and relationship/family stability, (4) emotional satisfaction (and regulation), (5) a validating relationship, (6) resolution of conflicts, and (7) emotional closeness and intimacy. Constructing the hierarchy also includes building in basic self-management skills first; more complicated skills that require a solid foundation come later on in therapy.

For example, if a couple's list of presenting complaints includes conflicts about money, child-rearing issues, recent partner abuse and violence, and conflicts around sex and emotional distance, then violence is addressed and resolved initially (as described earlier), prior to addressing any other issues. Once the violence in the relationship is stopped, then the other, less severe issues presented by the couple are addressed, with the more severe conflicts in the treatment target hierarchy addressed first. The following identifies the general kinds of targets and the order in which they are addressed, in couple DBT.

Increase Safety

As discussed previously, a violent partner may need to be referred for individual treatment if there has been recent violence or the threat of violence. Furthermore, when domestic violence has occurred or is a risk factor, the therapist needs to take additional steps to ensure client safety (Fruzzetti & Levensky, 2000; Fruzzetti & Jacobson, 1992). It may be necessary to develop a safety plan if one client needs to escape a threatening interaction with his or her partner. This may include, for example, having a set of spare keys, hidden cash, a prepacked suitcase, or other preparations, in case the client needs to move quickly to a safe environment.

In addition to addressing domestic violence to improve safety, both suicidal and nonsuicidal self-injury may be present in one (or both) partners in couples with BPD. Sometimes it becomes clear that a partner is *positively reinforcing* self-harm, often with increased positive attention, warmth, and/or soothing. Thus, it may be necessary to target *moving the partner's reinforcing behaviors.* In practice, the target would be to urge the non-self-harming partner to provide warmth, attention, and soothing on a regular basis to the partner who self-harms, no longer providing the differential reinforcers that follow self-harm. Similarly, one partner may be quite critical and hostile toward the other, reducing this negativity only when the partner becomes acutely distressed, suicidal, or engages in self-harm or other dysfunctional behaviors. In such cases, the partner's reduced aversive behaviors actually *negatively reinforce* the self-harm or other problem behaviors (i.e., the self-harm functions to reduce the partner's aversive responses). In these cases, the therapist would target *removing* the negative or aversive responses altogether.

For example, Jillian typically describes her husband Kevin as distant and disconnected, preferring to play softball or golf, or to go bowling with his friends or watch sports at a local bar, than spend time with her. She reports that when she tries to "be close" to Kevin and spend time with him at home, he often retreats to the TV to watch the sports channel. This leaves Jillian feeling unloved and lonely, which often escalates into other intense, negative emotions and leads to self-injurious thoughts, urges, or behaviors. When Jillian begins to engage in these dysfunctional behaviors, Kevin becomes more attentive and involved, in fact providing some of the warmth and attention that Jillian had craved. The attention Kevin gives to Jillian during these dysfunctional episodes reinforces her self-harm. However, were he to simply remove that warmth, Jillian would be left with none at all. Consequently, the target is to have Kevin spend time with Jillian on a regular basis ("move" the reinforcer), so that she is not dependent on suicidality or urges to self-harm to have Kevin's love and attention. For example, Kevin may agree to spend 45 minutes with Jillian on most days, and to keep his attention (and warmth) focused on her during that time. Jillian might agree that when she begins to have self-injurious thoughts, she will not turn to Kevin for support, but will instead use self-management techniques she has learned from therapy or call others for support (e.g., friends or her individual therapist), thus not putting Kevin in the position of reinforcing her self-harm.

Alternatively, James sometimes becomes extremely judgmental, angry, and critical of Liza, to the point that he screams at her and tells her many things that are "wrong" with her. After a dose of James berating her, Liza often becomes "stuck" in his criticism, feels very ashamed and worthless, abandoned, and becomes increasingly suicidal. James can see the shift in her and typically stops his criticism, gets quite scared, and may even apologize for his mean behavior. Thus, his intense criticism elicits her negative emotion (primarily shame), and by stopping his criticism only after Liza becomes suicidal, James is, in fact, negatively reinforcing her suicidality. Here, the target would be get James to stop expressing his dislikes with such negative intensity ("remove" the negative reinforcer), thereby reducing Liza's suicidal behavior and potential.

Reduce Invalidation

Once safety has been established in the relationship, the next target for difficult couples is to decrease the invalidating behaviors of one or both partners. "Invalidating" behaviors convey judgments (e.g., right vs. wrong, self-righteousness) and assert that valid thoughts, feelings, or desires are instead wrong, illegitimate, or otherwise invalid, or they are used to criticize or express contempt for the other person (Fruzzetti & Iverson, 2004; Fruzzetti et al., 2007). This step involves identifying the most corrosive invalidating responses, those that are most responsible for hurt feelings, further negative responses (negative escalation), and destructive conflict.

Reducing invalidating responses requires a number of secondary targets; that is, the partner first has to be willing to give up his or her "self-righteousness" and to "step down" in a conflict situation, because it is more important to be effective in the relationship than to be "right." Once the partner is willing, he or she still has to recognize when emotions are rising and conflict is intensifying, and to use some alternative skill instead of criticizing and invalidating the other partner (regardless of the legitimacy of the criticism). These alternative skills include learning mindfulness and being able to focus on long term-goals (e.g., having an improved relationship and enhanced self-respect) rather than noticing and acting on only short-term goals (e.g., impulses to say something invalidating that might allow the partner to feel self-righteous). In reality, this is another self-control or self-management target, albeit with behaviors that are less dangerous (invalidating verbal responses) and not directly tied to safety issues.

Relationship Reactivation: Increase Time Together, and "Being Together" When Together

Often couples have so many aversive interactions that they become increasingly distant, resulting in decreased and limited time together. As partners argue more, they avoid each other more, and even the positive and neutral things in their relationship fall away. Because of this decrease in positive interactions, the proportion of *all* of their time together that is negative increases greatly. Thus, relationship reactivation is another treatment target.

It is important for couples to share time and experiences together. However, these experiences should be mutually satisfying to both partners, at least overall. Illustrative activities include spending time with friends and/or family, joint participation in recreational activities, sharing intellectual pursuits and spiritual experiences, or simply sitting in the same room in the evening while engaging in various activities. It is important for the couple to include a variety of activities, and not to focus too much on talking, especially on "hot" or recurrent problem topics. Many couples have significant differences in both verbal skills and comfort with intense or extended verbal interactions. In this approach, the talking comes later, after safety has been established, negative interactions have been reduced, and positive time together has been restored.

Part of what makes closeness grow is a sense of "we-ness" in a couple, the idea that one is part of something bigger, the couple, and has both an individual identity *and* a couple identity. One way to increase this sense of being in the relationship is by increasing mindfulness of the other person, or "relationship mindfulness." Partners using this

skill do not even necessarily have to spend more time physically with each other to engage in relationship reactivation: It may be sufficient simply to increase awareness of themselves as a couple in situations in which they are connect in some way (e.g., they both may be in the kitchen, but doing different things). Simply being more aware of each other may enhance their "we-ness" and provide moments of positive emotions in the relationship.

Increase Accurate Expression and Validation

Many people with BPD have difficulty identifying and labeling their emotions, which leads to inaccurate expression of the emotions they are feeling, ultimately resulting in partner invalidation (Fruzzetti et al., 2005). Partners with BPD (and other very distressed partners) often initially express more judgments and secondary emotions, such as anger and shame, instead of more accurate and descriptive primary emotions, such as disappointment, loneliness, or fear. When a client expresses judgments and secondary emotions, the partner often responds in an invalidating way that leads the interaction into an escalating argument between them (see Figure 20.1). To express emotions accurately, one must possess the skills necessary to do so, and be in a supportive and validating environment that encourages and reinforces effective emotional expression. Therefore, some treatment targets during this phase in therapy include developing the skills to be aware of one's own emotions and to express them in a descriptive way, as well as to become increasingly aware of one's partner's emotions and more validating.

For example, rather than saying, "You're such a jerk. I can't believe you forgot my mother's birthday dinner is tonight, after I just reminded you yesterday. What the hell is wrong with you!" it would be more effective and accurate (and would likely make one feel more vulnerable) to say, "My feelings are hurt and I'm really disappointed because you forgot her birthday dinner." The latter is a more accurate expression of legitimate feelings, whereas the former is filled with judgments ("jerk") and secondary emotions (anger) that are likely to leave one's partner feeling attacked. Moreover, it is almost impossible to validate the other's disappointment when one is under attack, so the critical partner's emotions are very likely to be invalidated, further escalating the conflict.

The focus of this step in teasing out primary emotions overlaps considerably with the work of

Greenberg and Johnson (1988; Johnson, Chapter 4, this volume). However, from the DBT perspective, the reciprocal roles of inaccurate expression (including secondary emotions) and invalidation (especially of primary emotions) are posited as the central features in the maintenance of chronic emotional dysregulation and BPD. Consequently, from this view, multiple skills are required to help regulate partners and turn the dysfunctional transaction (inaccurate expression ↔ invalidation) around, and into a more stable and constructive transaction (accurate expression ↔ validation). These skills are a centerpiece of the DBT approach (see below). In addition, extreme partner behaviors such as suicide attempts or self-harm are contraindicated in emotionally focused couple therapy (Greenberg & Johnson, 1988) but commonly encountered and addressed in DBT with couples, as noted earlier.

Manage Conflict

"Problem solving" refers to issues in the relationship that can be addressed, resolved, and "forgotten," at least for a while. "Problem management" refers to how to handle problems that cannot be solved but instead require continued attention and validation. At this point in therapy, couples should have established safety and stability in their relationship through self-management skills, decreased invalidating conflict cycles, increased time together, and increased accurate emotional expression and validation cycles. Because of these changes in the relationship, the partners should be less reactive and better able to discuss sensitive problem issues in their relationship. Problem management includes defining the problem, analyzing the problem, and looking at acceptance as an alternative to change. Defining the problem is necessary for resolving couple problems, because often partners in conflict may be fighting over the same issue or over two separate but related issues.

Many times partners in severely distressed relationships engage in interaction patterns that impede effective communication. Because partners often engage in negative patterns or engage–distance patterns, changing these interaction patterns is an important target that aids in effective problem management. Couple mindfulness skills (see below) can help partners slow down in their interactions and refocus on their long-term relationship goals. Radical acceptance and emotion regulation skills can help to decrease individual reactivity and increase accurate descriptive expression of emotion. Improving such skills helps couples to discuss sensitive topics in effective, intimacy-enhancing ways.

Increase Closeness and Intimacy

At this point, clients have learned how to communicate more effectively and deal with daily life problems, but often they still struggle with isolation and a lack of intimacy. Often the next logical treatment target is for clients to enhance the amount of closeness and intimacy in their relationship, but not at the expense of also maintaining autonomy. Thus, this last target involves finding a balance, or a synthesis, of the tensions between intimacy and autonomy (Fruzzetti, 2006).

Many clients with BPD report fears that increasing individuality will not only be painful but also decrease the overall current level of intimacy in their relationships. At the same time, partners of some individuals with BPD express feelings of being overwhelmed by the attachment needs of their partners, often leading to feelings that their own independence is being threatened or severely limited. Previously, sharing activities together was addressed as a way to reactivate the relationship, but in addition to spending time together, it can also be highly beneficial to balance time together with time alone, to synthesize autonomy and intimacy. Engaging in independent activities can lead to three positive outcomes for the relationship: (1) An energized and satisfied partner is much more pleasurable to be around and also has more energy to give to the other partner and the relationship; (2) nonshared activities allow each partner to share verbally and discuss those activities with the other; and (3) partners feel less stress and obligation to confine their interests only to shared activities, resulting in a greater appreciation for the variety of both partners' interests. Intimacy can be used to support autonomy, and autonomy can infuse the relationship with novelty and excitement that contributes more to sharing and results in enhanced closeness.

Thus, as partners begin to establish their autonomy, it is important for them also to encourage emotional intimacy with one another. To maintain both autonomy and intimacy, it is important for couples to do three things: (1) maintain a balance between time apart and time together; (2) support one another in independent activities; and (3) discuss and support each other's time apart.

Once couples have learned all these skills, the next step is generalization of these skills effectively to maintain a healthy, stable relationship outside therapy. Couples may choose to take a temporary break from therapy to monitor their relationship on their own. During this break, couples often find it helpful to make note of situations in which they found it difficult to use their skills or to behave effectively. When the partners returns to therapy, they can discuss these difficult situations and possible solutions. The partners can then take another break from therapy to try their skills on their own.

To synthesize this dialectic of intimacy and autonomy, couples learn several skills: (1) acceptance or behavioral tolerance in regard to partner problem behaviors that are not likely to change in the near future; (2) mindfulness to understand the "problem" behavior in context, to learn that critical attention not only worsens problem behavior but also introduces negativity into the couple interaction; and (3) radical acceptance of the partner's problem behavior, and recontextualizing the partner and the relationship to broaden the context in which the problem behavior occurs. When these skills are practiced, along with relationship mindfulness and validation, a possible negative interaction can be changed into opportunities to increase intimacy and closeness.

As clients learn to implement skills such as emotion regulation, radical acceptance, accurate expression, and validation, they strengthen not only their individual autonomy but also their couple intimacy, because they are learning to work collaboratively to communicate more effectively and to understand one another.

COUPLE SKILLS

Most partners, minutes or hours after an argument in which they behaved badly, recognize that their responses were not only ineffective and hurtful, but also, paradoxically, resulted in getting *less* of what they wanted (e.g., more closeness and understanding, more support, more collaboration, a better relationship). The reality is that, on the one hand, such partners often already know what they need to do to be effective. On the other hand, they often do not have the skills to manage their emotional arousal and to do what is needed to become more relationally effective. Many partners know at least a little about clear expression and active listening (or similar skills and constructs) but are not able to use these more skillful alternatives, especially when their negative emotional arousal is at a painful level.

For these reasons, couple DBT focuses more attention on the skills needed to regulate emotions, to increase awareness of genuine or heartfelt goals (e.g., having a better relationship) even when the urge to be nasty is present, and to match the form and function of communication, so that expression is more accurate, making it easier for partners to understand and validate each other. This approach focuses on creating a variety of effective ways to validate the inherently valid things that partners express.

There is a lot of flexibility in how these skills are taught, as we mentioned earlier. Skills may be taught formally, in a more classroom-oriented environment in groups, or while doing chain analyses, if the therapist identifies one or more skills that are lacking and would result in a less destructive transaction. In this section, we highlight the main skills taught in DBT for couples.

Mindfulness and Relationship Mindfulness

In DBT, mindfulness and relationship mindfulness are the first skills couples are taught (Fruzzetti, 2006; Linehan, 1993b). Mindfulness in general includes being able to focus attention and awareness, and to be aware in a descriptive (rather than judgmental, or "right–wrong") way. Being mindful of one's partner includes simply becoming aware of him or her, and noticing and describing him or her physically, along with whatever behaviors and feelings, thoughts, and attitudes that can be observed rather than inferred. Being mindful of one's partner does not include attaching judgments to the things one notices and describes. Often, a partner may start to notice the behavior of the other ("She's talking on the phone with her sister and not paying attention to me"), describe how he or she feels ("I feel disappointed, and a bit lonely"), then immediately attach a judgment to what he or she noticed and described (e.g., "She's selfish and insensitive" or "He doesn't really care about me") that then transforms the energy from the primary emotion to a secondary emotion ("I'm angry"). The result may be an inaccurate expression (e.g., withdrawal in a huff, which does not accurately express loneliness) or an attack (resulting immediately in less warmth and soothing attention). Partners often automatically and unknowingly jump to judgments about each other. Mindfulness skills allow partners to slow down their reactivity; to become more aware of a situation, and their genuine emotions and desires in that situation; and to help them simply to notice and describe (more accurate expressions) rather than to become judgmental and ineffective.

Noticing and describing are open responses that lead to a desire to know more about the partner and understand him or her better; in contrast, judging is a closed response that is full of assumptions; no more information is sought or processed, because the individual has already reached a "final judgment." Although being judgmental is a form of thinking, mindfulness provides a different approach to dealing with judgments than might be found in traditional cognitive therapy. In a mindful approach, the partner's target is always first to be aware of a judgment, then to turn attention to noticing and describing both the thing being judged (e.g., the other partner, what he or she did) and one's own experience (e.g., sensations, emotions, desires). The consequence is that emotional arousal does not rise to dysregulated levels. A mindful approach does not include challenging negative thoughts or judgments per se, or changing thoughts according to rational rules.

Mindfulness comprises three "whats" (*what* to do to be mindful) and three "hows" (*how* to do it), developed by Linehan (1993b), who adapted mindfulness as taught by Thich Nhat Hanh (1975) into psychological and attention skills. With couples, the "whats" include (1) *notice/observe*—just notice, become aware of, your own experience or that of the other person; (2) *describe*—attach words to the experience; and (3) *participate*—let go of self-consciousness or self-talk (including worry thoughts) and just engage in the experience or activity. The "hows" include (1) *be nonjudgmental*—let go of ideas of "shoulds" and "rights" and "wrongs"; (2) *act one-mindfully*—focus on only one thing at a time, in the present moment, such as one's own experience or that of the partner, and so forth; and (3) *act effectively*—remember that this is someone you love.

Relationship mindfulness is a key skill in couple DBT. In addition to letting go of judgments and being emotionally present, relationship mindfulness also focuses on the clients "being 'together' when they are together" (Fruzzetti, 2006, p. 39). There are three ways for couples to be together:

1. Passively together: Partners are physically present, but not interacting or really aware of one another. Attention is focused on the individual tasks in which each partner is engaged.
2. Actively together: Partners are engaged in an activity together, such as watching a movie or taking a walk. Attention is focused primarily on the activity, but partners are minimally aware of each other, and may increase their awareness of each other without sacrificing the activity.
3. Interactively together: Regardless of other activities going on, partners' attention is focused primarily on each other. Both partners feel that they are engaging in an activity together and intimately sharing an experience.

Relationship mindfulness allows partners to be more aware of each other, regardless of the activity or how much verbal communication is exchanged. Partners are encouraged to notice when they are passively together and to try to become more actively together, and to notice when they are actively together and try to become more interactively together. Mindfulness and relationship mindfulness are taught and emphasized throughout the therapy.

Emotion Self-Management

Partners in distressed relationships must manage their own emotional arousal if they are to change dysfunctional patterns of interaction successfully. To increase self-control, clients must be committed to this target (being "effective" rather than being "right"). To be able to control their emotions in highly arousing situations, clients must commit to practicing emotional self-management and emotional self-regulation before they find themselves in such highly arousing situations. Practicing the management of emotions enhances these capabilities, so that they may eventually feel "automatic."

At times, a person may feel justified in responding to his or her partner in a critical or invalidating way, because he or she "deserved it." However, behaving in this way does not improve conflict management; rather, it leads to overall distress in the relationship. If both partners are mindful of the relationship, they will see that they are engaging in harmful and invalidating behaviors, and that unless one of them decides to step back and break this cycle, it will continue. It is important for partners to use mindfulness to remind themselves that they love and cherish each other and their relationship, and that invalidating behaviors do not help their relationship. A person may feel that he or she surrenders by "giving in" and letting the partner attack him or her and not attacking back. However, partners must increasingly realize that engaging in an invalidating conflict is a "lose–lose" situation. They lose control of their own emotions while simultaneously hurting the partner, doing more damage to the relationship, and getting less and less of what they want. By stopping the cycle, partners enter into a "win–win" situation by maintaining their own self-control and self-respect, and not damaging the partner or the relationship. It is much harder for clients to stop the cycle and to think mindfully about being effective in difficult situations than simply to react to the situation without thinking about the effects of their behavior. This is why partners need to be fully committed to managing their emotions and stopping the process of invalidation early in the chain of a potentially damaging situation.

To decrease the likelihood of getting in a damaging argument, partners need to anticipate their impulsiveness by identifying potential triggers and rehearsing how they will respond to them. By anticipating potential destructive triggers, partners can be better prepared to handle them effectively by down-regulating their emotional arousal. One strategy for achieving this is for the partner to distract him- or herself from the situation until arousal decreases, by going for a walk, saying a short prayer or a calming verse, doing slow, deep breathing or something soothing, such as listening to music or taking a bath. Once partners identify possible triggers, and possible ways to handle their reactions to those triggers, they can mentally rehearse and prepare for times when those difficult situations arise. Another strategy in situations of emotional and conflict escalation is to remember the question, "Will responding this way get me what I really want in the world, a close and loving relationship?" Many other skills may be utilized to change overlearned, automatic, negative responses (Fruzzetti, 2006; Linehan, 1993b).

Not only is it important for couples to be committed to effective practice and to anticipate their triggers and impulses, but it is also important to learn to manage destructive urges. To control destructive urges, partners can visualize the expected negative outcomes that are likely to occur if they act on their urges. By thinking about possible negative outcomes, partners learn to balance the short-term outcomes (acting on urges may make them feel better initially) with the long-term outcomes (acting on urges will most likely lead to long-term damage). Partners can also learn simply to notice the urge without acting on it. Urges subside over time, and this reduction can be facilitated by simply "noticing" the urges. Doing this can make acting on the urge seem less desirable. If, however, the urge does not subside by simply noticing the urge, the partner has given him- or herself the choice to act rather than to react automatically. Couples can also recall and visualize the positive outcomes of "riding out the urge." Unlike the previously discussed strategy that uses partners' *desires to avoid negative situations* as a motivation, this method helps partners use their *desire to achieve positive outcomes* as a motivation to regulate themselves more effectively.

Accurate Expression

To increase understanding and validation, partners are taught how to express their emotions accurately. To express him- or herself accurately, a partner must know what he or she wants, feels, thinks, and so forth. Partners are taught to use mindfulness to identify what they want, feel, and think. Mindfulness can help partners realize that they are unsure of what they want or that they simply need more time to identify their goals.

Couples typically inaccurately express emotions in one of two ways. The first ways is to express secondary emotions instead of primary emotions, as discussed earlier. Expressing secondary emotions usually leads to misunderstanding and invalidation (see Figure 20.1).

For example, Tracey decided she wanted to take Tim out for a date on their 1-year anniversary. She asked him to be home by 6:00 P.M. to make their reservation, and he agreed. However, on the way home, Tim got stuck in snarled traffic and had accidentally left his cell phone at the office. While Tracey was waiting at home for him, she became very worried, wondering where Tim was. After an hour, she assumed that Tim had forgotten about their date and had gone to the gym after work instead—something that he did regularly. She decided that was probably why he was not at the office and not answering his cell phone. By the time Tim arrived home at 7:15, Tracey was very angry. When he walked in the house, excited to see her and feeling bad he was late for their dinner, Tracey met him with a grimace and a biting remark about him being "selfish" and that she "can't count on him for anything." Tim then became defensive and the argument escalated from there. However, if Tracey had simply noticed and described the situation, without attaching judgments, she could have more effectively and accurately expressed to Tim that she had been very worried and concerned because he was not home when he said he would be, and disappointed that they had missed their date. Tim would likely have validated her disappointment and been able to soothe her, along with explaining what had actually happened. They probably would have gone on their date, just a bit later, and had a pleasant time.

The second way partners inaccurately express their emotions is by overvaluing or undervaluing the importance of a topic and of their feelings about it. A person who makes negative self-judgments often undervalues him- or herself and what he or she wants by downplaying the importance of the topic or his or her feelings about it, so that the partner may be unable to know or to understand its significance. On the other hand, people sometimes overvalue or overstate the importance of matters out of fear that their partners will not take their desires seriously. However, if a person presents too many issues as being of maximum importance, it is difficult for the partner to know what really is relatively more important to that person.

It is also important for clients to learn how to match their goals with an effective strategy to help them accurately express emotions. If the goal is to "sort out feelings," the strategy would be to describe both the situation and reactions to it. If the goal is to communicate, the strategy would be to use mindfulness to describe emotions, wants, and opinions. If the goal is to get the other person to change, the strategy would be to describe the situation or problem mindfully, to express clearly what one desires, and to work collaboratively on a solution to support and encourage each other. If the goal is to support the partner, one should validate him or her on multiple levels. Finally, if the goal is to correct an injustice, the goal would be to describe the situation, the emotions surrounding the situation, then negotiate possible solutions. All of these skills and strategies aid accurate expression, which in turn allows partners to validate each other's emotions and experiences.

Validation

"Validation" is identifying and clearly communicating one's understanding and acceptance of another's feeling, thoughts, behavior, or experiences. Validation is not appeasement, advice, or agreement. It simply conveys that one accepts and understands the experiences of the partner. Validation helps couples to encourage accurate emotional expression, to build trust, to reduce negative emotional arousal, and to make difficult situations and discussions tolerable. There are several different ways to validate a partner verbally (Fruzzetti, 2006; Fruzzetti & Iverson, 2006; Fruzzetti et al., 2007): (1) simply paying attention and actively listening (relationship mindfulness, therefore, is also often validating); (2) acknowledging the other's feelings or desires descriptively (nonjudgmentally); (3) asking questions about the partner's perspective or experience to seek clarification; (4) understanding mistakes and problems narrowly, in the context of the partner's life given his or her history and experiences (i.e., we are defined by a good deal more than our mistakes); (5) normalizing the partner's experience, trying to understand how his or her feelings or desires make perfect sense (i.e., "Wouldn't almost anyone feel that way in that situation?"); (6) being genuine by treating the partner as an equal, with respect and care (not as fragile, nor as incompetent or unworthy); and (7) self-disclosing one's own vulnerability to match the other's vulnerability.

There also are ways to validate one's partner nonverbally, for example, by (1) responding to the partner in a way that takes him or her seriously (e.g., if one partner wants company, the other may join him or her in an activity to validate this desire); and (2) providing support and nurturance, asking oneself, "How would I want to be treated in this situation?" By using mindfulness, relationship mindfulness, accurate expression, and validation skills, the couple is likely to experience enhanced satisfaction and likely reduce much potential conflict. In addition, these skills make it possible for partners to engage in problem solving and problem management.

Problem Management Skills

Now that couples have learned skills to communicate effectively, it is important for them to learn skills to effectively manage difficult problems that are not easily resolved. There are some problems for which there are no obvious solutions, and many times it is necessary for partners simply to accept their situations for now, realizing that it may not be currently solvable. This acceptance, is referred to as "radical acceptance," involves not trying to change the other partner's behavior, tolerating one's own disappointment (including letting go of judgments and anger), and accepting the fact that the problem behavior may continue to be bothersome.

However, when change does seem to be a feasible option, several skills are involved in negotiating solutions. These steps include (1) focusing on one conflict at a time; (2) brainstorming possible solutions; (3) negotiating an agreement; (4) committing to an agreement; and (5) reevaluating the effectiveness of the agreement and modifying it as needed. Although these steps are similar to those found in more traditional behavioral approaches (e.g., Jacobson & Margolin, 1979), all these steps rest on the foundation of accurate expression and validation, and generation of a solution per se is not the goal. Rather, the goal is an improved relationship marked by closeness and understanding. Thus, accepting the existence of a problem and recognizing that it may, at least temporarily, be intractable can be as valuable an outcome as resolving the problem. This process helps partners work together to reach mutually satisfying decisions about how to handle problem situations. By approaching the situation skillfully, the conflict resolution process, which previously might have been emotionally volatile and difficult, can now be managed in an effective manner in which both partners communicate clearly, validate one another, and work together to solve a problem (or accept it as not currently solvable). Such improved processes ultimately play a large role in increasing closeness and intimacy between the partners.

Closeness and Intimacy

Clearly, spending mindful time together; being able to express emotions, desires, and thoughts accurately; and being validated help to foster closeness. However, when couples have encountered an excess of escalating conflict in their relationship they also have been hurt emotionally and are still sensitive to distancing and emotional separation. Effective conflict resolution can serve to bring partners closer together, but some problems just cannot be solved, or at least not at the moment. Thus, radical acceptance of undesirable situations or behaviors can not only be a solution to unsolvable conflict but also bring partners together.

Being able neither to solve nor to accept problems leads to frustration, bitterness, blame, judgments, and increased distance. If one partner will not, or cannot, accept a partner's behavior or a relationship situation that is not likely to change, the relationship will most likely continue to be plagued frustration and unhappiness. In situations in which problem behaviors are likely to be maintained, it can be helpful for clients to attempt to accept the behavior. The first step in acceptance is for one partner to stop putting energy into the attempt to change the other partner to get what he or she wants, because these efforts do not work. These types of behaviors include nagging, complaining, negative looks, and so forth. If the partner can successfully curtail these change-seeking behaviors for a period of time, it is likely that he or she will experience some disappointment simply because the situation is not what he or she wants.

To keep from getting stuck in disappointment, it is necessary for the partner to validate the disappointment (it makes sense to be disappointed when one does not get what one wants) and to soothe the pain. The partner needs to treat him- or herself kindly, often in ways similar to how he or she would treat others going through a sad or disappointing time, and then become active in the relationship again. Becoming active helps to distract the partner from his or her negative emotional experience and also helps to create more positive experiences.

Another approach to help clients learn to tolerate and accept one another involves having both partners keep a log of their attitudes and emotions after they "tolerate" a problem behavior. As partners begin learning to accept problem behaviors, they most likely continue to experience frustration toward each other. Each time a partner "tolerates" a problem behavior by not engaging in change-oriented behavior, that partner keeps a log of how he or she feels after the encounter, and how long these feelings of frustration lasted. This exercise helps partners to see how much time and energy their desire to change is costing them, and how little it works. It can help them to see more accurately the effort they expend thinking about the problem behavior, perhaps along with an enhanced awareness of other, more satisfying aspects of their lives that they are missing. The log helps partners weigh the costs and benefits of their habitual ways of trying to change each other.

As partners strive to accept one another's difficult behaviors, a few techniques can help them to engage more fully in life and accept one another. Recontextualizing the partner's problem behavior (understanding it in the context of the partner's life) may help a client to see the problem behavior in a different, more beneficial way. Focusing on the "bigger picture," and on what they like about each other, may help partners accept, understand, and even appreciate the problem behavior.

Couples can also benefit when each partner finds legitimate, alternative meanings for the other behavior. This strategy is similar in some ways to "reframing" a problem but involves considerable mindful attention to the reframe. By carefully looking at each other's lives, histories, and experiences, partners are better able to understand why they act the way they do. This approach is very similar to finding things to validate about the partner and his or her behaviors. Although partners may not like certain behaviors, if they are better able to understand why they occur, then it is easier to accept them.

Often couples in distressed relationships experience increased amounts of misunderstanding and become judgmental. To increase intimacy and mutual acceptance, partners can benefit from "minding the gaps" in their relationship and in their closeness. When partners experience gaps in the understanding of one another, faulty assumptions and judgments often follow. If partners can learn not to reach conclusions too quickly and not to make judgments about each other, they can be curious, interested, or confused instead of angry and attacking.

OTHER TREATMENT STRATEGIES

Several additional treatment strategies employed in DBT with couples are typically used throughout the treatment process, in every phase and type of session, so they constitute important components of the therapist's repertoire.

Therapist Mindfulness

In part because mindfulness and relationship mindfulness are core skills for clients, it is also important for therapists to adopt a mindful, nonjudgmental stance and actively practice from this perspective. This is important in part because many people respond to partners who display extreme reactivity in invalidating ways, and this only exacerbates their difficulties. In addition, maintaining a nonjudgmental perspective promotes collaboration with both partners, and models acceptance (personifying the treatment, in a sense). Having an effective consultation team (discussed below) facilitates achieving and maintaining a mindful approach, because colleagues are also committed to understanding and accepting, rather than blaming, clients for their difficulties.

In addition, clients with BPD and related problems sometimes engage in extreme behavior that can frustrate their therapists (as well as their partners), even pushing them to react countertherapeutically. Suicide attempts, nonsuicidal self-injury, substance abuse, extreme expressions of anger or shame, and other impulsive behaviors can be taxing. By consistently practicing mindfulness, the therapist is able to focus on assessing, understanding, and validating (the valid parts) rather than distancing, criticizing, blaming, or threatening when challenging situations come along. Mindfulness leads to understanding and acceptance, then to validation, which helps

to deescalate mutual negative emotional arousal. This deescalation in turn promotes effective therapeutic interventions and minimizes dropouts and treatment failures.

Skills Generalization

As described earlier, there are many skills for partners to learn in this approach. Skill training is always done in session. Unfortunately, at least in some ways, clients' arousal in session is often much lower than it is in difficult situations *in vivo*. Thus, being able to transfer (i.e., generalize) the skills learned in therapy to difficult situations at home requires direct and sustained efforts.

Fortunately, after completing several detailed chain analyses, the therapist is likely to have a good sense of the situations (both the interpersonal context and the level of emotional arousal present) in which skills are needed. Thus, the therapist may engage in many different types of rehearsal with one or both clients in anticipation of difficult situations at home. Similarly, the therapist may assign homework for partners to continue to practice or rehearse at home, but under slightly lower arousal conditions, thereby enabling partners to become more and more skillful and better able to use the new, more skillful approach, even when the conversation or situation feels provocative.

In addition, the therapist may make him- or herself available by telephone between sessions for quick (e.g., 5-minute) "coaching" calls. In these kinds of phone calls, the therapist may remind the partner (or both partners in a three-way call) what he or she has been practicing and is committed to doing differently, and may offer support and "cheerleading."

Dialectical Strategies

Although many parts of the treatment include one or more dialectical elements, there are additional ways the therapist can provide the treatment dialectically (Fruzzetti & Fruzzetti, 2003b). For example, the therapist can practice thinking dialectically. This might involve noticing every time he or she is pushing for change, and balancing that by offering acceptance as an equally acceptable goal (and vice versa). The therapist can model "both–and" rather than "either–or" thinking (e.g., "Both George and Martha have legitimate points in different ways" rather than "Either it happened the way he says or the way she says"). And, when stuck, by asking "What are we missing?" the therapist can look for imbalances or polarizations (transforming acceptance vs. change, intimacy vs. autonomy, emotion vs. rationality, pros vs. cons, into both–and rather than either–or perspectives) and try to depolarize and synthesize both partners into a more useful stance.

In addition, the therapist can vary his or her communication style, demonstrating at times a warm, supportive, accepting, and/or reverent approach, and at other times a more confrontative, matter-of-fact, change-oriented, and/or irreverent approach (Linehan, 1993a).

Session Management Strategies

Sessions with reactive partners can sometimes be a challenge to manage effectively. Consequently, being able to utilize the dialectical strategies just described in the service of managing the session is important. For example, the therapist must be able to block partners from escalation of emotion when needed, while continuing to validate why that escalation urge makes sense. Similarly, the therapist must be able to invalidate the invalid actions partners take, while simultaneously finding other aspects of the same behavior to validate. For example, one partner may perceive that the other is lying to make him or her feel bad or look bad to the therapist, and may loudly and destructively express a lot of anger about this. The other partner may simply be describing his or her beliefs, perhaps in an unmindful and selectively descriptive way (but without lying or intentionally trying to distort the story). The therapist may need to separate the partners (briefly, or perhaps even for the rest of the session), and find genuine ways to validate each person's experience and perspective, while also making it clear that destructive behavior and selective reporting are damaging and not acceptable.

Sometimes one or both partners may become too aroused about a particular topic to participate effectively. In these circumstances, separating partners for part of a session or even for several sessions, so that they spend individual time with therapist, may be useful. When arousal is too high, people feel out of control, and their ability to remember or learn new things is reduced. Thus, it may be counterproductive to try to "push through" when arousal has risen to a particular level. These situations include the following:

1. One or both partners' affect is too high to be useful, the usual "traffic control" strategies are not working, and each partner is at that mo-

ment a trigger for the other's escalating arousal.

2. One partner, who is trying and practicing new approaches to the couple interaction but is not yet very skillful, is talking about the other partner in rather negative ways; in this situation, the criticized partner is spared the bludgeoning, and the practicing partner is spared being "reined in" publicly by the therapist.

3. Sometimes the therapist wants to push a client very hard to change something but not humiliate him or her in front of the partner or give the other partner "ammunition" with which to criticize later.

4. Conversely, the therapist may want to validate one partner's experiences quite strongly (e.g., sadness, fear, hopelessness, etc., following an episode of individual dysfunction, such as self-harm by the partner), without eliciting further shame or defensiveness on the part of the other partner.

Team Consultation

It should be clear by now that a great deal of "balancing" work is done with highly reactive partners. It may be impossible to do what is needed, staying emotionally balanced and nonjudgmental, in isolation. A treatment team in DBT is essential both to help therapists continue to improve their own skills and to apply skills effectively in often difficult (and sometimes novel) situations, and to help provide emotional support to reduce stress and burnout (Fruzzetti, Waltz, & Linehan, 1997). When working with couples with a BPD member or similar problems, a treatment or consultation team should meet between sessions. In these meetings, the therapists accept a dialectical approach and commit to practicing mindfully, both with clients and with each other. Thus, in this emotionally supportive environment, each therapist can seek consultation, learning how to improve his or her therapeutic repertoire, while simultaneously receiving support and validation, and allaying stress and burnout.

CONCLUSIONS

This chapter has provided an overview of some of the problems of couples in which at least one partner has BPD or related difficulties, and how these problems make couple therapy challenging, but also how these difficulties are common to many other distressed couples. By providing a conceptualization that leads to compassion and understanding, the therapist may be able to communicate this acceptance by validating, and balance acceptance with efforts to help partners change in important ways. The treatment target hierarchy was detailed, as were the skills and strategies needed to help partners regulate their emotions, reduce their destructive behaviors, express themselves more accurately, validate each other, and thus generate more peace and intimacy in their relationship.

SUGGESTIONS FOR FURTHER READING

Fruzzetti, A. E. (2006). *The high conflict couple: A dialectical behavior therapy guide to finding peace, intimacy, and validation.* Oakland, CA: New Harbinger Press.— This book provides a step-by-step guide for both couples and therapists about how to manage emotions in order to improve couple interactions and increase satisfaction.

Fruzzetti, A. E., & Iverson, K. M. (2006). Intervening with couples and families to treat emotion dysregulation and psychopathology. In D. K. Snyder, J. Simpson, & J. Hughes (Eds.), *Emotion regulation in couples and families: Pathways to dysfunction and health* (pp. 249–267). Washington, DC: American Psychological Association.—This chapter highlights the small steps involved in regulating emotion, how they can quickly be dysregulated as a result of lack of emotion management skills and invalidating social and family responses, and some of the interventions to improve the process.

Fruzzetti, A. E., Santisteban, D., & Hoffman, P. D. (2007). Dialectical behavior therapy for families. In L. Dimeff & K. Koerner (Eds.), *Adaptations of dialectical behavior therapy* (pp. 222–244). New York: Guilford Press.—This chapter describes different applications of DBT with couples, parents, and families across a variety of settings, and may be useful in particular to therapists knowledgeable about DBT.

Fruzzetti, A. E., Shenk, C., & Hoffman, P. D. (2005). Family interaction and the development of borderline personality disorder: A transactional model. *Development and Psychopathology, 17,* 1007–1030.—This article looks in detail at different ways to understand the development of BPD, with emphasis on a transactional model that includes both individual vulnerabilities and invalidating family responses.

REFERENCES

Bateman, A., & Fonagy, P. (2001). Treatment of borderline personality disorder with psychoanalytically oriented partial hospitalization: An 18-month follow-up. *American Journal of Psychiatry, 158,* 36–42.

Fruzzetti, A. E. (1996). Causes and consequences: Individual distress in the context of couple interactions. *Journal of Consulting and Clinical Psychology, 64,* 1192–1201.

Fruzzetti, A. E. (2002). Dialectical behavior therapy for borderline personality and related disorders. In T. Patterson (Ed.), *Comprehensive handbook of psychotherapy: Vol. 2. Cognitive-behavioral approaches* (pp. 215–240). New York: Wiley.

Fruzzetti, A. E. (2006). *The high conflict couple: A dialectical behavior therapy guide to finding peace, intimacy, and validation.* Oakland, CA: New Harbinger Press.

Fruzzetti, A. E., & Fruzzetti, A. R. (2003a). Borderline personality disorder. In D. Snyder & M. A. Whisman (Eds.), *Treating difficult couples: Helping clients with coexisting mental and relationship disorders* (pp. 235–260). New York: Guilford Press.

Fruzzetti, A. E., & Iverson, K. M. (2004). Mindfulness, acceptance, validation and "individual" psychopathology in couples. In S. C. Hayes, V. M. Follette, & M. M. Linehan (Eds.), *Mindfulness and acceptance: Expanding the cognitive-behavioral tradition* (pp. 168–191). New York: Guilford Press.

Fruzzetti, A. E., & Iverson, K. M. (2006). Intervening with couples and families to treat emotion dysregulation and psychopathology. In D. K. Snyder, J. Simpson, & J. Hughes (Eds.), *Emotion regulation in couples and families: Pathways to dysfunction and health* (pp. 249–267). Washington, DC: American Psychological Association.

Fruzzetti, A. E., & Jacobson, N. S. (1990). Toward a behavioral conceptualization of adult intimacy: Implications for marital therapy. In E. Blechman (Ed.), *Emotions and the family: For better or for worse* (pp. 117–135). Hillsdale, NJ: Erlbaum.

Fruzzetti, A. E., & Jacobson, N. S. (1992). Couple assessment. In J. C. Rosen & P. McReynolds (Eds.), *Advances in psychological assessment* (Vol. 8, pp. 201–224). New York: Plenum Press.

Fruzzetti, A. E., & Levensky, E. R. (2000). Dialectical behavior therapy with batterers: Rationale and procedures. *Cognitive and Behavioral Practice, 7,* 435–447.

Fruzzetti, A. E., & Mosco, E. (2007). *Dialectical behavior therapy adapted for couples and families: A pilot group intervention for couples.* Unpublished manuscript, University of Nevada, Reno.

Fruzzetti, A. E., Santisteban, D., & Hoffman, P. D. (2007). Dialectical behavior therapy with families. To appear in L. Dimeff & K. Koerner (Eds.), *Dialectical behavior therapy in clinical practice* (pp. 222–244). New York: Guilford Press.

Fruzzetti, A. E., Shenk, C., & Hoffman, P. D. (2005). Family interaction and the development of borderline personality disorder: A transactional model. *Development and Psychopathology, 17,* 1007–1030.

Fruzzetti, A. E., Waltz, J. A., & Linehan, M. M. (1997). Supervision in dialectical behavior therapy. In C. E. Watkins, Jr. (Ed.), *Handbook of psychotherapy supervision* (pp. 84–100). New York: Wiley.

Fruzzetti, A. R., & Fruzzetti, A. E. (2003b). Dialectics in cognitive and behavior therapy. In W. T. O'Donohue, J. E. Fisher, & S. C. Hayes (Eds.), *Cognitive behavior therapy: Applying empirically supported techniques in your practice* (pp. 121–128). New York: Wiley.

Giesen-Bloo, J., van Dyck, R., Spinhoven, P., van Tilburg, W., Dirksen, C., van Asselt, T., et al. (2006). Outpatient psychotherapy for borderline personality disorder: Randomized trial of schema-focused therapy vs. transference-focused psychotherapy. *Archives of General Psychiatry, 63*, 649–658.

Greenberg, L. S., & Johnson, S. M. (1988). *Emotionally focused therapy for couples.* New York: Guilford Press.

Greenberg, L. S., & Johnson, S. M. (1990). Emotional change processes in couples therapy. In E. Blechman (Ed.), *Emotions and the family: For better or for worse* (pp. 137–153). Hillsdale, NJ: Erlbaum.

Gunderson, J. G., & Hoffman, P. D. (Eds.). (2005). *Understanding and treating borderline personality disorder: A guide for professionals and families.* Washington, DC: American Psychiatric Publishing.

Hoffman, P. D., Buteau, E., & Fruzzetti, A. E. (2007). Borderline personality disorder: NEO-Personality Inventory ratings of patients and their family members. *International Journal of Social Psychiatry, 53*, 204–215.

Hoffman, P. D., Buteau, E., Hooley, J. M., Fruzzetti, A. E., & Bruce, M. L. (2003). Family members' knowledge about borderline personality disorder: Correspondence with their levels of depression, burden, distress, and expressed emotion. *Family Process, 42*, 469–478.

Hoffman, P. D., & Fruzzetti, A. E. (2005). Psychoeducation. In J. M. Oldham, A. Skodal, & D. Bender (Eds.), *Textbook of personality disorders* (pp. 375–385). Washington, DC: American Psychiatric Publishing.

Hoffman, P. D., Fruzzetti, A. E., & Buteau, E. (2007). Understanding and engaging families: An education, skills and support program for relatives impacted by borderline personality disorder. *Journal of Mental Health, 16*, 69–82.

Hoffman, P. D., Fruzzetti, A. E., Buteau, E., Penney, D., Neiditch, E., Penney, D., et al. (2005). Family connections: Effectiveness of a program for relatives of persons with borderline personality disorder. *Family Process, 44*, 217–225.

Jacobson, N. S., & Christensen, A. (1996). *Acceptance and change in couple therapy: A therapist's guide to transforming relationships.* New York: Norton.

Jacobson, N. S., & Margolin, G. (1979). *Marital therapy: Strategies based on social learning and behavior exchange principles.* New York: Brunner/Mazel.

Linehan, M. (1993a). *Cognitive-behavioral treatment of borderline personality disorder.* New York: Guilford Press.

Linehan, M. (1993b). *Skills training manual for treating borderline personality disorder.* New York: Guilford Press.

Linehan, M. M. (1997). Validation and psychotherapy. In A. Bohart & L. S. Greenberg (Eds.), *Empathy and psychotherapy: New directions to theory, research, and practice* (pp. 353–392). Washington, DC: American Psychological Association.

Nhat Hanh, T. (1975). *The miracle of mindfulness: A manual on meditation.* Boston: Beacon Press.

Robins, C. J., & Chapman, A. L. (2004). Dialectical behavior therapy: Current status, recent developments, and future directions. *Journal of Personality Disorders, 18*, 73–89.

Straus, M. A., Hamby, S. L., Boney-McCoy, S., & Sugarman, D. B. (1996). The revised Conflict Tactics Scales (CTS2): Development and preliminary psychometric data. *Journal of Family Issues, 17*, 283–316.

Zanarini, M. C., Frankenburg, F. R., Hennen, J., & Silk, K. R. (2004). Mental health service utilization by borderline personality disorder patients and Axis II comparison subjects followed prospectively for 6 years. *Journal of Clinical Psychiatry, 65*, 28–36.

CHAPTER 21

Couple Therapy and the Treatment of Sexual Dysfunction

BARRY W. MCCARTHY
MARIA THESTRUP

BACKGROUND

Masters and Johnson (1970) were the founders of modern couple sex therapy. Their 2-week intensive, male–female cotherapy team model is almost extinct, but two of their concepts form the essence of contemporary sex therapy. First, sexual dysfunction is best conceptualized, assessed, and treated as a couple issue. Second, sexual comfort, skills, and functioning can be learned. A crucial third concept in modern sex therapy is the psychobiosocial approach to understanding, assessing, and treating sexual dysfunction (Metz & McCarthy, 2007a). Sexual exercises are the preferred modality for helping couples develop a comfortable and functional sexual style. Sexual exercises (McCarthy & McCarthy, 2002; Wincze & Barlow, 1996) have been greatly expanded from the original sensate focus format to include exercises involving bridges to sexual desire, nondemand pleasuring, and erotic scenarios, as well as exercises for specific male and female sexual dysfunctions.

Although the culture, especially the mass media, is saturated and obsessed with stories of great sexual performance and ultimate ecstasy, the reality is that rates of sexual dysfunction, dissatisfaction, and trauma continue to be high (Laumann,

Gagnon, Michael, & Michaels, 1994). There has been significant growth in theoretical and clinical knowledge in the sexuality field, although the research base remains weak. A classification of sexual dysfunctions and disorders is included in the *Diagnostic and Statistical Manual of Mental Disorders* (American Psychiatric Association, 1994). However, the classification system is based on individual dysfunction and does not incorporate a relational diagnosis (Aubin & Heiman, 2004).

Models of Sexual Function and Dysfunction

Sexual dysfunctions are classified according to the triphasic model proposed by Kaplan (1974)—disorders of desire, arousal, and orgasm. The most common clinical complaints involve desire disorders, a category that was not considered in the original Masters and Johnson model. In the 1970s, "primary sexual dysfunction" predominated (i.e., a person has never been sexually functional). An example of primary sexual dysfunction is premature ejaculation, in which the man has always ejaculated prematurely. In the past 30 years, "secondary sexual dysfunction" has increased (i.e., a person was functional but is now dysfunctional). For example, a woman was previously orgasmic during partner sex but is now nonorgasmic. For both men and women, a common sexual dysfunction is secondary hypoactive sexual desire disorder.

Traditional causes of sexual dysfunction were lack of information, repressive attitudes, high anxiety, lack of sexual skills, and rigid sexual roles. Sexuality is best understood as a multicausal, multidimensional phenomenon with psychological, biological, relational, and cultural components (Leiblum, 2007). Rates of dysfunction and dissatisfaction remain high, but their causes and types have changed significantly. With the growth of sexuality courses and self-help books, lack of knowledge has been alleviated. Unfortunately, it has been replaced by unrealistic expectations and performance demands. The importance of sexuality for couple and life satisfaction is often overemphasized, resulting in confusion, dissatisfaction, and performance anxiety. The cultural milieu has gone from one extreme (repression, rigidity, lack of information and communication) to the other (sexual overload, confusion, intimidation about one's body and sexual performance, and emphasis on medical interventions, especially for male sexuality). There have been significant cultural shifts in the frequency of premarital sex, increases in sexually transmitted diseases, the HIV/AIDS epidemic, high divorce rates, and heightened sensitivity to sexual trauma (especially child sexual abuse). These changes have led to a counterreaction from religious and conservative groups, especially the "family values" movement, which advocates for abstinence-only sex education, focusing on celibacy until marriage and absolute fidelity in marriage.

With the introduction of Viagra in 1998 (Goldstein et al., 1998), a paradigm shift occurred in the conceptualization of male sexuality. Tiefer (1996) warned against the "medicalization of male sexuality," but this perspective is gaining momentum in the treatment of not only erectile dysfunction but also premature ejaculation. The movement to medicalize female sexuality (Rosen, Philips, Gendrano, & Ferguson, 1999) is now growing although it faces a strong countermovement (Kaschak & Tiefer, 2001).

The traditional marital/couple therapy approach was to view sexual dysfunction as symptomatic of an unresolved relationship problem (e.g., poor communication, power imbalances, struggles with emotional intimacy, family-of-origin conflicts). The focus was on individual and couple dynamics, with the assumption that once these were

dealt with, sexual issues would take care of themselves or be resolved with minimal intervention. There is little empirical support for this position, especially when the dysfunction is anxiety-based, with psychosexual skills deficits and a chronic avoidance pattern.

The couple therapy field has not given sufficient attention to sexuality and sexual dysfunction. Few couple training programs have courses, practica, or internships that include sex therapy as an integral component. Couple theory, research, and practice emphasize sexual trauma, not sexual dysfunction or sex therapy. Some writers have advocated the integration of couple and sex therapy (McCarthy, Bodnar, & Handal, 2004; Weeks, 2004; Schnarch, 1991).

Couple sex therapy is best understood as a subspecialty field. The clinician—whether trained as a psychologist, social worker, psychiatrist, couple therapist, pastoral counselor, or psychiatric nurse—must possess skills in individual therapy; couple therapy; the assessment of individual, couple, and sexual factors; and the ability to develop and implement sexual interventions. Sex therapy involves comprehensive assessment and treatment, with attention to a wide range of psychological, physiological, relational, cultural, and psychosexual skills factors. Of central importance is the clinician's comfort with prescribing, processing, and individualizing sexual exercises.

Unfortunately, the sex therapy field is not growing. Among young clinicians it is shrinking, especially in comparison to couple therapy. Few clinicians choose sex therapy as their primary professional identity. There are a number of reasons for this: National sexuality organizations are struggling in terms of membership and resources; there is no licensing for sex therapists; few insurance companies reimburse for sex therapy; there are few graduate sex therapy programs; and there are few funding organizations or financial resources for sex research (with the exception of drug companies). In addition, the controversy surrounding sexual trauma (Rind, Tromovitch, & Bauserman, 1998), especially recovered memories of sexual abuse, has made the field suspect, and less scientifically and professionally respected. Both the professional and the public look to medical interventions as a first-line therapy, particularly for erectile dysfunction and premature ejaculation.

The number of couples with sexual dysfunction or dissatisfaction has not decreased; if anything, it has increased. Of special concern is the nonsexual relationship. According to the criterion of being sexual fewer than 10 times a year, approximately 20% of married couples and 30% of unmarried couples who have been together at least 2 years have nonsexual relationships (Michael, Gagnon, Laumann, & Kolata, 1994).

Couples often find motivating a perspective that when sexuality goes well, it is a positive, integral component of a relationship, but not a major factor. A common clinical adage is that sexuality contributes 15–20% to a marriage, serving as a shared pleasure, a means to reinforce intimacy, and a tension reducer to deal with the stresses of life and marriage. Sexuality energizes the marital bond, facilitates special couple feelings, and allows each spouse to feel desired and desirable. When sexuality is dysfunctional or nonexistent, it plays an inordinately powerful role, perhaps 50–75%, draining the marriage of vitality and intimacy (McCarthy, 1997). Paradoxically, bad sex plays a more powerful negative role than good sex plays a positive role in a marriage. The most commonly cited reasons couples separate within the first 2 years of marriage (whether a first or second marriage) are fertility issues (e.g., unwanted pregnancy or infertility), an extramarital affair, or a sexual dysfunction—especially hypoactive sexual desire disorder.

ASSESSMENT IN COUPLE SEX THERAPY

History Taking

The primary assessment method in couple sex therapy is the semistructured sexual history (Risen, 2007). The protocol is a conjoint initial session that enables the therapist to assess the couple's motivation and appropriateness for sex therapy; to explore the sexual problem in the context of the relationship; to understand past attempts at resolution of the sexual problem and coexisting problems; to decide whether to conduct individual, couple, or sex therapy; to opt whether to use sex-enhancing medications; to explore medical problems (including side effects of medications); to decide whether there is a need to consult a urologist, gynecologist, psychiatrist, or endocrinologist; and to answer questions about the process of sex therapy. Sexual histories are conducted individually to obtain a clear, uncensored review of each partner's psychological, relational, and sexual development, as well as his or her attitudes toward, feelings about, and experiences with the partner. At the beginning of the session, the therapist tells the client,

"I want to know as much as possible about both the strengths and vulnerabilities in your sexual development and in this relationship. I ask you to be as frank and forthcoming as possible. At the end, I will ask whether there are sensitive or secret areas you do not want to share with your partner. I will respect your decision and not share information without your permission, but I need to understand as much as possible about you and your relationship if I'm going to be helpful."

The rationale for this format is that at least 50% of individuals (probably as many as 75–80%) have sensitive or secret material, either about the past or the present, that they would not have the courage to disclose in front of their partner. Without access to this material, the clinician might inadvertently enter into a sham therapy contract. The ideal scenario is for the client to give the clinician permission to share the material in the couple feedback session. It is then therapeutically integrated into a new, genuine individual and couple narrative. This is the most common outcome. If the sensitive/secret material would substantively undermine couple therapy and permission to disclose was not given, the clinician might suggest a therapeutic approach other than couple sex therapy.

The history taking follows a semistructured, chronological format, moving from general, less anxiety-provoking material to sensitive and anxiety-provoking issues. Open-ended questions are utilized. The clinician is supportive and nonjudgmental; he or she follows up and probes to elicit attitudes, experiences, feelings, and values. The goal is to understand fully the person's psychological, relational, and sexual history, including both strengths and vulnerabilities.

The first question—"How did you learn about sex and sexuality?"—allows exploration of formal education; religious background; parents as sex educators, and as marital and sexual models; as well as sexual experiences with siblings, neighborhood children, friends, and others. Social and sexual experiences as a child are addressed, including self-exploration/masturbation, comfort with body and gender, and sexual experimentation. Age and reaction to the first orgasmic experience (by oneself or with a partner) is explored.

The format of the questions facilitates disclosure. Yes–no questions are not used. Open-ended questions with the expectation of "yes" responses are utilized (e.g., "How and when did you begin self-exploration/masturbation—what were your feelings and reactions?"). This format is used to explore sexual experiences with members of the same sex, as well as extramarital affairs (e.g., "People often have sexual feelings, fantasies, and experiences with someone of the same sex. What have been your experiences?"). If the person has not masturbated, had same-sex experiences, or had extramarital affairs, it is easy to say "no."

A particularly important issue to explore is negative sexual experiences, including trauma. Once the client's age when he or she left home is established, the therapist asks, "As you review your childhood and adolescence, what was your most negative, confusing, guilt-inducing, or traumatic experience?" Toward the end of the history taking, the therapist asks about the most negative or traumatic sexual experience in the client's life. Although the therapist has spent 50–90 minutes reviewing the entire sexual history, as many as 25% of clients disclose significant new information. The therapist explores the client's cognitions and feelings both at the time of the traumatic incident and in retrospect. Especially crucial is whether traumatized clients see themselves as survivors or as victims (McCarthy & Sypeck, 2003).

A crucial assessment topic is that of past or current medical illnesses and medications. Sexuality involves physiological, as well as psychological and relational, factors. Ideally, the nonmedical therapist will have a consultative relationship with a sexual medicine subspecialist. Often one or both members of a couple have consulted a family practitioner, internist, gynecologist, urologist, psychiatrist, or endocrinologist. It is important to be aware of both partners' health and illness status, especially side effects of medications. There is substantial literature on the sexual side effects of antidepressant medications and strategies to reduce side effects (Ashton, 2007). Other psychiatric drugs, antihypertensive medications, and a number of other medications have been implicated in sexual dysfunction (Segreaves & Balon, 2003). With the introduction of Viagra in 1998, the use of sexual pharmacology for the treatment of male sexual dysfunction has dramatically increased. The potential benefits and pitfalls of medical interventions are discussed later in this chapter.

Couple Feedback Session: The Core Sex Therapy Intervention

The couple feedback session is a powerful method to promote understanding, increase motivation, and set the stage for change. It is scheduled as a 90-minute, or double, session with a threefold

focus: (1) establishing a new understanding of the problem, with a new individual and couple narrative that includes positive, realistic expectations; (2) outlining a change strategy that involves individual, couple, and sexual components; and (3) assigning the first exercise, with a specific plan for its implementation. The clinician gives feedback about each person's sexual development, noting strengths and vulnerabilities. The fundamental concept—each person is responsible for his or her sexuality, and the couple is an intimate team—is made personal and concrete.

The feedback session focuses and motivates the couple. It sets the stage for thinking of therapy as an integrated assessment/intervention program. Reactions to exercises, both positive and negative, provide crucial diagnostic information. For example, if nongenital pleasuring builds comfort with sensual touching and initiates turn taking, openness to the giver–recipient format, and utilization of feedback, but the process falls apart with the addition of genital pleasuring, the clinician becomes aware of one type of vulnerability (trap). If another couple does well as long as the woman is the initiator of the exercise and recipient of pleasure, but cannot function when the man is the recipient, or the man is too passive to be the initiator, the clinician explores a different type of vulnerability. Sexual exercises have both a diagnostic and an intervention function. Exercises provide feedback to address anxieties and inhibitions. Processing exercises allows the clinician and couple to individualize and refine subsequent interventions and exercises. Anxieties and vulnerabilities are addressed, with a focus on increasing sexual awareness, comfort, and psychosexual skills.

Many couples find the metaphor of building a sexual house helpful. The foundation of the house comprises trust, intimacy, awareness, and comfort. With nongenital and genital pleasuring, and the addition of erotic scenarios and techniques, they build on this foundation to establish a functional, satisfying couple sexual style.

THE PROCESS OF SEX THERAPY

The sex therapy format begins with weekly sessions, with the couple engaging in two to three homework exercises between sessions. The prime focus is on psychosexual skills exercises but may also include reading, discussion, and watching psychoeducational videotapes involving pleasuring, eroticism, or a specific dysfunction. The exercises follow a semistructured format (McCarthy & Mc-

Carthy, 2002) that is modified and individualized as the couple progresses. This format continues with exercises for the specific dysfunction. Exercises are refined and individualized as a result of the partners' experiences and their feedback to the therapist.

A core theme of sex therapy, in contrast to general couple therapy, is the focus on sexual attitudes, behavior, and feelings. Unlike other problems (e.g., dealing with emotional conflict, parenting, money), the therapist never directly observes the behavior; the partners never do anything sexual in the therapist's office or in front of the therapist. The code of ethics of the American Association of Sex Educators, Counselors, and Therapists (2004) specifically prohibits sexual interaction between a therapist and client.

Assigning, processing, and designing sexual exercises are core skills in sex therapy. Marital/couple therapists are usually more comfortable exploring feelings, family-of-origin dynamics, attitudes and values, and the context of couple intimacy than focusing on sexual behavior, with attendant feelings of anxiety, aversion, or eroticism. The primary goal of sex therapy is to establish a comfortable, functional couple sexual style, which means that each person is capable of experiencing desire, arousal, orgasm, and emotional satisfaction. Unless the clinician is willing and able to structure therapy to confront sexual problems directly and deal with anxieties, inhibitions, and/or skills deficits, the goal of developing a couple sexual style will probably not be achieved.

Therapy sessions are structured, especially at the beginning. The first agenda item is to discuss the previous week's experiences and exercises. The therapist emphasizes detailed processing, rather than asking whether the behavior occurred and accepting an overall evaluation. The therapy discussion involves a fine-grained analysis of initiation patterns, comfort levels, receptivity and responsivity to specific pleasuring techniques, interfering anxieties or inhibitions, and subjective and objective feelings of arousal. The therapist's own anxieties may center around a fear of appearing invasive or voyeuristic, eliciting erotic feelings or fantasies in the clients (or in him- or herself), and crossing ethical boundaries. Although these reactions do occur, there is no evidence that they are more likely to occur in sex therapy. Because of the therapist's heightened awareness of such matters, they may actually be less likely to occur. In processing sexual exercises, the clinician uses his or her best clinical judgment in eliciting a clear picture of progress and difficulties, so that therapy

is maximally effective. Therapist issues of boundaries, personal discomfort, or values are best dealt with in supervision with an experienced sex therapist.

Discussion of the coming week's exercises should not be left for the last 5 minutes, but should be integrated throughout the session. Individualizing exercises promotes sexual comfort, receptivity to sensual and erotic touching, and psychosexual skills and responsivity.

This process reinforces the one–two combination of personal responsibility for sexuality and being part of an intimate team. Each person is responsible for his or her desire, arousal, and orgasm; it is not the other partner's role to give him or her an orgasm. Sexuality is an interpersonal process. Ideally, the partners view each other as sexual friends, and one partner's arousal facilitates the other's arousal.

The sex therapist is active, especially in the early stages of therapy, and serves as a permission giver, sex educator, and advocate for intimate, erotic sexuality. As therapy progresses, structure and therapist activity decrease. The partners take increasing responsibility for processing experiences and feelings, creating their own agenda, moving to individualized and free-form sexual exercises, exploring personal and relational anxieties and vulnerabilities, and acknowledging strengths and valued characteristics. Therapy becomes less focused on psychosexual skills and focuses more on intimacy. The meanings of "intimacy" and "sexuality" are discussed, along with positive, realistic expectations. The challenge for couples, married or unmarried, straight or gay, is to integrate intimacy and eroticism into their relationship (Perel, 2006). The couple and the therapist collaborate in designing a relapse prevention program to maintain and generalize sexual gains.

The two most significant mistakes therapists make are (1) diverting the sexual focus and (2) prematurely terminating treatment when sex becomes functional. The therapist and couple may collude in avoidance because sexuality can be a sensitive and anxiety-provoking area, especially talking about erotic scenarios and techniques. Permission giving and providing relevant sexual information and sexual suggestions are helpful. However, dealing with specific inhibitions or avoidance—for instance, a man's fear of the "wax-and-wane" erection exercise (i.e., allowing the erection to subside, then resuming erotic stimulation to arousal and erection), or a woman's intimidation by the exercise to guide her partner's hand or mouth to increase eroticism—is therapeutically challenging.

It is essential that the clinician stay with the therapeutic strategy, process exercises, and maintain focus, without being invasive or voyeuristic. The line between facilitating sexual awareness/comfort and making the sexual situation clinical and self-conscious requires that the therapist be sensitive and skillful. Many clinicians and most clients would rather talk about nonsexual issues, such as conflicts with families of origin or the meaning of intimacy, than stay focused on sexual function and dysfunction. It requires clinical skill and judgment to decide when to stay sexually focused and when to switch the focus to other psychological or relational issues.

Learning to be sexually functional is easier than integrating sexual expression into the couple's life, particularly the ability to maintain gains and prevent relapse. Jacobson and Addis (1993) have reported high levels of relapse among couples in conjoint therapy, and there is every reason to believe that this applies to sexual dysfunction as well.

Ending therapy after the first sexually functional experience is not only premature, but it may also be iatrogenic. Even sexually functional couples occasionally have problems (about 5–15% of encounters) of dysfunction and dissatisfaction (Frank, Anderson, & Rubinstein, 1978). By its nature, couple sexuality involves variability in both function and satisfaction. The unrealistic expectation that each experience must include equal desire, arousal, orgasm, and satisfaction for both partners sets a performance demand that will inevitably lead to relapse.

An integral component of high-quality, comprehensive sex therapy is a relapse prevention program (McCarthy, 1999). Integration and relapse prevention involve acceptance of the role of touch and sexuality in the couple's everyday life. For example, how frequently do the partners express affection and sensuality, and is this valued in of itself or as a bridge to sexual arousal and intercourse? How important is sexual frequency, or is quality more important? How do they ensure that sexuality continues to play a 15–20% role in couple vitality and satisfaction? The key to maintaining therapeutic gains is positive, realistic (nonperfectionistic) expectations. Partners who accept a variable, flexible sexual style, and who realize it is normal to have occasional dysfunctional, unsatisfying, or mediocre experiences, will be inoculated against sexual problems associated with their own aging and that of the relationship. This is the focus of the "good enough sex" model (Metz & McCarthy, 2007a), in which intimacy is the ultimate focus, pleasure is as important as function, and mutual emotional acceptance serves as the couple context. Valuing variable, flexible sexual experiences (the "85% approach") and abandoning the "need" for perfect intercourse performance inoculates the couple against sexual dysfunction by overcoming performance pressure, fears of failure, and rejection. Good enough sex is congruent with the couple's genuine lifestyle and the couple values multiple purposes for sex and different desire and arousal styles.

COMMON SEXUAL DYSFUNCTIONS

Sexual dysfunction is more common among women than among men. The most common female dysfunctions are (1) hypoactive sexual desire disorder (HSDD), (2) nonorgasmic response during partner sex, (3) painful intercourse (dyspareunia), (4) female arousal dysfunction, (5) and primary nonorgasmic response. The most common male sexual dysfunctions are (1) premature ejaculation, (2) erectile dysfunction, (3) HSDD, and (4) ejaculatory inhibition.

The definition of "sexual function" is the ability to experience "desire" (positive anticipation and feel deserving of sexual pleasure), "arousal" (receptivity and responsivity to erotic touch, resulting in subjective arousal and lubrication for the woman and erection for the man), "orgasm" (a voluntary response that is a natural culmination of high arousal), and "satisfaction" (feeling emotionally and sexually fulfilled and bonded).

Sexual dysfunction often involves more than one problem and may be comorbid with a partner's dysfunction. The most common example of partner comorbidity is a male with secondary erectile dysfunction and hypoactive desire, and a female with primary hypoactive desire, and secondary arousal and orgasmic dysfunction. Dysfunction might not be constant, but it is predominant. For example, a woman with painful intercourse may have occasional comfortable experiences, or a male with ejaculatory inhibition may ejaculate intravaginally 30% of the time.

Female Sexual Dysfunction

Hypoactive Sexual Desire Disorder

Despite the number of books, chapters, and articles on HSDD (e.g., Basson, 2007; Hertlein, Weeks, & Gambescia, 2007; Kaplan, 1995), assessment and intervention strategies are not clear, and the outcome is often disappointing.

It had previously been assumed that if a woman has an orgasm, then everything is functional. However, a fine-grained analysis reveals that some women, though aroused and orgasmic once they are involved sexually, continue to experience low desire. The core components of desire are positive anticipation and a sense of deserving pleasure. Anticipation involves a number of factors—openness to touch, the presence of romantic or erotic thoughts and fantasies, emotional connection with her partner, a desire for orgasm, and responsiveness to the partner's desire. Contextual factors, such as an inviting milieu, a weekend away without children, or a romantic or fun night out, can facilitate anticipation.

The organizing therapeutic concept in dealing with HSDD is to have "his, her, and our bridges to sexual desire" (McCarthy, 1995). The initial romantic love/passionate sex desire found in premarital and extramarital sex does not maintain desire in ongoing relationships. Basson's (2000) breakthrough concept is "responsive female sexual desire" rather than the male model of desire—erotic fantasies and spontaneous erection. The responsive female sexual desire model posits that women are often neutral at first, but if open and receptive to touch and responsive either emotionally or physically to pleasure and sensuality (a subjective arousal level of 2 or 3), they then choose whether to experience desire and arousal.

Schnarch (1997) has challenged common therapy concepts regarding desire. He emphasizes the crucial role of individuation and autonomy in maintaining sexual desire. Schnarch also challenged the use of sexual exercises, believing that they promote an other-centered need for sexual validation, which subverts desire. Lobitz and Lobitz (1996) acknowledge the value of Schnarch's emphasis on autonomy but take this to the critical next step of being open to the partner's sexual feelings and preferences, and integrating these into the couple's sexual style. With integrated sexuality, each person's desire and arousal plays off that of the other. The major aphrodisiac is an involved, aroused partner. Use of sexual exercises in a mechanistic manner can be self-defeating. However, if the exercises are used in a manner that confronts avoidance and inhibitions, while facilitating the involvement of both partners in the process of giving and receiving pleasure, then they can be invaluable in the development of a positive, resilient couple sexual style. The desire exercises focus on

comfort, attraction, trust, and on partners designing their own sexual scenario (McCarthy & McCarthy, 2003).

Our culture idealizes spontaneous, nonverbal, intense erotic scenarios (the movie model). Such idealization creates unrealistic performance demands and expectations. Not surprisingly, marital sex is rarely shown in movies. Another unrealistic media theme is that both people are very turned on before touching. These scenarios make good entertainment but are poisonous for real-life couples.

One in three women complain of HSDD (Laumann, Rosen, & Paik, 1999); more than half of these complaints are secondary desire problems. With primary HSDD, the woman does not experience sexuality as a positive, integral part of her personhood. Primary desire problems can be caused by a number of factors—antisexual family learnings, poor body image, lack of experience with self-exploration/masturbation, childhood sexual trauma, fear of pregnancy or HIV/AIDS, a history of sexual humiliation or rejection, a fundamentalist religious background, or an antierotic value system.

The sexual history taking and processing of sexual exercises help to identify factors that inhibit desire. Common causes of secondary HSDD are disappointment or anger with the partner and negative sexual experiences (e.g., rape, unwanted pregnancy, painful intercourse, or being blamed for the partner's sexual dysfunction). Other possible causes include insufficient couple time, exhaustion due to child care, devaluation of marital sexuality, a belief that only intercourse counts as "sex," feeling pressured or coerced by her partner, feeling trapped in a boring sexual routine, fear of another pregnancy, and comparison of present sexual experiences with earlier experiences.

Couple exercises that can facilitate desire include building comfort with nudity and body image, taking turns initiating, identifying characteristics of the partner that the woman finds attractive, making one to three requests for change that increase attraction, establishing a trust/vulnerability position, identifying and playing out erotic scenarios, initiating erotic touching on a weekly basis, identifying external stimuli as turn-ons, utilizing role enactment arousal, and using a "veto" to stop an uncomfortable sexual experience (this is a crucial technique for persons with a history of sexual trauma).

A key concept in dealing with HSDD is that unless a woman feels she has the right to say "no" to sex, she is not able to say "yes" to sex. The therapy focuses on helping the woman learn to view her partner as an intimate, erotic friend who is aware of her needs and open to her requests. She needs to establish her "sexual voice." Female sexuality groups (Barbach, 1975), originally focused on teaching women to be orgasmic, have been expanded to deal with desire, arousal, and pain issues. The successful resolution of sexual dysfunction (e.g., learning to become aroused, orgasmic, or to eliminate pain) is of great value, but it is not enough. Orgasm alone does not build desire. Desire involves a complex interplay among cognitive, behavioral, emotional, and relational phenomena. Basson's (2007) integrative model of female sexual function and dysfunction, with its emphasis on responsive sexual desire, is of great value. Responsive sexual desire is equally important and valuable for male HSDD, especially for men over 50. The list of guidelines in Table 21.1, used for both males and females, is given to the couple as a handout.

Orgasmic Dysfunction

A common sexual complaint is that the woman is not orgasmic during intercourse. Typically, the man is more upset than the woman. He wants her to function the way he functions—to have one orgasm during intercourse without needing additional stimulation. This has traditionally been considered the "right" way to be orgasmic. In fact, one in three women who are regularly orgasmic with couple sex are not orgasmic during intercourse. This is not a dysfunction, but a normal variation in female sexual response. Female sexual response is more variable and complex than male sexual response. In truth, the majority of women who are orgasmic during intercourse use multiple stimulation, especially manual clitoral stimulation with the partner's fingers, her own fingers, or vibrator stimulation. A woman may be nonorgasmic, singly orgasmic, or multiorgasmic. Orgasms can occur with pleasuring/foreplay, during intercourse, or in afterplay. Feminist sexologists (e.g., Tiefer, 2004) have noted that concepts of sexual function and dysfunction are heavily influenced by the traditional male model, with a phallocentric obsession with intercourse as "real sex." The feminist sexual response model honors flexibility, variability, and individual differences in the meaning and experience of sexuality. Intimacy, pleasuring, playfulness, eroticism, manual–oral–rubbing stimulation, and erotic scenarios and techniques are in the normal range. Self-stimulation is encouraged during partner sex (Heiman & LoPiccolo, 1988). An example of the variability of female sexual response is that 15–20% of women have a multiorgasmic response pattern, most commonly with cunnilingus or manual stimulation.

As noted, being nonorgasmic during intercourse is a normal variation, not a dysfunction. Not being orgasmic at each sexual experience is also a normal variation. The therapist can set positive, realistic expectations about orgasmic response. An unrealistic performance demand of simultaneous orgasm during intercourse is self-defeating, as is belief that achieving orgasm during intercourse is the only "right" way to be sexual.

A positive, realistic expectation is that the woman develops a regular pattern of arousal and orgasm, with recognition of flexibility and variability. Dysfunction is the absence of orgasm by any means (primary nonorgasmic response), orgasmic response with self-stimulation but not partner sex, or infrequent orgasmic response (orgasm in fewer than 25% of experiences). Since the 1970s, there has been a decrease in primary nonorgasmic response due to increased awareness of female sexuality; the availability of female sexuality therapy groups and self-help books; increased use of vibrators, manual, and oral stimulation; and women taking a more active role in the sexual scenario. However, there has been an increase in secondary nonorgasmic response, partly due to performance demands and failure to incorporate the meaning and value of intimacy and eroticism in an ongoing relationship.

In assessing nonorgasmic response, several factors are crucial: the woman's attitudes toward sexuality and her body; awareness of her arousal–orgasm pattern; development of her "sexual voice"; awareness of what facilitates and inhibits desire and receptivity; inhibitions or resentments that interfere with responsivity and arousal; passivity; a history of sexual trauma; guilt over sexual secrets; and emotional and practical factors that block sexual expression. Orgasmic response is the natural culmination of comfort, pleasure, arousal, and erotic flow.

With secondary nonorgasmic response, it is crucial to assess carefully a wide range of personal, relational, physical, and situational factors that inhibit sexuality. Factors include side effects of medications (especially antidepressants); resentment toward or disappointment in the partner or the relationship; lack of time and energy due to competing demands from children, extended family, job, and house; feeling bored with a mechanical sexual

TABLE 21.1. Guidelines for Revitalizing and Maintaining Sexual Desire

1. The essential keys to sexual desire are positive anticipation and feeling that you deserve sexual pleasure in this relationship.

2. The change process is a one–two combination of personal responsibility and being an intimate team. Each person is responsible for his or her desire, with the couple functioning as an intimate team to nurture and enhance desire. Revitalizing sexual desire is a couple task. Guilt, blame, and pressure subvert the change process.

3. Inhibited desire is the most common sexual dysfunction, affecting two in five couples. Sexual power struggles and avoidance drain intimacy and vitality from the marital bond.

4. One in five married couples has a nonsexual relationship (being sexual less than 10 times a year). One in three nonmarried couples who have been together longer than 2 years has a nonsexual relationship.

5. The average frequency of sexual intercourse ranges from three times per week to once every 2 weeks. For couples in their 20s, the average sexual frequency is two to three times a week; for couples in their 50s, once a week.

6. The idealized romantic love/passionate sex type of desire lasts less than 2 years, and usually less than 6 months. Desire is facilitated by an intimate, interactive relationship.

7. Contrary to the myth that "horniness" occurs after not being sexual for weeks, desire is facilitated by a regular rhythm of sexual activity. When sex occurs less than twice a month, couples become self-conscious and fall into a cycle of anticipatory anxiety, tense and performance-oriented sex, and avoidance.

8. A key strategy is to develop "her," "his," and "our" bridges to sexual desire. This involves ways of thinking, talking, anticipating, and feeling that invite sexual encounters.

9. The essence of sexuality is giving and receiving pleasure-oriented touching. The prescription to maintaining desire is to integrate intimacy, pleasuring, and eroticism.

10. Touching occurs both inside and outside the bedroom. Touching is valued for itself. Both the man and woman are comfortable initiating. Touching should not always lead to intercourse. Both partners feel free to say "no" and to suggest an alternative way to connect and to share pleasure.

11. Couples who maintain a vital sexual relationship can use the touching metaphor that involves "five gears." First gear is clothes on, affectionate touch (holding hands, kissing, hugging). Second gear is nongenital, sensual touch, which can be clothed, semiclothed, or nude (whole-body massage, cuddling on the couch, touching while going to sleep or on awakening). Third gear is playful touch with intermixed genital and nongenital touching, clothed or unclothed, and may take place in bed, while dancing, in the shower, or on the couch. Fourth gear is erotic touch (manual, oral, or rubbing) to high arousal and orgasm for one or both partners. Fifth gear integrates pleasurable and erotic touch that flows into intercourse.

12. Personal turn-ons facilitate sexual anticipation and desire. These include the use of fantasy and favorite erotic scenarios, as well as sex associated with special celebrations or anniversaries, sex with the goal of conception, sex when feeling caring and close, or even sex to soothe a personal disappointment or loss.

13. External turn-ons (R- or X-rated videos, music, candles, visual feedback from mirrors, locations other than the bedroom, a weekend away from the kids) can elicit sexual desire.

14. Males and females with hormonal deficits may use testosterone injections, patches, or creams to enhance sexual desire, but only under medical supervision. Hormone replacement can be a positive resource but not a "stand-alone" intervention. The medical intervention needs to be integrated into the couple's sexual style of intimacy, pleasuring, and eroticism.

15. Medical problems and side effects of medication are a major cause of inhibited sexual desire. As a couple, consult your physician about medications and health behaviors.

16. Sexual desire is a psychobiosocial process. You need to use all of your psychological, physical, and emotional resources to promote openness to intimacy and sexuality.

17. Sexuality has a number of positive functions—a shared pleasure, a means to reinforce and deepen intimacy, and a tension reducer to deal with the stresses of life and marriage.

18. "Intimate coercion" is not acceptable. Sexuality is neither a reward nor a punishment. Healthy sexuality is voluntary, mutual, and pleasure-oriented.

19. Realistic expectations are crucial for maintaining a healthy sexual relationship. It is self-defeating to demand equal desire, orgasm, and satisfaction each time. A positive, realistic expectation is that 40–50% of experiences are very good for both partners; 20–25% are very good for one partner (usually the man) and fine for the other; 20–25% are acceptable but not remarkable; 5–15% of sexual experiences are dissatisfying or dysfunctional. Couples who accept occasional dissatisfaction or dysfunction without guilt or blaming and try again when they are receptive and responsive will have a vital, resilient sexual relationship. Satisfied couples use the guideline of "good enough" sex with positive, realistic expectations.

20. If the couple has gone 2 weeks without any sexual contact, the partner with the higher desire takes the initiative to set up a planned or spontaneous sexual date. If that does not occur, the other partner initiates a sensual or play date during the following week. If that does not occur and they have gone a month without sexual contact, they schedule a "booster" therapy session.

21. Healthy sexuality plays a positive, integral role in a relationship, with the main function to energize the bond and generate feelings of desirability and being desired. Paradoxically, bad or nonexistent sex plays a more powerful negative role in a relationship than the positive role of good sex.

pattern; or partner sexual dysfunction. Assessment continues in the treatment phase in response to exercises, processing during therapy, and exploring the meaning of "sexuality" and "sexual dysfunction" for the woman and relationship.

Therapeutic interventions for orgasmic dysfunction include encouraging the woman to develop her "sexual voice"; to use multiple stimulation during nonintercourse and intercourse sex; to identify "orgasm triggers" from masturbation and transfer these to partner sex; to increase comfort, emotional intimacy, and trust; to identify and play out erotic scenarios; to request and guide stimulation; to make the transition to intercourse at her initiation; and to give herself permission to let go and be orgasmic with manual, oral, or rubbing stimulation. When a woman's orgasm is viewed as a sign of a man's expertise, this creates performance anxiety. Women are not autonomous sexual responders; both female socialization and physiology support intimate, interactive sexuality. The man is viewed as her intimate, erotic friend. The optimal prescription for female orgasmic response is to integrate intimacy, pleasuring, and eroticism.

Traditionally, eroticism has been underplayed in female sexuality. Without a solid base of receptivity and responsivity, erotic techniques cannot "force" orgasm. Orgasm is the natural culmination of pleasure, arousal, erotic flow, and letting go. Her partner's attitudes, behavior, and feelings are integral to a woman's arousal. Often a man, under the guise of being a "sophisticated lover," is in fact manipulating the woman (i.e., her orgasm is to prove something for him). The woman is responsible for her orgasm, and the man respects her sexual voice and autonomy. Sex is about awareness and sharing pleasure, not a performance to satisfy an arbitrary criterion. As noted, a crucial therapeutic strategy is to reinforce the one–two combination of each person taking responsibility for sexuality, with the couple functioning as an intimate team.

Sex therapy strategies and techniques are most effective with anxiety-based dysfunctions, lack of awareness, and inhibitions. Therapeutic techniques include self-stimulation (with or without a vibrator), increased awareness, guiding a supportive partner, using multiple erotic stimulation, gaining confidence in one's arousal–orgasm pattern, and freedom to decide when and how to integrate intercourse into the couple's lovemaking style.

When dysfunction (especially secondary arousal dysfunction and/or nonorgasmic response) is confounded with negative emotions (disappointment, anger, alienation, distrust), treatment is more complex. Attention is focused on assessment/intervention at the systemic and meaning levels. An important technique is to help each person recognize the function of the sexual problem and do a cost–benefit assessment of the emotional and relational consequences of resolving the problem. Therapy sessions help clarify the functions and meaning of sexuality for the woman and the relationship (Heiman, 2007).

Female Arousal Dysfunction

Although much attention has been paid to male arousal dysfunction (erection), relatively little clinical or research attention has focused on female arousal dysfunction. The objective (physiological) measures of arousal are ease and amount of vaginal lubrication. The subjective measure is feeling "turned on." Both are variable and difficult to quantify (Basson, 2007). The introduction of Viagra has led to renewed interest in female arousal for researchers and clinicians.

When a woman enters therapy with the complaint of painful intercourse or nonorgasmic response, a careful analysis often reveals that the primary problem is lack of arousal. It is possible for a woman to have high desire and low arousal, or to be orgasmic but still have arousal dysfunction. The therapeutic focus is usually on desire or orgasm, but in fact arousal is a crucial component deserving assessment and intervention.

The key to understanding arousal is a careful assessment of the woman's receptivity–responsivity pattern. To what pleasuring scenarios and techniques is she most receptive? When is she open and responsive to erotic touch? What is the optimal timing and sequencing of erotic techniques? It is useful to think of sexual response on a 0- to 10-point scale (10 is orgasm): 1–3 refers to comfort and sensuality; 3–5 refers to pleasure; and 6–9 refers to arousal/erotic flow.

Traditionally, it is the male who controls "foreplay." The man stimulates the woman until he judges that she is ready for intercourse, then initiates intromission. In the treatment program for female arousal dysfunction, it is the woman who controls the type of stimulation and timing of transitions. For example, many women prefer prolonged nongenital pleasuring. Some women prefer taking turns in the pleasurer–recipient format, whereas others prefer mutual pleasuring. Attitudinally, the focus is on "pleasuring," not "foreplay." Intercourse is not necessarily the centerpiece of the pleasuring–eroticism process. In designing and processing exercises, the woman is encouraged to experiment with single versus multiple stimulation; taking turns versus mutual pleasuring; utilizing manual, oral, or rubbing stimulation versus intercourse; and using lubricants such as Astroglide, nonallergenic water-based lotions, or K-Y Jelly. She is actively involved in the pleasuring–arousal–eroticism process.

For those women who feel subjectively aroused but do not lubricate sufficiently, the preferred intervention is to use lubricants. This can be done in a comfortable, sensual manner, either using the lubricant prophylactically or as part of the pleasuring process. Being self-conscious or apologetic blocks erotic flow. A rhythm of comfort, pleasure, and eroticism is integral to overcoming female arousal dysfunction and orgasm dysfunction. The guidelines (in Table 21.2) to enhance female arousal and orgasm are given as a handout to women and couples.

TABLE 21.2. Guidelines for Female Arousal and Orgasm

1. You are responsible for your desire, arousal, and orgasm. Developing your "sexual voice" is a positive challenge. It is not the man's responsibility to "give you" an orgasm.

2. Together, a couple can develop an intimate, interactive sexual style that promotes desire, arousal, orgasm, and satisfaction for both partners.

3. Receptivity and responsivity to giving and receiving pleasurable and erotic touch is core to arousal and orgasm.

4. Arousal involves both subjective components (feeling responsive and turned on) and objective components (vaginal lubrication and physical receptivity to intercourse).

5. "Foreplay"—in which the man stimulates the woman to get her ready for intercourse—increases self consciousness and performance anxiety. The experience of "pleasuring"—which emphasizes mutuality and sharing—facilitates arousal.

6. Eroticism and arousal can lead to intercourse, but intercourse is not necessary for a satisfying sexual experience.

7. The prescription for satisfying sexuality is to integrate intimacy, pleasuring, and eroticism. Traditionally, female sexual socialization underplayed eroticism. Erotic scenarios and techniques are integral to female sexuality.

8. As you develop your "sexual voice," you increase awareness of the scenarios and techniques that enhance arousal. Use that awareness to make requests and guide your partner, verbally and nonverbally.

9. State your preferences—single versus multiple stimulation, taking turns versus mutual stimulation; when and how to transition from sensual to erotic stimulation; your emotional and practical conditions for a vital sexual relationship. Feel free to request erotic techniques (vibrator stimulation, your fingers or his for clitoral stimulation during intercourse, cunnilingus to orgasm).

10. You can initiate the transition from pleasuring to intercourse and guide intromission.

11. Women who prefer multiple stimulation during pleasuring/eroticism usually prefer multiple stimulation during intercourse. You can utilize additional clitoral stimulation with your hand or his, request breast or anal stimulation, fantasize, kiss, and/or switch intercourse positions.

12. Many women are interested in using medications, such as Viagra or testosterone, to enhance sexual response. Medication can be a valuable additional resource, but it is not a "magic pill." The sexual enhancement medication needs to be integrated into your couple sexual style of intimacy, pleasure, and eroticism.

13. Many women, especially after 40, use some form of estrogen and/or water-based lubricant to enhance lubrication and facilitate intercourse.

14. Only one in four women follow the traditional male pattern of one orgasm during intercourse without needing additional stimulation. Female sexual response is flexible and variable. A woman may be nonorgasmic, singly orgasmic, or multiorgasmic, and orgasm might occur during pleasuring, intercourse, or afterplay.

15. Sex is not a performance in order to have a G-spot orgasm, multiple orgasms, "vaginal" orgasm, extended orgasm, or whatever is the new fad. Each woman develops her own pattern of desire, arousal, and orgasm.

16. Orgasm is a 3- to 10-second experience. Orgasm is a natural result of giving yourself permission to enjoy arousal, eroticism, and letting go, so that arousal flows to orgasm.

17. The distinction between "clitoral" and "vaginal" orgasm is not scientifically valid. Whether orgasm occurs with manual, oral, rubbing, intercourse, or vibrator stimulation, the physiological response is the same. Subjective feelings of satisfaction vary depending upon preferences, experiences, and values.

18. Desire and emotional satisfaction are more important than orgasm.

19. It is unrealistic to expect arousal and orgasm during each sexual experience. You are not a sexual machine. Female sexuality is more variable and complex than male sexuality.

20. Remember, sexuality is not about proving anything to the partner, yourself, or anyone else. It is about experiencing and sharing intimacy, pleasure, and eroticism.

Painful Intercourse

The problem of painful intercourse is paradoxical. Whereas some cases are quite easy to resolve, others require the coordinated efforts of a gynecologist, sex therapist, and the most important member of the treatment team, a female physical therapist (because the intervention involves direct teaching and practice of control over pelvic floor musculature) with a subspecialty in female sexual health. The woman increases awareness and comfort with her genitalia, uses general relaxation and specific pelvic relaxation techniques, controls the type and pacing of genital stimulation, is comfortable using lubricants, initiates and guides intromission, and finds intercourse positions and types of thrusting that are comfortable. Involvement and arousal are the antidotes to passivity, hypervigilance about pain, and viewing intercourse as the man's domain.

Clinicians and researchers who deal with sexual pain recognize it as a complex psychobiosocial phenomenon that needs to be addressed in a multicausal, multidimensional manner (Binik, Bergeron, & Khalife, 2007). The new emphasis is on approaching sexual pain as a pain disorder rather than as a sexual dysfunction. Assessment often requires the participation of a gynecologist with a subspecialty in pain to assess syndromes such as vulvadinia, vaginal tears, vulvar vestibulitis syndrome, infections, sexually transmitted infections, poor vaginal tone, and medication side effects. Medical interventions include surgery, oral medications, and vaginal creams. A common therapeutic technique is exercising the pubococcygeal (PC) muscle, which increases awareness and strengthens the vaginal wall. Clinicians emphasize the efficacy of the PC muscle exercise, although empirical support is weak.

Couple sex therapy focuses on psychological and relational factors that facilitate comfort, pleasure, eroticism, and intercourse. This requires major attitudinal, behavioral, and emotional changes for both partners. It requires that she be assertive, and that he be open to her requests, guidance, and especially her rhythm for the sexual scenario. Comfort is the underpinning of desire and arousal. Pain, or fear of pain, sabotages sexual pleasure.

Vaginismus, spasming of the vaginal introitus that makes intercourse painful or impossible, is no longer considered a separate dysfunction but a variant of painful intercourse. As Donahey (1998) observed, many women who experience vaginismus have high anticipatory anxiety, are unaccepting of their bodies, and are intimidated by their partners' sexual desire and erection. The change process for painful intercourse may be slow, with a need for carefully crafted individual and couple interventions, especially comfort with vaginal insertion. Use of fingers (hers, and then his), graduated sizes of dilators, and insertion of the lubricated penis are stepwise interventions. Insertion is more comfortable when the woman is both subjectively and objectively aroused.

In summary, assessment and treatment of female sexual dysfunction require a broad-based approach to psychological, physical, relational, cultural, and psychosexual skills factors. The organizing concept is the woman as an aware, comfortable, and responsible sexual person—speaking with her clear "sexual voice." Couple interventions center around partners feeling and functioning as an intimate team in which the woman is an equal partner. Her anticipation and the feeling that she is deserving, and both partners' respect for her conditions for healthy sexuality are crucial in facilitating desire. Integrating intimacy and eroticism, and openness to requests and guidance, and focusing on erotic techniques (especially multiple stimulation and the woman guiding intercourse) are important for arousal. Awareness of her arousal–orgasm pattern, use of self- or partner stimulation during intercourse, multiple stimulation and orgasm triggers, and giving herself permission to be erotic and let go are important for orgasm. Developing afterplay scenarios, sharing intimacy, acknowledging emotional and sexual connection, and feeling bonded are important for satisfaction.

Male Sexual Dysfunction

With the exception of premature ejaculation, the great majority of male sexual problems are secondary. Males are generally eager to be in sex therapy when the problem is female dysfunction, but are reluctant and embarrassed when the problem is male dysfunction.

Male sexual socialization is antithetical to the strategies and techniques of couple sex therapy. In traditional socialization, the male is supposed to be the "sex expert," with no anxieties or inhibitions. Sexual performance is supposed to be totally predictable and perfect; sex is competitive, and no weaknesses or questions are tolerated; and masculinity and sexuality are highly related. The self-defeating concept is that a "real man" is willing and able to have sex with any woman at any time, in any situation (McCarthy & McCarthy, 1998). Males learn that desire, arousal, and orgasm are easy, predictable, and autonomous (i.e., a man needs nothing from a woman). Traditionally, males do not value intimate, interactive sexuality. This is a prime cause of secondary sexual dysfunction as men and their relationships age.

Sex therapy can help a man resolve a dysfunction. Even more importantly, therapy can help him learn healthy attitudes and skills, especially the value of intimate, interactive sex, setting the stage for relapse prevention and inoculation against sexual problems with aging.

Sex therapy concepts and techniques are more acceptable to women, but they are just as beneficial for men. When partners stop having sex, whether at 40 or 70, it is typically the man's decision (McCarthy, 1999). A major cause is feeling embarrassed and stigmatized because he has failed at the male sexual performance model. In therapy, he learns to view sexuality as pleasure, not as a performance; to value the woman as his sexual friend, not as someone for whom he performs or must prove something; to enjoy a variable, flexible couple sexual style rather than a rigid intercourse pass–fail test; and to regard sexuality as intimate and interactive, not as autonomous. The core concept is to adopt the "good enough sex" model of male and couple sexuality (Metz & McCarthy, 2007a).

Premature Ejaculation

Although premature ejaculation is the most common male sexual dysfunction, it is not easy to measure objectively. The most clinically useful assessment/definition of premature ejaculation focuses on the couple's subjective evaluation of pleasure and satisfaction rather than a strict time criterion (Metz & McCarthy, 2003). When the man ejaculates before intromission, at the point of intromission, with fewer than 10 thrusts, or within a minute of intercourse, almost all couples identify this as premature ejaculation. Most men begin their sexual careers with rapid ejaculation, and 30% of adult males complain of chronic premature ejaculation (Metz, Pryor, Nesvacil, Abuzzan, & Koznar, 1997). Strassberg, Brazao, Rowland, Tan, and Slob (1999) present evidence that for some men, a significant physiological component makes it difficult to learn ejaculatory control, and a significant number of these men relapse. A new trend, mimicking

the movement to medicalize erectile dysfunction, is use of a medication that facilitates ejaculatory control (Waldinger, 2004). However, medication should be regarded as an additional resource, not as a substitute for the couple learning ejaculatory control exercises.

The essence of the assessment/intervention program is to help the man break the connection between high arousal and quick orgasm. Contrary to "do-it-yourself" techniques to reduce arousal, such as wearing two condoms, applying a desensitizing cream to the glans of the penis, or using nonerotic thoughts, the focus in learning ejaculatory control is to maintain arousal while heightening awareness, relaxation, and psychosexual skills. The strategy is counterintuitive—practicing increased stimulation and arousal, while increasing comfort and control.

For the majority of males, premature ejaculation is a powerfully overlearned habit in both masturbation and intercourse. Relearning involves two processes. The first is the ability to discern the point of ejaculatory inevitability (after which ejaculation is no longer a voluntary function), and the second is to increase erotic stimulation while lengthening the time from arousal to orgasm. The major learning technique is the "stop–start" approach, which is easier to apply and more acceptable to the partner than the traditional "squeeze" technique.

Identifying the point of ejaculatory inevitability occurs through masturbation or manual stimulation by the partner. When the man is approaching the point of inevitability, he signals (either verbally or nonverbally) for the woman to cease stimulation. The urge to ejaculate decreases after 15–60 seconds, and stimulation is resumed. At first the stop–start technique may be used three or four times, but it becomes less necessary over time as the couple makes the transition into slowing down and altering stimulation.

Men (and women) have unrealistic expectations about the time spent in intercourse. A typical sexual scenario might last 15–45 minutes, with time spent in intercourse averaging from 2 to 7 minutes. Few intercourse experiences exceed 12 minutes. Men are intimidated by the fantasy goal of hour-long intercourse. Maintaining realistic expectations is crucial. Acceptance is difficult for the man whose expectations are based on male boasting, porn videos, and a competitive, performance-based norm.

A crucial concept is for the man to view the woman as his intimate sexual friend. A man typically emphasizes performance *for* the woman rather than sharing pleasure *with* her. The male hopes that if intercourse lasts longer, he will "give her an orgasm during intercourse." The man acts as if ejaculatory control is for her, not for him. The purpose of learning ejaculatory control is for the man to enhance pleasure and satisfaction. The entire sexual experience becomes more intimate and erotic.

Exercises are designed in a stepwise manner; the man learns ejaculatory control first with manual and oral stimulation, then with intercourse. The "quiet vagina" exercise involves minimal movement, controlled by the woman from the female-on-top position. The most difficult position to maintain control is the man on top, using short, rapid thrusts. A man often develops better ejaculatory control with circular thrusting; with longer, slower thrusting; or with the woman controlling thrusting. The partners work collaboratively to develop sexual scenarios and techniques that enhance pleasure and satisfaction. Throughout the process, the woman's sexual feelings and needs are important. Being intimate team members who clearly and comfortably communicate sexual feelings, techniques, and requests is integral to maintaining therapeutic gains.

A common result of unsuccessful treatment or "do-it-yourself" techniques is the development of erectile dysfunction. When the focus is on heightening awareness and pleasure, erectile functioning is not subverted. When arousal is decreased or self-consciousness raised, erectile problems or inhibited sexual desire are a likely outcome.

Erectile Dysfunction

With the introduction of Viagra in 1998, there has been a paradigm shift in the assessment and treatment of erectile dysfunction (ED) (Segreaves, 1998). The medical and lay public now view ED as a physical problem and Viagra (or the two other proerection medications: Levitra and Cialis) is considered the first-line intervention. Further assessment is typically undertaken only if Viagra is unsuccessful. Moreover, Viagra is usually prescribed by a family practitioner or internist rather than a sexual specialist.

Viagra is the first user-friendly medical intervention; it is much easier to accept taking a pill than to use an external pump, penile injection, MUSE (medicated urethral system for erections), or penile prosthesis. It has heightened public awareness of the ED frequency and ED as a side effect of surgery, illness, and medications, especially for men over 50. However, Viagra has resulted in the medicalization of male sexuality.

Althof (2003) stressed the crucial role of the sex therapist in assessing, treating, and motivating partners to integrate Viagra into their lovemaking style. McCarthy and Fucito (2005) have discussed the therapeutic and iatrogenic uses of Viagra and proposed an assessment/intervention approach that emphasizes couple sex therapy.

Erection is *not* solely a male concern, separate from the couple's experience. Viagra promises a return to the autonomous male model with predictable sex, while downplaying the woman's sexual feelings and role. Metz and McCarthy (2004) have presented a couple psychobiosocial model that emphasizes intimate, interactive sexuality, with a focus on pleasure and satisfaction. Marital sex may not be as frequent or intense as premarital sex, but quality, pleasure, and satisfaction can increase with time and age. A major transition for middle-aged and older males is being open to partner involvement and penile stimulation to enhance arousal and erection.

The frequency of at least mild ED for males over 50 is estimated to be more than 50%. ED is a multicausal, multidimensional phenomenon, with wide individual and couple differences. The simplistic "organic versus psychological" dichotomy of causation is recognized as scientifically invalid and therapeutically nonproductive. The present folklore suggests that 95% of erection problems are caused by physical factors is no more valid than the past folk wisdom that 90% of erection problems were caused by psychological or relational factors. Prostate surgery, poorly controlled diabetes, and spinal cord injury usually cause organic deficits. But even in a couple affected by such a disorder, an examination of psychological, relational, motivational, and psychosexual skills/factors is important to integrate Viagra or other medical interventions successfully into the couple's lovemaking style. When the man gets firm erections during masturbation, oral sex, sex with a partner other than his spouse, or a fetish arousal pattern, use of Viagra is unlikely to be successful and may be iatrogenic, because the core psychological and relationship problems are ignored.

The recommended assessment/intervention strategy is couple sex therapy, with a medical assessment of vascular, neurological, and hormonal functioning. Common health factors that interfere with erections are drinking, smoking, and drug abuse. In the individual sexual history, it is crucial to obtain an honest assessment of situations in which the man is functional. Being able to flag sensitive or secret material encourages honest reporting. A common pattern is that the man attains erections while masturbating, viewing pornography, or engaging in cybersex; in an affair (whether with a man or a woman); or in a variant erotic scenario with a prostitute. This information is vital in constructing an intervention strategy. The man who does not obtain an erection by any means requires a thorough medical assessment. The clinician assesses whether a desire problem preceded or followed the erection problem. A sexual secret—whether an affair, variant arousal, compulsive masturbation, or a sexual orientation issue—needs to be carefully explored for both function and meaning.

A question to explore during the woman's history taking is how she felt about sexuality before the ED began. How has the problem affected her sexual desire and arousal? In many cases, she blames herself for the erection problem (attributing it to her weight gain, lack of erotic skills, or his boredom with the relationship) and/or sees it as a symbol of loss of love. In other cases, the woman has resented the man's sexual attitudes and behavior for years and is secretly glad he is not able to have erections and intercourse. In still other cases, the woman is hostile or verbally abusive about the ED. In contrast, a woman may be pleased, because the partner now devotes time and energy to pleasuring her. The woman's attitudes and feelings both before and since the ED are carefully assessed. ED makes some men more open to receiving and giving sensual and erotic stimulation. Unfortunately, most males with ED avoid any affectionate or sexual contact, so that they do not have to face "the embarrassment of erectile failure." The arousal–erection guidelines in Table 21.3 are given to the couple as a handout.

The paradigm shift in the conceptualization of ED is more than the medicalization of the penis. It views erections as primarily, if not solely, the male's domain. In contrast, sex therapy emphasizes the one–two combination of personal responsibility and the couple functioning as an intimate team. In selected couples, Viagra is used during genital pleasuring exercises. A healthy cognition is that Viagra is an additional resource to facilitate maintaining an erection. With genital pleasuring exercises, it is important to reinforce the necessity of erotic stimulation to facilitate erection (it does not automatically occur because of Viagra) and the wax-and-wane exercise (when erotic flow is interrupted, the erection decreases, and it recurs with relaxation and stimulation). This reinforces for both partners that it is not just the pill that works magically; intimacy, pleasuring, and eroticism matter. This experience facilitates the integration of Viagra into the couple's lovemaking style.

Therapeutic gains made with Viagra must be generalized and maintained. The partners can use Viagra as a backup resource should they have a series of unsuccessful intercourse attempts. As in the treatment of female sexual dysfunction, we encourage the male to use self-stimulation in conjunction with partner stimulation. Many males are embarrassed to touch themselves when a partner is present—an inhibition that can be successfully confronted.

Exercises (Metz & McCarthy, 2004) are designed to rebuild comfort and confidence with arousal and erection. The cognition of "intercourse as a special pleasuring technique" is a significant change. This flexible, variable conceptualization of the "good enough sex" model is more easily accepted by the woman than by the man. Traditional male sexual socialization, cultural norms, urologists, and the media emphasize that "real sex is intercourse" and "intercourse is the only measure of treatment success." However, intercourse as the rigid 100% performance criterion is self-defeating.

A positive, realistic conceptualization is that intimacy, pleasure, and eroticism flow to erection and intercourse in about 85% of experiences. When intercourse does not occur, the couple can comfortably make a transition to one of two alternative scenarios—a sensual, cuddly scenario or an erotic, nonintercourse scenario resulting in orgasm for one or both partners. Whether erectile problems occur once a year or once a month, it is normal to have occasional dissatisfying or dysfunctional sexual experiences. If this fact is not accepted, a man is "one failure away from square one." Clinging to the adolescent expectation of easy, automatic, 100% predictable erections is self-defeating. Even when using Viagra each time, men cannot live up to such perfectionistic criteria (McCarthy & Metz, 2007).

Hypoactive Sexual Desire Disorder

For the great majority of males, HSDD is a secondary dysfunction. HSDD affects approximately 15% of men and increases with age. The most common cause is another sexual dysfunction (ED or ejaculatory inhibition) that becomes chronic and severe over time. The man becomes stuck in the

TABLE 21.3. Arousal and Erection Guidelines

1. By age 40, 90% of males experience at least one erectile failure. This is a normal occurrence, not a sign of ED.

2. ED can be caused by a wide variety of factors, including alcohol, anxiety, depression, vascular or neurological deficits, distraction, anger, side effects of medication, frustration, hormonal deficiency, fatigue, or not feeling sexual at that time or with that partner. As men age, the hormonal, vascular, and neurological systems become less efficient, so psychological, relational, and psychosexual skills factors become more important.

3. ED is a psychobiosocial problem with multiple causes, dimensions, and effects. To evaluate medical factors comprehensively, including side effects of medication, consult a urologist with training in erectile function and dysfunction.

4. Medical interventions, especially the oral medications—Viagra, Cialis, Levitra—can be a valuable resource to facilitate erectile function, but they are not magic pills. The partners need to integrate the medical intervention into their lovemaking style of intimacy, pleasuring, and eroticism.

5. Do not believe the myth of the male machine, ready to have intercourse at any time, with any woman, in any situation. You and your penis are human. You are not a performance machine.

6. View the erectile difficulty as a situational problem. Do not overact and label yourself as impotent or put yourself down as a failure.

7. A pervasive myth is that if a man loses his initial erection, then it means he is sexually turned off. It is a natural physiological process for erections to wax and wane during prolonged pleasuring.

8. In a 45-minute pleasuring session, erections will wax and wane two or more times. Subsequent erections, intercourse, and orgasm can be quite satisfying.

9. You do not need an erect penis to satisfy a woman. Orgasm can be achieved through manual, oral, or rubbing stimulation. If you have difficulty getting or maintaining an erection, do not stop the sexual encounter. Women find it arousing when the fingers, tongue, or penis (erect or flaccid) are used for stimulation.

10. Actively involve yourself in giving and receiving pleasurable and erotic touching. Erection is a natural result of pleasure, feeling turned on, and getting into an erotic flow.

11. You cannot will or force an erection. Do not be a "passive spectator" who is distracted by the state of his penis. Sex is not a spectator sport. It requires active involvement by both you and your partner.

12. Allow the woman to initiate intercourse and guide your penis into her vagina. This reduces the performance pressure and, because she is the expert on her vagina, is the most practical procedure.

13. Feel comfortable saying, "I want sex to be pleasurable and playful. When I feel pressure to perform, I get uptight and sex is not good. We can make sexuality enjoyable by taking it at a comfortable pace, enjoying playing and pleasure, and being an intimate team."

14. Erectile problems do not affect your ability to ejaculate (men can ejaculate with a flaccid penis). You can relearn ejaculation to the cue of an erect penis.

15. One way to regain confidence is through masturbation. During masturbation, you can practice gaining and losing erections, relearn ejaculation with an erection, and focus on fantasies and stimulation that transfer to partner sex.

16. Do not try to use a waking erection for quick intercourse. This erection is associated with REM (rapid eye movement) sleep and results from dreaming and being close to the partner. Men try in vain to have intercourse with the morning erection before losing it. Remember: Arousal and erection are regainable. Morning is a good time to be sexual.

17. When sleeping, you have an erection every 90 minutes—three to five erections a night. Sex is a natural physiological function. Do not block it with anticipatory anxiety, performance anxiety, distraction, or by putting yourself down. Give yourself (and your partner) permission to enjoy the pleasure of sexuality.

18. Make clear, direct, assertive requests (not demands) for stimulation that you find erotic. Verbally and nonverbally guide your partner in how to pleasure and arouse you.

19. Trying to stimulate your penis when it is flaccid is counterproductive. A man becomes distracted and obsessed with the state of his penis. Engage in sensuous, playful, nondemand touching. The basis of sexual response is relaxation and sensuality. Enjoy giving and receiving stimulation rather than trying to will yourself to have an erection.

20. Attitudes and self-thoughts affect arousal. The key is sex and pleasure, not sex and performance.

21. A sexual experience is best measured by pleasure and satisfaction, not whether you had an erection, how hard it was, or whether she was orgasmic. Some sexual experiences are great for both partners, some are better for one than for the other, some are mediocre, and others are unsuccessful. Do not put your sexual self-esteem on the line at each experience. The "good enough sex" model of sexual pleasure is much healthier than the perfect intercourse performance criterion.

cycle of anticipatory anxiety, tense and failed intercourse experiences, and sexual avoidance. Sex becomes an embarrassment rather than a pleasure. Although some men stop being sexual, the majority continue to masturbate, and some develop a secret life of pornography, cybersex, or prostitutes.

Primary HSDD is rare (less than 10% of men) because of the cultural link between masculinity and sexuality, as well as adolescent experiences with masturbation. Sex is viewed as a positive, integral part of being a male. Causes of primary HSDD can range from testosterone deficiency to rigid family or religious antisexual messages. The most common cause is a sexual secret, such as a variant arousal pattern (paraphilia), greater confidence with masturbatory sex than with couple sex, not dealing with a past sexual trauma, or conflict about sexual orientation. Approximately 2–5% of males have a paraphilia (Abel, Weigel, & Osborn, 2007). Most are benign, involving fetishes, cross-dressing, or cybersex. Noxious (deviant) paraphilias—exhibitionism, voyeurism, pedophilia, obscene phone calls—are illegal, cause trauma to others, and must be vigorously treated.

Conflicts regarding sexual orientation are in a different category. The emotional and sexual commitment to men is an acceptable sexual variation, and is in fact optimal for gay men. The scientific and clinical data strongly support the acceptance of homosexuality as a normal sexual variation, although this remains controversial (especially among conservative political and religious organizations). There is also major disagreement regarding the prevalence of homosexuality. The best estimate is that 25% of males have been orgasmic with a man in adolescence or young adulthood, and 10% have had major sexual involvement with men. Perhaps 4–6% of males have a "homosexual orientation," defined as an emotional and erotic commitment to sexuality with men.

Another subgroup of men with primary HSDD are afraid of sexual failure, have a history of sexual trauma, or are guilty or shameful about sexuality. The majority of primary HSDD involves a substitute sexual outlet rather than an absence of desire.

A man with HSDD who attends couple therapy is usually coerced by his partner. His goal is to avoid self-disclosure and therapy. He wants to keep his sexual life secret from his partner, as well as the therapist. Partner sex usually results in dysfunction, leaving him feeling embarrassed and defeated. It is crucial that the therapist be empathic, nonjudgmental, and not coerce the man to be sexual. The man feels alone and deficient; sexuality is his "shameful secret." The therapist's empathy and understanding of how the problem has developed and is maintained constitute a valuable intervention.

The man usually feels that his partner is his worst critic rather than an intimate sexual friend. The woman's role in assessment and treatment is crucial. She feels bewildered and rejected as a result of his HSDD and avoidance. Underneath the anger, she feels hurt, as well as abandoned. It is important to explore whether the woman has a sexual outlet—this could include either masturbation or an affair. Does she experience HSDD herself? If so, did her problem precede or follow the man's? Is the woman motivated to be an active, involved partner? Her sexual desire and arousal can facilitate the man's desire and arousal.

Male HSDD, whether secondary (usually linked to a dysfunction) or primary (usually caused by a sexual secret), is one of the most difficult problems to treat. A common sexual secret is that the man is engaged in an affair he is unwilling to give up. An active affair is a contraindication for couple sex therapy. Affairs require time and energy. Couple therapy typically fails when there is an active affair, primarily because the man lacks the motivation and focus to confront his HSDD in the marriage.

The presence of a sexual dysfunction does not necessarily make couple sex therapy the treatment of choice. Severe individual problems, such as untreated alcoholism, bipolar disorder, or panic disorder, can subvert sex therapy. Severe relationship distress (including partner abuse, lack of respect or trust, or conflict over money or children) can sabotage couple sex therapy. Traditionally, individual and/or couple therapy for such problems was recommended before proceeding with sex therapy. This decision requires high levels of clinical judgment, because the danger, especially with male HSDD, is that sexual avoidance becomes more severe and chronic. Rather than the traditional hierarchical model (treat alcoholism or depression first, relationship or communication problems second, and only then, sexual problems), we advocate a "both–and" therapy approach of addressing alcoholism and sexual issues in an integrated couple approach.

In successful treatment, each person develops bridges to sexual desire. The woman's responsiveness serves to reignite the man's sexuality (Mc-

Carthy, 1995). The man usually has an unspoken wish to return to the "good old days" when he was the sexual initiator and expert. However, this is self-defeating. Strategies and techniques for treating male HSDD are similar to those for treating female desire problems, but with a somewhat different focus. The permission-giving element is for the man to find a new "sexual voice" that emphasizes intimate, pleasure-oriented sexuality. Males are encouraged to use both internal and external cues to enhance sexuality, including fantasies; erotic stimuli, such as X-rated videos; elaborate and intricate pleasuring scenarios; multiple forms of stimulation during intercourse, and erotic non-intercourse scenarios. The man is encouraged to be aware of the multiple positive functions of sexuality for himself and the relationship.

Married men who have a secret life with prostitutes, compartmentalized affairs, cybersex, or compulsive masturbation are asked to assess carefully whether any elements of those experiences can be generalized to marital sexuality. Traditionally, the man's wife is kept in a circumscribed role. As one male said, "Since I pay the prostitute, it's her role to turn me on." His wife said, "I don't need your money, but I do need you to be there, open to my touch, and willing to share eroticism." The major aphrodisiac is an involved, aroused partner.

Ejaculatory Inhibition

Ejaculatory inhibition (EI) is the least common and most misunderstood male dysfunction. Usually the man can ejaculate with masturbation, and some man can ejaculate with manual or oral stimulation, but not during intercourse (or only rarely). Among young males, EI is mistakenly envied because the man is thought to be a "stud" whose lasting power ensures that the woman has an orgasm during intercourse. EI is frustrating for both the man and woman. The typical pattern is that he gets an erection and quickly proceeds to intercourse, but his level of subjective arousal is low and intercourse is not erotic. By thrusting mechanically, he hopes finally to "come." Most women find that after 15 minutes of thrusting, arousal and lubrication wane. Intercourse becomes emotionally frustrating and physically irritating. Nonerotic intercourse is not pleasurable for either partner.

The most common pattern is that men over 50 develop intermittent EI that is the result of reduced eroticism during intercourse. For males in their 20s, it is easy (often too easy) to reach or-

gasm; this is not true for males in their 50s. Thrusting alone is not enough. The man is stuck in the performance myth that a real man does not need additional erotic stimulation to reach orgasm. Once again, the key to successful treatment is for both partners to value intimate, interactive sexuality. More specifically, the man requests multiple forms of stimulation before and during intercourse and utilizes "orgasm triggers" (Metz & McCarthy, 2007b). Ejaculation is a natural result of high arousal, so the couple collaborates to increase subjective arousal. The woman's responsiveness and arousal reinforce the man's arousal. An important technique is delaying the onset of intercourse until the man is highly aroused. Traditionally, a man begins intercourse as soon as he achieves an erection, even if his subjective arousal level is 2. He is advised not to make the transition into intercourse until his subjective arousal level is a 7 or 8. Intercourse requires verbal and nonverbal communication, as well as an emphasis on the reciprocal effect of partner arousal and multiple forms of stimulation throughout the sexual experience. The technique suggestion is to utilize multiple forms of stimulation during intercourse and orgasm triggers (learned from masturbation) at high levels of arousal.

CASE ILLUSTRATION

This was the first marriage for 32-year-old Jeb and the second marriage for 31-year-old Maria. She was the custodial parent of her 8-year-old son from her previous marriage. Jeb had established a very good stepparent relationship with the boy, and both Jeb and Maria wanted another child.

It was Maria who called for the initial appointment. She and Jeb had been a couple for almost 4 years, lived together for over 3 years, and had been married for 19 months. Maria was considering leaving the marriage due to disappointment and frustration over their sexual relationship. Her dilemma was whether to become pregnant and then leave or to tell Jeb about her intense unhappiness and attempt to save the marriage. In the initial telephone consultation, the therapist urged Maria to set up the first appointment as a couple and engage in a four-session assessment process. Maria had four previous experiences with counseling/therapy, none of which she had found personally helpful. However, five couple counseling sessions, 1 year earlier, had helped Jeb accept that he would not be able to adopt Maria's son, because the biological father wanted to maintain parental rights. Maria's first therapy experience had been six sessions at a college counseling center. Her second experience had been a structured group program to fulfill requirements for a DUI (driving under the influence) program when she was 22. The third was a weekend retreat, followed by three couple sessions with the minister who had married Maria and Jeb.

At the first couple session, Maria and Jeb presented as a demoralized, alienated couple. It was clear that Jeb blamed himself for all the marital and sexual problems. However, Jeb very much wanted the marriage to work, and he also wanted a successful four-person family. He was aware of Maria's dissatisfaction and feared that she would leave him. Maria said she recognized that Jeb was a good person who had a successful career and was a wonderful stepfather. However, she was bitterly disappointed with their failed sexual relationship and felt that she could not accept this for the next 50 years. Maria had said to Jeb, "You're a good guy and good husband, but a sexual loser." Jeb accepted all the blame and said he would do anything to change, despite the fact that he was clueless regarding ways to improve their sex life. The last time they had tried to have sex, on their anniversary, 7 months earlier, Maria had had no desire and was very upset by Jeb's premature ejaculation.

The advantage of conducting the first session with both partners is that it sends a powerful and positive message about approaching marriage and sexual problem issues *as a couple*. It gives the clinician an opportunity to see how the partners interact, how they have previously attempted to address the problem, so that they do not repeat the same mistakes, as well as how motivated they are to address problems as an intimate team. At this session, the partners are asked to fill out a release of information form(s) to send to past and present individual therapists, psychiatrists, couple therapists, and ministers. The release of information form should mention that these individuals will be contacted within the next week. Waiting for a written report is like "waiting for Godot." Professionals will respond by phone, not in writing. It is important to hear other professionals' assessments of the individual and couple, their evaluation of the intervention, and suggestions about how to deal with the couple. It is fascinating to compare the couple's evaluation of the intervention with that of the professional.

The therapist usually ends the initial session by assigning the couple a short reading (no more than 20 pages, preferably 10) to reinforce the concept of each person taking responsibility for his or her sexual behavior and working as an intimate team member to resolve the problem. The reading does not cure problems, though it can help to reduce stigma and set reasonable expectations regarding the process of change.

The next step in the four-session assessment model is to interview each spouse separately regarding psychological, relational, and sexual history. The history begins with the following statement:

"I want to understand your strengths and vulnerabilities both before this marriage and within the marriage. I want you to be as blunt and forthcoming as possible. At the end, you can 'red flag' any sensitive or secret material, and I will not share it without your permission. However, I need to know this information in order to be as helpful as possible in resolving these problems."

Jeb had the first appointment and was extremely anxious and apologetic about himself, particularly regarding sexuality. Jeb had a lifelong problem of premature ejaculation, as well as a fetish arousal pattern to women's boots. Almost all of his sexual encounters had occurred when he was drinking heavily (Jeb needed "liquid courage" to be sexual). At the age of 23, Jeb had a particularly humiliating experience with a woman who said that he was "a pathetic excuse for a lover." Until he met Maria at 28, Jeb had avoided relational sex, engaging only with women he met at a bar. Jeb had wanted to get married and have children, and he felt that Maria was exactly what he needed. She was bright, attractive, prosexual, an excellent single parent, and interested in marriage and having another child. Her promarriage, prosexual attitude quickly won Jeb over. They began living together 6 months after they met, and everything seemed on track except the issue of premature ejaculation. Although it was a celebratory wedding with much support from family and friends, Jeb was aware of Maria's sexual disappointment and greatly reduced sexual desire. He felt worried and embarrassed, and retreated into Internet sex sites focused on the boot fetish. At the time of the interview, he was spending about $1,000 a month on cybersex. Jeb felt shameful and desperate, and was overwhelmed with the fear that Maria would leave him. Jeb originally wanted to "red-flag" his past and present sexual issues, especially the alcohol use and boot fetish. However, with some gentle prodding, he was willing to share this material during the couple feedback session. Jeb idealized Maria, put her on a pedestal, and was convinced that she had no psychological, relational, or sexual vulnerabilities.

The individual history conducted with Maria presented a very complex and ambivalent picture regarding sex and the marriage. Maria revealed several substantial strengths. She was smart, extroverted, prosexual, resilient, and an excellent single parent, with a strong desire for another child and a genuine respect and fondness for Jeb. However, she also revealed some notable vulnerabilities, including poor marital and sexual models; high sexual desire early in a relationship, giving way to disappointment in the man, resulting in HSDD; disappointment in Jeb and seeing him as a "sexual loser"; and the belief that their marriage was not viable. In addition, shortly after she became pregnant, Maria's first husband had revealed that he was gay, which reinforced her sensitivity about hidden agendas and disappointments. Maria had had three affairs since her marriage to Jeb, including "hookups" with two old boyfriends and an ongoing compartmentalized affair with a coworker. With a great deal of trepidation, Maria agreed that these sensitive/secret issues needed to be shared and processed if there was any chance of revitalizing trust and sex in the marriage.

The 90-minute couple feedback session began with a description of Maria's strengths and vulnerabilities. This was purposeful, to challenge Jeb's perception that he was the entire problem. They needed a new "her–his–our" narrative that was not only genuine but also motivating and hopeful. Maria felt relieved to have this information "on the table." She committed to using birth control to prevent pregnancy as they tried to rebuild their marriage and marital sexuality. She also committed to ending the work affair and to being transparent with Jeb. Most of the material that Maria shared was new to Jeb, and had the beneficial effect of taking Maria off the pedestal and presenting the sex problems as a couple issue. This information, including disclosure of extramarital involvement, was now open for processing as the couple therapy progressed. It was neither denied nor made the most important factor in the couple's relationship.

Jeb was very concerned about Maria's reaction to his history of performance anxiety, dependence on alcohol for sexual confidence, and misuse of funds for the Internet fetish site. In fact, Maria increased her understanding and empathy for Jeb's sexual struggles and was touched to hear how motivated he was to turn around the marital and sexual pattern. Jeb agreed to move the computer to the family room and to install an "Internet nanny" to block the fetish site. In addition, Jeb agreed to have no more than one drink before sex and to focus on learning psychosexual skills, especially for ejaculatory control.

Maria and Jeb were relieved that all of the issues were now clear. They would need to continue to process this material, because these were difficult issues. However, they were no longer afraid that "another shoe would drop." They were motivated and made a 6-month "good faith" commitment to revitalize their marriage and build a new couple sexual style.

The first homework "exercise" was to find at least one (preferably two) "trust position" to which they felt physically connected and safe. In subsequent psychosexual skills exercises, if either person became anxious or had a negative experience, he or she could use the "trust position" as a method to regroup. This exercise also served to begin rebuilding their couple trust bond.

In ongoing couple sessions, the first focus was to do a fine-grained analysis of the positive and negative attitudes, behaviors, and feelings the partners experienced during the exercises (ideally two or three) over the past week; the second focus was on their developing couple sexual style, and the role of intimacy and sexuality in their relationship, then discussing exercises and areas of focus for the coming week. Initial exercises focused on rebuilding sexual desire (comfort, attraction, trust, and each person's sexual scenario). For Jeb, the key was to stop apologizing for himself sexually and to stop avoiding touching and sexuality. Subsequently, they focused on Jeb learning ejaculatory control. For Maria, the focus was on rebuilding positive anticipation and a sense of deserving, so that sex might play a positive 15–20% role in the marriage. It was crucial that they value an integrated intimacy and eroticism, and confront disappointments and turn-offs.

Couple sex therapy involves four clients— each individual, the relationship, and the sexual relationship. It is an individualized, complex endeavor, and Maria and Jeb required the therapist to be actively involved to keep them motivated and focused. The trap for Maria was to become frustrated, disappointed, and critical. For Jeb, it was to become anxious, apologetic, and to focus on performing for Maria rather than sharing pleasure with her. Therapy sessions began on a weekly basis and after six sessions switched to biweekly sessions, for a total of 18 couple therapy sessions.

The most important couple exercises involved developing "his," "hers," and "our" bridges for sexual desire. For Jeb, the key for ejaculatory control was learning self-entrancement arousal, slowing down the sexual process, and doing circular thrusting from the woman-on-top intercourse position. For Maria, the issue was less about exercises and psychosexual skills, and more about trusting and valuing intimate, interactive couple sex.

Developing a relapse prevention program was a crucial therapy component for the couple. Jeb had to learn to make sure that a "lapse" did not turn into a "relapse." He had to accept that whether it occurred once a month or once a year, it was all right if he ejaculated rapidly. He did not need to apologize or worry.

Maria was now 4 months pregnant and needed Jeb's encouragement to "beat the odds" and maintain a healthy sexual relationship throughout the pregnancy. They learned to utilize the sitting/kneeling intercourse position for the third trimester and liked the position so much that it became a regular part of their sexual repertoire.

Maria and Jeb made an up-front agreement to prevent future extramarital affairs (McCarthy & McCarthy, 2003). Maria shared her personal vulnerabilities with Jeb, including how powerfully validating it was when a man came on to her. She shared how erotic she felt in a new relationship, particularly if life was boring or depressing. Maria agreed to talk to Jeb if there was a high-risk person or situation, rather than acting out the sexual impulse. Maria and Jeb had worked hard to build a functional, satisfying couple sexual style. They wanted to enjoy it, not to risk destabilizing the marriage or marital sex.

Jeb particularly valued the 6-month "check-in" sessions, which extended over a 4-year period (which is unusual; the norm is 2 years). At each follow-up session, they would set a new sexual goal for the next 6 months. Maria emphasized getting away as a couple, without the children, whether overnight or for a week, to revitalize their couple and sexual bond. Jeb emphasized adding something to their sexual repertoire, such as trying a new intercourse position; a new, sensual lotion; or being sexual in the shower. Jeb reveled in the role of confident, sexual husband.

OTHER CLINICAL ISSUES

Relapse Prevention Strategies and Techniques

Relapse prevention is often ignored in psychotherapy, including sex therapy. Metz and McCarthy (2004) have argued that relapse prevention strategies and techniques should be an integral component of sex therapy. The best prevention strategy is comprehensive, high-quality therapy that helps a couple develop a comfortable, functional sexual style and motivates the partners to maintain and generalize therapeutic gains. A relapse prevention program, like a sex therapy program, must be individualized. Common relapse prevention techniques are to keep the time allotted to a therapy session open, but, rather than attend therapy, have an intimacy date at home; schedule a pleasuring session every 4–8 weeks with a ban on intercourse; design a new sexual scenario every 6 months; and when there is a negative experience, to initiate a sensual or erotic date within 1–4 days. If the couple has not been sexual for 2 weeks, the partner with higher desire initiates a sensual or sexual experience; if that does not occur, the other partner initiates one the next week; if the partners have gone a month without a significant sexual experience, they schedule a "booster" session.

Additional response prevention strategies include the couple agreeing to take a weekend away, without the children, at least once a year. On occasion, the partners are sexual outside the bedroom. Sexuality cannot rest on its laurels; it needs time, attention, and energy. Perhaps the most important relapse prevention technique is establishing positive, realistic expectations. People wish that all sex would flow smoothly, yet the reality is that sexuality has natural variability. Among well-functioning, satisfied married couples, fewer than 50% of sexual encounters involve equal desire, arousal, orgasm, and satisfaction. Even more important is the fact that it is normal for 5–15% of sexual experiences to be dissatisfying or dysfunctional (Frank et al., 1978). Rather than seeing this as a source of panic or embarrassment, the couple can accept normal sexual variability. The best way to react to a negative, dysfunctional, or disappointing experience is to view it as a "lapse" and actively prevent it from turning into a "relapse." The strategy is to return to being sexual in 1–4 days, when both partners feel open, awake, and aware, anticipating a pleasure-oriented experience. There are specific "traps" to be aware of for each sexual dysfunction, so a relapse prevention program for ED (McCarthy, 2001) will have different components than a relapse prevention program for HSDD (McCarthy, Ginsberg, & Fucito, 2006).

Sex Therapy with Gay and Lesbian Couples

There are more data and clinical discussions of gay male sexual dysfunction than of lesbian sexuality. Rosser, Metz, Bockting, and Buroker (1997) suggest that more than 50% of gay men experience a sexual dysfunction or dissatisfaction. Rates of ED and EI appear to be the same or higher for gay versus straight men, with lower rates of premature ejaculation and HSDD. In Chapter 24, this volume, Green discusses couple therapy with gay and lesbian clients. A particular issue for same-sex couples is the relational context of sex. Is there a committed, monogamous relationship, or a loosely bonded, open relationship? Sexually open relationships were formerly widely accepted as healthy for gay couples (McWhirter & Mattison, 1984), but this concept has become questionable because of STD/HIV risks, as well as relationship instability.

Clinical guidelines require a commitment to monogamy during the course of sex therapy, although there is no empirical evidence to support it. The agreement to be monogamous during therapy is not because of moral issues; rather, couple sex therapy requires a time commitment and focus that would be subverted by extrarelationship involvement. An advantage gay men have is freedom to utilize a variety of erotic techniques—self-stimulation, erotic videos, one-way sexual scenarios, use of proerection medications, use of anal stimulation, and a proerotic value system (Nichols & Shernoff, 2007). Issues that interfere with treatment are comparisons with other partners; comparison with the stereotype of hot, problem-free sex; lack of commitment to work through difficult relationship and intimacy issues; pressure to perform for the partner; the assumption that if chemistry is present, than sex should be easy; and intimacy or erotic inhibitions.

A common issue for gay male couples involves high desire for recreational sex, but inhibited desire for intimate, interactive sexuality. In the therapy session, it is important to explore initiation patterns, erotic scenarios, affection outside the bedroom, and the meaning of couple sexuality. A particularly difficult issue is that of HIV/AIDS and safer sex. Will the partners jointly do an STD screen and HIV test? Will they commit to monog-

amy? If there is an incident of extrarelationship sex, will the man tell the partner and use condoms for 6 months until retesting?

Sexual exercises need to be modified and individualized for gay couples, but the basic format is transferable. However, pleasuring concepts might not be easily accepted. The combination of traditional male and traditional gay focus on goal-oriented sex (i.e., orgasm) has resulted in deemphasizing the importance of intimacy and pleasuring, though these can be of great value in a gay relationship. Of particular importance are comfort with and responsiveness to manual, oral, anal, and rubbing stimulation. In being specific about behavior and feelings, a common inhibition is challenged—"Gay men do it, they don't talk about it."

Awareness of the frequency of sexual dysfunction and dissatisfaction allows the partners to "normalize" their experience. The concept that being gay is optimal, and that each partner deserves to feel desire, arousal, orgasm, and satisfaction is a powerful antidote to internalized heterosexism and the sense of gay sex as "bad but exciting." There are few outcome data on the effectiveness of sex therapy with gay male couples (MacDonald, 1998).

There is even less scientific and clinical information on sex therapy with lesbian couples. Typically, lesbian couples seek out a female therapist. The most common complaint is HSDD. More lesbian women than straight women have a multi-orgasmic response pattern. This is hypothesized to be the result of greater awareness of female sexual response and use of cunnilingus.

With lesbian couples, there is less fear of STD/HIV, as well as freedom from fear of pregnancy. Some clinicians hypothesize that an overemphasis on cohesiveness at the expense of autonomy and initiation is a core factor in HSDD. Others hypothesize that traditional female socialization dampens sexual initiation and eroticism. Being overly solicitous of the partner's feelings and caretaking can inhibit desire, initiation, and eroticism. Sexual exercises encourage partners to take responsibility for their own sexuality and work as an intimate team to develop a comfortable, functional couple sexual style. Lesbian sexuality is facilitated by the cognition that each partner has a right to her "sexual voice." Issues of initiation and "bridges to desire" are particularly important. Each partner is encouraged to develop her bridges, and to realize that these do not need to be shared bridges.

A special emphasis is placed on exploring a level of intimacy that promotes sexual desire and initiation, taking turns initiating, exercises that emphasize pleasuring and eroticism, and promoting an erotic flow in which each person's arousal plays off that of the partner. The couple can experiment with focused versus multiple stimulation; pleasurer–recipient format versus mutual stimulation; one-way sex versus interactive sex; and manual, oral, rubbing, and vibrator stimulation. Traps of self-consciousness, not wanting to outperform the partner, tentativeness, and spectatoring are confronted.

Therapy with Unmarried Couples

Perhaps the best way to break up nonviable, unmarried partners is to put them in sex therapy; that is, the focus on intimacy and sexuality will destroy a fragile relationship. Rates of sexual dysfunction are higher in unmarried couples (in which the partners have been together more than 2 years) than in married couples.

Unmarried couples have a right to have their problems addressed. A therapeutic contract that focuses on mutually agreed-upon goals is crucial. For some, the assumption is that resolving the sex problem will result in marriage. For others, the sexual dysfunction is primary or chronic, and the man wants the partner to be a sexual friend, with the expectation that the relationship will last at least until the sexual dysfunction is resolved. The meaning of intimacy and commitment needs to be carefully explored, as well as the motivation for addressing the problem. For example, a divorced couple came to therapy to address the man's ED. The woman's motivation for therapy was guilt, because she had left him for another man. His motivation was to perform so well that she would return to the marriage. In that case (and others like it), couple sex therapy can be an iatrogenic intervention.

Couple sex therapy is an appropriate intervention when an unmarried couple experiences a sexual dysfunction that subverts satisfaction, and the partners are motivated to address the problem jointly. Rates of dysfunction, especially HSDD and nonsexual relationships, are higher. There has been little empirical support for the "commonsense" hypothesis that suggests the sex problem is caused by ambivalence and lack of commitment. Common causes are anticipatory anxiety, performance anxiety, lack of sexual awareness, poor psychosexual skills, unrealistic performance expectations, and low-quality sexual communication. The couple and therapist need to decide whether to focus on sexual dysfunction or to look broadly at attitudes, values, and emotional intimacy.

The couple is cautioned not to treat sex therapy as a test for a marriage. In other words, successful resolution of the sexual dysfunction does not mean that persons are viable marital partners. The person with the dysfunction does not owe the partner for his or her sexual help, nor is the opposite true. Moreover, an unresolved sexual problem does not mean that a couple cannot marry; sexuality is but one area of the relationship. There are no empirical data on therapy outcome and the decision to marry. Our clinical experience is that the majority of unmarried couples who attend sex therapy do not marry.

The successful resolution of the sexual dysfunction improves the relationship, but the partners' decision to commit to sharing their lives involves a very different dimension. In other cases, a breakdown in the sex therapy is often attributable to a relationship that is not viable. An example of the first type of outcome was a woman with primary nonorgasmic response, who learned to engage in self-stimulation to orgasm, then be orgasmic with partner sex. Although they had an intimate friendship and both partners enjoyed the relationship, religious, political, and life organization factors made it clear that this was a better dating relationship than a marriage. An example of the latter situation was a man with premature ejaculation, who was contemptuous of his depressed, professionally underfunctioning girlfriend, although she was a prosexual, responsive partner. Engaging in couple therapy and processing exercises was enough to highlight their incompatibilities and resulted in the termination of their cohabitating relationship. He continued individual sex therapy with a focus on masturbation training, guided imagery, and discussion about choosing a woman he trusted and found attractive, and with whom he was comfortable.

Women without partners can benefit from female sexuality groups. Sexuality groups for men without partners have been difficult to organize. Individuals with sexual dysfunction benefit from interventions that include exploring sexual history; masturbatory training; relaxation and guided imagery; establishing conditions for good sex; dealing with sexual health and contraception; setting positive, realistic sexual expectations; and choosing an appropriate partner.

Couple Sex Therapy When There Is a History of Sexual Trauma

The conceptualization, assessment, and intervention with persons who have undergone sexual trauma involve some of the most complex and controversial issues in mental health. The major types of sexual trauma are childhood sexual abuse, incest, and rape. Negative sexual experiences can be broadly defined to include dealing with an unwanted pregnancy; having an STD; experiencing a sexual dysfunction; being sexually humiliated or rejected; guilt about masturbation; shame or confusion about sexual fantasies; being exhibited to or peeped on; receiving obscene phone calls; or being sexually harassed. Negative, confusing, guilt-inducing, or traumatic sexual experiences are almost universal phenomena for both women and men, whether they occur in childhood, adolescence, adulthood, or old age. The model espoused by trauma theorists and therapists has emphasized dealing with the trauma and its aftereffects first, then, once these are resolved, focusing on couple sexual issues. The problem with this "benign neglect" strategy is that the longer the sexual hiatus, the stronger the cycle of anticipatory anxiety, tension-filled sex, and avoidance. Sexual avoidance reinforces anxiety and self-consciousness.

An alternative strategy proposed by Maltz (2001), and supported by McCarthy and Sypeck (2004), is to challenge the couple to be "partners in healing." A traumatized individual who is able to experience desire, arousal, and orgasm, and to feel intimately bonded, has taken back control of his or her life and sexuality. The person is a proud survivor, not a passive or angry victim. He or she accepts the adage "Living well is the best revenge." The partner plays an active role in the healing process; sexuality is voluntary, mutual, and pleasure-oriented. If the traumatized person vetoes something, the veto is respected and honored (i.e., the opposite of sexual abuse). A crucial concept is that one cannot say "yes" to sex until one is able to say "no."

The PLISSIT Model and Prevention

Annon (1974) has suggested an intervention model with four levels of clinician involvement. PLISSIT stands for "permission-giving, limited information, specific suggestions, and intensive sex therapy." Ideally, all couple therapists are aware of and comfortable with being permission givers, and provide accurate prosexuality information to individuals and couples.

Permission giving entails an accepting attitude toward sexuality as a positive component in the individual's and couple's life. Affectionate, sensual, and erotic expression is valued as a shared pleasure, a means to develop and reinforce intimacy, and a tension reducer to deal with the stresses of marriage and life. The clinician is comfortable and encouraging, so that the couple can explore erotic scenarios and techniques, as well as the meaning of intimacy and sexuality. The permission-giving therapist does not approach sexuality with benign neglect; sexuality is treated as a positive, integral component of the person's and couple's life. The clinician takes a prosexuality stance, not a neutral, value-free stance. The therapist is aware of and respects individual and cultural differences, while working within the couple's values system. The therapist acknowledges the integral role of sexuality in a relationship. A powerful permission-giving intervention is a consultation with a minister of the couple's faith, because almost all religions are prosexuality in terms of marriage.

In the limited information component, the therapist provides accurate, scientifically valid information about biological, psychological, and relational aspects of sexual function and dysfunction. He or she helps the couple to establish positive, realistic sexual expectations. Limited information includes referral to an appropriate subspecialist in dealing with issues such as infertility, diagnosis and treatment of an STD, hormone replacement therapy, or side effects of antidepressant or blood pressure medications. Limited information involves confronting sexual myths, including new myths of sexual performance and pressure to prove that a couple is "liberated." It also emphasizes the importance of developing a couple sexual style that is comfortable and functional for both people. This style includes acceptance that occasional dissatisfaction or dysfunctional sexual experiences are part of normal sexual variability. Contraception and safe sex are other integral components of limited information. Issues of initiation, sexual frequency, erotic scenarios and techniques, and sexual variations are covered. Couple therapists are comfortable with permission giving and limited information on a wide range of sexual topics.

The third component, specific sexual suggestions, is not necessarily part of the repertoire of a couple therapist. Referrals can be made to a sex therapist, physician, or individual therapist. Specific suggestions include pleasuring exercises, with a prohibition on intercourse; experience with initiation and saying "no"; stop–start ejaculatory control exercises; use of lubricants to facilitate female arousal; the wax-and-wane erection exercise; the use of a vibrator or self-stimulation for female orgasm during partner sex; and openness to afterplay scenarios and techniques.

Specific suggestions involve integrating sexual interventions into couple therapy. This assessment/intervention approach is diagnostic in determining whether couple sex therapy is warranted. Sometimes simply conducting a sexual history clarifies issues and helps to resolve the problem; at other times, it becomes clear that a referral for sex therapy is necessary. Some couple therapists are comfortable, skilled, and interested in integrating sex therapy into their therapeutic repertoires. The majority of couple therapists do not choose to adopt sex therapy as a subspecialty skill; they make a referral to a sex therapist, as they would to any subspecialist. Not every clinician can or should do sex therapy. The mental health clinician may choose to refer to a specialist because of a lack of interest, comfort, training, skill, or if the therapy conflicts with clinical or personal values (Levine, Risen, & Althof, 2003).

Sexual issues and problems are frequent sources of concern for both married and unmarried, straight, and gay couples. The couple therapist can promote healthy sexuality and act in a primary prevention manner by engaging in permission giving and providing personally relevant, scientifically and clinically helpful information. The clinician can engage in a secondary intervention by making specific suggestions to deal with a sexual problem in its acute stage. If a sexual dysfunction is chronic and severe, a referral for sex therapy is the appropriate choice.

SUMMARY

Sex therapy is a subspecialty skill. Intimacy and eroticism play a positive, integral role in sexual function and satisfaction. However, when sex is dysfunctional or absent, when there is an extramarital affair, or when fertility problems are present, sexuality can play an inordinately powerful negative role, draining the relationship of intimacy and vitality. Sexual problems are a major force in relationship disintegration and divorce. Couple sex therapy strategies and techniques enhance desire, arousal, orgasm, and satisfaction. The prescription for healthy, integrated sexuality is intimacy, pleasuring, and eroticism. The model of each person being responsible for his or her own sexuality, and the couple functioning as an intimate team, is the core concept.

SUGGESTIONS FOR FURTHER READING

Basson, R. (2007). Sexual desire/arousal disorders in women. In S. Leiblum (Ed.), *Principles and practice of sex therapy* (4th ed., pp. 25–53). New York: Guilford Press.—Provides a clinically relevant description of responsive sexual desire, a core concept in understanding the major sexual problem of HSDD.

McCarthy, B., & Fucito, L. (2005). Integrating medication, realistic expectations, and therapeutic expectations into treatment of male sexual dysfunction. *Journal of Sex and Marital Therapy, 31,* 319–328.—Description of the psychobiosocial model applied to erectile dysfunction.

McCarthy, B., & McCarthy, E. (2003). *Rekindling desire.* New York: Brunner/Routledge.—A book for couples to gain in-depth understanding of desire problems, as well as information about treatment and prevention.

McCarthy, B., & Metz, M. (2007). *Men's sexual health.* New York: Routledge.—This book presents the psychobiosocial model of male and couple sexuality with an emphasis on the "good enough sex" approach.

REFERENCES

Abel, G., Weigel, M., & Osborn, C. (2007). Pedophilia and other paraphilias. In L. VandeCreek, F. Peterson, & J. Bley (Eds.), *Innovations in clinical practice: Focus on sexual health* (pp. 157–175). Sarasota, FL: Professional Resource Press.

Althof, S. (2003). Therapeutic weaving: The integration of treatment techniques. In S. Levine, C. Risen, & S. Risen (Eds.), *Handbook of clinical sexuality for mental health professionals* (pp. 359–376). New York: Brunner/Routledge.

American Association of Sex Educators, Counselors, and Therapists. (2004). *Code of ethics.* Ashland, VA: Author.

American Psychiatric Association. (1994). *Diagnostic and statistical manual of mental disorders* (4th ed.). Washington, DC: Author.

Annon, J. (1974). *The behavioral treatment of sexual problems.* Honolulu: Enabling Systems.

Ashton, A. (2007). The new sexual pharmacology. In S. Leiblum (Ed.), *Principles and practice of sex therapy* (4th ed., pp. 509–541). New York: Guilford Press.

Aubin, S., & Heiman, J. (2004). Sexual dysfunction from a relationship perspective. In J. Harvey, A. Wenzel, & S. Sprecher (Eds.), *The handbook of sexuality in close relationships* (pp. 477–518). Mahwah, NJ: Erlbaum.

Barbach, L. (1975). *For yourself.* New York: Doubleday.

Basson, R. (2000). The female sexual response. *Journal of Sex and Marital Therapy, 26,* 51–65.

Basson, R. (2007). Sexual desire/arousal disorders in

women. In S. Leiblum (Ed.), *Principles and practice of sex therapy* (4th ed., pp. 25–53). New York: Guilford Press.

Binik, Y., Bergeron, S., & Khalife, S. (2007). Dyspareunia and vaginismus. In S. Leiblum (Ed.), *Principles and practice of sex therapy* (4th ed., pp. 124–156). New York: Guilford Press.

Donahey, K. (1998). Review of treating vaginismus. *Journal of Sex Education and Therapy, 23,* 266–267.

Frank, E., Anderson, A., & Rubinstein, D. (1978). Frequency of sexual dysfunction in "normal" couples. *New England Journal of Medicine, 229,* 111–115.

Goldstein, I., Lue, T., Padma-Nathan, H., Rosen, R., Steers, W., & Wicker, P. (1998). Oral sildenafil in the treatment of erectile dysfunction. *New England Journal of Medicine, 338,* 1397–1404.

Heiman, J. (2007). Orgasmic disorders in women. In S. Leiblum (Ed.), *Principles and practice of sex therapy* (4th ed., pp. 84–123). New York: Guilford Press.

Heiman, J., & LoPiccolo, J. (1988). *Becoming orgasmic.* Englewood Cliffs, NJ: Prentice-Hall.

Hertlein, K., Weeks, G., & Gambescia, N. (2007). The treatment of hypoactive sexual desire disorder: An intersystem approach. In L. VandeCreek, F. Peterson, & J. Bley (Eds.), *Innovations in clinical practice: Focus on sexual health* (pp. 75–92). Sarasota, FL: Professional Resource Press.

Jacobson, N., & Addis, M. (1993). Research on couples and couples therapy. *Journal of Consulting and Clinical Psychology, 65,* 85–93.

Kaplan, H. (1974). *The new sex therapy.* New York: Brunner/Mazel.

Kaplan, H. (1995). *The sexual desire disorders.* New York: Brunner/Mazel.

Kaschak, L., & Tiefer, L. (2001). *A new view of women's sexual problems.* Binghamton, NY: Haworth Press.

Laumann, E., Rosen, R., & Paik, A. (1999). Sexual dysfunction in the United States. *Journal of the American Medical Association, 281*(6), 537–544.

Laumann, F., Gagnon, J., Michael, R., & Michaels, S. (1994). *The social organization of sexuality.* Chicago: University of Chicago Press.

Leiblum, S. (Ed.). (2007). *Principles and practice of sex therapy* (4th ed.). New York: Guilford Press.

Levine, S., Risen, C., & Althof, S. (2003). *Handbook of clinical sexuality for mental health professionals.* New York: Brunner/Routledge.

Lobitz, W., & Lobitz, G. (1996). Resolving the sexual intimacy paradox. *Journal of Sex and Marital Therapy, 22,* 71–84.

MacDonald, B. (1998). Issues in therapy with gay and lesbian couples. *Journal of Sex and Marital Therapy, 24,* 165–190.

Maltz, W. (2001). *The sexual healing journey.* New York: HarperCollins.

Masters, W., & Johnson, V. (1970). *Human sexual inadequacy.* Boston: Little, Brown.

McCarthy, B. (1995). Bridges to sexual desire. *Journal of Sex Education and Therapy, 21,* 132–141.

McCarthy, B. (1997). Strategies and techniques for revitalizing a non-sexual marriage. *Journal of Sex and Marital Therapy, 23,* 231–240.

McCarthy, B. (1999). Relapse prevention strategies and techniques for inhibited sexual desire. *Journal of Sex and Marital Therapy, 25,* 297–303.

McCarthy, B. (2001). Relapse prevention strategies and techniques for erectile dysfunction. *Journal of Sex and Marital Therapy, 27,* 1–8.

McCarthy, B., Bodnar, L., & Handal, M. (2004). Integrating sex therapy and couple therapy. In J. Harvey, A. Wenzel, & S. Sprecher (Eds.), *The handbook of sexuality in close relationships* (pp. 573–593). Mahwah, NJ: Erlbaum.

McCarthy, B., & Fucito, L. (2005). Integrating medication, realistic expectations, and therapeutic expectations into treatment of male sexual dysfunction. *Journal of Sex and Marital Therapy, 31,* 319–328.

McCarthy, B., Ginsberg, R., & Fucito, L. (2006). Resilient sexual desire in heterosexual couples. *The Family Journal, 14*(1), 59–64.

McCarthy, B., & McCarthy, E. (1998). *Male sexual awareness.* New York: Carroll & Graf.

McCarthy, B., & McCarthy, E. (2002). *Sexual awareness.* New York: Carroll & Graf.

McCarthy, B., & McCarthy, E. (2003). *Rekindling desire.* New York: Brunner/Routledge.

McCarthy, B., & McCarthy, E. (2004). *Getting it right the first time.* New York: Brunner/Routledge.

McCarthy, B., & Metz, M. (2007). *Men's sexual health.* New York: Routledge.

McCarthy, B., & Sypeck, M. (2003). Childhood sexual trauma. In D. Snyder & M. Whisman (Eds.), *Treating difficult couples* (pp. 330–349). New York: Guilford Press.

McWhirter, D., & Mattison, A. (1984). *The male couple.* Englewood Cliffs, NJ: Prentice-Hall.

Metz, M., & McCarthy, B. (2003). *Coping with premature ejaculation.* Oakland, CA: New Harbinger.

Metz, M., & McCarthy, B. (2004). *Coping with erectile dysfunction.* Oakland, CA: New Harbinger.

Metz, M., & McCarthy, B. (2007a). The good enough sex model for couple sexual satisfaction. *Sexual and Relationship Therapy, 22,* 351–362.

Metz, M., & McCarthy, B. (2007b). Ejaculatory problems. In L. Vandecreek, F. Peterson, & J. Bley (Eds.), *Innovations in clinical practice: Focus on sexual health* (pp. 135–155). Sarasota, FL: Professional Resource Press.

Metz, M., Pryor, J., Nesvacil, L., Abuzzan, F., & Koznar, J. (1997). Premature ejaculation: A psychophysiological review. *Journal of Sex and Marital Therapy, 23,* 3–23.

Michael, R., Gagnon, J., Laumann, E., & Kolata, G. (1994). *Sex in America.* Boston: Little, Brown.

Nichols, M., & Shernoff, M. (2007). Therapy with sexual minorities. In S. Leiblum (Ed.), *Principles and practice of sex therapy* (4th ed., pp. 379–415). New York: Guilford Press.

Perel, E. (2006). *Mating in captivity.* New York: HarperCollins.

Rind, B., Tromovitch, D., & Bauserman, R. (1998). A meta-analytic examination of assumed properties of child sexual abuse using college samples. *Psychological Bulletin, 124,* 22–53.

Risen, C. (2007). How to do a sexual health assessment. In L. Vandecreek, F. Peterson, & J. Bley (Eds.), *Innovations in clinical practice: Focus on sexual health* (pp. 19–33). Sarasota, FL: Professional Resource Press.

Rosen, R., Philips, N., Gendrano, H., & Ferguson, D. (1999). Oral phenotalamine and female sexual arousal disorder. *Journal of Sex and Marital Therapy, 25,* 137–144.

Rosser, R., Metz, M., Bockting, W., & Buroker, T. (1997). Sexual difficulties, concerns, and satisfaction in homosexual men. *Journal of Sex and Marital Therapy, 23,* 61–73.

Schnarch, D. (1991). *Constructing the sexual crucible.* New York: Norton.

Schnarch, D. (1997). *Passionate marriage.* New York: Norton.

Segreaves, R. (1998). Pharmacological era in the treatment of sexual disorders. *Journal of Sex and Marital Therapy, 24,* 67–68.

Seagraves, R., & Balon, R. (2003). *Sexual pharmacology.* New York: Norton.

Strassberg, D., Brazao, C., Rowland, D., Tan, R., & Slob, A. (1999). Clomipramine in the treatment of rapid ejaculation. *Journal of Sex and Marital Therapy, 25,* 89–101.

Tiefer, L. (1996). The medicalization of sexuality. *Annual Review of Sex Research, 7,* 252–282.

Waldinger, M. (2004). Lifelong premature ejaculation. *British Journal of Urology, 93,* 201–207.

Weeks, G. (2004). The emergence of a new paradigm in sex therapy. *Sexual and Relationship Therapy, 20*(1), 89–103.

Wincze, J., & Barlow, D. (1996). *Enhancing sexuality: Client workbook.* Albany, NY: Graywind.

CHAPTER 22

Couple Therapy and Medical Issues

Working with Couples Facing Illness

NANCY BREEN RUDDY
SUSAN H. MCDANIEL

BACKGROUND

Medicine, like psychotherapy, has always been a hybrid of science and art. Time and training constraints can restrict the focus of health care professionals to only some biological aspects of a patient's illness experience—perhaps to an organ system, or to interrelated symptoms. Over the past half-century many health professionals (especially those in primary care) have shifted emphasis from biological processes toward integrating psychosocial facets of disease, with the "biopsychosocial model" as the gold standard of care (Engel, 1977; Frankel, Quill, & McDaniel, 2003; see Figure 22.1). The biopsychosocial model emphasizes the interrelatedness of biological, psychological, and community factors in health and disease. It applies systems theory to human functioning by recognizing how all of these levels simultaneously affect one another, and how health care intervention affects many levels of human experience. This shift has facilitated two major movements toward helping couples cope with medical problems.

The first change has been toward a broader recognition of the role of families in health and illness. Many in the discipline of family medicine treat the family rather than the individual or an organ system as the unit of care (Bloch, 1983; Doherty & Baird, 1983; McDaniel, Campbell, Hepworth, & Lorenz, 2005), acknowledging the reciprocal effects of family relationships and health and disease. Although some medical professionals from all specialties recognize the importance of these relationships, family medicine clinicians are trained to integrate family systems thinking into day-to-day health care by including fathers in prenatal care, spouses/partners or adult children in geriatric care, parents in adolescent care, and so forth. When the family is the center of health care, communication and other issues that are typically the purview of family therapists become the purview of medical professionals as well. Family medicine has been particularly welcoming to collaboration with family therapists, creating an inroad to treating families in the medical setting. Family therapists in medical settings have a "frontline" view of how couples cope with illness, and how psychotherapy can help couples face the challenges of illness (Rolland, 1994). Primary care medical settings increasingly offer on-site mental health services, furthering the role of psychosocial and interrelational elements of care (Blount, 1998; McDaniel et al., 2005; Ruddy, Borresen, & Gunn, 2008).

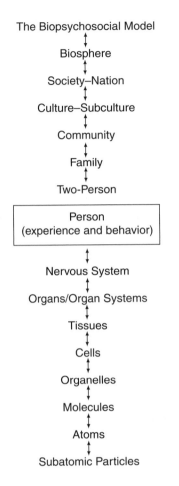

The Biopsychosocial Model

↑

Biosphere

↑

Society–Nation

↑

Culture–Subculture

↑

Community

↑

Family

↑

Two-Person

Person
(experience and behavior)

↑

Nervous System

↑

Organs/Organ Systems

↑

Tissues

↑

Cells

↑

Organelles

↑

Molecules

↑

Atoms

↑

Subatomic Particles

FIGURE 22.1. Systems hierarchy. From Engel (1980). Copyright 1980 by the American Psychiatric Association. Reprinted by permission.

The second major movement has been the growth of interdisciplinary clinics that specialize in treating specific diseases (Blount, 1998; Frank, Hagglund, & Farmer, 2004; Seaburn, Lorenz, Gawinski, & Gunn, 1996). Many specialty clinics for chronic illnesses such as cystic fibrosis, cancer, and diabetes offer family-oriented services and recognize the importance of family factors in achieving the best possible outcomes. Mental health professionals typically work in collaboration with other health professionals to identify families in need of services and to provide support and treatment. This support provides resources for medical professionals when they recognize a family struggling to cope with the stresses of a chronic illness. The common nature of these struggles is reflected in the many groups and associations that families

themselves have established to educate and support each other.

Finally, behavioral medicine has grown out of clinics that specialize in pain management and treatment, broadening the role of mental health professionals. Noting the impact of behavioral interventions on physical symptoms has lent further credence to the idea that mind and body are not only connected but also are both necessary elements to healing (Belar & Deardorff, 1995; Siegel, 1999; Campbell, 2003).

Family medicine practices and specialty clinics have created rich environments for the development of family therapy theory and techniques specifically designed for families and couples facing illness. In 1990, McDaniel, Campbell, Hepworth, and Lorenz published a book for physicians in training, *Family Oriented Primary Care* (second edition published in 2005), outlining a family systems approach to medical care. Two years later, McDaniel, Hepworth, and Doherty (1992) wrote a book for family therapists called *Medical Family Therapy*, describing how families often react and ultimately cope with illness, and how therapists can help them through this process. In 1994, in *Families, Illness, and Disability*, John Rolland described common patterns of family coping with different types of illnesses and health situations. These last two books provided foundation for psychotherapists working with families facing illness, and many books and articles have since then added to this work.

HEALTHY/WELL-FUNCTIONING VERSUS PATHOLOGICAL/DYSFUNCTIONAL RELATIONSHIPS

The Challenges of Chronic Illnesses

The poor and minorities are more likely to suffer from chronic illnesses (Dalstra et al., 2005; Lantz et al., 1998; Sorlie, Backlund, & Keller, 1995; Fiscella, 1999), and to have poor outcomes following critical illness (Alter et al., 2006; Van den Boss, Smits, Westert, & van Straten, 2002). Yet ill health knows no socioeconomic or racial bounds. Illness strikes both well-functioning and struggling couples, stressing the couple system at all levels.

One key factor that determines successful versus unsuccessful coping with illness is the couple's adaptability. In general, couples who adapt to the demands of the illness do well. Illness characteristics determine the adaptations a couple must make and the extent to which these adaptations affect day-to-day life. Some illnesses, such as mild diabetes, require lifestyle changes but do not necessarily force the couple to face mortality or to manage major role changes. Other illnesses can be more debilitating on a day-to-day basis, requiring major role changes and a larger care burden on the healthy partner.

Bill's neurologist referred Bill and Mary Ann because Bill's reluctance to accept help with his muscular dystrophy placed great stress on the marriage. Mary Ann was threatening to leave her husband of 30 years; she was clearly very frustrated at his refusal to use a wheelchair or other appliances that would assist his movement. Because of his refusal, Mary Ann more often had to lift or guide him, and even pick him up after his frequent falls. Bill also refused to stop driving; he had hit and hurt a woman in a parking lot. Mary Ann, for her part, had serious diabetes. Bill had had to inject her with insulin on two occasions in the past year to bring her out of a diabetic coma. She seemed to be doing better since being put on a pump. The spouses had to delay their appointment for psychological assessment because of their annual vacation on a Caribbean island without any medical care.

Clearly, Bill and Mary Ann had resisted accepting the extent of their own illnesses, and had not yet adjusted their roles to fit the demands of these chronic illnesses.

The course of an illness also affects how a couple must learn to cope. Some illnesses, such as muscular dystrophy, challenge couples by being unpredictable; any given day may be a "good day" or a "bad day." In other cases, an illness starts as an acute episode that everyone expects to "go away," and only over time is it clear that the illness is chronic and life is forever changed. Medical advances have altered the course of some imminently terminal diseases to chronic illnesses that can be managed (e.g., HIV, some cancers). Couples must balance hopeful optimism with realistic planning as they cope with such situations. They also may face derision from others who assume that their hopeful optimism is denial, believing that the heretofore terminal illness is still so. Still other illnesses, such as Parkinson's disease, take a progressive downward course, and couples must cope with the knowledge that it is likely only to get worse. This inevitability requires pacing and a high tolerance for uncertainty that often taxes even emotionally healthy couples.

Gregory was diagnosed with Parkinson's disease after some of his medical colleagues asked the family whether he had Parkinson's. Gregory and Anna had always been dedicated to each other throughout his active career and had raised five children. As Gregory's illness resulted in his slow deterioration, Anna cared for his every need. Their children and Gregory's fellow health care professionals suggested in-home care and respite, but Anna would allow it only when Gregory became psychotic and combative at night. When he improved, she would discharge the outside help. "I don't like strangers in my house," she said. Gregory agreed, and did not like Anna to be out of his sight. As the years went by and Gregory's functioning worsened, Anna became more and more fatigued, and their children began to worry about her health. During one confrontation with their physician, Anna admitted that for her, accepting outside help meant that Gregory was doing worse and would soon have to go to a nursing home, or even die. The longer she could do without help, she thought, the longer he would be with her.

Couples' Adaptations to Illness

Many types of adaptations may be necessary when a partner, such as Gregory, becomes ill. Couples must allow roles to shift. These shifts may first occur simply, at the "daily chores" level. However, broader role changes, including shifts in emotional/interactional roles, may need to occur over time. If the ill partner typically managed the emotional life of the couple, the partners may need to covertly or overtly renegotiate this role to maintain relational emotional health. For example, role strain takes on a different form when a woman becomes seriously ill during the early years of child rearing, if she has been the emotional center rather than the major breadwinner of the family. If she is the primary caregiver, the children may develop behavioral and mental health problems if her partner does not become much more attuned and responsive to their emotional needs. If she is the primary breadwinner, the family may experience financial difficulties unless her partner is able to increase his contribution to the family finances. Gender-related socialization may play a major role in a couple's ability to adapt (McDaniel & Cole-Kelly, 2003). Couples struggling with adaptation may benefit from referral for counseling or psychotherapy.

Gene was at a loss when Gretchen, his wife of 10 years, developed breast cancer. She had been the primary parent to their 5- and 7-year-old boys, and the link to the couple's social life while Gene worked hard to become a partner in a law firm. The onset of her illness challenged the couple's division of labor and resulted in frequent fighting. Gene felt resentment about added duties, guilt about his resentment, and fear for his wife's health.

Gretchen was overwhelmed with fear of dying and was largely paralyzed by this fear. She sensed that Gene was struggling to manage everything and felt guilty that she was not able to do more for her family. Gene and Gretchen avoided talking about her illness and its effects on their family. Occasionally, tempers would flare, resulting in terrible arguments. They had never discussed difficult issues before Gretchen's illness, and they were ill-equipped to handle this challenge. Gretchen's primary care physician, sensing that she was struggling to cope with her illness, suggested that she see a therapist. The therapist asked directly about the effect of Gretchen's illness on her marriage. Gretchen acknowledged the difficulties and agreed to invite her husband to the next session. Although both were nervous about the appointment, they experienced a great deal of relief when they had a venue to discuss how difficult the illness had been, and to learn new means of coping. Just learning that other couples struggled in similar ways in the face of an illness was very helpful.

Shifting role issues may be particularly difficult to resolve when other family members avoid communicating about family issues with the ill person out of fear of stressing him or her and exacerbating the illness. Also, if the ill family member was previously the person who initiated conversations about family matters, he or she may not have the physical or emotional energy to corral the family for dialogue, thus impeding the resolution of relationship issues.

Couples facing major health care issues may need to make major lifestyle changes. Dietary changes, smoking cessation, activity level changes, schedule changes for administration of medicines, and/or other changes in daily routine both affect and are affected by family members. Family members can help or hinder the ill person's attempts to make lifestyle changes. Sometimes family members may themselves need to make changes (e.g., one partner stops smoking to help the ill partner manage breathing problems). The couple's ability to adapt to these changes as a unit, and to discuss the issues these changes create, is one factor in determining overall coping (Doherty, 1988; Harkaway, 1983).

The couple needs to find a way to communicate about all the stresses the illness places on both partners, and to find support. This sense of "communion" (McDaniel et al., 1992) both mitigates the conflict that is bound to arise at a stressful time and gives both partners a sense that they are there for each other. In addition, couples often need to reach out to other people who have experienced similar challenges—both to normalize their experiences and to obtain means of coping that have worked for others.

The couple must determine which aspects of the illness experience they can and cannot control. The reality that some aspects of the illness are immutable can lead to a debilitating sense of overall helplessness. Family members who generate a sense of "agency" by differentiating between uncontrollable and controllable issues, and focus on controlling the aspects of the illness that they can typically cope much better (McDaniel et al., 1992).

Couples must find meaning in the illness. Both the individual with the illness and the partner commonly ask, "Why me?" Like any challenge, illness is an opportunity for reflection and change. The process of reflection and change often provides the answer to this question. Finding meaning in the illness gives the couple a sense of peace and acceptance (Rolland, 1994; McDaniel et al., 1992).

The couple must grieve for the many losses associated with the illness. Loss issues are most overt with terminal illness, when the couple must cope with the anticipated loss of life (McDaniel & Cole-Kelly, 2003; Rolland, 1994). Partners often avoid discussing death out of a desire to protect themselves and each other from this grim reality. Even a well partner's mortality fears are roused by watching a close loved one die. It seems likely that partners who are able to discuss the ultimate loss productively are better prepared to make critical decisions at the end of life, and that the surviving partner may be better able to cope after the death of the other partner. Even non-life-threatening illnesses are accompanied by many other, less obvious losses. The partners need to grieve for the loss of their preillness life and the patient's loss of functioning. The ill person may lose the ability to work, to drive, to walk, or to live independently. His or her increasing dependence may limit sharply the activities of the partner as well. Partners may lose the ability to be sexually intimate. They need to grieve actively for the change in functioning they experience.

Another source of stress that affect overall coping is the couple's interactions with the health care community. Couples who have negative, preconceived ideas about and experiences with medical care professionals may have difficulty establishing a good, collaborative relationship with the health care team. The variability in care quality between different health care professionals can affect the couple's expectations and their sense of connection and partnership with the health care team. The couple and the health care team must learn to work together with a shared mission to return the ill partner's health or to maximize his or her quality of life (McDaniel & Hepworth, 2004).

Donald was diagnosed with prostate cancer at the age of 73. His family physician Dr. Marks had a difficult time telling him that cancer cells were found outside the prostate capsule, because Donald was the same age as Dr. Marks's father. At first Dr. Marks minimized the danger, but when Donald's wife pushed him for more information about prognosis and treatment, he acknowledged there was a significant risk that the cancer could be eventually terminal. Dr. Marks discussed the case with the psychologist on his team, who helped him see how he could use his attachment to Donald to do the best possible job of caring for him through this difficult time. At Christmas that year, Donald and his wife wrote a card to Dr. Marks, saying how much they appreciated his partnership with them in caring for Donald's illness.

Problematic Patterns

The stress of illness can set the stage for the development of maladaptive patterns. Caregivers can become overwhelmed and resentful of their duties. In many families, caregivers experience difficulty obtaining support for themselves—because either they do not ask directly or other family members are unable or unwilling to help. Research indicates a high level of depression in caregiving partners (Beeson, 2003; Schultz, O'Brien, Bookwala, & Fleissner, 1995; Tsai & Jirovec, 2005). In addition, some research has indicated that caregiving stress negatively impacts the caregiver's immune system, even years after the caregiving tasks are completed (Kiecolt-Glaser et al., 2003).

The stress of illness can also exacerbate premorbid maladaptive patterns. Communication difficulties, old resentments, patterns of over- or underfunctioning, and other problems can become entrenched or intensified just when adaptability and support are most needed. Partners who have achieved a comfortable balance between closeness and distance suddenly must work closely together under unusually stressful conditions.

Rolland (1994) encourages therapists to assess for "relationship skews" that occur when one person is debilitated by illness and the other must fill the vacuum. The resulting power differential can lead to resentment and tension within the couple, and a sense that the illness "belongs" to one person rather than being a burden to be shared by all.

Paradoxically, given the need for caregiving, illness breeds isolation. The reduction in activities, the need for caregiving, and other factors often preclude socializing. In addition, friends and family members may withdraw because they do not know how to support the couple or are overwhelmed by their own emotional reactions to the illness. Again, this emotional distancing occurs just when both individuals within the couple most need support. Even within a couple, the illness can increase emotional distance. Some partners find that an illness is like having "an elephant in the living room" that they cannot discuss. It is not uncommon for each member of the couple to avoid talking, because he or she believes the other "can't handle" talking about the illness. Protecting oneself in the guise of protecting a loved one is a common dynamic. Also, as mentioned earlier, many illnesses and their treatments interfere with sexual intimacy, creating yet another way a couple cannot feel "normal" and emotionally close.

Each individual within the family must find his or her own way to cope with the illness. Sometimes different levels of acceptance and coping mechanisms clash, resulting in conflict. For example, whereas one family member may withdraw in an attempt to shield self and others from his or her own pain, others feel abandoned by the distance. Denial is another coping strategy that family members may use differently. Denial can be healthy, helping one to tolerate massive stressors. However, too much denial can be problematic, particularly when it interferes with appropriate treatment or lifestyle alterations. Couples with differing levels of denial may experience conflict if one person feels that the other is making too much of a small issue, while the other feels that critical issues are being ignored. Denial may be more common and detrimental when family members face an illness with an unclear prognosis or treatment plan.

Karl was diagnosed with a rare bone cancer at the age of 39. His family physician Dr. Jackson had a difficult time telling him that his cancer was likely to be fatal. She waited for the oncologist and the surgeon to tell this young patient about the implication of his illness. However, no one made this clear. Karl came to Dr. Jackson and seemed to indicate in a roundabout way that he wanted to know what his tests showed. Dr. Jackson thought about Karl, his wife Debra, and their 2-year-old twins. She told Karl that it was important for them to talk about his illness, and to schedule an appointment when they could get a babysitter and his wife could come along. In the meantime, Dr. Jackson told her psychologist collaborator (S. McDaniel) about the meeting, and asked that she join them, because of the sensitivity and importance of what needed to be said. Dr. Jackson was concerned that Karl was not ready to hear his terminal diagnosis. She said that she knew little about Karl's family, his wife, and the wife's understanding of Karl's illness. The psychologist encouraged her to start with a brief genogram (so they would know which family members were available, where they lived, and the family's previous experience with illness), then ask the spouses what they knew about the illness. Within a few days, Karl, Debra, and the two professionals met. The genogram was quite helpful in assessing the family's support network. When Dr. Jackson asked the spouses what they knew about the illness, Karl responded that he knew he was dying, although no one had told him this directly. He said that his wife refused to accept this. When Debra anxiously turned to Dr. Jackson for reassurance, Dr. Jackson told her the difficult news: "Karl is right. He has a cancer that's not curable." Debra began crying and said angrily, "Well, how much time does he have? Six years? Six months?" Dr. Jackson responded, "We don't know for sure, but it's likely to be closer to 6 months." Debra began wailing, then turned to her husband: "But my plan was to grow old with you. You can't leave me now."

The session lasted 45 minutes, with the psychologist encouraging the couple to ask questions of Dr. Jackson, to talk to each other, to begin planning how best to use the time they had left, and to think about how to communicate with the twins. In fact, Karl had already begun making a videotape, talking to the twins about his own life and his wishes for theirs. The session ended without a dry eye in the room.

Sometimes differing levels of acceptance and understanding of the illness may underlie the appearance of denial in the family (McDaniel et al., 2005). Even nonterminal illnesses require an acceptance process, much like the stages that patients go through in accepting a terminal diagnosis (McDaniel et al., 1992). Each family member progresses through this process at his or her own speed. The acceptance process can be facilitated or hampered by the characteristics of the illness. An illness that remits and returns may force the family to endure the acceptance process many times over. An illness that does not coincide with the course and prognosis predicted by health care providers also may confound the family. Differing levels of acceptance can create conflict secondary to mismatched expectations, coping behaviors, and degrees of readiness to make decisions and take action. Conflict is particularly likely when family members must make treatment or end-of-life decisions collectively.

As couples shift their roles in response to the demands of the illness, problems can ensue if the "illness role" becomes rigid and entrenched. The person with the illness begins to identify him- or herself as an "ill person" and to maximize dependence on others. The healthy partner identifies with the caregiver role and does not encourage greater independence on the part of the ill person. At extremes, the ill person continues to play the sick role when no longer necessary, or the caregiver actively creates illness (or the illusion of illness) in the formerly ill partner. The dynamic amplifies the effect of the illness, because the ill person may not take advantage of periods of improved health. Often people who have chronic illness need support and encouragement to "try out their wings" when they are feeling better. Partners whose illness-related roles are very entrenched cannot adapt to health or take advantage of "good times."

Some role rigidity can be rooted in gender issues (McDaniel & Cole-Kelly, 2003). Illness often causes partners to respond to gender-based "caregiver" and "ill person" roles. Women may rigidly assume the caregiver role in the face of illness and be hesitant to ask for or accept assistance when it is needed. Men may feel inadequate as a caregiver or lack the necessary skills. Traditional coping mechanisms of "female" emoting versus "male" action may not meet the needs of each member of a couple, and may clash with the demands of an illness. The traditional gender roles mirror the concepts of "agency" and "communion," both of which are essential to coping with illness. The challenge is to help the partners balance their needs for each and adapt this balance to the demands of the illness. The health care system may not support couples in which partners have assumed nontraditional gender roles, assuming that the woman has been the caregiver and the man, the primary wage earner. They may fail to recognize how a non-gender-stereotyped couple may have different concerns. Finally, the ill person's adjustment to the illness may be affected by gender as well. Men's socialization to avoid showing weakness may make acknowledging and managing the illness more challenging, but it may also insulate men from taking on a rigid "sick role." Women may have less difficulty accepting the illness but more difficulty adjusting to health once the illness is cured or managed more effectively.

The stress of an illness, like any major stressor, has ramifications for the family's development, and vice versa. Late-life illness is more consistent with normal development; therefore, it may be somewhat less stressful. Illness that occurs out of the normal individual or family life cycle can have larger ramifications (the primary wage earner becomes ill in middle age, the primary child care provider becomes ill when the children are young, etc.). Life-cycle tasks should be considered during assessment of the family's response to illness. A family may become "stuck" at the lifestyle stage at which the illness started or was most acute. The lack of continued development can result in myriad problematic patterns for the couple and family.

Couples also must make adaptations when they are faced with the disability or illness of a child. Clearly, raising a child with a developmental disability or a chronic illness can be a challenge. Despite these challenges, research regarding marital satisfaction in couples with disabled children has been mixed, with some results indicating a negative effect on marital satisfaction, and others indicating no effect or a positive effect (Stoneman & Gavidia-Payne, 2006). Similar disparate results have been obtained in studies of couples facing the chronic illness of a child (Gaither, Bingen, & Hopkins, 2000). There is some evidence that both childhood disability and chronic illness increase role strain (Quittner et al., 1998), and decrease the couple's sense of coherence (Oelofsen & Richardson, 2006). Studies examining the impact of a child's critical illness or accident indicate that marital functioning is negatively impacted at the time of the event, but it is less clear whether this impact is lasting (Shudy et al., 2006). However, marital therapists should be alert to the health status of the couple's children, and how this might be affecting the family's stress level and marital functioning.

THE PRACTICE OF COUPLE THERAPY

Structure of the Therapy Process

Couple therapists may need to expand the treatment system to include the ill person's partner, because patients with illness often present alone. Often, it is helpful to expand the participants to include all who affect, or are affected by, the illness. Session attendance plans should be fluid to accommodate changes as the patient and his or her partner identify more and more relevant people as treatment progresses. Individual sessions may help the therapist respond to particular stressors or to explore an issue more thoroughly. Clearly, people outside the biological family may become involved. Including important non-family-members can facilitate assessment and increase the family's

sense of social support. Finally, members of the health care team obviously affect the illness and (perhaps less obviously) may be affected by the illness as well. Including members of the health care team, even when the interface between the couple and the team is not problematic, can be very helpful. Joint appointments attended by members of the health care team give the family members opportunities to ask questions about the illness. This may alleviate fears among family members that someone is hiding critical information.

Dr. Giancomo, Alice's neurologist, attended the last 15 minutes of the first family session. In response to the psychologist's request, he described Alice's hospitalization, the tests she took, and the certainty of the health care team that she did not have epilepsy. Instead, he said, she was experiencing stress-induced, nonelectrical seizures. He praised the family for having the courage to come to psychotherapy and said he was certain that Alice and her husband Bob would benefit from their work with the psychologist.

Collaboration with health care providers also gives therapists who are unable to prescribe psychotropic medication built-in consultants regarding these issues. Psychotropic medication can be particularly helpful when depression or anxiety significantly impair the patient's functioning. Giving patients information about psychotropic medication and helping them decide whether and when they feel it could be helpful is another opportunity for agency.

Health care professionals should be included when problematic patterns develop between the couple and the treatment team. Resolving or improving problematic interactions with the treatment team also can create a sense of agency. Health professionals also benefit from learning about the family's coping, and how the team can improve the care of this patient and family.

Alice and Bob's family physician, Dr. Romero, attended the sixth session with the spouses, after they had discussed Bob's mood swings and the possibility of antidepressant medication. After making records of his moods and their effect on his family life, Bob was more open to the possibility of medication, as well as psychotherapy. Dr. Romero participated in the first part of a session to describe potential benefits and side effects. Soon thereafter, he prescribed medication for Bob, who benefited considerably.

Some therapists who work primarily with families facing illness choose to work in a health care setting. This context changes the structure of therapy in a number of ways. The therapy room may be an exam room or space adjacent to medical office, making it easier for physicians such as Drs. Giancomo and Romero to participate in a session. The therapist may engage patients during medical appointments or be part of the "medical treatment team." Many therapists who work in medical settings have noted that patients and their partners who seek psychotherapy in a medical setting may be at a different level of "readiness for change" (Prochaska & DiClemente, 1983). They may attend psychotherapy based on treatment team expectations or recommendations rather than an insight regarding the need to resolve emotional or relational issues. The medical professional, rather than the patient may be the "customer" for the psychotherapy. Under these circumstances, the therapist needs to recognize the potential for motivational issues and assess the couple's willingness to attend therapy. If the partners really are not interested in psychotherapy, the therapist can consult with the health care provider regarding the concerns driving the referral, and how the health care professional can prepare the couple for referral. If the couple agrees to continue, the therapist may need to adjust expectations and pacing, and begin with basic psychoeducation about how therapy can help the couple cope.

Another result of practicing in close alignment with medical professionals is a different pace of therapy than is often seen in other settings. Because patients usually go to their health care providers on an "as-needed" basis, they may seek psychotherapy only when they feel it is immediately necessary. This pattern can disrupt the typical "joining/assessment–midphase–termination" cycle of psychotherapy. However, it can parallel the course of an illness in ways that help the therapist understand the couple's different needs at different times. It is common that patients are seen one or two times a month rather than every week. Sometimes, especially with severely somatizing or otherwise complex patients, it can be helpful to have a physician serve as a cotherapist (McDaniel, 1997; McDaniel et al., 2005). The physician's biomedical expertise can facilitate discussion of the illness itself. Moreover, the physician's understanding of the dynamics of the health care team can help the therapist and couple to understand any issues they have with the care or the professionals.

Therapists also can utilize family members or other social supports as link therapists (Landau, 1981). A "link therapist" is a social support who is able to connect with all factions of the family and facilitate communication among them to create movement toward consensus and joint functioning. This technique is particularly helpful when a family or couple has fragmented in the context of the illness, or when some family members cannot or will not attend therapy sessions.

Role of the Therapist

One means of empowering the couple is to take a collaborative stance toward the therapy. Although the therapist may have expertise in helping couples cope with illness in general, the members of each couple are the experts on their own illness experience. The therapist can normalize reactions that patients sometimes find confusing or painful (e.g., anger), facilitate communication and dialogue, and help the couple find a sense of agency and communion. A collaborative stance minimizes the likelihood that the partners will experience psychotherapy as disempowering or as imposed upon them, the way they may experience other aspects of the overall treatment plan.

In part because of the collaborative nature of this work, therapists tend to be quite active. Couples often need encouragement to discuss these challenging topics. As is the case for physicians, any self-disclosure in medical family therapy must be thoughtful, brief, focused on the patient's issues, and generally limited (McDaniel et al., 2007). A therapist who has personal experience with the couple's illness must be careful to separate his or her own experience from the couple's unique illness experience. Therapists also need to be generally conscious of their own illness experiences and health beliefs, and of the ways these affect the therapy. In many ways, the use of his or her own family-of-origin experiences concerning health and illness may inform the therapist, just as other family-of-origin experiences can be helpful or hindering in all types of psychotherapy (McDaniel et al., 1992).

Theresa was referred for psychotherapy because she was having difficulty coping with multiple family problems. It quickly became apparent that she had coped with stress somatically for much of her life. Her husband Larry agreed to attend psychotherapy with her, primarily out of frustration about how her many illnesses affected the family. One major issue acknowledged by both Theresa and Larry was a rift between Theresa and their adult daughters. Larry frequently felt caught between "the girls" and his wife. Both were angry that their daughters were not more understanding of their mother's physical problems. The therapist (N. B. Ruddy), who was about the same age as their daughters, discussed her own experience with her mother's cardiac illness that had resulted in a heart transplant. She noted that even though she understood that her mother was not to blame for her illness, there were times when it was difficult not to feel at least "cheated" because her mother was not healthy. This seemed to help Theresa and Larry look at the situation as their daughters might have experienced it. They began to recognize how this sense of loss for the daughters might be particularly strong given that their mother had often been unable to mother them when they were younger as well.

Some therapists are more likely than others to enjoy and thrive in the health care environment. Therapists who understand and are drawn to the complex interplay of biological, psychological, and relational elements of the illness experience are more likely to enjoy helping couples cope with illness. Therapists who enjoy working as part of a team, and are willing to collaborate with other health care professionals, also may thrive in a more medicalized environment. Clearly, anyone who has very negative feelings about the medical profession or health care system may struggle to recognize the positive experiences of others. They may be less likely to enjoy the collaborative aspects of this work, less able to tolerate issues that press their "antimedicine" buttons, and perhaps more likely to become triangulated when a couple experiences difficulties with the medical system. Accessibility of peer consultation is important for all medical family therapists.

Assessment and Treatment Planning

Overall, therapists should be aware that illness might be a part of the context for any couple's presenting concern. Either patients or therapists can fail to make the connection between a history of illness and current need for treatment. Every couple that presents for couple therapy should be asked whether either partner is now ill, or has previously had a significant illness. Often patients who are referred for assistance in coping with an illness present alone. In such a case, it is the therapist's job to broaden the focus to the couple and family. The first step in accomplishing this is to ask questions that bring others' perspectives and experiences into the dialogue, even if they are not physically present. We list questions that can facilitate this in Table 22.1.

Assessment of the family and relational levels is consistent with the biopsychosocial model. To remain true to this model, therapists must also as-

TABLE 22.1. Questions to Elicit Patient's and Family Members' Illness Perceptions

For the patient

1. What do you think caused your problem?
2. Why do you think it started when it did?
3. What do you think your sickness does to you? How does it work?
4. How severe is your sickness? Will it have a long or short course?
5. What are the chief problems your sickness has caused for you?
6. What do you fear most about your sickness?
7. What kind of treatment do you think you should receive?
8. What are the most important results you hope to receive from this treatment?
9. Should we expect complications?
10. What has been your extended family's experience with illness?
11. Has anyone else in your family faced an illness similar to the one you have now? If so, what was its course?
12. What is your and your family's past history of recuperation?
13. What might make healing now a struggle for you?
14. Do you see yourself as having much to live for?

For family members

15. What changes in family responsibilities do you think will be needed because of the patient's sickness?
16. If the patient needs care or special help, what family members are going to be responsible for providing it?
17. If the illness is already chronic or appears likely to become chronic, what are the patient's and family members' plans for taking care of the problem over the long term?

Note. The first eight questions are taken from Kleinman, Eisenberg, and Good (1978). Questions 9 and 10 are adapted from Seaburn, Lorenz, and Kaplan (1993). Questions 11 through 14 are adapted from Friedman (1991). Questions 15 through 17 are from Shields, Wynne, and Sirkin (1992).

sess the impact of the biological processes, and social and community issues. Often a therapist must work with other professionals to understand better the biological and social context of an illness. Therefore, collaboration with other health professionals is critical—both in gathering information about the illness, its treatment, and prognosis; and in understanding the patient's relationships with the health care system.

Helping the couple create a time line of the illness is very helpful. A "time line" should include family history with this or other illnesses, because scripts about illness are often part of a family's "lore." This is particularly true when an illness is common to many family members or has a significant genetic component. Beyond specific illnesses in the family, it is helpful to hear how the family traditionally has dealt with illness and its history with the health care system. Again, these can be sources of expectations, fears, and myths that lead to seemingly "noncompliant" behavior and are relevant to adapting to the illness. Stretching the time line to include the family's expectations of the future is also useful. If the illness is terminal, it is helpful to assess the couple's (and each individual's) acceptance level. Even if the illness is not anticipated to result in death, it almost certainly has already caused, and will continue to cause, numerous permanent and temporary losses. Assessing the couple's awareness and anxiety about these losses, and partners' ability to tolerate overt conversation about them, is essential.

Maria was referred for psychotherapy with one of us (N. B. Ruddy) to help her cope with her declining health related to chronic obstructive pulmonary disorder. In addition, her physician was frustrated, because Maria continued to smoke even as her lung functioning deteriorated. Her family was frustrated with her, because they did not believe Maria was being honest with them about her illness, and did not trust that she was caring for herself in the best manner. In a family meeting with her husband and three of her four children, the therapist, and her physician Dr. Grange, the children discussed their experience of Maria's surviving ovarian cancer a decade earlier. Maria, her husband, and the extended family had colluded to hide her cancer from the children, and had never told them directly that she was expected to die. Thus, the children had been confused by mixed messages about their mother's illness. Now, as they faced a new illness experience with their mother, they did not trust their parents to be honest with them.

Multiple family meetings and ongoing psychotherapy helped Maria and her husband begin to share more openly with their adult children, and helped the children understand their parents' earlier behavior and trust them more. Family members once again needed to process the likelihood that Maria's illness would ultimately be terminal, although they recognized that her downward course would take years.

The therapist should also investigate the couple's preillness level of functioning. As noted earlier, the stress of an illness can exacerbate preexisting problems; it can also disorganize an otherwise healthy couple relationship. Understanding the partners' lives before the illness provides a context for the current situation and gives the therapist a sense of how much adaptation the cou-

ple has already made. Acknowledging the steps that they have already taken to cope with the illness can help partners to recognize how they have taken control over what feels uncontrollable.

When the ill person is incapacitated, this discussion can also shed light on his or her personality and functioning prior to the illness. In noting issues that might be exacerbated by the illness, the therapist should also note the strengths the partners bring to their struggle. Often these strengths form the basis of maximizing the couple's quality of life and adaptation.

George and Joanne sought couple therapy after George had a heart attack and could no longer work. George had always been a workaholic. Joanne had coped by developing an active social life that did not include George. Now that George was not working, Joanne experienced his presence as an interference. Their "comfortable distance" no longer worked. Couple therapy helped them to realize how their preillness pattern was now maladaptive, and how they needed to find a new balance. In addition, George developed more outside interests, and he respected Joanne's need for privacy and distance at times.

Eliciting the couple's illness story allows the therapist to assess the partners' interactions with the health care system. These interactions can be either a source of great comfort or a source of enormous frustration, pain, and anger. Often the couple has had a mix of experiences with different providers and institutions. If the illness story includes a long, arduous diagnostic process, misdiagnosis, or delayed diagnosis, the couple may mistrust health care professionals, including couple therapists.

Examining the couple's life-cycle issues is another useful assessment tool (Carter & McGoldrick, 1999). Are illness and debilitation normal aspects of the couple's stage of development, or has the illness struck out of sequence? What challenges does the couple face as part of normal development that might be intensified by the illness? Understanding how the couple has navigated other life-cycle challenges can help the therapist maximize the partners' natural coping strengths to manage this challenge as well. For example, the members of one couple had a lengthy discussion regarding the usefulness of the process they used when their children were young to divide tasks of caring for the husband's ailing mother.

Intrinsic to this discussion of assessing a couple is the assumption that the couple benefits from the assessment. Overt conversations about the losses and challenges the couple faces, time lines, life-cycle discussions, collaboration with medical professionals, and genograms all help the therapist better understand the family. However, they also help family members better understand themselves and put their current situation in a coherent context. The processes of telling one's illness narrative, and hearing how other family members have experienced the illness, are therapeutic in and of themselves.

Goal Setting

The primary goal for couples facing illness is to adapt to the changes that illness has thrust upon their lives. Couples may need assistance in forming smaller goals that enhance their overall adaptation. Common smaller goals include resolution of preexisting issues that block partners' ability to adapt and work together as a team, finding meaning in the illness, taking control over the controllable aspects of the illness, accepting the uncontrollable aspects for what they are, and learning to live around the illness. Most couples need to improve their ability to communicate about things in general, as well as about the illness in particular. In addition, many couples need assistance in communicating with the health care system.

Two general goals that underlie successful adaptation are "agency" and "communion" (McDaniel et al., 1992). Adapting Bakan's (1969) general usage of the term to an illness context, Totman (1979) used "agency" to describe active involvement in and commitment to one's own care. Couples can feel overwhelmed and powerless in the face of illness, resulting in increased passivity. The health care system and "patient" or "illness" roles may also reinforce this passivity. Patients who manage to take control over what is controllable, and to accept what is not controllable, tend to adapt and accept more easily. Patients need a sense of support and community around them. Because illness can be very isolating, the therapist should focus on increasing social support. Psychotherapy facilitates communion by helping family members join together via a dialogue about these experiences. The therapist can attempt to draw in family members who may have distanced themselves either prior to or in response to the illness. Finally, he or she can help the family connect with other families facing similar challenges.

Alice had a history of seizures and depression. After hospitalization for seizure evaluation, Alice's neurologist said that she had nonelectrical seizures that he felt were rooted in marital and family problems. He sent Alice and her family to a family psychologist (S. H. McDaniel). In the first session, Alice stated that her goal was "to have everyone in the family stop blaming her and stop being so dependent" on her for household chores. With her agreement, the psychologist suggested that Alice's goals were to stop accepting blame for the family's problems, and to stop babying her adult children and her husband. Alice's husband Bob stated that his goal for therapy was to help his wife "in whatever time she had left on this earth." After comments by his wife and daughter about his needing antidepressant medication, Bob acknowledged that he had serious mood swings, but said, "They have no effect on our family life." With Bob's agreement, the psychologist suggested that Bob's goals were to help his wife physically and emotionally, and to evaluate the effect of his mood swings on the family.

As is true in many couples, Alice experienced too much communion and not enough agency, whereas Bob had too much agency and not enough communion. Therefore, one therapeutic goal was to achieve a balance between agency and communion for the individuals and the family. Helgeson (1994), in a review of the research on agency and communion, found that either unmitigated agency or unmitigated communion is associated with negative health outcomes.

Emotionally focused therapy with couples facing illness emphasizes helping couples "normalize and validate each partner's experience, to help partners process their emotional experiences, to externalize negative interaction cycles, and to help partners seek safety, security, and comfort from each other (i.e., create a more secure attachment bond)" (Kowal, Johnson, & Lee, 2003, p. 304). This model targets the couple's underlying attachment needs, and how these needs relate to the health and wellness of the couple.

Process and Technical Aspects of Couple Therapy

McDaniel et al. (1992), in their work on medical family therapy, discuss a number of key concepts and techniques in helping families cope with serious illness. The first is to recognize the biological dimension of a couple's or family's problems. In some forms of family therapy, the family's labeling of one member as "sick" is seen as part of the problem. In medical family therapy, the therapist accepts the family's definition of the problem as a medical illness. Including physicians in one of the initial encounters to explain the illness, its prognosis, and its probable course ensures that therapist, patient, and family members all have the same information about the illness. This dialogue can demystify the illness for family members and give them the opportunity to ask questions.

In the context of an ambiguous diagnosis or course of illness, it is important to be open to many possible explanations for the patient's symptomatology. It is easy to "pigeonhole" a patient into a medical, psychological, or relational diagnosis. Both biomedical and psychosocial factors can be given too much weight. It is not uncommon to find that relational and intrapsychic issues exacerbate even the most biomedical of illnesses. Sometimes a patient is referred simply because the health care team has been unable to find a biomedical explanation for his or her symptoms. Under these circumstances, it can be tempting to assume that the issues are primarily psychosocial, or at least "stress-related." Patients sometimes experience this stance as negation of their illness experience, the suggestion that their symptoms are "all in their head." Ambiguous ailments that do not fall easily into a diagnostic category (and may therefore not fall into a clear treatment plan category) can be particularly challenging for couples. They may feel blamed for the illness, confused because they do not understand the source of the problem, or frustrated because they are not sure how to proceed.

Theresa and Larry struggled to understand why Theresa so often experienced illnesses for which the medical community did not have ready diagnoses and treatments. Theresa vacillated between being angry with her medical team and feeling guilty that she kept getting sick. Only after a great deal of treatment did she and her husband begin to discuss the link between stress and illness in a productive, nonblaming way. Larry and their daughters tended to believe either that Theresa was "really sick" (e.g., the physicians had a diagnosis, prognosis, and treatment), or that "it was all in her head." Because she had to "prove" her illness with physicians' testimonials or medical test results, Theresa's utilization of medical care and diagnostic testing was even greater. Slowly Larry came to accept that all illness is both biological and psychological, and stopped trying to categorize Theresa's illnesses. Removing this pressure enabled Theresa to begin to discuss and to change her lifelong pattern of avoiding conflict and emotional upset by channeling her difficulties into somatic symptoms.

The second concept of medical family therapy is to elicit the illness story. The illness story/time line helps the therapist understand the couple's journey, and helps the partners recognize how illness has affected their lives. Many partners have not had the opportunity to review their entire experience with an illness from the appearance of the first symptoms to the present. Physicians who gather a biomedical history understandably focus on only certain aspects of the experience. Family members and friends may feel comfortable hearing only certain elements, or they may have attempted to avoid hearing the story. The partners find that just telling their story to an empathic listener very therapeutic. In organizing the time line, the therapist should ask about the onset of the illness; illness symptoms; diagnostic process and diagnosis; treatments that have been suggested, been tried, or that are desired; the patient's and family members' emotional and practical responses to the illness; and the patient's current condition. Gathering genogram information allows the therapist to solicit an illness story that may have unfolded over generations, and to understand better the family's general scripts about illness.

In one of the first couple sessions Larry and Theresa attended, the therapist completed a genogram. Although Larry was aware that Theresa's father had died of gastrointestinal (GI) cancer, he did not know that six of her father's seven siblings had also died of GI cancer. Theresa recounted how horrifyingly painful her father's death had been, and her fear that she too would contract a GI cancer. She also stated that she had been advised to have her GI tract scoped whenever she "felt any kind of twinge," because of her strong family history. Her story helped the therapist, Larry, and Theresa herself understand why she was quite focused on body sensations, particularly those from her abdomen, and why she immediately looked to her medical care providers to reassure her that she would not succumb to her father's dreadful fate. Given Theresa's script about cancer, the therapist also made sure that her physician reeducated her about worrisome versus benign GI symptoms, and about modern cancer treatment.

Therapists who help couples cope with medical illness need to respect defenses, remove blame, and accept unacceptable feelings. A couple facing an illness is in crisis. As in any crisis intervention treatment, the partners' current coping mechanisms need to be left intact until they develop new strategies. This is particularly true of their use of denial. Denial that gives a couple enough hope to face the next day, while not interfering with appropriate treatment or planning for the future, is adaptive. In addition, a couple facing illness can be particularly sensitive and vulnerable to perceived criticism, because there is often a latent sense of guilt about the illness. If family members feel they are being criticized, and are ambivalent about the psychotherapy referral, it is highly unlikely that they will engage in treatment. A strong dose of support in the context of helping the couple examine and change maladaptive patterns is generally much more likely to result in a positive outcome.

Much of the latent sense of guilt over illness stems from ideas about fairness and personal responsibility. People want to believe that bad things, such as illness, do not happen randomly; someone must have done something to cause this terrible thing. The context of this general cognitive schema and the links between lifestyle, behavior, and illness often result in family members' attributing illness to something they or their health care team did or did not do. Facilitating a dialogue about these fears allows the family to accept the illness, relieves the patient or others of inappropriate blame, and uses rituals to heal wounds from real relational or behavioral causes of the illness.

Mary Jane harbored the fear that she had miscarried in her third month because of a fall she had taken in her second month. Her therapist (S. H. McDaniel) convened a meeting that included Mary Jane, her husband John; and her obstetrician Dr. Eisen to discuss the cause of her miscarriage. Dr. Eisen reassured Mary Jane that it was unlikely that her fall was related to her miscarriage, and told her that one in five pregnancies end in miscarriage. Furthermore, he was able both to sympathize with the couple's loss and to reassure John and Mary Jane that their future pregnancies would have as good a chance of completion as those of any other couple.

Partners in any couple have negative feelings about each other that are difficult to discuss and process even under the best of circumstances. What was once difficult can seem impossible to a couple facing illness. Although this avoidance can reduce squabbles over relatively unimportant issues, it can also preclude resolution of important issues and increase emotional distance within the couple. Medical family therapy can help family members accept unacceptable emotions, particularly those that tend to emerge under the stress of illness. For example, the well partner may begin to resent the needs of the ill partner, and may feel guilty about this resentment. Both normalizing this process and helping the partners discuss their "unacceptable" feelings are therapeutic.

Medical family therapy strives to maintain and facilitate communication. The desire to protect one another can create or exacerbate poor communication among family members, resulting in a general sense of loneliness or isolation. It is often helpful for the family to realize that any

member's secretiveness is usually well intentioned. Also, each member of a couple must recognize and acknowledge his or her own secretive behavior. Often one partner notices when the other is secretive, but is not aware of how his or her own secretive behavior blocks communication. As they begin to discuss painful issues, the therapist can help partners recognize how open communication fosters a sense of support and teamwork. Medical family therapy gives family members a venue in which to discuss these important issues safely, and it normalizes their desire to protect each other by avoiding difficult feelings.

The medical family therapist can also work to improve communication between the couple and the health care system. The therapist can use his or her expertise in collaborating with health care professionals to coach both members of the couple in preparing questions for medical appointments and asserting themselves appropriately. When there are issues with the medical professionals, the therapist can hold a joint meeting to facilitate communication in the moment. Meetings that include medical care providers also help to reduce the likelihood of the medical family therapist becoming triangulated with the couple and the other professionals. Also, the therapist should maintain open communication with other members of the health care team, both to provide a model for the couple and to avoid creating parallel processes of poor communication among the team, the couple, and the therapist.

Dr. Loren came to one of us (S. H. McDaniel) and said she felt caught, because her 65-year-old patient Jack Brown told her that he did not want his wife Jane to know that he was dying. He feared that "she could not handle it." Meanwhile, privately, Jane told Dr. Loren that she did not want her to share her husband's terminal diagnosis with him, because he was "not yet ready to hear it." The therapist suggested a family conference, and met with the couple and Dr. Loren. At the therapist's suggestion, Dr. Loren opened the meeting by asking both spouses what they knew of Jack's illness and what questions they had about prognosis and treatment. Within a few minutes, Jack and Jane each reported what they knew (which was remarkably similar information) and moved on to discuss pain management and hospice care.

Medical family therapists must place current issues in a developmental context (Carter & McGoldrick, 1999; McDaniel et al., 1992; Rolland, 1994). The therapist and couple must attend to matters involving both individual and family development, development of the illness and its ramifications, and the interaction between the illness and developmental needs of the individual and family—while not allowing the illness to "take over." Gonzalez, Steinglass, and Reiss (1989) describe this as putting illness in its place. Medical family therapists can help families keep "illness in its place" by encouraging the couple and family to maintain routines, rituals, and traditions, and to create space for each family member to get his or her own needs met as much as possible.

Lorena and Joe Williams sought therapy to help them cope with Lorena's breast cancer. They had two children, both in their late teens. Their older daughter had planned to attend college out of state. However, with her mother's diagnosis, she announced to the family that she planned to attend the local community college, which would allow her to be closer to her mother and to help the family. Lorena and Joe did not want her to make this sacrifice, because they felt it might prevent her from living up to her potential. In therapy, they were able to discuss how they wanted to approach their daughter about this. This dialogue was an opportunity for them to discuss the sacrifices everyone was making because of the illness. Lorena acknowledged her guilt about this, and Joe discussed his sadness that there was nothing he could do to protect his wife from her ordeal.

As we have noted, increasing the patient's and couple's sense of agency optimizes coping. Couples often need assistance to differentiate between controllable and uncontrollable factors, to take charge of the controllable issues, and to accept the uncontrollable issues. Therapists can facilitate this process by encouraging the couple to discuss treatment decisions and share their preferences with the health care team. When the couple or patient disagrees with or does not adhere to medical advice, the therapist can help the couple and the health care team understand this behavior as an attempt to gain control. The therapist can help the couple work through "resistance," or disagreement, by emphasizing the temporary nature of all decisions. This approach can help free the members of the couple (or the health care team) to "try out" a suggestion they are ambivalent about trying, or allow them to reconsider hard-line stances in the future.

Judith became more and more fatigued, until finally she went to her doctor for a physical. She told both her husband and her doctor that she was sure it was "nothing." However, her white blood cell count was very high. Unfortunately, this started a diagnostic process that went on for almost a year before Judith was found to meet the criteria for non-Hodgkin's lymphoma. During this time, Judith actively searched the Internet and the library for information about her condition. She took lists of questions to her physician, trying to make the most efficient use of each appointment. She focused on what she could do to increase a sense of agency in a highly uncertain and stressful situation.

To avoid replicating the loss of control that patients often experience with illness and in the health care area, the therapist should avoid giving advice or pushing couples in a specific direction. Rather, the therapist should encourage couples to gather information and help them to discuss options and make decisions. Putting the responsibility and power of decisions firmly in the couple's court facilitates a sense of agency and avoids creating a parallel process in which the couple is "nonadherent" with the therapist as well.

As their final general technique, McDaniel et al. (1992) advise therapists to "keep the door open"—a principle that medical family therapy shares with most time-limited, brief psychotherapy (Budman & Gurman, 1988). Family members consult with the therapist on an as-needed basis. Accepting their time line for seeking psychotherapy supports the partners' decision-making skills and sense of agency. In addition, because the medical professional will continue to be involved, the couple does have a sounding board for issues, and may be referred back for further treatment if the medical professional and couple feel it may be helpful. Conducting follow-up—either by seeing the patient during a medical visit if the physician and therapist share space, or by placing a phone call or writing a letter 6–12 months after termination—can set the stage for the couple to return if needed.

John Bell and Gerry Sanders had been long-term partners when Gerry suffered a serious heart attack. Both men had difficulty with the lifestyle changes encouraged by Gerry's cardiologist and his family physician. Gerry's heart condition really required him to change his diet, decrease his stress, and increase his exercise regimen. Because both physicians knew these changes were much more likely to happen if the partners worked on them together, so all parties worked with a therapist (S. H. McDaniel) to develop a plan that was possible for the couple. These goals were accomplished in six sessions over a 3-month period. Because maintenance was of great importance, the couple agreed to return at 3-, 6-, and 12-month intervals for booster sessions.

Rolland (1994) has focused specifically on the effect of illness on intimacy. He notes that illness challenges both physically and emotionally the "intimacy homeostasis" a couple has evolved over time. The first challenge to this homeostasis is the real and anticipated losses associated with illness. Rolland notes that loss is not always associated with negative emotions, and that a direct focus on the loss may not be the most helpful course. Rather, he suggests that the therapist help the couple see the threatened loss as an opportunity to live more fully in the present, and to broaden the partners' experience of intimacy. Rolland suggests, "In general, couples adapt best when they revise their closeness to include rather than avoid issues of incapacitation and threatened loss" (p. 237).

The second challenge to intimacy involves changes the partners must make in how they communicate. Rolland notes that partners must find a "functional balance" in their communication. In other words, they must discern which fears, feelings, and thoughts need to be shared (no matter how difficult this may be), and which are best kept to themselves. Like McDaniel et al. (1992), Rolland (1994) notes that illness challenges couple communication in many ways. Many of the new issues and adaptations that must be addressed are difficult to discuss, because so many of the fears, feelings, and thoughts are overwhelming or shameful, and the partners want to protect each other. A therapist can help the couple by normalizing these intense experiences, and by helping the partners to share their experiences rather than allowing them to create distance. Rolland notes that the anger that accompanies illness can be particularly challenging for couples.

Rolland also stresses rebalancing relationship skews. If the illness is seen as only one person's problem, the relationship will be redefined around inequality in the couple. The inequality in health can generalize to inequalities in power and control, resulting in decreased intimacy, resentment, guilt, and emotional distance. To avoid this, Rolland suggests that the members of the couple redefine the illness as "our" problem. This acknowledges the very real changes that both partners experience as a result of the illness, and allows them to discuss and challenge their preconceptions about "appropriate" roles of the ill and well partners. A couple may need assistance in breaking out of roles and scripts about illness based on family-of-origin experiences with illness.

Karen and Joel had a very unstable marital relationship. Both partners attributed many of their difficulties to Karen's longstanding mood disorder. After much struggling, Karen started to take a mood stabilizer that was very helpful to her. However, the couple's dynamics in relating to her illness continued to be a problem. Joel harbored a great deal of resentment about old incidents, particularly about some financial difficulties related to Karen's mood swings. He often stated that all of the problems had been "Karen's fault," and that there was nothing he could do to improve their relationship. He refused to take any responsibility for difficulties, including financial problems that were related to his behavior. He clearly felt powerless to help Karen, and was torn between his love for her and his anger about how difficult their lives were. Even when Karen's condition stabilized, he had difficulty shifting out of this powerlessness. Ultimately, the couple separated and divorced. Only with distance and individual therapy did Karen recognized how her illness was a large factor in her "lightning rod" position in many relationships. She acknowledged that her relationship with Joel had been based on her being "the sick one" and Joel's being the "victim" of her illness. Joel began to recognize his own culpability in the problems and worked to create a more balanced relationship with his next partner.

Illness can be like a new, unwanted family member. Like any other family member, the illness itself can be the third point in triangulation of conflicts, reducing the couple's ability to resolve issues as a dyad. Also, when the illness is the source of resolution of some problem (albeit an unhealthy resolution), the illness becomes necessary. This can interfere with restoring health and increase the likelihood that relational issues or secondary gains support symptoms. When the illness becomes a central point in the couple's dynamics, the therapy must help the couple realign the relationship to make this third point of the triangle less necessary. The demise of Karen and Joel's relationship after Karen improved illustrates what can happen when the illness is central in how the partners relate to each other.

Couples often need assistance in drawing a boundary around the illness, so that the relationship ultimately does not become defined by the illness. The very real changes that illness necessitates can make partners feel that their entire lives and relationship will never be the same again, and will change only for the worse. They can become so focused on the illness and its effects that they see themselves as separate from the healthy world. As Rolland (1994) states, "Living a normal life is external to the relationship and illness that is within" (p. 242). To counteract these insidious assumptions and their effects, Rolland suggests some simple strategies for compartmentalizing the illness. The partners can agree upon times when the illness is the focus of their communication, and other times, when it is "off limits." The boundary can be placed geographically, prohibiting discussion of the illness in certain places, such as the bedroom. The couple can be encouraged to maintain social contacts and to continue preillness social routines as much as possible.

Rolland also notes that members of a couple need to be able to adapt their functioning to the level required by the illness. There will be crisis periods when the illness is central and all-consuming. However, the therapist can help the partners recognize when they can return to a lifestyle more consistent with their preillness functioning. To feel safe engaging in more emotionally or physically strenuous activities, they may need specific information about the illness or the ill person's current level of health and ability to tolerate stress. An overt discussion of resuming their sex life, for example, is particularly helpful, because many partners are embarrassed to ask about this and fear that physical intimacy is contraindicated.

Jerry and Marta came to therapy because they were having difficulty adjusting to life after Jerry's heart attack. Jerry had smoked heavily and was unable to stop, until the day he was hospitalized with chest pain and an eventual myocardial infarction. Marta came to the hospital every day, then, as Jerry said, "watched him like a hawk" thereafter. He had not had a cigarette since the hospitalization, and Marta was trying to learn to cook low-fat foods, but Jerry was complaining about the taste and threatening to start smoking again. Before focusing on the needed lifestyle changes, the therapist (S. H. McDaniel) spent two sessions discussing how scary the heart attack experience had been for them both. In the second session, for the first time, Jerry broke down and cried, admitting how worried he was about whether he would live to see his grandchildren. Marta, with support from the therapist, was able to listen and to empathize with her husband's fears. Jerry had always been the strong, silent type, so expressing his feelings was a new experience for both partners. In the fourth session, the therapist asked when they planned to resume their sex life. Jerry was relieved that she brought the subject up, and said that both he and Marta were worried about the possibility of his "dying like Nelson Rockefeller." The therapist asked Jerry's family doctor to stop by during the next session to reassure them and to answer any questions about sexual activity. She also encouraged them to continue developing all aspects of their communication.

The stress of illness can exacerbate difficulties in the couple's emotional regulation, resulting in an "emotional rollercoaster." Watson and McDaniel (2005) outline a seven-step approach to address emotional reactivity in couples facing illness. They recommend that the therapist help the couple to do the following:

1. Discuss the pragmatic and emotional impact of the illness.
2. Determine how emotional reactivity affects each area of concern, and which areas cause the most anxiety and distress.
3. Refocus on the internal response to the illness and its meaning, rather than on how it impacts on daily living.
4. Discuss emotional reactions, and the internal processes associated with them.
5. Connect the emotions to each person's personal history and vulnerabilities.
6. Facilitate separation of reaction to the current situation from reactions to historical triggers.
7. Develop alternative, adaptive responses to current stressors and triggers.

As couples review various issues via this process, they increase differentiation and decrease reactivity, increasing their ability to adapt to the demands of the illness and their sense of agency and communion.

A number of other general psychotherapy techniques can be applied usefully to therapy with couples facing illness. Many authors have discussed the role of psychoeducation in helping couples cope with illness (McDaniel et al., 1992; Miller, McDaniel, Rolland, & Feetham, 2006; Rolland, 1994). Psychoeducation prepares couples for possible changes in mood, energy level, behavioral inhibition or disinhibition, and other expected areas related to illness. Reviewing possible relational challenges helps the couple understand "normal" change and recognize potentially unhealthy changes. Therefore, psychoeducation can set the stage for the couple to engage in preventive work before patterns become embedded, or the relationship becomes very damaged. When partners discuss the challenges ahead of time, they can "know the enemy," predict which issues are likely to be most challenging for them, and agree on a plan for preventing and managing these issues before they become too problematic.

Many patients and their partners are either unfamiliar with psychotherapy or may seek it only because their physician suggested it. Therefore, it is often necessary to begin by educating the couple about the process of psychotherapy. For example, the therapist helps the patient and partner understand how psychotherapy encounters will be different from medical encounters, and what skills psychotherapists have to assist them.

A couple's therapist should actively assist the partners in developing and maintaining communication, especially a social and support network. The partners need assistance in recognizing family members and friends who can support them, and "permission" and encouragement to access these groups. Just as they do not want to burden each other with problems, partners may shut out possible sources of support because they fear that asking for help will alienate or overburden others, or be seen as a sign of weakness. Sometimes partners fear creating inequity in their social relationships, or feel that others do not understand how the illness is affecting them. Under these circumstances, they may be most comfortable reaching out to support groups that focus on the particular illness, or on couples facing illness in general. Finally, the therapist, through collaboration with the medical professionals and other team members, can assist the family members in maximizing their benefit from the available professional supports.

Curative Factors/Mechanisms of Change

Although it is not welcome, illness does create an opportunity for growth. Couples may be able to face intrapsychic and existential issues that they might otherwise have avoided. Clearly, different illnesses create different opportunities, but almost all illnesses increase partners' awareness of the fragility of life and of simple, daily pleasures that they previously took for granted. Illness can make partners appreciate each other in new ways—both because it may force them to contemplate life without each other, and because they must work as a team and support each other. Illness also can force partners to explore new ways of relating to each other as old patterns become less functional. The couple must broaden its repertoire of interactional patterns to accommodate the illness. Therapy facilitates adaptation in interactional patterns and perceptions by making the adaptations overt, and facilitating discussion of the elements of successful adaptation. Therapy empowers the couple to increase agency by taking control over the situation and making informed, planful decisions. Sometimes partners who learn to take a proactive stance toward the illness begin to take more a more proactive stance in other areas of life as well. When the partners begin to view these adaptations as a positive force in their lives, they find meaning in the illness and develop a greater sense of cohesion. The growth catalyzed by illness can result in a more satisfying relationship overall.

Therapists who attend to biological, psychological, and social context factors are more likely than those who neglect these areas to facilitate positive change with couples facing illness. Even when illness is not the presenting concern, it is critical that therapists attend to these factors, and to the roles that health and illness play in the lives of all couples. Collaboration with health care professionals is very valuable in couple therapy, even in the absence of significant illness. Often such professionals have a long-term view of a couple, understanding the couple's current situation in the context of a much richer history that can only be gathered through a long-term relationship. In the context of illness, collaboration with health care professionals is essential. Broadening the "treatment team" to include the family and natural support systems also facilitates a sense of communion and positive outcome. Our model maintains a focus on healthy adaptation and on the strengths couples bring to the challenging transitions imposed by illness. Together, these elements form the essential core of successful couple therapy related to illness. Clearly, this approach integrates many models and applies them to the specific instance of relational difficulties related to illness. The metaframeworks of the biopsychosocial model and collaborative family health care can be layered over established couple treatments.

Treatment Applicability and Empirical Support

This model was developed from work with couples facing illness. However, much of it can be applied to couples facing any major life transition. Most couples who present for psychotherapy are in transition. The stress of the transition may cause the presenting problems, or it may merely have exposed preexisting issues that must be resolved for a couple to progress successfully.

Using the multiple lenses implicit in the biopsychosocial model allows therapists to assess and intervene sensitively, and to help create change. Though all illnesses force transition and adaptation, some are particularly challenging for couples. For example, illnesses that have a genetic component can force a couple to make difficult decisions about childbearing. Genetic illnesses can also create a sense of guilt in the partner who "brought" the illness into the family (Miller et al., 2006). Survivor guilt may occur in family members who have been spared the genetic problem (McDaniel & Speice, 2001). Other health problems directly related to developmental challenges (e.g., infertility) can clearly challenge couples as they attempt to make the transition to parenthood. Infertility assessment lends itself to blame and divisiveness, as the members of a couple seek to determine who has "the problem" that prevents them from bearing children (McDaniel et al., 1992).

Many couples who seek therapy in the context of a medical illness face other significant challenges. As appropriate, this model can be augmented with programs specifically designed to treat substance abuse/dependence or major mental illness. This model can be helpful to families coping with these issues as well, because of the many parallels between adaptations families must make to chronic physical illness and adaptations in the face of major psychiatric illness or substance abuse.

Working with couples facing medical illness does engender some ethical issues that are less likely to appear in other couple work (McDaniel et al., 1992; Seaburn, McDaniel, Kim, & Bassen, 2005). First, therapists working in a medical setting are likely to encounter different norms regarding confidentiality. They must navigate maintaining an appropriate level of confidentiality while collaborating with medical professionals, who are freer with information about patients than mental health professionals tend to be. Couple therapists may also become involved in treatment plan negotiations, particularly when a couple and medical care providers disagree on the best course of treatment. Therapists may encounter ethical issues about end-of-life decisions and advanced directives about treatment should a patient become incapacitated. Many other medical–ethical issues may arise in treating couples coping with controversial medical procedures such as abortion, fertility treatments, transplantation, and genetic testing. Therapists themselves may need consultation to cope with these challenging issues, or at least a place to process their own reactions and feelings about them.

CONCLUSION

It is not accidental that marriage vows include the words "in sickness and in health." Illness is one of the most difficult challenges a couple can face. Couples coping with illness are often on an emotional roller coaster full of unexpected twists and turns. Couple therapists who take a biopsychosocial view of their work are in a unique position to help these couples cope. Although psychotherapy for couples facing illness uses many skills from more general crisis intervention and transition-oriented therapies (Seaburn, Landau-Stanton, & Horwitz, 1995), several important skills and intervention principles are specific to this work. When illness is even a part of a couple's situation (even when it is not the stated presenting problem), it is critical that the therapist address issues related to the illness. This may require collaborating with the medical community; learning about disease progression as it relates to functionality and behavior; providing specific psychoeducation; normalizing difficulties; and helping the couple find a sense of meaning, agency, and communion.

SUGGESTIONS FOR FURTHER READING

Campbell, T. L. (2003). The effectiveness of family interventions for physical disorders. *Journal of Marital and Family Therapy, 29*, 263–281.

Fisher, L. (2006). Research on the family and chronic disease among adults: Major trends and directions. *Families, Systems, and Health, 24*, 373–380.

McDaniel, S. H., & Cole-Kelly, K. (2003). Gender, couples and illness: A feminist analysis of medical family therapy. In T. Goodrich & L. Silverstein (Eds.), *Feminist family therapy* (pp. 267–280). Washington, DC: American Psychological Association.

McDaniel, S. H., Hepworth, J., & Doherty, W. J. (1992). *Medical family therapy: A biopsychosocial approach to families with health problems.* New York: Basic Books.

Ruddy, N. B., Borresen, D., & Gunn, W. (2008). *The collaborative psychotherapist: How to create reciprocal relationships with medical professionals.* Washington, DC: American Psychological Association.

Watson, W. H., & McDaniel, S. H. (2005). Managing emotional reactivity in couples facing illness: Smoothing out the emotional roller coaster. In M. Harway (Ed.), *The handbook of couples therapy* (pp. 253–271). New York: Wiley.

REFERENCES

Alter, D. A., Chong, A., Austin, P. C., Mustart, C., Iron, K., Williams, J. I., et al. (2006). Socioeconomic status and mortality after acute myocardial infarction. *Annals of Internal Medicine, 144*, 82–93.

Bakan, D. (1969). *The duality of human existence.* Chicago: Rand McNally.

Beeson, R. A. (2003). Loneliness and depression in spousal caregivers of those with Alzheimer's disease versus non-caregiving spouses. *Archives of Psychiatric Nursing, 17*, 135–143.

Belar, C. D., & Deardorff, W. W. (1995). *Clinical health psychology in medical settings: A practitioner's guidebook.* Washington, DC: American Psychological Association.

Bloch, D. (1983). Family systems medicine: The field and the journal. *Family Systems Medicine, 1,* 3–11.

Blount, A. (1998). *Integrative primary care.* New York: Basic Books.

Budman, S. H., & Gurman, A. S. (1988). *Theory and practice of brief therapy.* New York: Guilford Press.

Campbell, T. L. (2003). The effectiveness of family interventions for physical disorders. *Journal of Marital and Family Therapy, 29,* 263–281.

Carter E., & McGoldrick, M. (1999). *The expanded family life cycle.* Needham Heights, MA: Allyn & Bacon.

Dalstra, J. A., Kunst, A. E., Borrell, C., Breeze, E., Cambois, E., Costa, G., et al. (2005). Socioeconomic differences in the prevalence of common chronic diseases: An overview of eight European countries. *International Journal of Epidemiology, 34,* 316–326.

Doherty, W. J. (1988). Implications of chronic illness for family treatment. In C. Childman, E. Nunnally, & F. Cox (Eds.), *Chronic illness and disability* (pp. 193–210). Newbury Park, CA: Sage.

Doherty, W. J., & Baird, M. (1983). *Family therapy and family medicine: Toward the primary care of families.* New York: Guilford Press.

Engel, G. L. (1977). The need for a new medical model: A challenge for biomedicine. *Science, 196,* 129–136.

Engel, G. L. (1980). The clinical application of the biopsychosocial model. *American Journal of Psychiatry, 137,* 535–544.

Fiscella, K. (1999). Is lower income associated with greater biopsychosocial morbidity?: Implications for physicians working with underserved patients. *Journal of Family Practice, 48,* 372–377.

Frank, R., Hagglund, K., & Farmer, J. E. (2004). Chronic illness management in primary care: The cardinal symptoms model. In R. Frank, S. H. McDaniel, J. Bray, & M. Heldring (Eds.), *Primary care psychology* (pp. 259–276). Washington, DC: American Psychological Association.

Frankel, R., Quill, T., & McDaniel, S. H. (2003). *The biopsychosocial approach: Past, present, future.* Rochester, NY: University of Rochester Press.

Friedman, E. (1991, June). *Managing crisis: Bowen theory incarnate.* Audiotape of a presentation at a Family Systems Theory seminar, Bethesda, MD.

Gaither, R., Bingen, K., & Hopkins, J. (2000). When the bough breaks: The relationship between chronic illness in children and couple functioning. In K. B. Schmaling & T. Goldman Sher (Eds.), *The psychology of couples and illness: Theory research, and practice* (pp. 337–365). Washington, DC: American Psychological Association.

Gonzalez, S., Steinglass, P., & Reiss, D. (1989). Putting illness in its place: Discussion groups for families with chronic medical illness. *Family Process, 28,* 69–87.

Harkaway, J. (1983). Obesity: Reducing the larger system. *Journal of Strategic and Systemic Therapy, 2,* 2–16.

Helgeson, V. S. (1994). Relation of agency and communion to well-being: Evidence and potential explanations. *Psychological Bulletin, 116,* 412–428.

Kiecolt-Glaser, J. K., Preacher, K. J., MacCallum, R. C., Atkinson, C., Malarkey, W. B., & Glaser, R. (2003). Chronic stress and age-related increases in the poinflammatory cytokine IL-6. *Proceedings of the National Academy of Sciences USA, 100,* 9090–9095.

Kleinman, A., Eisenberg, M., & Good, B. (1978). Culture illness, and care: Clinical lessons from anthropological and cross-cultural research. *Annals of Internal Medicine, 88,* 251–258.

Kowal, J., Johnson, S. M., & Lee, A. (2003). Chronic illness a couples: A case for emotionally focused therapy. *Journal of Marital and Family Therapy, 29*(3), 299–310.

Landau, J. (1981). Link therapy as a family therapy technique for transitional extended families. *Psychotherapia, 7,* 1–15.

Lantz, P. M., House, J. S., Lepkowski, J. M., Williams, D. R., Mero, R. P., & Chen, J. (1998). Socioeconomic factors, health behaviors, and mortality: Results from a nationally representative prospective study of U.S. adults. *Journal of the American Medical Association, 279,* 1703–1708.

McDaniel, S., Campbell, T., Hepworth, J., & Lorenz, A. (2005). *Family oriented primary care, second edition.* New York: Springer.

McDaniel, S. H. (1997). Trapped inside a body without a voice: Two cases of somatic fixation. In S. H. McDaniel, J. Hepworth, & W. J. Doherty (Eds.), *The shared experience of illness: Stories of patients, families and their therapists* (pp. 274–290). New York: Basic Books.

McDaniel, S. H., Beckman, H., Morse, D., Seaburn, D., Silberman, J., & Epstein, R. (2007). Physician self-disclosure in the primary care visits: Enough about you, what about me? *Archives of Internal Medicine, 167,* 1321–1326.

McDaniel, S. H., & Campbell, T. L. (2000). Consumers and collaborative family healthcare. *Families, Systems, and Health, 18,* 133–136.

McDaniel, S. H., Campbell, T. L., Hepworth, J., & Lorenz, A. (2005). *Family oriented primary care* (2nd ed.). New York: Springer-Verlag.

McDaniel, S. H., & Cole-Kelly, K. (2003). Gender, couples and illness: A feminist analysis of medical family therapy. In T. Goodrich & L. Silverstein (Eds.), *Feminist family therapy* (pp. 267–280). Washington, DC: American Psychological Association.

McDaniel, S. H., & Hepworth, J. (2004). Family psychology in primary care: Managing issues of power and dependency through collaboration. In R. Frank, S. H. McDaniel, J. Bray, & M. Heldring (Eds.), *Primary care psychology* (pp. 113–132). Washington, DC: American Psychological Association.

McDaniel, S. H., Hepworth, J., & Doherty, W. J. (1992). *Medical family therapy: A biopsychosocial approach to families with health problems.* New York: Basic Books.

McDaniel, S. H., & Speice, J. (2001). What family psychology has to offer women's health: The examples of conversion, somatization, infertility treatment, and genetic testing. *Professional Psychology: Research and Practice, 32,* 44–51.

Miller, S., McDaniel, S., Rolland, J., & Feetham, S. (Eds.). (2006). *Individuals, families and the new era of genetics: Biopsychosocial perspectives.* New York: Norton.

Oelofsen, N., & Richardson, P. (2006). Sense of coherence and parenting stress in mothers and fathers of preschool children with developmental disability. *Journal of Intellectual and Developmental Disability, 31,* 1–12.

Prochaska, J., & DiClemente, C. (1983). Stages and process of self-change of smoking: Toward an integrative model of change. *Journal of Consulting and Clinical Psychology, 51,* 390–395.

Quittner, A. L., Espelage, D. L., Opipari, L. C., Carter, B., Eid, N., & Eigen, H. (1998). Role strain in couples with and without a child with a chronic illness: Associations with marital satisfaction, intimacy, and daily mood. *Health Psychology, 172,* 112–124.

Rolland, J. (1994). *Families, illness, and disability: An integrative treatment model.* New York: Basic Books.

Ruddy, N. B., Borresen, D., & Gunn, W. (2008). *Working together: The psychotherapist's toolbox for collaborating with medical professionals.* Washington, DC: American Psychological Association.

Schultz, R., O'Brien, T., Bookwala, J., & Fleissner, K. (1995). Psychiatric and physical morbidity effects of Alzheimer's disease caregiving: Prevalence, correlates and causes. *Gerontologist, 35,* 771–791.

Seaburn, D. B., Landau-Stanton, J., & Horwitz, S. (1995). Core techniques in family therapy. In D. Mikesell, D. D. Lusterman, & S. H. McDaniel (Eds.), *Integrating family therapy: Handbook of systems theory and family psychology* (pp. 5–26). Washington, DC: American Psychological Association.

Seaburn, D. B., Lorenz, A., Gawinski, B. A., & Gunn, W. (1996). *Models of collaboration: A guide for family therapists practicing with health care professionals.* New York: Basic Books.

Seaburn, D. B., Lorenz, A., & Kaplan, D. (1993). The transgenerational development of chronic illness meanings. *Family Systems Medicine, 10,* 385–394.

Seaburn, D. B., McDaniel, S. H., Kim, S., & Bassen, D. (2005). The role of the family in resolving bioethical dilemmas: Clinical insights from a family systems perspective. *Journal of Clinical Ethics, 20,* 525–530.

Shields, C., Wynne, L., & Sirkin, M. (1992). Illness, family theory, and family therapy: I. Conceptual issues. II. The perception of physical illness in the family system. *Family Process, 31,* 3–18.

Shudy, M., de Almeida, M. L., Ly, S., Landon, C., Groft, S., Jenkins, T., et al. (2006). Impact of pediatric critical illness and injury on families: A systematic literature review. *Pediatrics, 118,* S203–S218.

Siegel, D. (1999). *The developing mind: How relationships and the brain interact to shape who we are.* New York: Guilford Press.

Sorlie, P. D., Backlund, E., & Keller, J. B. (1995). U.S. mortality by economic, demographic, and social characteristics: The National Longitudinal Mortality Study. *American Journal of Public Health, 85,* 949–956.

Stoneman, Z., & Gavidia-Payne, S. (2006). Marital adjustment in families of young children with disabilities: Associations with daily hassles and problem focused coping. *American Journal on Mental Retardation, 111*(1), 1–14.

Totman, R. (1979). *Social causes of illness.* New York: Pantheon Books.

Tsai, P. F., & Jirovec, M. M. (2005). The relationships between depression and other outcomes of chronic illness caregiving. *BMC Nursing, 4,* 3.

Van den Boss, G. A. M., Smits, J. P., Westert, G. P., & van Straten, A. (2002). Socioeconomic variations in the course of stroke: Unequal health outcomes, equal care? *Journal of Epidemiology and Community Health, 56,* 943–948.

Watson, W. H., & McDaniel, S. H. (2005). Managing emotional reactivity in couples facing illness: Smoothing out the emotional roller coaster. In M. Harway (Ed.), *The handbook of couples therapy* (pp. 53–271). New York: Wiley.

Couple Therapy in Broader Context

CHAPTER 23

Gender Issues in the Practice of Couple Therapy

Carmen Knudson-Martin

"Gender" refers to the meaning that members of a culture attribute to being male or female. It is an organizing category ascribed at birth and recreated through ongoing social interaction. As such, gender affects nearly every aspect of our lives and results in different expectations, roles, behaviors, and statuses for women and men. Gender-stereotypical behavior has been found to work against intimacy and relationship success (Johnson, 2003). However, the issues associated with gender often exist beneath the surface and are easily overlooked clinically. Despite increased awareness regarding the salience of gender to couple life, many therapists still do not address the social-contextual aspects of gender. In this chapter, I take the position that addressing gender is a critical aspect of successful heterosexual couple therapy and offer a framework for dealing with gender that can be integrated with most other models of therapy. The approach is described in more detail in Knudson-Martin and Mahoney (in press).

GENDER AS CONTEXT FOR COUPLE LIFE

Most contemporary couples want to be able to develop intimate, mutually rewarding relationships (Sullivan, 2006). They believe that each partner should benefit from intimate relationships and have more or less equal power to shape the relationship in ways that meet personal and relational needs, goals, and desires. However, numerous studies show that few couples are yet able to achieve these ideals (Hochschild, 1989; Horst & Doherty, 1995; Knudson-Martin & Mahoney, 1998; Sullivan, 2006; Zvonkovick, Greaves, Schmeige, & Hall, 1996). Instead, they recreate gender-defined patterns that are legacies from another era. These patterns are subtle; they seem natural. But they waylay attempts to develop intimate relationships (Steil, 1997).

Gendered differences in current behavior have historical roots in relationship patterns and structures that accorded men higher status than women. In the past, women depended upon men for their identities and livelihood, and were expected to be subservient and attentive to them. Men were acknowledged as the legitimate authorities in households and were expected to maintain their position, provide protection for their dependents, and avoid emotional vulnerability. Though relationship ideals have changed, many stereotypical gender patterns persist (Knudson-Martin & Mahoney, 2005). They influence couple behavior, especially when they remain beyond conscious awareness.

Stereotypical gender behavior occurs with particular frequency among distressed couples (Beavers, 1985; Gottman, 1994; Johnson, 2003). These couples become locked into repetitive, gender-defined patterns that escalate feelings of anger, disappointment, and incompetence. Freedom from old gender constructions makes available to couples a wider range of responses and relationship options. Thus, helping couples move beyond culturally based gender patterns is an important component of relational success.

The Contextual Legacy of Marital and Family Therapy

The pioneers of family therapy challenged the status quo. They encouraged therapists to look outside the individual for explanations of relationship and mental health problems. Most of these early family therapists did not question the gendered assumptions and ways of behaving that define many aspects of couple relationships. However, addressing gender is a logical outcome of the contextual legacy of marital and family therapy.

When heterosexual women and men form intimate relationships, they bring socially created inequalities and perceptions with them. What couples perceive as individual choices arise within this gendered context. Even when partners hold egalitarian ideals and say that their relationships are not gender-based, gender inequalities can have a profound impact on how decisions are made, the ways couples communicate, and how partners attend and respond to each other (Knudson-Martin & Mahoney, 2005).

During the 1980s, feminism provided a contextual lens from which second-generation family therapists began to examine how gender is socially constructed and reproduced through day-to-day interaction. This lens highlighted the social embeddedness of gender inequality and helped to make visible that which we could not see—gender processes so much a part of the culture that they had become taken-for-granted "reality."

Feminist-informed works showed how early models of family therapy overlooked societal influences that privileged male voices and characteristics, and proceeded *as though* male and female partners were equal, independent of social forces. Among the most notable was Virginia Goldner's (1985, 1988) explication of how power and gender organize family structure. New texts and the *Journal of Feminist Family Therapy* provided models for practitioners that incorporated and respected the experience of women. *The Invisible Web* (Walters, Carter, Papp, & Silverstein, 1988), *The Family Reinterpreted* (Luepnitz,1988), and *Women in Families* (McGoldrick, Anderson, & Walsh, 1989) were among the most influential books in this domain.

Feminism suggested that what therapists do is not and cannot be neutral. Practice as usual meant that old constructions of gender were supported and reproduced. Movement toward more equitable practice required conscious attention to the ways normative, gendered aspects of the social context are part of major relational and mental health issues, such as physical and sexual violence, substance abuse, depression, eating disorders, and marital distress.

During the 1990s feminist scholarship began to recognize multiple female voices and examine how gender intersects with other social categories, such as race, ethnicity, social class, and sexual orientation (e.g., Bograd, 1999; Laird, 2000). Social constructionists developed new, explicitly political approaches to therapy that could bring forth and counteract culturally based gender inequality. These new approaches helped to provide the tools to deconstruct the influences of societal injustices and to liberate women and men from constraining cultural narratives.

Gender is now understood in more pluralistic ways than it was a quarter-century ago. Essentialist ideas of stable, dualistic gender categories are giving way to more fluid, participatory ones (see Laird, 1998). Gender itself is often recognized as a socially constructed category. Many different kinds of genders and gendered experiences are acknowledged. An individual's "gendered" characteristics may change from one setting to another. For example, what it means to be a woman may be different for an African American woman than for a Hispanic woman. It may also change when the woman leaves work and comes home.

Isn't Everything Different Now?

It is easy to assume that knowledge about gender has been translated into practice, or that gender inequality has been corrected in women and men's lives. However, recent research shows that despite changing gender ideals, inequality continues to limit and shape relationship patterns and to influence the onset, symptoms, and course of mental health problems (e.g., Knudson-Martin, 2003b; Sullivan, 2006). Moreover, several studies indicate that only those marital and family therapists who explicitly define themselves as "feminist" are likely to attend to gender equality issues in their work (Haddock, MacPhee, & Zimmerman, 2001; Leslie & Clossick, 1996). For example, they may treat men and women as though they are "equals," with the same options and choices in a relationship, or fail to identify the impact of societal-based power differences on the structure of family life. In the next section I suggest that failure to attend to gender issues in therapy may be due to how "gender differences" are defined and to a failure to recognize the institutional aspects of power (Knudson-Martin & Mahoney, 1999).

BEYOND DIFFERENT WORLDS

Thirty years ago, Hare-Mustin (1978) cautioned therapists to recognize both alpha and beta biases when dealing with gender. "Alpha biases" cause us to ignore important differences between women and men. "Beta biases" cause us to exaggerate them. As therapists attempt to overcome the early failure of the field to address gender, a beta bias that reinforces a false dichotomy between women and men has become common.

It is now popular to think of men and women as inhabiting different worlds; that men and women naturally think and behave in very different ways. The problem with this perspective is that it emphasizes the differences between women and men without much attention to how such differences come to be, and overlooks the substantial variations in how men and women actually live (Kimmel, 2004). The "different worlds" approach tends to view gender as an intrinsic, stable set of characteristics that define the essential nature of women and men. Yet there is tremendous variation in how couples do or do not live out gender stereotypes. Thus, how therapists resolve the nature–nurture debate regarding gender differences has important clinical implications. A useful model of gender differences helps to explain the conditions under which some couples reproduce gender stereotypes that limit their options and other couples expand their choices.

Nature versus Nurture

Gender studies have brought to light important differences in the meaning, timing, and symptoms reported by women and men (Anderson & Holder, 1989; Knudson-Martin, 2003a). Women are two to three times more likely than men to experience depression and anxiety. Onset of schizophrenia is later for women. Women and men respond differently to psychotropic medications and require different dosages for the same body weight (Padgett, 1997). These differences need to be understood and incorporated into models for treatment.

Virtually all scholars agree, however, that the differences between women and men are small compared with the similarities, and that variations within the genders are greater than those between them (Kimmel, 2004; Lindsey, 1997; Hyde, 2005). Hyde's review of 46 meta-analyses supports the conclusion that women and men are statistically similar on nearly all the psychological variables studied. Hyde's analysis emphasized the importance of considering the social context in "creating, erasing, or even reversing psychological differences" (p. 588). Based on these findings, she argues that there are "serious costs to overinflated claims of gender differences" (p. 589).

Biological explanations for observed gender differences tend to obscure the impact of social experience on gender. Focusing on differences in how women and men are "wired" encourages societal and interpersonal inequalities to remain invisible and invites an essentialist perspective (i.e., that differences are natural and can not be changed; Hare-Mustin, 1978; Knudson-Martin & Mahoney, 1999; Rhode, 1997). Biological explanations do not invite us to explore possibilities for changing gender stereotypes or ask us to identify and address relational inequalities.

Confounding the nature–nurture debates are ways that ideas and research regarding human biology have been influenced by cultural constructions that emphasize individualism and rationality, and use the male body and psyche as the norm (Angier, 1999). For example, until recently scientists ignored the positive value of emotion and created an artificial distinction between cognition and feeling in brain functioning (Atkinson, 2005). And though tending to others is a common response to stress among females (in contrast to flight or fight), the physiological processes involved in affiliation have received little scientific study (Taylor, 2002). Furthermore, most conventional views of genetic and biological influences have been linear and deterministic (Quartz & Sejnowski, 2002); that is, that genes and brain structures *cause* behavior.

An integrated, process view of gender suggests a more circular relationship among biology, relationships, and the environment (see Knudson-Martin, 2003a). This view emphasizes mutual influences between these factors and holds more potential for change. As family therapists, our influence on gender is directed primarily toward interpersonal and social processes.

Gender as Interpersonal and Social Process

Social constructionists sometimes describe individual thought and action as social or cultural performances. Individuals perform or "do gender" in relation to others (Gergen, 1999; Laird, 1998). Even "private" thoughts are constructed in terms of their meaning within the larger collective and personal relationships. Individuals act out gendered scripts or roles—"appropriate" male or female behavior—that they have adopted through interaction with parents, peers, language, religious organizations, the media, and other social institutions. These scripts get reinforced or modified as individuals take in new messages. Gender scripts touch many aspects of love and intimacy. In American culture they keep alive the beliefs that women should seek relationship and connection, and that men should protect their independence and maintain control (see Tannen, 1990).

Gender scripts are part of larger societal discourses. These cultural systems of meaning constrain what is possible and shape individual experience (Gee, 2005). Language is the mechanism though which individual experience is mediated within larger societal discourses (Gergen, 1999). It structures how we know ourselves and what we conceive as possible. Thus, individual identities, such as male or female, are located within these larger societal discourses (Sarbin, 2001). Similarly, individual emotional experience, such as romantic attraction, love, anger, or grief, is constituted within particular discursive accounts (i.e., cultural stories) in which gender is often paramount. For example, gender discourses may invite a man to feel angry if his needs are not met, or a woman to feel responsible if her partner is upset. On the other hand, equality discourse may stimulate a woman to feel hurt if her partner does not listen to her. In a complex and changing society, people are typically embedded in many intersecting and sometimes contradictory discourses.

However, language does not simply constrict individual experience. It also actively creates the social worlds within which we live (Gergen, 1999). According to Sullivan (2006), language and changes in gender patterns are part of a complex causal loop. To conceive of new relationship forms

we must have words for them. New language and new ways of thinking about issues are important parts of the change process. Once the language defining an issue changes, new ways of evaluating it are also likely to emerge. Thus, Sullivan believes that the increasingly egalitarian gender ideals expressed in virtually all Western societies represent an important, if incomplete, gender change.

Unfortunately, old gender patterns are not so easily cast off. Despite their inherent flexibility, gender practices become institutionalized, and are made into tradition and experienced as taken-for-granted realities. Furthermore, ideas about gender nearly always become embedded in a society's systems for allocating social power. Those with more power learn that they are entitled to have their expectations met. Those in less powerful positions learn to accommodate. Stereotypical gender communication patterns arise within this context (Tannen, 1994).

Even though old gender patterns are being challenged in many aspects of societies, couple life, to a large extent, remains organized around persistent gender structures. Strong pressures at individual, interactional, and institutional levels can pull couples back toward old gender-stereotypical behaviors (Risman, 1998). Yet how couples deal with gender and power is integral to individual well-being (Steil, 1997) and relationship success. This means that gender and power are at the core of the struggles that contemporary partners face as they love each other and form families.

Approaches to couple therapy will recreate or challenge existing gender stereotypes. When working from the view that women and men come from different worlds, see the world through different lenses, and develop different styles of relating (e.g., Gilligan, 1982; Gray, 1994), therapists typically attempt to help heterosexual couples understand gender differences, so that they can adapt to these differences and communicate in spite of them. Unfortunately, in so doing, they may perpetuate unequal relationships that limit their clients' ability to achieve the intimacy they desire.

The approach presented here helps therapists and couples move away from culturally embedded gender stereotypes that perpetuate gender equality. In this approach, the therapist raises conversation about relational processes that women and men otherwise fall into automatically, without conscious intention. Assessment and the development of relational goals are guided by a model of relationships that includes a broader range of life trajectories. Relationships are thought of in terms of equality rather than gender difference. Within a framework of equality, a diversity of options for women and men are possible (Krolokke & Sorensen, 2006).

EQUALITY: A FRAMEWORK FOR RELATIONAL HEALTH

Although a feminist concern for gender equality and a therapeutic concern for the well-being and stability of relationships have not always been seen as compatible, these two are closely connected. Gottman's long-term research on marriage reveals old gender scripts in couple communication processes. Men frequently stonewall issues raised by wives, making it difficult for women to influence them. Though wives may be upset or critical, they tend to engage in the men's concerns (Gottman, Coan, Carrere, & Swanson, 1998). The effect of this disparity is dramatic. Among men who were unwilling to be influenced by their wives, Gottman et al. found an 81% chance of divorce.

Coltrane's (1996) study of men also shows that egalitarian family organization enhances couple stability. He suggests that the act of caring for children in itself changes men, because it stimulates development of greater sensitivity and nurturing behavior. In a study of gender equality, and individual and relational well-being, Steil (1997) found that equal power was important to relationship satisfaction for both women and men. Her analysis suggested that when both partners believe they are able to influence the other, they use direct communication strategies that enhance intimacy and lead to increased relational satisfaction and personal well-being for both partners.

However, attaining equality can be elusive. Women and men lack the language and images that would help them translate loosely defined ideals into equality in day-to-day life. Latent and invisible male power also remains structured into many couple relationships. Latent power is embedded in social norms and values that make it difficult to imagine an alternative (Komter, 1989). Partners automatically do what men and women stereotypically do. Similarly, invisible power is the power to prevent issues from being raised. There is no conflict, because the person with less power simply anticipates what the more powerful person wants and accommodates. Historically, women have been socialized to this adaptive position. Latent and invisible power differences between heterosexual partners are institutional in nature and operate almost independently of the will of the individuals involved (Lips, 1991).

Dimensions of Equality

Focusing on the relational processes that constitute equality helps therapists and couples recognize the institutional gender scripts and power differences that organize couple life. It provides a framework from which couples can evaluate their relationships and make conscious decisions about previously below-the-surface gender and power issues. Examining gender equality involves four dimensions: comparative status, accommodation patterns, attention to other, and well-being (Knudson-Martin & Mahoney, 2005, in press). It includes roles and the division of labor, but extends beyond these to the very heart of how intimate partners relate.

Comparative Status

If partners hold equal status in a relationship, they are equally able to shape the relationship in ways that sustain their well-being. This is related to perceptions of entitlement. Because traditional gender socialization encourages women more than men to define their own needs in relation to others, women and men may enter relationships with different implicit statuses. Men may feel more entitled than women to pursue their personal goals and have their needs met. This does not necessarily mean that either partner consciously believes a man's needs and interests should be more important than a woman's. But if women are less confident of their entitlement or silence their own needs and interests, and men take them for granted and express them, an imbalance of entitlement results. This translates into different comparative statuses between partners.

Therapists need to examine the extent to which partners feel equally entitled to express and attain personal goals, needs, and wishes. How able is each partner to express these? How able is one partner to influence the other? Whose interests shape what happens in the relationship? How are low-status tasks such as housework addressed? To what extent are decisions determined by gender traditions? In equal relationships both partners should feel equally entitled to pursue their personal goals either in the short or long term and also equally responsible for maintaining the relationship.

Accommodation Patterns

Accommodation to one's partner is a necessary part of couple life. If partners equally influence the relationship, accommodation is mutual. There is no latent or invisible power that influences one partner to accommodate more readily than the other. When relationships are not equal, accommodation by the lower status person may feel natural or expected. Women are socialized more than men to accommodate and to direct their behavior in anticipation of the partner's wants or needs, with neither men or women being aware of what is happening. To men who have been taught to maintain their independence, accommodating may feel like being controlled. Although women frequently accommodate without being aware that they are doing so, the social context may invite men to overestimate men's amount of accommodation.

The therapist should examine the extent to which each partner bends to accommodate the other. Who accommodates to whom? Under what circumstances? How do couples explain these choices? Are they made intentionally? Whose interests and needs are reflected in daily schedules and decisions? How do couples accommodate the family and work roles of each partner? How are gender and power reflected in these accommodation patterns, and how do societal processes outside the couple relationship influence accommodation patterns?

Attention to Other

Part of the egalitarian model for relationships is an expectation that partners will be emotionally present for and support each other. In an equal relationship both partners are attuned to the needs of the other. Partners are equally responsive to stresses impacting the other. However, attention to the other is influenced by differences in power. Powerful persons may be less likely to notice or respond to the state of others. Institutional differences in power and socialized gender differences impact this dynamic in contemporary couple relationships.

The therapist needs to examine who attends to whom in the relationship. How attuned and interested are partners to the needs and perspectives of the other? How likely is each to notice the partner's needs and feelings? How responsive are partners to each other's states? How do partners take initiative toward the care and well-being of the other? Does one respond to the other without being asked? How well and in what circumstances does each listen to the other? In what ways does each partner show empathy for the other's experience and attend to the other's emotional needs? Look for examples that show who notices what the other needs, and consider how women and men respond to and care for the other.

Well-Being

In equal relationships burdens are shared, and the well-being of each partner is supported equally both in the short term and over the long haul. However, considerable research documents that women continue to bear the main responsibility for nurturing family members and managing family life (e.g., Coltrane & Adams, 2000; Zimmerman, Haddock, Ziemba, & Rust, 2001). Women also tend to get poorer jobs and to have lower incomes. Couple relationships frequently reflect these differing allocations of power and resources. At the same time, men may lack positive emotional connections and struggle with the dependencies inherent in relationships (Brooks, 2003).

The therapist should examine whether a relationship supports the psychological health of both partners, or if one person's sense of competence, optimism, and well-being comes at the expense of the other's physical or emotional health. Does one partner seem to be faring better than the other? Do relationship patterns equally support the physical and emotional health of both partners, or does the structure cause one person to be more physically stressed or fatigued than the other over the long term? Does the relationship support the economic viability of each partner?

Attaining Equality

For most couples, development of an egalitarian relationship is likely to be an ongoing process. Research on gender equality in marriage distinguishes the conditions under which some couples are able to achieve equality (Blaisure & Allen, 1995; Cowdery & Knudson-Martin, 2005; Deutsch, 1999; Knudson-Martin & Mahoney, 1998, 2005; Matta & Knudson-Martin, 2006; Quek & Knudson-Martin, 2006; Rabin, 1996; Risman, 1998; Schwartz, 1994). These studies show that gender equality is most likely to occur when women's work is valued, when partners are aware of gender influences and consciously counteract them, when partners are able to tolerate conflict and embrace two voices in the relationship, and when women and men develop new skills and competencies.

Though most studies of gender equality have focused on white, middle- and professional-class couples, more recent research (e.g., Knudson-Martin & Mahoney, 2005; Lim, 1997; Quek & Knudson-Martin, 2006) has examined culturally diverse populations. These studies suggest that the interpersonal processes creating relationship equality appear to be similar across groups. Knudson-Martin and Mahoney (2005) found examples of equal relationships among European American, African American, Hispanic, and Asian couples in their qualitative study of couples in California. These processes transcended time and were also present among white, East Coast couples interviewed in 1982. Interest in equality was widespread even among religious couples who held traditional views of gender roles.

Though the basic processes constituting gender equality appear similar across diverse populations, the meanings that couples bring to gender and power issues are embedded in the larger social context. For example, collectivist values influence equality development in Singapore (Quek & Knudson-Martin, 2006). African American couples have adapted gender roles to take into account their unique social context (Boyd-Franklin & Franklin, 1998; Hill, 2005). Immigrants also adapt gender structures to meet their changing economic and cultural circumstances (Lim, 1997). Thus, gender equality evolves at the intersection of multiple social contexts.

The ability to sustain relationship equality across all these contexts requires creative problem solving and ways of communicating that defy gender stereotypes and transform the power relationship between women and men. Mutuality, which, according to Jordan (2004), involves profound respect and responsiveness to the other, is at the core of equality. However, successfully helping couples make progress toward equality in their individual relationships requires more than attention to interpersonal systems. It is necessary to address the socially created aspects of gender.

A MODEL FOR POSTGENDER PRACTICE

Postgender practice asks, "What would be possible if gender did not unconsciously organize relationship options?" It makes the hidden aspects of gender visible and helps couples move beyond limited

gender stereotypes. At the same time, it emphasizes respect for clients' decision-making processes. The clinician plays a facilitative, cultural broker role rather than a directive one. Focusing on gender in the early years of relationship formation and when children are young is especially powerful and often does not require many sessions. Working with gender in more entrenched relationships, or when other serious mental health issues are involved, takes longer but can be a key to getting beyond the impasse and creating a healthier relationship context.

The model outlined below does not address every aspect of couple therapy. It is best thought of as a gender-informed lens to be applied with other clinical approaches. It draws on gender research and feminist scholarship, with particular attention to the impact of the social context on couple issues. However, it is not necessary to identify primarily as a feminist to apply a perspective that moves beyond the limits of gender stereotypes. Readers are encouraged to consider what would be required to integrate a postgender lens into their work. Therefore, decisions about whom to include, frequency, and duration of treatment may vary depending on one's approach.

Consciously attending to the sociopolitical context of treatment is the most critical aspect of postgender therapy. Approaches that take what Minuchin, Lee, and Simon (2003) call a "non-interventionist" position (i.e., solution-focused, collaborative language systems) may require more change from therapy as usual than more active modalities (e.g., structural, experiential, emotionally focused, narrative). On the other hand, like social constructionist and postmodern approaches, the model presented here also focuses on reducing the power of the therapist. The postgender therapist is deeply interested in and respectful of the client's context. Thus, the approach is equally relevant when working with very religious and rural couples, or with dual-career professional couples. The goal is not to make all couples alike; it is to consider how gender and power issues contribute to the presenting issues and limit possible solutions, particularly when the couple seeks a relationship based on intimacy and mutual well-being.

The Sociopolitical Context of Treatment

Like clients, therapists are socialized within a context that takes many gender patterns for granted. These can limit what we see, what we define as problems, and what we consider possible. To the extent that aspects of gender remain invisible to the therapist, he or she will not be able to recognize them in therapy or to help couples move beyond them. For example, I have watched many therapy sessions in which the man interrupted or contradicted the wife and the therapist accepted his version of reality, without being consciously aware of doing so. When couples describe gender stereotypical patterns, such as the mother attending to the child, therapists often pass this by without question or reflection. There are hundreds of ways that all therapists get caught in old gender scripts. Despite years of studying this topic, I still am chagrined at the pieces I sometimes miss. For example, one day I was scheduling an appointment with a banker and his wife, who was a stay-at-home mother. I asked him about his schedule and ignored hers, assuming that she would accommodate us. Gender awareness requires deliberate attention and ongoing self-reflexivity.

Attention to the sociopolitical context also recognizes that treatment delivery systems are embedded within societal institutions that are not neutral, and that may not equally support or value women or other persons with less power. Many of the theories and assumptions in clinical approaches tend to reinforce gender inequality. For example, they may value characteristics, such as "clear" thinking and autonomy, that are often associated with masculinity but pathologize more "feminine" qualities, such as focusing on the needs of others. An important part of postgender practice is recognizing and validating typically "feminine" activities, such as attending to the details of relationships and contributing to the well-being of others.

Though validating attention given to others seems logical and appropriate in couple therapy, therapists frequently not only overlook it but also approach it as a problem. For example, recently I used a new training tape to help teach a particular theoretical approach to therapy. In the case, the woman felt intense pressure to be responsible at work and in her extended family. The husband wanted more of her time and felt hurt by her ministrations to others. Though each partner was given tasks to do, the assignments focused on how *she* could give him more time and how he could interpret *her* behavior in a less hurtful way. There was no suggestion of what he might do to help her or any acknowledgment of the positive contributions her responsible behavior provided to others. Her "excessive" responsibility was personalized and pathologized as "inappropriate" guilt rather than placed in the context of societal proscriptions

requiring that women "give." Yet the husband's desire to be the focus of her attention was passively accepted, and apparently was considered "normal" or "appropriate" rather than being questioned or labeled as "excessive."

In this example, the therapist unwittingly colluded with constructions of gender that were invisible in the therapy because they seemed normal. He failed to identify the ways in which the gendered social context contributed to the couple's problems. Yet the meanings surrounding the couple's conflict were heavily influenced by culturally prescribed gender expectations for women "to attend" and men to be "attended to." These gendered scripts created an imbalance in the give and take of in the relationship. A postgender therapist would be attentive to these culturally constructed gender processes and serve as a "broker" between the couple and institutionalized gender to create new relationship options.

Therapist as "Cultural Broker"

How women and men relate to each other arises within specific cultural contexts. But cultures are not static, unchanging sets of rules that people adopt (Laird, 2000). Rather, culture is performed, created, and adapted as people play it out on a day-to-day basis and within changing circumstances. As "cultural brokers," we therapists help clients bring together the old and the new. It is our job to bring these varying, and often contradictory, elements to the surface, so that clients can put them together in ways that work to enhance their relationships and well-being. In this process, we help clients create a language and framework for evolving models of gender, equality, and relationship, and help them see their situations within larger cultural patterns that affect many women and men.

Though some psychoeducation about gender and power processes may be woven into the therapeutic process, the postgender therapist avoids an authoritative "teaching" stance and takes steps to minimize the generally inherent power differences between therapists and clients. As a collaborative consultant whose job is to help clients negotiate a changing gender landscape, the therapist helps couples examine their issues through a contextual lens that may be new to them, and that provides information when it is therapeutically useful in the particular case.

For example, when there is a disparity within the couple in partners' ability to relax at home,

I might share the research finding (Larson & Richards, 1994) that most women find it difficult to relax because they are concerned about other family members. I might also share a story about a male friend who was confused when his partner said she could not read because he was always at home. Sharing this information places the couple's issue within a larger social context in which others struggle with the same issues.

One of my favorite accounts of the therapist working as a cultural broker in relation to gender equality is Garcia-Preto's (1998) account of bridging gender worlds with Latina women. She respectfully connects with these women around cultural values such as motherhood and virginity, then helps them retain aspects of these values that are important to them while also resisting limitations imposed by culturally defined gender scripts. Though, in this example, Garcia-Preto is working with individual women and their family-of-origin relationships, this kind of work can also be done with couples.

Individual Sessions in Postgender Therapy

The role as cultural broker is relevant whether participants attend therapy together or are seen individually. However, a postgender therapist attends to who is doing the work of change for the relationship. Seeing partners together makes it easier to identify gender processes between partners. Individual sessions can sometimes help either partner reflect on his or her gendered experiences. Decisions about working individually should be made carefully. From a gender-equality perspective, it is important to expect both partners to be responsible for relationship maintenance.

Thus, when Eduardo came to see me because he wanted to work on improving his connection to Maria, his wife of 17 years, I first asked Maria to join us. She reported that she had put herself aside for many years and was more interested in personal development at this point in time. So, in this case, working first with Eduardo, I helped him take more responsibility for what he could do to connect emotionally with Maria. He also discovered that, like many similarly socialized men, he wanted to be close to his wife but expected that she would do the emotional work to facilitate it. Once Eduardo took steps to correct this imbalance, Maria was more willing to participate in couple therapy.

I responded differently when Rhea came in to learn how not to upset her husband. I helped her probe what she thought it would take for Rhea not to upset Roger. When the solution appeared to be "letting go" of issues that were important to her, I decided that continuing to see her individually would have perpetuated the imbalance already in the relationship. So, I told her that though I could refer her to someone who would work with her alone, I did not think I could ethically work with just one of the partners in their relationship. Two weeks later Rhea and Roger came in together.

Certainly there are many cases in which one partner, most often a woman, seeks therapy in the hope of making her marriage better. If it is not possible also to engage the partner in couple therapy, a postgender therapist may decide to take the case but make the one-sided nature of the work visible and a part of the therapy.

Psychotropic Medications in Postgender Therapy

A postgender therapist frames psychotropic medications within the context of reciprocal influences among gender, interpersonal relationships, and the larger society. Physiological symptoms, such as depression, are not separate from interpersonal and sociopolitical contexts (see Knudson-Martin, 2003a). Medication may not be necessary if the client's position in these contexts can be changed. For example, Barbara called to make an appointment for herself, saying that she "couldn't cope anymore" and that she was "depressed." I invited her husband Jim to attend the initial session. He immediately expressed his concern that "maybe she needs to be hospitalized" or put on medication. Yet Barbara's symptoms disappeared entirely in only a few sessions once she and Jim began to address how they could more equally share child care burdens.

On the other hand, medication can sometimes facilitate a client's ability to make difficult changes. In this case, rather than medication as the source of change, it is important that the therapist help to create a framework that empowers clients. For example, Sonja and Aaron were referred to me for couple work by an Employee Assistance Program (EAP) provider who also referred Sonja to a physician for antidepressants. Sonja felt hopeless and would have been unable to generate motivation to attempt change in her relationship without the medication. The challenge was also to engage Aaron in his part of the relational work and not to collude with his tendency to focus on her medication as the solution, and overlook his part in the problem.

Out-of-Session Contact

The meaning of "out-of-session contact" depends on the power relationships between the partners. A partner's attempted out-of-session calls frequently reflect less power in the relationship and reliance on indirect influence tactics. For example, a woman in a male-dominant relationship called an hour before the session and left a message containing information she did not feel she could safely share directly in the session. In another case, Greta called during a particularly stressful time because she did not trust her own judgment. Because Greta consistently took a one-down position in the relationship, my response was to reinforce her right to her perspective and to schedule an appointment for both partners that focused on their anxiety around the power shift that comes with having two voices in the relationship.

Creating an Alliance

As in all couple work, an alliance with each partner, and with the couple as a unit, is important to the ultimate success of the therapy. Gender–power issues are integral to this process in three ways:

1. Each partner must feel understood. Hearing each person's story through a gender lens can facilitate connecting with each person's unique emotional experience.
2. The therapist must position his or her relationship with the couple such that silenced voices are supported and made safe.
3. The therapist must join with the couple as a unit, such that gender influences are external to them.

For example, if a wife complains that her husband does not listen to her, and he reports frustration regarding what she wants of him, I would seek to understand empathically the gender context in which not being heard is so painful for the woman and in which the man is so genuinely puzzled about her expectations. I might also respond that nearly every couple I see struggles with issues like these, and explain that expectations for women and men have changed so much over the years that most of us do not have good models for how to create the kinds of relationships we want. I would also recognize that the listening issue is probably related to the gendered nature of power in their relationship and ensure that the woman's voice is not inadvertently diminished in the session. Making the issue one of social change preserves the dignity of each

partner and helps them join together to create relational change.

Attributes of a Successful Postgender Therapist

Postgender practice requires that the therapist be engaged with clients in ways that bring hidden gender and power elements to the surface, yet avoid a prescriptive stance. The seven traits listed below help therapists in this process:

1. *Self-reflexive*: Therapists must examine how their own expectations regarding appropriate behavior for women and men limit what they see, and how the cultural and therapeutic context permits the expression of some ideas but not others.
2. *Active*: Overcoming gender bias and old gender stereotypes requires conscious and active engagement by the therapist in identifying hidden gender issues. Being passively "neutral" perpetuates hidden power differences.
3. *Curious*: Therapists open new avenues for therapeutic conversation by being curious about how couples developed taken-for-granted patterns, such as a wife organizing her time around her husband's schedule. Curiosity not only suggests that cultural patterns are not inevitable but it also shows respect for clients as the decision-makers.
4. *Empathic*: To work effectively with gender issues, the therapist must seek to understand each partner's experience within his or her particular constellation of social contexts. Empathy evolves from putting oneself in the partners' contexts. It invites acceptance of each person, while helping both partners expand their options.
5. *Strengths focused*: Therapists must systematically look for strengths not regularly acknowledged in the dominant culture. For example, the capacity for fusion, typically framed as a problem, is one of the strengths common to women and often coexists with high levels of ego strength (Menchner, 1997).
6. *Differentiated*: Therapists need to be able to help partners tolerate uncertainty and conflict as they let go of familiar gender patterns. Therapists must not avoid anxiety by moving too quickly to solutions in which one partner simply accommodates or takes on most of the responsibility for change.
7. *Visionary*: Postgender therapists must see be-

yond stereotypes to a wider range of possibilities. They must assume that men, as well as women, are capable of being relational. Speaking of gender patterns as "habits" rather than "traits" conveys the sense that women and men can develop new ways of relating.

Postgender Assessment and Treatment Planning

Assessment and treatment planning from a postgender perspective must begin with a focus on the social context of the therapy. Though assessment is ongoing and never separate from intervention,

Figure 23.1 provides a framework for initial case conceptualization that begins by examining how sociopolitical contexts shape what the therapist sees, and how these contexts (1) inform the emotional experience of each partner, (2) structure the relative status and well-being in the relationship and each partner's ability to accommodate and attend to the other, and (3) limit each partner's range of available skills. As the therapist raises questions that probe these issues, previously taken-for-granted gender and power structures are made visible. Through discussion of these issues and their relational ideals, treatment goals specific to the couple can be identified.

Social Context
- How do my expectations for women and men inform what I see and consider normal in this case?
- Do I privilege "masculine" traits such as autonomy and rationality over "feminine" ones such as connection and emotional expressiveness?
- In what kinds of contexts is the couple embedded (e.g., ethnic, economic, religious, etc.)?
  What gender scripts are within the couple's social contexts?
  How much institutional power does each partner hold as a result of his or her societal position?
- What power differences exist between the therapist and the couple?

Emotion
- How are individual feelings and reactions within the relationship framed by gender?
- What gender discourses and structures within the larger social context inform the emotional experience of each partner?
  How do these influence how partners perceive themselves?
  How do these influence expectations of the partner and the relationship?
- Which emotional issues are particularly salient from a gender perspective?
  How are these related to conflict in the relationship?
  How are these related to intimacy and attachment in the relationship?

Structure
- Do partners hold equal status in the relationship?
  Do partners feel equally entitled to express and attain personal goals, needs, and wishes?
  How able is each to influence the other?
  How are low-status tasks such as housework addressed?
- To what extent does each partner accommodate the other?
  Who accommodates whom? Under what circumstances?
  Whose interests and needs are reflected in daily schedules and decisions?
  How do partners accommodate the family and work roles of each?
- How do partners attend to each other?
  How likely is each to notice and respond to the partner's needs and feelings?
  Do partners take initiative toward the care and well-being of the other?
  How well and in what circumstances do they listen to each other, show empathy, and attend to their partner's emotional needs?
- Does the relationship equally support the physical, emotional, and economic well-being of each partner?

Skills
- How able are partners to tolerate conflict and make room for two voices?
- How are communication skills limited by gender?
- How are each partner's competencies limited by gender?
- What new skills or habits will help partners mutually support each other?

FIGURE 23.1. Assessment for gender and power in couple relationships.

For example, when Barbara and Jim (discussed earlier) came in regarding Barbara's depression, I observed that Jim appeared to be vital and energetic, whereas Barbara was on the verge of breakdown. In that first session I wondered out loud, "How is it that you are so stressed and Jim is doing so well?" Though the couple had just told me that their relationship was good, this simple question opened the floodgate. Barbara began to express anger that all her spare time was spent taking care of the children and household, while Jim, though a "good" father, went skiing or golfing on his days off. In this case, Jim immediately moved the discussion toward a goal of how to balance the stress in the relationship.

In addition to the questions listed in Figure 23.1, two other assessment guides are also helpful. Each can be used as a basis for questions that raise social-contextual gender and power issues, and can also be used with couples directly for psychoeducation or for research.

- Relational Assessment Guide (RAG; Silverstein, Bass, Tuttle, Knudson-Martin, & Huenergardt, 2006). The first part of the guide helps frame ways to relate to others within the larger social context. It then allows the therapist to classify each partner on two dimensions closely related to gender: power and focus. "Power" refers to whether one approaches relationships with internalized expectations of hierarchy or equality. "Focus" refers to how the self is experienced in relationships on a continuum from autonomy to connection. The RAG is useful in taking multicultural differences into account. This assessment format can be found in the December 2006 *Family Process* journal.
- The Power Equity Guide (Haddock, Zimmerman, & MacPhee, 2000). This guide includes 39 questions through which the therapist and couple assess power differentials between the partners, and between the therapist and the clients. It includes questions on decision making, communication and conflict resolution, work/life goals, housework, finances, sex, and relationship maintenance, as well as characteristics of the relationship. It is described in detail in the April 2000 *Journal of Marital and Family Therapy*.

Postgender Treatment Goals

Treatment goals specific to the couple are developed collaboratively. However, as in the example

with Barbara and Jim, the kinds of questions asked in the initial assessment play an important part in the development of goals around the issues presented by the couple. They are useful whether the presenting issues are described as relational problems, such as poor communication, conflict, or falling out of love, or individual problems, such as depression, anxiety, or impulse control. The following general goals for the therapist guide this process and subsequent sessions:

1. Identify the ways gender invokes meaning and emotion in couple relationships.
2. Create a context through which couples can address previously invisible aspects of gender and power in their relationships.
3. Help couples develop a framework for evaluating equality in their relationships.
4. Help couples seeking intimacy, open communication, and mutuality move beyond gender-stereotypical behavior toward relationship equality.
5. Help women and men expand relational skills and competencies limited by gender stereotypes.

Three Levels of Postgender Work

The strategies and techniques used in postgender therapy involve three levels: emotion, structure, and skills. Though these do not necessarily play out in a linear fashion (i.e., the therapist may be dealing with elements of each throughout the therapy process), there is a conceptual order from which to approach them. "Emotion" arises within cultural and interpersonal contexts that ascribe meaning to experience. Thus, gender plays a major role in shaping emotion. "Structure" refers to the gendered relationships patterns that evolve between intimate partners. These patterns typically develop without conscious awareness but become the ongoing context through which partners know themselves and each other. "Skills" also develop within a social context. Change in the gender structures organizing couple relationships usually requires changes in what people do and the development of new skills. This provides the context for new emotional experience.

Emotion

Before a therapist can help couples expand beyond gender-defined skills or create new gender patterns, he or she must tune into each partner's gender/cultural experience at the emotional level. Entry into another person's experience is an attitude as well as a skill. It requires a conscious desire to experience the perspective of the client and involves active listening, questioning, and empathic reflection. This is different from "therapy as usual," in that conscious attention is given to the gender/cultural context within which the emotion arises.

To contextualize emotion, the therapist draws on knowledge of societal and cultural patterns, such as gendered power structures and ideals for masculinity and femininity that touch all people's lives in a particular society to some extent, then seeks to know the unique personal experience of the client within this larger context. The ability to grasp each partner's unique contextual experience communicates respect and assures clients that they are understood. It is also likely that key underlying emotional issues in the relationship will become visible. Seeking to empathically identify each partner's emotional experience is an essential part of the initial sessions. However, it may take a number of sessions before key pieces of the gender story become fully visible.

For example, in the earlier case of Eduardo and Maria, Maria's resistance to participating in couple therapy at first seemed to suggest that she was oriented more toward personal autonomy than toward connection. This struck me as unusual, because institutional gender norms encourage women to orient to others. Eduardo, a kindergarten teacher, also transcended gender stereotypes and reported doing most of the caretaking for their 8-year-old son. As I came to understand Eduardo's emotional experience empathically, I "got" how alone he felt. He felt different from other men and experienced little respect from society in general. Though he actively supported Maria's career, he had also been socialized to expect her to be emotionally available to him on demand. When she was not, he felt ashamed and alone.

But there was more to their gender stories. After several joint sessions in which I focused on understanding Maria's experience as a woman, she finally shared that before they married, she had agreed to have sex with Eduardo even though this violated her own moral values. This sense that, as a woman, she must accommodate to the man, had been repeated many times in the early years of their marriage. She experienced her efforts to resist him now as a sign of personal accomplishment. Though Maria and Eduardo had moved beyond gender-stereotypical roles, their emotions were embedded within contradictory and changing cultural discourses for gender. Addressing these allowed the therapy to move forward.

Structure

Equal power is an important foundation for emotional intimacy and mutual well-being (e.g., Beavers, 1985; Horst & Doherty, 1995; Steil, 1997). To help couples create more equal relationship structures, the therapist must first identify the ways in which institutional gender inequalities may be organizing relationships. The goal is not necessarily to change the overall structure of the couple relationship, but to make power issues visible, so that their consequences can be openly addressed. For example, Wang Lu and Luisa both believed that he should be "head of the family," but Luisa felt discounted and frustrated from trying to organize family activities around his schedule. As their relationship improved, Wang Lu retained his leadership position, but Luisa gained a stronger, more valued voice in their relationship, and he learned to be more attentive and responsive to family members in carrying out his role.

Identifying power issues involves asking questions that address equality, such as how decisions are made, who accommodates to whom, and whose interests take priority. It also involves observing what happens, and what is said and not said in the therapy room. Whose version of reality prevails? How easily does one partner back down? How are the contributions of each valued? For example, Simon called for help regarding Carlene's compulsive spending (see Knudson-Martin, 2003b). When I asked them to discuss their issues, Carlene stated her opinion. But when Simon gave his view, she agreed that he was right. Simon spoke with more certainty than did Carlene and would immediately explain to Carlene why she was wrong.

The postgender therapist takes an active role in addressing observed power differences. This includes identifying and naming these issues as they arise and taking steps in the session to help the couple relate from more equal positions. Therefore, it is important to make sure that Carlene's point of view was validated in the session, and to help Simon acknowledge her perspective. Similarly, when another husband said that he listened to his wife "when I think it is important," I named this as a power issue by saying, "So you get to decide what's important?" This raised his awareness of a power position that he did not want to hold.

The therapist needs to consider how underlying power disparities may be contributing to other problems in the relationship and make this an explicit part of the treatment plan. When Carlene could more openly express her ideas about money, the compulsive spending stopped. In the case of Rhea's depression, the relationship had become organized almost completely around Aaron's schedule (he was a farmer) and his interests. Therapy centered on how to make room for Rhea. As a first step, Rhea focused on sometimes cooking foods that she liked. Aaron gradually learned to plan some couple activities around her interests.

Skills

To maintain changes in the structure of their relationships, most couples need to expand their skills and develop new habits. Old gender scripts reduced a lot of conflict by providing ready-made answers about who should make decisions, whose needs should take priority, or who should do certain tasks. As partners become more equal and share power, they need help to tolerate the conflict and anxiety that arises as they step out of old patterns.

It was extremely difficult for Rhea to cook something new that her family might question. This act raised emotions of guilt (for not doing gender as she had been taught) and exhilaration (that she could value her preferences). In the process of learning new skills, it would have been easy to send the message that the giving she did was "wrong." Though, like Carlene and Rhea, women may need to learn how to limit the habit of accommodating so readily, it is also very important that they also be acknowledged for their positive contributions to others.

In creating an equal relationship, it is critical that men, as well as women, learn to access their caring for their partners to more readily attend and accommodate to them. For example, Aaron and Simon both loved their wives but had not learned how to express this caring by listening to them or noticing their needs. The therapist first needed to believe that these men had the capacity to orient toward others, then look for ways to help the men expand their attending skills. For example, Rhea was deeply unhappy in the marriage. She longed for Aaron to notice how she felt and share some of his feelings with her. However, he typically responded to her attempts to raise these issues with him by telling her she was unreasonable, or by getting angry. Her expectations made him feel incompetent. Helping Aaron show empathy to Rhea was a key to creating a relational context that supported Rhea's mental health and improved satisfaction for both partners.

MECHANISMS OF CHANGE

From a postgender perspective, relationships and personal well-being are improved as partners move beyond the limits imposed by gender stereotypes. Steil's (1997) study of the links between gender equality, personal well-being, and relationship satisfaction helps to explain why changing gender patterns creates positive relational change. Her results show that a partner who perceives that he or she can influence the other is likely to use direct influence strategies. This increases reported intimacy and relationship satisfaction for both women and men. Beavers (1985) observed that when power in the relationship is unequal, the "top dog" cannot afford to be vulnerable. Fear of showing weakness therefore limits open communication and the capacity for intimacy. Similarly, the "underdog" must hold back thoughts, feelings, and needs for fear of upsetting the balance in the relationship.

In postgender therapy, partners are not asked to give up their "natures." Instead, as they free themselves from cultural and societal aspects of gender, individual differences and expanded choices are possible.

TREATMENT APPLICABILITY

The approach outlined here is not meant to stand alone to address all the issues in couple therapy. Rather, it calls attention to the social context of relationship problems as gender intersects with other sociopolitical forces, such as race, ethnicity, religion and socioeconomic and legal status. The model suggested here shows how gender issues are relevant at multiple levels of clinical focus (i.e., emotion, structure, and skills) and are potentially important aspects of nearly all kinds of presenting issues. The examples in this chapter included mental health issues, such as depression, as well as marital conflict or dissatisfaction, as the impetus for therapy.

There is considerable evidence to support the need to address gender in couple therapy. The research cited in this chapter suggests that gender disparities in the larger society frequently result in inequality in couple relationships, and that this takes a toll on both women and men. Though a number of studies have found more relationship equality when women's work is valued (e.g., Risman, 1998; Knudson-Martin & Mahoney, 2005; Matta & Knudson-Martin, 2006), the effects of gender are pervasive and not resolved simply by access to resources such as money and education. Tichenor's (2005) in-depth study of couples in which wives earn more than their partners shows that the power to influence and organize the relationship remains deeply determined by gender, and that women cannot "buy" equality.

In their analysis of a national probability sample, Amato, Johnson, Booth, and Rogers (2003) found that equal decision making was a critical factor in explaining relationship quality and stability. Though relationship quality has been related to health for both women and men (Sternberg, 2001), research continues to indicate that husbands more often than wives report being understood and affirmed by their spouses, and that this is related to depression in women (e.g., Lynch, 1998; McGrath, Keita, Strickland, & Russo, 1990). This gender discrepancy in the benefits of marriage, first identified by Bernard (1973), means that hidden power issues in couple relationships have important health consequences and may account for recent findings that most divorces are now instigated by women (Coontz, 2005).

A number of feminist family therapists have offered in-depth case analyses that illuminate how addressing gender in couple therapy can be helpful (e.g., Silverstein & Goodrich, 2003; Walters et al., 1988). However, despite the considerable evidence documenting how gender issues contribute to relationship problems, research that examines the impact of gender-informed practice on the outcome of couple therapy or which methods are most effective in dealing with gender issues remains to be conducted.

The case example that follows illustrates how attending to gender was central to helping a couple improve their relationship and identifies an important power imbalance that needed to be addressed. The specific interventions necessarily reflect my style of practice. Other therapists may apply a postgender lens using somewhat different techniques, but would purposefully address these sociopolitical issues and help the couple overcome some of the limits of gender-stereotypical relationship processes.

CASE ILLUSTRATION

Dave (white, age 34) called for couple therapy, citing irresolvable conflict, particularly around his wife Sonja's (white, age 33) desire to move from California to New Mexico. They had been married 10 years and had two children. He was concerned that Sonja might be emotionally unstable. The

couple was willing to be observed by students in exchange for seeing a faculty member at a low fee. Initial assessment focused collaboratively on each aspect of the guide in Figure 23.1.

Getting Started: Forming a Collaboration

Social Context

Dave and Sonja approached the first session of therapy from a one-down position. Dave, a foreman for a concrete company, viewed the world hierarchically. He liked being boss on the work site but otherwise experienced little social power. He approached me deferentially, repeatedly saying that he came to learn what he was doing wrong. Sonja, who had left home at age 16 to have a child, also viewed me as an authority figure. She had experienced some counseling as a young woman and believed our team had knowledge she and Dave needed.

As a PhD-trained professional with students observing, I entered the therapy with considerable power. I hoped to reduce this hierarchy, but I also had to acknowledge my power and use it respectfully. The couple faced numerous problems related to their lower socioeconomic position. To afford a house, Sonja and Dave had purchased a home in a crime-ridden neighborhood. Their shy, 14-year-old son Benjie had been beaten up in school. Their 16-year-old daughter Sophie told Sonja that she was regularly offered drugs. They were juggling potential foreclosure on their house and other bills that they could not pay.

Dave and Sonja fit many of the stereotypes for women and men. Without conscious attention to gender and power issues, I would have viewed Sonja as highly reactive. She got upset quickly and vacillated between tears and anger. On the one hand, she seemed desperate for Dave to pay attention to her; on the other, she insisted that he do what she wanted. She could probably have qualified for a number of labels: "histrionic," "enmeshed," "dependent," or "low self-esteem." Dave seemed more reasonable. Though he needed better "communication skills," it was easy to give him credit (as a man) just for being at the therapy sessions. He commuted long hours and had to get up very early the next morning. In contrast to Sonja, he seemed solid and steady.

It was important to begin the therapy in a way that positioned me as equally supportive of both partners and minimized the power distinctions between us. I needed to recognize and validate Sonja's overlooked strengths and contributions to Dave's well-being and the family. I needed also to understand empathically each partner's gendered experience in a world quite different from mine and not to assume that Dave was less emotional or able to express caring than Sonja. Both needed credit for taking on adult responsibilities at young ages and persevering in the face of many obstacles.

Emotion

Dave and Sonja feared they were headed for divorce. As I listened, I tried to understand their experience through a gender lens. Thus, as Sonja adamantly insisted that a move would be good for the family, I reflected on her emotion surrounding her role as mother: "You care deeply about Benjie and Sophie." At this, tears began to stream down her face. Not only did this help get at some of the emotion underlying the couple's conflict but it also gave me an opportunity to validate Sonja's considerable strengths as a nurturing mother. Dave agreed and commented that she was a "giver." When I asked if she gave to him as well, he unhesitatingly agreed, and noted that she probably did not get as much back from him.

Contextualizing Sonja's experience in relation to gender helped me understand empathically why she was so invested in moving, and it opened the door to acknowledging her many contributions to the family. Similarly, when Sonja turned away from Dave in frustration, I drew on my understanding of her as a woman to comment, "You want him to value your opinion. When he doesn't, you don't feel loved." Sonja appeared grateful to be understood, responding, "Exactly. I don't need him to agree, but he could act as if I mattered."

On the other hand, Dave kept arguing "the facts" and insisted that Sonja did not understand "reality." Despite his hierarchical, "I know what is true," stance toward Sonja, I tried to understand him as the man who wanted to know what he was doing wrong. Because Dave had a hard time accessing or naming his feelings in session, I offered a possible description in a hesitating, open form that would allow him to correct my term: "Does it make you feel ... incompetent?" I chose this word because I know that feeling incompetent is uncomfortable for men socialized to believe they should have the answers.

Dave seemed to feel relieved that I understood his experience. I felt him begin to connect with me and the therapy. He stopped arguing and explained how hard he tried to get Sonja to understand "the situation." Because Sonja believed he was more invested in work than in her and the

family, I asked whether he felt competent at work. "Yes," he said, "I do—a lot more competent than at home." We agreed that helping him to feel more competent and Sonja to feel more valued were important goals.

Structure

As I listened to their story, I assessed their relative status and well-being, and their patterns for accommodating and attending each other. My first observation was that there appeared to be two strong voices. Though they thought the conflict was a problem, I suggested that it was positive and used it as an opportunity to bring equality into our discussion:

> "You know, I see a lot of couples and often there is no conflict, because one person accommodates all the time. But their relationships are in trouble, because to be an equal partnership, both people have to be able to express their opinions. You seem good at this. What do you think it is about you that makes room for two voices?"

Framing conflict as a positive facilitated a shift from battling and hostility. Dave commented that when they were first married, Sonja had not expressed herself. He seemed proud and supportive of Sonja as they described how she had learned to take initiative for herself and her children since ending an earlier, abusive marriage. We were also able to credit Dave: "You must have been doing something right ... to help her feel that it was safe to express herself." Framing conflict positively in the context of equality helped us develop another goal: to be better able to make decisions together.

As we looked in more detail at what happened when they made decisions and related to each other day by day, it became clear that Sonja's newfound assertiveness was fragile, and though Dave supported her equality in theory, in practice, he held considerable invisible power in their relationship. He gained status as "a good man" in comparison to Sonja's previous experiences. She trusted that he would never hit her and was grateful that he had taken on responsibility of her children as though they were his own. Yet Dave had the final say in decisions. Their conflicts arose only, as in the case of the move, when Sonja refused either to go along or to drop a subject. Sonja was expected to pay the bills, but Dave made financial decisions without consulting her. Unconsciously, he felt more entitled than Sonja to doing and getting what he wanted.

Both partners declared that they loved each other, but the disparity in attending to each other was pronounced. Like many women, Sonja felt hurt and rejected when her input was discounted. Dave was frustrated by the time talking took. He did not see how it would help them find a solution. Sonja longed for more emotional connection with Dave. She spent a lot of time trying to be responsive to his needs. But she got angry when he did not seem to want time with her. They agreed that helping each of them to feel loved and respected was an important goal.

Skills

The pressure to learn new skills to improve their marriage came from Sonja. She tearfully reported that if they did not, she would have to leave the marriage. Dave agreed that they could not continue as they were. Though each held equality as an ideal, neither partner had a clear model for how to live as equal partners. Therefore, subsequent therapy focused on developing more equal communication and decision-making processes, with particular attention to helping Dave demonstrate his caring and, while validating the legitimacy of Sonja's concerns, helping her to manage her anger constructively and acknowledge her right to make choices.

Moving toward Equality

We met weekly for 8 weeks, then every 2 or 3 weeks for 4 more months. In each session, I was attentive to creating a context through which Sonja and Dave could (1) externalize gender and power issues, (2) contextualize emotion, (3) equalize power, and (4) develop new habits and skills.

Externalize Gender and Power

It was important to consider Dave's rather limited attending skills in the context of his experience as a man. The men at work listened to him and did what they were told. He was embarrassed when Sonja called him at work. He believed he was much more family-oriented than most men. Therefore, we talked about how expectations for men and women are changing. Dave was encouraged to his examine own ideals, which, he insisted, included being more engaged in the family, and to consider how old models for men got in the way. The power difference that allowed Dave to overlook Sonja's perspectives and emotional needs was framed outside him in the larger social context.

Contextualize Emotion

It was important to remain tuned in to the gender/cultural experiences of both Sonja and Dave. For example, in response to their children's recent crises, Sonja had quit her job as a sales clerk. When I asked her what quitting work meant to her, she said it was a "huge sacrifice." Sonja felt valued and appreciated at work, and though she had been paid very little, she wanted to expand herself professionally. When she raised this issue with Dave, he suggested that she go back to work. Missing in this exchange, and so important for the therapist to understand empathically, was how deeply gender socialization compelled Sonja to believe she must sacrifice for her children. She wanted Dave to acknowledge this and appreciate her gift.

As we tuned into the emotion behind Sonja's desire to move, she tearfully reported that when they were first married, she had moved because of Dave, even though this meant taking the children from a safe and supportive environment. In this, as in so many things, she automatically had done what Dave wanted. To her, this was love. When Dave did not listen to her now, she felt unimportant to him. She needed to feel important and able to influence the relationship.

Equalize Power

It was important that I identify and redirect inequality when it occurred in the session. Dave regularly spent money on items he wanted. Thus, when he unconsciously assumed the right to define economic "reality," instead of immediately turning to explore his side of the issue, I first made the inequality visible:

SONJA: I found a way we could afford a weekend getaway.

DAVE: (silence) We can't do that.

THERAPIST: It sounds like it's important to Sonja. Was it your intention to ignore her ideas?

Then I offered Dave an opportunity to acknowledge Sonja as an equal partner, even if he did not agree with her:

DAVE: Well, I don't want to ignore her, but she just doesn't get reality.

THERAPIST: It seems to me that Sonja has put a lot of thought into this. Have you noticed that?

DAVE: Yes, she spends a lot of time on the computer comparing prices. She finds good buys, too.

Interrupting inequality when it occurs challenges gender-based communication patterns and provides an opportunity to explore new relationship options. An important way to equalize power in this relationship was to help Dave be more attentive to Sonja's concerns. Therefore, I assumed that Dave did care about Sonja, and I helped him consider how to respond to her from that place:

THERAPIST: It seems to me that you care a lot about Sonja and don't mean to hurt her. What did you notice about how she felt when you didn't listen to her ideas?

DAVE: ... (confused) What do you mean?

THERAPIST: What do you think it felt like to her?

DAVE: Not good.

THERAPIST: Is there something you might like to say to her instead ... something that lets her know you care about her ... that you are interested in what matters to her?

Dave's habit of not tuning in to Sonja was not intentional. But since Sonja did try to understand Dave, it resulted in an imbalance of power to influence the other.

Reinforce New Habits

Dave did listen to others at work. Therefore, developing the habit of listening to Sonja was more a change of position than a skill. Validating and highlighting the times when he was attuned to Sonja was important. Similarly, Sonja had learned to discount herself, then get angry at others. A key aspect of the ongoing therapy included active efforts to validate and highlight direct expression of her concerns, particularly in contrast to silence, tears, or anger. For example, when Dave said she needed to be more firm with Sophie, Sonja carefully responded, "I know I sometimes need to be more firm, but I think it's important to keep her talking about what she's doing." This clear and direct expression of her opinion needed to be reinforced.

THERAPIST: You sound clear that you want to keep communication open.

SONJA: [lengthy explanation of why] I think it's important, yes I do!

THERAPIST: You said this very clearly to Dave ... and I didn't hear anger.

SONJA: Well, it was hard ... but I'm feeling more confident.

THERAPIST: What is it like to speak with confidence?

SONJA: (smiling) Good ... good, but I'm not sure, you know.

It was also important to help Dave support her new skill.

THERAPIST: (to Dave) Was it helpful to you that Sonja was clear?

DAVE: Well, I still think she should be more firm with Sophie.

THERAPIST: Yes, you value being firm. But I wonder if it was helpful to know where Sonja is coming from ... if that's easier than her getting mad at you.

DAVE: Ya ... she's got a point too. You don't want Sophie just going behind our backs.

From here, we were able to move into a discussion of what it takes to be clear with each other. As both partners began to try out habits and skills different from their gender socialization, each sometimes felt uncomfortable. They described successfully discussing an issue at home:

THERAPIST: What was it like to stay with the issue like that?

DAVE: Uncomfortable. I wanted us to get done!

THERAPIST: But you stuck with it.

DAVE: Well. We have to get through this ...

SONJA: I liked it. But I was afraid he would leave (tears).

Thus, as Dave and Sonja tried out new ways of relating, their anxieties surfaced. They needed support and validation as new skills gradually became habits. Help them to tolerate conflict was particularly important.

New Possibilities

Sonja and Dave did not leave the therapy with all their problems solved. However, they reported renewed hope that they could solve their problems together. They reported decision-making processes that involved both of them and fewer angry outbursts. They decided to put their house on the market, and to continue to explore how to make the family work for all of them. Each also described personal changes that challenged gender stereotypes and reflected more equal power in the relationship:

DAVE: I've learned not to focus so much on my own interests. ... I've got to take into account all of them. I think I can do that, but I have to think it through ... see how it goes.

SONJA: I feel so much better about myself. I have more confidence. I think we can work it out. But whatever happens, I'll be OK.

Like most men, Dave did not intentionally seek to hold the power in the relationship. He responded positively to invitations to be more attuned to Sonja. Sonja learned to give up the habit of accommodating, then resenting Dave for it. Both benefited from increased intimacy and confidence in their ability to solve problems together.

ACKNOWLEDGMENTS

The framework for practice presented in this chapter was developed in collaboration with Anne Rankin Mahoney, Professor Emerita, Sociology Department, University of Denver and Douglas Huenergardt, Professor and Director of the Doctorate in Marital and Family Therapy (DMFT) program at Loma Linda University.

SUGGESTIONS FOR FURTHER READING

Case Studies

Brooks, G. (2003). Helping men embrace equality. In L. Silverstein & T. J. Goodrich (Eds.), *Feminist family therapy: Empowerment in social context* (pp. 163–176). Washington, DC: American Psychological Association.—This case example shows how working with a man's perception that he needed to be strong and invulnerable was central to successful couple therapy.

Goodrich, T. J., Rampage, C., Ellman, B., & Halstead, K. (1988). The standard pairing. In *Feminist family therapy: A casebook* (pp. 88–112). New York: Norton.—This classic case illustrates how to work with a couple that demonstrates gender stereotypical "complementarity."

Research Articles

Hyde, J. S. (2005). The gender similarities hypothesis. *American Psychologist, 60,* 581–592.—This comprehensive review of 46 meta-analyses shows that males and females are similar on most psychological variables and cautions therapists against inflated claims of gender differences.

Knudson-Martin, C., & Mahoney, A. (2005). Moving beyond gender: Processes that create relationship equality. *Journal of Marital and Family Therapy, 31,* 113–129.—This qualitative study of couples across two time cohorts identifies the processes that facilitate relationship equality and minimize drift back to stereotyped gender patterns.

Books

Knudson-Martin, C., & Mahoney, A. (Eds.). (in press). *Transforming power: How couples move from gender legacy to gender equality.* New York: Springer.—This research-based guide identifies the subtle ways gender and power undermine relationships and qualitatively examines how to help couples across a range of cultural contexts transcend the gender legacy and transform power.

Rabin, C. (1996). *Equal partners, good friends: Empowering couples through therapy.* London: Routledge.—Rabin examines the connection between inequality in marriage and marital distress and provides a clinical treatment model for couple therapists.

REFERENCES

Amato, P. R., Johnson, D. R., Booth, A., & Rogers, S. (2003). Continuity and change in marital quality between 1980 and 2000. *Journal of Marriage and Family, 65,* 1–22.

Angier, N. (1999). *Woman: An intimate geography.* New York: Random House.

Anderson, C., & Holder, D. (1989). Women and serious mental disorders. In M. McGoldrick, C. Anderson, & F. Walsh (Eds.), *Women in families: A framework for family therapy* (pp. 381–405). New York: Norton.

Atkinson, B. J. (2005). *Emotional intelligence in couples therapy.* New York: Norton.

Beavers, W. R. (1985). *Successful marriage: A family systems approach to couples therapy.* New York: Norton.

Bernard, J. (1973). *The future of marriage.* New York: Bantam Books.

Blaisure, K., & Allen, K. (1995). Feminism and ideology and the practice of marital equality. *Journal of Marriage and the Family, 57,* 5–19.

Bograd, M. (1999). Strengthening domestic violence theories: Intersection of race, class, sexual orientation, and gender. *Journal of Marital and Family Therapy, 25,* 275–290.

Boyd-Franklin, N., & Frankin, A. J. (1998). African-American couples in therapy. In M. McGoldrick (Ed.), *Revisioning family therapy: Race, culture, and gender in clinical practice* (pp. 268–281). New York: Guilford Press.

Brooks, G. (2003). Helping men embrace equality. In L.

Silverstein & T. J. Goodrich (Eds.), *Feminist family therapy: Empowerment in social context* (pp. 163–176). Washington, DC: American Psychological Association.

Coltrane, S. (1996). *Family man: Fatherhood, housework, and gender equality*. Oxford, UK: Oxford University Press.

Coltrane, S., & Adams, M. (2001). Men's family work: Child-centered fathering and the sharing of domestic labor. In R. Hertz & N. Marshall (Eds.), *Work family: Today's realities and tomorrow's visions* (pp. 72–99). Berkeley, CA: University of California Press.

Coontz, S. (2005). *Marriage, a history: From obedience to intimacy or how love conquered marriage*. New York: Viking.

Cowdery, R. S., & Knudson-Martin, C. (2005). Motherhood: Tasks, relational connection, and gender equality. *Family Relations, 54*, 335–346.

Deutsch, F. (1999). *Halving it all: How equally shared parenting works*. Cambridge, MA: Harvard University Press.

Garcia-Preto, N. (1998). Latinas in the United States: Bridging two worlds. In M. McGoldrick (Ed.), *Revisioning family therapy: Race, culture and gender in clinical practice* (pp. 330–346). New York: Guilford Press.

Gee, J. P. (2005). *An introduction to discourse analysis: Theory and method* (2nd ed.). New York: Routledge.

Gergen, K. (1999). *An invitation to social construction*. Newbury Park, CA: Sage.

Gilligan, C. (1982). *In a different voice: Psychological theory and women's development*. Cambridge, MA: Harvard University Press.

Goldner, V. (1985). Feminism and family therapy. *Family Process, 24*, 31–47.

Goldner, V. (1988). Generation and gender: Normative and covert hierarchies. *Family Process, 27*, 17–31.

Gottman, J. (1994). *Why marriages succeed or fail*. New York: Simon & Schuster.

Gottman, J. M., Coan, J., Carrere, S., & Swanson, C. (1998). Predicting marital happiness and stability from newlywed interactions. *Journal of Marriage and the Family, 60*, 5–22.

Gray, J. (1994). *Men are from Mars: Women are from Venus*. New York: HarperCollins.

Haddock, S., MacPhee, D., & Zimmerman, T. (2001). AAMFT master series tapes: An analysis of the inclusion of feminist principles into family therapy practice. *Journal of Marital and Family Therapy, 27*, 487–500.

Haddock, S., Zimmerman, T. S., & MacPhee, D. (2000). The power equity guide: Attending to gender in family therapy. *Journal of Marital and Family Therapy, 26*, 153–170.

Hare-Mustin, R. (1978). A feminist approach to family therapy. *Family Process, 17*, 181–194.

Hill, S. A. (2005). *Black intimacies: A gender perspective on families and relationships*. Walnut Creek, CA: AltaMira Press.

Hochschild, A. (1989). *The second shift: Working parents and the revolution at home*. New York: Viking.

Horst, E., & Doherty, W. (1995). Gender, power, and intimacy. *Journal of Feminist Family Therapy, 6*, 63–85.

Hyde, J. S. (2005). The gender similarities hypothesis. *American Psychologist, 60*, 581–592.

Johnson, S. M. (2003). The revolution in couple therapy: A practitioner–scientist perspective. *Journal of Marital and Family Therapy, 29*, 365–384.

Jordan, J. V. (2004). Toward competence and connection. In J. Jordan, M. Walker, & L. Hartling (Eds.), *The complexity of connection: Writings from the Stone Center's Jean Baker Miller Training Institute* (pp. 11–27). New York: Guilford Press.

Kimmel, M. (2004). *The gendered society* (2nd ed.). Oxford, UK: Oxford University Press.

Knudson-Martin, C. (2003a). Gender and biology: A recursive framework for clinical practice. *Journal of Feminist Family Therapy, 15*(2/3), 1–21.

Knudson-Martin, C. (2003b). How to avoid gender bias in mental health treatment. *Journal of Family Psychotherapy, 14*(3), 45–66.

Knudson-Martin, C., & Mahoney, A. (1998). Language and processes in the construction of equality in new marriages. *Family Relations, 47*, 81–91.

Knudson-Martin, C., & Mahoney, A. (1999). Beyond different worlds: A "postgender" approach to relational development. *Family Process, 38*, 325–340.

Knudson-Martin, C., & Mahoney, A. (2005). Moving beyond gender: Processes that create relationship equality. *Journal of Marital and Family Therapy, 31*, 113–129.

Knudson-Martin, C., & Mahoney, A. (in press). *Transforming power: How couples move from gender legacy to gender equality*. New York: Springer.

Komter, A. (1989). Hidden power in marriage. *Gender and Society, 3*, 187–216.

Krolokke, C., & Sorensen, A. S. (2006). *Gender communication theories and analysis: From silence to performance*. Thousand Oaks, CA: Sage.

Laird, J. (1998). Theorizing culture. In M. McGoldrick (Ed.), *Re-visioning family therapy: Race, culture, and gender in clinical practice* (pp. 20–36). New York: Guilford Press.

Laird, J. (2000). Gender in lesbian relationships: Cultural, feminist, and constructionist reflections. *Journal of Marital and Family Therapy, 26*, 455–468.

Larson, R., & Richards, M. (1994). *Divergent realities: The emotional lives of mothers, fathers, and adolescents*. New York: Basic Books.

Leslie, L., & Clossick, M. (1996). Sexism in family therapy: Does training in gender make a difference? *Journal of Marital and Family Therapy, 22*, 253–269.

Lim, I. (1997). Korean immigrant women's challenge to gender inequality at home: The interplay of economic resources, gender, and family. *Gender and Society, 11*, 31–51.

Lindsey, L. (1997). *Gender roles: A sociological perspective* (3rd ed.). Upper Saddle River, NJ: Prentice-Hall.

Lips, H. (1991). *Women, men, and power*. Mountain View, CA: Mayfield.

Luepnitz, D. (1988). *The family interpreted: Feminist theory in clinical practice*. New York: Basic Books.

Lynch, S. (1998). Who supports whom?: How age and gender affect the perceived quality of support of family and friends. *Gerontologist, 38*, 231–238.

Matta, D., & Knudson-Martin, C. (2006). Couple processes in the co-construction of fatherhood. *Family Process, 45*, 19–37.

McGoldrick, M., Anderson, C., & Walsh, F. (1989). *Women in families: A framework for family therapy*. New York: Norton.

McGrath, E., Keita, G. P., Strickland, B., & Russo, N. F. (1990). *Women and depression: Risk factors and treatment issues*. Washington, DC: American Psychological Association.

Mencher, J. (1997). Intimacy in lesbian relationships: A critical reexamination of fusion. In J. Jordan (Ed.), *Women's growth in diversity* (pp. 311–330). New York: Guilford Press.

Minuchin, S., Lee, W., & Simon, G. (2003). *Mastering family therapy: Journeys of growth and transformation* (2nd ed.). New York: Wiley.

Padgett, D. (1997). Women's mental health: Some directions for research. *American Journal of Orthopsychiatry, 67*, 522–534.

Quartz, S., & Sejnowski, T. (2002). *Liars, lovers, and heroes: What the new brain science reveals about how we become who were are*. New York: HarperCollins.

Quek, K. M., & Knudson-Martin, C. (2006). A push towards equality: Processes among dual-income couples in a collectivist culture. *Journal of Marriage and Family, 68*, 56–69.

Rabin, C. (1996). *Equal partners, good friends: Empowering couples through therapy*. London: Routledge.

Rhode, D. (1997). *Speaking of sex: The denial of gender inequality*. Cambridge, MA: Harvard University Press.

Risman, B. J. (1998). *Gender vertigo: American families in transition*. New Haven, CT: Yale University Press.

Sarbin, T. (2001). Embodiment and the narrative structure of emotional life. *Narrative Inquiry, 11*, 217–225.

Schwartz, P. (1994). *Peer marriage: How love between equals really works*. New York: Free Press.

Silverstein, L., & Goodrich, T. J. (Eds.). (2003). *Feminist family therapy: Empowerment in social context* (pp. 17–35). Washington, DC: American Psychological Association.

Silverstein, R., Bass, L. B., Tuttle, A., Knudson-Martin, C., & Huenergardt, D. (2006). What does it mean to be relational?: A framework for assessment and practice. *Family Process, 45*, 391–405.

Steil, J. (1997). *Marital equality: Its relationship to the well-being of husbands and wives*. Newbury Park, CA: Sage.

Sternberg, E. (2001). *The balance within: The science connecting health and emotions*. New York: Freeman.

Sullivan, O. (2006). *Changing gender relations, changing families: Tracing the pace of change over time*. Boulder: Rowman & Littlefield.

Tannen, D. (1990). *You just don't understand: Men and women in conversation*. New York: Ballantine Books.

Tannen, D. (1994). *Gender and discourse*. New York: Oxford University Press.

Taylor, S. (2002). *The tending instinct: How nurturing is essential to who we are and how we live*. New York: Holt.

Tichenor, V. J. (2005). *Earning more and getting less: Why successful wives can't buy equality*. New Brunswick, NJ: Rutgers University Press.

Walters, M., Carter, B., Papp, P., & Silverstein, O. (1988). *The invisible web: Gender patterns in family relationships*. New York: Guilford Press.

Zimmerman, T. S., Haddock, S. A., Ziemba, S., & Rust, A. (2001). Family organizational labor: Who is calling the plays? In T. S. Zimmerman (Ed.), *Balancing family and work: Special considerations in feminist therapy?* (pp. 65–90). New York: Haworth Press.

Zvonkovic, A., Greaves, K., Schmeige, C., & Hall, L. (1996). The marital construction of gender through work and family decisions. *Journal of Marriage and the Family, 58*, 91–100.

CHAPTER 24

Gay and Lesbian Couples in Therapy

Minority Stress, Relational Ambiguity, and Families of Choice

ROBERT-JAY GREEN
VALORY MITCHELL

Imagine that you are invited to write a chapter titled "Therapy with Heterosexual Couples" for the fourth edition of the *Clinical Handbook of Couple Therapy*. Where to begin? At the very least, this invitation requires you to make broad generalizations about the entire client population of heterosexual couples in North America, if not the world. No small challenge.

A request for such a chapter also implies that other chapters in the handbook will not deal sufficiently with heterosexual couples in therapy. It is *your* job alone to explain how general theories of couple therapy need to be altered to fit the characteristics of heterosexual couples:

- Are certain kinds of clinical problems more frequently found among heterosexual couples in therapy?
- Does the status "legally married" (which is unique to heterosexual couples under Federal Law in the United States) increase or diminish relationship problems?
- What different goals are required when doing therapy with heterosexual couples?
- What strategies would you suggest for building an effective therapist–client relationship when a couple is heterosexual?

- Taking into account a couple's heterosexuality, what change-oriented techniques are especially suitable in therapy?
- How might a couple's heterosexuality require special adaptations in the way particular approaches to couple therapy are practiced (cognitive-behavioral, structural–strategic, emotion focused, psychodynamic, integrative, etc.)?
- Given that so many married couples enter therapy in a crisis following the discovery of a spouse's affair, how can therapists help couples cope with this aspect of the heterosexual lifestyle?

As these questions illustrate, it is extremely difficult to make generalized statements about heterosexual couples in therapy. Answers to such questions are elusive, and the risk of stereotyping is high. Heterosexual couples usually are *not* viewed as a unitary cultural group based on their sexual orientation. Rather, being in the majority, heterosexual couples blend in. Their distinctive ways go unnoticed, apparently not needing further dissection because they are so common.

Just as this field has no book about European American families in therapy but excellent books about African American families in therapy

(Boyd-Franklin, 2003), Latino families in therapy (Falicov, 1998), and Asian American families in therapy (Lee, 1997), the field is not likely any time soon to see a book with the title *Heterosexual Families in Therapy*. However, heterosexual couples are no less a subculturally bound, norm-driven, singular group than are same-sex couples (who show just as much intragroup diversity in all the sociodemographic and psychiatric ways imaginable).

Our purpose in this "thought experiment" is to demonstrate that in learning about "therapy with gay and lesbian couples," one must at least tacitly understand that heterosexual couples also occupy a distinct social status, with expectations, norms, and sanctions affecting their functioning. One must grasp that, just like coupled homosexuality, coupled heterosexuality has certain built-in advantages and stresses. Most important, one has to comprehend the myriad ways heterosexual relationships are shaped by historical traditions, given legal legitimization, and offered widespread social supports, rendering them simultaneously more secure and stable but also more constrained than lesbian and gay relationships.

FOCUS OF THIS CHAPTER

The bulk of the literature on couple therapy presumes a heterosexual status among couples seeking treatment. The consequence is that many couple therapists are uncertain about how to conceptualize and intervene actively in the problems of lesbian and gay couples. Surveys have shown that nearly half of all members of the American Association for Marriage and Family Therapy (AAMFT) report that they do *not* feel competent treating lesbians or gay men in therapy (Doherty & Simmons, 1996). Nevertheless, a very large majority of such therapists (72%) state that at least 1 out of every 10 cases in their practices involve lesbians or gay men (S. K. Green & Bobele, 1994). Data from these and other surveys imply that many mental health professionals are treating same-sex couples without adequate preparation, and their clients may suffer the consequences (Garnets, Hancock, Cochran, Godchilds, & Peplau, 1991).

We are not implying that one needs a whole new theory of therapy to work effectively with same-sex couples. Homosexuality and heterosexuality are not opposites. However, therapists who work with same-sex couples (which means almost all couple therapists) should be aware of the unique challenges facing lesbian and gay couples.

In this chapter, we group these special developmental challenges facing same-sex couples under three broad categories: (1) coping with lesbian and gay minority stress; (2) resolving relational ambiguity in the areas of commitment, boundaries, and gender-linked behaviors; and (3) developing a "family of choice" (a cohesive network of social support).

Most lesbian and gay couples manage these tasks successfully on their own. In fact, research on community, nonclinical samples of lesbian, gay, and heterosexual couples indicates that same-sex couples are generally functioning as well, or better than, heterosexual couples (Green, Bettinger, & Zacks, 1996; Gottman, Levenson, et al., 2003; Gottman, Levenson, Swanson, et al., 2003; Kurdek, 2004, 2005; Peplau & Fingerhut, 2007). However, in this chapter, we focus on same-sex partners who are not coping well with the typical developmental hurdles. These couples may enter therapy to deal with lesbian–gay-specific issues such as conflicts over how to handle prejudice in one or both partners' families of origin, or how "out" they should be in their communities. Still other such couples begin therapy with common psychiatric symptoms (e.g., depression in one partner) that turn out to be strongly linked to antigay prejudice in their families or work, ambiguity in a partner's commitment, and/or lack of social support from friends.

The therapist's first task is to assess whether and to what extent a given couple's problems are connected to these special challenges of being lesbian or gay versus to other generic couple issues, such as basic attachment styles, communication patterns, or conflict negotiation strategies. Although it is important always to assess for the three factors emphasized in this chapter, it is equally important to remain open to the possibility that a given same-sex couple's problems have little or nothing to do with the partners being lesbian or gay. In this process, therapists face the twin dangers of either overestimating or underestimating the importance of lesbian–gay-specific factors in the etiology of a particular presenting problem.

In what follows, we describe how therapists can help same-sex partners cope with minority stress, make their couple commitments and relationship roles less ambiguous, and build a more closely knit network of social support. For each of these issues, we describe problem-specific dynamics and related therapeutic techniques, then discuss how therapists (especially heterosexual therapists) can prepare themselves personally and professionally for this kind of work.

MINORITY STRESS

The most salient characteristic that distinguishes lesbian and gay couples from heterosexual couples as a group is that *all same-sex couples are vulnerable to similar kinds of prejudice, discrimination, and marginalization by persons and institutions outside of their relationships.*

Research consistently shows that antigay attitudes (sometimes called "homophobia") are associated with conservative social attitudes overall, and with gender role traditionalism and fundamentalist religious beliefs in particular (Herek, 1998). Males tend to be more homophobic than females. Studies also reveal that heterosexuals—including couple and family therapists—who have more direct contact with lesbians and gay men as friends, family members, and/or clients express more accepting attitudes about homosexuality (S. K. Green & Bobele, 1994; Herek, 1998).

"Internalized homophobia" occurs when lesbian and gay persons have acquired society's antigay attitudes and direct those negative attitudes toward the self. It is associated with lesbian–gay persons' devaluation of self (lowered self-esteem), higher rates of concealing sexual orientation, greater depression in response to homophobic prejudice, higher levels of suicidality, increased HIV risk-taking behaviors, and mental health and substance abuse problems (Malyon, 1982; Meyer & Dean, 1998; Shidlo, 1994).

It is axiomatic that all openly lesbian and gay people, including members of couples, have had to counter and unlearn internalized homophobia to some extent to achieve a measure of self-acceptance and to form a same-sex relationship. However, in many couples, one or both partners may continue to have internalized homophobia, which frequently contributes to the demise of couple relationships in direct or indirect ways. In the context of couple therapy, an important aspect of internalized homophobia is that some lesbian and gay clients nihilistically believe the cultural stereotype that enduring love relationships between same-sex partners are wrong or impossible to achieve. These clients may unconsciously sabotage their relationships in a kind of self-fulfilling prophecy, pessimistically giving up too quickly rather than trying to work through the inevitable impasses in a long-term relationship. Therapists

can help such clients challenge negative stereotypes about lesbian and gay relationships, and achieve a greater degree of freedom to commit to same-sex couplehood.

The combination of external and internalized sources of prejudice creates "minority stress" for all lesbian and gay people at various points in their lives (Meyer, 2003). This kind of stress typically reaches a crescendo in adolescence, when the individual begins self-identifying as lesbian, gay, or bisexual, but still has not disclosed these feelings to others (Savin-Williams, 1996). Beyond adolescence, most lesbian and gay people continue to experience some degree of prejudice and fear of discrimination throughout their adult lives, depending on their locations and life circumstances (Bepko & Johnson, 2000).

A couple's sexual orientation affects that couple's relationship to almost all other entities in society—family, work, school, medical care, insurance, the legal system, housing, religious institutions, government, and so on. The very right of same-sex persons to associate with one another in a romantic/sexual relationship was against the law in many states until recently (the so-called "sodomy" statutes, which were not overturned by the U.S. Supreme Court until June 2003). Even now, the civil rights of lesbian and gay couples are challenged almost every year by court cases, ballot initiatives, legislative proposals, and regulatory revisions at all levels of government (Hartman, 1996). As of this writing, with President Bush's promise to veto the Employment Non-Discrimination Act (ENDA) that recently passed the U.S. House of Representatives, it still is legal in 31 states for lesbian and gay people to be summarily fired from their jobs or discriminated against in hiring and promotion decisions, simply because of their sexual orientations.

Thus, in most areas of the United States, same-sex couples are still vulnerable to housing and employment discrimination and to physical harm if they are out and visible; or if they conceal their relationships, they live with fear of discovery. Discrimination and fear of discovery each may undermine the couple's relationship if the partners do not have internal ways of countering the social stigma of homosexuality or a social support system to buffer that stress. Although there are pockets of increasing political support for same-sex couples, and although the U.S. Bureau of the Census has begun counting households headed by same-sex partners, the overall message from the mainstream of American politics to lesbian and gay couples is something like: "We don't want you to exist, so we simply decline to acknowledge or support your relationships in the way we support heterosexual relationships." In this way, much of the discrimination is presumptive and exclusionary rather than overtly aggressive, and it contributes to a feeling of marginality and invisibility for lesbian and gay couples.

In this context, to engage in a committed couple relationship becomes both a personal and a political act for lesbian and gay people, who were literally outlaws in many states until the U.S. Supreme Court decriminalized homosexual relations in 2003. No matter how mundane their everyday suburban lives, Rozzie and Harriet's couplehood remains at variance with the dominant social and political status quo. They are caught in a cultural vortex of conflicting attitudes—support from some quarters, neglect from most, overt hostility from others. In Massachusetts they can get married, but nowhere else in the United States is such a marriage recognized. In most circumstances in the United States and around the world, they still risk being gawked at if they hold hands in public. In other circumstances, they will be verbally or physically attacked for such benign displays of everyday couplehood.

Although same-sex couples do not encounter intolerance or hatred at every turn, they experience enough of it personally, vicariously (by identification with other lesbian–gay victims of discrimination), and through the media to remain vigilant for its occurrence. It is almost impossible for a person to grow up in this society without internalizing some negative attitudes and fears about his or her own homosexual feelings and the dangers of discrimination against lesbian–gay people. Social scientists are only beginning to understand the mechanisms that lesbian–gay people employ to cope with such "minority stress" (Meyer, 2003).

Most relevant for formation of couple relationships, the difficulty accepting one's homosexuality (internalized homophobia) and/or the fear of being exposed as lesbian or gay discourage many lesbian and gay people from forming lasting couple bonds. In many areas of the United States and in almost all Asian, Latin American, African, and all Islamic countries, it is safer to remain closeted and to restrict one's sexual/romantic encounters to brief, anonymous interludes than to commit to a same-sex relationship and risk the greater likelihood of public exposure. To reach the latter level of "outness," lesbian and gay partners must live in more accepting communities and successfully

challenge in their own minds the negative views they were taught about homosexuality.

The vulnerability to these external dangers renders lesbian and gay couples vigilant for discrimination, especially in unfamiliar surroundings. If each partner has reached a high level of self-acceptance about being lesbian or gay, this external stress is manageable, unless, of course, it involves physical violence. However, to the extent that partners are still dealing with internalized homophobia themselves, their relationship can be threatened by even subtle forms of prejudice and discrimination, and by the vigilance necessary to protect against it.

For example, realistic fears about holding hands and being affectionate in certain public contexts can stimulate a partner's internalized homophobia, leaving him or her feeling defective, ashamed, bad, unworthy, sick, sinful, depressed, and so forth. Or, in certain work environments, the necessity to self-monitor what one says and how one acts may leave a partner feeling constantly stressed and blaming his or her sexual orientation for causing this problem rather than locating the problem's cause in society's ignorance. When partners' internalized homophobia is triggered in these ways, it sometimes translates into couple difficulties, including (1) inexplicable arguments (e.g., frustration is displaced onto the partner, or self-hatred turns into criticism of one's partner); (2) sexual desire or performance difficulties (caused by inhibition or guilt); and (3) depression and withdrawal from the partner (feeling unworthy, or feeling ambivalent about committing to a lesbian or gay relationship). For couples in which these dynamics are operating, the stated goals of couple therapy (agreed upon collaboratively with the clients) should include reducing or eliminating the partners' internalized homophobia.

Interventions to Counter Minority Stress

Successfully countering antigay prejudice and internalized homophobia requires attributing them to societal ignorance, prejudice, fear, and the human tendency to conform to dominant norms. It also requires exposure to and social support from other lesbian–gay people whose behavior counteracts negative stereotypes about homosexuality.

In a sense, all of the techniques discussed in this chapter can help clients cope with external or internalized antigay prejudice. However, we present some very specific strategies below. In this aspect of the work, therapists should make use of feminist, gay-affirmative, multicultural, and narrative family systems therapy principles.

The two central ideas in applying feminist theories of therapy to same-sex couples are the notions of cultural "resistance" and "subversion." These concepts have been well articulated by Brown (1994, p. 25):

> In feminist theory, resistance means the refusal to merge with dominant cultural norms and to attend to one's own voice and integrity. ... Each act of feminist therapy ... must have as an implicit goal the uncovering of the presence of the patriarchy as a source of distress so that this influence of the dominant can be named, undermined, resisted, and subverted. ... Awareness and transformation mean teaching of resistance, learning the ways in which each of us is damaged by our witting or unwitting participation in dominant norms or by the ways in which such norms have been thrust upon us.

In terms of applying these concepts of resistance and subversion to the treatment of lesbian and gay couples, one starts with the basic awareness that by loving someone of the same sex, lesbians and gay men are violating the most basic gender norms of the society. Cultural resistance entails helping clients examine all the oppressive social influences in their lives, influences that pressure them not to engage in same-sex love and to regard their capacity for same-sex love as bad, sinful, disturbed, inferior, and so forth. This includes a careful, detailed reconstruction of the various messages they received about homosexuality (in their families, in school, in their neighborhood, in their religious institutions, through the media, and from members of their specific racial/ethnic group) as they were growing up.

The therapist should explore with clients their internalization of traditional gender norms, as well as the overt prejudice and discrimination they continue to face in their current social networks (family, neighbors, coworkers) and from the "impersonal" institutions of society (the media, the government, insurance companies, employment settings, health care institutions, religious communities, etc.). Most important, the therapist should counter these oppressive messages, neutralizing society's condemnation of same-sex love and framing it as a normal human variation, not reinforcing (in subtle or unsubtle ways) its pejorative framing by the larger society. Thus, the therapist functions as a celebrant and witness of constructive lesbian and gay relationships, acknowledging their legitimacy and worthiness of equal support.

This approach is an elaboration of what has become known as "gay-affirmative therapy." As Malyon wrote in first describing this approach in 1982:

> Gay-affirmative psychotherapy is not an independent system of psychotherapy. Rather, it represents a special range of psychological knowledge which challenges the traditional view that homosexual desire and fixed homosexual orientations are pathological. ... This approach regards homophobia, as opposed to homosexuality, as a major pathological variable in the development of certain symptomatic conditions. (pp. 68–69)

Gay-affirmative therapy involves actively challenging society's negative attitudes towards homosexuality that contribute to the problems of lesbian and gay couples. The partners are encouraged to dispute, deconstruct, and subvert society's prejudicial views rather than continue to internalize or be limited by them. In a sense, the work is similar to what narrative therapists have described as externalizing the problem (in this case, viewing homophobia as the oppressive problem rather than viewing one's sexual orientation as the problem), and what cognitive therapists have sometimes called "disputation" of irrational beliefs.

In some couple therapy cases, partners are at markedly different levels of accepting their sexual orientations. Individual therapy may be indicated for the partner with a great deal more internalized homophobia than the other, especially if he or she seems ashamed to explore these aspects of self in the presence of the partner. However, if both partners are at roughly the same stage on this dimension, it is most helpful to see them together in conjoint sessions, because both will benefit by self-exploration in one another's presence.

In addition to this work of deconstructing internalized homophobia in the sessions, therapists should encourage clients to engage in various forms of participation in lesbian–gay community organizations, including political advocacy, if it fits their sensibilities (i.e., the cultural "subversion" aspect of liberationist therapies). For example, one client (who had played a musical instrument in her high school band) was encouraged to join the San Francisco Lesbian/Gay Freedom Band, which marches in the local Pride Parade and performs in other venues throughout the city. Another client, because of his skills in accounting, was encouraged to join the finance committee of the Board of Directors of a local lesbian–gay youth agency.

Acts such as these constitute an important way in which lesbian and gay clients with internalized homophobia can stand up (in solidarity with others) for their right to exist, meet others who can model high levels of self-esteem and empowerment, and contribute to the reduction of antigay attitudes in the larger society. These acts of lesbian–gay community participation are both a form of subversion of the heteronormative status quo and a legitimization of the self, implicitly naming society's prejudice (rather than the self) as the problem that needs to be eliminated.

Depending on the kind of discrimination that same-sex partners face, coping successfully may require (1) working actively for change in one's current social environment; (2) changing to a different social environment (literally relocating geographically or quitting one's job to escape an intransigent or dangerously antigay situation); (3) re-attributing the cause of one's distress to different factors (e.g., attributing one's distress to external prejudice and ignorance rather than to personal inadequacy); or (4) reconciling to the fact that some discriminatory situations cannot be changed, then focusing on other areas in one's life as sources of hope and fulfillment.

Therapists can help couples determine which course of action is most effective given the context. However, when confronted with similar levels of external prejudice, same-sex couples with more internalized homophobia tend to be more derailed by antigay incidents. Thus the therapeutic work often focuses simultaneously on partners' internalized homophobia *and* on ways to cope with discrimination in the external environment.

RELATIONAL AMBIGUITY

A key concept in couple and family systems theory has been the notion of boundaries, especially interpersonal boundaries between individuals, generational boundaries between the partners and their families of origin, and boundaries between the couple and the social network surrounding it. Minuchin (1974) defined family boundaries as "the rules defining who participates and how" (p. 53). It is just as important to consider who or what is excluded from participation in a subsystem as considering who or what is included.

Also basic to the notion of boundaries is the way a relationship is defined by the participants (i.e., what kind of relationship is this?—a best friendship, a social acquaintanceship, a romantic involvement, a lifelong primary commitment, a temporary dating relationship, a mainly sexual encounter, etc.). With lesbian and gay couples in

therapy, we frequently observe a lack of clarity in how they define their couplehood to themselves and to others. We believe this is partly because lesbian and gay couples (in contrast to legally married, heterosexual couples) lack a socially endorsed, legally framed, normative template for how couplehood should be. Overall, partners do not know what they can expect from a same-sex relationship, because there is no socially or legally prescribed kind of couplehood for them, and no prevailing way of being a same-sex couple. The popular film, *Brokeback Mountain*, illustrates these "definition of the relationship" problems in the extreme.

Boss's (1999) concept of "boundary ambiguity" is very relevant here: "a state in which family members are uncertain in their perception about who is in or out of the family and who is performing what roles and tasks within the family system" (Boss & Greenberg, 1984, p. 536). We extend the concept of boundary ambiguity to situations that might best be labeled "ambiguous commitment," where one or both partners' intentions or degree of joining in the relationship remain in doubt. Ambiguous commitment is prevalent in same-sex couples in therapy, partly because partners' decisions to be together are not usually preceded by an extended courtship or engagement phase, demarcated by a commitment ceremony, governed by statutes for legal marriage, approved by the partners' respective families of origin, or (in most cases) solidified by becoming coparents to children.

Relationships that we are characterizing by the phrase "ambiguous commitment" are closest to having what Boss, Caron, Horbal, and Mortimer (1990) describe as "physical presence" but "psychological absence." The partners are physically in the relationship (physically present), but the extent and exact nature of their psychological commitment to the relationship is unclear.

In addition, terminations of lesbian and gay couple relationships are sometimes characterized by ambiguous loss, partly because of the absence of formal divorce proceedings that clearly demarcate the ending. The absence of a legal ritual formalizing divorce may increase the likelihood that boundary ambiguity will occur and last longer during transitions out of some lesbian and gay couple relationships. In Boss et al.'s (1990) terms, these relationships are closest to having "physical absence" but "psychological presence." The partners are out of the relationship (e.g., may no longer be living together or defining themselves publicly as a couple), but the extent and nature of their ongoing commitment to the relationship is still in doubt. With some lesbian or gay couples in therapy, this ongoing connection with an ex-partner seems to interfere with starting a new couple relationship, or with a new partner's sense of primacy over the former partner.

What is strikingly different for same-sex couples is that almost all of the usual expectations that heterosexuals bring to marriage (e.g., monogamy, pooled finances, dividing instrumental/expressive and household roles somewhat along gender lines, caring for each other through serious illness, moving together for each other's career advancement, providing and caring for one another's families in old age, mutual inheritance, health care power of attorney rights in the event of a partner's mental or physical incapacity) do not necessarily apply to same-sex couple relationships unless discussed and explicitly agreed to in writing by the partners. Typically, same-sex couples do not clarify these expectations before moving in together, and discrepancies in their visions of the relationship only become apparent when unspoken expectations are suddenly breached, which can be shocking and hurtful to the partners.

Although contemporary heterosexual couples also experience uncertainty about what being a couple means to them, it is a matter of degree. Clinical observation suggests that same-sex couples, as a group, experience more boundary and commitment ambiguity than do married couples. For example, committed heterosexual couples typically take a wedding vow to stay together "in sickness and in health till death do us part." This vow to take care of each other is also a promise to family members, friends, and other witnesses, including, in most cases, to "God as a witness."

By contrast, it is unclear when or whether most same-sex partners can have the same expectations of their relationship. Do same-sex partners implicitly make this vow when they move in together? After being together for 2 years or 10 years? Can there be equivalent vow making for same-sex couples who cannot get legally married in all but one state (Massachusetts) and even then not in the eyes of the federal government? Is a vow made in private the same psychologically as one made in public? Is a promise made in a public "commitment ceremony" that is not recognized by the state and/or federal government the same as a promise made against the backdrop of legally enforceable marriage laws?

Lacking a preordained prescription for what being a same-sex couple means, lesbian–gay partners must develop some basic parameters and rules for themselves as a couple. Inevitably, they rely to some extent on earlier observations of successful and unsuccessful heterosexual marriages, and try to apply some of these lessons to their relationship. However, the same-sex composition of the couple and the unusual position of lesbians and gays in society throw into doubt how relevant these heterosexual models might be. At the very least, same-sex partners cannot conform to sex-typed gender roles without encountering the special problems that ensue when both partners enact the same gender roles in the relationship.

Absence of Gender-Linked Roles

Composed of two women or two men, same-sex couples cannot rely on the usual gender-linked division of tasks in areas such as financial decision making, relationship maintenance (talking about feelings and problems), earning money, doing housework, preparing meals, taking the lead in sex, arranging their social life, or taking care of children and elderly relatives, if applicable. The fact that both partners are the same sex holds the possibility of greater equality if neither is attached to traditional gender roles, but it also increases the ambiguity about who is supposed to do what in the relationship and in the management of the household (Mitchell, 1996). As a result, most same-sex couples go though a long period of trial and error before settling on "who does what" in their relationship (Carrington, 1999).

Furthermore, to the degree that both partners were socialized into and still adhere to traditional gendered behavior for their sex, they may develop more conflicts or certain deficiencies in their relationship (Roth, 1989). In general, whereas women are socialized for more caring, connection, and cooperation, men are socialized for more independence, competition, and dominance. Although the majority of lesbians and gay men at least partially defy traditional gender prescriptions (Green et al., 1996), a minority of lesbians and gay men still conform to traditional gender roles in all respects except for their sexuality. Such gender conformity produces predictable problems in this particular subset of same-sex couples: (1) Both women try to please the other too much and neglect to communicate their own needs (i.e., the so-called problem of "fusion" in the lesbian relationship; Krestan & Bepko, 1980); (2) neither man will relocate for the other's job offer; (3) both men want to be the leader in sex; (4) neither woman feels comfortable initiating sex; (5) neither of the men is able to depend on or nurture the other in times of distress; (6) the woman who earns more money than her female partner feels guilty and disempowers herself in other areas; or (7) one man's career success leaves the other feeling inadequate as a man (Green, 1998). In other words, these problems arise not because the relationship is composed of two women or two men, but because some pairs of lesbian women or gay men still adhere to traditional gender roles, which multiplies gender-related deficits in their particular relationships (Wade & Donis, 2007).

Furthermore, in sharp contradiction to old cultural stereotypes, only a small minority of lesbian or gay partners divvy up relationship roles such that one plays the traditional "husband" role, while the other plays the traditional "wife" role. The ideal for most lesbian and gay couples is equality of power, and sharing of the instrumental and emotional tasks usually associated with the male or female role (Carrington, 1999). To achieve this kind of compatibility without fixed complementarity requires gender flexibility from both partners. The division of labor has to become a more conscious, deliberative process than it is for heterosexual couples.

This is not to say that contemporary heterosexual couples never struggle with such issues, but that a majority of them still devolve—sometimes despite their egalitarian aspirations—toward traditional, gender-linked roles in the areas of housework, child care, care of elderly relatives, cooking, and so on (Hochschild, 1989). Lesbian and gay couples cannot rely on these gender-linked divisions to figure out who does what in the household or with regard to care of other relatives.

Furthermore, the greater variety of relationship arrangements that are acceptable within the gay community (e.g., many such couples never live together, others have nonmonogamous relationships by agreement; shorter relationships are normative; raising children is viewed as entirely optional) leaves open the possibility that the lesbian–gay couple's commitment could be quite different than that of most married couples. Thus, the acceptance of nontraditional couple arrangements of all sorts within the lesbian–gay community seems to thrust each same-sex couple into a longer period of uncertainty and negotiation regarding its definition of personal couplehood.

Legalization of Same-Sex Couple Relationships

The rapidly changing situation regarding legalization of same-sex couple relationships is adding to the uncertainty for some couples. Consider the fol-

lowing: Homosexuality between consenting adults was finally decriminalized by the U.S. Supreme Court in 2003, then suddenly, in 2004—only 1 year later—same-sex marriages were being performed legally in Massachusetts. This left many surprised lesbian and gay couples asking themselves—and being asked by friends and family members—whether they were going to marry, and having to justify those intentions internally and publicly. Lesbian and gay couples had suddenly gone from being *outlaws to in-laws* in the space of a year!

Although one would think that the recent advent of enhanced domestic partnerships and/or civil unions in 10 states, and legal marriage in Massachusetts, would help to reduce some same-sex couples' relational ambiguity, the definitions of those legal statuses have also been unstable, sometimes adding to relational ambiguity. For example, California first enacted a Domestic Partner Law in 1999, that provided little more than hospital visitation privileges to same-sex partners. In 2003, however, the state legislature expanded the scope of the law to include many of the rights and responsibilities common to marriage in California (including community property laws and inheritance rights). Domestic partners who had registered before 2005 were required to dissolve their legal partnerships if they did not want their relationships to be governed by the new law, requiring many couples to reconsider their level of commitment to one another.

Similarly, uncertainty exists for same-sex couples who got married in Massachusetts beginning in 2004. Although the state legislature in Spring 2007, upheld the constitutionality of same-sex marriages in Massachusetts at least until 2012, this decision could be overturned by a contrary future decision by the Massachusetts Supreme Court, or by the U.S. Supreme Court, or even by a federal amendment banning such marriages. Furthermore, no other state or the federal government recognizes marriages performed in Massachusetts. In other words, even same-sex couples who have attained legal status for their relationships cannot be certain that their rights to that status will remain constant in the future or be upheld across jurisdictions.

Most important is to realize that 42 states have passed Defense of Marriage Acts (DOMAs), prohibiting those states from honoring same-sex marriages performed elsewhere. Twenty-six of these states also have passed constitutional amendments defining marriage as only between a man and woman, rendering courts in those states unable to consider the constitutionality of same-sex marriage bans. *Thus, for the vast majority of U.S. citizens in same-sex couples, there still is no legal status of any kind available for their relationships.* Even in states with civil unions, domestic partnerships, or in Massachusetts (where same-sex marriage is permitted) none of the 1,138 federal protections, rights, and benefits of marriage (such as Social Security benefits for surviving spouses) are available to same-sex couples (General Accounting Office, 2004). The lack of legal protections leaves same-sex couples especially vulnerable and stressed during times of serious illness, mental incapacity, or death of a partner—the very times when such protections are most needed psychologically (Herdt & Kertzner, 2006; Herek, 2006).

Also related to the question of legal issues and relational ambiguity, in the last 10 years we have witnessed a dramatic upsurge in the number of same-sex couples having children via adoption or through the use of alternative insemination or surrogacy (Mitchell & Green, 2008; Patterson, 2005). On the one hand, in some jurisdictions, the lack of legal guidelines for parental custody can add to the relational ambiguity these couples and their children face. On the other hand, the commitment to having children together dramatically reduces couples' relational ambiguity, usually requires the creation of legal agreements to clarify custody of the children, and provides a very strong incentive for couples to stay together, creating an implicit set of mutual obligations and responsibilities. In general, the presence of children is likely to stabilize many same-sex couple relationships, increasing their longevity and the amount of support they receive from family-of-origin members.

Most impressive are recent survey data collected by D'Augelli and colleagues on the marriage and parenting aspirations of a sample of lesbian–gay youth (ages 15–22) in the New York metropolitan area (D'Augelli, Grossman, & Rendina; 2006; D'Augelli, Rendina, Grossman, & Sinclair, 2008):

- Ninety-two percent of lesbian youths and 82% of gay male youth wanted to be in a long-term. monogamous relationship in 10 years.
- Seventy-eight percent of lesbian youth and 61% of gay male youth said it was "very" or "extremely" likely they would marry a same-sex partner, if legally possible.
- Sixty-six percent of lesbian youth and 52% of gay male youth said it was "very" or "extremely" likely they would be raising children in the future.

These findings suggest that the numbers of committed same-sex couples will dramatically increase over the next decade, and that large numbers of them will be raising children. Not only will these trends likely alter in positive ways the support that same-sex couples receive within the lesbian and gay community, but they also will exert increased pressure on society as a whole to recognize same-sex couples and coparents as being legally equivalent to their heterosexual counterparts.

Techniques to Counter Relational Ambiguity

Overall, the lack of a prescribed definition and parameters for couplehood, the same-gender composition of the couple, and the lack of a consistent legal framework to govern formation and dissolution of couple relationships leaves many lesbian–gay couples in a sea of uncertainty, unless they work out the rules and agreements for their relationships on their own. Although most same-sex couples are able to achieve clarity on many of these issues over a period of time (typically in about 10 years, based on our clinical experience), a significant number of same-sex couples (especially in the early years of a relationship) seem to founder.

There are no formulaic solutions for resolving these ambiguities in same-sex couple relationships. Nor should their resolution necessarily look like heterosexual marriages, in which many of these uncertainties are settled by law and tradition. In general, however, a couple tends to function best when there are clear agreements about their commitment and boundaries, and when the couple's relationship is given higher priority than any other relationship (in terms of emotional involvement, caregiving, honesty, time, and influence over major decisions). From the therapy standpoint, regardless of couples' presenting problems, asking the following kinds of questions and arriving at clear answers can be helpful to many same-sex couples:

- How do you define being "a couple" (what does it mean to you that you are a "couple")?
- What has been your history as couple?
- How did your becoming a couple affect your relationships with other family members, friends, the lesbian–gay community, and the straight community?
- What are the rules in your relationship regarding monogamy versus sex outside the relation-

ship? What are the rules in terms of safer sex practices with each other and/or with others (explicitly in terms of exact sexual practices to prevent HIV transmission)?

- What are your agreements with one another about monthly finances, current or future debts, pooling versus separation of financial resources, ownership of joint property, and other financial planning matters?
- Who does what tasks in the relationship and in the household, and how is this division or sharing of tasks decided? Are you satisfied with the current division or sharing of these tasks?
- What do you see as your obligations to one another in terms of caring for one another in illness, injury, or disability?
- Are you viewing this as a lifetime commitment? If so, have you prepared legal health care power of attorney documents and wills to protect one another's interests in case of serious illness or death?

Clarifying the extent and nature of partners' emotional commitments to one another is central to the work with same-sex couples in the early stages of their relationship. Sometimes this clarification involves resolving partners' conflicts of allegiance between the couple relationship and other family members, friends, or ex-partners. At other times, it involves spelling out what promises and reassurances each partner is willing to give—caregiving, time, monogamy, or other guarantees—that might increase both partners' sense of security, durability, and potential longevity of the relationship.

For couples who view their relationships as entailing a lifetime commitment, therapists should strongly encourage drawing up appropriate legal documents (especially health care power of attorney and wills/trusts). *A Legal Guide for Lesbian and Gay Couples* (Clifford, Hertz, & Doskow, 2007) is an excellent resource book for this purpose. Partners' inhibitions about obtaining legalized couple status (if domestic partnerships, civil unions, or marriages are available in their state of residence) should be explored. If it is in keeping with their sensibilities, couples can be encouraged to have a commitment ceremony and a formal exchange of vows covering some of these issues. A helpful book for this purpose is *The Essential Guide to Lesbian and Gay Weddings* (Ayers & Brown, 1999).

If one or both partners' gender conformity is creating problems in a same-sex couple, therapists can help by reviewing the clients' original gender role socialization experiences and challenging limitations associated with current gender role behavior, much as one might do with heterosexual partners in relationships. Similarly, if ambiguity or dissension exists about who does what in the household or the relationship, then the therapeutic work includes making sure these emotional and instrumental tasks are clarified and distributed equitably, as well as challenging any polarization of roles or dominance–submission patterns that might be destructive to the relationship over the long run.

If ambiguity exists in the monogamy agreement, this also should be spelled-out, based on full exploration of the underlying emotions and motivations of the partners. In particular, many gay male couples have had "nonmonogamous relationships by agreement" in the past, but the rates seem to be declining (Blumstein & Schwartz, 1983; Campbell, 2000; Solomon, Rothblum, & Balsam, 2004). This previous research has shown that for gay male couples with nonmonogamy agreements, it typically is not sex with outsiders per se that becomes problematic, rather it is any ambiguity in their agreements about it (including secrecy, lying, lack of clarity about the parameters, or inconsistent adherence to the parameters—all of which can trigger feelings of insecurity about the primary commitment). Thus, if a couple in therapy chooses to have an open relationship, the specific behavioral rules for sex outside the relationship should be specified in detail and agreed upon beforehand (in terms of who, what, when, where, how often, with how much communication about each encounter, and with what limitations; Shernoff, 2006).

In dealing with relational ambiguity of the kinds described earlier, homework assignments or in-session exercises that involve negotiating relationship expectations/agreements may be useful. Such vows (in addition to the legal contracts mentioned earlier) require that the partners address specific issues and come up with specific behavioral agreements for the future. Any intervention that helps the partners clarify expectations and agreements in contested areas, or in areas that have never been discussed (e.g., finances or monogamy) reduces relational ambiguity. This in turn increases partners' feelings of secure attachment and belief in the permanence of their union, anchoring their relationship in tangible definitions of what it means that they are a couple.

FAMILIES OF CHOICE

Unlike members of racial, ethnic, and religious minority groups, children who become lesbian and gay rarely have parents who share their same sexual minority status. Being different from other family members in this way has profound consequences for the development of almost every lesbian and gay person. For example, because heterosexual parents have never suffered sexual orientation discrimination themselves, even the most well-meaning among them are not able to offer the kind of insight and socialization experiences that would buffer their child against antigay prejudice and its internalization.

By contrast, when children and parents mutually identify as members of the same minority group (e.g., Jews, African Americans), the children are explicitly taught—and parents implicitly model—ways to counter society's prejudice toward their group. Typically, such parents and children are involved together in community institutions (religious, social) that are instrumental in supporting the child's development of a positive minority identity, and parents take a protective stance toward their children's experiences of oppression in majority cultural contexts.

However, parents of future lesbian–gay children are typically unaware of their child's minority status; therefore, they are unlikely to seek out community groups that would support the development of a positive lesbian–gay identity. In fact, rather than protecting their child against external prejudice, parents often show subtle or not-so-subtle signs of antigay prejudice themselves. Instead of being on the same side as their child against the external dangers, the parents' antigay attitudes and behavior may be the greatest external danger of all for the child.

Relatively large numbers of lesbian–gay adults in the United States—especially members of conservative religious families or of immigrant families with traditional values—still remain closeted from one or both parents who have strong antigay attitudes. In terms of couple relationships, this secrecy requires either distancing from family-of-origin members, lest the secret be revealed, or foregoing couple commitments to stay connected with family-of-origin members.

Although most parents do not completely reject their lesbian–gay children after the disclosure, the level of acceptance that offspring receive is highly variable and usually somewhat qualified (Savin-Williams, 2001). Generally, even though they may attempt to be accepting, heterosexual parents are unable to identify fully with their lesbian–gay children's lives and loves in the same way they identify with their heterosexual children's lives and loves. Thus, for the majority of lesbian and gay adults, the levels of family "acceptance" they receive may more aptly be described as levels of "tolerance."

Parents may resign themselves to the fact of their child's sexual orientation but still not feel comfortable with it, and they may keep it a secret from their own friends, coworkers, and extended family members. They may invite their child's partner to holiday events but still not treat the partner the same way a heterosexual sibling's spouse is treated as "real family." More typically, the couple may seem integrated into the life of the family of origin, but no mention whatsoever is made of the fact that this couple is lesbian or gay and is subject to minority stress, which creates a kind of wall of silence on this important issue. Of course, there are exceptional families of origin that reach very high levels of acceptance of their lesbian–gay offspring, but the modal pattern still remains more akin to peaceable tolerance than to full understanding and acceptance.

As a result of this qualified acceptance, same-sex couples frequently turn to their lesbian–gay friends for greater levels of mutual support and identification. Ideally, these friendships are woven together into a so-called "family of choice" (an interconnected system of emotional and instrumental support over time; Weston, 1991). This kind of friendship circle provides the couple with a sense of social embeddedness and continuity that many families of origin fail to provide for their offspring in same-sex couple relationships.

When assessing a couple's social support, most family therapists in the past focused almost exclusively on the partners' family-of-origin relations and neglected to take friendships as seriously. This is a grave oversight when working with lesbian and gay people, because both family and nonfamily sources of support can be relevant, and often the friendship sources are much more significant.

Creating a Sociogram of the Couple's Social Support Network

In evaluating a same-sex couple's overall social support from both family and nonfamily sources, it frequently helps the therapists and clients to do a sociogram, as well as a family genogram, to map out the people in the couple's social network. Because the formats for drawing genograms are well-known (McGoldrick, Gerson, & Petry, 2007). We will focus here only on a format for doing a sociogram with lesbian–gay couples.

The therapist can draw a simplified sociogram as five concentric circles, labeling these from innermost to outermost circles as follows (then writing in the names of the couple's relevant network members in the appropriate concentric rings):

THE COUPLE (the innermost circle)
VERY CLOSE/SUPPORTIVE TIES (including usually two to six closest people, such as best friends or closest family member)
CLOSE/SUPPORTIVE TIES (including other close friends or family members)
INSTRUMENTAL TIES/ACQUAINTANCES (which typically includes ongoing work associates who are not close friends, ongoing acquaintances with whom the partners might get together a few times a year, or perhaps family members with whom the partners do not have very close ties)
OTHERS (the outermost circle—a miscellaneous category that might include neighbors who are not close friends, former coworkers who were not close friends, members of organizations to which the couple is connected, family members from whom the couple is very disengaged, old acquaintances who are rarely encountered, etc.)

After writing the names of relevant network members in the appropriate rings based on the partners' input, lines can then be drawn to depict which network members are also connected to each other (with sotlid lines indicating close/supportive connections, dotted lines indicating loose connections). All the rings together make up the couple's social network. The people in the innermost two or three rings comprise the couple's emotionally supportive relationships. These people would only constitute a social support "system" or "family of choice" if they also were close and supportive with one another (solid lines between them).

In general, lesbian and gay couples tend to have less interconnected social networks than heterosexual couples. Their lesbian–gay friends and their heterosexual family members and friends may meet only rarely, if at all. Even their lesbian–gay friends may hardly know one another, because these friendships usually have to be found out-side of everyday situations, such as work settings, schools, or churches, where many heterosexuals meet their friends, and where these friends already know one another. The tendency toward social segregation of the straight and gay worlds generally—and between the straight and gay segments of an individual's social network—usually requires that same-sex couples have to expend more deliberate effort to create an integrated social support system that has family-like qualities. The ideal would be to integrate family members, lesbian–gay friends, and heterosexual friends into a cohesive support system.

Family-of-Origin Support

In assessing family-of-origin support, therapists should examine three distinct issues—family members' general support for the clients as individuals, family members' support specifically related to the clients being lesbian or gay individuals, and family members' support for the same-sex couple. Toward these ends, the following kinds of questions have proven useful:

1. When did you first become aware that you might be lesbian or gay?
2. How do you think this "differentness" may have affected your relationships with family members as you were growing up?
3. If you have *not* come out to certain family members, what factors led to this decision? Are there any ways that remaining closeted with your family is affecting your couple relationship positively or negatively?
4. If you have come out to certain family members, describe the process, including what preceded, happened during, and has followed the disclosure up to the present time?
5. If you have introduced your partner to your family-of-origin members, how have they treated your partner up until now? How have you responded to their treatment of your partner and of the two of you as a couple?

Although a full discussion of family-of-origin interventions related to adults' coming out and getting family support is beyond the scope of this chapter, the first step in any such effort involves helping the lesbian or gay person work through any residual internalized homophobia (as described earlier). When adult children can accept their own sexual orientation and choice of partner, dealing with the family is emotionally much easier, and clients can then cope with family members' antigay attitudes more dispassionately, planfully, assertively, and with fewer setbacks to the couple's functioning.

Disapproving family members quickly sense any internalized homophobia of a lesbian–gay offspring and often exacerbate the lesbian–gay person's self-doubts with critical comments and attempts to diminish the importance of the couple relationship. The offspring with internalized homophobia sometimes colludes with this process by not bringing the partner home on visits or rarely mentioning the partner in the family member's presence. In contrast, when the lesbian–gay person reaches a high level of self-acceptance and can calmly manifest that level in the family's presence, the family members either adapt to and become more accepting of the individual's sexual orientation and choice of partner, or the lesbian–gay person makes family relationships less salient, sometimes decreasing the amount of contact.

Therapeutic interventions in family-of-origin relations can include (1) Bowen-type coaching assignments, in which the client takes steps toward differentiation of self in the family of origin without the therapist present (Iasenza, Collucci, & Rothberg, 1996; McGoldrick & Carter, 2001); (2) conjoint family therapy sessions, with all family-of-origin members together in the therapist's office (Framo, 1992); or (3) a combination of both methods. Therapists should be cautious about doing any coaching assignments or conjoint sessions with the family of origin until the lesbian–gay person has reached a reasonably sustainable level of self-acceptance. After that point, the client's talking directly with family members about self and partner issues will be much more successful, regardless of whether the therapist is present during those encounters.

Building a Family of Choice

In helping couples build a "family of choice," therapists should encourage them to take a very proactive, deliberate stance toward the goal of developing an ongoing social support system of about six to eight individuals. The therapist should discuss this goal with the partners explicitly, sharing with them some of the research findings on the importance of friendship support for the psychological well-being of lesbian–gay individuals and couples.

Many same-sex couples in therapy spontaneously report feeling isolated and wish they had more and closer friendships, especially with other same-sex couples, and they immediately grasp the importance of developing a stronger support system. Defining some of the traits of a strong social support system for them (size, accessibility, frequency, quality, reciprocity, stability, interconnectedness of network members) in lay terms is itself very helpful in orienting the couple to the task at hand. Therapists can normalize both the need for this kind of support and the necessity for being proactive, especially for clients who are geographically or emotionally distant from their families of origin.

In our experience, the terminology "families of choice" resonates somewhat more strongly with lesbian couples than with gay male couples. Some couples (more male couples) may find this family metaphor and language hyperbolic, or they may have negative reactions to the idea of being part of anything called "a family" if their own family of origin has been rejecting. With this latter group of couples, one can use the phrase "social support system" or sometimes "sense of community," because these phrases connote both the warm/nurturing and the reciprocal/interconnected aspects of the goal we are discussing. Therapists should also convey that a social support system or family of choice ideally includes supportive family members, as well as friends.

The couple has to take two basic steps in building a personal support system: (1) developing or maintaining a reciprocally supportive relationship with each individual who would be a member of the couple's support system; and (2) "knitting" these individuals together into an integrated system of support. The first step is already familiar to all therapists, who have much experience helping clients develop new friendships and deepen existing ones. The couple's relationships with individuals in the support system must be reasonably close before the second step of creating cross-ties among those individuals can be accomplished.

If the couple's existing number of friendships is small, the perennial questions arise about where to meet people and how to move the friendships forward. Other than work settings, ideal venues for meeting potential friends in urban environments are lesbian–gay social, recreational, religious, charitable, self-help, educational, artistic, musical, or political organizations. The best strategy is for both partners to become very active together in one well-established organization, attend its events regularly to become "fixtures" in that organization, and take on positions of leadership or active committee involvement that require repeated interaction with the same people over months or years. In smaller or rural communities with fewer lesbian–gay organizations, the local gay bar may still be the best venue for starting friendships. Many such bars are the focal point for lesbian–gay social life in their locales, regularly celebrating patrons' birthdays, life transitions, and holidays; raising funds for people in special need; and so forth.

The great advantage of meeting new people through existing lesbian–gay organizations is that those organizations already have some degree of interpersonal cohesion or "groupness," so that the couple may be able to become an integral part of a preexisting social support system. Therapists who work with lesbian–gay couples should familiarize themselves with lesbian–gay organizations in their communities, or at least know where to suggest that clients find such information.

If one's close individual relationships are accrued at different times from different settings, more effort has to go into weaving these dispersed relationships into a more cohesive unit. The only way to increase the cohesiveness of a fragmented support system is for the couple to actively and persistently take the lead in physically bringing together the disconnected individuals or subgroups. One route is for the client couple to take charge of arranging repeated social events and invite all members of their support system to these events. Some extraverted couples have great success becoming the "social directors" of their support systems—arranging group tickets for movies, plays, concerts, setting up hikes, picnics, boat rides, ski trips, vacation rentals, and group volunteer efforts in the community; and so on. More intimacy is achieved when the partners invite everyone to their home for holiday events, brunches, Sunday dinners, movie nights, and so forth. A long-term lesbian or gay couple's relationship and home can become powerful anchors for close friends and family on the holidays or regular weekly or monthly get-togethers.

Couples who can sustain this effort to build a cohesive support system find that other members of their support system "spontaneously" start to develop autonomous dyadic friendships, getting together on their own. Ultimately, these members start organizing ways to bring together the larger support system, along with some of their other individual friends. The two key ingredients for reaching this goal are simply for the couple to maintain the closeness of the individual relationships, then to bring these individuals together as frequently as possible. Given that structure, the emotional in-

terconnections among other members of the support system tend to happen spontaneously starting at around 6 months into the effort.

It generally takes about 1 year to knit a disconnected collection of about six to eight individual relationships into the beginnings of a functional social support system with a sustainable life of its own beyond the original couple's involvement. After that, it requires significantly less effort to keep the system going. However, new people must continually be introduced, because some members inevitably withdraw because of other interests, demands, geographical relocation, or deaths.

In the ways described here, couple therapists should begin to view friendship sources of social support as being at least as important as family-of-origin support for lesbian–gay persons' mental health and couple functioning. Many aspects of the therapy with same-sex couples—taking a history; mapping the relevant people in the couple's life; formulating the problem; setting goals; deciding whom to include in sessions; and referrals to adjunctive therapeutic, educational, and support services—should reflect this expanded social network focus.

THERAPIST ISSUES

The single, most important prerequisite for helping same-sex couples is the therapist's personal comfort with love and sexuality between two women or two men. Therapists who are not comfortable with such love and sexuality may actually increase lesbian and gay clients' minority stress and unintentionally exacerbate their problems.

This statement does not mean misguided, blind approval of everything a lesbian or gay person does, or avoidance of dealing directly with lesbian or gay couples' destructive patterns of behavior. It does not mean superficial acceptance or patronizing overprotectiveness with clients. It requires familiarity with lesbian and gay culture, the ability to identify empathically with (but still remain sufficiently "objective" about) the behavior of lesbian and gay clients, and genuine personal ease ("comfort in your bones") when dealing with lesbian–gay partners' emotions for one another. It also requires an ability to ask and talk about homosexual sex in explicit terms with couples who are having sexual difficulties. We believe that with sufficient good will, motivation, and openness to learning and feedback, most therapists can achieve this level of preparedness for therapy with lesbian and gay couples.

To prepare mental health professionals to work with lesbian and gay clients, the American Psychological Association (2000) published a superb set of treatment guidelines that can serve as starting point for those who wish to learn more. In the field of couple and family therapy, many of the central ideas about lesbian–gay issues can be found in the review by Laird (2003), the book edited by Laird and Green (1996), a special section of the *Journal of Marital and Family Therapy* (Green, 2000), and two books on couple therapy (Bigner & Wetchler, 2004; Greenan & Tunnell, 2002). There also are two excellent publications about straight therapists working with lesbian–gay clients (Bernstein, 2000; Siegel & Walker, 1996).

Although such readings are vital, there is ample evidence that heterocentric stereotypes persist among mental health professionals even after they presumably know (or should know) the basic information about lesbian and gay issues (Garnets et al., 1991; Johnson, Brems, & Alford-Keating, 1995). Didactic information is not sufficient to override unconscious prejudice that has been acquired over a lifetime. Working effectively with lesbian and gay clients involves more than just good intentions, significant reading, and the perfunctory kinds of preparation that are common now in this field. Affective and attitudinal learning is at least as important.

Guarding against Heterocentric Bias: Countertransference

If heterocentric biases were fully conscious, therapists could counteract them through rational self-monitoring. Unfortunately, therapists tend "not to know what they don't know." Hence, some therapists believe they are sufficiently knowledgeable about lesbian–gay issues without having immersed themselves in the clinical and research literature (Green, 1996) and without having received sustained supervision from lesbian–gay-knowledgeable colleagues. Even lesbian and gay therapists are not immune to heterocentric assumptions or antigay reactions. The main advantage that lesbian and gay therapists have is extensive exposure to ordinary, nondistressed lesbian–gay persons and relationships, which helps to disconfirm prejudicial stereotypes maintained in the larger society.

The field of family therapy is just beginning to build culturally attuned treatment models for working with lesbian and gay couples and families (Bigner & Wetchler, 2004; Greenan & Tunnell, 2002; Laird & Green, 1996). On a personal level, the first step is to acknowledge that heterocentric assumptions are inevitable for all members of our society, including couple therapists. The goal is to make these assumptions conscious and examine them in the light of existing psychological knowledge and professional ethics. Below we discuss a few additional steps that every therapist can take to deal with heterocentric bias/countertransference issues.

Examine Unconscious Biases and Assumptions

How do we personally view lesbian and gay people's lives, and do our views fit with recent research findings? What are the emotional cues of bias in this area? In general, the signs of bias among professionals tend to be subtle and comprise inchoate feelings of discomfort, ambivalence, pessimism, anxiety, or "reactive" eagerness to please and appear "expert" when working with lesbian–gay clients. The antidote to acting out such bias is to become comfortable with "not knowing," retaining a willingness to learn from clients, taking a collaborative stance, and making space for discussion of cultural discrepancies and misunderstandings between oneself and one's clients. The optimal attitude is one of nondefensive humility about the true limits of one's training, personal experience, and expert knowledge, while still retaining professional integrity and realistic confidence.

Personal Immersion in Lesbian–Gay Culture: Becoming "Bicultural"

The research on homophobia and the clinical literature on heterosexual therapists working with lesbian–gay clients both point to the positive effects of more social contact to reduce prejudice (Bernstein, 2000; S. K. Green & Bobele, 1994; Siegel & Walker, 1996). Heterosexuals (including therapists) who have more interaction with lesbians–gays as personal friends, colleagues, family members, and clients report significantly fewer heterosexist attitudes. High levels of immersion in lesbian–gay culture involve taking concrete actions to work against heterosexism in one's own family, friendships, professional settings, and communities. On the political level, couple therapists can contribute by participating in local chapters of Parents, Families, and Friends of Lesbians and

Gays (PFLAG; *www.pflag.org*). It is important to acknowledge that although unbiased psychotherapy and psychological research have made positive contributions, the gay equal rights movement has made the single greatest contribution to the psychological well-being of lesbian and gay couples. For lesbians and gays, the political is very personal, and working toward the elimination of antigay prejudice and discrimination in one's social networks, community institutions, work settings, and local and state laws is good preparation for doing therapy with lesbian and gay couples.

Training through Workshops and Case Consultation

Few practicing therapists have had as much as a semester-long course on lesbian–gay issues or been supervised by an expert on lesbian–gay therapy. At a minimum, clinicians should read the available literature and seek continuing education in training workshops to make up for this deficit in their graduate education. Most important, therapists who are not knowledgeable about lesbian–gay couple therapy should seek expert consultation early in treatment, especially if progress with a couple seems slower than desirable. Given that mental health graduate programs provide minimal preparation, we recommend that therapists seek at least one expert consultation (in person or by telephone) about every same-sex couple they treat, until they feel competent to provide culturally attuned care.

Sharing Power in Sessions

When working with lesbian–gay populations, it is important to acknowledge and respect mutual expertise, which includes sharing the power to interpret. A couple's therapist should be willing to discuss in layperson's terminology all assessment results, treatment goals, and therapeutic plans in a collaborative manner with clients, soliciting the partners' active input. The key is to guard against making unwarranted assumptions and to check out one's perceptions about lesbian–gay issues with the clients themselves. If a therapist believes that the therapeutic goals for a given couple should include resolving internalized homophobia, reducing relational ambiguity, and building a family of choice, he or she should discuss these objectives in layperson's terms with the partners. Their understanding and shared commitment to these stated goals should be achieved before proceeding.

CONCLUSION

A summary of the material presented in this chapter appears in Figure 24.1.

We wish to emphasize again that generalizations about lesbian–gay couples as a group do not apply uniformly to *all* same-sex couples in therapy. In particular, this chapter has not covered specialized therapeutic issues for same-sex couples of color, interracial couples, or couples in which one or both members are bisexual or transgender (for these topics, see especially Firestein, 2007; Fox, 2006; Greene & Boyd-Franklin, 1996; Liu & Chan, 1996; Lev, 2004; Mason, 2006; Morales, 1996). These same-sex couples often are subject to much higher levels of antigay discrimination from their families and communities, and usually experience significantly more difficulty integrating their social networks into a coherent whole.

Furthermore, this chapter focuses on same-sex partners who have particular kinds of clinical problems related to the unique position of lesbians–gays in this society. Readers should keep in mind that such couples in therapy do not represent the majority of lesbian and gay couples who are not distressed. In the past, the mental health fields have shown a tendency to blur the distinction between well-functioning and distressed lesbian–gay couples, and to assume that all same-sex couples are like the dysfunctional couples described in the clinical literature. For example, the notions of "fusion in lesbian couples" and "disengagement in gay male couples"—which are from clinical work with distressed couples (Krestan & Bepko, 1980)—became a kind of legend about all lesbian and gay couples. However, research with community, nonclinical samples has since clarified that lesbian couples in general are extremely cohesive but not fused, and that gay male couples are actually more cohesive than heterosexual married couples, not more disengaged (Green et al., 1996; Mitchell, 1988).

To the extent that we have offered generalizations about same-sex couples in therapy, we also wish to underscore that such statements are valuable only insofar as they serve as initial hypotheses in a new case—as ideas to be tested and either retained or discarded depending on one's observations in that particular case. Descriptions of dysfunctional same-sex couples in this chapter should be taken as statements of "possible characteristics you may find" rather than universal truths about lesbian and gay couples in therapy. The particulars of real clients in treatment always should super-

Challenges/Risk Factors	Potential Couple Problems	Therapeutic Interventions	Outcome Goals
I. Antigay prejudice in the community and larger society creates minority stress	(a) Internalized homophobia—fear and ambivalence about committing to a same-sex couple relationship (b) Partner conflicts over how out the couple will be with family, at work, and in the community	(a) Externalizing the homophobia—viewing societal ignorance and prejudice (not homosexuality) as a problem (b) Negotiating any outness conflicts between partners based on realistic constraints/dangers	(a) Self-acceptance of lesbian/gay identity; comfort in committing to a same-sex couple relationship (b) Maximizing involvement in social contexts where the couple can be out
II. Lack of normative and legal template for same-sex couplehood	Relational ambiguity (unclear couple commitment, boundaries, expectations, and obligations); insecure attachment in current relationship	Exploration and collaboration about what being a couple means to them (roles, boundaries, mutual obligations); explore creating legal documents, legalized relationships	Commitment clarity, operating as a team, primary commitment to each other, longer-term planning ability, secure attachment in current relationship
III. Same-sex composition of couple (problematic only if partners are gender conforming)	(a) Problems of emotional fusion and avoidance of conflict in female couples (b) Problems of emotional disengagement or competition in male couples	Reviewing partners' traditional male or female gender socialization in families of origin and current social contexts. Encouraging resistance and subversion of conventional gender role expectations in the relationship.	Androgynous, gender-flexible, egalitarian sharing of emotional and instrumental tasks in the relationship. Collaborative rather than avoidant or competitive approaches to conflict resolution
IV. Lack of social support for the couple relationship	Social isolation; lack of couple identity in a defined community; inability to get emotional support, advice, and instrumental help from a support system	Coaching to build "families of choice" (cohesive social support networks with interconnections among network members)	Embedded couple identity and community of care (social network cohesion, reciprocity of support, higher levels of emotional and instrumental support)

FIGURE 24.1. Same-sex couples in therapy: Challenges, problems, interventions, goals.

sede abstract generalizations about categories of clients. Otherwise, therapy with same-sex couples would become little more than imposing on them yet another set of stereotypes.

SUGGESTIONS FOR FURTHER READINGS

American Psychological Association. (2000). Guidelines for psychotherapy with lesbian, gay, and bisexual clients. *American Psychologist, 55,* 1440–1451.

Bigner, J., & Wetchler, J. (Eds.). (2004). *Relationship therapy with same-sex couples.* Binghamton, NY: Haworth Press.

Greenan, D., & Tunnell, G. (2002). *Couple therapy with gay men.* New York: Guilford Press.

Laird, J., & Green, R.-J. (Eds.). (1996). *Lesbians and gays in couples and families: A handbook for therapists.* San Francisco: Jossey-Bass.

REFERENCES

American Psychological Association. (2000). Guidelines for psychotherapy with lesbian, gay, and bisexual clients. *American Psychologist, 55,* 1440–1451.

Ayers, T., & Brown, P. (1999). *The essential guide to lesbian and gay weddings.* Los Angeles: Alyson.

Bepko, C., & Johnson, T. (2000). Gay and lesbian couples in therapy: Perspectives for the contemporary family therapist. *Journal of Marital and Family Therapy, 26,* 409–419.

Bernstein, A. C. (2000). Straight therapists working with lesbians and gays in family therapy. *Journal of Marital and Family Therapy, 26,* 443–454.

Blumstein, P., & Schwartz, P. (1983). *American couples: Money, work and sex.* New York: Morrow.

Boss, P. (1999). *Ambiguous loss: Learning to live with unresolved grief.* Cambridge, MA: Harvard University Press.

Boss, P., Caron, W., Horbal, J., & Mortimer, J. (1990). Predictors of depression in caregivers of dementia patients: Boundary ambiguity and mastery. *Family Process, 29,* 245–254.

Boss, P., & Greenberg, J. (1984). Family boundary ambiguity: A new variable in family stress theory. *Family Process, 23,* 535–546.

Boyd-Franklin, N. (2003). *Black families in therapy: Understanding the African American experience* (2nd ed.). New York: Guilford Press.

Brown, L. S. (1994). *Subversive dialogues: Theory in feminist therapy.* New York: Basic Books.

Campbell, K. M. (2000). *Relationship characteristics, social support, masculine ideologies and psychological functioning of gay men in couples.* Unpublished doctoral dissertation, California School of Professional Psychology, Alameda, CA.

Carrington, C. (1999). *No place like home: Relationships and family life among lesbians and gay men.* Chicago: University of Chicago Press.

Clifford, D., Hertz, F., & Doskow, E. (2007). *A legal guide for lesbian and gay couples* (14th ed.). Berkeley, CA: Nolo Press.

D'Augelli, A. R., Grossman, A. H., & Rendina, J. (2006, May). *Lesbian, gay, and bisexual youth: Marriage and child-rearing aspirations.* Paper presented at the Family Pride Academic Symposium, University of Pennsylvania, Philadelphia.

D'Augelli, A. R., Rendina, H. J., Grossman, A. H., & Sinclair, K. O. (2007). Lesbian and gay youths' aspirations for marriage and raising children. *Journal of LGBT Issues in Counseling, 1,* 77–98.

Doherty, W. J., & Simmons, D. S. (1996). Clinical practice patterns of marriage and family therapists: A national survey of therapists and their clients. *Journal of Marital and Family Therapy, 22,* 9–25.

Falicov, C. J. (1998). *Latino families in therapy: A guide to multicultural practice.* New York: Guilford Press.

Firestein, B. (Ed.). (2007). *Becoming visible: Counseling bisexuals across the lifespan.* New York: Columbia University Press.

Fox, R. (Ed.). (2006). *Affirmative psychotherapy with bisexual women and bisexual men.* Binghamton, NY: Haworth Press.

Framo, J. L. (1992). *Family-of-origin therapy: An intergenerational approach.* New York: Brunner/Mazel.

Garnets, L., Hancock, K. A., Cochran, S. D., Godchilds, J., & Peplau, L. A. (1991). Issues in psychotherapy with lesbians and gay men: A survey of psychologists. *American Psychologist, 46,* 964–972.

General Accounting Office. (2004). *Defense of Marriage Act: Update to prior report, GAO-04-353R.* Retrieved October 23, 2004, from *www.gao.gov/new.items/d04353r.pdf.*

Gottman, J. M., Levenson, R. W., Gross, J., Frederickson, B. L., McCoy, K., Rosenthal, L., et al. (2003). Correlates of gay and lesbian couples' relationship satisfaction and relationship dissolution. *Journal of Homosexuality, 45,* 23–43.

Gottman, J. M., Levenson, R. W., Swanson, C., Swanson, K., Tyson, R. & Yoshimoto, D. (2003). Observing gay, lesbian, and heterosexual couples' relationships: Mathematical modeling of conflict interaction. *Journal of Homosexuality, 45,* 65–91.

Green, R.-J. (1996). Why ask, why tell?: Teaching and learning about lesbians and gays in family therapy. *Family Process, 35,* 389–400.

Green, R.-J. (1998). Traditional norms of the male role. *Journal of Feminist Family Therapy, 10,* 81–83.

Green, R.-J. (Ed.). (2000). Gay, lesbian, and bisexual issues in family therapy [Special section]. *Journal of Marital and Family Therapy, 26,* 407–468.

Green, R.-J., Bettinger, M., & Zacks, E. (1996). Are lesbian couples fused and gay male couples disengaged?: Questioning gender straightjackets. In J. Laird & R.-J. Green (Eds.), *Lesbians and gays in couples and families: A handbook for therapists* (pp. 185–230). San Francisco: Jossey-Bass.

Green, S. K., & Bobele, M. (1994). Family therapists' response to AIDS: An examination of attitudes, knowledge, and contact. *Journal of Marital and Family Therapy, 20,* 349–367.

Greene, B., & Boyd-Franklin, N. (1996). African American lesbians: Issues in couples therapy. In J. Laird & R.-J. Green (Eds.), *Lesbians and gays in couples and families: A handbook for therapists* (pp. 251–271). San Francisco: Jossey-Bass.

Hartman, A. (1996). Social policy as a context for lesbian and gay families: The political is personal. In J. Laird & R.-J. Green (Eds.), *Lesbians and gays in couples and families: A handbook for therapists* (pp. 69–85). San Francisco: Jossey-Bass.

Herdt, G., & Kertzner, R., (2006). I do, but I can't: The impact of marriage denial on the mental health and sexual citizenship of lesbians and gay men in the United States. *Sexuality Research and Social Policy, 3,* 33–34.

Herek, G. M. (Ed.). (1998). *Stigma and sexual orientation: Understanding prejudice against lesbians, gay men, and bisexuals.* Thousand Oaks, CA: Sage.

Herek, G. M. (2006). Legal recognition of same-sex relationships in the United States: A social science perspective. *American Psychologist, 61,* 607–621.

Hochschild, A. (1989). *The second shift: Working parents and the revolution at home.* New York: Viking.

Iasenza, S., Colucci, P. L., & Rothberg, B. (1996). Coming out and the mother–daughter bond: Two case examples. In J. Laird & R.-J. Green (Eds.), *Lesbians and gays in couples and families: A handbook for therapists* (pp. 123–136). San Francisco: Jossey-Bass.

Johnson, M. E., Brems, C., & Alford-Keating, P. (1995). Parental sexual orientation and therapists' perceptions of family functioning. *Journal of Gay and Lesbian Psychotherapy, 2,* 1–15.

Krestan, J.-A., & Bepko, C. S. (1980). The problem of fusion in the lesbian relationship. *Family Process, 19,* 277–289.

Kurdek, L. A. (2004). Are gay and lesbian cohabiting couples really different from heterosexual married couples? *Journal of Marriage and the Family, 66,* 880–900.

Kurdek, L. A. (2005). What do we know about gay and lesbian couples? *Current Directions in Psychological Science, 14,* 251–254.

Laird, J. (2003). Lesbian and gay families. In F. Walsh (Ed.), *Normal family processes: Growing diversity and complexity* (3rd ed., pp. 176–209). New York: Guilford Press.

Laird, J., & Green, R.-J. (Eds.). (1996). *Lesbians and gays in couples and families: A handbook for therapists.* San Francisco: Jossey-Bass.

Lee, E. (Ed.). (1997). *Working with Asian Americans: A guide for clinicians.* New York: Guilford Press.

Lev, A. I. (2004). *Transgender emergence: Therapeutic guidelines for working with gender-variant people and their families.* Binghamton, NY: Haworth Press.

Liu, P., & Chan, C. (1996). Lesbian, gay, and bisexual Asian Americans and their families. In J. Laird & R.-J. Green (Eds.), *Lesbians and gays in couples and families: A handbook for therapists* (pp. 137–152). San Francisco: Jossey-Bass.

Malyon, A. K. (1982). Psychotherapeutic implications of internalized homophobia in gay men. In J. Gonsiorek (Ed.), *Homosexuality and psychotherapy: A practitioner's handbook of affirmative models* (pp. 59–69). New York: Haworth Press.

Mason, M. (2006). *The experience of transition for lesbian partners of female to male transsexuals: A phenomenological dissertation.* California School of Professional Psychology, Alliant International University, San Francisco, CA.

McGoldrick, M., & Carter, B. (2001). Advances in coaching: Family therapy with one person. *Journal of Marital and Family Therapy, 27,* 281–300.

McGoldrick, M., Gerson, R., & Petry, S. (2007). *Genograms: Assessment and intervention* (3rd ed.). New York: Norton.

Meyer, I. H. (2003). Prejudice, social stress, and mental health in lesbian, gay, and bisexual populations: Conceptual issues and research evidence. *Psychological Bulletin, 129,* 674–697.

Meyer, I. H., & Dean, L. (1998). Internalized homophobia, intimacy, and sexual behavior among gay and bisexual men. In G. M. Herek (Ed.), *Stigma and sexual orientation: Understanding prejudice against lesbians, gay men, and bisexuals* (pp. 160–186). Thousand Oaks, CA: Sage.

Minuchin, S. (1974). *Families and family therapy.* Cambridge, MA: Harvard University Press.

Mitchell, V. (1988). Using Kohut's self psychology in work with lesbian couples. *Women and Therapy, 8,* 157–166.

Mitchell, V. (1996). Two moms: Contribution of the planned lesbian family to the deconstruction of gen-

dered parenting. In J. Laird & R.-J. Green (Eds.), *Lesbians and gays in couples and families: A handbook for therapists* (pp. 343–357). San Francisco: Jossey-Bass.

Mitchell, V., & Green, R.-J. (2007). Different storks for different folks: Lesbian and gay parents' experiences with alternative insemination and surrogacy. *Journal of GLBT Family Studies, 3,* 81–104.

Morales, E. (1996). Gender roles among Latino gay/bisexual men: Implications for family and couples relationships. In J. Laird & R.-J. Green (Eds.), *Lesbians and gays in couples and families: A handbook for therapists* (pp. 272–297). San Francisco: Jossey-Bass.

Patterson, C. J. (2005). *Lesbian and gay parenting: Summary of research findings.* Washington, DC: American Psychological Association. (Available online at *www.apa.org/pi/parent.html*)

Peplau, L. A., & Fingerhut, A. W. (2007). The close relationships of lesbians and gay men. *Annual Review of Psychology, 58,* 405–424.

Roth, S. (1989). Psychotherapy with lesbian couples: Individual issues, female socialization, and the social context. In M. McGoldrick, C. M. Anderson, & F. Walsh (Eds.), *Women in families: A framework for family therapy* (pp. 286–307). New York: Norton.

Savin-Williams, R. C. (1996). Self-labeling and disclosure among gay, lesbian, and bisexual youths. In J. Laird & R.-J. Green (Eds.), *Lesbians and gays in couples and families: A handbook for therapists* (pp. 153–182). San Francisco: Jossey-Bass.

Savin-Williams, R. C. (2001). *Mom, Dad, I'm gay: How families negotiate coming out.* Washington, DC: American Psychological Association.

Shernoff, M. (2006). Negotiated nonmonogamy and male couples. *Family Process, 45,* 407–418.

Shidlo, A. (1994). Internalized homophobia: Conceptual and empirical issues in measurement. In B. Greene & G. Herek (Eds.), *Lesbian and gay psychology: Theory, research, and clinical applications* (pp. 176–205). Thousand Oaks, CA: Sage.

Siegel, S., & Walker, G. (1996). Connections: Conversation between a gay therapist and a straight therapist. In J. Laird & R.-J. Green (Eds.), *Lesbians and gays in couples and families: A handbook for therapists* (pp. 28–68). San Francisco: Jossey-Bass.

Solomon, S. E., Rothblum, E. D., & Balsam, K. F. (2004). Pioneers in partnership: Lesbian and gay male couples in civil unions compared with those not in civil unions and married heterosexual siblings. *Journal of Family Psychology, 18,* 275–286.

Wade, J. C., & Donis, E. (2007). Masculinity ideology, male identity, and romantic relationship quality among heterosexual and gay men. *Sex Roles, 57,* 775–786.

Weston, K. (1991). *Families we choose: Lesbians, gays, kinship.* New York: Columbia University Press.

CHAPTER 25

African American Couples in Therapy

Nancy Boyd-Franklin
Shalonda Kelly
Jennifer Durham

BACKGROUND

The African American community is tremendously diverse in terms of socioeconomic class, educational level, religion, geographical region, level of identification with African American and mainstream American culture, racial identity, degree of experience with racism, etcetera. Therapists may encounter Black couples from the Caribbean (Brice-Baker, 2005; Menos, 2005) or Africa (Kamya, 2005; Mc-Goldrick, Giordano, & Garcia-Preto, 2005) as well as African Americans. In addition, 7% of all African Americans are involved in interracial relationships (LaTaillade, 2006). This chapter focuses only on African American couples. Readers who treat other couples of African descent are encouraged to read the references cited earlier.

Our definition of a "couple" includes nonmarried partners. Many African American clients and families, viewed by clinicians as "single parents," in fact have a partner living in the home. Franklin (2004) has argued that mental health providers often treat African American men in nonmarried partnerships as if they are "invisible." Therefore, we encourage therapists to include such partners as a part of couple and family therapy. Given the diversity of the African American community,

therapists should avoid stereotyping and are encouraged to view the material presented in this chapter as a "camera lens" that furthers our ability to understand African American couples, but must be adjusted for each new client and couple seen in therapy (Boyd-Franklin, 2003).

Racism, Discrimination, and Economic Burdens on African American Couples

It is very important for therapists to understand the impact that racism and discrimination may have on the couple relationships of African Americans, even if couples do not articulate these issues in therapy (Boyd-Franklin, 2003; Kelly, 2003). Clinicians must take into account the ways in which racism and discrimination may contribute to lower marriage rates and higher divorce rates (Tucker & Mitchell-Kernan, 1995), as well as the other research findings regarding Black couples that are discussed below. Without this contextual understanding, therapists may develop a deficit perspective on African American couple relationships that can negatively influence the treatment process.

It is very well documented that African American couples have faced significant challenges in making their relationships work. Teachman, Tedrow, and Crowder (2000) and McKinnon (2003) have demonstrated that Black men and women are less likely to marry than their White counterparts. Risk factors include the shortage of Black men due to incarceration, drug use, and high homicide rates; high unemployment rates; and poverty (Tucker & Mitchell-Kernan, 1995; Taylor, Jackson, & Chatters, 1997), as well as exposure to racism and discrimination (Kelly, 2003; LaTaillade, 2006).

U.S. Census Bureau 2001 data indicated that 43% of African American men and 41% of African American women had never married as compared to 27.4% of White men and 20.7% of White women (McKinnon, 2003). African Americans also report greater marital dissatisfaction (Broman, 2005) and have higher separation and divorce rates than their White counterparts (Tucker & Mitchell-Kernan, 1995). Also, rates of remarriage are lower: 66% of White women remarry within 10 years of divorce compared to only 32% of Black women (Cherlin, 1992). Black couples are significantly more likely to enter marriage with children as compared to their White counterparts (Karney, Kreitz, & Sweeney, 2004), and this is known to be a risk factor for divorce in all relationships.

To place these statistical disparities in perspective, therapists must first acknowledge that racism and economic marginalization have placed undue burdens on African American couple relationships that often are not experienced by White couples (Boyd-Franklin, 2003; Boyd-Franklin & Franklin, 1998; Franklin, 2004; Kelly, 2003; Kelly & Floyd, 2001, 2006; LaTaillade, 2006). For some African Americans, experiences with discrimination and factors such as their internalized racism and/or displacement of these experiences may lead to negative, unsupportive behaviors within their relationships (Kelly & Floyd, 2001, 2006). Boyd-Franklin (2003) and Boyd-Franklin and Franklin (1998) have given numerous clinical examples of the ways in which racism or discrimination can create anger or frustration that is then displaced onto a partner in a couple relationship. LaTaillade, Baucom, and Jacobson (2000) found that African American couples who reported experiences of racism and discrimination were more likely to exhibit verbal aggression and violence than positive communication patterns. Kelly and Floyd (2001, 2006) have also demonstrated that experiences with racism can be internalized, thus negatively affecting trust and marital satisfaction among African American married and nonmarried couples.

It is not surprising, therefore, that data from a nationally representative sample show that African Americans are more likely to report lower levels of marital quality than their White counterparts (Broman, 2005).

In addition to the burdens associated with racism and discrimination, Tucker and Mitchell-Kernan (1995) have shown that economic marginalization and higher poverty levels can place considerable strain on some Black couple relationships and account for a portion of the relationship between high divorce rates and the decline in marriages among African Americans. A lack of economic resources can contribute to decreases in marital quality for Black husbands in lower income groups (Clark-Nicolas & Gray-Little, 1991). For example, whereas African Americans as a whole endorse fewer male dominance ideologies than Whites, Black men more often support such ideologies than do Black women, and this ideological gap is further widened when Black women's income increases (Bryant & Beckett, 1997). It is likely that the resultant socioeconomic, status-exacerbated differences in values and role expectations can lead to relationship conflicts for Black couples, particularly given the often sexist mainstream American expectations that the male will be the primary provider.

The aforementioned difficulties do not diminish research that indicates African American couples value marriage (Gibson, Edin, & McLanahan, 2003; LaTaillade, 2006) and it continues to be a desirable goal for many unmarried African American couples (Tucker & Mitchell-Kernan, 1995). For some, marriage is perceived as evidence that they have achieved middle-class status (Edin, 2000). Moreover, married African Americans have tended to show more life satisfaction than their unmarried counterparts (Beale, 1997).

The Importance of Home as a Safe Place for African Americans

"Home" is the place where couples of all ethnic and racial groups look to nurture their relationships. Home has taken on an additional significance for African Americans (Burton, Winn, Stevenson, & Clark, 2004; Hooks, 1990). For functional African American couples and families, home is a safe place where they can recover from experiences with racism and discrimination that so many encounter on a regular basis (Clark, Anderson, Clark, & Williams, 1999), and nurture coping mechanisms and psychological resilience. This is particularly challenging for African Americans, because incidents of racism and discrimination can be subtle and ambiguous (Carter, 2007; Jones, 1997), and are more easily denied. Such events may be encountered on a daily basis and have been described as "microaggressions" by Franklin (2004), Franklin, Boyd-Franklin, and Kelly (2006), Pierce (1995), and Sue (2003). African American couples who have not been able to create a safe place in their homes or relationships are at great risk for disharmony and family problems (Burton et al., 2004).

Strengths in African American Couples and Families

LaTaillade (2006) and Kelly (2003) have noted that many African American couples have managed to survive and thrive despite being more likely than other couples to face race-related stressors. A number of cultural strengths contribute to the resilience and survival of couples, including strong extended family and kinship support, religion and spirituality, and positive racial and ethnic identity. Extended family supports have been an identified protective factor in African American families for generations (Boyd-Franklin, 2003; Hines & Boyd-Franklin, 2005; LaTaillade, 2006). Hatchett, Veroff, and Douvan (1995) demonstrated that African American women who have ongoing contact with their extended family have more stable marriages. Their research has also shown that African American couples without these supports are more likely to experience marital or relationship instability.

Many therapists have been trained to view couples as distinct, independent entities, separate from their families of origin and their extended families. In communal cultures (e.g., African American, Caribbean, and Latino), this perspective can often cause therapists to overlook very important family dynamics. For many healthy African American families, extended family contact is very frequent, often on a daily basis. Every family member offers help to other family members, not only through love and support but also in more concrete manifestations, such as child care and financial support. In these families, boundaries and roles are clear, and the couple feels empowered and supported by the family. Extended family membership often includes "adoption" by the family of a spouse or partner and continues despite separation or divorce. It is very important for clinicians to understand the ways that extended family involvement may positively impact couple relationships and even be integral to healthy African American

families. This may provide a model to guide their interventions with couples experiencing challenges in their relationships. Unfortunately, clinicians' perspectives on African American couples are often based on the deficit focus of the research literature described earlier, or on past experiences treating couples who may have presented with conflicts between extended family values and their own couple relationships.

African Americans who have a great deal of contact with family and extended family members can experience extreme pain when this contact is abruptly discontinued. Such "emotional cutoff" (Bowen, 1976; Nichols & Schwartz, 2001) may lead to serious conflict in the couple relationship. Another conflict arising from extended family involvement may occur when one member of the couple is very involved with his or her extended family. Although this type of close-knit family involvement may have initially been attractive, the partner who is not as involved with the extended family may begin to resent this and feel that the couple relationship is being neglected. This is particularly likely given the pedestal upon which the ideal couple relationship is placed in mainstream American society, rendering it more important than, and separate from, extended family relationships.

It is also important to emphasize that many African Americans do not limit their "family" to biological relatives. Many families include godmothers, godfathers, "play mamas, play daddies, play aunts and uncles," close friends, neighbors, and members of their Church as "family" (Boyd-Franklin, 2003, p. 59; Hines & Boyd-Franklin, 2005). This can be very important when other close "family" members help to provide support during troubled times and/or when there is friction between key family members and the couple.

Another relevant strength has been the importance of religion and spirituality in the lives of African Americans (Bowen-Reid & Harrell, 2002; Boyd-Franklin, 2003; Hines & Boyd-Franklin, 2005; Kelly & Floyd, 2006; LaTaillade, 2006; Taylor, Mattis, & Chatters, 1999). Generations of African Americans, who endured the Middle Passage, slavery, racism, discrimination, segregation, etcetera, have utilized their spiritual beliefs to survive. Such beliefs have been a very important factor in the psychological resilience of Black people (Boyd-Franklin, 2003; Hines & Boyd-Franklin, 2005).

For some African American couples and families, church involvement is associated with positive well-being and close family relationships (Ellison, 1997). Kelly and Floyd (2006) found that in one sample of 93 married African American men, religious well-being was associated with increased marital trust. Also, married African American men have been found to score higher on religiosity variables than their unmarried counterparts (Taylor et al., 1999). LaTaillade (2006) theorized that participation in a church may serve positive psychological and social functions in the relationship. For example, the church's provision of emotional support and the prevalence of "couple ministries" can help to empower and to assist couples in overcoming relationship stressors (Boyd-Franklin, 2003; LaTaillade, 2006). On the other hand, religious differences can present issues in Black couples, particularly if one member of the couple is deeply involved in his or her religion or church and the other is not.

It is important that therapists not approach religion or spirituality in a stereotypical manner. Many African American individuals may be deeply spiritual and have a personal relationship with God or a higher power (Boyd-Franklin, 2003), but may not be "religious" or have a formal church affiliation. Therapists are encouraged to explore each partner's definition of spirituality and how he or she uses it as a resource in life.

There is tremendous diversity among African Americans in terms of religion. Religious groups with significant African American membership include Baptist, Methodist, African Methodist Episcopal (AME), Church of God in Christ, Catholic, Episcopalian, Lutheran, Presbyterian, Pentecostal, Seventh Day Adventist, and Jehovah's Witnesses. In addition, a growing number of African Americans are members of the Nation of Islam, other Muslim groups (e.g., Sunni Muslims; McAdams-Mahmoud, 2005), or practice African religions. Boyd-Franklin (2003) discusses the diversity in African American religious practice in depth.

Therapists should be aware that some African Americans express psychological distress in spiritual terms (Boyd-Franklin, 2003). In the African tradition, the psyche and the spirit are one (Nobles, 2004). They are not considered separate entities. In addition, many African Americans use their spirituality to address issues of depression, anxiety, death, loss, grief, etcetera. Spirituality and religion can provide a great deal of comfort and support during periods of emotional distress.

When they need counseling, many African Americans are more likely to go to their family members or to seek counseling from their pastors, ministers, or other members of their "Church families" (Boyd-Franklin, 2003). Therapists routinely obtain information release forms from their clients but often neglect to do so when clients are also receiving pastoral counseling. Support of the pastor may be very useful in treating a couple and influential in the partners' decision to continue treatment. Moreover, relationships that clinicians build with pastors and other key church personnel, such as deacons, may be tapped, so that distressed African American couples may be referred for therapeutic services if necessary.

Racial or Ethnic Identity

One aspect of the diversity among African Americans is their understanding of their own racial or cultural identity. Franklin, Carter, and Grace (1993) described Cross's (1978) stages of racial identity, which include "preencounter," in which the person may be very identified with White society; "encounter," in which the person has had a challenging experience related to race or racism; "immersion/emersion," in which the person responds to this encounter with anger and becomes more identified with an idealization of Black culture and often harbors a great deal of anger toward Whites; "internalization," in which the person has a strong Black identity and has been able to recognize strengths and weaknesses in both Black and White cultures; and "internalization/commitment," or active involvement in giving something back to the Black community. Boyd-Franklin (2003), Carter (1995, 2007), Cross (1991), Helms, (1990), and Helms and Cook (1999) have also explored and elaborated on these stages of racial identity development.

A strong, positive racial identity may protect many African Americans against the negative consequences of racism, discrimination, and microaggressions (Boyd-Franklin, 2003). Couples may experience their level of ethnic or racial identity as a strength or protective factor (Bell, Bouie, & Baldwin, 1990; Kelly & Floyd, 2006; LaTaillade et al., 2000; LaTaillade, 2006) and use it to increase communication in their relationships (LaTaillade, 2006). Kelly and Floyd (2006) found a positive association between Afrocentricity, a positive, pro–African American racial attitude, and spousal trust of African American men who were less religious or had higher socioeconomic statuses.

The partners may have racial identity differences, and it is not unusual for the resulting divergent views to cause couple conflict (Kelly, 2003). The differences may lie dormant until the partners begin to raise children together, and may then be forced to confront their different messages to their children regarding racial identity development. Couples with different levels of racial identity can also disagree about issues related to racism. Indeed, preliminary data from a small, nonrepresentative sample of middle-class African American couples indicate that those partners frequently disagree about whether incidents in their lives are due to racism, and how they should address these issues (Kelly, 2007).

ISSUES IN THE TREATMENT OF AFRICAN AMERICAN COUPLES

Responses to Therapy in the African American Community

Diversity among African Americans is also reflected in a wide rage of responses to therapy. A number of factors can complicate an African American couple's initial response to treatment and resistance to the treatment process. One issue relates to perceptions among some members of the African American community that therapy is an intervention solely for "sick or crazy people" (Boyd-Franklin, 2003). Another common phenomenon is rooted in the long legacy of experiences with racism, discrimination, and other forms of oppression, wherein many African Americans bring a "healthy cultural suspicion" (Boyd-Franklin, 2003) to the treatment process, particularly in cross-racial situations. Many couple therapists are unprepared for this suspicion when it presents in initial therapy sessions.

It is very important that therapists working with African American couples understand this dynamic and not personalize this initial response or react defensively. It is also imperative that therapists take the time to establish therapeutic rapport and trust in the first session with their clients. Many well-meaning couple therapists can unwittingly alienate African American couples from the treatment process by bombarding them with assessment and intake questionnaires, before a therapeutic relationship has been established (Boyd-Franklin, 2003; LaTaillade, 2006). This can lead to high levels of early attrition after the initial session. This response is related to a strong tendency of many African American families to maintain a great deal of privacy or secrecy in terms of "family business" as a survival strategy particularly in

response to fears that might threaten the family. In fact, many African Americans are taught to avoid discussing personal family issues outside the family (Boyd-Franklin, 2003). This prohibition can be even more intense when intimate couple issues are being discussed. Given these challenges, "joining" becomes a crucial element of the therapeutic process.

Many couple and family therapists have discussed the importance of "joining," or establishing therapeutic rapport with all clients (Nichols & Schwartz, 2001). This process is even more crucial when working with African American clients because of the initial concerns and resistance described earlier. Therapists should take the time to get to know each member of the couple gradually and to emphasize their strengths. This is important, because many African Americans are aware of the negative stereotypes that are often applied to their relationships and family life. If the therapist is relaxed, warm, welcoming, validating, respectful, and strengths-focused, and conveys interest in each of their lives, the likelihood of creating a therapeutic relationship with both members of the couple is greatly increased.

Raising the Issue of Racial or Cultural Differences in Treatment

Therapists often err on one of two extremes in terms of the question of raising cultural or racial differences or similarities in treatment. Some therapists have been taught not to raise these issues in treatment until they are mentioned by their client(s); therefore, they are very uncomfortable in initiating this discussion. At the other extreme are therapists who, through their training in multicultural approaches, are aware that these issues need to be raised; therefore, they raise them prematurely, before a therapeutic relationship has been established. A number of multicultural scholars and researchers have discussed the need to raise cultural differences in treatment (Bean, Perry, & Bedell, 2002; Boyd-Franklin, 2003; Kelly, 2003; LaTaillade, 2006; Sue & Sue, 2003). Bean et al. (2002) emphasized that it is particularly important for non–African American therapists to invite clients to "discuss their feelings about being seen by a therapist from outside their ethnic group" (p. 155). It is crucial, however, that therapists be careful about the timing of this intervention. If effective joining has occurred in the first session and a relationship has begun to form, then raising this issue of racial or ethnic differences in future sessions can help to facilitate continued joining by addressing an issue that is often very present in the minds of African Americans in treatment (Boyd-Franklin, 2003).

Each client's response to the race or ethnicity of the therapist may vary according to his or her stage of racial identity development, as described earlier. For example, a client or couple in the preencounter stage of racial identity development may be very White-identified and may prefer a White therapist. It is often a surprise to Black therapist to realize that a Black couple may be uncomfortable working with him or her. Similarly, a client in the immersion/emersion stage of racial identity development may be very angry with White people and may find it very hard to work with a White therapist. A client in the internalization stage might have a strong sense of his or her own racial identity, and may initially express a preference for a Black therapist but may be able to work with a culturally competent therapist of a different racial or cultural background.

Impact of Race-Based Stressors on Couple and Family Relationships

Although race-based stressors, such as experiences of racism, economic strain, and power discrepancies, have been noted to strain Black couple relationships (Boyd-Franklin & Franklin, 1998; Kelly, 2003), sometimes it is difficult for the couple to identify and acknowledge the impact of such stressors. It is often easier for a couple to acknowledge a manifestation of their problem within a child. Therefore, a child may be presented as the identified client, who is reacting to the discord within the couple system. In this instance it may be helpful for the clinician to use an approach that first addresses the presenting problem of the child, then moves gradually to the couple's issue. This is illustrated by the case of Jill and Allen.

Jill and Allen, an African American couple, had been married for 12 years and lived in a middle-class, somewhat diverse suburb with their son Wesley, age 9, and daughter Lauren, age 6. They sought therapy due to a marked escalation in sibling conflict. The children who had interacted rather nicely until a year ago were having altercations that often became physical.

The couple described themselves as being happily married, and their children as being locked in a pattern of rejection, provocation, retaliation, and sibling rivalry, for which they wanted assistance. Wesley, who had interacted well with his sister in the past, had become more likely to avoid and ignore her. This led Lauren to provoke him with teasing and attention-seeking behav-

ior, such as using his things. Wesley would then retaliate, and a fight would ensue. Allen and Jill reported that this never-ending cycle was disruptive and had begun to impact the school functioning of their children.

Closer examination of the presenting problem indicated that Allen had started a new job, with increased responsibility and time away from home, approximately 18 months prior to the change in the children. He was the only Black manager in his division and often was the recipient of belittling and exclusionary tactics at work that he felt were race-related. This put even more pressure on him not to be invisible and to assert his presence during work-related social events. Socializing with his White colleagues for business purposes left Allen feeling drained and isolated. To compensate for these feelings, he began to increase the amount of time he spent with other Black males, through membership in church groups and his fraternity. His strong need to be around other Black men who might be experiencing similar circumstances left even less time for Allen to spend with his wife. She interpreted his behavior as a withdrawal from her and began engaging in attention-seeking behaviors, such as an escalation in spending. This only made Allen feel more isolated from her, because the upgrade in lifestyle depended on a job he did not like. Jill and Allen had not acknowledged a change in their relationship. Although the children were the identified clients, race-based stressors were impacting the relationship between Jill and Allen, and the children were mimicking the dynamics between their parents.

When such situations occur, it is often necessary to begin addressing the problem as it has been framed by the client(s). Even though it was clear to the clinician that the problem was rooted in the couple's relationship, it would have hindered the joining process, or sent the couple elsewhere, if the clinician did not first address the sibling discord. In this instance, a behavior modification plan was designed for the children first. The need for the couple to act as a team was used to segue into work with the couple alone. The clinician then encouraged Allen and Jill to explore how they each might support the other in the implementation of the plan, while simultaneously reinforcing their functioning as a unified couple.

Once the couple was able to demonstrate supportive behavior with the plan, this became the foundation and model for a broader exploration of support. At this time, Jill was encouraged to articulate feeling shut out, and Allen was able to share some of his thoughts about work. He spoke of feeling trapped and degraded because of what he described as the "racism on his job." He explained that this was initially difficult to share with his wife, because he did not want to be perceived as weak. The therapist was able to help the couple to understand the impact that the race-related stressors Allen was experiencing were having on the relationship. To realign the couple in a more unified way, the therapist utilized a "racism reframe" (Boyd-Franklin & Franklin, 1998), in which she told the couple that the racism Allen was experiencing on his job was threatening to destroy their relationship. She encouraged them to join together to support Allen in coping with these stressors. They began to communicate more openly about these issues in a number of their sessions. The couple progressed to the point that supporting one another in the face of challenges related to race became the theme of their work, as opposed to the squabbles of their children. Once they began to develop their partnership as a couple, the children's fighting decreased. When the pattern of mutual support between Jill and Allen was established, the therapist helped them to apply it to other aspects of their relationship.

Addressing the negative impact of race-based stressors on a couple relationship may be complicated. The previous example illustrates how the stressor may not even be acknowledged by the couple and can cause symptoms that are perceived to be outside of their couple relationship. The process involved in working through this complex situation involved four basic steps.

Step 1 involved addressing the presenting symptom of the children's behavior. Although the therapist was aware that this was not the root of the problem, it was an opportunity for joining, building trust and a therapeutic rapport with the couple, and segueing to the second step. In Step 2, the therapist helped the couple to build a stronger relationship and to address the presenting symptom as a unit. They began to develop the parenting skills and techniques needed to work together, while experiencing the positive impact of giving and receiving support.

The first two steps laid the foundation for the third step, wherein the shift from the presenting issue actually occurred. Step 3 involved reframing the presenting problem to include race-based stressors. Utilizing the "racism reframe," the therapist helped both members of the couple to see that Allen's experiences with racism on his job were threatening to destroy their relationship. The couple was then encouraged to unite together to support each other through these experiences. Step 4 involved strengthening the couple unit to acknowledge and to address race-based stressors when they occurred in the future, and strengthening the partners' resistance to these stressors. They then learned to apply this pattern to other challenges in their relationship as they arose.

Extended Family Involvement

As indicated earlier, extended family involvement is a strength in many African American families. Because many couples initially present their problems rather than their strengths in therapy, it is important for therapists to have a view of positive extended-family involvement. This can then be used as a guide in treatment with African American couples who are experiencing difficulties in their relationships. The following case illustrates these issues in the lives of a young couple.

Barbara (29) and Wade (40), an African American couple referred for treatment by Barbara's girlfriend, had met through an Internet dating service about 2 years earlier, and were currently living together and engaged to be married in a few months. They came for therapy because of a number of serious stressors.

Barbara, an elementary school teacher, was the first member of her family to go to college. Wade, a construction worker, had dropped out of high school. He had been married and was divorced in the year he met Barbara. He had two young children, John (6) and Karla (4). In their first session, they reported that they loved each other very much, but that they were feeling overwhelmed. They had been planning their wedding, and a number of issues had begun to emerge. They had begun to question whether they should get married.

Wade was the son of a drug-involved, single mother. His grandmother had raised him after his mother died of a drug overdose when Wade was young. He had been very close to his grandmother, who had died suddenly of a heart attack 2 years earlier. It was clear as he talked about her that Wade was still mourning her loss. He had never known his father. He had married at 19 and had recently divorced. Wade's ex-wife was very angry with him because of the divorce and his plans to marry Barbara. Although he regularly paid child support, she had refused to allow the children to see him for the last 6 months. He missed his children and was feeling very depressed. Barbara was concerned, because she felt that Wade had a tendency to withdraw from her and everyone when he was depressed. She felt that she could not "reach him."

Barbara was the older of two children. Her younger brother had died at age 5. She was very close to both her parents and loved them very much, but felt burdened by the fact that all of her parents' hopes had been directed toward her. Her parents were extremely hardworking. Both had grown up in Brooklyn, New York. They had met in high school. When Barbara's mother became pregnant with her, she had dropped out of high school in her junior year. Shortly thereafter, her father also dropped out of school to get married and to get a job. He had worked for a local supermarket most of his life, and her mother was receiving workman's compensation as a result of a work-related accident that left her unable to work for a number of years. Barbara's parents had always struggled financially and had sacrificed a great deal to send her to City College in New York. They were so proud when she graduated from college and became a teacher.

When Barbara had first begun dating Wade, her parents were very angry and disappointed. They objected to Wade on many levels. They had sacrificed so much to send Barbara to college, and they felt he was not "good enough" for their daughter, that she was marrying "beneath her." Furthermore, his status as a high school dropout was painfully reminiscent of their own earlier experiences. His prior marriage and divorce also concerned them. Her parents were afraid that so much of Wade's salary was given in child support that he and Barbara would not be able to provide for any children that they might have in the future. They were also upset about the couple's choice to live together before marriage.

Things had become very tense between Barbara and her parents, particularly when she announced that she and Wade were getting married. Her father refused to attend the wedding and was pressuring her mother not to attend either. Her mother felt very torn but had "sided with" her husband. Barbara was distraught. Their wedding was only a few months away, and she could not imagine not having her parents present. She had always dreamed of her father walking her down the aisle.

Both members of the couple were under a great deal of pressure, individually and together, and they found themselves fighting a great deal and blaming each other for these "family problems." The therapist joined with both of them in the first session and listened to their concerns. She asked at one point whether they loved each other. Both reported that they did, but that being together had just become "too hard." They were considering breaking up.

Consistent with a strength-based approach, the therapist reflected their concerns but also observed that they seemed to have a great deal of love for each other. Both members of the couple glanced at each other and seemed to soften somewhat. She then asked what had attracted them to each other initially. Barbara reported that she had always felt that Wade was a hard worker and very devoted to his children. It took Wade a bit longer, but he finally responded that he felt that Barbara was "a good looking woman" and very smart. He liked her ambition and her goals for the future. At the end of that session, their affect had begun to change, and they seemed more connected to each other.

In the next session, the therapist asked each partner to share his or her goals. Rather than have them share them with her, the therapist moved their chairs together and asked that they share them with each other. Barbara talked about her desire to get a master's degree eventually, and her hope to have children with Wade. Wade reported that he honestly could not think about future goals, because he was so "down" about the situation with his children. The therapist asked him to share with Barbara his hopes regarding his children. He told her that, as she knew, he had always wanted to get custody of his children, but that he was feeling very hopeless about his chances. His ex-wife would not even allow him to visit them. He told Barbara that he felt like a failure, and he was spending all of his money on a lawyer to fight for the right to see his children.

In the week following this session, Wade went back to court and, although he was not given full cus-tody, he was given visitation rights with his children. In the next session, his mood had improved. He had seen his children the weekend before, and he was feeling slightly better. He reported that his ex-wife refused to allow his children to attend his wedding, and that the judge had not forced the issue. He was still very angry about this. The therapist helped him to share all of this directly with Barbara. She praised him for being able to open up in this way. Barbara expressed her relief that Wade was beginning to talk to her about his concerns. The therapist worked with them for a number of sessions on improving their communication.

"Family" was extremely important to both members of the couple. The therapist had offered to meet with Barbara and her parents or with Wade's and his ex-wife, but both were horrified at either prospect. Searching for other sources of support for the couple, the therapist helped them to do a genogram or family tree. Both came from rather large, close, extended families. The therapist was surprised that neither partner had mentioned any of these family members prior to this session. Barbara shared that she had a number of aunts, uncles, and cousins who lived close to her. The therapist, knowing how important it was to her to have her father "give her away," asked if there was anyone else who could "walk her down the aisle." She thought for a long time and then she shared that her "godfather," her father's best friend since childhood, had been trying to "talk some sense" into her father and had been insisting that he attend his daughter's wedding. Her godfather had actually offered to "give her away" if her father did not. Although she was very sad and angry about her father's refusal, she agreed to talk with her godfather.

Wade also had several cousins who were very close to him. A number of them were in the wedding party. He also shared that a person named "Aunt Lou," who was not a blood relative, had been his grandmother's best friend. He shared that she had always been a "play mama" to him. The therapist helped them to see that they were not alone and that they had many people who loved and cared about them. Hoping to open up other sources of support, the therapist encouraged Wade and Barbara to speak to their extended family members about their dilemmas and to ask for their support.

As the wedding date approached, they both became increasingly upset as it became clear that Barbara's parents and Wade's children might not attend the ceremony. They had had a number of angry arguments about this. The therapist helped them to talk about this together. They were both feeling "very down" about these realities. She then asked the partners to share with each other any aspects of the wedding or the reception about which they were excited. Both had a large number of friends who would attend the wedding. The therapist told them how fortunate they were to have so many people who loved and cared about them. She asked what else they had planned for their wedding. They reported that they had been thinking about writing their own vows, but "hadn't gotten around to it." The therapist encouraged them each to write down a few thoughts to share with each other in the next session.

In the next session, both Barbara and Wade had written such beautiful vows that they were both a bit tearful by the end of the session. The therapist took out a piece of paper and placed it on her desk. She drew a circle for each of them. She then drew circles for Wade's ex-wife and each of his kids, and for each of Barbara's parents. She told them that these represented all of the people that they were upset with or concerned about. She then took a black magic marker and drew a dark circle around the two of them. She told them that it was obvious to her that they loved each other, but they needed to visualize themselves as a strong unit together and to remind themselves that as long as they had each other, they could deal with anything. They needed to see themselves as the center of all of these family members and support each other through these crises in their lives. Both were very pensive as they left the session.

In the next few weeks, the therapist saw several changes in Barbara and Wade. They had a number of discussions about the wedding. The therapist once again showed them the picture with the circle drawn around them, and asked them how they could make their wedding special and memorable even though some of the people they wanted to be there might not attend. They took more interest in planning their ceremony and even decided to "jump the broom," an old African American tradition, at the end of the service.

Two weeks before their wedding, the couple came in very hesitantly and seemed reluctant to ask the therapist a question. They were not sure whether she would agree, but that they would be honored if she would attend their wedding ceremony, because she had made such a difference in their lives. The therapist was torn. She had been trained to maintain "clear boundaries" between herself and her clients. As the session proceeded, she realized how important this was to the couple and agreed to attend.

On the day of their wedding, just before the ceremony, Barbara's godfather arrived, bringing her father and mother with him. At the last moment, her parents asked Barbara's forgiveness, and her father asked to walk her down the aisle. As she watched their ceremony, the therapist knew that they had learned to "hold onto each other" even when there was conflict with the other people in their families, and to support each other through whatever turmoil they would face in the future.

This case is an excellent example of many of the presenting issues of African American couples. Like this couple, many African Americans come from very close, "enmeshed" (Minuchin, 1974) extended family networks. Some of these family members may use "emotional cutoff" (Bowen, 1976; Nichols & Schwartz, 2001) as a strategy to control their loved ones. Moreover, sometimes one partner may encourage the other to use emotional cutoffs with other family members, leaving the other partner feeling torn between the couple relationship and the extended family.

It is very important that therapists recognize the "both–and" aspects of these situations, which means that partners can realistically have a strong relationship with each other and with their extended family members. Family connectedness is a very important value and strength in African American families. When this is disrupted, it can be extremely painful. Both Barbara and Wade felt "cut off" from people they loved. Although they were very sad and angry about these estrangements, they still felt the need for connectedness. The therapist had to work to help them to address all sides of this issue: their love, sadness, and anger. She also had to help them to communicate these feelings more effectively to each other. By helping them to "draw the circle around their relationship," the therapist had bestowed upon them a lifetime lesson. Given the complexity of their relationship within their large extended families and Wade's role as a remarried father, there would always be many different and often conflicting family messages and needs.

Therapists who have been trained to prioritize the couple relationship may not fully understand extended family involvement in the lives of some African American couples. They may then unintentionally encourage further cutoff between the couple and the extended family. The "both–and" reframe allows both points of view to be included in the treatment process. Some couples, like Wade and Barbara, can negotiate keeping a strong couple boundary, while also maintaining their other family relationships. Other couples may need assistance to find concrete methods to support both their couple and extended family relationships. Traditional problem-solving interventions provide an excellent means to help these couples make close and healthy couple and extended-family relationship goals a reality.

By doing the genogram with the couple and asking about their support systems, the therapist had tracked a cultural strength and helped to remind the partners that they were not alone with their problems. She uncovered not only "blood" relatives but also "family" members who, though not directly related, were extremely important in their lives (i.e., Barbara's godfather and Wade's "play mama"). This is an important lesson for clinicians who work with African American couples. If we know to ask about them, these individuals can serve a therapeutic and supportive function.

Although Wade and Barbara would both mourn the fact that some of their loved ones might not attend their wedding, they felt embraced by the support of their friends and other family members. Moreover, such members often have their own culturally sanctioned ways of solving problems that can be utilized by the couple, such as Barbara's godfather, who had done important work toward reconciling Barbara and her father.

This case also illustrates an important lesson about boundaries. In African American communities, it is not unusual for the minister to offer pastoral counseling and to be very present at all of the important events in the lives of his or her congregation. When an African American couple has established a strong therapeutic relationship with a therapist, it is not unusual for them to ask the clinician to attend important rituals (funerals, weddings, baptisms, baby dedications, etc.). It is important in these situations for therapists to consider the meaning of this gesture to their clients, and at times to relax their rigid "boundaries" around the process of therapy. This is particularly important for those who may be supervising African American therapists, who may live in the same communities as their clients and attend the same churches, or who may see their clients in other contexts.

Research has shown that whereas only 35% of White women and 40% of Latina women enter marriage with children, 77% of African American women do so (Karney et al., 2004), and these children may often be from prior relationships. As a consequence, child-related dilemmas, particularly those concerning ex-"baby mamas" or "baby daddies," are very common presenting concerns for African American newlyweds. Therapists must be prepared to help African American couples to negotiate these dilemmas and to communicate openly about their concerns.

This case also illustrates a historically rooted and growing pattern in the Black community, in which more educated women partner with less educated men. In the past, Black families often educated their daughters to protect them from the dangers of sexual harassment and victimization that often accompanied domestic employment situations (Boyd-Franklin, 2003). Part of this gender difference in education can be attributed to the "shortage of Black men." This shortage can refer to the relative lack of Black men, because of factors such as imprisonment, drugs, and death, as described earlier, or to the relative lack of Black men of comparable socioeconomic status

(Kelly, 2003; Stockard & Tucker, 2001; Tucker & Mitchell-Kernan, 1995). Therefore, many Black women who want to have children and families of their own are choosing to partner with or to marry men who have less education and job status. Although this is becoming more common in the Black community, it can be a major issue for some Black women in their extended family and friend networks, particularly because it goes against the larger society's often sexist values that the man should be of a higher status than the woman.

Religion and Spirituality

Some African Americans, especially those who are deeply religious, may view therapy as "antispiritual" and express concerns that therapy may undermine their religious beliefs (Boyd-Franklin, 2003). Although the mental health field is beginning to change on this issue, clinicians should be aware that only within the last 10 years has a discussion of religious or spiritual beliefs been considered acceptable in therapy. Prior to that time, it was common for mental health providers to label or pathologize their clients as demonstrating "religiosity," if they mentioned their spiritual beliefs in therapy (Boyd-Franklin, 2003).

Due to their importance in African American culture, religion and spirituality often play a major role in couple relationships. It has become increasingly common for African Americans to request treatment by a "Christian therapist" or a Black Christian therapist. Therapists who are not Christian, or who do not share their clients' religious or spiritual beliefs, are often surprised by such requests. It is often helpful to encourage the couple to come in for one session and discuss their concerns about religion, spirituality, and race or ethnicity in treatment. A therapist can offer to refer the couple to a Christian therapist if they remain uncomfortable. Similarly, when partners have requested treatment by a therapist from their cultural, racial, or religious group, a therapist who lacks this background may encourage a couple to come for one session. At the end of the first session, after the therapist has joined with the couple and established therapeutic rapport, he or she can return to the issue of racial, cultural, or religious differences. Often, if the therapist is culturally (and religiously) sensitive, the couple will be willing to continue the work with him or her. If not, it is important for the therapist to be aware of other clinicians, who may be more similar to the couple, and to facilitate a referral.

Healthy African American couples understand and value the role of religion and spirituality, and respect differences, although religious differences can present issues in Black couples, particularly if one member of the couple is deeply involved in religion or in the church, and the other is not. Religious and spiritual beliefs can also be important therapeutic tools in the treatment of African American couples. The following vignette illustrates this process with a couple whose members considered the church to be an integral part of their lives:

Martha (66) and Carl (69), an older African American couple, were referred by a friend. They had met at Church 4 years earlier and had married after dating for 2 years.

Initially, Martha called requesting therapy. In the first session, the couple seemed very uncomfortable. They reported that they had been hoping for a "Black Christian therapist." The therapist, a White woman, was not particularly religious and was concerned about her ability to treat this couple. She invited Martha and Carl to "give the therapy a try" for one session to see whether they felt comfortable working with her. If not, she promised to try to help them to find a Black Christian therapist.

In the session, the therapist inquired about how they met. Martha replied that she had grown up in the same Baptist Church and had been a member for her entire life. Carl had retired 4 years earlier and had moved from his home in New York City to an "adult community" in New Jersey. They met when Carl joined the church and became a member of the church choir. Martha had been a member of the choir "for years." Both had been married before, and each had adult children and grandchildren. Both were very connected to their families.

The partners shared that they had both dreamed of retiring early and having the opportunity to travel and "see the world." When Martha had retired 9 months earlier, they had had a big celebration and invited their family and "Church family" members. Shortly after Martha's retirement, however, her mother (age 86) had a stroke. She was unable to care for herself, and Martha had brought her home from the hospital to stay with them.

Thinking that this was a short-term arrangement, Carl was very supportive initially. Martha's mother received physical, speech, and occupational therapy in their home. After 6 months, there was no improvement in her condition. Her speech was still very slurred, she was confined to a wheelchair, and she was unable to care for herself. Her doctor told Martha and Carl that, given her age, she was not likely to regain full functioning. He recommended a nursing home. Martha was devastated and refused to put her mother in a nursing home. Carl was torn—he understood Martha's feelings, but was

angry as he saw their dreams for their retirement slipping away. They had begun to have very angry arguments.

The therapist normalized each person's feelings and began working to help them to communicate their feelings more openly. Each reported feeling very sad and "stuck" in terms of this dilemma. The therapist was impressed by the fact that despite their disagreements, they obviously loved and cared about each other. She reflected those feelings to them in the session. At the end of the session, she asked them how they had felt working with her, a White therapist. They both reported that they had felt comfortable and agreed to come back. She explored the initial request for a Black Christian therapist, and both Carl and Martha stated that although they would both prefer someone of their own culture and faith, they would "take a chance on her." The therapeutic alliance had begun.

In the next session, Carl shared that he was very angry with both Martha and her family. He reported that Martha was the "superwoman" in her family. She did everything and took care of everyone. He was upset because they all seemed to assume that Martha would be the one to "take in Mama." The therapist inquired about their families and spent the next few sessions constructing genograms with both of them. Martha was the oldest of three children. Her sister lived with her family in Atlanta, and her brother lived in Los Angeles. Prior to the stroke, her mother had been very independent and had been living on her own in the same town in which Martha and Carl resided. She had also been a member of their Church for most of her life. Martha's daughter lived in New York City and had three children of her own. During this discussion, Carl reiterated that Martha "took care of everyone." Martha countered that everyone else was far away or "busy with their own lives," and she was the only one available to "take care of Mama."

Carl was an only child. His parents had died when he was a young man. He was close with his extended family, but most of them lived in the South, and he saw them mainly at family reunions each summer. He had one daughter, a single parent, who was raising her two children in Cleveland, Ohio. He was very close to her, and his grandchildren and made frequent trips to visit.

When the therapist discussed the case in supervision, her supervisor, a Black woman, encouraged her to ask more about their "Church family," because the couple had reported such a high degree of involvement with them. The mother was still as active in the Church, as much as her condition allowed, attending services in her wheelchair when Martha and Carl brought her with them. The therapist inquired about the supports that they had in their Church. They reported that their minister and his wife were very supportive, and that the other members of the choir were "like family." Members of the deacon and deaconess boards often "came by the house to visit with and pray with Mama." Many church members were "prayer warriors," who had prayed for Martha's mother when she had first had her stroke and had offered to help. The therapist explored the kinds of help that had been offered. Martha shared that some of the other "seniors" in the Church had offered to drive her mother to some of the senior activities in the Church, so that she could "get out of the house."

Carl reported that all of this was true, but that Martha had been reluctant to accept such offers of help. Martha countered that she did not want to "place a burden" on anyone. The therapist asked how common these services were in their Black Church, because this concept was new to the therapist. Both Martha and Carl agreed that this was the norm, particularly among the senior citizens. It was common for Church members to pick up seniors and drive them to Church, if they were no longer able to get there on their own. The therapist asked Martha and Carl to talk together in the session about the ways the members of their church might help them with "Mama" and give them a little bit of time to do things together. They finally agreed that they would ask one of the senior "sisters" in the Church, who was a close friend of Martha's mother, to come and visit with her one Sunday after Church. The therapist explored what the partners would like to do with their free time. They reported that they used to enjoy going into New York City to a show. With the therapist's help and encouragement, they agreed to try to arrange this time. In the next few sessions, the therapist reinforced the fact that they needed time "for themselves" as a couple, and introduced the concept of "respite time," when they would ask someone from their family or their "Church family" to help out for a few hours.

As their relationship began to improve, the therapist spent a number of sessions working on communication between the partners. In one session, Carl reported that although things were better between them, they had not gone out together except for the one trip to the city. He still found himself resenting the fact that they could not travel as they had once planned. He again raised the question of a nursing home for Martha's mother. She burst into tears and said that she could never do that to her mother, who had always been there for her. The therapist asked Carl how he felt about Martha's mother. He said that he actually liked her very much and they got along well, but he honestly resented the fact that they could no longer "have a life." The therapist explored what he meant by this, and Carl told her about his dream of traveling with Martha. She asked him to talk with Martha about this. Martha again cried and explained that she wanted that too, but "somebody had to take care of Mama."

The therapist was feeling discouraged and asked for the help of her supervisor. At the supervisor's urging, the therapist asked Carl and Martha how they both solved other difficult situations. They reported that they usually prayed, but that their prayers for help in this situation had not been answered. The therapist told them to hold hands and pray together that evening and every evening before their next session for someone who might help them out, so that they could take a short trip together. She asked them to come back and share the answer that

they received. In the next session, they reported that they had not received an answer. The therapist asked them to reach out to their family and Church family members, and ask them to pray with them for someone to help out and give them a short break.

In the next session, both Carl and Martha were all smiles. Members of the church had offered to "give them breaks" so that they could "get away" for weekends together. Her sister had offered to come and "take care of Mama for a week," so that they could take a longer trip to the Caribbean. In future sessions, the therapist helped them, particularly Martha, to ask for help and to support each other in the process. At her supervisor's suggestion, she told them that although they had always prayed, they had prayed alone. By praying together, and by asking for the help and prayers of others, their prayers had become more powerful and they had received answers. She encouraged them to remember this in the future as they faced new challenges.

This case illustrates many aspects of the religious and spiritual connections of Black families and the ways in which they can be utilized in couple therapy. The therapist, a young White woman without a church or religious affiliation, was initially very concerned and intimidated by the request for a "Black Christian therapist." To her credit, she did not personalize this as a rejection of her. She encouraged the couple to stay for the first session and see how they felt at the end. She also offered to try to help them to find a "Black Christian therapist" if they were not comfortable at the end of the session. This showed her respect for them, and her willingness to take their request seriously.

Many therapists of other cultural and racial backgrounds may construct a genogram of "blood" family members with a couple, but they often overlook the importance of the "Church family." As this case illustrates, Black Churches have many different networks of support, particularly for the "seniors" in the community. Caring for elders is a deeply held value in African American families, and many persons react with horror, as Martha did, to the idea of "placing Mama in a nursing home." Even Black families who lack the option Martha and Carl had as a retired couple caring for an elderly relative at home will feel a great deal of anguish and guilt if forced to place a family member in a nursing home. This dilemma is common enough that some Black Churches have established their own nursing home facilities to help these families. Still others have developed formal and informal outreach services to support homebound seniors and their family members. With her supervisor's help, this therapist was able to ask about the sources of help that the church provided and assist the couple, particularly Martha, to ask for and accept such help.

Carl's observation that Martha was the "superwoman" who took care of everyone in her family is also illustrative of a deeply ingrained and positively reinforced pattern for many African American women, in which someone like Martha becomes the family caretaker and the "switchboard" (Boyd-Franklin, 2003) for family communication. This can become a burden for them and can become a problem in their couple relationships. The therapist struggled to find a way to address this and to empower Martha to accept help from others without inadvertently siding with Carl in the couple's arguments. The use of the "prayer metaphor" (Boyd-Franklin, 2003) was a culturally and spiritually familiar reference for the couple. It accomplished many things simultaneously. It showed the therapist's respect for their spiritual belief system. By asking them to join hands and pray together at home, the therapist began a pattern that could be applied successfully to future situations. The request for them to pray together also reinforced their couple bond. When their prayers alone did not produce the results that they wanted, she encouraged them to ask for the prayers of others. This is a very common request in African American families and "Church families," when "prayer warriors" are often called upon to pray for special needs and requests. This provided a face-saving way for Martha to ask for and receive help, and it addressed Carl's need for more opportunities for the couple to spend time together and to travel.

Infidelity in an African American Couple

Infidelity is a very difficult treatment issue with couples of any ethnic or racial background (Finkel, Rusbult, Kumashiro, & Hannon, 2002). It is a particularly complicated issue in the Black community. Many of the stereotypes projected onto Black men and women since slavery have been sexualized images (Boyd-Franklin, 2003; Franklin, 2004). In addition, Black men have faced severe discrimination. Franklin (2004) has described an "invisibility syndrome"—a paradoxical reality in which society often sees the stereotypes and not the real person. Some Black men assert their manhood in the face of experiences with racism by adopting what Majors and Billson (1992) termed the "cool pose." Often this definition of manhood

involves their appeal to women. In addition, some Black men have experienced multiple periods of job loss and instability due to the institutional racism inherent in "last hired, first fired" policies (Boyd-Franklin, 2003). During these times, the desire to "prove their manhood" may be expressed by sexual acting out. It is important for therapists to understand these realities but not to allow their use as an excuse mechanism for the violation of trust in a relationship. The following case illustrates many of these dilemmas.

Adam (32) and Carol (31), an African American couple, came for treatment after Carol caught Adam in bed with another woman. They had been married for 10 years and had been together since high school. Adam worked as a truck driver and was often away from home on long-distance assignments. Carol worked in a local department store as a sales clerk. They had two children, Shayna (9) and Michael (7). Carol complained that although she knew that Adam loved his children, he was away so much that she felt that she was raising their children alone. There had been problems in their marriage for a number of years, and Carol had suspected that Adam had affairs with women when he was away from home. She had confronted him repeatedly but was always met with his denials. Two months prior to coming for treatment, Adam had lost his job due to a "downsizing" in his company. The next week, Carol had developed a severe migraine headache at work and had returned home early to find Adam in bed with another woman. She was furious and had angrily "thrown them both out of the house."

Carol had refused to allow Adam back into the house, and he had been living for 2 months with his sister and her family. Carol requested the appointment and reported that Adam, who had refused to come in the past, was "desperate now," because he wanted to reunite with her and their children.

The atmosphere in the first session was very tense. The therapist, having heard about the infidelity from Carol during the initial phone call, was very careful to join with both members of the couple. She asked where they were born and talked briefly about where each of them had been raised. It was also clear that both were concerned about their children, who were very upset by their parents' separation. Carol and Adam were especially worried about their son, Michael, who had "taken the separation very hard." He cried often for his father and had begun to act out angrily at home with his mother and in school.

When the therapist explored the concerns that had brought the couple to therapy, Carol immediately raised the infidelity. She reported that she wanted a divorce. Adam was very upset, and said that he thought they were coming for therapy to work on their relationship. Carol agreed to work on their relationship but indicated that she was not very hopeful about their marriage.

She reported that she was "sick of him messing around with other women." Her anger and hurt were evident. The therapist stated that she understood each of their positions and thought that they could benefit from therapy whether or not they decided to continue their marriage. They would always be coparents and need to have ongoing contact for the sake of their children. She indicated that it was obvious they both cared about their children.

In the second session, the therapist discussed with Adam the importance of refraining from any relationships or sexual encounters outside of their couple relationship during the time that they were in treatment. He agreed, but Carol expressed her doubt that he would be able to deliver on his promise. In the third session, the therapist explored the history of the couple's relationship. Carol reported that Adam had always "played around with other women," even in high school, but she had thought that he would "outgrow it." Adam reported that he loved Carol and that those women "did not mean anything" to him. Carol responded angrily, and they began arguing with each other in the session. The therapist acknowledged Carol's anger, which became a major focus of the session. Conflict resolution techniques were used to help the couple address the issue.

In the next session, the therapist asked the partners what initially had attracted them to each other. Adam reported that Carol was the one girl in high school who "would not give him the time of day." He pursued her and they began dating during his senior year and her junior year in high school. Carol reported that Adam was very good looking and one of the most popular boys in school. The therapist also asked more about their experiences when they were growing up. They shared more about their families of origin.

Carol stated that she did not want to end up like her mother and her sister. The therapist asked her about that comment. Carol reported that her mother had been a single parent, with "no one" to help her. Her father had left her mother before Carol was a year old. Her older sister had a different father. She also indicated that her older sister had become pregnant as a teenager, and Carol was determined to avoid this. She stated she had always been told that there was a "shortage of Black men out there" and she had tried to "put up with Adam" for the sake of her children, but that she was "fed up" with his behavior.

In the next session, the therapist pursued Adam's family background. He had grown up in a family in which his father "played around with other women." His mother had "thrown him out a number of times but had always taken him back." The therapist pointed out that people often learn what to expect as a couple by watching their parents' relationships. This seemed to be a new concept for them, and Carol and Adam explored it more in detail. The therapist helped them to complete their family genograms in the next two sessions. These patterns and messages were evident throughout both of their families. The therapist reframed the therapy as an

opportunity for the couple to change their family scripts and to create a new kind of relationship. It was an opportunity to see whether they could repair their relationship, work on forgiveness, and improve their communication patterns and parenting relationship. Both members of the couple agreed.

A number of sessions explored their communication styles. It became clear that they did not discuss their issues and problems, and often acted them out. In a number of sessions, the partners were encouraged to talk to each other about their problems. When the issue of infidelity was explored, Carol poured out her hurt and anger and asked Adam directly why he "did this" to her. She felt that he did not respect her at all. Adam questioned that and told her that he did love and respect her, but that he "couldn't stop" himself.

The therapist helped them to explore this issue. When she asked why he felt this way, Adam was silent. He said that he "could not talk about it." Carol became very angry and accused him of "pulling away like he always does." The therapist tried a number of times to help the couple to talk about this issue. She was concerned that Adam might not return for the next session. Therefore, she asked Carol's permission to speak to Adam alone. The therapist, eager not to create another "secret" in their relationship, added that she would help Adam to share his concern with Carol.

In their time alone, Adam was very embarrassed. He told the therapist that he just could not talk about what had happened to him. The therapist asked whether it concerned Carol. He said no, that it had happened long before he met her. The therapist told him that she thought that Carol was afraid that she had "done something." After a long pause, Adam finally revealed that when he was about 8 years old, his older brother had come into his bed one night and "raped" him. He had been angry with his brother for years and had never told anyone. His brother had been killed in a car accident while a teenager, and this had remained an unresolved area for him. He told the therapist that girls had always found him "cute," and because he had been determined to prove that he "was a man," he had always gotten involved with as many girls as he could.

The therapist acknowledged how difficult it had been for Adam to share this with her and told him that it had taken a great deal of courage. She asked him whether he thought that he could tell Carol, with her help. Initially, he was very embarrassed and reluctant to describe this incident. The therapist helped Adam to see that this experience had interfered with his relationship with Carol for years, and that she was afraid she had done something to cause this behavior. With the therapist's encouragement, he agreed to have Carol rejoin the session. With the therapist's help, Adam was able to share this experience with Carol. Adam became very tearful during this session, and Carol cried with him.

In the next two sessions, the partners discussed the ways that this experience might have affected their relationship. These very intense sessions led to reconciliation between the partners. Adam moved back into the home. They spent a couple of sessions talking about their concerns about their children, particularly their son, Michael. About 2 months later, a woman called the house claiming to have a relationship with Adam. He denied it at first, but later admitted to having had sex with her on one occasion. He claimed that this was not a relationship, and that the woman meant nothing to him. Carol was again furious. She told Adam in a session that she cared about him and was very sorry about his experience with his brother, but she could not "do this any more." She told him that she wanted a divorce. All attempts to explore the possibility of continuing to work on the relationship were met with Carol's firm resolve. Carol again insisted that Adam move out of the house. The therapist encouraged both of them to spend some time thinking about this before the next session. In the next few sessions, the therapist explored the possibilities with the couple. Adam literally begged Carol to reconsider, but she remained firm. The therapist encouraged Adam to pursue individual therapy to explore the impact of the sexual abuse on his view of himself as a man. Adam was hesitant at first, but she helped him to see that this would continue to be an issue in his life and in his future relationships. He finally accepted a referral and agreed to individual treatment.

In the next session, Carol reported that she had already consulted a lawyer. Concerned that the divorce process and antagonistic lawyers would make their situation worse, the therapist encouraged the partners to go for divorce mediation. They agreed. She also encouraged them to continue to come for a number of sessions to work out and establish a solid coparenting relationship for the sake of the children. Adam and Carol agreed. They came regularly for 3 more months and worked out their visitation schedule. In addition, they had a number of sessions with the therapist and their children. The therapist helped them to establish clear agreement about their parenting behavior, particularly in terms of addressing Michael's anger and acting out. They agreed to talk with the children together and to assure them that the separation and divorce had nothing to do with them. Both parents also told the children that they loved them, and assured them of their continued love even though they would not be together. The therapist also encouraged Adam to spend some time with the children individually to continue a special relationship with each child. Michael's acting-out behavior began to decrease.

This case, like all experiences of infidelity, was extremely difficult. The therapist felt that even though the partners did not continue in their marriage, there was a sense of resolution in their lives, and they were able to lay the groundwork for a more positive coparenting relationship in the future.

As indicated earlier, some Black men who feel demeaned by society may resort to sexual liai-

sons to "prove" their manhood. This was particularly apparent after Adam lost his job, and it was further complicated by the fact that his brother had raped him at a young age. These kinds of experiences present many complications for some Black couples. Carol was furious at Adam's repeated, and often denied, experiences of infidelity. She knew of Adam's behavior when they were dating in high school. Like many Black women, however, she was also well aware of the "shortage of Black men" described earlier. In many ways, this reality caused Carol to tolerate his behavior even though she was hurt and furious. She was afraid that, like her mother and her sister, she would "end up with no one." It is very important that therapists understand this dynamic in African American couples, and help Black women and men to address these concerns (Boyd-Franklin, 2003; Boyd-Franklin & Franklin, 1998).

The multigenerational family transmission process (Bowen, 1976; Boyd-Franklin, 2003) is also very striking in this case. In families of all cultural backgrounds, patterns in prior generations can repeat in the current generation. In Carol's family, the legacy of women raising children alone was often repeated. She was determined to break the cycle in her family by "getting married and staying married," but sadly, this had trapped her in a very painful marital situation. On the other hand, Adam's father also had had multiple affairs with women. Adam had learned not to take his mother's threats seriously. Therefore, he was very surprised when Carol "threw him out of the house." It was helpful to both members of the couple to explore together the ways their family legacies had influenced their views of couple relationships and their behavior in marriage. If done in later sessions, after trust has been established, therapists may find that this type of a genogram (or family tree) exercise is extremely helpful with African American couples.

CONCLUSION

This chapter has provided an overview of the impact of racism, discrimination, and economic hardship on the quality of Black couple relationships. Despite these challenges, Black couples bring to treatment many strengths that are often underutilized, such as extended families, religion, spirituality, and a positive racial identity. Therapists are cautioned to refrain from applying a deficit perspective to couple issues that are integrally related to the status of African Americans in society. Clinicians who incorporate the culturally competent view of Black couples presented in this chapter will be able to join and establish rapport more effectively with them and to impact the process of therapeutic change positively.

SUGGESTIONS FOR FURTHER READING

Boyd-Franklin, N. (2003). *Black families in therapy: Understanding the African American experience.* New York: Guilford Press.

Franklin, A. J. (2004). *From brotherhood to manhood: How Black men rescue their relationships and dreams from the invisibility syndrome.* Hoboken, NJ: Wiley.

McGoldrick, M., Giordano, J., & Garcia-Preto, N. (Eds.). (2005). *Ethnicity and family therapy.* New York: Guilford Press.

REFERENCES

Beale, R. L. (1997). Multiple familial-worker role strain and psychological well-being: Moderating effects of coping resources among Black American parents. In R. J. Taylor, J. S. Jackson, & L. Chatters (Eds.), *Family life in Black America* (pp. 132–145). Newbury Park, CA: Sage.

Bean, R. A., Perry, B. J., & Bedell, T. M. (2002). Developing culturally competent marriage and family therapists: Treatment guidelines for non-African-American therapists working with African-American families. *Journal of Marital and Family Therapy, 28,* 153–164.

Bell, Y. R., Bouie, C. L., & Baldwin, J. A. (1990). Afrocentric cultural consciousness and African-American male–female relationships. *Journal of Black Studies, 21,* 162–189.

Bowen, M. (1976). Theory in the practice of psychotherapy. In P. J. Guerin (Ed.), *Family therapy: Theory and practice* (pp. 42–90). New York: Gardner Press.

Bowen-Reid, T. L., & Harrell, J. P. (2002). Racist experiences and health outcomes: An examination of spirituality as a buffer. *Journal of Black Psychology, 28,* 18–36.

Boyd-Franklin, N. (2003). *Black families in therapy: Understanding the African American experience.* New York: Guilford Press.

Boyd-Franklin, N., & Franklin, A. J. (1998). African American couples in therapy. In M. McGoldrick (Ed.), *Re-visioning family therapy: Race, culture, and gender in clinical practice* (pp. 268–281). New York: Guilford Press.

Brice-Baker, J. (2005). British West Indian families. In M. McGoldrick, J. Giordano, & N. Garcia-Preto (Eds.), *Ethnicity and family therapy* (3rd ed., pp. 117–126). New York: Guilford Press.

Broman, C. L. (2005). Marital quality in Black and White marriages. *Journal of Family Issues, 26,* 431–441.

Bryant, S. A., & Beckett, J. O. (1997). Effects of status resources and gender on role expectations of African American couples. *Smith College Studies in Social Work, 67,* 348–374.

Burton, L. M., Winn, D., Stevenson, H., & Clark, S. L. (2004). Working with African American clients: Considering the "homeplace" in marriage and family therapy practices. *Journal of Marital and Family Therapy, 4,* 397–410.

Carter, R. T. (1995). *The influence of race and racial identity in psychotherapy: Toward a racially inclusive model.* New York: Wiley.

Carter, R. T. (2007). Racism and psychological and emotional injury: Recognizing and assessing race-based traumatic stress. *Counseling Psychologist, 35(1),* 13–105.

Cherlin, A. J. (1992). *Marriage, divorce, remarriage.* Cambridge, MA: Harvard University Press.

Clark, R., Anderson, N. B., Clark, V. R., & Williams, D. R. (1999). Racism as a stressor for African Americans: A biopsychosocial model. *American Psychologist, 54,* 805–816.

Clark-Nicolas, P., & Gray-Little, B. (1991). Effect of economic resources on marital quality in black married couples. *Journal of Marriage and the Family, 53,* 645–655.

Cross, W. E., Jr. (1978). The Thomas and Cross models of psychological Nigrescence: A review. *Journal of Black Psychology, 5,* 13–31.

Cross, W. E., Jr. (1991). *Shades of black.* Philadelphia: Temple University Press.

Edin, K. (2000). What do low-income single mothers say about marriage? *Social Problems, 47,* 112–133.

Ellison, C. G. (1997). Religious involvement and the subjective quality of family life among African Americans. In R. J. Taylor, J. S. Jackson, & L. M. Chatters (Eds.), *Family life in Black America* (pp. 117–131). Thousand Oaks, CA: Sage.

Finkel, E. J., Rusbult, C. E., Kumashiro, M., & Hannon, P. A. (2002). Dealing with betrayal in close relationships: Does commitment promote forgiveness? *Journal of Personality and Social Psychology, 6,* 956–974.

Franklin, A. J. (2004). *From brotherhood to manhood: How Black men rescue their relationships and dreams from the invisibility syndrome.* Hoboken, NJ: Wiley.

Franklin, A. J., Boyd-Franklin, N., & Kelly, S. (2006). Racism and invisibility: Race-related stress, emotional abuse and psychological trauma for people of color. *Journal of Emotional Abuse, 6,* 9–30.

Franklin, A. J., Carter, R. T., & Grace, C. (1993). An integrative approach to psychotherapy with Black/African Americans: The relevance of race and culture. In G. Stricker & J. Gold (Eds.), *Comprehensive handbook of psychotherapy integration* (pp. 465–479). New York: Plenum Press.

Gibson, C., Edin, K., & McLanahan, S. (2003, June). *High hopes but even higher expectations: The retreat from marriage among low-income couples* (Working Paper No. 2003-06-FF). Princeton, NJ: Center for Research on Child Well-Being.

Hatchett, S., Veroff, J., & Douvan, E. (1995). Marital instability among black and white newlyweds. In M. B. Tucker & C. Mitchell-Kernan (Eds.), *The decline in marriage among African Americans* (pp. 177–218). New York: Russell Sage Foundation.

Helms, J. E. (1990). *Black and white racial identity: Theory, research, and practice.* Westport, CT: Greenwood Press.

Helms, J. E., & Cook, D. A. (1999). *Using race and culture in counseling and psychotherapy: Theory and process.* Boston: Allyn & Bacon.

Hines, P., & Boyd-Franklin, N. (2005). African American families. In M. McGoldrick, J. Giordano, & N. Garcia-Preto (Eds.), *Ethnicity and family therapy* (3rd ed., pp. 87–100). New York: Guilford Press.

Hooks, B. (1990). *Yearning: Race, gender, and cultural politics.* Boston: South End Press.

Jones, J. M. (1997). *Prejudice and racism* (2nd ed.). New York: McGraw-Hill.

Kamya, H. (2005). African immigrant families. In M. McGoldrick, J. Giordano, & N. Garcia-Preto (Eds.), *Ethnicity and family therapy* (3rd ed., pp. 101–116). New York: Guilford Press.

Karney, B. R., Kreitz, M. A., & Sweeney, K. E. (2004). Obstacles to ethnic diversity in marital research: On the failure of good intentions. *Journal of Social and Personal Relationships, 21,* 509–526.

Kelly, S. (2003). African American couples: Their importance to the stability of African American families and their mental health issues. In J. S. Mio & G. Y. Iwamasa (Eds.), *Culturally diverse mental health: The challenges of research and resistance* (pp. 141–157). New York: Brunner-Routledge.

Kelly, S. (2007). *How African American couples cope with racial issues.* Unpublished manuscript, Rutgers University, New Brunswick, NJ.

Kelly, S., & Floyd, F. J. (2001). The effects of negative racial stereotypes and Afrocentricity on black couple relationships. *Journal of Family Psychology, 15,* 110–123.

Kelly, S., & Floyd, F. J. (2006). Impact of racial perspectives and contextual variables on marital trust and adjustment for African American couples. *Journal of Family Psychology, 20,* 79–87.

LaTaillade, J. J. (2006). Considerations for treatment of African American couple relationships. *Journal of Cognitive Psychotherapy: An International Quarterly, 4,* 341–358.

LaTaillade, J. J., Baucom, D. H., & Jacobson, N. S. (2000, November). *Correlates of satisfaction and resiliency in African American/white interracial relationships.* Paper presented as part of the symposium (J. J. LaTaillade, Chair), The Influence of Culture and Context of the Intimate Relationships of African Americans, at the annual convention of the Association for Advancement of Behavior Therapy, New Orleans, LA.

Majors, R., & Billson, J. M. (1992). *Cool pose: The dilemmas of black manhood in America.* New York: Simon & Schuster.

McAdams-Mahmoud, V. (2005). African American Muslim families. In M. McGoldrick, J. Giordano, & N. Garcia-Preto (Eds.), *Ethnicity and family therapy* (3rd ed., pp. 138–150). New York: Guilford Press.

McGoldrick, M., Giordano, J., & Garcia-Preto, N. (Eds.). (2005). *Ethnicity and family therapy* (3rd ed.). New York: Guilford Press.

McKinnon, J. (2003). *The black population in the United States: March 2002.* Retrieved August 3, 2004, from *www.census.gov/prod/2003pubs/p20-541.pdf.*

Menos, J. (2005). Haitian families. In M. McGoldrick, J. Giordano, & N. Garcia-Preto (Eds.), *Ethnicity and family therapy* (3rd ed., pp. 127–137). New York: Guilford Press.

Minuchin, S. (1974). *Families and family therapy.* Cambridge, MA: Harvard University Press.

Nichols, M.P., & Schwartz, R. (2001). *Family therapy: Concepts and methods.* Boston: Allyn & Bacon.

Nobles, W. (2004). African philosophy: Foundations of black psychology. In R. Jones (Ed.), *Black psychology* (4th ed., pp. 47–64). Hampton, VA: Cobb & Henry Press.

Pierce, C. M. (1995). Stress analogs of racism and sexism: Terrorism, torture, and disaster. In C. V. Willie, P. P. Reiker, B. M. Kramer, & B. S. Brown (Eds.), *Mental health, racism, and sexism* (pp. 277–293). Pittsburgh: University of Pittsburgh Press.

Stockard, R. L., & Tucker, M. B. (2001). Young African American men and women: Separate paths? In L. Daniels (Ed.), *The state of black America 2001* (pp. 143–160). New York: National Urban League.

Sue, D. W. (2003). *Overcoming our racism: The journey to liberation.* San Francisco, CA: Jossey-Bass.

Sue, D. W., & Sue, D. (2003). *Counseling the culturally diverse: Theory and practice* (4th ed.). New York: Wiley.

Taylor, R. J., Jackson, J. S., & Chatters, L. M. (1997). *Family life in Black America.* Thousand Oaks, CA: Sage.

Taylor, R. J., Mattis, J., & Chatters, L. M. (1999). Subjective religiosity among African Americans: A synthesis of findings from five national samples. *Journal of Black Psychology, 25,* 524–543.

Teachman, J. D., Tedrow, L. M., & Crowder, K. D. (2000). The changing demography of America's families. *Journal of Marriage and the Family, 62,* 1234–1246.

Tucker, M. B., & Mitchell-Kernan, C. (1995). Trends in African American family formation: A theoretical and statistical overview. In M. B. Tucker & C. Mitchell-Kernan (Eds.), *The decline in marriage among African Americans* (pp. 3–26). New York: Sage.

CHAPTER 26

Legal and Ethical Issues in Couple Therapy

Michael C. Gottlieb
Jon Lasser
Georganna L. Simpson

Individual therapists are subject to a variety of ethical and legal standards but, for the most part, the rules governing such treatment are relatively unambiguous, such as maintaining confidentiality and working for the welfare of one's client. When practitioners choose to work with couples, they encounter vexing ethical issues and legal challenges unique to this therapeutic modality. The introductory section of this chapter briefly provides some historical context, followed by a review of basic principles of biomedical ethics. We conclude that section with assumptions grounded in systems theory. The next section reviews unique ethical challenges faced by couple therapists, along with available alternatives and recommendations for practice. The final section concerns some of the legal issues that may arise in this practice niche and the available alternatives for coping with them.

BACKGROUND

Psychotherapy began as an individual matter. The early psychoanalysts were physicians who, basing their practice on a medical model, worked for the benefit of their patients. For example, in their ef- forts to guard confidentiality zealously, it was not uncommon to exclude family members, who were often seen as obstacles to the therapeutic endeavor.

In the 1950s, practitioners from various disciplines began experimenting with a variety of relational therapies, such as the interdisciplinary group at the Mental Research Institute in Palo Alto, California (e.g., Broderick & Schrader, 1991; Gurman & Frankel, 2002). Although many considered such practices to be unique and groundbreaking, more traditional therapists viewed these activities as unethical, because they believed that therapists should not treat more than one member of a family.

Recalling this history now seems quaint. Relational therapy, in one form or another, is now practiced by a majority of mental health practitioners (Norcross, Hedges, & Castle, 2002), and a significant body of research has shown that various forms of marital and family therapy are both safe and effective (e.g., Pinsof, Wynne, & Hambright, 1996; Prince & Jacobson, 1995; Shadish, Ragsdale, Glaser, & Montgomery, 1995). Nevertheless, these treatment modalities present ethical and legal challenges that have received little attention in the literature.

PRINCIPLES OF BIOMEDICAL ETHICS

We base our ethical discussion on a system commonly referred to as principle-based or "prima facie" ethics. These terms refer to a system developed by English philosopher W. D. Ross (1877–1940), who tried to resolve the problems associated with both utilitarian and deontological theories of philosophy. According to Ross, the best ethical theory rests on certain basic moral principles he referred to as "prima facie duties." By this he meant that an obligation would be maintained unless it was overridden by a superior one (Knapp & Vande-Creek, 2006). There is now common agreement that there are five such principles: autonomy, nonmaleficence, beneficence, justice, and fidelity (for a detailed discussion of these principles, see Beauchamp & Childress, 2001).

"Autonomy" refers to freedom of choice; that is, people are free to choose their own course of action so long as they are responsible for their own behavior. Autonomy includes both the right to act as a free agent and the idea that if we wish to be treated as autonomous persons, we should treat others in the same manner (Kitchener, 1984). From this principle, various ethical standards can be derived, such as respect for a client's privacy and providing informed consent.

The concept of "nonmaleficence" is derived from the medical principle of *primum non necere*, or "above all do no harm." This obligation requires that one not cause intentional harm or act in a way that risks causing harm. Although marital therapy does not entail the same risks as thoracic surgery, our work is not benign and, as we will see, certain unavoidable iatrogenic risks inhere in this treatment format.

"Beneficence" refers to the fact that we should work for the betterment of others. In other words, we are required not only to avoid harm but also to contribute to the welfare of others (e.g., American Psychological Association, 2002, Principle A) and to work for social justice (e.g., ethical principles; National Association of Social Workers, 1996). As we see below, when therapists have couples as clients, working for the benefit of both partners can be very challenging.

Ethics scholars' use of the term "justice" generally refers to the Aristotelian notion that we should treat others as equals and unequals unequally, but only in proportion to their relative differences (Kitchener, 1984, p. 49). For example, such issues arise in couple therapy when decisions must be made regarding a disproportionate allocation of limited family resources.

The final principle, "fidelity," or "professional–patient relationships," includes elements such as the obligation of veracity, or truth telling (Beauchamp & Childress, 2001, p. 284). For example, fidelity is one of the bases for our obligation to provide informed consent. But what are we to do when certain therapeutic techniques require deception? Another aspect of fidelity is the notion that we must place the welfare of clients above that of our own and work for their benefit. In a legal sense, this creates a fiduciary duty between the therapist and the couple, but the goal of fidelity can be quite difficult to achieve when couples present with opposing interests that are not readily solvable.

SYSTEMS THEORY

Couple therapy can be performed with a variety of theoretical approaches, as this volume demonstrates. We choose to base our discussion on the principles of systems theory, because we believe the ethical challenges that couple therapists face are best understood from this perspective.

Systems theory is not a unitary concept; thinking in this area has evolved and expanded in a variety of directions, and has been applied to the understanding of biological, social, and cultural systems. Discussion of all of these notions is beyond the scope of this chapter. Here, we focus on the most basic and widely held systemic assumptions that directly impinge on marital therapy.

1. In its most basic formulation, systems theory holds that a group of interrelated parts functions as a larger unit of analysis (Becvar & Becvar, 2006). Systems theory maintains that families, like other systems, are greater than the sum of their parts, and that change in one part of the system can create changes elsewhere.

2. Systems theory emphasizes the contextually based nature of human behavior. Rather than maintaining a focus on individuals in a decontextualized manner, as do certain individual therapy approaches, systems theory focuses on interdependence and the notion that, based on the circumstances in which we find ourselves, our behavior varies. Because our primary relationships establish a basic relational context for our behavior, we assume that working with couples is a more eco-

logically valid and effective approach to relational problems.

3. Human behavior cannot be understood in a logical or linear fashion, such that we can explain C if we know how A caused B. Rather, systems theory emphasizes the circular and recurring nature of behavior, which makes the search for ultimate causes impossible. As a result, systems approaches to therapy entail interrupting dysfunctional behavioral patterns to provide an opportunity for healthier ones to emerge.

4. Systems theory does not explain how behavior changes. Rather, it teaches us how behavior remains the same; that is, presenting problems often represent a way couples have found to maintain problems rather than to solve them. Systems-oriented practitioners understand that the solution for the couple may lie in addressing issues of which they are unaware by disrupting dysfunctional interactional patterns rather than helping clients to understand them better.

5. "Triangulation" refers to the notion that when two persons are in conflict, each will try to align with a third person (or, at times, with a philosophical principle, value, or standard) to avoid or to gain assistance with the stressful dyad (Nichols & Schwartz, 1998; e.g., by increasing that person's influence in the dyad). For example, a husband might intensify his relationship with his son as an alternative to addressing a problematic relationship with his wife. Minuchin (1974) noted that this structure frequently places children in the uncomfortable position of being unable to satisfy both parents, because alignment with one is seen as an attack on the other. Systems-oriented practitioners remain mindful of this idea and work to maintain neutrality, because failing to do so may erode therapeutic effectiveness.

ETHICAL CHALLENGES

As we noted earlier, many psychotherapists viewed any type of multiperson therapy as unethical when it was first introduced. Now, over 50 years later, treating couples is considered common practice (Norcross et al., 2001), but it still presents us with unique ethical challenges that individual therapists do not encounter. To date, seven challenges have been identified that apply to couple, family, and group therapy. Below we describe these issues and the dilemmas they can create, list the alternatives that pertain to each, and provide recommen-

dations where possible (the first three issues were originally identified by Margolin [1982]).

Definition of the Client

The Problem

In any form of multiperson therapy, a practitioner's first and most important question is, "Who is the client?" Another way to ask this question is, "To whom am I primarily responsible?" Is the obligation to the couple, or to a more broadly defined "system," such as the members of a couple and a parent who lives in their home and provides care for the children? Or might it be the person for whom treatment is sought, such as the "identified patient?" Alternatively, should we consider treating the member who brings the couple into therapy even though he or she feels that the problem lies with the other?

The concern regarding defining the client is based on the systemic assumption that any intervention, even with an individual, may have an affect on one or another family members (Minuchin, 1974). Such a possibility can cause significant problems, because any intervention on behalf of one member may not be in the interest of another. Consider the following example:

John and Mary Smith present for marital therapy. Mary has decided to leave the relationship and agreed to marital therapy in response to John's request to give it "one last try." Although John is willing to do anything to keep her, Mary's motivation to pursue treatment is at best ambivalent.

This is an all-too-common scenario for couple therapists, and it creates a fundamental ethical dilemma. How is the practitioner to work on behalf of both parties when they have competing goals and actions that might benefit one but harm the other? To expand the problem only a bit further, what about the children? Whereas the therapist has no legal duty to nonclients, systems-oriented therapists cannot ignore the potential adverse impact that a divorce might have upon the children (see Lebow, Chapter 15, this volume).

A similar problem arises in the following example:

Susie and Bill Jones bring their son Bill Jr. for individual psychotherapy. Whereas Susie believes that Bill Jr. is distressed, Bill Sr. believes he is underdisciplined and blames Susie for the problem. After an initial assessment, the practitioner recommends couple therapy for Bill and Susie, based on the assumption that Bill Jr. is the symptom bearer of the marital conflict. Bill Sr. responds, claiming that any problems in the family are Susie's fault, and he is unwilling to participate in any relational counseling.

In this example, the practitioner is left in a difficult situation. If he or she proceeds with treatment but does not include Bill Sr., treatment efficacy may be compromised, and Bill Jr. could deteriorate even further. On the other hand, if the therapist adheres to his or her initial recommendation, and Bill Sr. refuses to involve himself, the family might receive no services.

Alternatives

There are a number of alternatives available to the couple therapist that may resolve these questions. Following the first example, the potential for competing interests requires that the therapist make a thorough clinical assessment of the situation before agreeing to proceed. For example, he or she may determine that Mary's motivation is insufficient to proceed with marital therapy despite John's wishes. If so, agreeing to work with the couple, and being equally responsible to both, would be quite inadvisable, because the course of treatment is unlikely to be effective and is potentially harmful to one or both of them.

Alternatively, Mary might agree to a time-limited period of evaluation/exploration to determine whether she might find some hope for proceeding with a longer-term commitment to the treatment process. In this case, the therapist could accept the couple as the client for this limited purpose, so long as the agreement is reviewed at some predetermined point in the future.

What if Mary is unwilling to engage in either of these alternatives? Rather, she states that she is only leaving the marriage as a result of John's problems. She plans to move out and contends that were John to receive help, she might be willing to return after he has demonstrated progress in her eyes. In this situation, the therapist might agree to work with John individually, using Mary as a collateral resource assisting in the treatment, and if the treatment went well, Mary might agree to return for couple therapy later. (We address related situations in a later section on change of format.)

The second example presents similar conflicts. It would be inappropriate for the therapist to exert pressure on Bill Sr. to comply with treatment recommendations. Doing so would be coercive

and potentially harmful. Alternatively, accepting his terms may very well perpetuate the problems that brought the family for treatment in the first place. Finally, the therapist may determine that proceeding under any circumstances risks greater harm than doing nothing at all.

Recommendations

These examples present complex and vexing dilemmas regarding whether to proceed with the couple therapy, and if so, on what basis? Unfortunately, little guidance is available. The American Association of Marital and Family Therapy (AAMFT) code of ethics does not address this issue, and the *Ethical Principles and Code of Conduct* (American Psychological Association, 2002) devotes only one paragraph to it:

> §10.02(a) When psychologists agree to provide services to several persons who have a relationship (such as spouses, significant others, or parents and children), they take reasonable steps to clarify at the outset (1) which of the individuals are clients/patients and (2) the relationship the psychologist will have with each person. This clarification includes the psychologist's role and the probable uses of the services provided or the information obtained.

This standard contains a number of issues that deserve closer explanation. First, the paragraph assumes that the practitioner has agreed to provide services. As a conservative matter, we must assume that this agreement was preceded by an initial evaluation. It is not advisable to initiate treatment without first making a professional assessment of the presenting problem and recommending a course of treatment. Second, after the plan is presented, a discussion should ensue regarding to whom the practitioner will be responsible. Treatment should not proceed until such agreements are made. To do otherwise creates unnecessary risk for therapists and clients alike. Third, after determining who is to be a client, there may remain a question about what relationship the practitioner will have with other family members. If for example, a family member agrees to serve as a collateral resource, the practitioner must make clear that he or she has no fiduciary obligation to that individual. Fourth, the practitioner must provide a thorough explanation of the advantages and disadvantages of the chosen course. Finally, the American Psychological Association code of conduct omits an important procedural detail.

Because making these agreements is a matter of informed consent, the practitioner must engage in this process as early as is feasible as a matter of respect for autonomy and to avoid harm [AAMFT, 2001, §1.2; American Psychological Association, 2002, §10.01(a)].

We recognize that it may be unappealing to some to engage in such procedures at the outset of a professional relationship. Although such feelings are understandable, we cannot overemphasize the importance of resolving these matters, and taking as much time as is needed to do so, before initiating treatment.

Confidentiality

The notion of confidentiality dates from the Hippocratic Oath (Beauchamp & Childress, 2001, p. 304). It is based on the assumption that clients will only reveal personal information if they have a reasonable expectation that it will remain private and under their control. As a result, confidentiality is a prerequisite to all mental health treatment, and most ethics codes are relatively clear regarding how, and under what circumstances, information may be disclosed to third parties. All 50 states have a statute providing for a psychotherapist–patient privilege, but it takes very different form from state to state. It ranges from stating that the privilege is the same as the attorney–client privilege (e.g., New York and Pennsylvania),[1] to creating a separate act with detailed provisions (e.g., Illinois). Other states (e.g., Maine, New Hampshire, North Carolina, and Virginia) have created a balancing test, making the privilege less reliable. One way or another, the privilege is always held by the patient and must be exercised by the therapist on the patient's behalf, and generally covers communications and records made in the course of treatment. Unfortunately, these ethical standards and laws have limited applicability in couple therapy.

The Problem

The expectation of confidentiality gradually expanded from the doctor–patient relationship to many other types of professional relationships, such as priest–penitent, attorney–client, and ultimately to mental health professionals and their clients. However, all of these protected relationships involved conversation between two persons. In fact, English Common Law held that anything said in the presence of a third party was, by definition, not confidential, and we know of no juris-

diction that has held otherwise. How, then, is a couple therapist to proceed when the couple cannot be ensured confidentiality?

Alternatives

The couple therapist has a choice between two basic alternatives. The first is to treat information provided by each member of the couple in individual sessions as confidential. If there are conjoint sessions, information provided to the therapist during individual sessions would remain confidential. This alternative solves the ethical–legal problem, because the therapist has two individual clients. This option may be more appealing for those who practice from a more traditional or psychodynamic perspective, but it presents two serious disadvantages. First, this alternative requires that the therapist keep information from the other member of the couple to whom he or she is equally responsible. The confidentiality obligation continues even in situations where the information would be vital to the unwitting partner, such as an extramarital affair or the existence of a sexually transmitted disease. By withholding such information, the practitioner risks harming the very person to whom he or she is primarily obligated. Second, treatment effectiveness may be reduced, because information obtained from one member of the couple cannot be used in conjoint sessions with the other. Hence, the therapist's inability to share and use information may reduce the effectiveness of the relational portion of the therapy.

The second alternative is to adopt the opposite position and refuse to keep any information confidential, even if the practitioner conducts individual treatment sessions. This "no secrets" policy is appealing because of its straightforwardness. Taking this position also has the advantage of supporting the couple's relationship, since the therapist reduces the risk of inadvertently aligning with one partner by withholding information from the other. While superficially appealing, this alternative also involves the significant disadvantage that potentially important information will be withheld. For example, little progress can be expected in a situation where the couple is working on "communications issues," while one partner maintains an undisclosed extramarital affair. This is a serious problem, because the therapist, had he or she known of the affair, most certainly would have treated the family quite differently. Therefore, a "no secrets" policy risks compromising treatment effectiveness and harming other family members when vital information is withheld.

In addition to the two alternatives noted earlier, two special circumstances deserve note. First, a therapist might have a "no secrets" policy but agree to keep certain information confidential. This is a common practice when treating children. For example, parents may be given information regarding their child but not necessarily be provided personal details that the child would prefer to remain private. Also, it is common to excuse children from family therapy discussions that involve purely adult matters, such as finances or the couple's sexual relationship. Therefore, keeping certain information confidential is an appealing compromise, especially because it already occurs with some frequency. The dilemma however lies in the question of where to draw the line. How is a therapist to decide in advance which information will be held in confidence and which will not? What criteria would he or she employ in making such a decision? Furthermore, keeping certain information in confidence risks having the therapist become triangulated into the couple's conflict by the member who knows that the information he or she disclosed will not be revealed.

Second, there may be times when a practitioner keeps certain information confidential on a temporary basis. Consider the following:

Helen and Robert Brown present for marital therapy complaining of long-term conflict regarding a number of basic issues. After a few sessions, the therapist meets with each partner individually. Despite the therapist's "no secrets" policy, Robert reveals a previously undisclosed and ongoing extramarital affair. He wants to keep the secret from Helen long enough for the therapist to help him tell her.

This scenario places the practitioner in a very difficult situation. There is little question that he or she has an obligation to inform Helen of the affair. On the other hand, agreeing to keep the secret temporarily might facilitate the disclosure and contribute to a better outcome. However, this means that the therapist would withhold vital information from Helen, who is also a client and to whom he or she is equally obligated.

To make matters worse, what if Robert changes his mind and decides not to reveal the affair to Helen? The therapist can neither inform Helen without violating Robert's confidentiality nor continue the therapy, knowing that Helen is being deceived. In this situation, a therapist might contemplate withdrawing from the case, but he or she should not do so without first considering two issues. First, termination may prompt Helen to speculate about the therapist's reason(s) and could lead to the secret being revealed against Robert's wishes. Second, the therapist must terminate in a way that does not risk abandoning either member of the couple.

Recommendations

There is no ready solution to the problem of managing confidentiality in couple therapy. All available alternatives entail risks that cannot be avoided. One alternative is for the therapist to make decisions on a case-by-case basis using his or her clinical judgment. We contend that doing so is inadvisable, because the therapist will inevitably become confused regarding which rules apply to which couples, raising the possibility of inadvertent disclosures and potential harm.

Unfortunately, therapists are left to make judgments about such matters in the absence of any empirical data to provide guidance. Given the limitations inherent in each approach, we recommend that practitioners establish policy regarding confidentiality based on their theoretical orientation, the population served, and practice niche (for further information, see "Record Keeping"). Such a policy does not avoid all the problems we have mentioned, but we contend that establishing an ethics policy reduces adverse outcomes for two reasons. First, the practitioner who works from only one stance is more likely to be more consistent in his or her approach. Second, the practitioner is more alert to the inherent problems in adopting a particular policy, and more able to deal with them should they arise (for detailed recommendations, see Gottlieb, 1997).

Therapeutic Neutrality

Therapists who treat individuals are expected to be supportive, encouraging, and advocate for the benefit of their client. How does one do this when there are two clients?

The Problem

Systems theory teaches that when treating a couple, the therapist must remain neutral to avoid being triangulated into a dysfunctional family system (Epstein & Loos, 1989; Stancombe & White, 2005). If the therapist violates neutrality and aligns with one family member at the expense of another, treatment effectiveness may be diminished or even lost. Despite this seemingly obvious recommendation, there is no consensus regarding how neutrality should be maintained.

Alternatives

First, the therapist may adopt the position that there will be no conflict of loyalties as long as he or she works for the good of the couple. This is an appealing alternative, in that it would seem to be the best way to avoid conflict. Unfortunately, things are seldom so simple. Consider the following:

Sandra McCall and Lisa Ellsworth come to treatment regarding a conflict over family resources. Sandra and Lisa have sacrificed themselves and their economic resources to no avail in an attempt to help their son Robert, who has a chronic, severe, disabling, and rare medical condition. They were recently informed that a new medical procedure might help Robert. Because it is still experimental, their insurance carrier will not cover the cost of treatment. The only available funds are those in their daughter Jill's college fund. Sandra wants to use the remaining funds to try and help their son, whereas Lisa feels that Jill has already sacrificed enough for her brother and should not be penalized further.

In this example, it is hard to imagine how the therapist could maintain neutrality and work for the good of family members with such deeply held and opposing values.

A second alternative is that the couple therapist may align him- or herself with one or another member of the couple at different times throughout the course of treatment. This approach, sometimes referred to as "multipartiality" (Stancombe & White, 2005), is exemplified by the work of Salvador Minuchin. Although this position is appealing, it is not without its disadvantages. First, one must frequently align with one member of the couple or another. Maintaining neutrality in this way requires much skill. It can be difficult for the therapist, because it requires great personal flexibility, intense concentration, and an ability to repair relational ruptures, so that neither member of the couple feels attacked or ignored for very long. For a therapist with a large number of couples in his or her practice, this approach can be quite tiring. A second problem is that multipartiality assumes that the couple will come to understand the continual shifting of allegiances as indicative of the therapist's neutrality. Such an assumption presumes a certain degree of insight and intellectual

sophistication that all couples may not possess. Finally, unless the therapist is careful, this approach risks premature termination. For example, as we noted in our assumptions, systems-oriented practitioners understand that the solution may lie in addressing issues of which the couple is unaware, and that doing so may disrupt interactional patterns. Such disruptions can be unpleasant. If such an intervention occurs at the end of a therapy session, the member of the couple who feels unsupported by the therapist may feel resentful and later work to sabotage the treatment.

Third, one may take the position of maintaining no alliances at all, declaring loyalty only to achieving the goals presented by the couple. Such "absolute neutrality" may help to maintain a focus on the presenting problem and enhance treatment effectiveness. On the other hand, accepting information provided by the couple at face value risks ignoring potentially critical clinical information. For example, many couples present with "communication problems," but experienced therapists know that such euphemisms can mask far more serious problems. If the therapist accepts the presenting problem at face value and makes no independent assessment, he or she might overlook serious but unvoiced problems, such as substance abuse, chemical dependency, and/or intimate partner violence (IPV). A second problem in having "no alliances" is its value-free assumption. This alternative may be appealing to social constructionist and narrative therapists, but we contend, as have others, that value-free practice is difficult, if not impossible, to achieve (Patterson, 1958; Vachon & Agresti, 1992; Wachtel, 1993; for an interesting discussion of this issue, see Tjeltveit, 2006).

Finally, there are at least two circumstances in which its may be necessary for even the most devoted systems therapist must abandon therapeutic neutrality. The most obvious example is that of child abuse or neglect. To qualify for funding under the Child Abuse Treatment and Prevention Act, all 50 states have passed some type of statute that mandates reporting of suspected maltreatment of a child to the authorities. If a therapist has reason to believe that one member of the couple may be mistreating a child, he or she can no longer remain neutral and must act to protect the child. Although taking such action clearly risks a rupture in the therapeutic relationship, some research has indicated that this outcome is not inevitable (Watson & Levine, 1989; Weinstein, Levine, & Kogan, 2000).

A second exception to maintaining neutrality arises in cases of IPV. There are a wide variety of views on whether therapists should even see couples under these circumstances, and if so, which criteria should be used in making the determination (e.g., Dutton & Corvo, 2006; Trute, 1998). Although a discussion of this issue is the beyond the scope of this chapter, we note it here, because there are times when a member of the couple may be victimized, and the therapist must act to protect him or her. This issue is addressed in more detail by O'Leary (Chapter 16, this volume).

Recommendations

There is general agreement that neutrality is a prerequisite to therapeutic effectiveness, but there is no consensus on how it should be maintained, and we are unaware of any empirical data that support one position over another. Therefore, practitioners must find an approach that works, consistent with the population they serve, their theoretical orientation, and "practice niche." As we noted earlier, adhering to one position consistently remains the preferred choice for effective risk management (Gottlieb, 1997).

In addition to navigating the murky waters of neutrality, we must recognize that neutrality must at times be abandoned to protect vulnerable populations. Many data suggest that sizable percentages of practitioners resist making such reports (e.g., Flaherty et al., 2006). Although such decisions can be extremely difficult, there are times when following the law must supersede ethical guidelines, because failing to do so can incur criminal penalties (e.g., Florida, Oklahoma, and Texas; for further reading on conflicts between ethics and the law, see Knapp, Gottlieb, Berman, & Handelsman, 2007).

Iatrogenic Risk

As a matter of public policy, the work of mental health professionals is considered beneficial both to individuals and society (e.g., "the mental health of our citizenry, no less than its physical health, is a public good of transcendent importance"; *Jaffee v. Redmond*, 1996). We consider ourselves to be healers, and for the most part we reward society's expectations of us with good work. On the other hand, counseling and psychotherapy are not always benign processes; discomfort and/or harm can result when practitioners are ignorant, incompetent, and/or distressed. But all forms of

psychotherapy entail some iatrogenic risk, that is, some discomfort may be unavoidable even when treatment is provided competently and is successful (e.g., Kitchener, 1984; for a detailed discussion, see Beauchamp & Childress, 2001). Hence, practitioners must weigh potential discomfort and harm against expected long-term benefits for each client they choose to treat.

The General Problem

When a therapist agrees to treat a couple, assessing potential iatrogenic risk becomes more complex; the therapist has two tasks. First, he or she must make a risk–benefit assessment for each member of the couple, as would an individual therapist. Second, if the outcome of the individual assessment for both parties is favorable, he or she must then perform a similar analysis based on interactional or relational factors. This problem was elegantly articulated by O'Shea and Jessee (1982), who defined "iatrogenic risk" as a situation in which "a previously asymptomatic family member may become symptomatic during or subsequent to therapy" (p. 15).

If we are to treat couples, this risk seems unavoidable in cases such as that of the Smiths. However, two considerations mitigate this problem. First, O'Shea and Jessee's definition was based on a theoretical assumption from systems theory; it is good advice, because it suggests a conservative course. However, recent data suggest that such an adverse impact is not always the case (Liddle, 2004). Although this is encouraging news, it does not preclude the need for the assessment we noted earlier.

Second, individual risk–benefit assessments may yield troubling findings. Consider the following:

Molly and Larry Short request couple therapy due to significant communications problems. Molly asserts that Larry does not understand her and is verbally abusive. Larry claims that Molly responds to him in ways that are incomprehensible to him. He denies ever mistreating Molly and is unable to understand what he did that so upset Molly, despite his ongoing efforts to comply with her wishes and understand her point of view.

Given the potential seriousness of this situation, the therapist decides to perform individual assessments. The assessments revealed that whereas Larry was generally functioning well, Molly had posttraumatic stress disorder due to severe child abuse, of which Larry was only vaguely aware.

What is a couple therapist to do in such a situation? A variety of treatment plans may be derived on the basis of one's theoretical orientation, but even the most devoted systems therapist must consider the possibility that therapy from an experienced and skilled individual therapist is the preferred course for Molly, and that any type of relational therapy may need to be postponed.

Specific Iatrogenic Risks

In addition to the general problem noted earlier, systems-oriented couple therapy also presents specific iatrogenic issues based on certain theoretical approaches. In this section we discuss some of the problems that can arise when using these treatment modalities.

UNWITTING COERCION

Couple therapists see themselves as helpers and healers, who intend to hurt no one and certainly do not view themselves as coercive agents. Unfortunately, there are circumstances in which clients may be coerced into therapy without the practitioner's knowledge. This problem can arise in a variety of clinical situations, but one of the greatest dangers may arise in cases of undisclosed IPV.

Ann and Jeff Carter presented for couple therapy. Both complained of chronic conflict. Ann complained that Jeff was easily angered over minor matters, and Jeff said that Ann was becoming too independent and less concerned with his needs. The therapist decided to help by improving communication between them, but after a number of weeks, they had made no progress. Only by virtue of an offhand remark did the therapist become suspicious that Jeff was physically abusing Ann, who had not disclosed the mistreatment in his presence.

This is a vexing situation in which the therapist may have unwittingly supported Jeff's coercion and abetted his abuse. However, couple therapists are not clairvoyant, and it is often very hard to identify IPV at the outset of treatment. Routinely screening for IPV is a prudent measure, and we recommend it, but even if Ann had been asked about such a problem, there is some likelihood that she might have denied it.

STRATEGIC AND PARADOXICAL STRATEGIES

One important way to reduce iatrogenic risk is by providing thorough informed consent prior to the initiation of treatment (e.g., AAMFT, 2001,

§1.2; American Psychological Association, 2002, §10.01), but this requirement presents a significant ethical challenge for strategic therapists and others who wish to use paradoxical strategies and other sorts of interventions that, at least to some in the field, may be considered to be deceptive.

Such techniques, firmly grounded in the systemic notion of the need to disrupt dysfunctional interactional patterns, have a long history and can be effective in many clinical situations (Beutler, Moleiro, & Talebi, 2002; Seltzer, 1986). They employ counterintuitive and/or seemingly contradictory instructions that often are intended to confuse clients. Seltzer defined "paradoxical strategies" as "a therapeutic directive or attitude that is perceived by the client, at least initially, as contrary to therapeutic goals, but which is yet rationally understandable and specifically devised by the therapist to achieve these goals" (p. 10). For strategic approaches to be effective, the therapist must play his or her cards close to the chest, not revealing the intention behind the instructions. Furthermore, these approaches are indicated and are most helpful only in situations in which symptoms are under voluntary control, and couples have a documented history of resistance to more direct instructions (Gurman, 1982; Rohrbaugh, Tennen, & Press, 1981). Hence, providing informed consent by explaining the therapist's intentions with such couples would likely reduce treatment effectiveness (Brown & Slee, 1996). For example, Hampton (1991) contended that "informed consent must be reasonably tempered when using paradoxical strategies in the interest of promoting client welfare, as full disclosure could result in premature termination and client harm" (p. 53).

A second problem involves harm that may arise from improper use of these techniques. We have seen inexperienced and/or frustrated therapists use these approaches to act out their own anger against an uncooperative couple. It is unclear to us why strategic approaches seem so vulnerable to misuse in such circumstances, but their use under these conditions is contraindicated and potentially dangerous. Out of an abundance of caution, those who are not thoroughly trained in these approaches should obtain consultation prior to using them (Huber & Barth, 1987).

NOT KNOWING

Narrative therapy is rooted in the postmodern and social constructivist traditions (e.g., Gergen,

1985, 2001). The unique contribution of this body of work is its emphasis on the cultural and political influences that form the ecosystemic context for individual and relational problems (Lyddon, 1995). Some who practice within this theoretical orientation employee a technique referred to as "not knowing," in which the therapist eschews an expert position. Anderson and Goolishian (1992) defined it as means of maintaining neutrality, in which "the therapist's actions and attitudes express a need to know more about what has been said, rather than convey preconceived opinions and expectations about the client, the problem, or what must be changed" (p. 29). This technique and attitude may be helpful in normalizing certain problems, but it also contains certain risks, at least in certain circumstances. For example, some cultures have strong traditions of collectivism, self-sacrifice, and respect for authority (e.g., Smith, 2004). When persons from such backgrounds seek couple therapy, they may be inclined to seek concrete advice from a practitioner. If told that they are the experts about their own situation, they may feel dismissed, confused, and leave treatment, concluding that couple therapy has nothing to offer them. We recommend that one's theoretical orientation not take precedence over client welfare, and that when specific, treatment-relevant questions are asked, they should be answered as a matter of respect for a client's autonomy (for further reading on diversity issues, see Sue & Sue, 2003).

Recommendations

There are iatrogenic risks inherent in all therapeutic approaches, and systems-oriented couple therapy is no exception. From this brief discussion, it should be clear that there is no way to avoid all of these pitfalls. Rather, one must be alert to the specific iatrogenic risks that exist within one's practice niche and take appropriate steps to avoid or mitigate them when they arise or are suspected. Being alert for IPV, monitoring one's resentful feelings toward a couple, and offering concrete recommendations, where indicated, are all prudent ways to minimize risk and enhance client welfare.

Change of Format

The term "change of format" was first used by Margolin (1982) as an example of frequently encountered problems of confidentiality in couple

therapy. She noted that ethical dilemmas can arise when a therapist who had been treating an individual changes the format to work conjointly with the individual and his or her spouse, or vise versa. Later, Gottlieb (1986) operationally defined this term as "a circumstance in which the formal definition of the client changes after the initiation of treatment such that the responsibility of the therapist is altered." He then identified three specific ethical issues that arise in these circumstances (Gottlieb, 1995). Before reviewing these, consider the following example:

Jennifer Cooper called a couple therapist for assistance. Based on a telephone screening, an initial conjoint assessment session was recommended for Jennifer and her husband. Jennifer agreed and said that she and her husband Mike would be there. At the appointed hour Jennifer appeared by herself. She explained that Mike was suddenly called away on business, and she thought she could use the time for some of her own issues. The therapist agreed to see her, with the understanding that couple therapy remained the initial treatment plan. Another five individual sessions ensued before Mike arrived.

Confidentiality and Change of Format

Assuming that Mike is to be incorporated into the treatment process, how is the therapist to manage the information he or she has already obtained from Jennifer? Ideally, Jennifer would have agreed to a "no secrets" policy from the outset. If so, she would have no objection to the therapist sharing with Mike any information she had disclosed. However, after a number of treatment sessions, she may now be reluctant or even unwilling to share certain information with Mike.

This problem might have been resolved at the first session had Jennifer been asked to sign a release giving the therapist permission to share information with Mike. Had this been done, the therapist might feel free to proceed unencumbered. However, can the therapist safely presume that Jennifer will remember all the information she has revealed? Is it possible that she forgot about this agreement and shared with the therapist information she did not want Mike to know? Because the therapist cannot know Jennifer's feelings about this issue, it would be prudent for him or her to review the agreement, as well as some of the information that had been revealed, to ensure that the "no secrets" policy, is still in force. If after this review, Jennifer remains comfortable with the arrangement, it may be safe to proceed with couple therapy. But it is also possible that, after this discussion, Jennifer might assert her right to confidentiality. If so, the therapist would have little choice but to refuse to proceed with couple therapy, because he or she has good reason to believe that therapeutic neutrality cannot be maintained because of the need to keep secrets. The couple would need to be referred elsewhere, and Jennifer and the therapist would have to decide whether to proceed with individual therapy, in addition to couple therapy.

Professional Responsibility and Change of Format

As we noted earlier, the practitioner has an obligation to clarify the nature of the professional relationship with each person involved and to maintain equal professional responsibility for all clients (see the sections "Definition of the Client" and "Therapeutic Neutrality"). In the preceding example, how is the therapist to incorporate Mike into an ongoing individual therapy that he or she intends to change to conjoint treatment? For example, what risks are entailed in shifting from the previous position of exclusive responsibility to Jennifer to a new position of neutrality and equal responsibility for both partners? Is there a risk that Jennifer will feel betrayed by the therapist who used to be aligned with her? On the other hand, will Mike be apprehensive about entering a situation in which he fears that Jennifer and the therapist may already be aligned against him? How would the therapist persuade Mike of his or her neutrality? Finally, will the therapist risk alienating Jennifer when he or she spends a disproportionate amount of time at the outset establishing a relationship with Mike?

Iatrogenic Risk and Change of Format

As we noted earlier, when providing individual therapy to a married person, that person's spouse may deteriorate as he or she improves. In the case of Jennifer and Mike, the reverse must also be considered. For example, Jennifer may have made gains during the individual treatment sessions. If the therapist agrees to the change of format, he or she risks loss or deterioration of the progress Jennifer has made. In such a case, the therapist might unintentionally harm the person to whom he or she was primarily obligated.

Recommendations

Change of format is hardly new to mental health practitioners. As we noted earlier, children are often excused from family therapy when adult matters are discussed. When children are seen in individual therapy, one or both parents may often be incorporated into the process at the end of a session. Hence, changing format is commonplace and generally is considered helpful. Nevertheless, some guidelines may be useful in facilitating the process.

First, the therapist should make clear his or her systems perspective, even during an initial telephone call. Among other things, informing the prospective client of a "no secrets" policy should be a major consideration. Once treatment has begun, we recommend that the therapist maintain a focus on sharing rather than concealing information as a matter of respect for their relationship. Second, it is the responsibility of a couple therapist to be aware of the literature regarding the risks and benefits of individual versus couple therapy. Moving from an individual to a conjoint format is not risk-free, and the practitioner must remember that his or her primary obligation is to the existing client. Even if the client agrees to conjoint therapy, the wise therapist will ask how the client anticipates he or she will feel when the spouse joins them. Once conjoint treatment begins, it is highly advisable that the therapist ask the original client periodically how he or she feels about the change in format. Third, the couple therapist needs to remain mindful of potentially having additional responsibilities to the incoming spouse. We recommend that the therapist review the agreement with the original client and determine whether the incoming spouse understands it and wants to proceed. If so, the therapist should take as much time as is necessary to join with the new client before proceeding conjointly. Finally, making these decisions is not always a clear-cut matter. It is always advisable to provide clients with ample opportunity to discuss the risks and benefits of all treatment alternatives and time to think about them in advance.

Live Supervision

Live supervision, which has been an integral part of couple therapy since its inception, has many advantages, and it has now become a powerful teaching tool from which many benefit. Originally, live supervision was practiced relatively unobtrusively. Soon, telephones were installed to allow supervisors to communicate with therapists only when necessary to minimize disruption (Haley, 1976). The next stage led to a wide variety of experiments in an effort to improve the quality of interventions (e.g., Selvini-Palazzoli, Boscolo, Cecchin, & Prata, 1978; Minuchin & Montalvo, 1967). These experiments led Gottlieb (1995) to comment that "these developments have created a situation in which a method of training has become a form of therapy in which families are no longer treated by an individual but by a group" (p. 565). From an ethical perspective, he asked, "Who is the therapist? Or Who is professionally responsible for the family?" (Gottlieb, 1995, p. 565). He concluded that use of this treatment modality gave rise to three general ethical issues.

Professional Responsibility

The couple therapist has an obligation to clarify his or her own professional role, as well as that of the other members of the team (e.g., American Psychological Association, 2002, §10.02) as a matter of informed consent (e.g., AAMFT, 2001, §1.2; and American Psychological Association, 2002, §10.01). In "vertical models" (Gottlieb, 1995), lines of responsibility are clear-cut. For example, in training situations, a student therapist informs the couple about his or her status, and that the supervisor behind the one-way mirror is ultimately responsible for their care.

"Horizontal models" (e.g., Selvini-Palazzoli et al., 1978) create additional problems when no clear lines of authority are established. For example, who is to be contacted in case of emergency? How are decisions to be made if a team member disagrees with the others? How are lines of responsibility established? Who is ultimately responsible for the care of the couple?

Informed Consent

What is a couple told in advance about live supervision? For example, some couples may be reluctant to engage in this process out of legitimate concerns regarding privacy. If so, are alternative treatment options offered? If the service is offered for free or at low cost, would the partners feel some degree of pressure to remain if they could not obtain similar services elsewhere, without incurring additional cost or inconvenience? A second con-

cern surrounds interruptions from the team (e.g., Smith, Smith, & Saltz, 1991). How does the couple have confidence in a therapist who appears to need the supervision of so many others (Bullock & Kobayashi, 1978)?

Iatrogenic Risk

Social psychologists have known for many years that people make more extreme or riskier decisions in groups, especially when the group comprises like-minded individuals, than they would as individuals. This well-documented phenomenon is termed the "risky shift" (Hinsz & Davis, 1984). (More recently it has also been referred to as "choice shift" or "group polarization.") The obvious implication of this effect is that a team may recommend more extreme measures than would an individual therapist. If so, they risk harming the couple (Gottlieb, 1995). Furthermore, the probability of the team making more risky decisions increases in ambiguous situations (Elmes & Gemmill, 1990). Risk is also increased in situations when social status plays a role in the process, because lower status and less experienced trainees are more likely to defer to senior colleagues (Schaller, 1992). Should this effect change the way live supervision is conducted? Is there a way to control the group's influence?

Recommendations

Live supervision has been transformed from a teaching tool to a therapeutic technique. This change arose as a natural evolution of the field, but little research has been done to demonstrate its effectiveness (Kivlighan, Angelone, & Swafford, 1991), and little attention has been paid to the ethical issues it presents.

To some degree, the issues presented by live supervision are less worrisome today. The experimentation of the 1980s is over, and the advent of managed care has significantly restricted reimbursement for practitioners, making live supervision less practical due to its added expense. For example, two of use (Gottlieb and Simpson) live in an urban area of nearly 6 million people but are aware of only two locations in which live supervision is available to students. Furthermore, many of the problems noted here have been addressed and resolved by thoughtful trainers, who have taken these concerns into account (Personal communication, Dr. Shelly Riggs, May 12, 2007).

We feel that a useful way to think about the ethical issues involved in live supervision is to ask how we would like to be treated if it were offered to us. In that spirit we have the following recommendations.

Because live supervision is not something with which most clients are familiar, we recommend that, as a matter of informed consent, agency policies be explained fully. At a minimum, the couple should know the identities of the therapist and team members, their level of training and experience, who will be responsible for their care, and who is to be contacted in case of emergency. Finally, a couple that is uncomfortable with this format should be offered other treatment options with which the partners are more comfortable.

In our view, vertical models, in which lines of authority and decision making are unambiguous, are safer. If group members are to have an equal say in decision making, a senior practitioner should monitor the process and act to contain more risky recommendations. Finally, all these matters should be memorialized in a written agency policy that is provided to practicum students, interns, supervisors, and clients. Explaining these policies should be part of every annual trainee orientation and ongoing staff development.

Record Keeping

Record keeping is a necessary professional responsibility, because it improves the quality of care and provides for continuity of treatment (e.g., American Psychological Association, 2002, §6.01; AAMFT, 2001, §3.7). As with many other ethical principles, our record-keeping requirements come from the medical tradition, in which a physician has one patient and maintains an individual record.

The Problem

Unlike individual therapists, couple therapists have two clients, and interventions are generally relational in nature. But may a therapist keep one record for both clients (hereafter referred to as a comingled record), or should he or she keep two separate, individual records? A number of years ago, the Texas State Board of Examiners of Psychologists (TSBEP) published an opinion regarding record keeping in couple therapy, stating that "Separate patient files should be kept on each of the couple. Co-mingling of records should be

avoided" (*TSBEP Newsletter*, Spring 1992, p. 2). As one can imagine, this opinion was met with a firestorm of criticism from the marriage and family therapy community, and it was later rescinded. Even though this proposal was eventually withdrawn, ethical dilemmas surrounding comingled records continue.

Issue

A major problem with comingled records occurs when a couple therapist receives a request from a client to release information. For example, what if the partners have ended their relationship or divorced, and one of them requests individual therapy from another practitioner? In such a case, it is typical for the couple therapist to receive a release from one member of the couple to transmit information about him or her to the new therapist. But the couple therapist cannot release the entire record without first obtaining permission from the other member of the former couple. Releasing the entire record without permission would violate the couple therapist's obligation to maintain the confidentiality of the other member of the couple. This issue often arises when couples previously seen in treatment decide to divorce and litigate matters regarding child custody. In such cases, one or the other member of the former couple may seek the couple therapist's records to use to his or her advantage in the lawsuit. But what if the other member of the former couple refuses to allow the couple therapist to release the record? If so, he or she is now caught in the dilemma of trying to help one member of the former couple at the possible expense of the other.

Recommendations

There is no doubt that maintaining comingled records presents both ethical and legal difficulties that individual therapists do not encounter. Nevertheless, for those who choose to practice relational therapies, we contend that a comingled record is preferable to two individual ones. The more important reason is that a comingled record is the one place where interactional data can be preserved. Because relational therapies are based on interpersonal interventions, the comingled record is the only place where such clinical notes can be made, thereby providing the greatest benefit to the couple (Gottlieb, 1993).

As with the other ethical dilemmas we have discussed, there are no straightforward answers to the problems presented by keeping comingled records, but many problems associated with them can be prevented by a thorough informed consent procedure at the outset of treatment. Specifically, it is necessary that the couple therapist inform the couple that the record cannot be released without the written permission of both parties, and that he or she take as much time as is needed to explain the process and requirements for releasing information to others.

In response to these dilemmas, one may ask why it is not simpler to avoid all these problems by redacting all references to the other member of the couple, then sending the record to the requesting party. In fact, at least one state requires it:

> Licensees who release confidential record relating to a patient or client that also contain confidential information relating to a second patient or client that the licensee obtained through the provision of services to that second individual, and who lack consent or other legal authority to disclose the second individual's identity and/or records, must remove all identifying and confidential information relating to the second individual before releasing the records. [Texas State Board of Examiners of Psychologists, 2006, §465.12(f)]

We do not know how many other states have such provisions in their regulations, but we consider redacting a record undesirable. First, it is very difficult to protect the identity of the other party without redacting very large portions of the record; doing so may leave very little that would be of any use to another practitioner. Furthermore, the remaining information may be misleading, because it was obtained in a conjoint rather than an individual format. Because behavior is contextually based, it is not prudent for a new therapist to assume that his or her client will present in a manner similar to that reflected in the comingled record.

Finally, what if the other member of the couple cannot be located? This is less of a problem when married couples with children divorce, so long as they maintain family ties. But many therapists see couples who choose to not marry and/or are unable to do so. When these couples separate, there are fewer ties that would help the couple therapist locate the former partner. We are unaware of any law or regulation that specifically addresses this issue, but we recommend that the therapist always assert the privilege on behalf of the missing member of the couple and refuse to release their records without a court order. Because

this void leaves couple therapists in a very difficult position, we recommend that a local attorney be consulted before releasing the information.

With regard to custody litigation, laws vary widely. Some states (e.g., Texas and Alabama) specifically prevent the assertion of the privilege in custody matters and compel the disclosure of the records. Others (e.g., Indiana and Kentucky) hold that an affirmative request for custody places a party's mental health into question; therefore, the privilege is automatically waived. In still other states (e.g., New York and Kansas), courts have held that the children's paramount interests trump the parties' individual privilege. Finally, some states (e.g., Michigan, Mississippi, and Missouri), even in matters involving custody, uphold the privilege and prohibit disclosure of information. We would prefer to offer clear guidance on this matter, but given differing legal requirements across the states, the reader is well-advised to consult a knowledgeable attorney to be informed regarding the law in his or her jurisdiction before engaging in relational therapies.

If asked, most lawyers would advise practitioners to not keep comingled records as a matter of prudent risk management due to the complexities they create. This would especially be so when legal disputes arise (see the following section for a detailed discussion of how to manage these situations). Nevertheless, we contend that maintaining comingled records is ethically appropriate and clinically indicated, because it captures contextually based interactional data that are vital to successful relational counseling. Although it is not without its challenges, we contend that keeping individual records would lead to a loss of the very information that would be vital to helping a couple (Gottlieb, 1993).

In concluding this section, we would be remiss if we did not take a moment to discuss the importance of adequate record keeping. Many misguided practitioners continue to believe that *de minimus* record keeping somehow protects them from professional and legal liability. In our view, nothing could be further from the truth. We simply wish to remind the reader that couple therapists have fiduciary obligations to their clients. Keeping thorough records is both our ethical obligation and the best way to provide good care. Furthermore, in the event of an ethics complaint and/or civil law suit, a sound record can be the next best thing to a friendly witness (for further reading regarding the importance of record keeping, see Bennett et al., 2007).

LEGAL ISSUES

As licensed professionals, couple therapists function within the legal system. Yet many know little about how the system operates and are often frightened by it. In this section, we review some typical situations that may arise when treating couples and offer general suggestions for how they may be addressed to provide good care, protect clients' rights, and practice good risk management. Please note that our recommendations should not be construed as legal advice. Therapists should always consult an attorney familiar with the law in their jurisdiction whenever legal questions arise.

Dealing with Subpoenas

At one point or another, couple therapists are likely to receive subpoenas for comingled records. Practitioners who receive such subpoenas are well advised to remember that releasing information without a client's permission may expose them to both state regulatory board complaints and civil suit. In this section, we address how one should deal with such requests. We consider how to provide information to a client's attorney, then address how to protect information in adversarial situations. We conclude with how best to manage testifying about one's clients when it becomes necessary to do so.

Subpoenas

A "subpoena" is a writ that commands a person to appear before a court and subjects him or her to a penalty for failing to comply; if it includes a request for records, it is referred to as a *subpoena duces tecum* (for further reading, see Committee on Legal Issues, 1996). As we noted earlier, it is not unusual for a couple therapist to receive such a subpoena. Upon receipt of such an order, one should never assume that it should automatically be obeyed.

WHEN NO RELEASE IS INCLUDED
FOR AN INDIVIDUAL CLIENT

It is often the case that subpoenas are sent with no release from the client or former client. To our knowledge, there is no jurisdiction that would allow the couple therapist to release information about a client without a release, because doing so would violate the client's right to keep the information confidential.

When no release is included, the couple therapist is well advised to call the sender of the subpoena, usually a lawyer, and respectfully decline to release the information, explaining that no release was included. Making a note of this conversation in the record is a must, and it is best to follow the telephone call with a letter to the requesting attorney, reminding him or her of the telephone conversation, and restating the reason the therapist is unable to release record. Absent a release, the therapist should provide no information to the attorney. For example, one might say:

> "I'm sorry, but absent a competent waiver [the legal term for a release], I am unable to tell you whether the person named in the subpoena is or ever was a client of mine."

The attorney will generally understand and accept this explanation; often this omission is an oversight, and a release follows. If a release is not forthcoming, the couple therapist should do nothing further, other than to notify the client of the action taken.

WHEN A RELEASE IS INCLUDED
FOR AN INDIVIDUAL CLIENT

It would seem that in this situation, one could send the record without further concern; typically, this may be the case, but we recommend an additional step. Even though a release has been enclosed, we suggest first calling the client to inform him or her of receipt of the subpoena and asking whether he or she knew about it, and to explain his or her understanding of what the release entails. Explain the general obligation to maintain confidentiality and determine the client's wishes, noting that the client still has the right to rescind the release if he or she so chooses. If the client agrees to releasing the information, explain to him or her the risks and benefits of doing so. One might go so far as to mention that previously disclosed, specific and/or sensitive information is contained in the record. Because the client may not remember giving the therapist this information when he or she signed the release, the reminder may prompt a change of mind. If the client chooses to rescind the release, the therapist must respond to the subpoena as discussed earlier, noting that the release has been withdrawn. The therapist should also encourage the client to call his or her lawyer to explain the reasons for the change.

Regardless of the outcome of this conversation, the therapist should follow the conversation with a letter to the client explaining his or her understanding of the client's position. We recommend including a place for the client to sign the letter indicating his or her acknowledgment of the therapist's understanding, that the therapist has discussed his or her concerns with the client, and that the client understands those concerns. After following this procedure, if the client still wishes the therapist to share information with his or her lawyer, then document the conversation in the record and proceed to the step below.

WHEN PERMISSION IS RECEIVED

Once these steps have been taken and permission is received, the therapist should call the attorney, identify him- or herself, explain the reason for the call, and offer his or her cooperation as the client has requested. It is always advisable, before sending the record, to determine what information the lawyer is seeking. For example, he or she may only want certain information that the therapist can provide verbally. In this situation, it may not be necessary to send the record, and the client's privacy can be preserved to the maximum degree possible. If the attorney wishes to have the entire file, then we recommend that he or she be made aware that the therapist's compliance with that wish may present certain risks and benefits to the client. For example, if the record contains personal and/or sensitive information that is not relevant to the legal matter, the attorney should be made aware of its existence in the hope that he or she may be able to protect it.

Finally, we would be remiss if we did not mention that lawyers often ask questions that therapists cannot answer. For example, "Well, Doctor, don't you think that my client would be the better parent of the two?" Unfortunately, some therapists, out of a boundless desire to help and/or ignorance, answer such a question, even though they should not. In this example, only a court-appointed custody evaluator can answer that question. For a therapist to do so exceeds the boundaries of his or her competence (e.g., American Psychological Association, 2002, §2.01) and is unethical (for a more detailed treatment of this issue, see Greenberg & Shuman, 1997; Committee on Ethical Guidelines for Forensic Psychologists, 1991). It is also likely that testifying to such a conclusion in court will lead to a blistering cross-examination and the likely exclusion of the testimony (see Federal Rule of Evidence 702; *Kumho Tire Co., Ltd. v. Carmichael*, 526 U.S. 137, 119 S. Ct. 1167 [1999]; and *Daubert v. Merrell Dow Pharmaceuticals, Inc.*, 509 U.S. 579, 113 S. Ct. 2786 [1993]). It is not rare for a state regulatory board complaint to follow. Therefore, therapists are well advised to provide information only to the extent that their data permit.

A RELEASE IS INCLUDED FOR ONE MEMBER BUT NOT ANOTHER

If the client was a couple and a subpoena is accompanied by a release from only one of them, the couple therapist should follow the recommendations given earlier, as if no release were obtained. The attorney should be informed that the records are comingled; therefore, the records cannot be provided without releases from all the persons who were clients. If the attorney asks who else was seen as a client, he or she must be reminded that the therapist is not free to disclose that information.

MAKING EFFORTS TO PROTECT THE RECORD

It is not unusual for a couple therapist to receive a subpoena when his or her former clients choose to separate or divorce and child custody is an issue. Unfortunately, the previously recommended steps are not always adequate if an attorney threatens to get a court order to obtain the records. If so ordered, the therapist is required to tender the records, but he or she may take certain steps to prevent having to provide them.

First, we recommend contacting the member of the couple whose release was not included in the subpoena and determining his or her wishes. In some cases, he or she will be unaware of the subpoena and instruct the therapist not to turn over the record. Because the couple therapist has some reason to believe that the requesting attorney will file a motion to compel the therapist to produce the record, he or she is well advised to have the client who has not signed the release contact his or her attorney. By doing so, the attorney for the client who did not sign the release has the opportunity to file a Motion to Quash the subpoena and/or a Motion for a Protective Order. If either of these motions is sustained, the record is protected.

If the client's attorney fails to file such motions, some lawyers recommend that the therapist retain his or her own attorney to file them. This alternative is seldom necessary, and it is expensive. On the other hand, doing so clearly indicates that the therapist has done everything he or she can to protect the client's confidential information.

If such a motion is overruled, the attorney may ask for an *in camera* review of the records by the trial court. In this way, the judge has the opportunity to decide whether certain information can be protected.

By following these steps, the therapist has done everything he or she can to protect the client's record. But, if all the above efforts fail, and the court orders the records to be produced, then the therapist must surrender them. Therefore, the therapist should already have made a copy of the complete file to provide to the court, if the need arises. While failing to cooperate at this juncture means that the therapist risks being cited for contempt of court, cooperating, while perhaps undesirable from the therapist's perspective, assures the therapist that no complaint against him or her can be sustained. One can never be sanctioned for following a court order.

The importance of thorough documentation of all the actions taken cannot be overemphasized. Verbal communications with the client or an attorney should be followed up with a letter. In doing so, the therapist can avoid miscommunications or misunderstanding of his or her position and understanding of the client's position. Having an attorney review such letters is always a good idea.

Testimony

Couple therapists may be called to testify in court for a variety of reasons. In some cases, they do so willingly in an effort to help a client. In other cases, they are subpoenaed to testify despite their efforts to avoid it. We discuss these two possibilities below.

Voluntary Testimony

Most therapists are unfamiliar with their role in the legal process, appropriate courtroom demeanor, and legal procedures. As a result, they may feel apprehensive regarding their testimony, even when trying to help a client. In these cases, it is wise for the therapist to review with the lawyer the questions that will be asked and what to expect from cross-examination. Once the therapist understands what information will be requested, he or she should meet with the client before the trial to review the testimony that will be presented. (This step should also be taken in the case of compelled testimony, discussed below.) This step is vital, because the therapist will often be asked to reveal information that he or she never gave, and did not intend to give, to the client. Therefore, providing this information beforehand helps the client to know what to expect at trial and works to preserve the therapeutic relationship. The client needs to understand that the therapist must answer the questions and is not allowed to refuse to answer. Some of this information may be very distressing to the client, and discussing it beforehand is the best the therapist can do to minimize harm.

Compelled Testimony

Sometimes therapists are called to testify with no release and against their will. If called in such a situation, the therapist may wish to retain counsel to make the necessary motions to protect both the therapist and the client. If the therapist chooses not to retain counsel, then after being sworn in and qualified, it will be necessary for the therapist to refuse respectfully to answer any questions about the client based on the fact that he or she has received no release and the requested information is privileged. At that point, the lawyer who is doing the questioning will ask the court to order the therapist to testify. If the court makes such a ruling, the therapist is released from his or her confidentiality obligation and may testify without fear of recrimination. If it is unclear whether the court has ordered the therapist to testify, it is appropriate for the therapist to ask the court specifically if that is what is being ordered. Once the judge has clarified the ruling, the therapist may testify safely. (For a general review of the process and requirements of expert testimony see Barsky & Gould [2002, pp. 147–187].)

After Testifying

We have every reason to believe that clients will be distressed after listening to their therapist testify about them in open court, even when it is done in the most supportive and caring manner. Therefore, we recommend that the therapist schedule a debriefing session as soon after the testimony as possible. Doing so sends a clear message that the therapist is doing whatever he or she can to preserve the therapeutic relationship in adverse circumstances.

Boundaries of Competence

As we noted earlier, therapists create great risks for themselves if they testify to matters for which they lack scientific support. Therapists are entitled to have opinions regarding a variety of matters, including signs and symptoms of mental and emotional disorders, diagnosis, prognosis, treatment choice, course, and anticipated expense. Going beyond these issues means sailing into treacherous waters. For example, therapists cannot have opinions regarding relative parenting capacity or whether a child has been sexually abused. Doing so hurts the parties involved, is disrespectful to the justice system, and is a formula for personal disaster. (For those unfamiliar with these issues, we recommend a detailed reading of Greenberg & Shuman [1997], who outline with great clarity the differences between therapeutic and forensic roles.)

CONCLUSION

After reading this chapter, some readers may feel deterred from practicing couple therapy because it presents unique legal and ethical challenges that individual therapists do not face. In our view, such a decision would be unfortunate. Our clients live within social and relational contexts that, when taken into account, can enhance treatment effectiveness and enrich their lives. We hope that by providing this information, we have assisted the reader in negotiating these issues, so that he or she can provide these services more safely and effectively.

NOTE

1. Full legal citations for all examples listed are available from the authors upon request.

SUGGESTIONS FOR FURTHER READING

Committee on Legal Issues. (1996). Strategies for private practitioners coping with subpoenas or compelled testimony for client records or test data. *Professional Psychology, 27,* 245–251.

Greenberg, S. A., & Shuman, D. W. (1997). Irreconcilable conflict between therapeutic and forensic roles. *Professional Psychology, 28,* 50–57.

Knapp, S. J., & VandeCreek, L. D. (2006). *Practical ethics for psychologists.* Washington, DC: American Psychological Association.

REFERENCES

American Association of Marriage and Family Therapy. (2001). *AAMFT Code of Ethics.* Washington: Author.

American Psychological Association. (2002). Ethical principles and code of conduct. *American Psychologist, 57,* 1060–1073.

Anderson, H., & Goolishian, H. (1992). The client is the expert: A not-knowing approach to therapy. In S. McNamee & K. J. Gergen (Eds.), *Therapy as social construction* (pp. 25–39). London: Sage.

Barsky, A. E., & Gould, J. W. (2002). *Clinicians in court: A guide to subpoenas, depositions, testifying, and everything else you need to know.* New York: Guilford Press.

Beauchamp, T. L., & Childress, J. F. (2001). *Principles of biomedical ethics* (5th ed.). New York: Oxford University Press.

Becvar, R. J., & Becvar, D. S. (2006). *Family theory: A systemic integration* (6th ed.). Boston: Allyn & Bacon.

Bennett, B. E., Bricklin, P. M., Harris, E., Knapp, S., Vandecreek, L., & Younggren, J. N. (2007). *Assessing and managing risk in psychological practice: An individualized approach.* Rockville, MD: The Trust.

Beutler, L. E., Moleiro, C., & Talebi, H. (2002). Resistance in psychotherapy: What conclusions are supported by research? *Journal of Clinical Psychology, 58,* 207–217.

Broderick, C. B., & Schrader, S. S. (1991). The history of professional marriage and family therapy. In A. S. Gurman & D. P. Kniskern (Eds.), *Handbook of family therapy* (Vol. 2, pp. 3–40). New York: Brunner/Mazel.

Brown, J. E., & Slee, P. T. (1989). Paradoxical strategies: The ethics of intervention. *Professional Psychology: Research and Practice, 17,* 487–490.

Bullock, D., & Kobayashi, K. (1978). The use of live consultation in family therapy. *Family Therapy, 5,* 245–250.

Committee on Ethical Guidelines for Forensic Psychologists. (1991). Specialty guidelines for forensic psychologists. *Law and Human Behavior, 15,* 655–665.

Committee on Legal Issues. (1996). Strategies for private practitioners coping with subpoenas or compelled testimony for client records or test data. *Professional Psychology: Research and Practice, 27,* 245–251.

Dutton, D. G., & Corvo, K. (2006). Transforming a flawed policy: A call to revive psychology and science in domestic violence research and practice. *Aggression and Violent Behavior, 11,* 457–483.

Elmes, M. B., & Gemmill, G. (1990). The psychodynamics of mindlessness and dissent in small groups. *Small Group Research, 21,* 28–44.

Epstein, E., & Loos, V. E. (1989). Some irreverent thoughts on the limits of family therapy. *Journal of Family Psychology, 2,* 405–421.

Flaherty, E. G., Sege, R., Price, L. L., Christoffel, K. K.,

Norton, D. P., & O'Connor, K. G. (2006). Pediatrician characteristics associated with child abuse identification: Results from a national survey of pediatricians. *Child Maltreatment, 11*, 361–369.

Gergen, K. J. (1985). The social constructionist movement in modern psychology. *American Psychologist, 40*, 266–275.

Gergen, K. J. (2001). Psychological science in a postmodern context. *American Psychologist, 56*, 803–813.

Gottlieb, M. C. (1986, November). *Selected topics in the ethics of marital and family therapy.* Paper presented at the annual meeting of the Texas Psychological Association, Dallas, TX.

Gottlieb, M. C. (1993, Spring). Co-mingling of patient records: What's a family psychologist to do? *Family Psychologist,* 19–20.

Gottlieb, M. C. (1995). Ethical dilemmas in change of format and live supervision. In R. H. Mikesell, D. Lusterman, & S. H. McDaniel (Eds.), *Integrating family therapy: Handbook of family psychology and systems therapy* (pp. 561–570). Washington, DC: American Psychological Association.

Gottlieb, M. C. (1997). An ethics policy for family practice management. In D. T. Marsh & R. D. Magee (Eds.), *Ethical and legal issues in professional practice with families* (pp. 257–270). New York: Wiley.

Greenberg, S. A., & Shuman, D. W. (1997). Irreconcilable conflict between therapeutic and forensic roles. *Professional Psychology: Research and Practice, 28*, 50–57.

Gurman, A. S. (1982). Using paradox in psychodynamic marital therapy. *American Journal of Family Therapy, 10*, 72–74.

Gurman, A. S., & Fraenkel, P. (2002). The history of couple therapy: A millennial review. *Family Process, 41*, 199–260.

Haley, J. (1976). *Problem-solving therapy: New strategies for effective family therapy.* San Francisco: Jossey-Bass.

Hampton, B. (1991). Ethical issues in the practice of strategic therapy. *Psychotherapy in Private Practice, 9*, 47–59.

Hinsz, V. B., & Davis, J. H. (1984). Persuasive arguments, theory group polarization and choice shifts. *Personality and Social Psychology Bulletin, 10*, 260–268.

Huber, C. H., & Baruth, L. G. (1987). *Ethical, legal, and professional issues in the practice of marriage and family therapy.* Columbus, OH: Merrill.

Jaffee v. Redmond, 135 L.Ed.2d 337 (1996).

Kitchener, K. S. (1984). Intuition, critical evaluation and ethical principles: The foundation for ethical decisions in counseling psychology. *Counseling Psychologist, 12*, 43–55.

Kivlighan, D. M., Angelone, E. O., & Swafford, K. G. (1991). Live supervision in individual psychotherapy: Effects on therapists intention use and client's evaluation of session effects and working alliance. *Professional Psychology: Research and Practice, 22*, 489–495.

Knapp, S., Gottlieb, M., Berman, J., & Handelsman, M. (2007). When law and ethics collide: What should

psychologists do? *Professional Psychology: Research and Practice, 38*, 54–59.

Knapp, S. J., & VandeCreek, L. D. (2006). *Practical ethics for psychologists.* Washington, DC: American Psychological Association.

Liddle, H. A. (2004). Family-based therapies for adolescent alcohol and drug use: Research contributions and future research needs. *Addiction, 99*, 76–92.

Lyddon, W. J. (1995). Cognitive therapy and theories of knowing: A social constructionist view. *Journal of Counseling and Development, 73*, 579–585.

Margolin, G. (1982). Ethical and legal consideration in marital and family therapy. *American Psychologist, 37*, 788–801.

Minuchin, S. (1974). *Families and family therapy.* Cambridge, MA: Harvard University Press.

Minuchin, S., & Montalvo, B. (1967). Techniques of working with disorganized and low socioeconomic families. *American Journal of Orthopsychiatry, 37*, 880–887.

National Association of Social Workers. (1996). *Code of ethics.* Washington, DC: Author.

Nichols, M. P., & Schwartz, R. C. (1998). *Family therapy: Concepts and methods.* Needham Heights, MA: Allyn & Bacon.

Norcross, J. C., Hedges, M., & Castle, P. H. (2002). Psychologists conducting psychotherapy in 2001: A study of the division 29 membership. *Psychotherapy: Theory, Research, Practice and Training, 39*, 97–102.

O'Shea, M., & Jessee, E. (1982). Ethical, value, and professional conflicts in systems therapy. In J. C. Hansen & L. L'Abate (Eds.), *Values, ethics, legalities, and the family therapist* (pp. 1–21). Rockville, MD: Aspen.

Patterson, C. H. (1958). The place of values in counseling and psychotherapy. *Journal of Counseling Psychology, 5*, 216–223.

Pinsof, W. M., Wynne, L. C., & Hambright, A. B. (1996). The outcomes of couple and family therapy: Findings, conclusions, and recommendations. *Psychotherapy: Theory, Research, Practice and Training, 33*, 321–331.

Prince, S. E., & Jacobson, N. S. (1995). A review and evaluation of marital and family therapies for affective disorders. *Journal of Marital and Family Therapy, 21*, 377–401.

Rohrbaugh, M., Tennen, H., & Press, S. (1981). Compliance, defiance and therapeutic paradox: Guidelines for strategic use of paradoxical interventions. *American Journal of Orthopsychiatry, 51*, 454–467.

Schaller, M. (1992). In-group favoritism and statistical reasoning in social influence: Implications for formation and maintenance of group stereotypes. *Journal of Personality and Social Psychology, 63*, 61–74.

Seltzer, L. F. (1986). *Paradoxical strategies in psychotherapy: A comprehensive overview and guidebook.* Oxford, UK: Wiley.

Selvini-Palazzoli, M., Boscolo, L., Cecchin, G., & Prata, G. (1978). *Paradox and counterparadox: A new model for the family in schizophrenic transaction.* New York: Aronson.

Shadish, W. R., Ragsdale, K., Glaser, R. R., & Montgomery, L. M. (1995). The efficacy and effectiveness of marital and family therapy: A perspective from meta-analysis. *Journal of Marital and Family Therapy, 21*, 345–360.

Smith, C. W., Smith, I. A., & Saltz, C. J. (1991). The effects of supervisory interruptions on therapists and clients. *American Journal of Family Therapy, 19*, 250–255.

Smith, T. B. (2004). *Practicing multiculturalism: Affirming diversity in counseling and psychology.* Boston: Allyn & Bacon.

Stancombe, J., & White, S. (2005). Cause and responsibility: towards an interactional understanding of blaming and "neutrality" in family therapy. *Journal of Family Therapy, 27*, 330–351.

Sue, D. W., & Sue, D. (2003). *Counseling the culturally diverse: Theory and practice.* New York: Wiley.

Texas State Board of Examiners of Psychologists. (2006). *Psychologists' Licensing Act and rules and regulations of the Texas State Board of Examiners of Psychologists.* Austin, TX: Author.

Tjeltveit, A. C. (2006). To what ends?: Psychotherapy goals and outcomes, the good life, and the principle of beneficence. *Psychotherapy: Theory, Research, Practice and Training, 43*, 186–200.

Trute, B. (1998). Going beyond gender-specific treatments in wife battering: Profeminist couple and family therapy. *Aggression and Violent Behavior, 3*, 1–15.

Vachon, D. O., & Agresti, A. A. (1992). A training proposal to help mental health professionals clarify and manage implicit values in the counseling process. *Professional Psychology: Research and Practice, 23*, 509–514.

Wachtel, P. L. (1993). *Therapeutic communication: Principles and effective practice.* New York: Guilford Press.

Watson, H., & Levine, M. (1989). Psychotherapy and mandated reporting of child abuse. *American Journal of Orthopsychiatry, 59*, 246–256.

Weinstein, B., Levine, M., & Kogan, N. (2000). Mental health professionals' experiences reporting suspected child abuse and maltreatment. *Child Abuse and Neglect, 24*, 1317–1328.

Index

Figure numbers are indicated by *f*. Table numbers are indicated by *t*